Cancer of the
Head and Neck

Cancer of the Head and Neck

Edited by

James Y. Suen, M.D., F.A.C.S.

Professor and Chairman
Department of Otolaryngology and Maxillofacial Surgery
University of Arkansas College of Medicine
Little Rock, Arkansas

and

Eugene N. Myers, M.D., F.A.C.S.

Professor and Chairman
Department of Otolaryngology
University of Pittsburgh School of Medicine
Professor of Oral Pathology
University of Pittsburgh School of Dental Medicine
Chief, Department of Otolaryngology
Eye and Ear Hospital of Pittsburgh
Pittsburgh, Pennsylvania

Churchill Livingstone
New York, Edinburgh, London, and Melbourne   1981

Distributed in the United Kingdom by Churchill Livingstone,
Robert Stevenson House, 1-3 Baxter's Place, Leith Walk,
Edinburgh EH1 3AF and by associated companies, branches
and representatives throughout the world.

First published 1981
Printed in U.S.A.

ISBN 0-443-08045-3

7 6 5 4 3 2 1

Library of Congress Cataloging in Publication Data
Main entry under title:

Cancer of the head and neck.

   Bibliography: p.
   Includes index.
   1. Head—Cancer. 2. Neck—Cancer. I. Suen,
James Y. II. Myers, Eugene N. [DNLM: 1. Head and
neck neoplasms.   WE 707 C215]
RC280.H4C35   616.99′491   80-25286
ISBN   0-443-08045-3

Dedication

This book is dedicated to:

My parents, Yee Gow and Mary Suen, whom I love and respect for their sacrifices so that I could have opportunities they never had;

My children, Brent Yee and Tiffany Anne, for the happiness they bring to me and for their patience and understanding during the preparation of this book;

Carol Anne, whom I admire for her courage and fortitude;

Richard H. Jesse, who has dedicated his life to improving the care of the patient afflicted with cancer of the head and neck;

Alando J. Ballantyne, my mentor and friend, whose surgical brilliance never ceases to amaze me; and

My patients, whose strength and courage have been an inspiration to me.

J.Y.S.

This book is dedicated to my wife, Barbara, and my children, Marjorie Rose Myers and Jeffrey Nicholas Myers, all of whom are a constant source of joy and inspiration to me; my parents, Dr. and Mrs. David Myers, whose dedication to patient care has been a way of life; and to Dr. John Conley, with whom I learned the principles of head and neck surgery.

E.N.M.

Contributors

Mohamed A. Aramany, D.M.D., M.S.
Professor of Prosthodontics, University of Pittsburgh School of Dental Medicine; Professor of Otolaryngology, University of Pittsburgh School of Medicine; Director, Division of Maxillofacial Prosthodontics, Eye and Ear Hospital of Pittsburgh, Pittsburgh, Pennsylvania
Maxillofacial Prosthetic Rehabilitation

Daniel C. Baker, M.D.
Assistant Professor of Surgery (Plastic Surgery), New York University School of Medicine; Assistant Attending Surgeon, Institute of Reconstructive Plastic Surgery, Manhattan Eye, Ear & Throat Hospital, New York, New York
Cancer of the Salivary Glands

Shan Ray Baker, M.D.
Assistant Professor, Department of Otorhinolaryngology, University of Michigan Medical School, Ann Arbor, Michigan
Cancer of the Lip

Alando J. Ballantyne, M.D., F.A.C.S.
Professor, Department of Head and Neck Surgery, University of Texas System Cancer Center, M.D. Anderson Hospital and Tumor Institute, Houston, Texas
Reconstructive Procedures

Alberto Banfi, M.D.
Professor of Radiology, University of Milan School of Medicine; Director, Division of Radiology, Istituto Nazionale Tumori, Milan, Italy
Hodgkin and Non-Hodgkin Lymphoma Presenting in the Head and Neck

John G. Batsakis, M.D.
Chairman, Department of Pathology, Maine Medical Center, Portland, Maine
Histopathological Considerations

Oliver H. Beahrs, M.D., F.A.C.S.
Professor of Surgery, Mayo Medical School; Head of Section of Head and Neck and General Surgery, Mayo Clinic and Mayo Foundation, Rochester, Minnesota
Cancer of the Thyroid Gland
Cancer of the Parathyroid

Stephen P. Becker, M.D., F.A.C.S.
Assistant Professor, Department of Otolaryngology and Maxillofacial Surgery, Northwestern University Medical School, Chicago, Illinois
Cancer of the Nasal Cavity and Paranasal Sinuses

Hugh F. Biller, M.D., F.A.C.S.
Professor and Chairman, Department of Otolaryngology, Mount Sinai School of Medicine, New York, New York
Cancer of the Larynx

James D. Billie, M.D., D.M.D.
Chief Resident, Department of Otolaryngology and Maxillofacial Surgery, University of Arkansas College of Medicine, Little Rock, Arkansas
Dental Considerations in the Head and Neck Cancer Patient

Gianni Bonadonna, M.D.
Director, Division of Clinical Oncology F (Medical Oncology), Istituto Nazionale Tumori, Milan, Italy
Hodgkin and Non-Hodgkin Lymphoma Presenting in the Head and Neck

Warren C. Boop, Jr., M.D., F.A.C.S.
Professor of Neurosurgery, University of Arkansas College of Medicine; Chief of Neurosurgery Section, Veterans Administration Medical Center, Little Rock, Arkansas
Methods of Pain Control

John A. Brunner, III, M.D.
Assistant Professor, Department of Anesthesiology, University of Arkansas College of Medicine, Little Rock, Arkansas
Anesthetic Considerations

George Choa, M.D., B.S., F.R.C.S. (Ed.), F.A.C.S.
Honorary Lecturer in Otolaryngology, Department of Surgery, University of Hong Kong, Hong Kong
Cancer of the Nasopharynx

Paul B. Chretien, M.D., F.A.C.S.
Chief, Tumor Immunology Section; Assistant Chief, Surgery Branch, National Cancer Institute, Bethesda, Maryland
The Chemotherapy and Immunotherapy of Head and Neck Cancer

John Conley, M.D., F.A.C.S.
Professor Emeritus of Clinical Otolaryngology, Columbia University College of Physicians and Surgeons; Chief of Head and Neck Service, St. Vincent's Hospital and Medical Center, New York, New York
Cancer of the Salivary Glands

William M. Cooper, M.D., F.A.C.P.
Clinical Professor of Medicine, University of Pittsburgh School of Medicine, Pittsburgh, Pennsylvania
Preoperative and Postoperative Medical Considerations

Edward M. Copeland, III, M.D., F.A.C.S.
Professor of Surgery, University of Texas Medical School at Houston; Professor of Surgery, University of Texas System Cancer Center, M.D. Anderson Hospital and Tumor Institute, Houston, Texas
Nutritional Management of Patients with Head and Neck Malignancies

John M. Daly, M.D.
Assistant Professor of Surgery, University of Texas Medical School at Houston; Faculty Associate, Department of Surgery, University of Texas System Cancer Center, M.D. Anderson Hospital and Tumor Institute, Houston, Texas
Nutritional Management of Patients with Head and Neck Malignancies

James M. Dowaliby, II, M.D., F.A.C.S.
Clinical Assistant Professor of Surgery (Otolaryngology), Yale University School of Medicine; Attending Surgeon (Otolaryngology), Hospital of St. Raphael and Yale-New Haven Hospital, New Haven, Connecticut
The Incurable Patient

Stanley J. Dudrick, M.D., F.A.C.S.
Professor and Chairman, Department of Surgery, University of Texas Medical School at Houston; Consultant in Surgery, University of Texas System Cancer Center, M.D. Anderson Hospital and Tumor Institute, Houston, Texas
Nutritional Management of Patients with Head and Neck Malignancies

Janet A. Fisher, R.N., B.S.N.
Registered Nurse Practitioner, University of Arkansas College of Medicine, Little Rock, Arkansas
Methods of Pain Control

Jack L. Gluckman, M.D.
Assistant Professor, Department of Otolaryngology and Maxillofacial Surgery, University of Cincinnati College of Medicine, Cincinnati, Ohio
Cancer of the Oropharynx

Helmuth Goepfert, M.D., F.A.C.S.
Professor and Vice-Chairman, Department of Head and Neck Surgery, M.D. Anderson Hospital and Tumor Institute, University of Texas System Cancer Center, Houston, Texas
Carcinoma of the Hypopharynx and Cervical Esophagus

Hermes C. Grillo, M.D., F.A.C.S.
Professor of Surgery, Harvard Medical School; Chief of General Thoracic Surgery, Massachusetts General Hospital, Boston, Massachusetts
Tumors of the Cervical Trachea

Karen Jean Hannahs, R.N., B.S.N.
Clinical Nurse Practitioner, Department of Otolaryngology and Maxillofacial Surgery, University of Arkansas College of Medicine, Little Rock, Arkansas
Nursing Care of the Head and Neck Cancer Patient

Donald F. N. Harrison, M.D., F.R.C.S., F.R.A.C.S.
Professor of Laryngology and Otology, University of London, London, England
Unusual Tumors

Jill A. Hooper, R.N., B.S.N.
Clinical Nurse Practitioner, Department of Otolaryngology and Maxillofacial Surgery, University of Arkansas College of Medicine, Little Rock, Arkansas
Nursing Care of the Head and Neck Cancer Patient

John P. Hubert, Jr., M.D.
Chief Resident Associate in Surgery, Mayo Graduate School of Medicine, Rochester, Minnesota
Cancer of the Thyroid Gland
Cancer of the Parathyroid

Matthew J. Jackson, D.M.D., M.S.D.
Assistant Clinical Professor of Restorative Dentistry, Tufts University School of Dental Medicine; Chief of Prosthodontics, Veterans Administration Medical Center, Boston, Massachusetts
Dental Considerations in the Head and Neck Cancer Patient

G. Thomas Jansen, M.D.
Professor and Chairman, Department of Dermatology, University of Arkansas College of Medicine, Little Rock, Arkansas
Cancer of the Skin

Richard H. Jesse, M.D., F.A.C.S.
Professor of Surgery and Chief, Department of Head and Neck Surgery, University of Texas System Cancer Center, M.D. Anderson Hospital and Tumor Institute, Houston, Texas
General Considerations

Paul D. Kiernan, M.D., F.A.C.S.
Chief Resident Associate in Surgery, Mayo Graduate School of Medicine, Rochester, Minnesota
Cancer of the Thyroid Gland
Cancer of the Parathyroid

Charles J. Krause, M.D., F.A.C.S.
Professor and Chairman, Department of Otorhinolaryngology, University of Michigan Medical School, Ann Arbor, Michigan
Cancer of the Lip

Noel W. Lawson, M.D.
Associate Professor, Department of Anesthesiology, University of Arkansas College of Medicine, Little Rock, Arkansas
Anesthetic Considerations

William Lawson, M.D., D.D.S.
Associate Professor, Department of Otolaryngology, Mount Sinai School of Medicine, New York, New York
Cancer of the Larynx

John S. Lewis, M.D., F.A.C.S.
Chief, Otolaryngology Service, Roosevelt Hospital; Associate Attending Surgeon, Head and Neck Service, Memorial Sloan-Kettering Cancer Center, New York, New York
Cancer of the External Auditory Canal, Middle Ear, and Mastoid

Raleigh E. Lingeman, M.D., F.A.C.S.
Professor and Chairman, Department of Otolaryngology, Indiana University School of Medicine, Indianapolis, Indiana
Evaluation of the Patient with Head and Neck Cancer

Roberto Molinari, M.D.
Director, Division of Clinical Oncology C (Head & Neck), Istituto Nazionale Tumori, Milan, Italy
Hodgkin and Non-Hodgkin Lymphoma Presenting in the Head and Neck

Eugene N. Myers, M.D., F.A.C.S.
Professor and Chairman, Department of Otolaryngology, University of Pittsburgh School of Medicine; Professor of Oral Pathology, University of Pittsburgh School of Dental Medicine; Chief, Department of Otolaryngology, Eye and Ear Hospital of Pittsburgh, Pittsburgh, Pennsylvania
Maxillofacial Prosthetic Rehabilitation
Management of Complications

Victor L. Schramm, Jr., M.D.
Assistant Professor, Department of Otolaryngology, University of Pittsburgh School of Medicine, Pittsburgh, Pennsylvania
Management of Complications

Donald A. Shumrick, M.D., F.A.C.S.
Professor and Chairman, Department of Otolaryngology and Maxillofacial Surgery, University of Cincinnati College of Medicine, Cincinnati, Ohio
Cancer of the Oropharynx

Barbara A. Sigler, R.N., M.N.Ed.
Oncology Nurse Clinician, Department of Otolaryngology, University of Pittsburgh School of Medicine, Pittsburgh, Pennsylvania
Nursing Care of the Head and Neck Cancer Patient

Mark I. Singer, M.D.
Assistant Professor, Department of Otolaryngology, Indiana University School of Medicine, Indianapolis, Indiana
Evaluation of the Patient with Head and Neck Cancer

George A. Sisson, M.D., F.A.C.S.
Professor and Chairman, Department of Otolaryngology and Maxillofacial Surgery, Northwestern University Medical School, Chicago, Illinois
Cancer of the Nasal Cavity and Paranasal Sinuses

Ronald H. Spiro, M.D., F.A.C.S.
Associate Attending Surgeon, Head and Neck Surgery Section, Memorial Sloan-Kettering Cancer Center, New York, New York
Cancer of the Oral Cavity

Charles H. Srodes, M.D., F.A.C.P.

Clinical Assistant Professor of Medicine, University of Pittsburgh School of Medicine, Pittsburgh, Pennsylvania

Preoperative and Postoperative Medical Considerations

Elliot W. Strong, M.D., F.A.C.S.

Chief, Head and Neck Surgery Section, Memorial Sloan-Kettering Cancer Center, New York, New York

Cancer of the Oral Cavity

James Y. Suen, M.D., F.A.C.S.

Professor and Chairman, Department of Otolaryngology and Maxillofacial Surgery, University of Arkansas College of Medicine, Little Rock, Arkansas

Cancer of the Neck

C. C. Wang, M.D.

Professor of Radiation Therapy, Harvard Medical School; Radiation Therapist and Head, Division of Clinical Services, Department of Radiation Medicine, Massachusetts General Hospital; Consultant Radiation Therapist, Massachusetts Eye and Ear Infirmary, Boston, Massachusetts

General Principles of Radiation Therapy of Head and Neck Tumors

Kent C. Westbrook, M.D., F.A.C.S.

Professor, Department of Surgery, University of Arkansas College of Medicine, Little Rock, Arkansas

Cancer of the Skin

Stephen J. Wetmore, M.D.

Assistant Professor, Department of Otolaryngology and Maxillofacial Surgery, University of Arkansas College of Medicine; Chief, Otolaryngology Section, Veterans Administration Medical Center, Little Rock, Arkansas

Cancer of the Neck

Gregory T. Wolf, M.D.

Assistant Professor, Department of Otorhinolaryngology, University of Michigan, Ann Arbor, Michigan. Formerly Special Assistant for Surgical Oncology, Division of Cancer Treatment; Project Officer, Head and Neck Contracts Program, Cancer Therapy Evaluation Program, National Cancer Institute, Bethesda, Maryland

The Chemotherapy and Immunotherapy of Head and Neck Cancer

John E. Wright, M.D., F.R.C.S.

Consultant Ophthalmic Surgeon, Director of Orbital Clinic, Moorfields Eye Hospital, London, England

Cancer of the Eye and Orbit

Preface

The concept of the "Health Care Team" reaches its ultimate expression in the management of the patient with cancer of the head and neck. It has long been recognized that highly skilled professionals and technicians must work together in order to accomplish any meaningful objectives, as the complexity of technology has eclipsed the possibility of one individual being able to comprehend an entire field of knowledge. The incorporation of a variety of professional and paraprofessional persons into the Health Care Team, while unfortunately not significantly improving the cure rate in most head and neck cancers, has accomplished a great deal in reducing the morbidity and mortality consequent to this type of surgery and has markedly improved the quality of life for this group of patients.

Each team must have a leader, and our concept is that the surgeon specializing in head and neck cancer, no matter what his basic surgical specialty field, should be the leader of this team. This book is oriented as a surgical textbook but does not ignore medical therapy and other important aspects of overall patient care. The key to the team functioning well is communication, and it is incumbent upon the leader of the team to emphasize both vertical and horizontal lines of communication.

In the last two decades, we have witnessed an exciting evolution in the management of head and neck cancer. Surgical management of these patients has improved considerably; however, it would appear that the surgical extirpative procedures have been pushed to their fullest extent. We have witnessed the development of team management of skull base tumors, which has combined the expertise of the head and neck surgeon and the neurosurgeon to approach these tumors in a combined intracranial and extracranial manner. The concept of immediate reconstruction utilizing regional pedicle flaps was introduced and has gone through an enormous evolutionary phase with the development of multiple new regional flaps. At the same time, the older concept of using skin grafts in reconstruction has been reintroduced.

An exciting area of development is in new techniques of reconstruction to restore the phonatory apparatus in patients who have undergone laryngectomy. At the present moment, this area is in the same developmental stage as regional pedicle flaps were two decades ago. It is anticipated that although one technique will not be satisfactory for all, a variety of techniques will be available, as is true in other areas of reconstruction of the head and neck.

These developments have transpired in the two decades of our experience and we anticipate that future developments will be equally as exciting. We are hopeful that the great concentration of effort and interest in this field and the new techniques in surgery, radiation therapy, and chemotherapy will not only improve the quality of life but will also result in an improvement of the cure rate for head and neck cancer. We are dedicated to keeping this book current to reflect the improvements in this field.

James Y. Suen
Eugene N. Myers

Acknowledgments

My deep appreciation to Mary Janes and Dee Gee Phipps for their many hours of labor in preparing the manuscripts. Mary Janes's dedication and humor gave the project life. Jack Diner gave many hours of his life preparing and helping with the illustrations; I am indebted to him. There are no words kind enough or generous enough to express our gratitude to Jan Drake, our editorial assistant and coordinator, who did a superb job. Jan's talents and abilities are infinite. And finally I wish to thank the staff at Churchill Livingstone, especially Donna Balopole, for their outstanding assistance.

J.Y.S.

My appreciation to Marge Norris, my administrative assistant, for her organizational abilities during the entire time of this project, and to Sherree Schroeder and Nancy Rudis for their help in processing the manuscripts. I would also like to acknowledge the help of Melanie Feduska and Bruce Johnston for their assistance in helping to reference this book. My appreciation also to Barbara A. Sigler, R.N., M.N.Ed., Nurse Oncologist, for her overall assistance in this project.

E.N.M.

Contents

1 | General Considerations

Richard H. Jesse, M.D.

INTRODUCTION

While not among the five leading causes of death from cancer in the United States, cancer of the head and neck is a particularly threatening experience for the patient, his family, and friends. Cancers in this area are disabling and fatal if untreated, but even if treated a patient faces possible loss of sensory organs, disability from loss of physiological function, sometimes a drastic change in personal appearance, and often death.

The cancers considered here are those arising in the upper aerodigestive tract: lips, oral cavity, nasal fossa and paranasal sinuses, nasopharynx, oropharynx, hypopharynx, larynx, cervical esophagus, and cervical trachea. The major and minor salivary glands and the thyroid glands are also included. Skin cancer, melanoma, and lymphomas, as well as patients with cervical metastases and undetectable primary cancer, are specifically excluded from the scope of this discussion in accordance with the National Cancer Institute's formulation of the Head and Neck Cancer Control Network Program.

Approximately 80 percent of the cancers occurring in this area are squamous cell carcinomas. The various histologic types of salivary gland cancer, soft tissue sarcomas, thyroid cancer, and an occasional bone sarcoma constitute the majority of the remaining 20 percent.

EPIDEMIOLOGY

An exact figure of the total number of patients in the United States with a newly diagnosed primary cancer originating in the head and neck is difficult to determine because cancer does not have to be reported. Publications of the National Cancer Institute,[2] the American Cancer Society,[3] and data from tumor registries approved by the American College of Surgeons estimate that the number of new head and neck cancer patients was 67,000 in 1978, of which one-third to one-half will succumb to the disease. The 1977 estimates included 24,000 cancers of the oral cavity and pharynx, 9,200 cancers of the larynx, and 8,200 cancers of the thyroid. If one excludes the cancers of the central nervous system and the eyes, the lymphomas, and the cutaneous melanomas, one arrives at an estimated annual figure of 45,000 newly diagnosed head and neck cancers of those types covered in this chapter.

The age-adjusted incidence rates per 100,000 population for all the cancers under consideration are approximately 17.2 for white males, 5.6 for white females, 13.2 for black males, and 5.2 for black females. These head and neck cancers comprise about 5 percent of the incidence of cancer in males and about 2 percent of the cancers in females. The incidence of cancer originating within the oral cavity and pharynx is two times higher than cancer of the larynx and ten times higher than cancer of the thyroid. Cancer of the thyroid occurs three to four times more commonly in females than in males. Cancer of the lip rarely occurs in a black person. Cancers of the nasal cavity and paranasal sinuses comprise only about 4 to 5 percent of the total.

There is a rather wide geographic distribution among patients with cancers of the buccal cavity and pharynx.[5] These cancers occur 25 percent more commonly among the population in the southern and western United States and the Latin American area on the border of the United States and Mexico than among the population in the northern and eastern portions of the United States. Cancers of the larynx, however, seem to have no geographic predilection.

The average age for the entire group of head and neck cancer patients is approximately 59 years at the time of diagnosis, and the type of histology of the cancer is related to the patient's age. Patients with cancers of the salivary glands, thyroid, paranasal sinuses, and those with sarcomas of the soft tissue and bone are likely to be younger than 59 years, whereas those with squamous cell carcinomas of the oral cavity, pharynx, and larynx are typically older than the 59-year average.

International comparisons between the United States and other countries as to the incidence of head and neck cancer are difficult to obtain because of the differences in reporting. The death rate for patients with head and neck cancer per 100,000 population in France, Switzerland, Ireland, South Africa, Italy, and Scotland is greater than in the United States, whereas the rate in England, the Scandinavian countries, West Germany, Japan, and Israel is lower than that in the United States. One might infer from this information that in those countries in which there is a high alcohol consumption, the death rate is higher. It is difficult to determine from the data whether these deaths are specifically related to cancer of the head and neck or whether they reflect general death rates. Cancer of the nasopharynx is extremely high in native born and first generation Chinese. Beginning with the second generation, there appears to be less difference in incidence.

SURVIVAL

Overall patient survival at 5 years is 67 percent when the disease is classified as local, whereas it is only 30 percent with regional disease. The 1972 death rates for head and neck cancer per 100,000 population were 4.67 for males as compared to 1.5 for females. These figures had changed only slightly from those published in 1952. The lower death rate for females may be related to the fact that females are more likely to present themselves to the physician at a time when the cancer can be classified as local.

The average cure rates for squamous cell carcinoma of the oral cavity and pharynx decrease as the site of origin of the cancer becomes lower in the aerodigestive tract. Carcinoma of the lip is cured in approximately 84 percent of the patients, floor of mouth 45 percent, tongue 36 percent, oropharynx 24 percent, and hypopharynx 13 percent. Patients with cancer of the nasopharynx have a 29 percent survival rate, those with cancer of the nasal cavity 42 percent, and those with cancer of the larynx 63 percent. The relatively high patient survival in patients with cancer of the vocal cord is related to the fact that symptoms occur when the lesion is small. Survival for patients with cancer of the salivary gland varies widely depending upon which gland is the site of origin. There is a higher incidence of malignant disease in minor salivary gland sites and in the submandibular gland than in the parotid gland. Five-year survival figures quoted for these cancers are not valid, since recurrence after this length of time appears rather frequently. True survival rates for these cancers would be more accurately reported at periods from $7^1/_2$ to 10 years.

ETIOLOGIC FACTORS

The aerodigestive tract serves as a conduit for air, fluid, and food to the body and thereby comes directly in contact with a broad range of possibly carcinogenic agents. Other than some direct information on carcinogens gathered from studies on a few specific occupations in manufacturing plants, the etiologic factors that can produce cancer in the general population in

TABLE 1-1. ETIOLOGY OF HEAD AND NECK CANCER—SPECIFIC SITES

Site	Carcinogens	Other factors
Skin	Inorganic arsenics in drugs, water, or occupational environment Ultraviolet rays of sun, ionizing radiation Polycyclic aromatic hydrocarbons, coke ovens, gas workers Chloroprene (neoprene) in synthetic rubber	Burns Riboflavin deficiency Syphilis—lip
Nose and sinuses	Wood dust (furniture industry) Shoe industry (leather manufacturing) Textile workers Radiochemical (Thorotrast) Radium dial painters and chemists (osteogenic sarcomas) Mustard gas Nickel refining Isopropyl oil Bcme-bis (chloromethyl) ether-alkalating agent (produces esthesioneuroepithelioma in animals)	?Chronic sinusitis ?Cigarette smoke
Nasopharynx	Nitrosamines (n-nitrosodimethylamine)	Epstein-Barr virus Genetics: Chinese 25 times for Kwangtung province Vitamin C deficiency Salted fish
Oral cavity	Cigarettes, reverse smoking Ethyl alcohol Snuff, chewing tobacco, betel nut Textile industries Coke ovens Leather manufacturing	Syphilis—tongue Nutrition: vitamin B, riboflavin deficiencies
Hypopharynx—Larynx	Cigarettes Asbestos (ship builders) Mustard gas Polycyclic aromatic hydrocarbons (coke ovens) Ethyl alcohol Wood exposure	Nutrition: riboflavin deficiency
Esophagus	Ethyl alcohol Cigarettes	Nutrition: riboflavin, nitrosamines Race and nationality: Eskimos Iranians, blacks
Thyroid	Radiation exposure	Iodine deficiencies Genetics
Salivary glands	Radiation	Genetics: Eskimos

the United States have not been well researched. Occupational exposures have been studied and show a positive correlation between various factors and head and neck cancer. These are summarized in Table 1-1.

Both tobacco and alcohol are well established as risk factors for developing cancer of the oral cavity, pharynx, and larynx. The incidence of precancerous lesions and cancer of the buccal mucosa, alveolar ridge (gum), and floor of the mouth in those who have dipped snuff or chewed tobacco for 40 years or more is well known. These cancers tend to be indolent, verrucal, and remain at a noninvasive stage for a long period of time. Cancer may occur in individuals who use a pipe in one position within the mouth, developing at the site where the hot tobacco smoke is directed at the mucosa. In some series, 85 percent of patients with head and neck cancer have been found to use some form of lighted tobacco.

A careful medical history, which has as part of its aim the determination of the amount of tobacco smoked, will show that a high proportion of these patients with head and neck cancer admit to smoking one pack of cigarettes daily or its equivalent. The same careful history taken relative to alcohol consumption is somewhat harder to elicit, particularly among white females, because the social stigma associated with the heavy consumption of alcohol often prevents them from being truthful. However, when the physician combines the history given by the patient with that given by the family, he finds that at least 60 percent of the head and neck cancer patients consume three drinks daily. It can generally be determined in patients consuming mixed drinks that the amount of alcohol is "eyeballed" into the glass and no measuring jigger is used. It is probably safe to assume that 75 percent of cancers of the oral cavity, pharynx, and larynx are associated with heavy tobacco or alcohol consumption or both. There is evidence of a synergistic interaction between alcohol and tobacco. Whereas each factor alone accounts for a two-fold or three-fold increase in risk, jointly they can

increase risk more than 15 times that experienced by individuals who neither smoke nor drink.[6] It appears, therefore, that cancer of the oral cavity, pharynx, and larynx could be decreased to 25 percent of its present incidence if alcohol and tobacco were not excessively used.

A viral etiology has been proposed for nasopharyngeal cancer. Studies of antibodies to the Epstein-Barr virus have been done and, while they are not conclusive, they show that there may be some relationship. Sophisticated histopathology and virology studies that should provide further evidence on this point are underway. Cancers of the thyroid gland occur more frequently in those who had received small doses of radiation therapy 20 years or more previously for acne, enlarged thymus, chronic tonsillitis, or middle ear disease. Cancer of the parotid gland and cancer and hyperplasia of the parathyroid glands have also been linked to radiation exposure. There is an increasing incidence of cancer of the paranasal sinuses in individuals who have had diagnostic procedures using the radiochemical dye Thoratrast.

MULTIDISCIPLINARY APPROACH

The implications of head and neck cancer for the patient and his family are so complex that the time has long since passed that one individual physician can manage the entire problem. The entire spectrum of patient care including patient education, diagnosis, examination, treatment planning, treatment decisions, rehabilitation, social problems, and psychological problems requires an integrated team. Team members always include the patient, his family, his own physician, the surgeon, radiotherapist, medical oncologist, nurse, dietitian, and social worker. The team may also include experts in maxillofacial rehabilitation, in speech and hearing problems, and social agencies adjacent to the patient's home environment.

The patient with head and neck cancer

has a desperate problem, and the treatment for his illness often demands radical measures to achieve cure or relief of symptoms, prolongation of useful life, and assistance with death if it becomes inevitable. Specific goals for optimal therapy include eradication of the cancer, satisfactory posttreatment physiological function, and acceptable cosmetic appearance. The correct treatment for an individual patient is the particular therapeutic approach that most nearly achieves these goals. Selection of the correct therapy requires an accurate and detailed assessment of not only the cancer, but also of the patient's psychological make-up, his work goals, and his own personal needs. The treatment team must have knowledge of the various applicable treatment regimens and the wisdom to choose the optimal therapeutic course for an individual patient. This evaluation involves three groups of variables: tumor factors, patient factors, and physician factors.[8]

Tumor Factors

Cancers arising in certain anatomic sites such as the lip, oral tongue, buccal mucosa, and floor of the mouth are relatively accessible and may be handled easily by surgery or by radiation therapy. Lesions of the retromolar trigone, faucial arch, pyriform sinus, oropharynx, and hypopharynx are more difficult to manage surgically, often requiring resections that will produce marked compromise in physiological function. Lesions of the vocal cords and supraglottic larynx can generally be managed by radiation therapy in the early stages, while in the later stages surgery or combined therapy may be necessary. Because of its location, nasopharyngeal cancer is difficult to remove surgically; therefore, its treatment is primarily by irradiation. Cancers of the salivary gland or thyroid gland are primarily surgical problems, although in some instances it appears that postoperative radiation therapy may increase the patient's survival. The sarcomas, particularly those in children, are often in relatively inaccessible areas and seem to be controlled as well by a combination of chemotherapy and radiation therapy. The sarcomas of soft tissue and bone in adults are generally treated with surgery, irradiation, and chemotherapy.

The size and extent of the primary tumor is equally important as site in determining the type of treatment to be employed. A rough guide to the size and extent of the primary tumor is present in most of the classification systems in use within the United States today. The most widely used classification is that of the American Joint Commission on Cancer Staging and End Results Reporting, 1978.[1] This classification system was developed by representatives from the multidisciplinary groups concerned with the treatment of head and neck cancer and was tested by the retrospective input of thousands of case histories of treatment and end results. In general, small cancers without metastases (T1 or T2, and N0) do not require multiple modality treatment. The incidence of second primary cancers in surviving patients is so high that it is better to save the alternative treatment modality for the future when it may be needed. For the larger primary tumor (T3 or T4), the advantages of multimodal therapy outweigh the disadvantages and it probably should be employed.

Regional metastasis remains primarily a surgical problem in patients classified N0 or N1. As the extent of cervical metastasis increases (N2 or N3), indicating either multiple nodal involvement, fixation, or extension into the soft tissue of the neck, the addition of radiation therapy to extirpative surgery has repeatedly shown to prevent most recurrence within the neck.

The primary lesion and regional metastases in patients with strong evidence of distant metastases should be treated only palliatively. The treatment team should be aware, however, that a suspected metastatic lesion may represent a curable second primary cancer. The amount of treatment given to the local or regional disease depends upon the team's evaluation of whether or not the suspected metastases will cause the patient's demise prior to the lesion interfering with physiological function and cosmetic appearance. In general, radiation therapy is the most appropriate form of treatment for palliative purposes.

Patient Factors

A head and neck cancer cannot be considered separate and apart from the patient in whom it occurs. The patient factors include age, general health, dental health, social habits, psychological make-up, socioeconomic factors, previous therapy, and the patient's individual needs. Patients with a history of ascites or a history of myocardial infarction within 3 months should not be operated upon if at all possible. It is generally a mistake, however, to withhold necessary surgery from any other patient, because almost invariably he will get into difficulties from his cancer before the noncancerous disease severely disables him.

An evaluation of the patient's smoking and drinking habits, particularly as to his ability to stop these activities, is essential in the formation of the treatment plan. It is desirable to have him stop both, but if the team had to choose, they should recommend the cessation of smoking. A patient who in the opinion of the treatment team will not curtail these activities should probably be selected for primary surgical therapy rather than radiotherapy if at all possible, since tobacco and alcohol applied to radiated mucosa often cause it to breakdown. If this breakdown happens over bone, radiation necrosis results.

The socioeconomic factors play a definite role in therapy selections. This is particularly true if a single modality treatment is recommended. If the end results of surgical or radiation therapy are probably going to be essentially the same, a patient who wishes to continue his working life and meet the public may, for example, select radiation therapy over surgery because he feels that surgical extirpation may cause disruption of physiological function and/or cosmetic appearance and may destroy his ability to make a living. On the other hand, a patient who would have to receive radiation therapy for 6 to 8 weeks at a facility located a long distance away from home might choose to have a surgical procedure if it requires only a week or two away from his home and job. The choice of therapy is also influenced when the patient is afraid of one type of therapy because of past experience with a family member or acquaintance who has supposedly had a bad experience.

Finally, treatment cannot be administered to a patient against his will and he may choose to have no therapy for a lesion that is considered by the team to be curable. In these cases the team members should consult with the patient in a calm manner. They have the responsibility of pointing out the natural progress of his disease and how it will disturb him in the future. The treatment team must respect his personal desires and should not threaten the patient even though they think he is making a mistake.

Physician Factors

The tumor must be treated by a doctor or a group of doctors, and the physicians responsible for making the therapeutic decision must be familiar with the various alternative regimens applicable to an individual patient. In any geographic area within the United States, the skills and experience of the head and neck surgeon, radiotherapist, and medical oncologist vary tremendously. Surgical specialties are fairly well represented throughout the country, although the number of highly trained head and neck cancer surgeons is limited. The radiotherapists who are expert in administration of high dose therapy to other parts of the body may have had limited experience with a variety of head and neck cancer cases. The medical oncologists naturally tend to concentrate their skill in the areas other than the head and neck, in which the cure rate may be higher. Their experience in the head and neck area may, therefore, be limited. The availability of interested dentists expert in evaluating the teeth of patients who are to undergo radiation therapy and the availability of maxillofacial prosthodontists are also factors that must be taken into consideration. Unless all health care professionals involved have a reasonable degree of experience, they would probably do their patient a favor by referring him to a more experienced group. Assuming that the skill of the members of the decision-making team are equal, they must then meet to discuss the patient and develop an appropriate course of treatment. This plan should be adhered to, but should be flexible enough to allow for changes in treatment if new tumor or patient factors become manifest.

GENERAL CONSIDERATIONS IN TREATMENT PLANNING

The advantages of surgery include eradication of the primary cancer, an accurate histologic assessment of the extent of the primary tumor, an accurate assessment of the extent of regional metastases, and the possibility of immediate reconstruction of surgical defects. The disadvantages of surgery include the possibilities of not detecting occult extensions of cancer cells at the periphery of the tumor, loss of physiological function, cosmetic disfigurement, and of performing a surgical procedure upon a patient with associated potentially lethal diseases.

The advantages of radiation therapy include the ability to treat large areas of cancer, the eradication of subclinical extension at the periphery of the tumor, the decreased chance for functional disturbances, and the fact that anesthetics are not required in patients with other potentially lethal diseases. The disadvantages of radiation therapy include the relative radioresistance of anoxic cells in large cancers; the disability associated with xerostomia, which is usually permanent and often severe; the occurrence of anorexia and weight loss secondary to loss of taste; and the possibility of nerve and soft-tissue damage as the result of high dose therapy.

Chemotherapy has the theoretic advantage over surgery and radiation therapy of producing a systemic effect on cancer cells that may have escaped from the regional area. It may also be used to decrease the size of the primary tumor so that it can be more easily treated by one of the other modalities; this is particularly true for embryonal types of sarcomas in children. Chemotherapy has the disadvantage of not producing a 100 percent kill, at least with the present drugs.

A complete dental evaluation is necessary before any radiation therapy is administered to the oral cavity. Repair of diseased or damaged teeth, extraction of nonsalvagable teeth, evaluation of exostoses, and the institution of a sodium fluoride prophylaxis program should be mandatory. There is strong proof that such a fluoride program is of utmost importance in preventing subsequent osteoradionecrosis of the mandible.[4]

SPECIFIC TREATMENT PLANNING

If multiple modality treatment is decided upon, each member of the team must be certain of the exact part he or she is to play in the patient's treatment. Since the treatment of a patient is by a team, individual egos must be absorbed into the team concept. Certain principles of cancer treatment that were taught to surgeons and radiotherapists during training may have to be modified in order to support the team concept. An example would be the surgeon who has been taught that he must resect the tumor with a 2 cm "normal" margin. If radiotherapy is to be added to surgery, 2 cm surgical margins are unnecessary, since the cells at the margin of the resection are those most easily destroyed by radiation. Conversely, whereas a radiotherapist is taught that a dose of 7,000 rads in 7 weeks is the recognized norm for the treatment of a palpable and visible tumor, the dose can be lowered if the surgical extirpation removes the gross disease leaving perhaps a minimum of occult cancer cells. A constant review of patient records, concentrating mainly on the failures, will provide the treatment team with an accurate assessment of whether or not they are attaining their goals.

SOUND CLINICAL MANAGEMENT

Sound clinical management is collectively developed over years of cumulative experience in the setting in which the treatment team finds itself. What can be accomplished in one hospital or geographic area may not necessarily be duplicated in another area because of the differences and the factors enumerated above. However, there are certain sound management principles that are applicable to all patients. Deviation from these principles may at times be permissable for certain experienced treatment teams.

It would be impractical to attempt an exhaustive listing or discussion of these departures from sound management principles; however, some should be addressed. In a large referral center, one sees many patients whose results might have been different if sound management principles had been diligently practiced. The pitfalls to avoid can be listed and discussed as they relate to the proper progression of investigation and treatment management. These can be categorized as follows: unsound practice during patient's initial symptoms, unsound practice during investigative stage, unsound practice during treatment stage, and unsound practice in assessing treatment results.

Unsound Practice During Patient's Initial Symptoms

A primary care physician may, on the average, see one patient with head and neck cancer for every 3 years he is in practice. This lowers his index of suspicion for cancer to practically nil. He does not, therefore, impress upon the patients the necessity of returning within a few weeks if his treatment for their symptoms has not effected an im-

provement. Antibiotics are prescribed almost universally at the patient's first visit. A second course of antibiotics is frequently prescribed in the face of unchanging symptoms without a thorough reexamination. This delays referral of the patient to a physician specialist, which leads to a delay in cancer diagnosis and treatment. A mass, especially one that is asymptomatic, should be observed for a maximum of 2 to 3 weeks while the patient is under prescribed treatment. If there is no significant improvement in the mass, the patient should be referred to a physician who specializes in cancer management.

Unsound Practice During Investigative Stage

The next group of examples of unsound management practice can be shared by the primary care physician or dentist, the medical or dental specialist, and too often by the patient himself. If the primary care practitioner suspects cancer, he must share this concern with the patient. This often frightens the patient and even though the doctor has made arrangements to refer him to a specialist, the patient does not keep this appointment. All too often the patient will not seek help until the cancer becomes painful or interferes with normal physiological functions. When the patient finally arrives at the referral center, he often blames the primary care physician for the delay rather than blame himself. A primary care practitioner who refers a patient to a specialist would be wise to check to be sure that the patient kept his appointment. The physician can protect himself from legal problems and can help the patient by trying again to allay his fears and to persuade him to accept the referral.

Many mistakes are made in the adequate taking and evaluation of a biopsy. Biopsies of the primary lesion usually should be of an incisional rather than excisional type, unless the excisional biopsy is the definitive procedure. Too often, excisional biopsies are done with inadequate or questionably adequate margins. Often the pathologist has not been alerted to check margins, resulting in confusion relative to adequacy of treatment. Frequently, reexcision with unnecessarily large margins or high dose radiation therapy over large fields is the necessary treatment to settle the confusion. This may be overtreatment for a lesion, but the treatment team must react in an aggressive manner to avoid recurrence. A much better choice of biopsy is the incisional type. A deep incisional biopsy that obtains tissue below any piled-up keratin covering is necessary. The area selected for biopsy should be close to the center of the lesion, unless much necrotic tissue is present. In the latter case, the area should be just peripheral to the necrotic area.

Open biopsy of a mass in the neck prior to completing exhaustive regional and general physical examination is another pitfall that is all too common. The procedure may severely limit or alter the treatment the patient receives when an adjacent primary cancer is found, because incisions have been improperly placed or cancer cells have been disseminated. Since problems within the neck must be considered in treatment planning, node biopsy, if necessary at all, should be performed by the treatment team.

Another common error usually made by the treatment team is to ignore any histologic material that may already be available relative to present or past problems the patient may have had. All materials should be reviewed by the pathologist member of the team. The working diagnosis, which may have been established years ago, may have to be changed when old histologic material is compared with recently acquired biopsies.

Lastly in this category is the practice of some to perform special x-ray studies, particularly those of the larynx, pharynx, and sinuses, after extensive biopsy procedures have been done. Biopsy alters the mucosa and bone detail and can cause the radiologist to misinterpret the film. Biopsy procedures should be performed only after the specified x-rays studies have been completed.

Unsound Practice During Treatment Stage

Fewer common departures from sound surgical management are seen now than were a few years ago, since surgeons now receive better training in oncologic principles. By far the most prevalent problem is the surgeon who, due to lack of experience, tailors the scope of the surgical procedure to his ability rather than to the requirements imposed by the cancer. This can only be changed when training programs realize that not enough head and neck cancer exists to make experts, by experience, out of more than 20 surgeons yearly. The tendency in training programs with minimal material is to teach the trainees "operations." The trainees then see a patient with cancer of the head and neck for whom they prescribe an "operation," independent of the procedure dictated by the presenting tumor or what they might learn during the surgical procedure. They, therefore, have done the operation correctly, but upon the wrong patient. Until these training programs are modified, practices—such as enucleation of a mass in the parotid rather than protidectomy with facial nerve dissection, enucleation of malignant thyroid cancer instead of subtotal or total thyroidectomy, and inadequate search for the primary in a patient with a mass in the neck for which no obvious primary lesion exists—will continue to occur.

The final unsound management practice commonly seen during the treatment phase is that of compromising the ablative portion of the surgical resection in order to accommodate reconstructive techniques. Procedures are often planned and flaps raised or delayed prior to the ablative portion of the procedure, and at the time of extirpation, cancer is found in an area that will interfere with the repair. Unless the surgeon has properly prepared his patient for this eventuality, his tendency is to proceed with a poor repair or to limit the extirpation, with the latter resulting in margins that will probably contain cancer.

Since the American Board of Radiology recently changed its requirements to permit a certifying examination in the practice of radiation therapy fewer mistakes are made in this field. It is still possible, however, to complete training in radiation therapy at a center with a minimal number of patients with cancer of the head and neck. Radiotherapists coming from these programs are not only inexperienced in the radiation treatment of cancer of the head and neck, but they have been denied the opportunity of working with surgeons, dentists, and chemotherapists in a team approach. An example of this type of problem stemming from such training is observed in irradiated patients who have never had the benefit of a dental caries-fluoride program and who develop osteoradionecrosis.

Unsound Practice in Assessing Treatment Results

A few problems relative to properly assessing treatment results are still seen. The first is the team failure to appreciate that a cancer that has been recently treated may contain cells the viability of which even the pathologist cannot determine. Biopsies taken from a shrinking or nongrowing tumor mass within 3 months from the completion of radiation therapy mean very little. Also related is the misconception that there is a direct relationship between the rate of disappearance of a tumor being irradiated and the ultimate result. If surgery is to be added to radiation therapy, it should be part of the treatment plan from the beginning and should be performed regardless of biopsies of recently irradiated tissue or regression rates during radiation therapy. Finally, the treatment team should realize that the mucosa of the majority of patients with squamous cancer has a very high possibility of developing a second cancer, approaching 30 percent for patients with the original cancer in the pharynx and oropharynx.[7] Three years after the initial treatment, the patient has a higher probability of developing a second cancer than of having his first cancer recur.

INSTITUTIONAL COMMITMENT TO CANCER

The services that support the treatment team, the patient, and his family are so important that it is difficult to properly handle head and neck cancer patients in institutions not sensitive to these problems. A very minimal requirement is that the cancer program within the hospital be approved by the American College of Surgeons. This at least assures that there is a proper organization within the medical staff, educational activities dealing with cancer, and an active tumor registry.

Tumor registries have three important functions in addition to the most obvious one of providing statistics for state and national agencies. Firstly, by determining the stage of the cancer at the time the patient appears for treatment and comparing this figure with a previous time period, a registry can tell a community served by the hospital whether there is a greater need for public or professional education. Secondly, the registry can tell the treatment team whether or not they are improving their results. Thirdly, and perhaps most importantly, the properly managed registry gives the treatment team and the patient assurance of a lifetime of follow-up and alerts both parties that the time for check-up is due.

Specified tumor units, particularly head and neck cancer units, are important if the volume within the hospital warrants it. For example, nursing on an oncology unit is very different from general nursing on a pediatric unit. The type of nurse who is attracted to the oncology unit must have different goals and personality make-up from that of a pediatric nurse. Patients operated on and/or irradiated for cancer of the head and neck are often cosmetically unacceptable, particularly during intermediate repair stages; in addition, they often smell, they often drool, and many cannot eat properly. They require constant cleaning and attention, which is most easily performed in a specialized treatment room where built-in power spray and suction units are available. The nurses on this unit must be able to teach spouses and relatives how to perform self-care functions in home environments. This often requires that specialized equipment be rented or loaned during the home convalescent period. Many educational and specific patient related conferences need to be held between the nursing, dietetic, and social worker staffs and constant leadership from the surgeon members of the treatment team must be provided. It is foolish to believe that the physician will spend the time necessary to overcome the problems of institutions that are neither approved by the American College of Surgeons nor have specialized oncologic wards. Patients with head and neck cancer should therefore probably not be treated in such institutions, but should be referred to teams working within institutions where optimal facilities exist.

REFERENCES

1. American Joint Committee for Cancer Staging and End Results Reporting. 1978. Manual for Staging of Cancer. American Joint Committee, Chicago.

2. Axtell, L. M., Asire, A. J., and Myers, M. H., Eds. 1976. Cancer Patient Survival. U.S. Department of Health, Education and Welfare, Bethesda, Maryland.

3. Cancer Facts and Figures. 1977. American Cancer Society, New York.

4. Daly, T. E., Drane, J. B., and MacComb, W. S. 1972. Management of problems of the teeth and jaws in patients undergoing irradiation. American Journal of Surgery, 124: 539.

5. MacComb, W. S., and Fletcher, G. H., Eds. 1967. Cancer of the Head and Neck. Williams and Wilkins, Baltimore.

6. Rothman, K. J. 1978. Epidemiology of head and neck cancer. Laryngoscope, 88: 435.

7. Sugarbaker, E. V., and Jesse, R. H. 1979. Second primary carcinoma of the "Foregut": High risk of the head and neck cancer patient. (In preparation).

8. Westbrook, K. C.: 1972. Evaluation of Patients with Head and Neck Cancer. In M. D. Anderson Hospital, Ed.: Neoplasms of the Head and Neck. Year Book Medical Publishers, Chicago, 39.

2 | Evaluation of the Patient with Head and Neck Cancer

Raleigh E. Lingeman, M.D.
Mark I. Singer, M.D.

INTRODUCTION

In all disciplines in medicine, thorough histories and painstaking, methodical physical examinations support the diagnostic impression and provide direction for the treatment plan. Based upon this information, special studies are considered; these may include radiographic requests, special scans and isotope studies, echography, cytology, endoscopy, and finally biopsy. After all the data is collected and reviewed and the diagnosis is made, the patient's disease is staged, the modality of treatment is recommended to the patient, and the management of the problem is pursued.

HISTORY TAKING

History taking of a patient with possible head and neck cancer is similar to history taking of any patient in general medicine. More mistakes occur in history taking from errors of omission than from errors of commission. Too often the examiner is not a good listener and may be so hurried that he does not obtain and assemble facts from what has been learned from the patient. If time is spent listening to the patient, clues can be obtained that will lead more readily to an accurate diagnosis. The examiner must have a thorough knowledge of the various disease processes affecting the head and neck. After the patient presents a narrative of the problem, it is necessary for the examiner to direct the patient with more specific questions. The patient may minimize and deny important symptoms that could provide the physician with important clues leading to the diagnosis.

The family history must be reviewed, since a history of multiple members of the family having cancer may indicate an inherent weakness of the patient's immune system against cancer. Previous neoplastic disease must be noted, because patients who have had one cancer will have a greater chance of having the second primary tumor. A specific history of exposure to carcinogens is desirable. This includes the use of tobacco and alcohol with respect to both amount and duration. A long-standing presence of infectious disease should be carefully noted. Although the presence of infection and use of alcohol and tobacco have not been determined with certainty to cause cancer, most investigators agree that there is a direct correlation between these agents and the development of squamous cell carcinoma in the head and neck.

It is important to seek information concerning the patient's psychosocial status. Many of the patients with head and neck cancer have severe personality disorders, are alcoholics, and may have been institutionalized for treatment of emotional disorders. Specific reference to each of these situations should be made in order to be able not only to present the diagnosis and plan of management to the patient, but to be better able to manage his emotional status during the treatment program. Information should also be obtained about the status of the patient's family unit or support system and their interrelationships, since radical surgery for head and neck cancer may inflict severe functional disabilities upon the patient. This may then place the burden for the patient's care directly upon the remaining family members.

The nutritional status of the cancer patient must be evaluated. Progressive loss of weight may be due to distant metastases to vital organs or to nutritional deficiencies due to difficulty in swallowing, pain, excessive alcohol intake, concurrent medical diseases, or another primary cancer. It is necessary to correct marked nutritional deficiency prior to undertaking treatment whether it be surgical or radiation therapy, or a combination of these modalities.

The most common symptoms of cancer in the head and neck are pain, bleeding, obstruction, and the presence of a mass. Pain may represent the very first sign of a change from normal. The pain may be local and result from an ulceration in the oral cavity or the pharynx. Pain may be referred to the orbit, skull base, or cranium. This referred pain occurs in nasopharyngeal tumors and in adenoid cystic carcinomas, which characteristically spread by perineural infiltration. Otalgia may be referred from the tongue, tonsil, hypopharynx, or larynx along the fifth, ninth, or tenth cranial nerve (Figs. 2-1 A and B). The severity of the pain usually can be estimated by making note of the analgesics utilized by the patient. Some patients will describe pain but will deny the need for medication, while others will emphasize the need for pain-relieving drugs which have been in daily use over a period of weeks and months for control of discomfort. Often the patient will deny having pain or using analgesics but the family may describe the patient's suffering and the extent of use of analgesics.

Persistent bleeding should alert the patient and the physician to the possibility of cancer. Bleeding can be very slight, but signs of its persistence are important. In patients with cancer of the nasal cavity and paranasal sinuses, bleeding is very often the first symptom noted by the patient. Such bleeding is rarely profuse.

Obstructive symptoms—such as difficulty in nasal breathing, voice changes related to progressive obstruction of the laryngeal segment of the airway, and difficulty in swallowing—are usually symptoms of advanced tumors and merit thorough investigation. Benign disorders occasionally produce similar symptoms.

The patient with a solitary mass in the neck who is 35 years of age or older should be considered to have cancer until proven otherwise. Approximately 85 percent of masses in the neck in adults are metastatic from the head and neck area. The patient should be questioned as to the duration of the mass, any fluctuation in its size, and the presence or absence of pain. The location of a mass in the neck will often suggest the site of the primary tumor; a mass occurring high in the cervical region and in the area inferior and slightly posterior to the ear will often represent metastasis from a primary tumor of the nasopharynx. Over 50 percent of the patients with nasopharyngeal cancer will present because of a mass in the neck, and at the time of diagnosis 80 percent of these patients will have palpable lymph nodes in the neck. The subdigastric nodes or junctional nodes of Fisch are the site of metastases from primary cancers somewhere in the oral cavity, oropharynx, or hypopharynx. However, cancers of the oral cavity may also involve the lymph nodes in the submandibular triangle. Masses in the midcervical region are commonly found to be associated with tumors of the hypopharynx, base of the tongue, larynx, and pyriform fossa. Metastatic disease of the thyroid gland will most often present along the deep jugular chain of nodes, commonly in the midcervical and lower cervical regions. Lower cervical nodes and supraclavicular

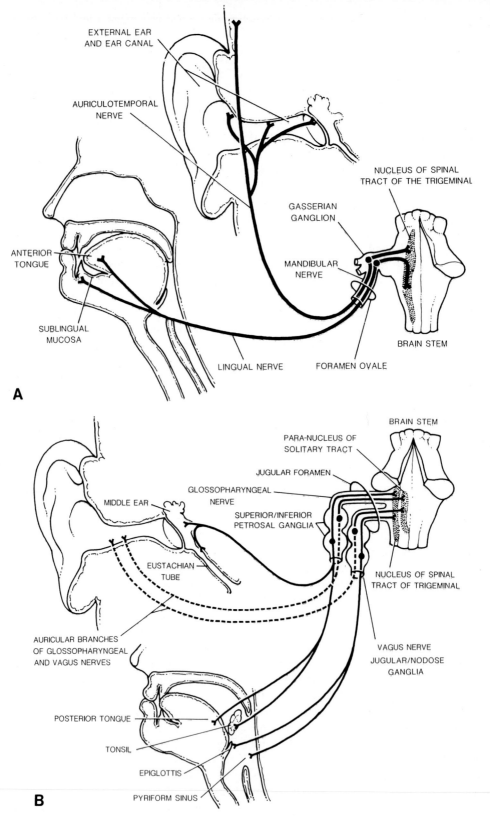

Fig. 2-1. (A) Referred ear pain along branches of the fifth cranial nerve. (B) Referred ear pain along branches of the ninth and tenth cranial nerves.

nodes are likely to be due also to a lesion in the chest or abdomen, and history taking should be directed to such areas as well.

PHYSICAL EXAMINATION

Examination of the head and neck requires that the patient be comfortably seated and the head supported by a rest. The physician either stands or sits by the patient. A source of bright light is essential for a thorough examination; either the reflection from a head mirror or the direct light from a headlight should be used. This permits freedom of the examiner's hands and a sharp focus of intense light in the line of vision.

A routine should be established for the examination to ensure that a complete evaluation is accomplished. Following observation of both the general appearance of the patient and of the head and neck, a suggested procedural format is to examine in sequence (by inspection and palpation) the skin and mucous membranes, underlying tissues, and the associated parts in the following regions:

1. Skin of the face and neck
2. Lips and oral cavity
3. Oropharynx
4. Hypopharynx and larynx
5. Nasopharynx
6. Nose
7. Ear
8. Neck and major salivary glands

GENERAL APPEARANCE AND SKIN

The patient should be observed at rest with notation made of evident weight loss, pain, or difficulty breathing or handling secretions. The skin of the face must be evaluated for abnormal color changes, nonhealing ulcers, and pigmented lesions. When appropriate, the scalp is also reviewed with these changes in mind. The face at rest is evaluated for ptosis of the eyelids; and facial nerve function should be noted with particular reference to asymmetry or loss of normal anatomic contours, such as the nasola-

bial fold or oral commissure. If areas of asymmetry are detected, notation should be made of which branch of the facial nerve is most likely involved. One must also ascertain that the lesion of the facial nerve is peripheral rather than central.

LIPS AND ORAL CAVITY

The vermilion border of the lips and the mucocutaneous junctions are inspected for symmetry, white areas, ulcers, crusted lesions, and localized swelling. The patient must remove all dentures, including partials, prior to the intraoral examination. The mouth is partially opened and the physician inspects and compares both sides. Examination should proceed from the gingivae and buccal areas superiorly and inferiorly. The presence of a painless lesion often is not appreciated by the patient but can be detected by careful inspection. White patches or erythematous lesions on the inside of the cheek should be noted for their configurations and locations and for whether they are bilateral. These lesions may represent underlying systemic diseases, chronic intraoral irritation, or frank premalignant changes. The orifices of Stensen's ducts should be noted in relationship to the second maxillary molar bilaterally, and estimation of the character of the salivary flow should be made. The palatal mucosa and tonsillar pillars are directly viewed by having the patient breathe deeply, making note of subtle changes in the color of the mucous membrane and surface texture. Regions of dryness, atrophy, or granularity should be noted.

The gingivae are inspected for change in color, for thickening, for friability, and for the appearance of white keratotic areas or ulcers. The status of the dentition is of great importance as an overall indicator of oral hygiene. Multiple caries, gingivitis, and periostitis may have a precancerous association. The presence of these conditions gives a clue as to the patient's self-image and tendency for self-neglect. Such conditions will require dental consultation prior to the initiation of therapy. Occlusal dysequilibrium may contribute to problems of mastication and atypical facial pain, and must be carefully noted in the physical examination. The presence of trismus should be noted and may indicate interference in the functioning of the pterygoid muscles by an inflammatory or localized infiltrative process. The pterygoid area should be palpated if trismus is present.

The tongue is examined at rest in the oral cavity and then with protrusion. While examining the tongue any difference in papillation should be noted. Gustatory sensation may be tested with standard salty, sour, bitter, and sweet reagents. There is a difference in sensory distribution between the anterior two-thirds innervated by the lingual nerve and posterior one-third innervated by the glossopharyngeal nerve. Deviation of the tongue to one side may indicate either fixation by tumor infiltration or an ipsilateral hypoglossal nerve paresis or paralysis (especially if there is associated atrophy). Fine lateral margin fasciculations may be an early manifestation of neurologic disease. Inspection of the lateral tongue margins and ventral surface is important because of the frequent neoplastic involvement of these locations. The presence of an exophytic growth, superficial ulceration, keratosis, and pain are frequent manifestations of neoplasia.

The sublingual examination should include the entire floor of the mouth extending posteriorly to the tonsillar pillars. In the midline, Wharton's ducts are noted and, as with Stensen's ducts, an estimation of the character of the salivary flow should be observed. The mucosa should first be dried with gauze or an air blower to ensure an accurate evaluation of salivary flow. Erythema of the papillae and erosions in this area are common signs of neoplastic degeneration. The tongue may be grasped with a piece of gauze and moved from side to side for better exposure of the lateral margins and floor of mouth structures.

The junction of the tongue with the an-terior tonsillar pillar is a site frequently involved by infiltrative cancer. The cancer may be indicated only subtly—by a color change or mucosal atrophy. Intraoral examination should include digital palpation for the detection of induration, tenderness, and ulceration. Bimanual examination of the floor of the mouth and the buccal region must be included for an assessment of the depth of infiltration and for possible adherence to neighboring structures, including the mandible and submandibular triangle contents.

OROPHARYNX

The oropharynx includes the tonsils, the soft palate, the lateral and posterior pharyngeal walls, and the base of the tongue. The base of the tongue is inspected using a laryngeal mirror and the area is carefully palpated. This region is a common location for an occult primary tumor, which may not be detected by inspection alone. Asymmetry of the tonsil, with the presence of a mass in the submucosa superior or posterior to the tonsil, is important and may suggest a parapharyngeal tumor originating either from the deep portion of the parotid gland or as an aneurysm or tumor of the vascular or neural structures in the carotid sheath. Cancers of the tonsil can be extremely subtle in their presentation.

HYPOPHARYNX AND LARYNX

The hypopharynx and larynx are examined with a large size laryngeal mirror; again the base of the tongue and the valleculae should be noted. The examination must also include observation of the epiglottis and false and true vocal cords as well as the adequacy of the airway and subglottic areas. The pharyngeal walls and the pyriform sinuses should be visualized. Cancers of the pharyngeal mucosa often present as ulcerations, and occasionally present as thickened, roughened masses or nodules on the mucosal surface. When cancer is present in the pyriform sinus, ulceration, edema, and fixation of the ipsilateral vocal cord are common accompaniments. Often the pyriform sinus does not open and an excessive amount of saliva will pool on the affected side. Pooling of saliva in an otherwise normal pyriform sinus may be suggestive of esophageal carcinoma. Exposure of the pharyngeal walls may be facilitated by phonation and deep breathing. The hyperexcitable gag reflex can usually be controlled by topical anesthesia, either 2 percent tetracaine hydrochloride (Pontocaine) solution, 4 percent cocaine solution, or benzocaine as an aerosol. Relaxation can be accomplished in the extremely anxious patient by small dosages of diazepam (Valium), administered intravenously.

Supraglottic lesions may be readily detected by their exophytic growth pattern. However, the epiglottic petiole is not easily observed by indirect means and a tumor in this area may not be visible utilizing this technique. Thickening or increased erythema of the aryepiglottic folds and false cords may be signs of an early carcinoma. The glottic region of the larynx may demonstrate areas of leukoplakia, erythema, or bulky exophytic masses that are sessile or even pedunculated. Impaired motion of the vocal cords may be the result of infiltration of the underlying thyroarytenoid musculature, of involvement of the cricoarytenoid joint, or of sheer bulk effect limiting the excursion of the cord. Stridor in the presence of glottic mucosal change should suggest subglottic involvement and narrowing of the laryngeal airway. This is difficult to see by reflected light but must be established promptly. Palpation of the larynx with loss of crepitus may indicate advanced infiltrative carcinoma. Laryngeal tenderness and limitation of movement on swallowing should also be noted.

It is not always possible to carry out a detailed indirect mirror examination of the larynx and hypopharynx. This may be due to a hyperactive gag reflex, a lack of patient cooperation, or certain anatomic features such as a large tongue, a thick, short, or rigid neck, or an overhanging epiglottis. The introduction of several types of direct laryngoscopes for office use has, in great measure, allowed the physician to overcome these problems. The Machida flexible fiberoptic laryngoscope[5] introduced transnasally or the Berci-Ward telescope[2] introduced transorally usually allows for complete inspection of these areas and also offers the opportunity for laryngeal photography. In the event that even the use of these instruments is unsuccessful in allowing for adequate examination of the patient who has symptoms referable to this area or who has a mass in the neck without an obvious primary tumor elsewhere, the patient should be hospitalized for direct laryngoscopy under general anesthesia.

NASOPHARYNX

The nasopharynx is examined by indirect visualization with the largest mirror possible. Although many patients can be examined without local anesthesia, supplemental anesthesia with Pontocaine or cocaine may be necessary. The soft palate can be retracted by intranasal catheters to permit direct or indirect visualization of the nasopharyngeal vault and retrotubal (lateral pharyngeal) recess. All areas of the nasopharynx are examined for suspicious areas of ulceration or exophytic growth. Direct nasopharyngeal telescopes and flexible fiberoptic instruments are important accessory tools for evaluation of the difficult patient or the very young. In addition to providing good visualization, they provide ready means for photodocumentation for future reference.

A nasopharyngeal mass lesion may be accompanied by unilateral middle ear effusion. Repeated careful examination and biopsy are required to eliminate the possibility of malignancy. A posterior cervical lymph node, unilateral middle ear effusion, and repeated epistaxis commonly accompany nasopharyngeal carcinoma. This examination should be carried out repeatedly in adult patients who have middle ear effusion without an obvious etiology.

NOSE AND PARANASAL SINUSES

The nasal skin and suprastructure of the external nose are carefully inspected. A nasal speculum is introduced to examine the interior of the nose—first without, and then if necessary with a vasoconstrictor—in order to fully visualize the structures within the nose. The examiner must observe all areas of crusting, ulceration, masses, and infection. Pooling of mucus may suggest underlying mechanical obstruction. Evaluation of the sinuses can be accomplished by means of appropriate radiographic studies. Palpation of the gingival-buccal sulcus, palate, and pterygoids is important in evaluation of sinus tumors. Hypesthesia of the maxillary division of the fifth cranial nerve and diplopia and proptosis are obvious manifestations of the tumor extending outside the antrum. The nasopharynx must also be carefully inspected in cases of maxillary sinus tumors, as infiltration of the nasopharynx is a contraindication to radical maxillectomy.

EAR

The external ear is observed for ulceration, skin pigmentation, crusting, signs of inflammation, and masses. The external meatus should be carefully cleansed of cerumen and the skin evaluated for chronic otorrhea, bleeding, and fissuring. Suspicious areas should be biopsied to rule out the possibility of an occult carcinoma of auricular skin. If the tympanic membrane is intact, the presence of a middle ear effusion must be noted. This can be confirmed by tuning fork testing, pneumotoscopy, standard air/bone audiometry, and impedance audiometry. As noted earlier, persistent unilateral middle ear effusion may be a sign of nasopharyngeal neoplasm.

Displacement of the auricle and/or induration surrounding the external meatus, tragus, and parotid tissues must be noted.

Neoplastic processes may extend via the fissures of Santorini through the ear canal into the parotid gland or retrograde from the parotid gland into the ear canal. Inspection of the meatus by palpation and otoscopy is important. Finally, in evaluation of the ear, notation of function of the seventh nerve should be routinely made. This is accompanied by palpation of the stylomastoid region. Facial nerve paralysis may be indicative of tumor involvement.

NECK AND MAJOR SALIVARY GLANDS

Examination of the neck should follow an established orderly plan. The examiner can carry out this part of the examination from a position either in front of, behind, or to one side of the patient. It must be borne in mind when searching for the primary tumor that although most malignant tumors of the neck are metastatic, there are tumors which do arise primarily in the cervical region. These include thyroid cancers, cancer of the parotid or submandibular salivary glands, and tumors of the lymphatic system and of soft tissues of the neck. Carotid body tumors, while uncommon, should be kept in mind during the examination.

Inspection of the neck begins with oblique lighting for demonstration of possible cervical asymmetry. The presence of scars, previous incisions, or other characteristics suggesting antecedent trauma are recorded. Prominent pulsations must be noted and an effort made to auscultate the carotid artery system for bruits indicating vascular narrowing. High flow through vascular tumors in this region may also be indicated by auscultation, with confirmation by palpating a thrill.

The neck is palpated over the anterior and lateral triangle and over the cervicooccipital area. This is accomplished usually by the flat of the hand with head support provided by the examiner's other hand. Masses should be noted relative to their movement with swallowing and tongue protrusion and to their possible attachment to the overlying skin or deep neck structures. Determination is made of the size of the mass, definition of the margins, tenderness to palpation, and as to whether solitary or multiple masses are present. The degree of firmness or fluctuation should be noted. Overlying skin changes such as dimples, inflammatory reaction, and atrophy are also observed. The topographic level in the neck must be carefully noted in relation to fixed structures such as the hyoid bone, digastric muscles, mandible, and transverse process of the cervical vertebrae. Masses at the angle of the mandible may be difficult to differentiate from the salivary glands. Bimanual palpation with the mouth open widely may be helpful for this assessment. The parotid is not readily palpable in the normal state, but the submandibular glands typically are and may usually be differentiated from cervical lymphadenopathy.

The thyroid is usually not palpable in the normal state, although occasionally the isthmus may be detected. Reflection of the sternocleidomastoid muscle from the overlying thyroid may permit early detection of a nodule. Tenderness and a bruit should also be reported in relation to the thyroid gland. Midline cervical adenopathy is also noted at this time.

Asymmetric enlargement of the cervical lymph nodes in the adult age group, generally over age 35 years, should be considered malignant until proven otherwise. Metastatic involvement of the neck most often is from a primary lesion arising from the mucous membrane of the nasopharynx, oral cavity, oropharynx, hypopharynx, or larynx, or from the thyroid gland. Masses in the supraclavicular fossa should be noted, recognizing that these often indicate primary disease in the chest or below the diaphragm. Scalene nodes are rarely palpable unless involved by metastatic disease. On the left the node of Virchow often indicates the presence of gastrointestinal malignancy.

A written description or a sketch with measurements provides a valuable future reference in the assessment of head and neck tumors. Preprinted diagrams and photographs are valuable additions to the patient's permanent medical record. Although each physician or department tends to adopt its own data forms for documentation, those contained in the *Manual for Staging of Cancer 1978* from the American Joint Committee for Cancer Staging and End Results Reporting provide an example of an excellent scheme for describing tumors of the larynx.[1]

PSYCHOSOCIAL EVALUATION

Evaluating the patient's psychosocial status may be more difficult than evaluating his physical status. Such an evaluation is, however, no less important. Many of the patients with head and neck cancer have substantial personality disorders and many are alcoholics. It is important during the history taking and physical examination to obtain some information about how well oriented the patient is to his environment, how appropriately he responds to questions and commands, and how he interacts with family or support members who accompany him. It is also important to get a feeling for how well motivated the patient is to overcome his disease. For instance, those who present with obviously far advanced disease may accept a treatment program but are not necessarily well motivated to survive. A patient's work record and marital history may also give important clues as to motivation. Proper evaluation of these spheres may not be possible in the initial examination but may become more apparent during the first few days of the patient's hospitalization.

Total evaluation of the patient requires a multidisciplinary approach. The liberal use of consultants is quite proper and should be accomplished prior to the institution of definitive therapy. The number and degree of involvement of consultants will vary but may include the following colleagues: medical internists, general surgeons, dentists, radiation therapists, medical oncologists, rehabilitation therapists, psychiatrists, pathologists, and of course social workers.

SPECIAL STUDIES

The information obtained from the patient's detailed history and the examination of the head and neck will direct the types of special studies required to complete the evaluation of the patient with head and neck cancer. These modalities are useful in attempting to stage the disease relative to its size, local extension, distant spread, and possible second primary cancer. Routine examination of all patients must include a chest x-ray.

Plain x-ray films of the paranasal sinuses, mandible, mastoid, and the base of the skull provide additional information should physical findings or symptoms suggest their involvement. The use of tomography to define location and extent of bone destruction in the paranasal sinuses, skull base, and temporal bone and involvement of the pterygopalatine space may be quite helpful. Tomography and contrast studies of the larynx, hypopharynx, and cervical esophagus may also provide useful additional information. Cine studies of the pharynx and larynx during swallowing are of special value for their use in the assessment of the dynamic function of velopharyngeal closure, cricopharyngeal relaxation or closure, and upper esophageal motility.

Although angiography is not a routine study in evaluating masses of the head and neck, its use is indicated in the differential diagnosis of the parapharyngeal space. Angiographic studies may outline the extent of mass, its association to vital structures, and its blood supply. The angiographic appearance of angiofibroma and chemodectoma is accepted as diagnostic and eliminates the need for open biopsy. It is useful to embolize feeder vessels to the angiofibroma thus decreasing the hazards of surgical excision.

Sialography is not usually helpful for the diagnosis of malignant tumors of the major salivary glands. This contrast study is of most value in differentiating solid tumors from the nonneoplastic inflammatory disorders.

Diagnosis of cancer by radioisotopic scanning is based upon the principle that various isotope-labeled compounds are incorporated into neoplastic tissues in a different manner than into normal tissues. Either the isotope concentrates in the neoplasm to a greater extent or neoplastic tissue is less capable of taking up the isotope. In the head and neck area, historically the thyroid was the first structure evaluated by this scanning method. The shape, size, nodularity, and functional status is assessed by scanning, which facilitates treatment planning. The preferred isotope is iodine 123 although technetium 99 may also be used. Technetium and gallium are also of some use for the scanning of major salivary glands but have yet to be of major value in differentiating benign from malignant disease.

In the evaluation of the head and neck cancer patient, certain organs are at risk for metastatic spread: commonly the lungs, bones, liver, and brain. If the patient's signs or symptoms warrant, the patient should be systemically evaluated by radionucleotide imaging. These studies may detect dissemination of an advanced head and neck cancer and save the patient from possible disabling surgery. The yield of positive radionucleotide studies is very low both in early cancer and in more advanced cancers if the patients are asymptomatic.

Diagnostic ultrasound or echography is helpful in the study of the thyroid gland. Ultrasound will differentiate a solid thyroid mass from a cystic lesion, which has a lower probability of malignancy. However, this differentiation does not definitively exclude the possibility of malignant disease. The use of computerized axial tomography (CT scanning) in the study of head and neck lesions has added another method for further definition of the head and neck tumor. CT scanning has a high resolution for differentiating soft tissue masses and bone destruction and is proving to be a valuable technique. These studies, however, are expensive and must be used judiciously as supplements to, rather than replacements for, conventional methods.

Endoscopy is an important procedure for more thoroughly evaluating a patient for disease of the upper aerodigestive tract. The open tube technique often requires general anesthesia for complete relaxation but provides excellent evaluation of the mucous membrane directly or with magnification. With the patient under continuous anesthesia, effective tissue sampling can be obtained through the open tube because of the adequate working space it affords. Furthermore its use facilitates management of secretions and hemorrhage. Problem areas for endoscopic evaluation are the epiglottic petiole, retrocricoid region, pyriform apices, laryngeal ventricles, glottis, and subglottis because of the possibility of concealed malignancy. On the other hand, the flexible fiberoptic endoscopes may make these recesses somewhat more accessible and may be well tolerated under local anesthesia. Problems limiting the use of these endoscopes include loss of optical resolution for evaluation of mucosal detail, difficulty in managing secretions and bleeding, and difficulty in obtaining adequate tissue specimens through the limited channels of the instrument.

There is a growing body of information about synchronous second primary cancers of the upper aerodigestive tract. Some surgeons feel that endoscopic evaluation of the larynx, hypopharynx, nasopharynx, esophagus, and tracheobronchial tree should be carried out as a routine part of the patient's evaluation.[3]

Biopsy and histologic tissue sampling is briefly reviewed in this section. Many cancers are visible to the examiner, while others may require further diagnostic procedures for their localization prior to biopsy. There are four methods of biopsy available to the examiner. The simplest technique uses punch forceps for removal of specimens of tissue from tumor located in accessible areas of the head and neck, such as the oral cavity, oropharynx, nasal walls, and nasopharynx. Anesthesia may be obtained by topical Pontocaine or cocaine or by infiltration with lidocaine for greater depth of anesthesia and possibly may be supplemented by a vasoconstrictor. The specimen must not be crushed and should be fixed at once in tissue preservatives (formalin, Bouin's solution).

A second method for biopsy involves the use of a needle, such as the Silverman needle, to remove a core of tissue to be submitted to the pathologist. Needle biopsy is most helpful in diagnosis of masses of the head and neck area, but the accuracy of the technique is determined by the experience and competence of the pathologist. A representative sample and adequate amount of tissue for interpretation must be provided for tissue section. Lymphoma and various types of sarcomas cannot be readily diagnosed by needle biopsy. Diagnosis with the needle technique is most accurate in metastatic epidermoid carcinoma to the neck.

A fine needle may be used with a vacuum to obtain an aspirate. This is smeared and stained for microscopic examination. The advantages of the use of the fine needle technique are claimed to be decreased chances for dermal or cutaneous implantation by the needle, while the main disadvantage is the necessity for a pathologist experienced in cytopathologic techniques.

A third method of biopsy is the incisional technique, which can be done under choice of local or general anesthesia. It is important not to violate or contaminate the surrounding tissues. Often the incisional biopsy may be combined with frozen section study.

Under a strict interpretation of the term, *biopsy* includes surgical excision such as parotidectomy, thyroidectomy, or wide local excision, which will determine the need for additional surgery or adjunctive treatment modalities. In the event the tumor is reported as malignant by the pathologist, and the opinion is definitive, the surgeon may then elect to proceed with a wide resection depending upon the histologic type and the biologic behavior of the tumor.

The establishment of a confirmed histologic diagnosis is essential before undertaking any of the therapeutic modalities of management available for the head and neck cancer patient. Repeated biopsies may be required before an accurate diagnosis is made. In the event of uncertainty or indecision on the part of the pathologist, it may be necessary to obtain the opinion of a consulting pathologist before undertaking any modality of treatment involving radical radiation therapy, surgery, or a combination of these methods.

Patients are often referred for definitive care by physicians who have already performed a biopsy. It is of the utmost importance to have the slides from the biopsy reviewed by the pathologist with whom the surgeon works. Simply accepting the written pathology report from the outside source will lead to mistakes in management. Many of the pathologists at community hospitals have limited exposure to neoplasms of the head and neck, and this leads to certain inaccuracies in diagnosis. Reviewing the slides, and at times obtaining tissue blocks from the outside source, will either upgrade, downgrade, or confirm the diagnosis and will save the patient the inconvenience of a repeat biopsy. Occasionally, definitive diagnosis cannot be established in this way and a repeat biopsy will be necessary.

Following the above techniques of evaluation, the patient's disease may be staged. This is an important aspect, as it allows for more accurate treatment planning, prognosticating, and later analysis of end results. The advent of TNM classification has helped in this task and the fine details of the system are discussed in many of the chapters of this book.

CONSIDERATIONS IN TREATMENT PLANNING

One of the most important facets relating to patient evaluation is that of dealing with the recommendations of the physician concerning management of the disease. Often the patient has suspected the underlying cause of the problem; nevertheless, it is the responsibility of the doctor, upon completion of a thorough review of the case, to inform the patient that a life-threatening condition exists. Because the diagnosis of cancer, and the subsequent discussion of therapeutic options, will most likely cause severe stress for the patient and the family, the question frequently arises as to whether or not to inform the patient of the presence of cancer. Most studies have demonstrated that patients are ultimately aware of the outcome of the diagnosis and that failure to initially provide honest feedback to the patient impairs the effectiveness of the doctor-patient relationship. In fact, most patients today assume that the word biopsy is synonymous with cancer.

Following assessment of the problem by the surgeon, it is imperative that the situation be reviewed with the patient. Too often, because of the considerable pressures brought to bear upon him by a busy medical practice, the physician does not allow sufficient time to properly convey to the patient the significance of the findings concerning the discovery of his serious head and neck cancer. Consequently, it is important to plan for adequate time for this discussion. It is advisable that the patient's family be present when this discussion is conducted and that questions be answered as completely as possible at this time. Most patients are under such terrible stress at this time that they may retain little of what has been told to them about their diagnosis and the recommended treatment. Having a family member present provides someone who will witness this conversation as well as help to reinforce the information for the patient.

In a discussion of the patient's problem, the surgeon must emphasize the probabilities rather than the absolutes, always leaving room for hope. The patient will expect the physician to make a recommendation as to the modality of treatment, but it remains the patient's prerogative to accept or to reject these recommendations. Having described the options, one method for the surgeon to assist the patient is to explain what he, the surgeon, would want done for himself or a member of his own family if faced with this particular problem in this position today. This is an effective means for explaining the importance of the recommended modality of treatment to the patient.

Patients will often bring up medical problems they have faced in the past and which pose as possible contraindications for the recommended surgery. Most head and neck surgeons are in agreement that there are no medical contraindications for cancer surgery. This philosophy was stated by Dr. Hayes Martin.[4] Martin considered this to be an entirely reasonable policy because the cancer itself is always fatal if untreated and if surgery—whether conservative or radical—offers the best chance of cure when compared to other methods, then it is logical to accept a reasonable operative risk rather than to accept the inevitable death from uncontrolled cancer. Experience proves that if the physician firmly believes in the soundness of the proposal and if he has given due consideration to the sensibility and sensitivity of the patient, he will have few refusals of the recommended modality of treatment even in the face of the most extensive operation.

It is essential that the physician develop a relationship with his patient predicated upon trust and confidence and that he instill in his patient a sense of maintenance of hope for the control of his disease. In addition, the physician, by building upon his trust, will find that his patient experiences less postoperative depression, avoids prolonged mourning for loss of an organ (as in laryngectomy), more easily accepts alterations in body image, and avoids severe loss of self-esteem that may occur as a result of radical surgery.

Patients and their families may request the opinion of a second surgeon and this should be encouraged. Many times the patient is not aware of other surgeons who may give him a competent opinion; it is the duty of the surgeon who initially examines the patient to refer him to surgeons in his locale who will provide competent medical advice or, if necessary, to medical centers in the general area where the patient may be certain to have a thorough evaluation and a competent opinion.

REEVALUATION

Periodic follow-up evaluations are an essential part of the total management of the patient with head and neck cancer. Early follow-up appointments following surgery will be necessary for psychological support and for such activities as suture removal, care of incompletely healed wounds, checking on nutritional status, and timely referrals for speech pathology or maxillofacial prosthodontics.

After this initial phase, examinations should take place at monthly intervals for the first year, every 2 months during the second year, every 3 to 4 months during the third year, and semiannually thereafter. The necessity for such intervals is that most recurrences (at least in squamous cell carcinoma) in the primary site appear within the first 12 months and most metastases to regional lymph nodes or to distant organs will have occurred within 2 years following treatment. Follow-up examination on an indefinite basis is necessary because of the tendency for patients with squamous cell carcinoma to develop second, third, and sometimes more, primary cancers in the upper and lower aerodigestive tract.

These periodic visits should consist of obtaining an interval history and performing a thorough examination of the head and neck. The patient's weight should be noted. A general physical examination and appropriate radiographs should be performed when indicated. Any findings deviating from normal expectations should be recorded.

Patients seen during these follow-up visits who complain of recurrence of the type of symptoms that they experienced prior to treatment, such as pain, hoarseness, or dysphagia, should be suspected of having recurrences of their tumors. New findings such as the appearance of a mass in the neck or any of the above symptoms should arouse suspicion of metastatic disease. It is in the patient's best interest to pursue a detailed examination including appropriate tests and biopsies to establish a diagnosis. There is a certain denial at times by the attending physician about the possibility of recurrence, as this represents a failure of the physician to cure the patient. Too often valuable time is lost before such a diagnosis is made and treatment instituted.

SUMMARY

The careful evaluation of the patient with head and neck cancer still depends primarily upon a detailed history and physical examination. Special studies may supplement this information and allow for more accurate staging of the disease. The use of consultation in specialized areas supports the concept of the team approach to management of these problems. Emphasis must be placed upon adequate psychological evaluation and a sound doctor-patient relationship based upon trust, confidence, and a forthright approach to the problem by the physician.

REFERENCES

1. American Joint Committee for Cancer Staging and End Results Reporting. 1978. Manual for Staging of Cancer. American Joint Committee, Chicago.
2. Berci, B. 1977. Present and future developments in endoscopy. Proceedings of the Royal Society of London (Biological Sciences), 195: 235.
3. Gluckman, J. L. 1979. Synchronous multiple primary lesions of the upper aerodigestive system. Archives of Otolaryngology, 105: 587.
4. Martin, H. E. 1957. Surgery of Head and Neck Tumors. Hoeber-Harper, New York.
5. Silberman, H. D., Wilf, H., and Tucker, J. 1976. Flexible fiberoptic nasopharyngoscope. Annals of Otology, Rhinology and Laryngology, 85: 640.

3 | Histopathological Considerations

John G. Batsakis, M.D.

The surgical pathology of cancer has become increasingly regional in nature and although general morphologic principles apply, the special requirements of anatomic regions are such that the relationship between pathologist and surgeon *must* be one of close cooperation and mutual education. To do otherwise is to place the pathologist and surgeon in a constant state of risk, or at least, promote an ill-judged complacency.

Even though founded on scientific principles, surgical pathology nonetheless remains an art; an art in which objectivity often yields to subjectivity. Surgical pathology's sister discipline, laboratory medicine, because of its relationship to more precise analytical data has reduced this subjectivity and consequently the error potential. Thus, to describe the role of the surgical pathologist in the management of cancer of the head and neck, I will use the laboratory medicine categories of *preanalytical, ana-*lytical and *postanalytical* in this chapter (Fig. 3-1).

In the preanalytical phase of the evaluation of cancer, it is imperative for the pathologist to have detailed clinical and radiologic information. At the least, a summary of these findings and prior histopathologic data should be provided by the clinician. No pathologist should be asked to provide a diagnosis in the absence of the clinical background. Perhaps Levene's quote from Stewart expresses this axiom best: "A pathological diagnosis is not a mere matching of microscopic pictures, it involves the whole evidence of the case, the natural history of the disease, and the pathologist's judgement."[34]

Even in the analytical phase of the diagnostic process, wherein the surgical pathologist uses the tools of his trade, clinical assistance and consultation is also required. Such interaction is outlined below under se-

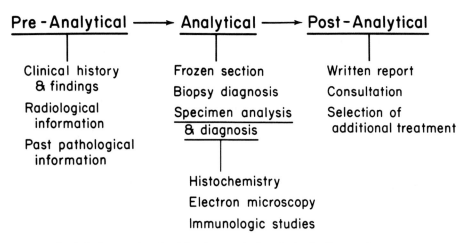

Fig. 3-1. Factors involved in the surgical-pathologic diagnostic process.

lected categories of the analytical aspects of surgical pathology. The consultative and educational circle is completed in the postanalytical phase, in which therapy is selected, based on pathologic and clinical findings.

CLASSIFICATION AND NOMENCLATURE

A knowledge of contemporary classification and taxonomy of tumors of the head and neck is indispensable to their proper management. The pathologist, in turn, should allocate a given lesion to a particular class and type as precisely as possible. This is easier said than done. In some areas of oncology there is a bewildering array of proposed classifications; some of which may be self-serving exercises. In the case of lymphoreticular neoplasia, the rapid evolution, changes and competitive classifications and subtypes almost guarantee confusion.[47, 53] Only time and *clinical* correlation will judge the usefulness of various classifications.

In general, classifications of disease and particularly neoplasia, follow three main lines: etiologic, histogenic, and those based on a subconscious or conscious recognition of normal cellular counterparts. Since the etiology of cancer is unknown, etiologic classifications relate almost exclusively to nonneoplastic diseases; Table 3-1, after Seifert and Donath,[48] outlines such a scheme for sialadenitis. Histogenic concepts are usually incorporated within the subjective forms of classification but may also stand alone as a basis for classification. Their basis is often hypothetical and correlation with clinical course is often lacking. One such histogenic classification is that used for salivary gland tumors wherein the tumors are considered to arise from reserve cells of the ductal system of the salivary gland unit.[43] A conceptualized diagram of tumors arising from the intercalated ducts is presented in Figure 3-2. Table 3-2 represents a form of classification (tumors of bone) based on a histologic basis;[2] this type of format is used for the majority of surgical diagnoses.

TABLE 3-1. ETIOLOGIC CLASSIFICATION OF SIALADENITIS

Bacterial sialadenitis
    Acute parotitis
    Chronic relapsing parotitis

Viral sialadenitis
    Epidemic parotitis ("mumps")
    Cytomegalic parotitis

Radiation sialadenitis

Electrolyte sialadenitis

Küttner tumor of submandibular gland

Immune sialadenitis
    Myoepithelial sialadenitis (lymphoepithelial lesion—Sjögren syndrome)
    Epitheliod cell sialadenitis (Heerfordt syndrome)

(Modified from Seifert, G., and Donath, K. 1976. Classification of the pathohistology of diseases of the salivary glands—review of 2,600 cases in the Salivary Gland Register. Beitraege zur Pathologie (Stuttgart), 159: 1.)

Taxonomic and nosologic classifications are used, in conjunction with the pathologist's armamentarium of analytical processes, when making surgical diagnoses. When using classifications, the pathologist

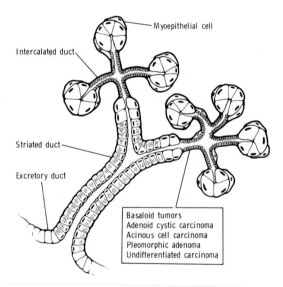

Fig. 3-2. Schematic version of a classification of salivary gland tumors based on histogenetic concepts. In this version the tumors listed are considered to arise from the intercalated duct reserve cell.

TABLE 3-2. CLASSIFICATION OF TUMORS OF SKULL AND BONES
OF THE FACE

Histologic Type	Benign	Malignant
Lymphoreticular	Histiocytosis	Plasmacytoma Myeloma Lymphoma Histiocytosis

Chondrogenic	Osteochondroma
	Chondroma
		Chondrosarcoma
		    Differentiated
		    Dedifferentiated
		    Mesenchymal

Osteogenic	Osteoma
	Osteoid osteoma
	Osteoblastoma
		Osteogenic sarcoma
		    Endosteal
		    Parosteal
		    Periosteal

Fibrogenic	Fibroma
	    Ossifying
	    Nonossifying
	Desmoplastic fibroma
		Fibrosarcoma

Odontogenic	Myxoma	(?) Myxosarcoma
Notochordal	—	Chordoma
Vascular	Hemangioma Vascular malformation Hemangiopericytoma	Angiosarcoma Hemangiopericytoma
Lipogenic	Lipoma	Liposarcoma
Neurogenic	Neurilemmoma Neurofibroma	Neurogenous sarcoma Other neuroectodermal tumors
Origin not established	Giant cell granuloma "Brown tumor" Cherubism Giant cell tumor Benign fibrous histiocytes	Malignant giant cell tumor Ewing sarcoma Malignant fibrous histiocytoma

(Modified from Batsakis, J. G. 1979. Tumors of the Head and Neck: Clinical and Pathological Considerations, 2nd edn., © (1979) Williams and Wilkins, Baltimore.)

should strive for uniformity in the criteria applied to morphologic and cellular subclassification. This reduces the principal difficulty when comparing often dissimilar data from series of cancer cases in the head and neck and elsewhere.

In former times, pathology was, and was preferred to be, isolated from clinical care. This led to Elisha Bartlett's opinion: "Therapeutics is not founded upon pathology. The former cannot be deduced from the latter. It rests solely upon exposure. It is, absolutely and exclusively, an imperfect art."[54] Now, however, the pathologic examination is integral to the planning of treatment and prognosis, and both pathology and therapeutics mutually benefit.

In the following, the interaction between surgeon and pathologist, if not emphasized, is strongly implied and indicates the changes in attitudes over the course of time.

THE BIOPSY

The main objective of a biopsy is to provide the pathologist with *representative* tissue for *diagnostic* purposes; however, as shown in Figure 3-3, the biopsied tissue is also capable of providing valuable information regarding treatment and prognosis.

The biopsy technique may be by excision, incision, aspiration cytology, needle biopsy (drill or core), or cellular means (imprint or exfoliative). Before discussing these methods in detail, however, certain generalizations are worth making. First, no pathologist can make a diagnosis of a disease from biopsy tissue that is not representative of the lesion. The methods of procurement, handling, and transport of the specimen are all vital. Material obtained by cautery is usually unsatisfactory for biopsy interpretation

because of the charring and distortion associated with the technique. Superficial or "nibbler" biopsies are subject to the risk of error. Necrotic lesions, if sampled in their center, may only show the retrogressive changes associated with the necrosis and the changes may not be representative of the lesions. In such instances, the biopsy should be taken with the scalpel and should include both normal and diseased tissues.

Second, quick placement of the biopsy specimen in the appropriate fixative will ensure preservation of important cytologic detail. Too often, improper fixation results in no diagnosis, an incomplete diagnosis, or worse, a wrong diagnosis. A universal fixative, suitable for both light and electron optic studies is highly recommended (see p. 39). If particular diagnostic studies are known to be needed, a priori consultation between pathologist and surgeon is required so as not to invalidate these studies by improper fixation.

Third, orientation of biopsy specimens,

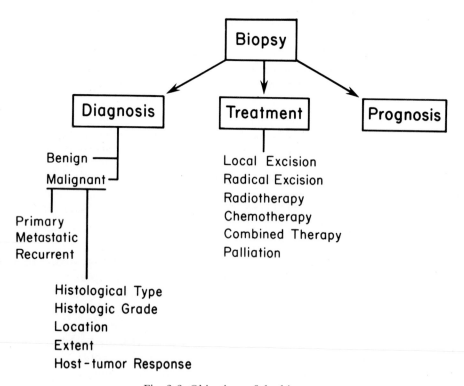

Fig. 3-3. Objectives of the biopsy.

especially for excisional biopsy material, is a requirement that is too often left to the surgical pathologist. Labeling of key dimensions with tags or through and through sutures facilitates the orientation and will negate the curling arising after excision. This simple measure will reduce tangential sectioning and diagnostic difficulty.

Frozen Section Diagnosis

The single most important purpose of the frozen section is to make a therapeutic decision. Academic curiosity never reasonably justifies a surgeon's request for frozen section diagnosis. I regard the frozen section as a consultation between physicians. As such it is imperative that a sound dialogue has been established between the surgeon and pathologist over the need for, limitations of, and consequences of the frozen section diagnosis.

Since frozen section examinations are to be used for immediate decision making, the indications for such examinations are as follows:

1. As an initial diagnostic procedure (no previous histopathologic diagnosis) for certain malignancies where a definitive radical procedure is to be carried out immediately.

2. For the diagnosis of any intraoperative tissue abnormality.

3. For the assessment of the margins of clearance in an operative surgical specimen (see p. 31).

4. For preliminary assessment of the extent of neoplastic involvement so as to plan effectively the therapy of choice.

5. To determine or confirm that a piece of tissue selected for frozen section is indeed relevant to the presumed clinical diagnosis.

Contraindications for and misuses of frozen section diagnosis are when the frozen section diagnosis carries no immediate therapeutic decision; the tissue is heavily calcified or ossified; the specimen is unique or of small size; or the diagnosis is used as an impatient substitute for examinations best performed on routinely processed material.

As Levene[34] points out, the difficulties inherent in the diagnosis are not contraindications to attempting a frozen-section, but are merely inhibiting factors. Other factors militating against successful diagnosis are frozen sections on lesions which even under optimum conditions require extensive study because of their complexity. These include the lymphoreticular disorders and granulomatous diseases. Since the purpose of needle biopsy is to obtain a diagnosis without resort to a formal operative procedure, it certainly is a contradiction to seek a frozen section diagnosis on such material if the surgeon is not prepared to immediately act on that diagnosis in a definitive therapeutic manner. Furthermore, the crush artefact usually attendant to these procedures and the possibility of nonrepresentative tissue compounds the difficulty of frozen section diagnosis.

Requests for frozen section diagnosis on tumors of the salivary glands require special introspection by the surgeon. The often variable appearance of such tumors in different areas introduces sampling error potential, and thus, in practice, extent rather than classification dictates the treatment. Unless a precise diagnosis modifies the surgical procedure, frozen section evaluation is no more than adjunctive. In this author's opinion, resection of the facial nerve is more dependent on the location and intimacy of the tumor to the nerve than upon histologic type. The plan then for surgical management of parotid gland malignancies is based primarily on clinical staging (with only partial modification of that plan) and ultimately prognosis by the histologic type of carcinoma.[51]

The use of frozen section consultations in surgery of the head and neck appears to be equal to the extent of use in general surgery.[4] The rate of error in general for frozen section diagnosis has ranged in published reports from 0.7 to 2.5 percent.[1, 12] Dehner and Rosai[12] report an accuracy rate of 96 percent on 1,187 individual nondeferred frozen sections. This figure is identical to Bauer's[4] data dealing exclusively with ear, nose, and throat frozen sections.

Improper surgical or pathologic sampling accounts for most frozen section errors. This deficiency in sampling often leads to the later discovery of diagnostic tissue in deeper cuts of the frozen section block. The latter has particularly vexed the present author, and the alert surgeon should always be aware of this possibility.

There is often a mistaken idea among surgeons that each frozen section should provide a precise histologic diagnosis. Any pathologist will agree that such a diagnosis is desirable, but in most operative situations, "benign" or "malignant" designations will be sufficient for the needs of the case. In that light, a deferred diagnosis, if not abused, is to be expected also by the surgeon. Dehner and Rosai[12] recorded a deferred diagnosis in 4 percent of 778 frozen section cases. As may have been expected, the majority of cases in this category are lesions of soft tissues and the lymphoreticular system. In our experience, deferred diagnoses also follow examination of head and neck frozen sections from patients with preoperative irradiation. Epithelial atypia, ulceration, atypical fibroangioblastic proliferation, and inflammation may follow irradiation and can complicate identification of residual tumor.

Finally, the dictum *scripta manent verba volant*—written words remain while spoken words fly away—applies for frozen section reporting. Dehner and Rosai[12] related the following reasons for the advisability of such a policy: it provides a permanent record for medical and legal purposes, it protects the pathologist and surgeon from possible misunderstanding at the time of verbal communication, and it provides a retrievable format for periodic evaluation of the procedure.

SURGICAL MARGINS

One of the axioms of "curative surgery" for cancer of the head and neck is that complete excision be performed with "adequate" margins. What constitute adequate margins varies from surgeon to surgeon and is influenced by the type of surgery (conservation or radical) and the site, size, and type of neoplasm.

Little relevant information is currently available about the significance of microscopic malignancy in the surgical margins.[6, 9, 33, 36] One thing is clear, however: extrapolation of information derived from study of different anatomic sites cannot be successfully made. Neoplasms from a given region or anatomic site appear to have their own natural history and biologic course.

Lee,[33] after studying carcinomas of the oral cavity, oropharynx, hypopharynx, and larynx, found inadequate tumor margins in 9 percent of 864 resections. Oral cavity carcinomas were excised inadequately most frequently (15 percent); hypopharyngeal and laryngeal lesions were least frequently excised inadequately (3 and 4 percent respectively). Of significance is Lee's finding that only 6 of 11 patients who were reexcised demonstrated tumor on histologic examination—a 50 percent accuracy rate.[33] Irradiation adversely affects estimation of margin adequacy. Lee[33] reporting on adequate margins from 607 cases found that local recurrences developed in 10 percent of cases initially treated surgically, in 17 percent of patients receiving combined therapy, and in 27 percent of radiation failure resections.

For T1, T2, and T3 squamous cell carcinomas of the oral cavity, oropharynx, and hypopharynx, the presence of positive margins is definitely associated with a higher rate of local recurrence than is that of negative margins (71 versus 32 percent in the series reported by Looser et al.[36]). The report of adequate margins of resection does not guarantee local control of disease, nor does it, in any way, predict the biologic behavior of the neoplasm. The correlation between positive margins and patient longevity is, however, very significant, since almost all of these patients die of their disease.

Conservative laryngeal surgery has allowed a thorough evaluation of the significance of surgical margins in carcinomas of the larynx. In contrast to squamous cell carcinomas of the oral cavity and upper digestive tract, in laryngeal carcinomas with positive margins there is a significantly lower incidence of local recurrence. In a study by Bauer et al.,[6] 39 of 111 patients undergoing hemilaryngectomy had positive margins. Fifteen of these margins were classified as close, 12 were grossly involved, and 12 showed intraepithelial carcinoma. None of the patients received any further treatment, and in a 5 to 12 year follow-up period only 7 of 39 (18 percent) developed local recurrences. Four of 72 patients (5.5 percent) with clear margins developed local recurrences.

Why recurrences appear in patients with adequate margins underscores our meager knowledge of neoplasia and the fallibility of microscopic evaluation. Two possible explanations may apply: a residual island distant to the adequate margin; and recurrence in a microscopic, multicentric focus (field cancerization).

The significance of margins is thus diminished by the capricious behavior of squamous cell carcinomas of the upper aerodigestive tract. Additionally, clinical stage bears heavily on the significance of a negative margin. For T1 and T2 carcinomas of the oral cavity, oropharynx, and hypopharynx, a 1.0 cm margin is advisable. The margin of safety is reduced to 0.5 cm for laryngeal carcinomas amenable to conservation surgery.

As indicated on page 29, I consider frozen section diagnosis to have a valuable and utilitarian role in the intraoperative assessment of margins of excision. Such frozen section specimens may be taken by two methods. The first relies on the pathologist, with the aid of the surgeon for orientation of the specimen. Depending on the size of the specimen and the nature of the malignancy, the pathologist may take serial full thickness samples or, alternatively, circumferential margins in addition to the base of the specimen. In the second method the surgeon provides *sequential* margins until the specimen is free of marginal neoplasm by frozen section examination. These two methods apply principally to cutaneous and readily excised mucosal lesions. Intraoperative assessment of margins in other areas, such as the upper airway and soft tissues, must rely primarily on the surgeon's selection of in situ samples after mobilization of the resected specimen; this allows two evaluations—one by the surgeon and the other by the pathologist on the submitted intact specimen. The in situ samples should correspond to margins and depth on the complete specimen, and the pathologist must be duly informed or alerted by appropriate tagging or labels. Any suspicious area should be clearly identified for pathologic examination, and pathologist-surgeon interaction should be at its maximum during any evaluation of adequacy of excision.

Needle Aspiration Cytology and Biopsy

A leading article in the British Medical Journal[32] divided the surgical world into two classes: "those who believe it is wrong to assault a tumor by anything less than its formal excision and those who are prepared to pass needles of varying sizes into it and reach either a cytopathologic or histomorphologic diagnosis ahead of definitive treatment." For the head and neck surgeon such a division is too rigid, but it nevertheless requires a critical review.

Decisions for needle biopsy of lesions of the head and neck require a thorough evaluation of the utility of the procedure. Distinction should also be made between needle aspiration with cytology and needle biopsy with tissue histopathology, but the criteria for utility apply equally. The components of utility may be divided into practical success, sensitivity, discrimination, and most important, how the procedure will influence clinical and therapeutic practice.

Practical success with needle aspiration cytology of tumors is related to the procurement of a satisfactory specimen by the operator and a reportable product by the cytologist. Depending on the clinician-cytologist combination and the tissue being sampled, unreportable specimens should be less than 10 percent and optimally less than 5 percent. For tumors of the head and neck, suitable specimens for examination have ranged from 70 to 95 percent of attempts.[18, 19, 35, 52] The higher percentage reflects data obtained by experienced workers. It is also to be noted that most reports with good results have been based on specimens aspirated by the cytopathologist himself, which generally implies appropriate specimen preparation, optimal fixation, and staining routines.

One of the major criticisms leveled at aspiration cytology has been the high false-negative rates in the presence of neoplastic disease. At this time, given the skill and experience of the cytopathologist, the false negatives are more attributable to the lack of an appropriate and representative sample.

Sensitivity and discrimination refer to the ability to detect malignancy when it is present and to identify clinically doubtful lesions as benign or malignant. In the breast and lung a greater than 90 percent sensitivity is achievable.[24] Percutaneous transthoracic aspiration biopsy has revolutionized the investigation of solitary pulmonary nodules; the accuracy rate is as high as 98 percent.[24] For primary lesions in the head and neck, however, rates for both sensitivity and discrimination are lower and vary according to site and class of tumors.[18, 19, 35, 50, 52] Table 3-3 from the study by Frable and Frable[19] relates thin-needle aspiration statistics for

tumors of salivary glands. Droese et al.[14] reported a diagnostic accuracy of 75.5 percent in their evaluation of fine-needle aspiration cytology in 194 samples of salivary gland tumors; Zajicek and Eneroth,[56] in their summary of 100 consecutive salivary gland carcinomas, recorded an accuracy rate of 70 percent. Lindberg and Akerman's[35] findings after aspiration cytology diagnosis in 461 patients (salivary gland tumors) can be summarized as follows: exact agreement with histopathology, 63 percent; good and not misleading agreement, 18 percent; false reports, 8 percent; and unsatisfactory specimens, 11 percent.

Schnurer and Widstrom[50] reported the accuracy rate of diagnosis using preliminary fine-needle biopsy in 303 patients undergoing thyroid surgery. Assessable cytologic material was obtained in 94 percent of cases, with a 93 percent agreement between the fine-needle biopsy and subsequent histologic diagnosis; 15 of 28 cases of carcinoma were diagnosed preoperatively (a 46 percent failure rate).

The utility of needle biopsy or aspiration must be judged, however, on more than correct assignment to diagnostic types. The final arbiter is how the technique influences the diagnostic sequence or therapy—but determining the usefulness of aspiration cytology is not easy, since the technique is intimately related to the management of an individual patient. Only after prospective studies which address the problem of utility will we have a valid answer.

At the present time, needle biopsy (as-

TABLE 3-3. MALIGNANT SALIVARY GLAND TUMORS—THIN NEEDLE ASPIRATION

Tumor Type	No. Cases	Correct Diagnosis (%)	False Positives (%)	False Negatives (%)
Adenoid cystic carcinoma	45	80	0	20
Acinous cell carcinoma	34	65	0	35
Mucoepidermoid carcinoma	18	62	0	38
Carcinoma ex pleomorphic adenoma	7	100	0	0

(Modified from Frable, W. J., and Frable, M. A. 1974. Thin-needle aspiration biopsy in the diagnosis of head and neck tumors. Laryngoscope, 84:1069.)

piration and tissue) for head and neck lesions satisfies the question of utility only for rapid confirmation of metastasis or recurrences from a previously known primary malignancy and biopsy of sites not readily accessible to the scalpel. For other proposed uses, such as the diagnosis of primary salivary gland tumors, proof of utility that leads to modification in the diagnostic or therapeutic sequence has *not* been established. With time and experience this attitude is subject to change but until then, it is my contention that needle biopsy for primary lesions is only one of several steps in the diagnostic evaluation, rather than an alternative, quicker method of reaching a diagnosis.

Exfoliative and Imprint Cytology

The diagnostic utility of examination of exfoliated cells from mucosal lesions of the upper aerodigestive tract is limited, and exfoliative cytology should never be a substitute for biopsy. Its role is adjunctive in the diagnostic process or for the monitoring of response to therapy. For the detection of presumptive lung *and* upper respiratory tract cancer in high-risk individuals, deep-cough sputum specimens may, on occasion, lead to the discovery of a small number of patients with tumors in the upper respiratory or alimentary passages.[39]

The adjunctive aspects of exfoliative cytology are perhaps best appreciated when one reviews its application for lesions in the oral cavity. False negative rates of over 30 percent and little or no correlation of the malignant cells to location, size, gross characteristics, and histologic differentiation of the neoplasm relegates the technique to a secondary or even lower level in the diagnostic sequence.[17, 42] A negative cytology report precludes neither malignancy nor other diseases.

Imprint and scrape cytology is dependent upon the transfer of cells from fresh tissues to glass slides by either touch (imprint) preparations or by scraping the cut surface of the tissue. The technique may be effectively used as an adjunct to frozen sections and especially for the evaluation of lymphomas or small-celled neoplasms that simulate lymphomas.

Since the imprint is a cytologic preparation, the relationship of cells to their stroma may be obscured or absent. Hence, an exact histologic diagnosis may not be possible and a distinction between benign and malignant cell composition may be sufficient.

In general, malignant lesions yield many more cells than do benign ones. An acellular touch preparation, if desmoplastic neoplasms are excluded, almost ensures that the process is benign. Benign epithelial tumors yield numbers of cohesive cells devoid of malignant features while imprints of most malignant tumors are composed of poorly cohesive clusters of cells and single atypical cells.

A variety of stains may be used but polychrome methylene blue is most common. Histochemical procedures such as a-naphthol acetate esterase methods can serve to distinguish histiocytes from cells with similar morphologic features, such as some epithelial cells.

In this author's opinion, touch preparations increase the accuracy of both frozen and permanent section diagnoses of lymph node specimens. In experienced hands, and with small or crushed specimens, the touch preparation may even exceed the permanent section in diagnostic accuracy.[7]

As it is with all cytologic preparations, false negative results bedevil the pathologist and surgeon. The false negative reports are generally due to either interpretative errors, such as may occur if the lesions are well differentiated and the morphologic changes of the neoplastic cells are subtle, or insufficient cells.

Histochemical Studies

Generally speaking, these studies are cytostructural analyses that are dependent upon the chemical or immunochemical reaction of cellular and extracellular constituents with reagents that range from organic dyes to antigens; these reactions are assessed by their chromogenicity or fluorescence. The limitations of these procedures are those inherent in the neoplasm itself: the use of improperly prepared tissues, and the technical difficulties of the techniques.

In head and neck oncology, histochemical analysis hopes to accomplish two ends: differential diagnosis and histochemical characterization of the cellular composition of the neoplasm. The analysis can be applied to both tissue sections and cytologic preparations.

From the diagnostic standpoint, one can regard histochemistry as an intermediate step between light and electron microscopy. In some instances, particularly in the differential diagnosis of supporting tissue neoplasms, histochemical stains may provide the correct classification. In melanomas the Fontana-Masson and dopa reactions are requisite steps in the diagnosis when pigmentation is not clear in routinely stained sections. False positive reactions are, however, fairly common with both stains, and furthermore both pigmented and nonpigmented melanomas can be tyrosine negative. Electron microscopy must then be used to locate the intracytoplasmic, membrane-bound ovoid structure representing melanosomes in various stages of development; these structures accurately identify the tumor.

For the differential diagnosis of small-celled neoplasms (esthesioneuroblastoma, rhabdomyosarcoma, lymphoreticular neoplasms), histochemical reactions are also an intermediate stage in the differential diagnosis. The Grimelius stain for neurosecretory products, if positive, eliminates muscle origin and the lymphomas.[21, 31] Surface markers, distinctive appearance on May-Gruenwald Giesma stains, and pyroninophilia support the diagnosis of lymphoreticular neoplasia.[29] The presence of glycogen within the cells favors rhabdomyosarcoma over the esthesioneuroblastoma. Depending upon the development of the cells, a phosphotungstic acid-hematoxylin (PTAH) stain can assist in identifying rhabdomyoblasts.

Here again, a negative reaction does not selectively exclude a diagnosis, and resort to electron microscopy may be required.

In the salivary glands, mucoprotein histochemistry and enzyme histochemistry have been a source of considerable investigations but these techniques have not been of particular diagnostic utility. There are variable quantities of both sialomucins and sulfomucins in salivary tissues, and there is a rather pronounced degree of mucin heterogeneity in man not merely from gland to gland but from acinus to acinus and indeed from cell to cell.[15, 23] Enzyme histochemistry (the phosphatases, glucuronidase, peroxidase, ATPase, etc.) of salivary tissues is very dependent upon the integrity of the cell and its functional state. This accounts for the variable data produced by studies.

Given the variability of reactive products and also variation in staining techniques, where does histochemical analysis fit into the diagnosis of salivary tumors? In this author's opinion, it has limited use. The demonstration of mucous cells will distinguish a high grade mucoepidermoid carcinoma from a squamous cell carcinoma but does little else. Even in this instance, care must be taken that the mucin is intracellular and that a suitable mucin stain is employed. The Alcian-blue critical electrolyte concentration technique (pH 2.5 with 0.1M $MgCl_2$) is far superior to other mucin stains.[23] Periodic acid Schiff (PAS) techniques provide pretty color contrasts but lack specificity (mucins, collagen, basement membranes, and granules are all stained). Combining the PAS technique with diastase digestion will permit characterization of intracellular glycogen but this too is dependent on functional status and fixation.[1, 37]

The choice of a fixing agent for the tissues to be examined is determined by the purpose for which the tissue is to be stained or preserved. Carnoy's solution (absolute alcohol, chloroform, and acetic acid) is one of the best penetrating and quickly acting fixatives known and for most histochemical studies is excellent.[37] However, 10 percent buffered neutral formalin is the most widely used because it is compatible with most staining techniques and, more importantly, formalin-fixed tissues can be used for electron microscopy. The fixative neither preserves nor destroys fats and, while not a fixative for carbohydrates, does preserve the proteins that in turn trap glycogen so that it is not easily dissolved.

In summary, the pathologist's histochemical battery should at least contain methods for the demonstration of mucins (Alcian blue), glycogen (PAS with diastase digestion), neurosecretory granules (Grimelius argyrohil technique; Figs. 3-4 and 3-5), supporting tissues (Mallory's PTAH), and a method for the demonstration of re-

ticulum architecture (Gomori, Snook, Wilder).[37, 41]

Electron Microscopy

Convincing arguments can be made for the wider application of electron microscopy as an aid to histologic diagnosis in problem cases in the head and neck. The high resolution of electron microscopy has made possible the examination of the most minute structures, but as a corollary the technique has greatly restricted the area that can be examined in a reasonable length of time. Often the proposed benefits of ultrastructural examination are offset by sampling

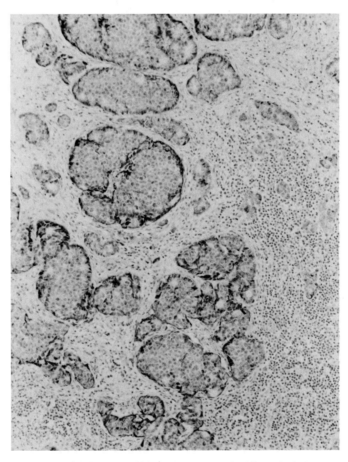

Fig. 3-4. Metastatic carcinoid from small intestine to cervical lymph node. The basilar darkly stained granules demonstrated by the Grimelius technique are secretory products. Figure 3-5, an electron micrograph of the same lesion, confirms the secretory granules.

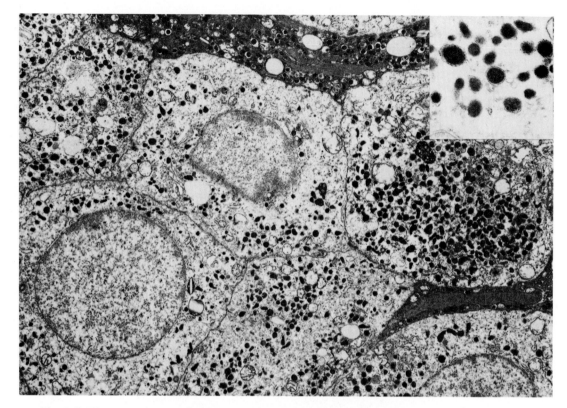

Fig. 3-5. Electron micrograph of the carcinoid in Figure 3-4. All cells contain electron dense secretory granules. The inset (upper right) clearly demonstrates the dense core granules with halos. This material was processed from buffered formalin. (Magnification × 6,000 and × 20,000.)

problems. In the end, a diagnosis of cancer is reached by looking at the patient and examining hematoxylin and eosin or similarly prepared light microscopic tissue sections and the electron photomicrographs —in that order.

The primary value of electron microscopy in the diagnosis of tumors lies in trying to identify in poorly differentiated neoplastic cells structural components that may be characteristic of the cell line from whence the neoplasm takes origin.[8, 22, 44] The elucidation of fine structure may be essential for the differential diagnosis of certain neoplasms, such as poorly differentiated, nonkeratinizing squamous cell carcinomas, achromatic melanomas, endocrine or neuroectodermal tumors, and lymphoreticular neoplasms. For example, lymphomas

can be separated from anaplastic carcinoma by the lack of cytologic features of epithelial cells.

In its simplest perspective, electronoptic evaluation differs little from lightoptic evaluation, since both require knowledge of normal structure and its variations. This may be illustrated by reference to the diagnosis of smooth muscle tumors. Benign, nontumorous smooth muscle cells have a characteristic ultrastructural appearance. Individual cells are usually invested with a basement membrane, and a variable number of pinocytotic vesicles can be identified in close proximity to the plasma membrane. In the cytoplasm there is a heavy concentration of microfilaments along with numerous electron dense bodies and marginal dense plaques. These dense bodies and plaques

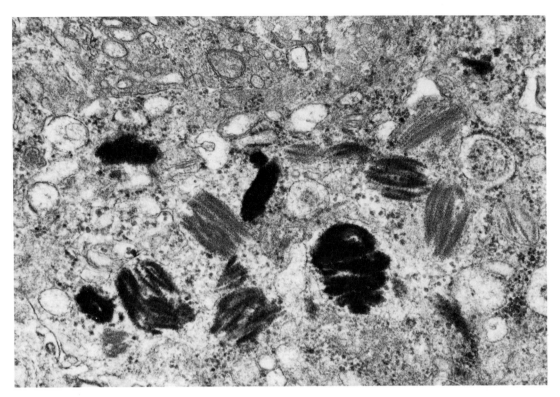

Fig. 3-6. The presence of the premelanosomes and melanosomes in this neoplastic cell specifically identifies the cell as a melanoma. (Magnification × 53,000.) Courtesy of Dr. James Sciubba.

are the most distinctive ultrastructural findings in smooth muscle and appear to be limited to these cells. The presence of these structures in a debated soft tissue tumor indicate the smooth muscle origin of the tumor; *their absence has little histogenetic significance.*

It must be appreciated that when cellular differentiation is of such a low order that *diagnostic* features are not clearly evident, the maternal cell of origin cannot be recognized. In such instances, a conclusion of high probability can be reached by analyzing the ultrastructure of the basal lamina, desmosomes, microvilli, tonofilaments, cytoplasmic filaments, secretory granules (size, shape, electron density), premelanosomes and melanosomes, glycogen, crystals, nuclear alterations, neurotubules and filaments, lipids, and endoplasmic reticulum.[8, 22, 44] These features, while although not entirely specific, aid in the diagnosis.

Perhaps the best example of this contribution of electron microscopy is in the differential diagnosis of poorly differentiated squamous cell carcinoma versus histiocytic lymphoma versus melanoma. The finding of prominent intracytoplasmic tonofilaments as well as desmosomal cell-to-cell attachments establishes the diagnosis of an epithelial neoplasm. Melanosomes and premelanosomes (intracytoplasmic) organelles with a fibrillar apparatus and periodic zigzag patterns and electron dense granular material (Fig. 3-6) confirm the diagnosis of melanoma. Lack of cellular contacts, other special features of the cell membrane for intercellular attachment, and other specific organelles are all features favoring a tumor of lymphoreticular origin. It should be noted here that there are no specific cytoplasmic features allowing an electron microscopic diagnosis of malignant lymphoma.

The ultrastructural finding of neurosecretory-like granules (measuring 1,100 to 1,400 Å) that have a distinctly electron dense core surrounded by a halo and a well-defined limiting membrane (Fig. 3-5) eliminates from diagnostic consideration undifferentiated epithelial neoplasms and lymphomas from neoplasms derived from progenitor neuroectodermal cells (i.e., esthesioneuroblastoma, oat-cell carcinoma, paragangliomas). A finer subclassification of these granules allows further distinction.[8]

Aside from the differential diagnosis of small-celled neoplasms, the contribution of electron microscopy to the differential diagnosis of soft-tissue tumors is perhaps the most valuable. Primordial or mature registered sarcomeres that have a distinct banding pattern serve to distinguish the rhabdomyosarcoma. Abundant intracytoplasmic microfilaments, poorly developed endo-plasmic reticulum, and specialized cell junctions and filopodia identify a cell as from a synovial sarcoma and not from neoplastic or nonneoplastic fibroblasts.

At this point, it is well to emphasize that we have been discussing *differential* diagnosis. Without prior knowledge of the light microscopic appearance of a neoplasm, electronoptic study cannot separate benign from malignant lesions. The light microscope remains the better tool for evaluation of malignancy.[44]

The nondiagnostic aspects of electron microscopy are valuable for clarification and classification of cellular and extracellular light microscopic observations. Elucidation of the subcellular characteristics of the oncocyte (Figs. 3-7 and 3-8) and "cysts" in the adenoid cystic carcinoma (Fig. 3-9) are just two examples of this type of use of the electron microscope.[28, 55] Classification of salivary tumors comprised wholly, or in part, of clear cells can be furthered by ultrastructural examination.[49] The problem of classification of these tumors results from the fact that the light microscopic descriptions encompass cell types of different origin and functional importance. Table 3-4 presents a listing and composition of salivary gland tumors characterized light-optically by a clear cytoplasm.

Resort to electron microscopy, because of time and expense, is justifiably left to the pathologist and not to the clinician. The clinician's responsibility, however, is not minimal, since satisfactory preservation of the cytoarchitecture is a prerequisite for identification of specific ultrastructural features essential for diagnosis. The desirable result is obtained when small tissue samples are fixed immediately after removal. Quality of tissue preservation bears an important relationship to the time interval between tissue removal and immersion of the tissue in fixative. Prolonged fixation is also disadvantageous for ultrastructural study. If electron microscopy is anticipated, phosphate buffered 2.5 percent gluteraldehyde is a suitable fixative. In many cases the need to perform ultrastructural

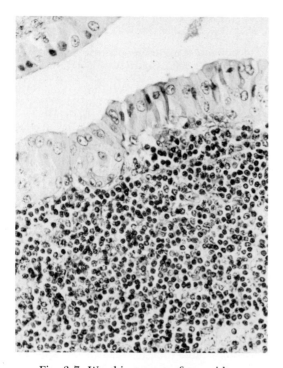

Fig. 3-7. Warthin tumor of parotid exhibiting the oncocytic columnar eosinophilic cells and accompanying lymphoid stroma. The character of the oncocyte is seen ultrastructurally in Figure 3-8. (Hematoxylin and eosin; magnification × 250.)

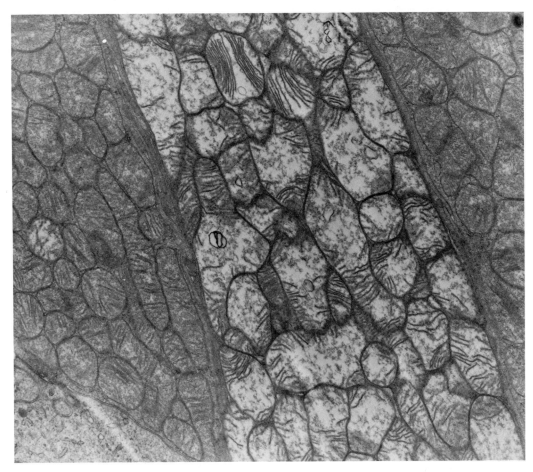

Fig. 3-8. Electronoptic appearance of an oncocyte from a Warthin tumor. The pink granularity of the cytoplasm on hematoxylin and eosin staining is due to the numerous and swollen mitochondria filling the cell. (Magnification × 35,000.)

studies cannot be anticipated; therefore, it is recommended that a universal fixative compatible with both light and electron microscopy be used routinely in fixing surgical specimens.[42] Phosphate buffered 10 percent neutral formalin and the Carson-Lynn fixative are advised.[42, 43] In selected instances, some diagnostic advantage can be gained even after retrieval of the specimens from paraffin embedded material.[44]

Histologic Grading and Histologic Staging

The histologic grading of neoplasms is not to be confused with typing and staging.

Typing of a neoplasm assigns it to its accepted class with appropriate nomenclature. The typing of Hodgkin and non-Hodgkin lymphoma is an example. Staging is the least subjective of the three and refers to the extent of microscopic involvement. Objective measurements of depth and/or volume of cutaneous melanomas is the paradigm of histologic staging for the head and neck surgeon.[38] The histologic grade of a neoplasm depends on the ability of the cell to differentiate. By differentiation is meant that property of a cancer cell that enables it to develop characteristics manifested by normal cells of the tissue from which it originates.

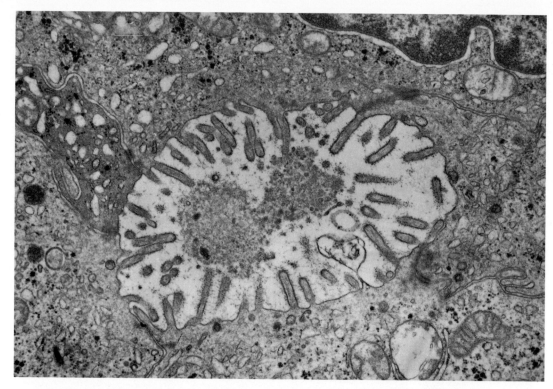

Fig. 3-9. True lumen in an adenoid cystic carcinoma. These lumina are outnumbered by the pseudocystic spaces in this carcinoma. Note the microvilli. (Magnification × 26,000.) Courtesy of Dr. James Sciubba.

TABLE 3-4. LIGHT-MICROSCOPIC CLEAR CELLS: SALIVARY TISSUES

Cell Type	Ultrastructure	Occurrence in Tumors
Undifferentiated (embryonic) duct cell	Few organelles Desmosomes	Monomorphic adenoma Clear-cell carcinoma
Storage cell (striated)	Glycogen granules Numerous mitochondria	Oncocytomas
Myoepithelial cell	Myofilaments Pinocytotic vesicles Lipofuchsin Hemidesmosomes	Salivary duct carcinoma Clear cell tumor Cellular pleomorphic adenomas
Clear epidermoid cell	Tonofilament desmosomes	Mucoepidermoid carcinomas Pleomorphic adenomas
Goblet cells	Mucous vacuoles Basal endoplasmic reticulum	Mucoepidermoid carcinomas
Sebaceous cells	Lipid Microvilli Desmosomes	Sebaceous gland lesions
Clear-cells in acinous carcinomas	Few organelles Electronoptically clear secretory granules	Acinous cell carcinoma

(Modified from Seifert, G., and Donath, K. 1976. Classification of the pathohistology of diseases of the salivary glands—review of 2,600 cases in the Salivary Gland Register. Beitraege zur Pathologie (Stuttgart), 159: 1.)

Grading and histologic staging have variable values depending on the type of neoplasm and current therapies available. The intended goal is to provide another predictive element for response to therapy and hence to prognosis. Emperically, grading is found to be of greater value in some classes of neoplasia than in others.

For most of the malignancies of the head and neck, neither histologic grade nor microscopic stage can stand alone as indicators for treatment or prognosis. On balance they yield, in most instances, to clinical stage. Neoplasms of the parotid gland provide us with an example of this point. With the exception of the division of mucoepidermoid carcinomas into high and low grades, attempts at a similar grading of other parotid gland carcinomas have not provided as reliable or consistent an indicator of biologic course as clinical staging.[3, 46, 51] However, it is becoming increasingly more apparent that for the majority of parotid gland malignancies and other mucosal lesions of the upper aerodigestive tract there is a considerable correlation between level of differentiation (grade) and clinical stage.

Exceptions to this grade-stage correlation certainly exist and it is for this reason that a renewed interest in histologic assessment of neoplasms has come forth. This renewed interest has been heightened by tumor-host relationships and their implications for treatment and long term prognosis for mucosal lesions of the head and neck.

In the application of histologic grading, the pathologist must resist the temptation to emphasize subclassifications that are clinically unimportant. For transferability, the grading must be kept as universally applicable as possible. Table 3-5 after Bauer[5] illustrates how such a grading scheme of squamous cell carcinoma can be used to relate to metastasis and survival.

Figure 3-10 presents another histologic grading scheme and divides the assessment of squamous cell carcinoma into two major categories: A, cellular and architectural features and B, tumor-host relationships. Evaluation of squamous cell carcinoma of the larynx using many or all of these features has been successfully done in retrospective studies and beginning work has been initiated for prospective studies.[26] By tabulation

TABLE 3-5. INFLUENCE OF DIFFERENTIATION OF SQUAMOUS CELL CARCINOMA AT VARIOUS SITES ON METASTASIS AND SURVIVAL

Location	Level of Differentiation	Metastasis Lymph Nodes (%)	Distant Metastasis (%)	5-Year Survival (%)
Lip	Well	6–12	Rare	80
Buccal mucosa	Well	50	Infrequent	50–65
Retromolar trigone	Well-moderate	65	Infrequent	55–60
Floor of mouth	Moderate	65	Rare	30–60
Base of tongue	Poor	75	10	25–40
Pyriform fossa	Poor	65–75	40–60	15–30
Posterior Nasal Space (Nasopharynx)	Poor	85–90	Frequent	25–35

(Modified from Bauer, W. C. 1974. Varieties of Squamous carcinoma—biologic behavior. Frontiers of Radiation Therapy and Oncology, 9:164, S. Karger AG, Basel.)

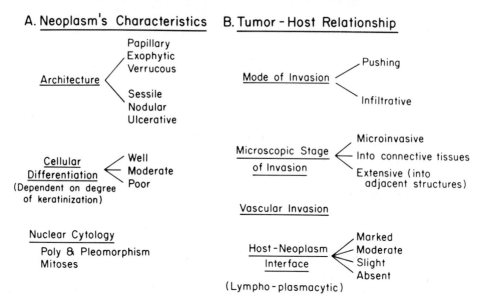

Fig. 3-10. Histological grading of squamous cell carcinoma.

of the items in Figure 3-10, a tumor profile can be added to clinical stage and its weight more scientifically entered in the total evaluation of a patient.[25]

For squamous cell carcinomas, the depth and mode of invasion (pushing versus infiltration) has, to date, permitted the most precise segregation of the high and low risk patients regarding the probability of lymph node metastases. Kashima[30] has related that the infiltrative pattern of invasion is three times more apt to be associated with metastases than is the pushing form of invasion.

The term *microinvasion* needs clarification in squamous cell carcinomas of the head and neck. This author defines it as follows: microinvasive squamous cell carcinoma is the earliest recognizable invasion by squamous cell carcinoma in which the depth of invasion is less than 1.0 mm. It may or may not arise in association with in situ carcinoma and may be uni- or multifocal. It is a diagnosis perhaps best reserved for excisional biopsy specimens, since a punch biopsy diagnosis may only indicate that microscopic lesion adjacent to unsampled more deeply invasive carcinoma.

Preliminary investigations on the cell-mediated immune reaction in the stroma of laryngeal carcinoma, as manifested by lymphocytic and plasma cell infiltration, show some promise. Sala and Ferlito[45, 46] have shown a correlation between histologic grade, lymphoplasmacellular response, and the 5-year survival. The immune response, however, seems to be a favorable prognostic sign only for well-differentiated carcinomas.

In a similar fashion, the biologic and prognostic implications of the morphologic aspects of the immune reactions in lymph nodes draining head and neck cancers have been evaluated.[16] These evaluations consider that most of the histologic changes in lymph nodes are related to immune responses of both humoral and cellular type and reflect the immunologic capability of the patient. By examining the lymph nodes that drain the cancer, it is considered possible to assess the quality and quantity of the immune response and its nature—humoral or cellular—and to draw therefrom reliable prognostic conclusions. Within the lymph nodes, the cortical area and medulla are associated with the humoral type of immune response, whereas the paracortex is related to the cell-mediated immune response. Histologically, four basic patterns of human lymph node morphology in relation to immunologic function may be seen: lymphocyte predominance, representing activation of the cell-mediated immune defense; germinal center predominance, representing activation of the humoral immune response; lymphocyte depletion, indicating an exhaustion of the immune response; and unstimulated immune response.[16]

While data presentations to date are far from conclusive, it is believed that a stimulated pattern, such as seen in lymphocyte predominance, positively affects the course of the disease and has a better prognosis than all other lymph node patterns. The lymphocyte predominance pattern is associated with a T-cell response, that is, effectors of an antineoplastic cellular immunity.[16] Fulfillment of the promise offered by such studies will be additive to the combined immunologic, clinical, and histologic assessment of the patient with cancer in the head and neck.

FUTURE DIRECTIONS

Over the past 15 years, oncologic pathology has undergone a remarkable expansion. Some of these events have been presented in this chapter. Electron microscopy, histochemistry, and fluorescence microscopy combined with improved biopsy techniques have brought the pathologist's role in diagnosis and management of head and neck cancer to a new plateau.

The limitations of diagnostic electron microscopy have been pointed out, and in some quarters application of ultrastructural study has already reached its peak. If electron microscopy, histochemical analysis, and fluorescence are relegated to static observations by the pathologist, no further progress can be anticipated. If, however, the theme of dynamic histology and tumor biology is espoused, surgical pathology will keep pace with the demands of progressive therapy and the surgical pathologist will continue to be a valued member of the cancer team.

Space allows but two examples of this type of dynamic histology: immunohistology, and in vivo kinetic analysis.

The use of labeled antibody molecules offers the potential of immunohistology for the investigation and diagnosis of tumors of lymphoreticular, endocrine, and other tissues. Many antigens including immunoglobulin and other plasma proteins, viruses, hormones, and tumor markers can be stained in conventional sections of tissues. Immunohistologic staining of such conventionally prepared sections has the advantage of applicability to specimens taken before the diagnostic indication for such staining is determined and is, therefore, useful for retrospective study.[13] In specially prepared tissue sections, the localization of antigen at ultrastructural sites opens entirely new vistas for electron microscopy. The impact of such applications is already being felt. If histologic antigen localization and microscopic assay can be also accomplished with histometry and microdensitometry, the limitations of present methods of tumor evaluation should disappear and be replaced by objective, quantitative measurements.[11]

The dynamics of tumor growth and related parameters, i.e., growth fraction, cell cycle times, and cell loss, can be assessed by the percent labelled mitoses technique and nuclear DNA content evaluation. Despite the inability of early efforts to predict therapeutic response in terms of cell kinetics by these techniques, their potential usefulness cannot be excluded. For instance, the characterization and identification of a possible residual cellular component in a neoplasm should be attainable on the basis of kinetic properties. In that light, an expansion of current technology (automated flow cytometry) may be able to recognize the proliferative state of cells before and during treatment.[40]

REFERENCES

1. Ackerman, L. V., and Ramirez, G. A. 1959. The indications for and limitations of frozen section diagnosis: A review of 1269 consecutive frozen section diagnoses. British Journal of Surgery, 46: 336.

2. Batsakis, J. G. 1979. Tumors of the Head and Neck: Clinical and Pathological Considerations. 2nd ed., Williams and Wilkins, Baltimore.

3. Batsakis, J. G., Chinn, E., Regezi, J. A., and Repola, D. A. 1978. The pathology of head and neck tumors: salivary glands, part 2. Head & Neck Surgery, 1: 167.

4. Bauer, W. C. 1974. The use of frozen sections in otolaryngology. Transactions of the American Academy of Ophthalmology and Otolaryngology, 78: ORL-88.

5. Bauer, W. C. 1974. Varieties of squamous carcinoma—biologic behavior. Frontiers of Radiation Therapy and Oncology, 9: 164.

6. Bauer, W. C., Lesinski, S. G., and Ogura, J. H. 1975. The significance of positive margins in hemilaryngectomy specimens. Laryngoscope, 85: 1.

7. Bloustein, P. A., and Silverberg, S. G., 1977. Rapid cytologic examination of surgical specimens. Pathology Annual, 12 (part 2): 251.

8. Bonikos, D. S., Bensch, K. G., and Kempson, R. L. 1976. The contribution of electron microscopy to the differential diagnosis of tumors. Beitraege zur Pathologie (Stuttgart), 158: 417.

9. Byers, R. M., Bland, K. I., Borlase, B., and Luna, M. 1978. The prognostic and therapeutic value of frozen section determinations in the surgical treatment of squamous carcinoma of the head and neck. American Journal of Surgery, 136: 525.

10. Carson, F. L., Martin, J. H., and, Lynn, J. A. 1973. Formalin fixation for electron microscopy: A re-evaluation. American Journal of Clinical Pathology, 59: 365.

11. Cooper, R. A. 1974. Dynamic histology and tumor biology—an overview. The role of the surgical pathologist in oncology. Frontiers of Radiation Therapy and Oncology, 9: 10.

12. Dehner, L. P., and Rosai, J. 1977. Frozen section examination in surgical pathology: A retrospective study of one year experience, comprising 778 cases. Minnesota Medicine, 60: 83.

13. Denk, H., Radaszkiewicz, T., and Witting, C. 1976. Immunofluorescence studies on pathologic routine material: Application to malignant lymphomas. Beitraege zur Pathologie (Stuttgart), 159: 219.

14. Droesse, M., Tute, M., and Haubrich, J. 1977. Punktionszytologie von Speicheldrusentumoren. Laryngologie, Rhinologie, Otologie und Ihre Grenzgebiete, 56: 703.

15. Eversole, L. R. 1972. The mucoprotein histochemistry of human mucous acinar cell containing salivary glands: Submandibular and sublingual glands. Archives of Oral Biology, 17: 43.

16. Ferlito, A., and Polidoro, F. 1979. Biological and prognostic implications of the morphologic aspects of immune reaction in lymph nodes draining head and neck cancers. A review. Journal of Laryngology and Otology, 93: 153.

17. Folsom, T. C., White, C. P., Bramer, L., Canby, H. F., and Garrington, G. E. 1972. Oral exfoliative study. Review of the literature and report of a three-year study. Oral Surgery, Oral Medicine, Oral Pathology, 33: 61.

18. Frable, W. J. 1976. Thin-needle aspiration biopsy. A personal experience with 469 cases. American Journal of Clinical Pathology, 65: 168.

19. Frable, W. J., and Frable, M. A. 1974. Thin-needle aspiration biopsy in the diagnosis of head and neck tumors. Laryngoscope, 84: 1069.

20. Geelhoed, G. W., Breslow, A., and McCune, W. S. 1977. Malignant melanoma: Correlation of long-term follow-up with clinical staging, level of invasion and thickness of the primary tumor. American Surgeon (Philadelphia), 43: 77.

21. Gould, V. E. 1977. Neuroendocrinomas and neuroendocrine carcinomas. APUD cell system neoplasms and their aberrant secretory activities. Pathology Annual, 12 (part 2): 33.

22. Gyorkey, F., Min. K.-W., Krisko, I., and Gyorkey, P. 1975. The usefulness of electron microscopy in the diagnosis of human tumors. Human Pathology, 6: 421.

23. Harrison, J. D. 1974. Minor salivary glands of man: Enzyme and mucosubstance histochemical studies. Histochemical Journal, 6: 633.

24. House, A. J. S., and Thomson, K. R., 1977.

Evaluation of a new transthoracic needle for biopsy of benign and malignant lung lesions. American Journal of Roentgenology Radium Therapy and Nuclear Medicine, 129: 215.

25. Jakobsson, P. A. 1975. Histologic grading of malignancy and prognosis in glottic carcinoma of the larynx. Canadian Journal of Otolaryngology, 4: 885.

26. Jakobsson, P. A., Eneroth, C.-M., Killander, D., Moberger, G., and Martensson, B. 1973. Histologic classification and grading of malignancy in carcinoma of the larynx. Acta Radiologica: Oncology, Radiation, Physics, Biology, 12: 1.

27. Johannessen, J. V. 1977. Use of paraffin material for electron microscopy. Pathology Annual, 12 (part 2): 189.

28. Johns, M. E., Regezi, J. A., and Batsakis, J. G. 1977. Oncocytic neoplasms of salivary glands: An ultrastructural study. Laryngoscope, 87: 862.

29. Kaschula, R. O., Staples, W. G., and Visser, A. E., 1978. Immunohistochemical characterization of Burkitt's lymphoma. South African Medical Journal, 53: 655.

30. Kashima, H. K. 1975. The characteristics of laryngeal cancer correlating with cervical lymph node metastasis (analysis based on 40 total organ sections). Canadian Journal of Otolaryngology, 4: 893.

31. Lack, E. E., and Mercer, L. 1977. A modified Grimelius argyrophil technique for neurosecretory granules. American Journal of Surgical Pathology, 1: 275.

32. Leading article (no author). 1978. Utility of needle aspiration of tumours. British Medical Journal, 1: 1507.

33. Lee, J. G. 1974. Detection of residual carcinoma of the oral cavity, oropharynx, hypopharynx, and larynx: A study of surgical margins. Transactions of the American Academy of Ophthalmology and Otolaryngology, 78: ORL-49.

34. Levene, A. 1977. Pathological aspects. Selected topics in tumor pathology. In Raven, R. W., Ed.: Principles of Surgical Oncology Plenum Medical Book Co., New York, 75.

35. Lindberg, L. G., and Akerman, M. 1976. Aspiration cytology of salivary gland tumors: Diagnostic experience from six years of routine laboratory work. Laryngoscope, 86: 584.

36. Looser, K. G., Shah, J. P., and Strong, E. W. 1978. The significance of "positive" margins in surgically resected epidermoid carcinomas. Head & Neck Surgery, 1: 107.

37. Luna, L. G. 1968. Manual of Histologic Staining Methods of the Armed Forces Institute of Pathology. 3rd edn. Blakiston Division McGraw-Hill, New York.

38. McDowell, E. M., and Trump, B. F. 1976. Histologic fixatives suitable for diagnostic light and electron microscopy. Archives of Pathology and Laboratory Medicine, 100: 405.

39. Neel, H. B., Woolner, L. B., and Sanderson, D. R. 1978. Sputum cytologic diagnosis of upper respiratory tract cancer. Annals of Otology, Rhinology and Laryngology, 87: 468.

40. Nervi, C., Arcangeli, G., Badaracco, G., Cortese, M., Morelli, M., and Starace, G. 1978. The relevance of tumor size and cell kinetics as predictors of radiation response in head and neck cancer. A randomized study on the effect of intraarterial chemotherapy followed by radiotherapy. Cancer, 41: 900.

41. Pearse, A. G. E. 1968. Histochemistry, Theoretical and Applied. 3rd edn. Vol. 1. J & A. Churchill, London.

42. Reddy, C. R. R. M., Kameswari, V. R., Prahlad, D., Ramulu, C., and Reddy, P. G. 1975. Correlative study of exfoliative cytology and histopathology of oral carcinomas. Journal of Oral Surgery, 33: 435.

43. Regezi, J. A., and Batsakis, J. G. 1977. Histogenesis of salivary gland neoplasms. Otolaryngologic Clinics of North America, 10: 297.

44. Regezi, J. A., and Batsakis, J. G. 1978. Diagnostic electron microscopy of head and neck tumors. Archives of Pathology and Laboratory Medicine, 102: 8.

45. Sala, O. 1976. Tumourhost relationship and its implications in the treatment and long term prognosis of laryngeal cancer. Critical observations on the TNM system of tumour classification. Acta Oto-Rhino-Laryngologica Belgica, 30: 371.

46. Sala, O., and Ferlito, A. 1976. Morphological observations of immunobiology of laryngeal cancer. Evaluation of the defensive activity of immunocompetent cells present in tumour stroma. Acta Otolaryngologica, 81: 353.

47. Schnitzer, B. 1978. Classification of lymphomas. CRC Critical Reviews in Clinical Laboratory Sciences, 9: 123.

48. Seifert, G., and Donath, K. 1976. Classification of the pathohistology of diseases of the salivary glands—review of 2,600 cases in the Salivary Gland Register. Beitraege zur Pathologie (Stuttgart), 159: 1.

49. Seifert, G. and Donath, K. 1978. Über das Vorkommen sog. heller Zellen in Speicheldrüsentumoren. Ultrastruktur und Differential diagnose. Zeitschrift Fur Krebforschung und Klinische Onkologie, 91:   165.

50. Schnurer, L. B. and Windström, A. 1978. Fine-needle biopsy of the thyroid gland. A cytohistological comparison in cases of goiter. Annals of Otology, Rhinology and Laryngology, 87:   224.

51. Spiro, R. H., Huvos, A. G., and Strong, E. W. 1975. Cancer of the parotid gland. A clinicopathologic study of 288 primary cases. American Journal of Surgery, 130:   452.

52. Stahle, J. 1960. Clinical cytology in otolaryngology. Aspiration biopsy (fine-needle puncture). Acta Otolaryngologica Supplement, 158:   187.

53. Strauchen, J. A., Young, R. C., DeVita, V. T., Anderson, T., Fantone, J. C., and Berard, C. W. 1978. Clinical relevance of the histopathological subclassification of diffuse "histiocytic" lymphoma. New England Journal of Medicine, 299:   1382.

54. Strauss, M. B., Ed. 1968. Familiar Medical Quotations. Little, Brown, Boston.

55. Tandler, B. 1971. Ultrastructure of adenoid cystic carcinoma of salivary gland origin. Laboratory Investigation, 24:   504.

56. Zajicek, J., and Eneroth, C.-M. 1970. Cytological diagnosis of salivary-gland carcinomata from aspiration biopsy smears. Acta Otolaryngologica Supplement, 263:   183.

4 | Preoperative and Postoperative Medical Considerations

William M. Cooper, M.D.
Charles H. Srodes, M.D.

INTRODUCTION

The operative procedure is of no value if the patient is either unable to tolerate the surgery and dies or is left in a physical state that is so altered that a reasonable quality of life cannot be maintained. The determination of the risk/benefit ratio of the contemplated surgical procedure is a complex task, requiring comprehensive knowledge of the patient's past medical history and current medical, surgical, and emotional problems, as well as baseline information on x-rays, cardiograms, blood chemistries, and urinalysis.

Emergency procedures, however, may need to be done without optimal preoperative evaluation and management. The internist must, in such cases, assess the risk in view of the patient's history, current status, likelihood of complication, and treatment goals and expectations and make a judgment based on his knowledge of the patient, however limited, and the nature of the intended surgery.

Seldom are patients with malignancies of the head and neck without significant medical problems. A careful review of preexisting and presently active medical disorders should be done. Certain disorders, such as hemophilia, severe hypertension, and end stage cardiorespiratory disease, may preclude surgical intervention or at least modify it significantly. Many patients, such as those with uncontrolled hypertension or acute bronchitis, require preparation for surgery that corrects the acute phase of their medical problem. Some, such as patients who have diabetes mellitus, may require careful and special monitoring in the perioperative period. The surgeon must participate in the decisions regarding medical care by providing an outline of the required operative procedures that includes some estimate of the demands on the patient. This chapter will deal with the major medical dilemmas that may interact with the surgical problems during the management of patients with head and neck cancer.

ARTERIOSCLEROTIC HEART DISEASE

Arteriosclerotic heart disease and hypertension are very common preexisting medical disorders, since most patients with head and neck cancer are in the older age group. Features that would preclude elective surgery in patients with arteriosclerotic heart disease include the presence of increasing angina, recent myocardial infarction, and the presence of uncontrolled congestive heart failure.[3] Important areas of history taking include tolerance to increased stress, a history of previous arrhythmia, episodes of pulmonary edema or chronic congestive heart failure, prior myocardial infarction, or the presence of angina. These data provide us with an estimate of the patient's tolerance to anesthesia and surgery.

Information with reference to the details of activity and tolerance to stress should be obtained by specifically determining the individual's habits and activities. For example, the patient with heart disease who is able to do her own housework, including washing, ironing, and climbing stairs, and shopping, including carrying groceries, should have a reasonable tolerance to any kind of surgery and anesthesia, unless, of course, an electrocardiogram reveals acute changes or there is evidence of congestive heart failure on physical examination. On the other hand, the patient who has severe angina or heart failure, even with a normal electrocardiogram (ECG) and chest x-ray, carries an increased risk for surgery. Logically, the patient who remains symptomatic despite medical management carries a greater risk than the untreated patient who potentially may be improved by proper medical management prior to surgery.

The stable patient should have his medication continued through surgery and the postoperative period. For example, the acute withdrawal of propranolol may be associated with exacerbations of angina or even precipitation of myocardial infarction. Patients are often receiving digitalis derivatives along with diuretics, nitroglycerin, or propranolol, and it is necessary to carefully monitor the electrolytes and often to measure the serum levels of digoxin to appropriately adjust the dosage.

Intraoperative or postoperative myocardial infarction due to the stress of anesthesia and surgery, transient hypotension, or hypoxia is not uncommon in the patient with arteriosclerotic heart disease. The patient cannot express the usual warning symptoms, and the symptoms may be attributed to other causes. It is of note that many of the serum enzymes used to assess myocardial infarction are not helpful after major surgery; however, the CPK (creatine phosphokinase)-MB is relatively specific for myocardial damage. Unexplained postoperative or intraoperative arrhythmias, hypotension, or congestive heart failure, should prompt consideration of possible myocardial injury or infarction. If the ECG shows a pattern of evolving infarction or the CPK-MB is

elevated, the patient should be monitored in the appropriate intensive care unit or coronary care unit, as there is a very high risk of life threatening arrhythmias or cardiogenic shock during the early postinfarction period.

The patient with arteriosclerotic heart disease may have arrhythmias from conduction abnormalities with atrial fibrillation and/or tachycardia, or bradyarrhythmias with varying degrees of heart block. Digoxin, quinidine, propranolol or related drugs may be used to control the former condition. The digoxin dosage is usually about 0.25 mg daily after an initial loading dose of 1.5 mg in a 24 to 48 hour period. The determination of digoxin levels allows for a more accurate titration of the medication to the patient's requirements. The dosage of quinidine for control of a tachyrhythmia may vary widely but the usual dosage is 1,200 mg per day. Quinidine levels when available are helpful in establishing the individual dose requirements. Propranolol dosage is usually instituted in the range of 80 to 100 mg per 24 hours in four divided doses and adjusted up or down as required in the individual patient.

VALVULAR HEART DISEASE

The patient with valvular heart disease may have an arteriosclerotic etiology, as in elderly patients with aortic stenosis or mitral regurgitation; but in a younger group, under 55, the probability of rheumatic or congenital heart disease is higher. The history of a valvular defect is extremely important. Younger patients with a history of rheumatic fever will require penicillin prophylaxis on a daily basis; and patients with valvular defects or congenital abnormalities as a rule will require antibiotic prophylaxis for subacute bacterial endocarditis when undergoing head and neck surgery. A currently suggested regimen is 1 million units of intramuscular (IM) crystalline penicillin given 1 hour before surgery along with 600,000 units of aqueous penicillin; following surgery, oral penicillin is administered in a dosage of 400 mg four times a day for 2 to 3 days. If the patient is unable to take oral medication, the penicillin should be given parenterally. For the patient who is allergic to penicillin, erythromycin with streptomycin can be substituted.

BLOOD PRESSURE PROBLEMS

Surgery should be delayed in patients who have hypertension that is acute and severe (diastolic greater than 110). The hypertension must be controlled, because of the increased risk of acute pulmonary edema, stroke, myocardial infarction, and hypertensive crisis associated with surgery in uncontrolled hypertension. Controlled hypertension is not a contraindication to surgery, but it is extremely important to have exact information on the drug or drugs the patient is using. This is essential because some antihypertensive agents may interact adversely with anesthetic agents. Certain antihypertensive agents, taken even for a short period, may cause rebound when discontinued. This may present further difficulties in management.[26]

The effect of antihypertensive medication on electrolyte levels must also be considered. Diuretics, which are the drugs most frequently used for control of hypertension, may cause significant hypokalemia and this may result in serious or life threatening arrhythmias, particularly in a patient who is also taking digoxin. Rapid normalization of potassium levels may be accomplished by the administration of parenteral potassium chloride in intravenous (IV) solutions, usually 40 mEq of potassium chloride in 1,000 cc of dextrose and water or of normal saline given over 3 to 4 hours and repeated until the potassium has reached its normal range. There is a close relationship between serum and total body potassium levels, with total body potassium of 100 to 300 mEq usually associated with serum potassium levels of 3 to 4 mEq per liter. Reductions in total body potassium of 300 to 500 mEq are usually associated with serum levels of 2.5 to 3 mEq per liter. Reductions in total body potassium of 800 to 1,000 mEq are associated with marked reductions of serum potassium concentration, typically in the range of 1.8 to 2.5 mEq per liter. A slower normalization of potassium levels can be carried out by the oral route in the form of potassium chloride or gluconate with a supplement of 30 to 60 mEq per day. Foods such as fruit juices, bananas, and eggs are high in potassium and are used to prevent the development of hypokalemia.

The drugs hydralazine, guanethidine, propranolol and colonidine may interact with anesthetic agents, and their use should be called to the attention of the anesthesiologist.

Occasionally, a patient with a large upper cervical neck mass overlying the carotid may experience hypotension and bradycardia (carotid sinus syncope) due to increased vagal tone from carotid sinus stimulation. This may also be caused by pressure on the carotid sinus during surgery, and in such cases can be reversed by relieving the pressure or injecting the bifurcation with Xylocaine. This condition may also be caused by a tight pressure dressing, in which case loosening of the dressings will correct the problem. When related to pressure from the tumor mass, atropine, isoproterenol, and occasionally a temporary pacemaker may be necessary until the mass can be reduced in size. Other causes of hypotension must always be considered; these include sepsis, hypovolemic states, overmedication with antihypertensive medications, and drugs (such as phenothiazines) that may cause major postural hypotension.

Poor prognostic signs that carry high surgical risks for cardiac patients are 1) history of poor exercise tolerance, 2) increasing angina, 3) chronic uncontrolled or acute congestive heart failure, 4) severe or uncontrolled hypertension, 5) bradyarrhythmias, 6) acute electrocardiographic changes of ischemia or injury, and 7) myocardial infarction within 6 months of surgery.[3, 16]

CHRONIC OBSTRUCTIVE LUNG DISEASE

The patient with respiratory insufficiency cannot adequately exchange gases to meet body needs during stress. Many of the patients undergoing head and neck surgery have underlying pneumoconiosis or chronic obstructive lung disease, secondary to smoking. Progression from respiratory insufficiency to respiratory failure when ventilation cannot support the body at rest is one of the risks during the immediate postoperative period. This may be caused or complicated by aspiration and atelectasis during the postoperative period. Assessment of the respiratory problem and anticipated pulmonary stress during and after surgery is essential to estimate the likelihood of postoperative complications and the patient's chances of survival. Actually, the patient is safest from the pulmonary standpoint during surgery, as the anesthesiologist is able to control the rate and depth of ventilation and the flow of oxygen.

Removal of a tumor obstructing the airway may markedly improve a patient's respiratory function and facilitate clearing of bronchial secretions, and it may be impossible to maximize pulmonary performance until after surgery. For instance, a patient with chronic aspiration and subsequent pneumonitis may have fever and signs of consolidation that will not improve until the obstructing tumor is removed and in such instances it is not feasible or desirable to delay surgery in an attempt to make the patient afebrile.

The history of any recent change in functional activity, the presence or absence of a productive cough, and a subjective experience of dyspnea are important. Inability to climb a flight of stairs or to blow out a match at a distance of 4 inches may give clinical evidence of respiratory insufficiency and complement the routine physical examination. Occasionally, the patient may have coexisting cardiac decompensation or anemia, which may accentuate respiratory insufficiency by increasing oxygen demands. From a laboratory standpoint, arterial blood gases and pulmonary function tests are important basic parameters. Arterial hypoxemia with a PO_2 of less than 44 mmHg portends significant complications and warrants attempts to maximize pulmonary function preoperatively. An elevated PCO_2 (e.g., 60 mmHg) is indicative of alveolar hypoventilation and respiratory failure. This combination of abnormalities when associated with acidosis may lead to coma and death.[2]

A patient with a history of alveolar hypoventilation may be particularly prone to the depressant effects of analgesics on the respiratory center, and a liberal administration of oxygen may further decrease this respiratory drive. In such cases, oxygen should be given with caution and with frequent monitoring of the arterial blood gases, particularly in the immediate postoperative period when seizure due to rapid lowering of the PCO_2 may occur.

In the patient with upper airway obstruction, pulmonary function tests may be misleading and not represent the underlying pulmonary reserve. The degree of upper airway obstruction can be ascertained by inspiratory and expiratory flow loops. If upper airway obstruction is not present, measurement of the maximal voluntary ventilation (MVV), the maximal expiratory flow rate (MEFR), and the forced expiratory volume (FEV_1) as a percentage of vital capacity are the most helpful parameters in chronic obstructive pulmonary disease.[7] A patient with an FEV_1 of less than 70 percent of total forced vital capacity or a maximal expiratory flow rate of less than 200 liters per minute is at high risk for significant postoperative respiratory failure (Table 4-1).[13]

When the primary problem is obstructive in nature, treatment goals are directed toward the liquefaction and elimination of bronchopulmonary secretions, the relief of bronchospasm, and the treatment of bronchitis with antibiotics. The therapy should include cessation of smoking, administra-

TABLE 4-1 RISK OF POSTOPERATIVE RESPIRATORY FAILURE

Spirometry	
Findings	Interpretation
Normal test	No increased risk
MVV greater than 50%, FEV_1 greater than 1.5 liters, normal arterial blood gases	Little increased risk if special precautions are taken
MVV 35% to 50% FEV_1 1 to 1.5 liters, normal $PaCO_2$, normal ECG, mild hypoxemia	Increased operative risk, contraindication to elective procedure
MVV less than 35%, FEV_1 less than 1 liter, normal $PaCO_2$	Greatly increased operative risk, contraindication to major elective surgical procedure
MVV less than 35%, FEV_1 less than 1 liter, increased $PaCO_2$	Extremely high risk, only mandatory surgery is justifiable

tion of antibiotics and bronchodilator drugs, inhalation of humidified gases with ultrasonic nebulizer, and use of chest physiotherapy. Intermittent positive pressure breathing (IPPB) is usually of little benefit and may actually increase the incidence of postoperative atelectasis.

In the postoperative period, frequent monitoring of the pulmonary status by physical examination, arterial blood gases, and periodic chest x-rays will help to identify problems promptly. Treatment with chest physiotherapy, deep breathing, and tracheal suctioning may alleviate the atelectasis and aid in clearing secretions. These are useful adjuncts as the patient often coughs ineffectively or requires significant analgesia, which further decreases the cough reflex. Attempts to minimize aspiration are often not completely successful because of the nature of the surgical procedure, and if heavy purulent secretions occur, associated with fever, antibiotics should be started after obtaining a blood culture and deep cough specimen for culture. Selection of the appropriate antibiotic frequently depends on local considerations, history of allergy, prior cultures, and individual physician preference. Ideally, however, the antibiotic is selected on the basis of culture and sensitivity.

FLUID BALANCE, ELECTROLYTES AND ACID BASE DISORDERS

Patients with neoplasms of the head and neck often experience interference with food intake, which leads to weight loss and negative nitrogen balance. This may result in a reduction in total plasma volume that renders the patient more susceptible to additional stress, blood loss, or hypotension. Even with a total body deficit of red blood cells, the patient's blood count may be normal because the plasma volume and red cell mass may be proportionately reduced. If volume depletion has occurred rapidly, there may, for a short period of time, be an increase in the hemoglobin and hematocrit levels because plasma volume losses have occurred at a greater rate than the loss of red blood cells. The patient who has persistent tachycardia, dizziness, or syncope upon standing should have a blood volume determination made and any deficit corrected preoperatively. The replacement may include red blood cells, 5 percent albumin, or normal saline depending on the major calculated deficit. Patients taking diuretics may have sodium or potassium depletion that requires preoperative correction. Patients who have been receiving parenteral hyperalimentation or tube feedings are prone to fluid and electrolyte abnormalities due to the hypertonicity of the nutrients. This is discussed in detail in Chapter 5.

Patients who have chronic renal disease, liver disease, or uncontrolled diabetes may have alterations in electrolytes and acid base balance, and these alterations may further complicate existing cardiac or pulmonary disorders. Arterial blood gas measurements and electrolyte measurements should be performed in these patients, and corrective action taken. Surgical intervention in a patient with electrolyte or blood gas abnormalities incurs a definite increase in risk to anesthesia as well as to the operation.

ENDOCRINE CONSIDERATIONS

Diabetes Mellitus

Under even optimal conditions, the control of blood sugar levels in the diabetic patient may be difficult. When one adds the frequently poor nutritional status, the stress of anesthesia, and the parenteral IV solutions containing glucose for long periods of time without oral intake, the problem becomes compounded; the issue becomes more one of avoiding catastrophic hypoglycemic responses, ketoacidosis, and hyperosmolar crisis and of allowing reasonable wound healing rather than of obtaining ideal blood glucose control. Infections antagonize the peripheral utilization of insulin, and some anesthetic agents alter significantly the metabolism of glucose. Halothane usually has little effect on the blood sugar level and for that reason is often the anesthetic of choice in the brittle diabetic. Preexisting diabetes may be aggravated by surgery, and latent diabetes may become clinically apparent following surgery.

No single approach to the management of diabetes in the surgical patient can be espoused as dogma; the glucose tolerance of patients varies considerably and often changes from day to day. Moreover, experts vary in their opinions as to the need for rigid control of blood sugar; however, some principles and guidelines for management are generally accepted.

A knowledge of the usual time for peak and duration of action of the various insulin preparations is important for adjustment of dose and management during the perioperative period. Regular insulin or CZI insulin given subcutaneously exerts its effect in about 30 minutes, reaches a peak in 2 to 4 hours, and has total duration of action of 6 to 8 hours. Intermediate acting insulin such as NPH or Lente begins to act in 3 to 4 hours, reaches a peak in 8 to 12 hours, and has a duration of action of 18 to 24 hours. Frequently, patients require a combination of short acting and intermediate acting insulin to provide some coverage throughout the 24 hour period. There is seldom a need for the extremely long acting insulin, and generally it should be avoided.[8]

Preoperatively, if the fasting blood sugar is between 150 and 300 mg percent, no change in insulin dosage need be made. With a fasting blood sugar below 100 mg percent, a reduction in dosage of insulin may help to avoid possible hypoglycemic complications. If the blood sugar is greater than 300 mg percent, frequently an increase in the daily dosage of insulin is necessary. As a general rule, gradual increases or decreases of insulin dosage, e.g., 3 to 5 units a day, will allow smoother regulation in diabetic control. In addition to following urine reductions, it is important to follow changes of insulin dosage with measurements of blood sugar at times of peak action of the insulin given. For instance, the patient whose NPH insulin has been increased from 40 to 45 units should have a blood sugar measurement 8 hours after the administration of the insulin. One of the principles of diabetic management in the perioperative period is to make fairly frequent measurements of the blood sugar so that one can anticipate problems or the need for changes in insulin dosage.

On the day of surgery, one method that allows for an extended period without eating yet provides some measure of coverage is to give one half of the total dosage of insulin as intermediate acting insulin in the morning at the same time as IV administration of 5 percent dextrose in water is started.[8] The blood glucose level should be obtained following surgery and depending on the glucose measurement, the remainder of the daily dosage may or may not be given. An alternative method of administering insulin is the perioperative period has been the use of the slow infusion of regular insulin at a rate of 1 or 2 units per hour. This method has resulted in equivalent control of the blood sugar. In the postoperative period, one should expect alterations in glucose tolerance and, therefore, in the insulin requirements.

The stresses of surgery, parenteral infusions of glucose-containing solutions, and occasionally wound or pulmonary infections will change the patient's requirements for insulin. Frequent urine reductions will show rough patterns of glucose control, but should not be substituted for periodic measurement of the actual blood sugar. Poorly controlled diabetes is a double-edged problem. The worse the control, the worse the wound healing; and conversely poor wound healing and intercurrent infections make diabetes more difficult to control. A rational, consistent approach to the management of diabetes will help the patient recover from surgery and avoid many serious complications.

Gout

Acute gouty arthritis is caused by the intraarticular precipitation of urate crystals and the subsequent inflammatory response evoked by the crystals. The exact mechanism by which urate crystals precipitate is not known; however, a common theory is that crystalization takes place at times of physical and/or emotional stress. Surgery is a common stress that may trigger attacks of acute gouty arthritis, with the most likely time of appearance of postoperative gout being 3 to 5 days following surgery. The uric acid level is usually above 7.4 mg percent, and the joints involved are usually in the lower extremities. In fact, 50 percent of all gouty attacks involve the great toe in a classical podagra. Any acutely inflamed, painful, erythematous joint, particularly in the lower extremity, should raise the possibility of acute gouty arthritis. Treatment may be instituted empirically, although the diagnosis is confirmed by the finding of urate crystals in the synovial fluid. Colchicine, 0.6 mg administered orally every hour for 6 to 8 hours, may give dramatic pain relief, and this can be considered a therapeutic confirmation of gout. If a patient is unable to eat, the IV route is preferred; colchicine, 1 to 2 mg in 20 ml of saline, injected slowly may provide prompt relief. This can be repeated in 4 to 5 hours. Alternative medications are the nonsteroidal antiinflammatory agents. Oral administration of indomethacin, 50 mg three to four times a day, or phenylbutazone, 100 mg every 4 to 8 hours for 2 or 3 days, may provide prompt and dramatic improvement in symptoms. It should be noted that allopurinol, which is an extremely useful agent for the management of hyperuricemia and prevention of gout, is of no benefit in acute gouty arthritis and, in fact, may exacerbate or even precipitate an attack. For long term management of gout, one may consider the use of allopurinol, beginning 2 to 4 weeks after the acute episode has resolved.

HYPERTHYROIDISM AND HYPOTHYROIDISM

Hyperthyroidism is an infrequent medical problem in the patient population with cancers of the head and neck. Occasionally, iatrogenic hyperthyroidism may occur due to overadministration of thyroid hormone by either the patient or physician. It should be remembered that the usual daily total replacement dose for a patient is only 2 or 3 grains of dessicated thyroid or its equivalent. An occasional patient has been reported with Graves disease following irradiation of the thyroid, but this is unusual.[6] Finally, one may have trouble on clinical grounds alone of distinguishing hyperthyroidism from alcohol withdrawal syndromes. Many symptoms, including agitation, tremulousness, tachycardia, fever, diaphoresis, insomnia, and heat intolerance, are common to both disorders. The syndromes can usually be separated by measurement of the serum thyroxin level (T-4) and by accurate history taking and other routine laboratory tests. If uncontrolled hyperthyroidism occurs, all but the most urgent surgical procedures should be avoided until control of the hyperthyroid state can be effected.

Hypothyroidism, on the other hand, is an insidious disease which frequently appears in the older age group and is often seen in association with head and neck cancer, either as a coincidental finding or subsequent to surgery and radiation.[11] The symptoms of hoarseness, lethargy, dry skin, weight gain, and constipation are often overlooked or felt to be secondary to another problem such as carcinoma of the larynx; and the physical signs may develop so slowly that they are missed by the patient, family, or physician. A high index of suspicion is important to diagnose occult hypothyroidism. To establish a baseline, thyroid function tests or at least a T-4 level should be part of the initial laboratory examination. If hypothyroidism is confirmed, thyroid replacement should be initiated prior to surgery and ideally, the patient should be euthyroid prior to proceeding with elective surgery. In moderately severe or severe hypothyroidism, replacement should be started with a low dose of T-3 (Cytomel, 5 to 10 μg per day with increases at 4 to 7 day intervals if no toxicity occurs). The hypothyroid individual tends to be hyper-responsive to small doses of thyroid replacement drug during the first few weeks and thus, full dose replacement thyroid supplements should be approached gradually. If surgery is urgently required in the patient with severe hypothyroidism, an IV dose of 100 μg of thyroxin (Synthroid) may be given and repeated in 12 hours after monitoring clinical

response for further therapy. If at all possible, surgery should be done under local anesthesia.

Patients who have had major surgical ablative procedures with removal of significant amounts of thyroid gland tissue or who receive therapeutic radiation doses encompassing the thyroid should be placed on thyroid replacement medication, the equivalent of 1 to 2 grains of thyroid extract a day, with thyroid functions measured annually.

HYPERPARATHYROIDISM AND HYPOPARATHYROIDISM

Hypercalcemia may be associated with epidermoid carcinomas of the head and neck in several circumstances: primary hyperparathyroidism, hyperparathyroidism as a secondary complication of therapeutic radiation to the neck region, tumor destruction of bone, or a parathormone-like material secreted from the tumor.[5] This latter form of "pseudo hyperparathyroidism" may be found in some patients with advanced epidermoid carcinoma and does not necessarily imply bone involvement. Primary hyperparathyroidism and pseudo hyperparathyroidism secondary to tumor excretion of a parathormone-like substance cannot usually be distinguished by routine clinical tests. Hypercalcemia due to direct bone involvement is usually associated with an elevated alkaline phosphatase and an elevated serum phosphate level and is accompanied by decreased or absent parathormone levels.

If the calcium elevation is slight (between 10.5 and 12 mg percent), the patient may be asymptomatic and require little therapy other than avoiding dehydration. Levels above 15 mg percent are often associated with mental obtundation, nephrocalcinosis, and at higher levels, coma. Calcium levels may be lowered by the use of hydration with or without furosemide, steroids, or phosphates. A more recent therapeutic maneuver has been the use of mithramycin. Mithramycin is an antibiotic, antineoplastic agent which has the ability, independent from its cytoxic properties, to decrease bone osteoclast activity and reverse hypercalcemia due to either primary hyperparathyroidism or neoplasm. The recommended dosage of 20 μg/kg given by slow IV infusion is a much lower dosage than that used in chemotherapy protocols and can be used every 3 to 4 days with relatively little likelihood of hematologic toxicity.

Hypoparathyroidism is most frequently seen as a complication of thyroid surgery or major ablative surgery (such as laryngopharyngectomy) because of either direct surgical trauma to the parathyroid glands or indirect interference with the blood supply to the parathyroids.[6] The resultant hypocalcemia leads to clinical symptoms of paresthesia and neuromuscular irritability with the concomitant positive Chvostek sign and Trousseau sign, and if acute drop in calcium level or profound hypocalcemia occurs, tetany, seizures, cardiac irritability with PVCs, ventricular tachycardia, and ventricular fibrillation may follow.

The ideal treatment of hypocalcemia related to hypoparathyroidism would be the administration of parathormone; however, this is not available at present and treatment consists of the administration of calcium and vitamin D. The goals of therapy are to maintain the calcium level within a low normal range. Rapid replacement of calcium can be achieved by IV administration of calcium gluconate, 10 ml of a 10 percent solution injected by slow IV push. Vitamin D from 50,000 to 150,000 units per day is usually necessary to support the blood calcium levels. Occasionally, the more expensive dihydrotachysterol in doses of 1.0 to 1.5 g per day is used. As soon as possible, oral calcium supplements should be started. The gluconate, lactate, carbonate, or chloride salt are usually interchangeable but occasionally calcium chloride is better absorbed from the gastrointestinal tract. Initial doses of calcium chloride are 6 to 8 g per day; calcium gluconate, 15 g per day; calcium lactate, 4 g three times a day along with lactose, 8 g three times a day. The dosages are then adjusted according to response. Although the postoperative hypocalcemia may be temporary, if it persists for more than 2 to 3 weeks, it is likely to be permanent and require serial measurements of the serum calcium level and continued administration of vitamin D and calcium.

MANAGEMENT OF DRUGS

An accurate drug history is extremely important in evaluating a patient for surgery. Specifically, one should inquire about the following drugs.

Steroids

Patients on these drugs for long periods of time have developed a number of complicating problems. One such condition not always recognized is vascular fragility with an increased bleeding tendency due to vitamin C depletion. Osteoporosis, glycosuria, and depression in immune mechanisms may all be produced by steroids, but the most important problem in the surgical patient is a relative adrenal insufficiency due to adrenal atrophy. These patients may not respond to the stress of surgical demands and may develop acute adrenal insufficiency with a shock-like picture. For this reason, patients on long-term steroids should be given supplemental steroids starting at the time of surgery. A recommended treatment is IV hydrocortisone administered during and following surgery, usually in the range of 200 to 400 mg a day during the period of acute stress; the dosage should then be tapered toward a baseline or physiological dose during the third, fourth, and subsequent postoperative days. An alternative program is to give one of the depocortisone derivatives such as triamcinolone or prednisolone in the dosage of 200 to 300 mg IM the night before surgery. This will allow slow absorption during the next 3 to 5 days.[1]

Propranolol

Propranolol is a beta blocking agent that blocks the sympathetic nerve stimulation of cardiac rate, output, and contractility. Many patients with angina, hypertension, and cardiac arrhythmias are receiving this drug. The action of propranolol may be prolonged in patients who have underlying liver disease. Patients with insulin dependent diabetes who are receiving propranolol may have hypoglycemia without the usual symptoms, as propranolol blocks many of the clinical manifestations of hypoglycemia. Propranolol should be avoided in asthmatic patients because it may produce bronchoconstriction and in patients with congestive heart failure because it causes decreased cardiac contractility.

Patients with arteriosclerotic heart disease who have been on long-term propranolol treatment may experience exacerbations of angina or even precipitation of myocardial infarction if the drug is abruptly discontinued. Therefore, the dosage of this drug should either be tapered slowly and discontinued prior to surgery or continued through surgery by parenteral administration. The major anesthetic risk in a patient on propranolol treatment is sustained bradycardia that is unresponsive to sympathomimetic drugs with resultant refractory heart failure.

Antiseizure Drugs

Patients with seizure disorders in the older age group frequently fail to report the use of these agents either because they come to regard them as "nonmedications" or may wish to conceal the stigma of a seizure disorder. If the patient does not report the use of the drug and the drugs are discontinued abruptly, acute episodes of seizure activity may quickly occur. Thus, antiseizure drugs should be continued through surgery and the postoperative period by parenteral administration and until the patient is able to resume oral medication.

The drugs most frequently encountered are phenylhydantoin (Dilantin) and phenobarbital, both of which are readily available in parenteral forms. Some of the agents that are not available parenterally can be temporarily replaced by Dilantin, phenobarbital or, less frequently, diazepam

(Valium). The interaction of various anesthetic agents must be considered in patients using these drugs, and the anesthesiologist must be made aware of their use.

Anticoagulants

The most commonly used group of long-term anticoagulants are warfarins, particularly Coumadin. If a patient is adequately anticoagulated with Coumadin, the prothrombin time is two to two-and-a-half times normal. Surgery at this level, particularly if bone resection is involved, will be associated with a significantly increased risk of bleeding. The prothrombin time can be rapidly returned to normal and the vitamin K dependent clotting proteins rapidly replenished by withholding Coumadin and giving vitamin K oxide intravenously or intramuscularly. Usually vitamin K oxide (Aquamephyton) in a dose of 10 to 20 mg given 12 to 24 hours prior to surgery will correct the clotting protein deficiency. Once vitamin K has been given, the patient cannot be anticoagulated with Coumadin for about 2 weeks.

If surgery will involve only soft tissues and the patient is at high risk for thrombosis if anticoagulation is stopped, then Coumadin should be stopped, low dose heparin should be instituted about 24 hours postoperatively and the oral Coumadin administration restarted later. It should also be recognized that aspirin may affect platelet aggregation for a prolonged period after ingestion. If at all possible, aspirin and aspirin-containing drugs should be avoided for 7 to 10 days prior to surgery.

There are a variety of other agents, too numerous to discuss in detail, for which adjustments in dose or route must be made during the perioperative period.

ALCOHOLISM

Alcoholism is one of the well established etiologic factors in the development of squamous cell carcinoma of the head and neck. Consequently, a large percentage of patients with these carcinomas will have complicating medical problems related to acute or chronic alcoholism. The chronic problems pertain to psychosocial issues as well as to chronic liver disease, peripheral neuropathies, and a damaged central nervous system. Laboratory parameters important to the evaluation of a patient with alcoholism are liver function tests and standard coagulation screening tests, such as platelet count, partial thromboplastin time, and prothrombin time.

The alcohol withdrawal syndrome, which includes symptoms ranging from mild tremulousness to delirium tremens, represents an exaggerated defense reaction by the body. As a direct CNS depressant, alcohol will cause compensatory mechanisms to facilitate an alert posture. Hence, upon the withdrawal of alcohol, the tremulousness, increased visual imagery, anxiety, and tachycardia are those compensatory mechanisms no longer balanced by the depressive effects of alcohol.

The time from cessation of alcohol to the manifestation of symptoms may be quite variable. The anxiety, agitation and mild tremulousness usually occur within the first 24 to 36 hours. Seizures (rum fits) as a withdrawal phenomenon most frequently take place within 24 to 48 hours, and delirium tremens is often preceeded by tremulousness and agitation; in some patients the severe manifestations may be delayed for 3 to 5 days following the cessation of drinking. One needs to be particularly aware of this complication if there is a history of prior alcohol withdrawal symptoms. If the patient is inebriated upon admission to the hospital and if the history suggests chronic, heavy use of alcohol, surgery should be delayed until the period of risk has passed. The patient should be hydrated and given thiamine, 100 mg intramuscularly initially and either orally or parenterally thereafter. Appropriate liver function tests, hematologic tests, and coagulation tests should be performed. Although some have recom-

mended continuing alcohol infusion to avoid withdrawal syndrome, it has been our practice to avoid this in patients who will be undergoing extensive surgical procedures.

The manifestations of alcohol withdrawal may complicate the postoperative period or be confused with other significant medical problems such as fluid overload, infection with fever, cardiac tachyrhythmias, hyperthyroidism, and other neurologic or psychiatric sequelae. Most important in the management of the alcohol withdrawal syndrome is the maintenance of adequate hydration, the administration of adequate calories and vitamin supplementation, and the suppression of CNS hyperactivity with sedation. Close monitoring of electrolytes is important because alcohol may be associated with a metabolic acidosis, specifically lactic acidosis with an excess accumulation of hydroxybutyric acid through a multiple inhibition of the Krebs cycle. This inhibition of multiple steps in the Krebs cycle may lead to a decreased bicarbonate, an increased anion gap, and often an associated hypoglycemia.

The most effective agents for sedation during the period of alcohol withdrawal syndrome are the benzodiazepines, which include diazepoxide, diazepam and oxazepam. Chlordiazepoxide (Librium) is a long-acting agent with pharmacologically active metabolites. Repeated doses result in accumulation of the drug and its metabolites in the body. An appropriate regimen consists of large doses of chlordiazepoxide in the range of 100 to 400 mg on the first day of treatment, followed by decreasing amounts thereafter, with reduction of 25 to 50 percent of the total dose each day. Oxazepam (Vistaril) is rapidly converted to an inactive metabolite and can be continued without reduction in dosage.[10]

Other agents occasionally useful in patients with alcohol withdrawal syndrome are lithium carbonate, which may diminish subjective symptoms of withdrawal; propranolol, which may reduce the severity of withdrawal tremor; and phenothiazines, although phenothiazines may lead to increase in the risk of postural hypotension and perhaps seizures. Dilantin or other drugs that prevent seizures are of uncertain value in controlling withdrawal seizures; in most patients who do not have a history of prior seizures, the benzodiazepines alone are probably sufficient to prevent withdrawal seizures. In patients who have had prior seizures, there may be some advantage afforded by the use if Dilantin, 100 mg three times a day. If seizures do occur, the Dilantin need not be continued past the withdrawal period.[10]

In summary, if at all possible, the patients at high risk of alcohol withdrawal syndrome should not undergo surgery until they are past the period of major risk of alcohol withdrawal syndrome or have been supported through the withdrawal period with hydration, sedation, and nutrition. Although at some institutions, patients are maintained during their hospitalization with an alcohol infusion, it is our policy to delay surgery until the period of risk from alcohol syndrome is over. The delay is additionally warranted because the stress of surgery itself may precipitate delirium tremens.

ANEMIA AND COAGULATION DISORDERS

Anemia

The routine complete blood count (CBC) done on automated equipment provides an excellent screen for anemia. If anemia is present, the indices on the report and perusal of peripheral blood smear frequently provide, with the addition of the patient's history and physical record, all the information needed on which to base a decision regarding intervention. The most efficient tissue oxygenation in the microcirculation takes place in a normal individual with a hemaglobin level of 10 g percent and a hematocrit level of 30 percent. The elderly patient with arteriosclerosis may need higher levels of oxygen carrying capacity. This means that surgery can be safely carried out in individuals with hematocrit levels no higher than 30 percent if major blood loss does not occur. It also follows that postoperatively a hemoglobin value of 10 g percent should not require transfusion unless acute or ongoing blood loss is occurring. Below these levels, however, there is a fairly rapid drop in tissue oxygenation efficiency, which may lead to symptoms of angina, confusion, or dyspnea. Considerations must also be given to maintenance of adequate tissue oxygenation to aid survival of regional pedicle flaps and to help in the prompt healing of large wounds. If symptoms are felt to be caused by anemia, transfusion is indicated but not dictated by an absolute level of hemoglobin. With acute symptoms, transfusion is usually indicated when the hemoglobin level is 9 g percent or lower.

In patients with chronic anemia, the correction should be with packed red blood cells, since the plasma volume is normal and the deficiency needed to be replaced is red cells. In patients with acute blood loss, both plasma or plasma equivalents plus red cells are needed to correct the deficit. Reconstituted whole blood (packed red blood cells plus fresh frozen plasma) or red blood cells plus 5 percent albumin will also support the patient. Fresh frozen plasma should be used if there is concurrent deficiency of clotting factors, e.g., an elevated prothrombin time or partial thromboplastin time. Prophylactic platelet transfusion should be reserved for patients with severe thrombocytopenia (less than 20,000 cu mm) or with active bleeding or anticipated surgery if the platelet count is below 50,000 to 80,000. Platelet transfusions of one donor pack per 8 to 10 pounds of body weight should be given and repeated, depending on the clinical circumstances. White blood cell transfusions are reserved for patients with established infections not responding to antibiotics who have an absolute neutrophil count of less than 500 per cu mm.

Coagulation Disorders

The finding of an underlying coagulation disorder is most often heralded by a history of unusual bleeding, easy susceptibility to bruising or bleeding following mild or minimal trauma, or excessive bleeding with dental extractions or surgery.[4, 15] The history of a family member or members with a bleeding disorder should raise the question of hereditary abnormality such as hemophilia, Von Willebrand disease, or hereditary hemorrhagic telangiectasia. Liver disease is a frequent cause of acquired, gross abnormalities of the clotting mechanism.

The screening coagulation studies should include platelet count; prothrombin time, which measures the extrinsic clotting system; and partial thromboplastin time, which measures the intrinsic system. These studies may all be normal and yet bleeding may occur on the basis of decreased vascular tone, a mild circulating inhibitor, or abnormal platelets. In general, it can be said that a prothrombin time of less than 50 percent, which fails to respond to parenterally administered vitamin K oxide, is indicative of a severe defect of vitamin K dependent factor synthesis in the liver and would be associated with serious risks of bleeding or hepatic decompensation from surgery and anesthesia. An abnormal partial thromboplastin time may occur as a result of a deficiency of any of the clotting proteins with the exception of factor VII, which is in the extrinsic system alone. It may also occur as a result of a nonspecific or specific circulating inhibitor of one or more of the clotting proteins. In this circumstance, direct quantitation of clotting proteins—including all the factors and procoagulants—is necessary in order that the specific substitution or correction of the defect can be accomplished.

One of the common causes of increased surgical bleeding may be the prior ingestion of aspirin, which may have occurred up to 7 to 10 days prior to surgery. Aspirin inhibits platelet aggregation and unusual bleeding may be noted, yet the standard tests of clotting function (platelet count, prothrombin time, partial thromboplastin time) may be normal. Patients should be advised to avoid aspirin preoperatively as mentioned previously.

DISSEMINATED INTRAVASCULAR COAGULATION

Disseminated intravascular coagulation (DIC) may be seen in the postoperative period due to sepsis, shock, or shower of embolic material. Patients with large tumor loads may have DIC because of liberation of tissue thromboplastic material due to tumor necrosis. These states of DIC may vary from a mild compensated state to an acute medical emergency leading to shock and death. The principle management of DIC is treatment of the underlying disorder. Serial measurements of clotting parameters, including fibrinogen, platelet count, and fibrinogen degradation products (FDP), help monitor the severity of DIC and its resolution. The use of heparin in these states is controversial and, if employed, should be managed in association with a comprehensive coagulation laboratory that is able to rapidly measure serially obtained clotting parameters.[4]

THROMBOPHLEBITIS AND PULMONARY EMBOLUS

Thrombophlebitis is a frequent postoperative complication which may lead to the cataclysmic consequence of life-threatening pulmonary emboli. Obesity, prolonged periods of bedrest, immobility, and venous insufficiency increase the tendency toward venous stasis and sludging. In addition, surgery per se leads to a relatively hypercoagulable state with increased thrombotic tendencies. Most pulmonary emboli emanate from thromboses in the deep veins of the lower extremities and they may often be unrecognized and asymptomatic until the development of an acute pulmonary embolus. This has lead to attempts to prevent lower extremity thrombosis in the perioperative and postoperative periods. Efforts should be directed towards early ambulation and the use of support stockings; for the immobile patient passive exercises of the lower extremities should be instituted. The low incidence of pulmonary embolism in patients undergoing head and neck surgery is probably due to the early ambulation possible in these patients. Recent studies show that "mini-dose heparin" may prevent the hypercoagulable state in the high risk patient. In patients with a prior history of pulmonary emboli, those with massive obesity, and those with venous insufficiency, for whom several days or more of bedrest are anticipated, heparin in a dosage of 5,000 units subcutaneously every 8 to 12 hours has been shown to decrease the incidence of thrombophlebitis and subsequent pulmonary emboli without increasing measurably the partial thromboplastin time or increasing the risk of bleeding unless there is also thrombocytopenia or other coagulation abnormalities present.

Thrombophlebitis of the lower extremity or pulmonary emboli require the use of therapeutic doses of heparin. The clinical concomitants of pulmonary emboli may not always be the classical syndrome of acute onset of chest pain, dyspnea, and hemoptysis but may merely be increased unexplained tachypnea and tachycardia. Important confirmatory findings are increased arterial hypoxemia and abnormal areas of perfusion on lung scanning that are normal on routine chest x-ray. Sometimes pulmonary arteriography is necessary to confirm the diagnosis.

The goals of anticoagulant therapy are to increase the partial thromboplastin time one-and-a-half to two times normal. Probably, this is accomplished most effectively and safely by continuous IV infusion with control flow pump. An arbitrary starting dosage is selected, usually between 25,000 and 30,000 units of heparin for 24 hours, and the rate adjusted to keep the partial thromboplastin time in the therapeutic range. If long term anticoagulation is required, Coumadin derivatives are instituted while the heparin dosage is gradually tapered over a 3 to 5 day period.

STRESS ULCERS

In the setting of major surgical trauma, particularly in patients with a prior history of ulcer disease, stress ulcers with gastrointestinal bleeding may occur. Recent evidence suggests that some protection may be afforded by the prophylactic administration of the H-2 receptor antagonist cimetidine in a dosage of 300 mg every 6 hours intravenously or orally.

CHANGE IN NEUROLOGIC STATUS

A sudden change in neurologic status, especially in the postoperative setting, requires careful and rapid evaluation. Dementia may be the result of simple sensory deprivation associated with normal aging and arteriosclerosis. A patient with borderline dementia, who in strange surroundings would have decreased sensory input due to wound dressings and/or analgesics, may lose orientation, have visual hallucinations, or evince vegetative or withdrawal behavior. This behavior may be due to simple sensory deprivation, and the patient will respond to increasing sensory input and reassurance.

Metabolic causes of acute changes in mental status include delayed alcohol withdrawal syndromes (including delirium tremens), hypercalcemia or hypocalcemia, diabetic ketoacidosis or nonketotic hyperasmolar coma, hyponatremia, hypo- or hyperkalemia, hepatic encephalopathy, anemia, or overmedication. Although there are often clinical clues to the type of metabolic encephalopathy, it is often prudent to measure certain parameters, such as hemoglobin, electrolytes, blood sugar, blood urea nitrogen (BUN) levels, calcium levels, and liver function tests. The patient's list of medication should be reviewed and those known to cause such problems discontinued.

Patients with chronic lung disease may tolerate surgery poorly. There may be significant drops on O_2 saturation and CO_2 retention with confusion as an early and primary symptom. The use of blood gas determinations in these clinical settings are to be encouraged for the accurate monitoring of these patients. Patients with normal pulmonary functions but severe cerebral atherosclerosis may also have striking alterations in mentation with small variations of O_2 saturation or CO_2 retention.

The possiblility of cerebral vascular accident should be considered if new focal neurologic signs appear, particularly if surgery involved clamping or manipulation of the carotid artery or if there have been intraoperative periods of hypotension. Unlike a patient with senile dementia or metabolic encephalopathy wherein global or general neurologic abnormalities occur, the patient with cerebral vascular disease embolic phenomena or metastatic disease will often have focal findings that are helpful in localizing the area of disease as well as the underlying cause.

The possibility of meningitis must be raised in a febrile patient if subarachnoid space has been violated during surgery. Lumbar puncture is mandatory. The fever itself may aggravate previous metabolic or vascular problems and create mental changes. The early diagnosis of meningitis is an extremely important determinant in the outcome of appropriate antimicrobial therapy. If neutrophils and organisms are seen in the spinal fluid gram stain, early appropriate antibiotic treatment can be instituted before culture and sensitivity results are available. CT scanning has been very helpful in the rapid differentiation of vascular abnormalities, cerebral atrophy, and brain abscesses.

SEPSIS

Any patient with sepsis evident preoperatively should have the organism identified, the antibiotic sensitivities determined, and the infection eradicated or controlled before any surgical intervention. Those patients with hidden infection or who require emergency surgery despite infection should have intensive parenteral treatment of such infections, as determined by organism identification and antibiotic sensitivities. Those patients with evidence of septicemia or showing symptoms of sepsis such as gram negative shock should not have treatment withheld pending cultures and sensitivity results, but treatment with drug combinations covering the widest and most likely bacteriologic spectrum should be started. We use Keflin, gentamycin, and carbenicillin; however, other combinations have been used for primary coverage. Once the bacteriologic sensitivities are determined, the antibiotic coverage can be sharpened to treat the specific infection.

Postoperative infection in head and neck surgery is common, not only locally because of unavoidable contamination but also from a pulmonary focus because of aspiration and mechanical obstruction. The question of antibiotic prophylaxis has been raised and is a matter of controversy.

SUMMARY

Recent advances in the surgical techniques and management of head and neck cancer, combined with radiation therapy and/or chemotherapy, offer the promise of increased salvage and improved function for these patients. The very nature of the disease and the difficulties imposed by the necessary treatment modalities underlie the importance of a careful medical evaluation in the team approach to the care of these patients and individualization of management programs. A few days spent in the careful preoperative patient assessment, medical evaluation, and health team communication are well justified for the prevention of postoperative complications, the psychological adjustment of the patient, the identification of family support systems, and the correction of underlying problems that may complicate the surgical procedure. The additional time spent in preoperative evaluation may actually decrease the period of inpatient convalescence as well as improve the quality of postoperative survival.

The psychological stresses of the disease, surgery, and convalescence have not been stressed in this chapter, as the important communication between the health care team, the patient, and family support systems is often on ontologic and kinetic bases and cannot be rigidly approached. This does not minimize the importance of the psychosocial factors in patient outcome.

This chapter has attempted to focus on the major medical complications and concurrent problems that may be faced in the care of the patient with head and neck cancer during the perioperative and convalescent period. The active and close cooperation between the surgeon and internist, as well as the communication with the rest of the health care team, represent one of the most important recent advances in the care of these patients.

REFERENCES

1. Axelrod, L., 1976. Glucocorticoid therapy. Medicine, 55:   39.

2. Diener, C. F., 1973. Evaluation of disability and assessment of operative risk. Medical Clinics of North America, 57:   763.

3. Goldman, L., Caldera, D. L., Southwick, F. S., Nussbaum, S. R., Murray, B., O'Malley, T. A., Goroll, A. H., Caplan, C. H., Nolan, J., Burke, D. S., Krogstad, D., Carabello, B., Slater, E. E.: 1978. Cardiac risk factors and complications in non-cardiac surgery. Medicine, 57:   357.

4. Lewis, J. H., Spero, J. A., Hasiba, U., 1977. Coagulopathies. Disease-A-Month, 23:   1.

5. Liston, S. L., 1978. Hypercalcemia and head and neck cancer. Bony metastases from tongue cancer. Archives of Otolaryngology, 104:   597.

6. Mossman, K. L., Scheer, A. C., 1977. Complications of radiotherapy of head and neck cancer. Ear, Nose and Throat Journal, 56:   145.

7. Olsen, A. M., 1967. Evaluation of surgical risk in patients with chronic obstructive lung disease and other respiratory handicaps. Medical Clinics of North America, 51:   341.

8. Rossini, A. A., Hare, J. W., 1976. How to control the blood glucose level in the surgical diabetic patient. Archives of Surgery, 111:   945.

9. Salzman, E. W., Deykin, D., Shapiro, R. M., and Rosenberg, R., 1975. Management of heparin therapy: Controlled prospective trial. New England Journal of Medicine, 292:   1046.

10. Sellers, E. M., Kalant, H. 1976. Alcohol intoxication and withdrawal. New England Journal of Medicine, 294:   757.

11. Shafer, R. B., Nuttall, F. Q., Pollak, K., and Kuisk, H. 1975. Thyroid function after radiation and surgery for head and neck cancer. Archives of Internal Medicine, 135:   843.

12. Sherry, S., 1976. Low-dose heparin for the prophylaxis of pulmonary embolism. American Review of Respiratory Disease, 114:   661.

13. Stein, M., Cassara, E. L., 1970. Preoperative pulmonary evaluation and therapy for surgery patients. JAMA, 211:   787.

14. Tisell, L. E., Carlsson, S., Lindberg, S., and Ragnhult, I. 1976. Autonomous hyperparathyroidism: A possible late complication of neck radiotherapy. Acta Chirurgica Scandinavica, 142:   367.

15. Tullis, James L. 1976. Clot. Charles C. Thomas, Springfield, Ill.

16. Wollam, G. L., Gifford, R. W., Jr., 1978. Four basic problems in controlling hypertension. Consultant, 18:   25.

5 | Nutritional Management of Patients with Head and Neck Malignancies

John M. Daly, M.D.
Stanley J. Dudrick, M.D.
Edward M. Copeland, III, M.D.

Because patients with oropharyngeal malignant neoplasms often have a history of smoking and dietary indiscretions and a high intake of alcohol, they usually have identifiable nutritional problems. They may be undernourished and have vitamin deficiencies at the time an oropharyngeal malignancy develops, and such underlying malnutrition may be potentiated by the anatomical location of the cancer if it results in obstruction or pain on deglutition. Patients with resectable or radiosensitive neoplasms should be optimally nourished so that adequate wound healing may occur and the incidence and severity of complications of surgery and radiotherapy may be minimized.[4] Protein-calorie malnutrition can result in impaired wound healing, reduced immunologic function, increased susceptibility to infection, and decreased tolerance to effective antineoplastic therapy. Clinical and experimental studies have demonstrated clearly that nutritional repletion prior to or during oncologic therapy can restore immunologic function to normal and reduce perioperative morbidity and mortality.[3, 5, 6] With the availability of special dietary supplements, tube feedings, and intravenous hyperalimentation, no longer should the nutritional needs of patients be neglected in the clinical practice of medicine.

Initiation of appropriate nutritional therapy for patients with head and neck cancer requires a thorough knowledge of nutritional requirements and the methods of assessment of nutritional status.[1, 2] A nutritional therapy team (Table 5-1) can perform an accurate nutritional assessment by history questionnaire, physical examination, and laboratory tests. Assessment of the individual's nutritional status can then be quantified and assigned a score. Knowledge of the patient's malignancy (type and stage), the anticipated method of treatment (surgery, radiation therapy, and/or chemotherapy), and the estimated length and degree of nutritional disability (length of time patient is unable to achieve optimal enteral alimentation) is mandatory prior to the initiation of a nutritional treatment program in order to assure that optimal therapeutic results are achieved with minimal morbidity.

TABLE 5-1 NUTRITIONAL THERAPY TEAM

Head and neck surgeon
Nutrition consultant (M.D. or Ph.D.)
Nurse
Senior dietician
Pharmacist

NUTRITIONAL REQUIREMENTS

Operative trauma initiates a complex series of events manifested as the metabolic response to injury. This response is more intense if postoperative complications such as pneumonia, sepsis, or wound infection develop. Patients undergoing major operative therapy have an acute increase in metabolic energy demands at a time when food intake is decreased or absent.[12] The demand for endogenous fuels can be intense. Stored carbohydrate in the form of glycogen is consumed within 24 hours; glucose demands are met subsequently by the breakdown of protein, particularly skeletal muscle and visceral protein, through the process of gluconeogenesis. Fat is also a major storehouse of energy but is better utilized during chronic starvation than during the acute phases of injury. The severity of the catabolic phase of illness and its duration depend upon the extent and type of operation or injury, the presence of significant infection, the length of time the patient is immobilized, the duration of inadequate nutrient intake, age, sex, previous nutritional status, and the effects of previously existing illness.

The well nourished, healthy patient who is subjected to a single, uncomplicated major operation usually responds well to a simple parenteral program designed to maintain adequate circulatory volume and to provide enough water, salt, potassium, and glucose to prevent dehydration, electrolyte imbalance, and excessive endogenous protein breakdown for gluconeogenesis. This perioperative need can be met with various 5 percent dextrose and electrolyte solutions, which are commercially available. Patients with head and neck malignancies, however, are often protein-calorie malnourished at the time they develop an oropharyngeal tumor, and surgical treatment often results in diminished oral intake for extended periods of time. In addition, radiation therapy frequently produces severe stomatitis, mucositis, and diminished salivary secretions. These adverse conditions result in decreased oral intake and consequent weight loss. Therefore, patients with head and neck malignancies who are malnourished prior to therapy enter a vicious cycle as oncologic treatment usually further impairs optimum nutritional repletion.

Metabolic rate gradually declines from childhood to old age, and is consistently lower in females than in males. Recommended daily dietary allowances for meeting energy and protein needs of nonstressed, previously well-nourished patients performing moderate activities are shown in Table 5-2. These figures serve as general guidelines in estimating maintenance requirements for average, *healthy* men and women. In patients with head and neck cancer either maintenance or anabolic calorie and protein levels are required depending upon the patient's nutritional status at the initial examination and the magnitude of therapy to be instituted. Caloric requirements for daily maintenance for each patient can be calculated from the Harris-Benedict Formula (see Table 5-3).[2, 9]

A simpler method for meeting caloric and protein needs is to supply calories at 35 kcal/kg/day for maintenance and at 45 kcal/kg/day for anabolism.[16] Nitrogen intake (protein ration divided by 6.25) should be approximately 1 g of nitrogen per 150 nonprotein calories in the average patient. This nitrogen to calorie ratio is approximated in most commercial tube formulas and when most standard hospital diets are blenderized.

NUTRITIONAL ASSESSMENT

It is the responsibility of the supervising physician to make an accurate assessment of the patient's nutritional status with the assistance of the nurse and dietician. Based on the patient's history (Table 5-4), the degree of recent weight loss and the patient's ability to ingest adequate quantities of nutrients orally are evaluated. This information provides a *qualitative* assessment of the patient's nutritional status and also determines to

TABLE 5-2 RECOMMENDED DAILY DIETARY ALLOWANCES (NORMAL ACTIVITY AND TEMPERATE CLIMATE)

	Age	Weight (kgm)	Height (cm)	Energy Needs (cal)
Males	11–14	45	157	2,700
	15–18	66	176	2,800
	19–22	70	177	2,900
	23–50	70	178	2,700
	51–75	70	178	2,400
	76+	70	178	2,050
Females	11–14	46	157	2,200
	15–18	55	163	2,100
	19–22	55	163	2,100
	23–50	55	163	2,000
	51–75	55	163	1,800
	76+	55	163	1,600

(From Committee on Dietary Allowances, Food and Nutrition Board. 1980. Recommended Dietary Allowances, 9th revised edn. National Research Council, Washington, DC. Reproduced with the permission of the National Academy of Sciences.)

TABLE 5-3 CALCULATION OF CALORIC REQUIREMENTS BY THE HARRIS-BENEDICT FORMULA

	Maintenance	Anabolism
Oral	1.2 × BEE* kcal†	1.6 × BEE kcal†
Intravenous	1.5 × BEE kcal†	1.8 × BEE kcal†

*BEE, Basal Energy Expenditure.
†BEE for male   = (66.5 + (13.7 × wt (kg)) + (5 × ht (cm)) − (6.7 × age (yrs)).
†BEE for female = (65.5 + (9.5 × wt (kg)) + (1.8 × ht (cm)) − (4.7 × age (yrs)).
Protein requirements per day can be calculated from the formula:

$$\text{Protein in grams} = 6.25 \times \frac{\text{caloric requirements}}{150}$$

TABLE 5-4 QUESTIONS FOR HISTORY TAKING

1. What is your normal weight? Weight two months ago? Weight now?

2. Are you able to eat three meals per day?

3. Has your clothing size remained the same?

4. Does food taste good?

5. Are you able to swallow without difficulty?

some extent the method of nutrient delivery required during the perioperative period. Our team has devised a nutrition scale of 4 points so that patients may be placed into nutritional categories: *good* (3 or 4 points), *fair* (2 points), and *poor* (0 or 1 point). The score from the nutritional assessment determines the amount of nutrition required (maintenance or anabolic). Based on the physical examination (Table 5-5), either 0, 1, or 2 points are awarded to the total nutri-

TABLE 5-5 PHYSICAL EXAMINATION

Measure		Good (2)	Fair (1)	Poor (0)
1. Weight (% ideal)*		90–100	80–89	< 80
2. Triceps skinfold thickness (mm)†	male	12.5	10–12.4	< 09.9
	female	16.5	12–16.4	< 11.9
3. Mid-upper-arm muscle circumference (cm)‡	male	25.0	20–24.9	< 20.0
	female	23.0	18–22.9	< 18.0
4. Mid-upper-arm circumference‡	male	29.0	23–28.9	< 23.0
	female	28.5	23–28.4	< 23.0
5. Ambulatory ability		walk 200' unassisted	walk 200' assisted	unable to walk

*See Appendix 5-1.
†See Appendix 5-3.
‡Arm muscle circumference = arm circumference − (0.314 × triceps skinfold thickness mm)

tional assessment score. If the majority of the five results (more than 2) fall into the poor category, then 0 points are awarded to the total patient score. If the majority of the results are in the fair category with one or two determinations in the poor category, then 0 points also are given. If, however, the majority of results are in the good category, but one or two results are in the fair or poor categories, then 1 point is awarded to the total patient score. If all five scores are in the fair category, 1 point is awarded. If all five results are in the good category, 2 points are awarded.

Results of laboratory values (Table 5-6) are also used in evaluating nutritional status during the initial assessment of the patient. The category into which the lowest two or

TABLE 5-6 LABORATORY VALUES (0, 1, OR 2 POINTS)

Test		Good (2)	Fair (1)	Poor (0)
1. Plasma hemoglobin (gm %)	male	14–17	11–13.9	< 11
	female	12–15	10–11.9	< 10
2. Serum albumin (gm %)		3.5–4.5	3.0–3.4	< 30
3. Serum iron (mg %)		75–175	50–74	< 50
4. Serum transferrin (mg %)*		>200	150–199	<150
5. Creatinine/height index (%)†		90–100	70–89	< 70
6. Cell-mediated immunocompetence (mm)‡ (Varidase, Candida, mumps, PPD, Dermatophytin)		>10	0–5	< 5

*An approximation of the serum transferrin value can be derived from the serum total iron binding capacity (TIBC) by the following formula: Serum transferrin = (0.8 × TIBC) − 43
†Creatinine/height index = 24 hour creatinine excretion of patient divided by 24 hour creatinine excretion of "normal" adult of same height (see Appendix 5-1).
‡Only one skin test must exceed minimum measurement for each category for patient to be grouped in either normal, fair, or poor category.

more test results fall determines the number of points awarded to the total nutritional score (good = 2, fair = 1, poor = 0).

Nutritional status, a subjective clinical term, can thus be determined more objectively with the use of a four point scale. *Good* nutritional status is defined when a total score of 3 or 4 points is awarded to the patient. *Fair* nutritional status is defined when a total of 2 points is awarded to the patient, while a total of 0 or 1 point defines *poor* nutritional status. Objective data can thus define a rather nebulous term and allow not only initial assessment of the patient, but repeated evaluations of the efficacy of nutritional therapy.

A simple, ready-to-use definition of malnutrition that can be memorized and readily applied clinically includes the following: a recent unintentional loss of 10 percent or more of body weight, a serum albumin level less than 3.4 g percent, and a negative reaction to a battery of recall skin test antigens. The combination of any two of these three criteria is an indication for nutritional repletion prior to therapy, and if these conditions develop post-therapy, special efforts at nutritional repletion are not only indicated, but may be necessary as a life-saving measure.

The magnitude of therapy that the cancer patient receives determines the degree of metabolic stress that the patient will undergo. Patients can be assigned arbitrarily to either high or low categories, depending on their treatment modalities (Table 5-7). The surgeon or radiotherapist who treats these patients must attempt to prepare them psychologically, metabolically, and physiologically for the recommended oncologic therapy.

Determination of the method of feeding patients depends upon the type of antineoplastic therapy used and the nutritional status of the patient. Attention to nutritional status at the initial interview and appropriate dietary counseling and vitamin supplementation will result in nutritional rehabilitation of most patients. Ideally, adequate oral feeding should be the ultimate goal in each patient, but often the type and magnitude of treatment precludes optimal enteral intake. Also, poor nutritional status may result in anorexia, lassitude, and muscle weakness, and thus further decrease oral ingestion of nutrients. Basically, standard hospital diets plus oral supplements and/or tube feedings should be administered to patients in good nutritional status under the direction of a dietitian. A functional gastrointestinal tract is the best means of insuring normal digestion and assimilation of foodstuffs; however, the gastrointestinal tract is not always available for use, and the delivery of adequate nutrients to the gut does not always result in rapid nutritional repletion because malnutrition may lead to malabsorption, diarrhea, and loss of enteral nutrients in the stool. If time permits, nutritional repletion may be accomplished by tube feeding maneuvers; however, nutritional rehabilitation via the gastrointestinal tract can be time-consuming, and the operative insertion of gastrostomy or jejunostomy tubes can impose an acute surgical stress upon the patient that will further delay nutritional repletion. Similarly, indwelling nasogastric tubes are unsatisfactory for

TABLE 5-7 MAGNITUDE OF THERAPY

High	Low
Total Glossectomy and Radical Neck Dissection	Radical Neck Dissection
Commando Procedure	Thyroidectomy
Laryngopharyngectomy	Hemiglossectomy
Cervical Esophagectomy	

long-term use because they often cause nasopharyngeal ulcerations, and esophagogastric reflux occurs around the tube. Nevertheless, short-term nutritional repletion of the moderately malnourished patient or nutritional maintenance of the previously healthy patient who cannot swallow can be quite satisfactory via a nasogastric feeding tube. For those patients whose gastrointestinal tracts are unavailable for nutrient administration or who need rapid nutritional repletion in order to initiate antineoplastic therapy promptly and safely, proper application of the technique of intravenous hyperalimentation (IVH) has allowed appropriate cancer treatment to be administered and in some cases has been life-saving.

TUBE FEEDINGS

Nasogastric

INDICATIONS

Although it is desirable to have patients voluntarily ingesting an adequate diet orally, a significant number of patients with head and neck malignancies are unable to do so. In general, it should be the physician's goal to utilize the alimentary tract for nutritional purposes if it is functioning adequately. Indications for nasogastric tube feeding must depend upon the patient's nutritional status (as determined by the initial nutritional assessment), the magnitude of therapy (degree of stress and length of nutritional disability), and the need for subsequent therapy required to eradicate the patient's malignancy. For example, a well-nourished patient undergoing a radical neck dissection (low magnitude of therapy) would require, under ordinary circumstances, only a brief interval of support with intravenous 5 percent dextrose in water and electrolytes. However, a malnourished patient who undergoes a laryngopharyngectomy either prior to or following radiation therapy and has an adequate, functioning gastrointestinal tract should be treated vigorously with

tube feedings to promote anabolism prior to and after operative therapy. However, there are several contraindications to tube feedings: partial or total intestinal obstruction; intestinal ileus; high intestinal fistulas; severe malabsorption and/or diarrhea; vomiting, secondary to mechanical obstruction, ileus, or chemotherapy; and depressed cough reflexes in debilitated patients with preexisting pulmonary disease.[15]

A number 14 or 16 French nasogastric tube may be inserted through one of the external nares to lie within the distal one-third of the esophagus (Fig. 5-1). Reflux esophagitis can be prevented if the large bore tube does not traverse the esophagogastric junction and render the esophagogastric sphincter incompetent. The tube should be replaced and repositioned via the opposite nostril at least every 10 to 14 days in order to prevent pressure necrosis of the nasal and nasopharyngeal mucosa. Most nasogastric tubes have markings spaced at equal distances along the tube to allow proper positioning of the tip of the tube 30 to 35 cm from the external nasal orifice (the esophagogastric junction is 40 cm from the nasal opening in the average adult male patient). When nasogastric tube feedings are required for longer periods, some patients can be taught to remove and reinsert the tube themselves. Proper tube placement is important, and if difficulty in insertion is encountered or doubt about location of the distal end of the feeding tube exists, roentgenographic confirmation of the tube location in the distal esophagus is indicated. Aspiration of the tube diet into the tracheobronchial tree can be especially dangerous in the malnourished patient who has depressed inflammatory and immunologic responses to infection and who does not have the ability to clear tracheobronchial secretions because of weak, ineffectual respiratory musculature. The threat of aspiration can be minimized by having the patient in an upright position during feeding, by preliminary testing for regurgitation with 5 percent dextrose infusion, by slow instillation of the tube feeding diet (best monitored by the patient), and by *not* feeding the pa-

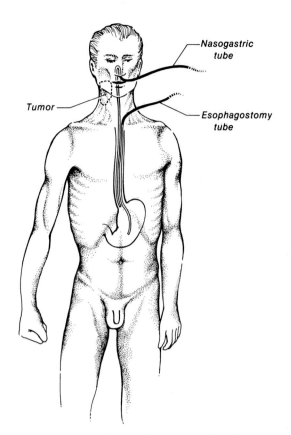

Fig. 5-1. Small, flexible nasogastric tubes provide ready access to the gastrointestinal tract, while establishment of an esophagostomy is an alternative for long-term feeding when necessary for nutritional maintenance.

tient while he is hiccoughing, asleep, or in the radiology department for diagnostic tests.

Often cancer patients object to tube feedings with large diameter feeding tubes because of previous unpleasant encounters with this method of treatment. However, a small, number 8 French pediatric feeding tube or silicone rubber tube has a greater degree of patient acceptability and reduces the risk of mucosal ulcerations. Small caliber tubes are flexible, however, and may be expelled upon regurgitation or coughing. This problem may be overcome by weighting the tubes with a small mercury bag or by inserting mercury into the lower segment of the tube and sealing it.[13] The soft, small caliber tubes are inserted more easily after being chilled with ice to impart some temporary rigidity. Alternatively, they can be coupled to a larger, more rigid tube by placing a gelatin capsule over the ends of the two tubes. Following passage of the tubes into the stomach, the gelatin capsule quickly softens or dissolves and the larger tube can be withdrawn, leaving the smaller tube in position. A problem with small diameter feeding tubes is that they can be easily occluded by viscid or blenderized diets. Crystalloid chemically defined diets obviate this problem, but they are more expensive to use.

The potential for aspiration of the formula must always be considered. Aspiration is especially hazardous in debilitated patients with depressed pharyngeal competence and inadequate cough reflexes. The incidence of this hazard can be decreased by slow drip delivery of the formula continuously from a bag or bottle rather than injecting larger volumes intermittently. Also, good positioning of the weighted tip of a small caliber, flexible tube in the duodenum or proximal jejunum can usually be accomplished by having the patient lie with his right side down for a time following initial placement of the tip of the tube in the prepyloric area. In this manner, aspiration of tube feedings can be minimized because the pylorus acts as a deterrent to regurgitation of the diet into the stomach.

Postcricoid ulceration of the larynx from the nasogastric tube is not uncommon. It may occur within 3 or 4 days and is very common with prolonged indwelling tubes. Pain in the laryngeal area is the primary symptom. These ulcers will not heal when the tube is in place and may require tube removal if pain becomes a problem.

Feeding Enterostomies

ESOPHAGOSTOMY

Occasionally, patients will be cured or will receive major palliation by an extensive head and neck procedure or radical radiation therapy that leaves the patient's deglutitory function disabled permanently. In some of these patients a tube may be inserted into the esophagus either through the pyriform sinus or through the wall of the cervical esophagus for long-term feeding as an alternative to nasogastric tubes (Fig. 5-1). Feeding esophagostomy is an alternative to jejunostomy for unobstructed patients who have had a prior subtotal gastrectomy or esophagogastrectomy. This procedure eliminates the psychological and social problems faced by a patient who would otherwise constantly have a tube protruding from his nose. While esophagostomy reduces the problem of aspiration, reflux esophagitis can still be a severe complication. Esophagostomy is probably contraindicated in the patient with previous radiation therapy to the neck area, as the radiation may complicate wound healing. This has, in some cases, resulted in carotid rupture.

GASTROSTOMY

In patients who require long-term gastrointestinal intubation for feeding, and in whom creation of a permanent esophagostomy is undesirable because of the patient's malignancy and treatment program, gastrostomy tube insertion is preferred. The gastrostomy tube has the advantage of being readily available, visible to the patient and easy to manipulate. Also, the stomach may retain its role as a reservoir for foodstuffs, and the dumping syndrome which sometimes follows diet administration into the duodenum or jejunum is minimized. Moreover, esophageal reflux is minimized because gastroesophageal sphincter function is not compromised.

Either a Janeway or Stamm gastrostomy is satisfactory (Fig. 5-2). For the patient who requires a *temporary gastrostomy,* a Stamm procedure is indicated. The operation to fashion the Stamm gastrostomy may be done through a midline upper abdominal incision. A number 30 to 36 French mushroom catheter is inserted into the middle one-third of the stomach midway be-

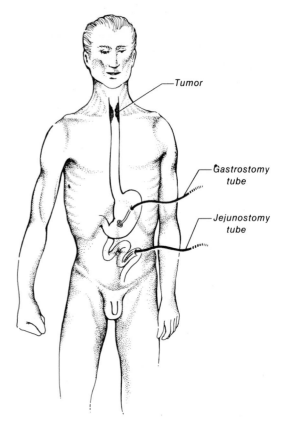

Fig. 5-2. A gastrostomy tube is readily available to the patient and its use allows the stomach to retain its role as a reservoir for foodstuffs reducing the incidence of the dumping syndrome.

tween the lesser and greater curvatures. Performed properly, this operation has minimal risk even in the malnourished patient and can be done using local or field block anesthesia.

Major surgical complications reported following gastrostomy tube insertion are bleeding from the gastrostomy site, separation of the gastric wall from the abdominal wall with subsequent peritonitis, inadvertent premature removal of the gastrotomy tube, and abdominal wound dehiscence. If the gastrostomy tube is accidently dislodged after the abdominal incisions have healed, it must be reinserted within 24 to 48 hours or the tract will constrict significantly or close, making simple reinsertion impossible. Surgical reinsertion is necessary if dislodgement of the tube occurs during the first 4 to 6 days postoperatively, because an adequate catheter tract has not yet been established by this time. The Stamm gastrostomy is a relatively easy surgical procedure, which can be performed under local, regional, or general anesthesia.

For the patient who requires a *permanent gastrostomy*, a Janeway gastrostomy should be considered. Although the operation technique is more complicated, this procedure is advantageous because it leaves a gastric mucosa-lined conduit from the stomach to the anterior abdominal wall through which a feeding tube can be inserted intermittently for infusion of the liquid diet. The tube can be removed when feeding instillation is completed. Occasionally, however, leakage of tube feedings will occur through the stoma if gastric emptying is delayed or gastric reservoir capacity is exceeded.

JEJUNOSTOMY

If insertion of a gastrostomy tube is impossible or impractical because of severe esophageal reflux or previous gastric resection, then a feeding tube can be placed in the proximal portion of the jejunum (Fig. 5-2). A number 12 to 16 French catheter is inserted into the jejunal lumen 30 cm from the ligament of Treitz. The tube exits the peritoneal cavity through an incision in the left lateral abdominal wall, and the jejunum is secured against the anterior abdominal wall at the exit site with several interrupted silk sutures.

Jejunostomy feedings may begin as soon as there is adequate wound healing and return of peristalsis (usually 3 days postoperatively). Initially, small amounts of glucose water or balanced salt solution should be introduced into the jejunostomy tube. If well tolerated, the diet can be advanced progressively from skimmed milk to a milk-base or water-base blenderized or commercially prepared diet, which may be infused continuously in amounts of up to 300 ml every 4 hours. Rapid entry into the

jejunum of hyperosmolar solutions may lead to the dumping syndrome. This potential problem can be prevented by infusing the formula initially at a slow rate and low concentration, and increasing first the rate and then the concentration. As with nasogastric tube feedings, continuous slow-drip infusion results in the best absorption with minimal bloating and diarrhea, but constant infusion over a 12 to 24 hour period may not be practical on a long-term basis. A potential problem with jejunal feeding is inadequate mixing of the diet formula with bile and pancreatic juice, resulting in poor digestion. This problem usually can be overcome with the use of pancreatic extract, medium chain triglycerides, and/or chemically defined diets containing protein hydrolysates or free amino acids that are absorbed easily in the absence of pancreatic extract or bile. Diarrhea may also be alleviated by reducing either the fat content or the carbohydrate content (especially lactose) of the formula.

The availability of commercial formulas that can be instilled through a small diameter catheter has made tube feeding feasible via a catheter inserted into the jejunum through a needle that has been tunneled through the layers of the bowel wall at laparotomy. Experience with this technique is still limited generally and is not recommended for use by a novice.

Tube Feeding Diets

When a patient with a normal gastrointestinal tract is unable to ingest adequate quantities of nutrients orally, it becomes obligatory to maintain his nutritional status with tube feedings. If a large diameter nasogastric tube has been placed for short-term nutritional support or a gastrostomy has been established, hospital prepared, blenderized diets are the most effective and economical formulas for providing adequate nutrients. A satisfactory blenderized diet in our experience is outlined in Appendix 5-2. This diet provides 2,765 kcal, 90 g protein, 145 g fat, and 275 g carbohydrate diluted with water to a volume of 3,465 ml. The ingredients of this diet should be warmed, homogenized in an electric blender, strained, and administered at body temperature. The formula should be stirred immediately before pouring it into the feeding tube in order to resuspend the solids which might have settled. Coffee and citrus juices are not integral constituents of the formula, but are given when desirable to simulate a more normal diet. Any excess formula may be refrigerated, rewarmed, and served at body temperature within 24 to 48 hours.

Many commercial liquid diets with varying nutrient substrates are also available for use in patients who require tube feeding (Table 5-8). Each commercially prepared formula has distinct advantages and disadvantages. For example, some patients are lactose intolerant because of an insufficiency of the small bowel mucosal enzyme lactase, and feeding these patients milk or commercial formulas containing lactose will result in malabsorption, bloating, and diarrhea. Milk intolerance also occurs in individuals following gastric or intestinal resection,

radiation enteritis, and other diseases that adversely affect normal intestinal function. If the patient is unable to tolerate lactose, a commercially prepared formula such as Isocal can be used. Occasionally, significant maldigestion or malabsorption of fat occurs, and a diet that is low in fat or that contains fat as medium-chain triglycerides may be useful. Medium-chain triglycerides are absorbed better than long-chain fatty acids when there are decreased amounts of conjugated bile salts or pancreatic enzymes in the upper small bowel or when damage to the endothelium of the intestinal mucosa inhibits resynthesis or transport of long-chain fatty acids. Again, knowledge of the exact nutrient sources in the commercially prepared formulas is essential for optimal nutritional treatment of patients receiving tube feedings.

A recent development has been the commercial production of nutritionally adequate, chemically defined ("elemental") diets that consist primarily of mixtures of purified L-amino acids, glucose, short or medium-chain triglycerides, and baseline

TABLE 5-8 COMPOSITION OF VARIOUS COMMERCIAL LIQUID DIETS

Composition	Compleat-B*	Isocal†	Ensure‡	Vivonex-HN§
kcal/ml	1.05	1.0	1.06	1.0
mOsm/l	350	468	460	800
N:kcal	1:169	1:131	1:155	1:127
% kcal (protein)	12.9	16	14	16.6
% kcal (carbohydrate)	49.6	48	54.5	84.1
% kcal (fat)	38.5	36	31.5	0.78
Protein source	Soy protein	Skim milk; beef	Casein; soy protein	Crystalline amino acids
Carbohydrate source	Glucose; corn syrup	Sucrose	Sucrose; corn syrup	Glucose; maltose
Fat source	MCT‖; soy oil	Corn oil; beef fat	Corn oil	Safflower oil

*Doyle Pharmaceutical Company, Minneapolis, MN 55416.
†Mead Johnson Laboratories, Evansville, IN 47721.
‡Ross Laboratories, Columbus, OH 43216.
§Eaton Laboratories, Norwich, NY 13815.
‖MCT, medium chain triglycerides.

requirements of electrolytes, trace minerals, and water and fat soluble vitamins exclusive of vitamin K (Table 5-8).[8] Almost complete absorption of these diets takes place in the proximal jejunum, and they may be used when digestion is impaired due to malabsorption or restricted absorptive surface area. They should initially be administered at 0.25 to 0.5 the recommended final osmolar concentration until the small bowel adapts to the high osmolarity and diarrhea ceases. When mixed at "full-strength," these formulas provide approximately 1 kcal/ml and have an osmolarity between 600 to 1200 mOsm. Tube feedings should begin with a 0.5 strength solution infused at 25 to 50 ml/hr. Adaptation may be slow, particularly if there has been a long period of malnutrition and intestinal disuse. Accordingly, changes in delivery rate and formula concentration must be very gradual. Once the patient has progressed from 50 to 100 ml/hr of 0.5 strength solution, a 0.75 or full strength solution is then substituted. Ideally, the diet should be infused at a constant rate. If nursing supervision is minimal and the gravity infusion method is used, it may be prudent to discontinue the feedings at night. Constant infusion pumps, however, may allow a safe infusion of these elemental diets around the clock.[10] In contrast to blenderized diets, additional free water is not needed with elemental diets unless evaporative or other dynamic losses are excessive, or if prerenal azotemia develops. The diet may be supplemented with additional electrolytes in patients with excessive electrolyte losses. Initially, patients may complain of abdominal cramps, distention, nausea, or mild watery diarrhea. These problems can be managed by slowing the rate of infusion or reducing the concentration of the elemental diet. Hyperosmotic diarrhea rapidly leads to prerenal azotemia, characterized by a disproportionately elevated blood urea nitrogen (BUN) level, a normal to slightly elevated serum creatinine value, hypernatremia, and hyperosmolarity. The development of prerenal azotemia should be aggressively managed by discontinuing the

elemental diet and administering parenteral fluids to replace volume and electrolyte losses.

During administration of commercial liquid diets, the urine should be checked routinely for glycosuria in order to insure that the administered glucose is being metabolized completely and is not being lost in the urine. Similarly, blood sugar, blood urea nitrogen, and serum electrolytes should be monitored two to three times weekly until the desired daily dietary ration is being tolerated. If significant glycosuria occurs and sufficient water and electrolytes are not provided exogenously, hypertonic dehydration and hyperosmolar coma can result. Hypernatremia, hyperchloremia, azotemia, and lethargy may result without glycosuria if adequate water replacement is not provided with the tube feedings. Additional metabolic monitoring of the patient should include daily body weights and strict intake and output measurements.

Method of Feeding

Selection of a method of feeding the patient with cancer of the head and neck is made when knowledge of the patient's nutritional status and type of oncologic therapy have been determined. Another factor which must be taken into consideration is the amount of calories and protein the patient ingests by the oral route during the first 48 hours in the hospital. This quantitative determination of oral caloric and protein intake can be calculated by the dietitian member of the nutritional therapy team. Patients in a *good* nutritional status category receiving either high or low magnitude therapy may be nourished orally or by tube at maintenance (35 kcal/kg) levels unless specific anatomic or physiological contraindications exist to these methods of feeding. If the oral route is inadequate, a small feeding tube should be positioned in the distal esophagus and the appropriate tube feeding instilled in amounts necessary to provide the calculated calorie and protein requirements. Calorie and protein intake measurements must be made on a daily basis to insure compliance with the assigned nutritional therapy. Patients placed in the *fair* nutritional status category undergoing low magnitude therapy can be treated in a fashion similar to the previous patient group. Those patients in the *fair* nutritional category who undergo high magnitude therapy must be fed at the higher (anabolic—45 kcal/kg) nutritional level. This subgroup of patients may require intravenous hyperalimentation. Patients placed in the *poor* nutritional category undergoing either high or low magnitude therapy require anabolic (45 kcal/kg) levels of nutrition. While the method of feeding may vary according to the patient's clinical situation, it is imperative that malnourished patients receive maximal nutritional support. Occasionally, both intravenous and enteral feeding may be utilized simultaneously to provide protein and calorie requirements.

Once nutritional and oncologic therapy are underway, daily and weekly measurements of each patient's progress should be made and recorded (Tables 5-9 and 5-10). Every 2 weeks, the patient's entire nutritional status score should be recalculated and feeding adjustments made accordingly (Table 5-11). All patients must be evaluated frequently for complications related to the method of feeding, response to and complications of oncologic therapy, and change in nutritional status.

INTRAVENOUS HYPERALIMENTATION

There is a subgroup of patients whose gastrointestinal tract may be unavailable for nutrient administration, or in whom nutritional replenishment via the gut may not be sufficiently rapid to achieve adequate nutritional restoration before the patient must undergo oncologic therapy. Under these circumstances, the use of intravenous hyperalimentation (IVH) is indicated. Intravenous hyperalimentation solutions can be formulated by mixing 350 ml of 50 percent

TABLE 5-9 DAILY MEASUREMENTS OF PATIENT'S PROGRESS

1. Body weight
2. Volume intake
3. Volume output
4. Protein intake
5. Caloric intake
6. Ambulatory ability

TABLE 5-10 WEEKLY MEASUREMENTS OF PATIENT'S PROGRESS

1. Body weight
2. Arm muscle circumference (cm)
3. Triceps skinfold thickness (mm)
4. Serum albumin (gm%), transferrin (mg%), and cholesterol (mg%); hemoglobin (gm%)
5. Serum electrolytes, creatinine, glucose, magnesium, phosphorus and calcium; BUN
6. Creatinine/height index
7. Patient acceptance of method of feeding
8. Approximate calorie (kcal) and protein (g) intake

dextrose with 750 ml of 5 percent protein hydrolysate and 5 percent dextrose, or by mixing 500 ml of 50 percent dextrose with 500 ml of an 8.5 to 10 percent crystalline amino acid solution.[3, 7] Each unit of IVH solution so prepared contains approximately 1,000 nonprotein calories. Electrolytes and vitamins are added to these base solutions in sufficient quantities to correct existing deficits and to satisfy maintenance requirements (Table 5-12). The usual electrolyte additives to solutions derived from amino acids are approximately 40 to 50 mEq of sodium chloride, 20 to 40 mEq of potassium acetate, 10 to 15 mEq of magnesium sulfate, and 15 to 20 mEq of potassium acid phosphate per liter. Amino acids in commercially available amino acid products may be in solution as the chloride, hydrochloride, or acetate salts. These preparations are acidic, and the in-

TABLE 5-11 CALCULATION OF PATIENT'S NUTRITIONAL STATUS SCORE

Name: Date:

Sex: Age:

Type of Malignancy: *Date Begun:*   *Date Ended:*
                                     Chemotherapy   Chemotherapy
                                     Surgery   Surgery
                                     Radiotherapy   Radiotherapy

History:

Normal wt (kg)
Current wt (kg)
Able to eat 3 meals/day (yes/no)
Swallows without difficulty (yes/no)
Clothing size remains the same (yes/no)

Physical Examination: *Total Score:*

Height (cm)
Ideal wt (kg) Appendix 5-1
Wt as % of ideal
Triceps skin-fold (mm)
Arm circumference (cm)
Arm muscle circumference (cm)
Ambulatory ability (good, fair, poor)

Laboratory Values: *Total Score:*

Hemoglobin (gm%)
Serum albumin (gm%)
Serum iron (mg%)
Serum transferrin (mg%)
Ideal urinary creatinine (mg)
Actual urinary creatinine (mg)
Creatinine/height index (% of ideal)
Cell-mediated immunity (good, fair, poor)

Grand Total Score:

Nutritional Status Category:

fusion of solutions which contain large amounts of sodium and/or potassium as the chloride salt may result in hyperchloremic metabolic acidosis. Consequently, sodium and potassium should be added as the acetate, lactate, bicarbonate, acid phosphate, or chloride salt as indicated by the patient's serum electrolyte concentration and acid-base status. Knowledge of the electrolyte and acid-base content of the base amino acid solution being used is required prior to any further additions of electrolytes thought necessary to maintain normal electrolyte and acid-base balance. Potassium, phosphorus, and/or magnesium rations, for example, are often reduced or omitted in patients with compromised renal function. Calcium and phosphate must be added to commer-

TABLE 5-12 USUAL COMPOSITION OF AMINO ACID SUBSTRATE SOLUTION

Base solution
   500 ml 50% dextrose plus 500 ml 8.5% crystalline amino acids

Additives
   40–50 mEq sodium chloride
   20–30 mEq potassium acetate
   10–15 mEq potassium acid phosphate
   15 mEq magnesium sulfate
   5 ml multivitamins* (M.V.I.)†
   1 g calcium fluconate*

*Added to only one unit of solution daily.
†M.V.I.—USV Pharmaceutical Corp. Tuckahoe, N.Y.

cially prepared amino acid solutions in order to maintain normal calcium and phosphorus metabolism. Hypomagnesemia and hypophosphatemia will often occur within 3 to 14 days of initiating IVH if sufficient quantities of these elements are not added. The severely malnourished patient treated with IVH has the greatest risk of developing serum deficiencies of phosphorus, magnesium, and potassium. One ampule of a mixture containing both fat and water soluble vitamins (Multi-Vitamin Infusion, [USV Pharmaceuticals]) should be added to 1 liter of IVH solution daily, and vitamin K, folic acid, and vitamin B_{12} must be administered regularly. Currently, 15 mg vitamin K and 15 mg folic acid are administered intramuscularly once a week. Every 3 weeks, 1 mg vitamin B_{12} is given intramuscularly. Serum albumin concentration should be maintained at a level greater than 3.4 g percent by daily administration of 12.5 to 25 g of albumin, which can be added directly to the IVH solution. After serum albumin concentration has been restored to normal, albumin infusion is discontinued.

Since several electrolyte mixtures must be added to the IVH solutions in the pharmacy, aseptic mixing under a laminar flow, filter air hood is essential for optimum safety. The additives should be placed in the IVH solutions immediately prior to infusion so that current electrolyte requirements are satisfied. The solutions should be refrigerated immediately after preparation and administered within the next 24 hours.

Technique

Intravenous hyperalimentation solutions are hyperosmolar (1,800 to 2,400 mOsm) and must be infused through a large diameter, high-flow blood vessel (preferably the superior vena cava) to prevent thrombophlebitis. An indwelling polyvinyl, Silastic or Teflon catheter directed into the superior vena cava via the percutaneous catheterization of a subclavian vein or an internal or external jugular vein is recommended. An internal or external jugular vein is acceptable for central venous catheterization, but the catheter dressings are cumbersome, uncomfortable, and insecure. Moreover a catheter introduced in these locations might interfere with the treatment plan for a patient with a head and neck malignancy. The subclavian vein is preferred for catheterization because of the ease in maintaining a sterile, occlusive dressing on the anterior chest wall. Either subclavian vein may be used safely unless a specific contraindication exists, such as the presence of ipsilateral giant emphysematous bullae, previous radical neck dissection, clavicular fracture, or radiation therapy through a lower neck portal.

The equipment for central venous catheterization should be readily available to reduce delay and enhance efficiency. Prior to attempting percutaneous subclavian venous catheterization, the patient should be placed in the Trendelenburg position. Hydrostatic dilation of the subclavian vein will occur, providing a larger target for the needle and increasing central venous pressure so that the risk of air embolization during the procedure is minimized. A rolled sheet is placed longitudinally under the thoracic vertebrae and between the scapulae. With the patient's shoulders depressed and extended over the roll, the subclavian vein becomes more accessible.

The skin over the clavicle, shoulder, neck, and upper chest is shaved widely and cleansed with an organic solvent to remove skin oil. The same area is then prepared with povidone-iodine solution and is draped with sterile towels. Local anesthetic is infiltrated into the skin, subcutaneous tissues, and periosteum at the inferior border of the midpoint of the clavicle. A two-inch long, 14-gauge needle attached to a 5 ml syringe is inserted through the skin wheal and advanced beneath the inferior margin of the clavicle in a horizontal (coronal) plane (Fig. 5-3). The needle tip is aimed for the anterior margin of the trachea at the level of the suprasternal notch. As the needle is advanced beneath the clavicle, slight negative pressure applied through the syringe will indicate the accuracy of the venipuncture by a return of blood. The needle should be advanced a few millimeters beyond the point at which blood first appears in the syringe to insure the placement of the entire beveled tip inside the lumen of the vein. At this point, the needle is rotated so that the bevel is aimed caudally. The patient is asked to perform a Valsalva maneuver to minimize the risk of air embolism. The syringe is then removed carefully while the needle is held firmly in place with a hemostat. An 8-inch long, 16-gauge radiopaque catheter is introduced through the needle and threaded its entire length into the vein (Fig. 5-4). If any difficulty is encountered during advancement of the catheter through the needle, the needle and catheter must be withdrawn carefully as a unit, and another attempt at venipuncture may be made. The catheter must never be withdrawn through the needle after the tip has passed beyond the end of the needle because transection and embolization of the catheter can result from this maneuver.

When the catheter has been advanced its full length, it is attached to a solution of

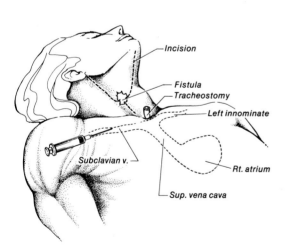

Fig. 5-3. A two-inch long, 14-gauge needle is inserted beneath the inferior margin of the middle of the clavicle and aimed for the anterior aspect of the trachea. A return of blood in the syringe indicates accurate subclavian venipuncture.

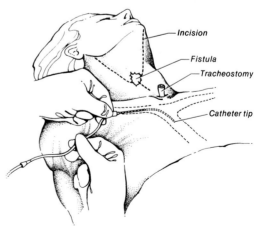

Fig. 5-4. With the bevel of the needle directed caudally in the direction of venous flow, the 16-gauge catheter is advanced into the superior vena cava.

isotonic saline or dextrose by sterile IV administration tubing. The needle and catheter are then withdrawn so that at least 1 cm of the catheter is visible, and the catheter is sutured in place just lateral to the skin puncture site (Fig. 5-5). Accurate position within the central venous system can be insured by lowering the solution bottle below the level of the patient and observing a prompt backflow of blood into the delivery tubing. A broad-spectrum antimicrobial ointment such as povidone-iodine is applied over the puncture site and a sterile, occlusive gauze dressing is fixed to the skin with tincture of benzoin and adhesive tape. The IV administration tubing is looped over the top of the dressing and secured again with adhesive tape to guard against accidental catheter dislodgement. A sterile plastic sheet is placed over the catheter dressing to further minimize the risk of contamination from stomal secretions in patients with draining pharyngocutaneous and/or tracheostomy stomata (Fig. 5-6). The catheter entry site is placed outside any designated radiation fields in those individuals who are to receive radiation therapy through lower neck portals. No tape is applied to skin of the neck or upper thorax that is included within a radiation portal in order to prevent skin bullae formation.

Conscientious adherence to this technique should ensure successful central ve-

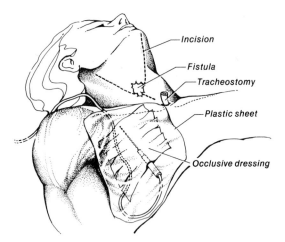

Fig. 5-6. An occlusive sterile dressing protects the catheterization site and secures the infusion tubing. A sterile plastic sheet is placed over the catheter dressing to further reduce the risk of contamination from stomal secretions. (Modified from Dudrick, S. J., and Copeland, E. M. 1974. Nutritional concepts in head and neck cancer. In Anderson Hospital, Ed.: Neoplasia of the Head and Neck. Copyright © by Year Book Medical Publishers Inc., Chicago, 325. Used by permission.)

nous catheterization. However, if air is aspirated into the syringe during needle advancement, entry of the needle tip into lung parenchyma is suggested, and the needle should be withdrawn. If the needle-syringe connection is air-tight and is not the source of the air leak, the patient should be observed for signs of respiratory embarrassment, and a portable chest roentgenogram should be obtained immediately. If, during insertion, bright red blood fills the syringe and moves the plunger of the syringe outward, the needle has probably entered the subclavian artery; the procedure should be terminated, and pressure should be applied over the artery for a minimum of 5 minutes.

After the subclavian venous catheter has been properly inserted and secured and before IVH is begun, a chest roentgenogram is obtained to verify the position of the catheter tip within the midportion of the superior vena cava. If the catheter has been directed into the internal or external jugular vein, scapular veins or internal mam-

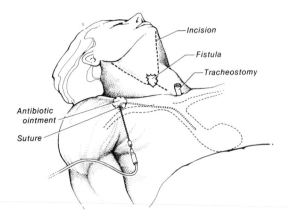

Fig. 5-5. The catheter is sutured to the skin lateral to the puncture site, and antimicrobial ointment is applied to maintain asepsis.

mary vein, it should be removed and replaced; otherwise, thrombophlebitis will usually occur promptly.

Catheter Care

Three times a week a nurse removes the catheter dressing and reprepares the skin around the catheter with an organic solvent and an antiseptic solution before reapplying the antimicrobial ointment and sterile dressing. The IVH delivery tubing is changed at this time. The catheter and delivery system should not be used for administration of blood or blood by-products, central venous pressure monitoring, bolus drug administration, or withdrawal of blood samples. A peripheral venous site is used for any simultaneously administered intravenous fluids other than IVH. Occasionally, simultaneous administration of other fluids through the IVH delivery tubing may, however, be necessary because malnourished patients often have very fragile peripheral veins, making peripheral infusion of the solutions impossible or impractical.

The need for rigorous aseptic management of the subclavian vein catheter is greatest in patients undergoing treatment for head and neck cancer because of the possibility of contamination from secretions from pharyngocutaneous fistulas and tracheostomy stomas. At the termination of IVH, each catheter is removed and immediately cultured for aerobic and anaerobic bacteria and fungi. If the patient is febrile at the time of catheter removal, a blood culture is taken through the catheter and simultaneously from a peripheral vein. Each febrile episode should be considered catheter-related, until proven otherwise, and if another source of fever cannot be identified, then the catheter should be incriminated empirically and removed. In order to prevent catheter contamination, dressings are changed as frequently as necessary, sometimes twice daily. If the catheter has been removed because of a febrile episode, a new catheter for administration of IVH should not be reinserted until 24 to 48 hours have elapsed after return of temperature to normal. Fever, per se, is not an absolute indication for discontinuing IVH. If an obvious source of infection other than the catheter is identified, it should be treated appropriately, and the catheter should be left in place. If, however, the elevated temperature does not respond to reasonable treatment, then the catheter should be removed. A positive blood culture is an absolute indication for removal of a subclavian venous catheter. In our experience, routine catheter changes have not been necessary, and the longest time that a single catheter has remained in place is 146 days.

Administration and Metabolic Monitoring

Intravenous hyperalimentation solutions should be delivered at a constant rate throughout each 24 hour period in order to promote optimum assimilation of the administered amino acids, dextrose, minerals, and vitamins. Although 2,000 ml of IVH can be given to many patients during the first day of nutritional repletion, these large dextrose dosages may result in hyperglycemia and excessive glycosuria in some patients, leading to hypertonic dehydration and coma. Once the patient is capable of metabolizing the amino acids and dextrose in 1,000 ml of IVH during a 24 hour period, the flow rate may be increased to 1,000 ml every 12 hours. Pancreatic insulin output will usually increase in response to the increased rate of dextrose infusion. Within the first 3 to 5 days of nutritional rehabilitation, the average adult will tolerate 3,000 ml of IVH daily. Those cancer patients who are extremely malnourished (nutritional category—poor) may not tolerate fluid volumes in excess of 2,000 ml per day, and until anabolism and weight gain are clearly established no more than 2,000 ml should be administered to these patients. Fractional urine sugar concentration should be determined every 6 hours. Although glycosuria may be noted when the infusion is begun initially, it will usually disappear within 24 hours. Manual regulation of the pediatric microdrip system usually is satisfactory for maintenance of a reasonably constant infusion rate, but infusion pumps may be more cost effective because they do not require flow readjustment by nursing personnel as often as a gravity drip system. A widely fluctuating rate of delivery of IVH will be signaled by glycosuria, and a constant flow rate should be reestablished. In patients with continuously elevated blood sugar concentrations resulting in excessive glycosuria, either exogenous insulin must be given, or the dextrose delivery rate must be reduced. Our recommendation is that additional insulin be added directly to the IVH solutions rather than given subcutaneously. While it is well known that crystalline insulin adheres to the bottle and administration tubing, the amount of insulin lost in this manner is insignificant. If the insulin is in the IVH bottle and the infusion stops, then insulin administration also stops. If insulin has been administered subcutaneously and infusion stops, marked hypoglycemia may result. Initial insulin dosages should be approximately 5 to 10 units per 1,000 ml and increased gradually until blood sugar levels return to 120 to 150 mg percent. Intravenous hyperalimentation administration should be tapered over a 24 to 48 hour period prior to completely discontinuing it. If these hypertonic solutions are stopped suddenly, rebound "insulin hypoglycemic shock" may occur. If rapid tapering is necessary, this can be accomplished over a 4 to 6 hour period, and a 10 percent glucose infusion is given through a peripheral vein after IVH is stopped. Prior to the administration of a general anesthetic, IVH should be tapered and discontinued. If the IVH were inadvertently stopped during anesthesia, hypoglycemia might occur, go unrecognized, and lead to potentially lethal complications or permanent brain damage.

Active rehabilitation should be instituted during nutritional therapy in order for muscle mass to be replenished and strength returned. Accumulation of lean body mass should not exceed more than 0.5 pound per day after the initial 48 to 72 hours of rehydration, during which time weight may increase 3 to 5 pounds. Following this period of rehydration, fluid retention must be assumed to have occurred if daily weight gain exceeds 1 pound per day. In this event, either a diuretic should be administered to the patient or the delivery rate of IVH should be reduced. Serum electrolyte, blood urea nitrogen, and blood sugar concentrations are determined every Monday, Wednesday, and Friday. Serum albumin, magnesium, calcium, phosphorus, creatinine, and liver function tests are determined weekly each Monday. A coagulation profile and complete blood count are obtained once weekly. Each day the patient's temperature, weight gain, adequacy of glucose metabolism, fluid and electrolyte intake, fluid output, and physical findings are reviewed. The results of these observations and determinations allow the physician to predict the proper composition and quantity of IVH for each patient for the next 24 hour period.

Clinical Experience in Head and Neck Cancer

Recently, the records of 70 consecutive malnourished patients with head and neck malignancies who received IVH were reviewed.[6] Intravenous hyperalimentation was indicated in order to prepare, maintain, and/or rehabilitate these patients nutritionally and metabolically so that chemotherapy, surgery, or radiation therapy could be completed and tolerated with maximum efficacy and safety (Table 5-13).

Fifty-three patients received IVH perioperatively (Table 5-14). Nineteen patients underwent laryngopharyngectomy, 16 patients underwent radical neck dissection, and 10 patients had reconstruction with thoracoacromial flaps. The patients required IVH for an average period of 36.6 days, and in the 15 patients who received IVH both pre- and postoperatively, average weight gain was 11.3 pounds. Intravenous hyperalimentation was used preoperatively for an average period of 16.1 days to insure adequate nutritional rehabilitation before

TABLE 5-13 REVIEW OF
HYPERALIMENTATION IN 70 PATIENTS
WITH HEAD AND NECK CANCER

Indications for IVH	Number of Patients
Perioperative support	29
Chemotherapy	16
Convalescent support	10
Radiation therapy	9
Enterocutaneous fistulas	6

TABLE 5-14 TYPES OF OPERATIONS
PERFORMED ON 53 PATIENTS
RECEIVING IVH PERIOPERATIVE
SUPPORT

Operation	Number of Patients
Laryngopharyngectomy	19
Radical neck dissection	16
Thoracoacromial flap	10 (1 bilateral)
Mandibulectomy	3
Glossectomy	3
Forehead flap	2

extensive surgical procedures. These patients required IVH postoperatively for an average period of 20.3 days until adequate nutrition could be maintained enterally. Fourteen patients received IVH only postoperatively for an average period of 36.8 days. The usual indications for IVH in these patients were complications of malnutrition, such as pneumonia*, poor wound healing, or malabsorption of enterally administered nutrients. We believe that many such com-

*Malnutrition leads to muscle weakness, including the intercostal and diaphragmatic muscles which in turn depress the cough reflex and ability to cough allowing for retained secretions and possibly pneumonia. Depressed immune function secondary to malnutrition also increases the chances for pneumonia.

plications could be avoided if proper attention were paid to preoperative nutritional repletion. As a rule, it is usually much easier to promote return of muscle strength, weight gain, significant rise in serum albumin concentration, and improvement of immune function by preoperative nutritional repletion rather than by waiting until malnutrition has become a severe problem postoperatively before electing to replenish the patient nutritionally. Nevertheless, in those patients in this series in whom IVH was used only postoperatively, weight gain was achieved, pneumonia and wound infection resolved, healthy granulation tissue appeared, and skin grafts and flaps could be used to cover denuded surfaces and to close fistula openings.

Sixteen patients received IVH as nutritional support in order to receive intensive chemotherapy with a variety of drugs used either singularly or in combination (Adriamycin, bleomycin, Cytoxan, methotrexate, 5-fluorouracil, vincristine, and vinblastine). These patients were not previously considered candidates for adequate chemotherapy because of the fear of complications that might result secondary to malnutrition. By utilizing IVH, each patient tolerated chemotherapy, and nausea, vomiting, diarrhea, and stomatitis were minimized. The average weight gain during chemotherapy and IVH was 9.8 pounds over an average period of 27 days. A 50 percent or greater reduction in tumor volume was obtained in 30 percent of the patients. Responding patients survived an average period of 6 months compared with 1 month for those patients who did not respond to chemotherapy.

In two patients, radiation therapy initially was contraindicated because of severe malnutrition. IVH was begun 7 to 10 days prior to beginning radiation therapy and was continued throughout the irradiation treatment period. Seven other patients developed severe stomatitis or pharyngitis while receiving radiation therapy, and anorexia, weight loss, and muscle weakness ensued. Because radiation therapy would have been stopped before a therapeutic or palliative dose was delivered, these patients were admitted to the hospital, rehydrated, and begun on IVH. In all but one patient, the planned course of radiation therapy was continued and completed. Intravenous hyperalimentation was administered for an average period of 34.8 days, average weight gain was 7.4 pounds, and the average radiation dose delivered during IVH was 3,250 rads. Eight of these nine patients had lesions that could be evaluated for therapeutic response, and a greater than 50 percent tumor regression occurred in five patients. Each patient gained in strength and experienced improvement in the symptoms of stomatitis and pharyngitis during radiation therapy.

Ten patients became severely malnourished after leaving the hospital following completion of their oncologic therapy. Each of these patients was readmitted to the hospital for nutritional supportive care. Their average weight gain was 8.7 pounds during an average period of 25.1 days of IVH. Nine of these patients were nutritionally rehabilitated and discharged from the hospital. Two of these nine patients required gastrostomy feeding tube insertion for long-term ambulatory nutritional maintenance, four patients were discharged on nasogastric tube feeding regimens, and three patients were discharged ingesting adequate quantities of food orally. One patient, who had been treated with radiation therapy to the tonsillar area 4 months previously, died of pneumonia while receiving IVH.

Rehabilitation after radiation therapy is important to strengthen the muscles of mastication and to prevent temporomandibular joint fibrosis. If the latter ensues, eating may become increasingly difficult and painful as jaw function becomes progressively more limited. This situation was encountered in five patients who received IVH for nutritional support while rehabilitation of jaw function was attempted.

Three patients had pharyngeal incompetence after either a partial glossectomy, posterior pharyngeal wall resection, or Commando procedure. Enough of the muscles of mastication remained so that pharyngeal incompetence was thought to be sec-

ondary to muscle weakness and reversible muscle injury. Weight gain of between 8 and 26 pounds was achieved in these patients, and with return of general body muscle strength and tone, swallowing function returned after 18 to 48 days of IVH.

Pharyngocutaneous fistula following radical head and neck surgery developed in six patients. Two of these fistulas closed spontaneously after 17 and 20 days of IVH. The remaining four fistulas were closed surgically after 12 to 47 days of IVH, and these patients gained an average of 15 pounds of weight during this time interval. Fistula management was easier after beginning IVH because mucosal and salivary secretions diminished when the nasogastric feeding tubes were removed.

Sepsis is the most frequent complication of the technique of intravenous hyperalimentation, particularly in the head and neck cancer group because of easy catheter contamination from nearby pharyngostomy and tracheostomy stomal secretions. Also, moist desquamation and superficial infection of the skin within irradiated fields increases the chance of subclavian vein catheter contamination. Eighteen percent of all catheters used in patients in the perioperative or convalescent support groups were contaminated upon removal. Four of these patients (10.3 percent) had simultaneous positive blood and catheter cultures associated with sepsis. In two patients, a subsequent source of infection that was responsible for the positive blood culture was identified, but in the remaining two patients, the catheter was incriminated as the source of sepsis. No patients receiving IVH as nutritional support during chemotherapy had organisms cultured from their catheters, even though these patients were often severely myelosuppressed. Three of nine patients in the radiation therapy group had pathogenic organisms cultured from their catheters; no patient had a positive blood culture and only one patient had a febrile episode. No complications or deaths secondary to catheter-related sepsis have occurred to date among these patients, but a constant vigil against catheter contamination must be maintained. Metabolic complications were few; one patient developed symptomatic hypophosphatemia that was manifested by psychotic behavior. His symptoms resolved with the infusion of an appropriate dosage of calcium and phosphate. Subclavian vein thrombosis occurred in one patient and was recognized by swelling of the arm ipsilateral to the subclavian vein catheter. The catheter was removed, edema resolved within 7 days, and heparin therapy was not necessary.

CANCER, NUTRITION, AND IMMUNITY

In the past 3 years, more than 1,000 patients have received IVH as adjunctive nutritional therapy for both benign and malignant diseases at the Hermann Hospital and the M.D. Anderson Hospital and Tumor Institute. Recently, the records of 406 consecutive cancer patients from the M.D. Anderson Hospital were reviewed.[3] Only 10 percent of patients in this series had head and neck malignancies; consequently, the head and neck cancer patient population made up only a small part of those patients who were candidates for IVH in a categorical cancer institution. Treatment categories were as follows: chemotherapy, 43 percent; general surgery, 24 percent; head and neck surgery, 10 percent; radiation therapy, 10 percent; fistulas, 6 percent; and supportive care, 7 percent. All of the patients in this series were adults, had a reasonable chance of responding to adequate oncologic therapy, and either fulfilled the criteria for nutritional depletion or were nutritionally healthy patients whose treatment plan would require multiple courses of chemotherapy, possibly combined with surgery or radiation therapy.

Two hundred and sixty courses of chemotherapy were given in conjunction with IVH to 175 patients. Hyperalimentation was used for an average period of 22.8 days; average weight gain was 5.6 pounds; tumor response rate was 27.8 percent, responding patients survived an average of

8.2 months, and nonresponding patients survived only 1.9 months. Catheter-related sepsis occurred in only 1.7 percent of patients, although 51.5 percent of patients had leukocyte depressions below 2,500 cells mm^3 that lasted for an average of 7.7 days. A positive correlation between nutritional status and response to chemotherapy was identified.

Thirty-five patients with carcinoma of the lung (excluding oat cell) who received the same treatment protocol (bleomycin, Cytoxan, 5-fluorouracil, methotrexate, and vincristine) were reviewed. Our nutritional therapy team was asked to evaluate and replenish 15 of these patients nutritionally prior to and during chemotherapy. Each patient had lost more than 15 percent of his body weight prior to IVH and chemotherapy. Seven patients responded to chemotherapy and experienced an average weight gain of 8 percent while receiving IVH. The nonresponding patients increased their weight an average of only 2 percent during IVH. The remaining 20 patients in this series were not treated by the nutritional therapy team. Twelve of these patients had lost more than 6 percent of their usual body weight and did not respond to chemotherapy. The other eight patients had lost less than 6 percent of their usual body weight, and six of these patients did respond to chemotherapy, whereas no nutritionally depleted patients responded. When nutritionally depleted patients were repleted with IVH, 47 percent responded to the chemotherapy. These results imply that responses are achieved in patients who are adequately nourished at the outset of chemotherapy or who are nutritionally replenished with IVH during chemotherapy.

Of the 100 general surgery patients, 68 percent underwent major ablative, curative resections, and 32 percent of the patients had major surgical procedures for palliation. The operative mortality for this entire group was only 4 percent. Thirty-nine patients required IVH in order to complete a planned course of radiation therapy, and 28 patients needed nutritional rehabilitation following an extensive course of radiation therapy or chemotherapy. Experience with the management of enteric fistulas in cancer patients was rewarding. Each patient was extremely cachectic at the outset of treatment; nevertheless, 44 percent of fistulas closed spontaneously, and 28 percent were successfully closed surgically. Those patients who achieved fistula closure were able to lead productive lives for at least a short period of time.

Complications from IVH in these 406 patients were few. Pathogenic organisms were grown from 19 of 428 consecutively cultured catheters. Simultaneous positive blood and catheter cultures were obtained in only ten patients (2.3 percent); in three of these ten patients, a primary source of septicemia other than the catheter was identified, and in the remaining seven patients (1.7 percent) body temperature returned to normal within 48 hours after catheter removal.

Clinical, epidemiologic, and laboratory studies have demonstrated that protein-calorie malnutrition results in a decrease in immune competence, especially established cell-mediated immunity.[2, 5, 6, 11, 19] Previously, indirect correlation between an increase in volume of malignant tissue and a decrease in immunity was proposed. Since a correlation between both intensity and duration of oncologic therapy and malnutrition exists, possibly a portion of the immune incompetence identified in cancer patients is a reflection of malnutrition rather than of increasing tumor volume. In an attempt to define the role of nutritional status in maintaining immune reactivity during oncologic therapy, 65 patients with a variety of malignant diseases were chosen for study based on their candidacy for intravenous hyperalimentation.[5] Response to chemotherapy was defined as a 50 percent or greater reduction in measurable tumor volume lasting for 30 days. Patients received an average daily dose of 2,500 ml of IVH for an average of 21.7 days.

On initial evaluation, 46 patients had negative reactions to skin tests; 29 (63 percent) converted skin tests to positive during an average period of 13.6 days of IVH.

Nineteen patients initially had positive skin test reactions; 14 (73.7 percent) remained positive during treatment with IVH.

In the radiation therapy patients, IVH was administered for an average of 23.8 days. The average weight gain was 6.2 pounds. Average serum albumin concentration before IVH was 2.9 g percent and rose significantly to 3.4 g percent at the termination of IVH. Even though nutritional repletion was considered adequate in this group of patients, only two of eight patients converted their skin test reactivity from negative to positive. One of these two patients was receiving radiation therapy to the head and neck region and the other was receiving radiation therapy to the mediastinum as treatment for carcinoma of the midthoracic esophagus. Six patients remained negative throughout radiation therapy, and two patients converted skin tests from positive to negative. As a rule, patients who were receiving radiation therapy to the thymus or a large segment of bone marrow or blood, for example the mediastinum or pelvis, failed to convert skin tests to positive during IVH or converted skin tests from positive to negative. It is possible that radiation therapy to these areas reduced the number or effectiveness of circulating T-lymphocytes that are responsible for establishing delayed hypersensitivity reactions.[10] Although skin test reactivity did not convert to positive in these patients, there were no complications secondary to radiation therapy, and nutritional rehabilitation was considered adequate in all patients.

In the supportive care group of patients, five patients converted skin tests from negative to positive during an average of 15.5 days of IVH. Three of 11 patients had skin tests remain positive throughout treatment with IVH. Subsequent treatment with either chemotherapy or radiation therapy in patients with positive skin test reactions was considered to have reverted to negative if at least one skin test had been positive initially, and all tests reverted to negative during treatment. Patients received an average of 2,500 kcal per day for an average time of 21.7 days.

Twenty-one patients in the chemotherapy group were initially skin test negative, and 16 of these patients (76 percent) converted to skin test positive after an average of 11.6 ± 4.8 days of IVH. Average serum albumin concentration in these patients was 3.2 ± 0.4 g percent at the initiation of IVH and rose to 3.5 ± 0.3 g percent by the time skin tests converted to positive. Average weight gained by the positive converters was 6.8 ± 3.2 pounds. The average weight gained in the nonconverting patients was 7.9 ± 2.3 pounds. Nonconverters had an average serum albumin concentration of 3.2 ± 0.4 g percent at the outset of IVH, which remained unchanged throughout intravenous nutritional therapy. Forty percent (6/15) of patients whose tumor could be evaluated and who converted skin tests to positive had a tumor response to chemotherapy, whereas 60 percent (3/5) of evaluable patients who retained positive skin test reactivity responded to chemotherapy. *No* patient responded to chemotherapy who did not convert to positive or maintain positive skin tests during IVH. All patients received IVH for 2 to 7 days prior to initiating chemotherapy, and were maintained on IVH throughout the course of chemotherapy until nutritional repletion was adequate and adequate oral intake was demonstrated by daily calorie counts.

In the surgery group, nine patients maintained positive skin test reactivity or converted skin tests to positive preoperatively, and each had an uncomplicated postoperative recovery. Of the five patients whose skin tests remained negative throughout IVH or converted to negative during IVH, three died postoperatively and two had prolonged ileus. Often, the patients who were negative reactors initially had become malnourished prior to treatment with IVH because of a decrease in food intake as a result of prior oncologic therapy or because the anatomic location of the cancer partially obstructed the gastrointestinal tract. Therefore, immune incompetence in many patients with solid tumors might often be a reflection of the degree of associated malnutrition and not necessarily the result of a circulating factor released by the cancer or a direct effect of the oncologic drugs on the immune system. When possible, restoring immune competence by nutritional repletion is desirable in the cancer patient, since—in this series of patients—positive reactors tolerated oncologic treatment better and had a better tumor response to chemotherapy.

CONCLUSIONS

Cancer cachexia should no longer be a contraindication to adequate oncologic treatment. Malnutrition is harmful to cancer patients because a cachectic patient has a narrower safe therapeutic margin for most surgery, chemotherapy, and radiation therapy. The cancericidal doses of these agents may be much closer to the lethal dose for normal tissues in the malnourished patient than in the well-nourished one. With optimal nutritional rehabilitation and maintenance, minimal treatment morbidity will result and patients who might have been denied possible curative surgical or radiation therapy because of the threat of major complications secondary to malnutrition may safely receive proper oncologic therapy. Nutritional assessment is necessary prior to initiation of oncologic treatment, and the results of such assessment must be reevaluated frequently so that nutritional status remains adequate during each phase of oncologic management. Ideally, nutritional therapy should be delivered by the enteral route unless this method becomes impossible due to adverse symptoms related to the head and neck cancer or to the oncologic treatment modality. Those patients requiring intravenous hyperalimentation should be admitted to the hospital, and IVH should be utilized prior to oncologic therapy until weight gain has begun and muscular strength is returning. Attention to proper metabolic, physiological, and nutritional repletion and maintenance can minimize the complications and maximize the results of all modalities of cancer therapy.

APPENDIX 5-1*

Reference Table for Men of Ideal Weight for Their Height of Urinary Creatinine/cm Body Height

Creatinine Coefficient—23 mg/kg/Body Weight

Height ft	in	cm	Medium Frame Ideal Weight lb	kg	Total mg Creatinine	mg Creatinine/cm Body ht/24 hrs
5	2	157.5	124	56	1288	8.17
5	2	160	127	57.6	1325	8.28
5	4	162.6	130	59.1	1359	8.36
5	5	165.1	133	60.3	1386	8.40
5	6	167.6	137	62	1426	8.51
5	7	170.2	141	63.8	1467	8.62
5	8	172.7	145	65.8	1513	8.76
5	9	175.3	149	67.6	1555	8.86
5	10	177.8	153	69.4	1596	8.98
5	11	180.3	158	71.4	1642	9.11
6	0	182.9	162	73.5	1691	9.24
6	1	185.4	167	75.6	1739	9.38
6	2	188	171	77.6	1785	9.49
6	3	190.5	176	79.6	1831	9.61
6	4	193	181	82.2	1891	9.80

Reference Table for Women of Ideal Weight for Their Height of Urinary Creatinine/cm Body Height

Creatinine Coefficient—18 mg/kg/Body Weight

Height ft	in	cm	Medium Frame Ideal Weight lb	kg	Total mg Creatinine	mg Creatinine/cm Body ht/24 hrs
4	10	147.3	101.5	46.1	830	5.63
4	11	149.9	104	47.3	851	5.68
5	0	152.4	107	48.6	875	5.74
5	1	154.9	110	50	900	5.81
5	2	157.5	113	51.4	925	5.87
5	3	160	116	52.7	949	5.93
5	4	162.6	119.5	54.3	977	6.01
5	5	165.1	123	55.9	1006	6.09
5	6	167.6	127.5	58	1044	6.23
5	7	170.2	131.5	59.8	1076	6.32
5	8	172.7	135.5	61.6	1109	6.42
5	9	175.3	139.5	63.4	1141	6.51
5	10	177.8	143.5	65.2	1174	6.60
5	11	180.3	147.5	67	1206	6.69
5	0	182.9	151.5	68.9	1240	6.78

*Adapted from Blackburn, F. L., Bistrian, B. R., and Maini, B. S. 1977. Nutritional and metabolic assessment of the hospitalized patient. Journal of Parenteral and Enteral Nutrition, 1: 11.

APPENDIX 5-2*

Regular Tube Feeding

This diet is used when the patient is unable to chew or swallow and must be fed by tube. It is adequate in all essential nutrients except niacin and thiamine.

Preparation of Formula

The ingredients should be warmed, homogenized in an electric blender, strained, and administered at body temperature. If the complete formula is not used at once, the remainder should be refrigerated, then heated to body temperature before serving. The containers of formula should be stirred before pouring into the tube in order to suspend the solids, which tend to settle to the bottom on standing. Citrus juice and coffee are not a part of this formula but are given to selected patients to simulate a more normal meal.

Suggested Daily Meal Plan†

Breakfast

1 cup citrus juice (as orange, grapefruit or tomato)
Coffee, ¹/₂ ounce cream, 2 teaspoons sugar
3 glasses *formula* containing 240 ml each;
  ¹/₂ cup warm strained cooked refined cereal (as farina, cream of wheat, cream of rice)
  1 cooked egg
  1¹/₂ cups warm milk
  ¹/₄ cup corn syrup
  1 tablespoon vegetable oil
  ¹/₂ cup water

Lunch and Supper (same)

1 cup juice
Coffee, ¹/₂ ounce cream, 2 teaspoons sugar
3 glasses *formula* containing 240 ml each:
  1 jar (3¹/₂ oz.) warm strained meat
  ¹/₂ cup warm strained vegetables
  2 cups warm milk
  2 tablespoons vegetable oil

COMPOSITION

Total (with juice & coffee)		Formula Only
Calories	2,765	2,150
Protein (g)	90	90
Fat (g)	145	130
Carbohydrate (g)	275	155
Volume (ml)	3,465	2,160

Milk-Free Tube Feeding

This formula may be used when the patient is unable to tolerate milk and develops diarrhea. It is adequate in all nutrients.

Isocal (Mead Johnson and Company, Evansville, IN) or an equivalent commercial formula is used when this feeding is required.

Suggested Daily Meal Plan†

Breakfast

1 cup citrus juice
Coffee, 2 teaspoons sugar
24 oz Isocal

Lunch and Supper (same)

1 cup juice
Coffee, 2 teaspoons sugar
24 oz Isocal

COMPOSITION

Total (with juice & coffee)		Formula Only
Calories	2,545	2,250
Protein (g)	72	72
Fat (g)	95	95
Carbohydrate (g)	350	280
Volume (ml)	3,420	2,160

†Prepared by the Dietetics Service, M.D. Anderson Hospital.

APPROXIMATE NUTRITIVE COMPOSITION OF TUBE FEEDING USED

	Regular tube feeding with juice and coffee	Regular tube feeding only	Milk-free tube feeding with juice and coffee	Milk-free feeding only six 12 oz cans
Total Volume in ml	3,465	2,160	3,420	2,160
Calories	2,765	2,150	2,545	2,250
Protein, g	90	90	72	72
Nitrogen, g	14.4	14.4	12.0	12.0
Fat, g	145	130	95	95
Carbohydrate, g	275	155	350	280
Calcium, g	1.88	1.77	1.84	1.35
Phosphorus, g	1.76	1.64	1.87	1.13
Sodium, g	1.32	1.29	1.32	1.12
Potassium, g	4.24	2.79	3.76	2.80
Iron, mg	16	14	21.6	20.4
Vitamin A, I.U.	12,202	11,695	6,780	5,610
Thiamine, mg	1.13	.90	4.52	4.3
Riboflavin, mg	3.16	2.93	5.13	4.9
Niacin, mg	12.8	9.1	59.8	56.4
Ascorbic acid, mg	120	40	481	336
Vitamin D, I.U.	577	577	450	450
Osmolarity, mOsm/kg water	—	355	—	355

*From Copeland, E. M. and Dudrick, S. J. 1976: Nutritional aspects of cancer. In Hickey, R. C. et. al., Eds.: Current Problems in Cancer. Copyright © 1976 by Year Book Medical Publishers Inc. Chicago.

APPENDIX 5-3

Technique for Measurement of the Triceps Skin-Fold and and Mid-Upper-Arm Circumference

Equipment

A skin-fold caliper with a standard contact surface area of 20 to 24 mm is used.[2] It should read to 0.1 mm accuracy and exert a constant pressure (10 g/mm²) through the whole range of skin-fold thickness at all distances of separation of the jaws.

Technique

The triceps skin-fold area is measured using the mid-point of the left arm while the arm is hanging freely.

Grasp firmly a lengthwise skin-fold and lift up slightly between finger and thumb of the left hand, care being taken not to include the underlying muscle.

The caliper is applied about 1 cm below the operator's finger at a depth about equal to the skin-fold while the skin-fold is still gently held throughout the measurement. Three measurements should be made and the results averaged.

The arm circumference is measured to the nearest 0.1 cm with a flexible steel or fiber-glass tape, which must be placed gently, but firmly, around the mid-left-upper arm to avoid compression of the soft tissues. The overlying subcutaneous fat is measured in the triceps region with the skin-fold calipers as described above.

From these two measurements, it is possible to calculate the inner circle, which is composed principally of muscle, with a small core of bone. It is usually assumed that the bone is relatively constant in size and the calculated value is termed the "mid-arm muscle circumference." The formula for the calculation of the mid-arm muscle circumference is:

Muscle circumference =

arm circumference − skin fold

REFERENCES

1. Bistrian, B. R., Blackburn, G. L., and Sherman, M., 1975. Therapeutic index of nutritional depletion in hospitalized patients. Surgery, Gynecology and Obstetrics, 141: 512.

2. Blackburn, F. L., Bistrian, B. R., and Maini, B. S., 1977. Nutritional and metabolic assessment of the hospitalized patient. Journal of Parenteral and Enteral Nutrition 1: 11.

3. Copeland, E. M., and Dudrick, S. J. 1976. Nutritional aspects of cancer. In Hickey, R. C. et. al., Eds.: Current Problems in Cancer. Year Book Medical Publishers Inc., Chicago.

4. Copeland, E. M., Guillamondegui, O. M., and Dudrick, S. J. 1979. Nutritional aspects of head and neck malignancies. In Conley, J. C., Ed.: Complications of Head and Neck Surgery. W. B. Saunders, Philadelphia, 308.

5. Copeland, E. M., Daly, J. M., Ota, D. M., and Dudrick, S. J. 1979. Nutrition, cancer and intravenous hyperalimentation. Cancer, 43: 2108.

6. Copeland, E. M., Daly, J. M., Ota, D. M., and Dudrick, S. (In press). Cancer, Nutrition and immunity. In Long, J. M. Ed.: Proceedings of the Symposium on "Metabolic Aspects of Critically Ill Patients." and American Medical Association, Chicago.

7. Dudrick, S. J., Willmore, D. W., Vars, H. M., and Rhoads, J. E. 1968. Long-term total parenteral nutrition with growth, development, and positive nitrogen balance. Surgery, 64: 134.

8. Freeman, J. B., Egan, M. C., and Millis, B. J. 1976. The elemental diet. Surgery, Gynecology and Obstetrics, 142: 925.

9. Harris-Benedict Standard of normal (total) calorie consumption per hour. 1962. In Documenta Geigy Scientific Tables. 6th edn. Geigy Pharmaceuticals, Ardsley, N.Y., 628.

10. Hoffmeister, J. A., and Dobbie, R. P. 1977. Continuous control pump-tube feeding of the malnourished patient with Isocal. American Surgeon, 43: 6.

11. Kenady, D. E., Chretien, P. B., Potvin, C., and Simon, R. M. 1977. Thymosin reconstitution of T cell deficits in vitro in cancer patients. Cancer, 39: 575.

12. Kinney, J. M. 1966. Proceedings of a Conference on Energy Metabolism and Body Fuel Utilization. Harvard University Press, Cambridge.

13. Keoshian, L. A., and Nelson T. S. 1969. A new design for a feeding tube. Plastic and Reconstructive Surgery 44: 508.

14. Law, D. K., Dudrick, S. J., and Abdou, N. I. 1973. Immunocompetence of patients with protein-calorie malnutrition. The effects of nutritional repletion. Annals of Internal Medicine, 79: 545.

15. Shils, M. E. 1978. Enteral nutritional management of the cancer patient. Cancer Bulletin, 30: 98.

16. Spanier, A. H., and Shizgal, H. M. 1977. Caloric requirements of the critically ill patient receiving intravenous hyperalimentation. American Journal of Surgery, 133: 99.

6 | Anesthetic Considerations

Noel W. Lawson, M.D.
John A. Brunner, III, M.D.

INTRODUCTION

The anesthesiologist plays no part in patient selection for head and neck cancer surgery. Once that selection is made, however, the anesthesiologist must play a prominent role, in cooperation with the surgeon and internist, in bringing the patient to optimum condition before surgery. The anesthesiologist's evaluation of risk must take into account the internist's assessment of the preoperative status of the patient and the nature of the surgery. An independent preanesthetic evaluation is then made regarding the effects that various anesthetic agents or techniques might have on preexisting pathology and concurrent medications.

The practice of anesthesia, aside from rendering the patient insensible to pain, is the practice of autonomic medicine. The anesthesiologist is responsible for managing the homeostatic alterations produced by anesthesia throughout the perioperative period. Anesthesiologists, by the nature of their training and their experience with the effects of potent anesthetics on existing pathophysiology, may offer a different viewpoint than that of the internist in preparing the patient for surgery. Additional studies or further consultation concerning the medical management or intended procedure may be requested. The surgeon should not take this as an affront but rather should recognize it as input from the anesthesiologist into the decision-making process. Current medical liability dictates such action but more importantly it is good medical practice.

The custom of classifying certain surgical procedures as minor because of their brevity or simplicity should in no way minimize the fact that the most common and serious difficulties associated with anesthesia occur during induction of and recovery from any general anesthetic. The nature or duration of surgery performed between these two events may have little bearing on these difficulties. There is no such thing as a minor anesthetic. Anesthesia for head and neck surgery imparts special technical as well as medical hazards to the patient. For example, the surgeon and anesthesiologist must share the airway, but with the anesthesiologist invariably sharing at a considerable distance from the surgical field. Communication between the surgeon and anesthesiologist as to their needs before and during the procedure is essential.

RISK

The contribution of anesthesia to surgical risk has been studied extensively. The grading of various disease manifestations has proven advantageous in providing data essential to the assessment of the risk of anesthesia and surgery. This advantage has been most noted in the area of cardiovascular disease. The American Society of Anesthesiology recognized early the need for a grading system to provide an estimate of anesthetic risk if for no other reason than clarity of communication (Table 6-1). The number of deaths attributable to anesthesia in patients in physical status 3 and 4 is four to five

TABLE 6-1 AMERICAN SOCIETY OF ANESTHESIOLOGISTS PREOPERATIVE PHYSICAL STATUS

Class 1

No organic, physiological, biochemical, or psychiatric disturbance. The pathology for which surgery is to be performed is localized and not systemic.

Class 2

Mild to moderate systemic disturbance caused either by the condition to be treated surgically or by other pathophysiological processes.

Class 3

Severe systemic disturbance or disease from whatever cause, even though it may not be possible to define the degree of disability.

Class 4

Severe systemic disorder already life-threatening, not always correctable by the operative procedure.

Class 5

The moribund patient with little chance of survival with or without surgery.

Emergency Operation (E)

Any patient in one of the classes who is operated upon as an emergency. The letter E is placed beside the numerical classification.

TABLE 6-2 NEW YORK HEART ASSOCIATION FUNCTIONAL CLASSIFICATION

Class I

Patients with cardiac disease but without limitations of physical activity. Ordinary physical activity does not cause undue fatigue, palpitation, dyspnea, or anginal pain.

Class II

Patients with cardiac disease resulting in slight limitation of physical activity. They are comfortable at rest. Ordinary physical activity results in fatigue, palpitation, dyspnea, or anginal pain.

Class III

Patients with cardiac disease resulting in marked limitation of physical activity. They are uncomfortable at rest. Less than ordinary physical activity causes fatigue, palpitation, dyspnea, or anginal pain.

Class IV

Patients with cardiac disease resulting in inability to carry on any physical activity without discomfort.

(Modified from Criteria Committee of the New York Heart Association, Inc. 1964. Diseases of the Heart and Blood Vessels: Nomenclature and Criteria for Diagnosis. 6th edn. Little, Brown, Boston.)

times that of patients in physical status 1 and 2.[2, 10] However, mortality from any cause—with or without surgery—would be expected to be higher in the former groups. Physical status, therefore, cannot be entirely equated with anesthetic risk. Furthermore, studies have shown that more than one-third of the deaths attributed to anesthesia could not have been predicted on the basis of preoperative physical status.[27]

The New York Heart Association Functional Classification (Table 6-2) is relevant to anesthesia. This classification relates to the reserve of the cardiac patient approaching surgery, but does not apply to other diseases as does the physical status. The Functional Classification has correlated well with overall surgical mortality in a large group of patients with heart disease who underwent noncardiac surgery. The principal drawback to using disease classification as a useful guide to operative risk is that it does not take into consideration differences in physician ability and in facility quality. It has been stated that risk estimations have been so inaccurate as to be little more than intuitive when applied to individual patients. For example, there are no data available relating cardiac disease specifically to anesthetic mortality. More surprising is the absence of available data relating anesthetic mortality to patients with heart disease presenting for heart surgery. Mortality instead is usually related to *total* mortality.

Estimation of risk is the probability of loss versus gain. When *total* mortality is considered, some informative risk statistics are available. However, one must recognize that statistics are much less meaningful when applied to the individual. These data related primarily to patients with cardiac disease presenting for non-cardiac surgery. We are now anesthetizing patients who because of their heart disease would not have been candidates for surgery 10 years ago. Many of the advances in anesthesia have come about because of the enthusiasm for coronary artery surgery during the past decade. These principles have had direct application to areas other than cardiac surgery. Better anesthetic management, improved surgical techniques, and better patient selection and preparation have led to a complete turnabout in our ability to offer the benefits of other surgical procedures to the cardiac patient.

An estimate has been made that 38 percent of all surgical patients over the age of 35 have evidence of heart disease, hypertension, or diabetes mellitus. Anesthesiologists and internists are frequently asked to estimate the capacity of patients with cardiac disease to undergo non-cardiac surgery. A number of reviews have been published delineating the attrition of surgical patients with coexisting heart disease. These data exclude open heart cases. An examination of these series is most striking because the data are quite similar even though collected years apart.

Surgical risk is greater in patients with coronary artery disease than in other forms of heart disease. Excluding all other factors, the perioperative mortality of patients with arteriosclerotic heart disease (ASHD) is twice that of patients without ASHD regardless of the surgical procedure[25] (Table 6-3). The perioperative mortality, however, is definitely age-related, since patients over the age of 70 with ASHD have two-fold increase in mortality compared to patients with ASHD under age 60. However, advanced age, alone, is not a contraindication to major surgery.

Patients over the age of 55 who have had a documented myocardial infarction have a 7 percent incidence of perioperative reinfarction with a mortality of 70 percent.[12, 21] In comparison, the incidence of perioperative myocardial infarction in patients over the age of 55 without a previous history of heart disease is less than 1 percent with a mortality of around 25 percent. The mortality from myocardial infarction in a general hospital is approximately 30 percent, and in a coronary care unit this may be reduced to 15 to 20 percent. Thus, myocardial infarction or recurrent infarction after anesthesia and a major operation is more serious and lethal than myocardial infarction alone.

The time between the occurrence of a myocardial infarct and surgery is of utmost importance in determining the probability of reinfarction after surgery; this risk is not age-related.[34] A 37 percent incidence of reinfarction was noted in patients who had operations occurring within 3 months of an infarction, and a 16 percent incidence was shown for the 4 to 6 month period (Table 6-4).[34] Beyond 6 months, the overall rate stabilizes at 5 percent or slightly higher for patients over the age of 55. As already pointed out, the mortality associated with this second infarct is quite high. It is recommended that all operations, except for life-threatening

TABLE 6-3 PERIOPERATIVE MORTALITY OF PATIENTS WITH AND WITHOUT ARTERIOSCLEROTIC HEART DISEASE (ASHD)*

Patients	Number of Operations	Mortality (%)
All ages—No ASHD	19,610	2.9
All ages—ASHD	3,144	6.6
>60 ASHD	2,675	7.2
>70 ASHD	2,852	14.1

*Data from Nachlas et al.[25] and a review of the literature.

TABLE 6-4 INCIDENCE OF
POSTOPERATIVE MYOCARDIAL
INFARCTION (MI) IN PATIENTS WHO
HAD PREOPERATIVE MI[34]

Time from Last MI to Surgery (Months)	Incidence of Postoperative MI (%)
≤3	37
4 to 6	16
>6	5

emergencies, should be deferred for the first 6 months. These data correlate with the finding that emergency procedures in patients with ASHD have a mortality twice that of the same procedures done on an elective basis. The cancer surgeon may then be faced with deciding the risk of delaying excision of a cancer versus cardiovascular risk. The anesthesiologist or internist can be very helpful in this regard.

An idea prevails among physicians that the duration of anesthesia and surgery is an additional risk factor. Several studies have examined this issue. These studies indicated superficially that mortality increased with the duration of surgery, but when individual procedures were compared as to duration, no correlation was found.[25, 31] Instead, the site of the operation had a greater influence on mortality than did duration. Predictably, thoracic and upper abdominal operations are followed by three times as many postoperative infarctions as are other operations. One must assume that greater impairment of ventilation and more frequent development of atelectasis occurs with thoracic and upper abdominal operations than with more peripheral surgical procedures. It is also of interest to note that myocardial reinfarction occurred most often (35 percent) on the *third* postoperative day.[34] This corresponds to the day when the greatest decrease in arterial oxygenation occurs in all postoperative patients. The mechanism of these phenomena remains unclear. These delayed infarctions do not remove the possibility of cause resulting from events initiated during anesthesia and surgery. Cardiac patients, especially those with a previous infarct, should be monitored after surgery and receive supplemental oxygen for 3 to 5 days as though they have had an infarction. Statistically, head and neck surgery imposes little additional risk to the cardiac patient as compared to procedures on major body cavities.[31] The mortality of head and neck surgery in the cardiac patients ranks favorably with other more peripheral procedures such as transurethral prostatectomy and orthopedic procedures. Duration of the surgical procedure, therefore, is not considered a significant factor.

The contribution of intraoperative hypotension towards mortality in patients with ASHD is a more nebulous issue than previously thought. A four-fold increase in the rate of myocardial infarction has been demonstrated when a significant fall in blood pressure occurs during surgery in patients at risk.[21] Similar findings demonstrate an 11.5 percent mortality in high risk patients becoming hypotensive during operation as compared to. an 8.5 percent mortality when no operative hypotension occurred.[25] One cannot, with certainty, attribute hypotension to the development of an intraoperative infarct. The hypotension may be the result rather than the cause of the infarction. The previous studies could not make this distinction. However, it is important to guard against a significant decline in pressure in patients with ASHD. This becomes even more important whenever the use of hypotensive anesthesia is contemplated. Blood flow to any organ, be it heart, brain, or kidney, becomes pressure dependent whenever (as occurs in arteriosclerosis) the vasculature can no longer autoregulate. Thus, hypotensive anesthesia is contraindicated in situations where the disease of an organ is characterized by fixed vascular resistance.

Only recently has it been appreciated that hypertension and tachycardia by increasing myocardial oxygen consumption are more common causes of intraoperative infarction than is hypotension.[19] Systolic blood pressure and heart rate are the two major determinants of myocardial oxygen consumption. A disparity between myocardial oxygen demand and supply produces the signs and symptoms of ischemia. Control of these parameters is the very basis of modern cardiovascular anesthesia contributing to the low mortality (< 1 percent) of coronary artery surgery. Thus, a stormy anesthetic induction or hypertension during intubation in the cardiac patient may cause the infarct, which is then attributed to the resultant hypotension.

CHOICE OF ANESTHESIA

The choice of anesthesia for patients presenting for head and neck cancer surgery depends upon a number of variables. This includes the familiarity of the anesthesiologist with a given agent as well as the pharmacologic properties of a specific agent and its effects on preexisting pathology. The duration and extent of the surgical procedure must also be considered. Several series of patients have been studied but no correlation in mortality has been found for patients receiving nerve blocks or local infiltration compared to patients receiving general anesthesia.[25] This is perhaps related to the fact that local anesthesia was selected for patients in the poor risk category.

The recent introduction of long-acting local anesthetics has made regional block anesthesia of the head and neck more practical. Regional anesthesia has its advocates for use in head and neck surgery but is of limited value in cancer cases. A superficial and deep cervical plexus block is a good block for soft tissue dissection of limited duration. However, such blocks are impractical for prolonged major head and neck procedures. Most patients cannot lie still for extended periods and will become restless. Many patients cannot tolerate the psychological stress of being awake, particularly if extensive bone resection is required. However, nerve blocks may be combined with general anesthesia to reduce the anesthetic requirements in poor risk patients.

The successful use of block anesthesia depends in great part upon the expertise of the anesthesiologist or surgeon and the emotional state of the patient. The cost of anxiety and pain is increased myocardial oxygen consumption, which may not be tolerated by the cardiac patient. It is important to understand that local or regional anesthesia may not be the safest anesthetic technique for poor risk patients. Instead, general anesthesia in some circumstances may be safer. Regional anesthesia lacks the reversibility of general anesthesia, and the agents themselves, like general anesthetics, may cause significant cardiovascular and respiratory depression when used in large amounts. General anesthesia has the advantage of airway control and quick reversibility. The potent inhalation anesthetics act directly to reduce myocardial oxygen consumption. In addition, they may be used to control the two major determinants of myocardial oxygen consumption—systolic blood pressure and pulse rate.

General anesthesia, as a rule, is usually indicated for most cases involving an area where local or nerve block anesthesia cannot be used safely. General endotracheal anesthesia may be provided by using a potent inhalation agent plus nitrous oxide and oxygen, a nitrous oxide-oxygen-narcotic-relaxant technique, or a nitrous oxide-oxygen-neuroleptanalgesia (narcotic-tranquilizer) and relaxant. The latter two techniques are often referred to as balanced anesthesia and could include the use of a regional block with a general anesthetic. Short-acting barbiturates such as thiopental sodium are commonly used to induce anesthesia. Thereafter, maintenance anesthesia is provided by one of the above methods. If airway obstruction is present before surgery, the anesthesiologist may elect a mask induction of anesthesia and maintain spontaneous ventilation until the endotracheal tube is in place. Mask inductions require absolute quiet in the operating room to avoid stimulating the patient into excitability during stage 2 anesthesia, which is otherwise avoided by the use of a barbiturate induction.

Ketamine and diazepam (Valium) are alternative agents used intravenously either alone or in combination with the barbiturates to induce general anesthesia. These agents may be utilized to avoid the myocardial depression inherent in the barbiturate induction. Ketamine is a nonbarbiturate "dissociative anesthetic" that rapidly induces unconsciousness when used in smaller doses than those required for surgical anesthesia. Elevations in blood pressure and heart rate accompanying its use make ketamine a less desirable choice when hypertension or cardiovascular disease is present. Hallucinations and disagreeable dreaming occur occasionally during emergence, but the incidence can be reduced by prior treatment with diazepam.

Diazepam, a benzodiazepine derivative, has become a popular drug to use as a supplement to the ultrashort-acting barbiturates for induction of general anesthesia. While larger doses of the drug will induce unconsciousness, the awakening time (particularly in the elderly, debilitated patient) is excessive because the effect of the drug can extend well beyond the immediate postoperative period. In the past, various desirable assets have been attributed to both ketamine and diazepam, including maintenance of protective airway reflexes and lack of respiratory depression. Most of these have not withstood extensive clinical scrutiny. Hazardous side effects are very real and must be considered against the possible risks of a conventional barbiturate induction.

Flammable anesthetics such as cyclopropane and ether have not been used for years due to the evolution of operating room electronics and electrocautery. Methoxyflurane was a popular anesthetic only a few years ago but is rarely used now because of a dose related nephrotoxicity. Today, halothane (Fluothane) and enflurane (Ethrane) are the two most commonly used potent inhalation anesthetics in combination with nitrous oxide and oxygen. However, these anesthetics sensitize the myocardium to the effects of epinephrine and may produce ventricular arrhythmias. Halothane is more dangerous in this regard than is enflurane. There is little danger, however, if the volume of epinephrine injected for hemostasis does not exceed 10 ml of a 1:100,000 solution or 20 ml of a 1:200,000 solution. One should not exceed 30 ml of either concentration in a 1 hour period. A new general anesthetic, isoflurane (Forane), is expected to be released soon that has many of the beneficial characteristics of halothane and enflurane but does not sensitize the myocardium to catecholamines. This anesthetic may prove to be of benefit to the head and neck cancer surgeon giving broader latitude in the use of epinephrine for hemostasis.

Intravenous narcotics are often used in modern anesthesia instead of the potent inhalation agents. Narcotics are commonly employed in cardiac anesthesia and for other poor risk patients because of their minimal cardiac depressant effects. These agents include morphine, Demerol, and the short-acting narcotic fentanyl (Sublimaze). They can be combined with nitrous oxide and a muscle relaxant to produce general anesthesia that may be reversed with naloxone (Narcan). One may elect to allow narcotic effects to continue into the postoperative period if continued mechanical ventilation is desired. Epinephrine may be used with these techniques without fear of myocardial sensitization. The hazards of narcotic anesthesia include unexpected episodes of hypertension not related to the level of anesthesia and the possibility of renarcotization in the postoperative period.

Narcotics may be combined with tranquilizers to produce anesthesia termed neuroleptanalgesia. Neuroleptanalgesia refers to a mental state controlled to the point that the patient may remain awake for a surgical procedure but will not appreciate pain. Neuroleptanalgesia employs a tranquilizer, droperidol (Inapsine), and a short-acting narcotic, fentanyl (Sublimaze), to produce this dissociative state of consciousness. These drugs may be combined as Innovar or administered individually as desired. The addition of nitrous oxide and a relaxant produces general anesthesia.

Muscle relaxation is not required in

head and neck surgery but long-acting muscle relaxants are often employed to control ventilation and to prevent patient movement at lighter levels of anesthesia. Total paralysis of the patient makes it impossible for the surgeon to use the nerve stimulator to locate the facial nerve during dissection around the parotid gland. If a relaxant technique is chosen, it is possible to use low relaxant doses and a nerve stimulator to keep the muscle twitch response visible. Under these circumstances, the surgeon should have no difficulty obtaining a response to direct nerve stimulation while achieving the desired relaxed anesthetic state. Preoperative communication can solve this dilemma.

BLOOD LOSS, BLOOD VOLUME AND VOLUME REPLACEMENT

Cancer patients use more blood products than do patients with any other disease, with the exception of those having hemophilia. Transfusion of blood components to the cancer patient is usually done for specific reasons, the most important being restoration of blood volume, maintenance of oxygen carrying capacity, restoration of cellular components such as platelets or granulocytes, and restoration of noncellular components such as fibrinogen and other coagulation factors.

Radical cancer surgery is often associated with massive blood loss and major fluid shifts. A review of the literature indicates that when radical cancer operations are divided into anatomic areas, a marked difference exists between the actual blood loss (isotopically verified) and the estimated blood loss. [36, 37] However, this difference was acceptable (± 10 percent of total blood volume) in patients undergoing head and neck surgery even though they required transfusions up to 6,000 ml of blood. Patients who had thoracic surgery were less accurately treated with blood replacement, and those undergoing abdominal cancer surgery were the most difficult to estimate. Abdominal

cases showed an error between actual and estimated blood loss of up to 49 percent (average 22.5 percent). Much of the discrepancy in loss versus replacement is the result of third space loss, which is not a major problem in head and neck surgery. To this extent, those involved in head and neck surgery enjoy an advantage in patient care not found in cancer surgery in other areas.

The surgeon must rely upon the judgment of the anesthesiologist as to the need for volume replacement during surgery. The anesthesiologist is attuned to the moment to moment blood loss as a matter of course in the monitoring of the patient's vital signs. Modern anesthesia has at its disposal a variety of techniques to monitor the needs for volume replacement. The availability of blood components permits the administration of the blood products or cystalloid to replace the deficit appropriately. The ability to discern the need for fluid volume and type is the hallmark of modern anesthesia, allowing surgery on patients today who would not have been surgical candidates a decade ago.

The management of the intraoperative blood loss and replacement is of great interest to the head and neck surgeon. The patient's total blood volume is composed of the red cell mass, the plasma volume, and clotting factors. There is a marked variation from patient to patient as to how much of a loss of whole blood components can be tolerated. The total blood volume is the most critical of these factors. For example, if blood volume is maintained, a patient can lose 40 percent of the red cell mass and up to 60 percent of the clotting factors with little clinical consequence. Most patients will tolerate an acute loss of 10 percent of their blood volume without need for replacement, but an acute loss of 20 percent of their blood volume is poorly tolerated and compensatory signs are usually evident. Chronic losses to this degree may not produce symptoms in the awake patient, but can become evident upon the induction of anesthesia. An example is the malnourished head and neck patient who is chronically hypovolemic. Vasodilitation or myocardial depression produced by anesthesia will block the usual compensatory mechanisms with resultant decompensation.

PREOPERATIVE BLOOD VOLUME ASSESSMENT

A preoperative assessment of the cancer patient's blood volume is mandatory in anticipation of volume management during surgery. Patients with head and neck neoplasms can present with varying degrees of blood volume and component disorders. Fortunately, these can be discerned by clinical means alone in the majority of cases. These patients will fall into four major groups, depending upon the extent to which the neoplasm has interfered with nutrition.

The first group are patients who, by history and physical examination, do not exhibit weight loss or debilitation. The hemogram is normal and no orthostatic circulatory changes occur upon examination. These patients may be considered normovolemic with a normal red cell mass, and no preoperative fluid therapy is necessary.

The second group of patients are those who also demonstrate no evidence of weight loss or orthostatic changes but who are anemic. In the absence of other hematologic evidence, the anemia will probably be related to malnutrition. These patients may also be considered normovolemic but may require transfusions of packed cells to achieve an acceptable preoperative hemoglobin level. Whole blood transfusion before surgery is inappropriate under these circumstances because of the danger of volume overload. Both this group and the first group of patients are characterized by a history of no weight loss and both are considered normovolemic, requiring only the correction of the anemia in the second group.

The third and fourth groups of patients are surviving under a more tenuous situation, as both groups are characterized by marked weight loss and/or debilitation. The similarity between groups three and

four stops at that point, however, and additional blood volume studies may be required to delineate volume status with certainty. Patients in group three are those with marked weight loss that can be attributed solely to malnutrition. Group four patients are those in whom there is marked nutritional wasting coupled with additional fluid or blood loss. Patients with head and neck cancer are less likely to be found in this latter category as this condition is more often related to neoplasms of the gastrointestinal tract. Nevertheless, it is important to make this differentiation because there may be wide variations in the preoperative blood volume status in these groups.

Blood volume measurements have shown that unless additional fluid loss was present preoperatively, nutritionally debilitated patients are rarely hypovolemic.[24, 36] No change is found in blood volume during experimental chronic starvation.[12] Instead, the blood volume of these nutritionally deficient patients is related to their observed weight. When the measured blood volume of cachectic patients is compared to their observed weight, blood volume is higher than that of normal subjects of the same weight. When the measured blood volume of patients is compared to their own usual normal weight, their blood volume is lower than normal. This is an important concept because it indicates that nutritionally debilitated patients, in the absence of sources of fluid loss, do not lose vascular volume to the same extent that they lose weight. Thus, debilitated patients may have a blood volume normal for the size of their vascular compartment, but the volume cannot be defined in terms of cc/kg as it can in normal patients. This may explain the diversity of findings in volume needs of cancer patients. On the other hand, cachectic patients with additional sources of fluid loss are almost always volume depleted before surgery.

The presence or absence of anemia in any of the groups of patients can be misleading in deciding upon the need for preoperative blood or volume therapy. A typical illustrative case is the patient who has a head and neck neoplasm and who also has cirrhosis of the liver. The physical examination may find some wasting, but no orthostatic circulatory changes. However, the hemogram would likely reveal an anemia. The first impression, in the presence of wasting and anemia, would be that this patient would at least need some packed cells before surgery. Actual blood volume measurements would instead show an expanded plasma volume and a normal red cell mass. The apparent anemia would be dilutional and, in fact, no properative volume or blood therapy would be required.

Volume Replacement

Intraoperative fluid management consists of replacing preoperative fluid deficits including that incurred from an overnight fast, intraoperative maintenance fluids, and blood lost or fluid translocated during surgery. Many different routines have been used over the years for the administration of intraoperative fluids during a wide variety of surgical procedures. These regimens have ranged from giving no fluid to giving only blood. Most patients survive with any regularly used regimen: some because of it and others despite it. Research capabilities in combination with the Vietnam War has resulted in a greater understanding of the fluid maintenance and replacement needs of surgical patients. These needs will vary with the site of the surgery as well as the anticipated blood and fluid shifts accompanying a particular procedure.

Balanced salt solutions clearly can restore plasma volume but a greater volume is required than when colloids are used.[16] Colloids remain in the vascular compartment whereas crystalloids redistribute between the intracellular, interstitial, and intravascular compartments. As a result of this redistribution, the ratio of the volume of balanced salt solution required to replace a given volume of blood loss in order to maintain a normal blood volume is 3:1.

The administration of colloids in the form of plasma or plasma substitutes has not been shown to have any definite advantage over the use of balanced salt solutions. They may clearly be indicated if significant decreases in plasma oncotic pressure are proven. The advantage of colloids in these circumstances is their ability to stay in the intravascular space. This intravascular confinement is also their main limiting factor because colloids do not correct the interstitial and intracellular fluid deficits known to occur during major surgical procedures. The controversy of colloid versus crystalloid may fade on the basis of economics alone. Colloids cost 20 times as much as an equivalent volume of crystalloid, and this factor should be considered as there is no clear cut advantage of one over the other.

The selection of the overall fluid therapy used during surgery is based on physiological necessities. These necessities will be judged against the patient's preoperative status and how the patient responds to anesthesia and surgery. Principles of fluid therapy must be applied to the specific problems of the patient actually being treated. Operations that are short and of little physiological consequence require minimal attention to fluid therapy. Operations such as those involving the extremities and head and neck surgery are less difficult to manage than operations within the major body cavities.

The choice of fluids will usually be a mixture of balanced salt solution and red cells. Frozen or washed red cells hold certain advantages if available. Volume replacement can then be made up of crystalloid or colloid. Massive and rapid blood loss will, of course, require whole blood. Provision should be made for maintaining total intravascular volume and oxygen carrying capacity as well as replenishing "third space" losses. Balanced salt solutions in combination with red cell replacement can do all of these things. The adult scheduled for elective head and neck surgery who has no fluid or electrolyte deficit should receive 500 ml of D5W to replace pure water loss that has occurred during the overnight fast. This should be started as soon as the patient is in the operating room. By the time the patient is prepared for the induction of anesthesia, approximately half of this volume should have been infused. Most patients, whether or not they have received drying agents in their premedication, will exhibit thirst. This thirst is the result of a slight increase in serum osmolality due to water restriction, continued loss through the kidneys, sweat, and exhaled moisture. The hypothalamus responds to the increase in osmolality by releasing antidiuretic hormone (ADH). The patient is, therefore, already in an early state of water retention before the surgery is started. This volume of D5W should suppress ADH secretion and avoid oliguria, barring other subsequent changes in the patient's volume status.

The addition of glucose is also beneficial for its protein sparing effect and ability to avert depletion of liver glycogen stores. Glycogen depletion can occur very quickly in the fasting and anxious patient. Evidence exists that the glycogen depleted liver is probably more susceptible to the hepatic effects of halogenated anesthetics.[7] Preoperative depletion of liver glycogen stores and the ADH effect will be exaggerated in those patients who have been without oral intake during their preoperative hospital stay. Thus, indications exist for the administration initially of free water plus glucose to the anesthetized patient who has no other fluid or electrolyte disorders. This practice may require modification in those patients with myocardial disease or diabetes.

Following the initial free water and glucose load, a balanced salt solution is utilized for the maintenance fluid regimen. Dextrose 5 percent in lactated Ringer's solution (D5LR) is infused at a rate of 6 to 10 ml/kg during the first hour of surgery. The normal 24-hour fluid intake of the 70 kg person is 2,000 ml/m² body surface area. The body surface area of the 70 kg person is 1.7 m². Therefore, the total 24-hour maintenance fluids usually consumed by the patient will be 3,400 ml. The usual fast imposed on the surgical patient during the night before surgery will result in a maintenance deficit of nearly half the usual daily water and salt requirements. This preoperative fluid deficit of fluid and water will be corrected by the end of the first hour of surgery when the above regimen is followed. The 70 kg person would have received by then about 1,500 ml of balanced salt solution. Once these maintenance requirements have been met, changes in vital signs and urine output may be assumed to be the result of blood loss of fluid translocation and can be treated appropriately.

One is reminded that these guidelines apply only to the patient in whom there are no preexisting fluid and electrolyte abnormalities. More extensive monitoring may be called for if the preoperative exam reveals altered circulatory hemodynamics. If the operation is continued into the second hour without undue loss of blood or tissue trauma, the rate of infusion is decreased in accordance with the urine output and vital signs. During more prolonged procedures, lactated Ringer's solution without dextrose may be substituted for D5LR.

Physiological changes leading to oliguria or anuria will occur when blood loss exceeds 10 percent of the patient's intravascular volume. These changes are primarily due to fluid translocation or actual blood loss. The total volume to be administered will depend upon the estimated blood loss and estimated loss of extracellular fluid due to the trauma of tissue manipulation. The rationale for the continued use of the balanced salt solution is that as intravascular volume is lost, fluid shifts into the intravascular compartment. This shift of extracellular fluid (ECF) is equivalent to the amount of blood loss. These losses are isotonic and maintaining the blood volume with D5LR for losses under 10 percent is justified to maintain ECF. This technique removes the primary stimuli for aldostersone secretion, and patients so treated will maintain a good urinary output throughout the operative period even though blood loss and replacement is in progress. Therefore monitoring the urine output is of further value in assessing ECF losses as well as intravascular losses. When the urine output diminishes in the absence of significant changes in blood pressure or pulse, one can assume an ECF deficit is present suggesting the development of subsequent hypotension. Patients given no salt during a major operation will retain a salt load, and water is given postoperatively because the salt will be retained (aldosterone effect) to correct for the ECF deficit (translocation) acquired during surgery. The administration of blood or colloid alone will not correct a deficit of functional ECF.

Balanced salt solutions should not be used as a substitute when the use of whole blood components is indicated. Whole blood or packed cell replacement is given consideration when the patient has lost 10 percent of his blood volume. Clinically, the blood loss is measured by weighing the freshly discarded sponges and drapes and by observation of the contents in the suction collection minus irrigation. This blood loss is continually compared to the patient's known or estimated blood volume. In the absence of fluid and electrolyte disturbances, the blood volume of the adult can be estimated to be 74 ml/kg of lean body weight. The normal 70 kg adult would therefore have an estimated blood volume of 5,180 ml or 5 liters. A 10 percent loss of this volume would be 500 ml, a volume only slightly greater than that lost when blood is donated. As previously noted, the estimation of blood volume on the basis of body weight is not a valid assumption when the patient has had significant weight loss. Hence, the determination of preoperative blood volume in this type of patient is of great value in the proper intraoperative management of fluid losses and shifts.

As a 10 percent loss is approached the decision as to whether there should be blood replacement will depend upon the anticipation of further blood loss during or after surgery, changes in the vital signs or pressure monitors, and the individual surgeon's proclivity towards hemostasis. Measurement of the hematocrit level may be helpful at this point to determine the *type* of volume replacement required. It must be emphasized, however, that this measure is of little value in assessing *volume* needs during active bleeding because during active bleeding the components of whole blood are lost equally and the hematocrit level will not change. Significant reductions of the hematocrit level are late signs of blood volume reductions and are the result of fluid shifts from the interstitial space into the vascular tree in the absence of other volume replacement. Small reductions of the hematocrit level are usually noted during surgery in the absence of active bleeding as patients' maintenance fluids are replaced at the start of the case. This is to be expected as a dilutional effect of rehydration. Decreases in the hematocrit level during active bleeding may be seen when crystalloids are used to maintain volume for the first 10 percent of the volume loss at the ratio of 3:1. Thus, the hematocrit level will indicate the need for red cell replacement and the vital signs will determine the volume. The combination of the two indicators will determine the need for whole blood (volume + oxygen carrying capacity) or packed red cells alone. If volume and cells are needed and only packed cells are available, the packed cells may be reconstituted with normal saline or plasma products and infused. This will handle the volume requirements and enhance the speed at which the infusion can be given as well. All transfusions should be administered through a blood warming device.

Great concern has been expressed over the use of balanced salt solutions during major surgical procedures. However, studies of humans and of experimental animals do not support this concern.[16] Electrolyte balance studies show that patients managed as previously described have only a small positive sodium balance at the end of the procedure and do not retain salt or water. Maintaining the circulating volume with salt containing solutions removes the stimulus for aldosterone secretion and thus prevents the salt and water retention, which was seen during the era of free water fluid management. Obviously the previously described regimen as to the use of balanced salt solutions will require alterations in those patients with other salt and water disturbances or cardiac disease.

Monitoring Volume Replacement

The rational use of fluids or blood products demands constant monitoring and careful interpretation of the information gained from the monitors. The development of electronic monitoring and advances in intravascular cannulation techniques over the past decade have contributed greatly to the safety of anesthesia and surgery. Despite the current development of electronic monitors, their use is intended not as a replacement for but as an adjunct to trained and intuitive clinical judgment. It is now clinically feasible to monitor routinely the arterial blood pressure by direct and indirect means. In addition, the central venous pressure (CVP), pulmonary capillary wedge pressure (PCWP), electrocardiogram, and core temperature can all be monitored. Rapid blood gas and electrolyte analysis also add to the monitoring capabilities. Electrodes for continuous intra-arterial blood gas determinations as well as for measuring tissue oxygenation and pH will soon be available. Many major surgical procedures can be done safely with noninvasive monitors. However, the poor risk patient may require varying degrees of invasive monitoring during surgery. The intensity of the monitoring will depend upon the patient's general condition and the extent of the contemplated surgery. Furthermore, these monitoring techniques will provide consistent and accurate continuation of patient monitoring from the surgical period into the recovery phase.

Current anesthesia practice dictates that the blood pressure, pulse, electrocardiogram, and core temperature be monitored continuously during even the shortest of surgical procedures. The reasons for monitoring the first three are obvious but the importance of temperature monitoring has only recently been appreciated. Patients under anesthesia lose their ability to regulate temperature. It is common for anes-

thetized adults to lose 3 to 4 °C of body temperature in an air-conditioned operating room. Less anesthesia is then required; and unless one is cognizant of the fall in temperature, an overdose of anesthesia might be given. Vasoconstriction occurs in response to the cooling and this can mislead the anesthesiologist as to the adequacy of volume replacement during surgery. Vasodilatation will occur with rewarming, turning what seemed to be adequate volume replacement during surgery into a hypotensive episode in the recovery room. Shivering will occur during recovery from anesthesia and can increase oxygen consumption by 300 percent above normal. This may not be tolerated by the patient with preexisting cardiovascular disease. Temperature monitoring should be a routine part of intraoperative monitoring not only to combat the effects of inadvertent hypothermia but to detect the occasional case of malignant hyperthermia that is uniformly fatal unless detected early in its course.[3]

A decade of experience in the use of CVP and PCWP monitoring has proven their usefulness and their limitations in assessing the volume requirements of the surgical patient.[15] Central venous pressure is a measurement of the right atrial pressure, which is the filling pressure of the right ventricle. The CVP is thus a direct reflection of the right ventricular end-diastolic pressure in the presence of an intact tricuspid valve. Right ventricular end-diastolic pressure is an index of preload, which determines resting myocardial fiber length. According to Starling's law, an increase in diastolic fiber length produces a stronger myocardial contraction in the nonfailing heart. Hypovolemia causes a fall in CVP resulting in a low cardiac output. The CVP has been advocated as a useful monitor in determining fluid requirements during major surgery or disease states in which the accuracy of fluid therapy is critical; but the use of the CVP is grossly over-rated. It may be helpful in determining volume needs only if the assumption can be made that both ventricles are functioning with equal efficiency and that no interposing pulmonary disease is present. When this premise breaks down, the CVP is not an accurate reflection of volume needs. The CVP measures right ventricular filling only and to relate CVP values to left ventricular filling pressure without recognizing these limitations is not only misleading but in some cases dangerous. Patients with myocardial dysfunction can have a high CVP even though they have a deficit in their extracellular fluid volume. Conversely serious overloads of volume can be given to normal patients without significant changes in the CVP.

The recent development of the flow-directed balloon-tipped (Swan-Ganz) catheter has been a major advance in the care of the poor risk patient. This catheter permits the indirect measurement of the left atrial pressure by measuring the PCWP.[17] The PCWP has been shown to be virtually identical to the left atrial pressure over the range of 6 to 35 mmHg. Thus, the PCWP reflects the filling pressure of the left ventricle just as the CVP reflects the filling pressure of the right ventricle. The measurement of the PCWP is advantageous in that left ventricular response to a given fluid load is immediately observed, obviating the dangers of the lag phenomenon when the CVP is used alone.

The balloon-tipped catheter can be introduced into the circulation by any of the routes commonly used for the CVP catheter. One may encounter some degree of trepidation over the use of the Swan-Ganz catheter as opposed to the CVP catheter. However, the immediate hazards of either CVP or PCWP catheter use are the same because the method of entry into the circulation is the same; but the information gleaned from the PCWP is of greater value (Table 6-5). The insertion of the catheter for the measurement of PCWP is simple and fast in experienced hands. It offers further advantage in that it can be inserted before or immediately after the induction of anesthesia. X-ray confirmation of placement is not an immediate necessity and it can serve

TABLE 6-5 INDICATIONS FOR CENTRAL MONITORING (CVP AND PCWP)*

Measurement of the CVP and PCWP
  Trauma
    Patients with cardiovascular disease undergoing major surgery
    Surgical procedures in which large volume shifts are anticipated

Lack of availability of peripheral veins

Rapid administration of blood and fluids

Hyperalimentation or long term parenteral feedings

Operations in which venous air embolism is a consideration (Head and neck operations in the sitting position)

Placement of transvenous cardiac pacemaker

Sampling site for mixed venous blood

Removal of blood for autotransfusion

Site for administration of potent vasoactive or caustic drugs.

*CVP, central venous pressure; PCWP, pulmonary capillary wedge pressure.

as a source of mixed venous blood gases. In addition, Swan-Ganz catheters now have a triple lumen that permits, with a single catheter insertion, assessment of biventricular function—CVP, pulmonary artery pressures, and PCWP. Thermal-dilution cardiac output determinations may also be done with this catheter, facilitating even further the care of the high risk surgical patient.

The introduction of the PCWP catheter is not without hazards (Table 6-6). Any intravascular monitoring technique introduces the possibility of local or systemic infection. Thrombosis around or embolus from the catheter is another rare but potential hazard. Meticulous attention to asepsis will avoid infection. The balloon of the catheter should remain deflated except when the PCWP (left atrial pressure [LAP]) is being measured. Maintenance of the line with heparinized crystalloid solution and removal of the catheter after 72 hours will prevent thromboembolic phenomenon.

The use of this degree of invasive mon-

TABLE 6-6 COMPLICATIONS OF PULMONARY ARTERY CATHETERIZATION FOR PCWP

Those encountered while performing central venous cannulation

Cardiac arrhythmias (usually transient and cease as balloon passes through pulmonary valve)

Thrombosis around catheter shaft

Knotting of catheter in the heart

Perforation of the pulmonary artery with catheter tip

Balloon rupture

Pulmonary infarction

Systemic sepsis

itoring is certainly not required in every major surgical case. However, patients who in addition to their head and neck disease have a history of myocardial dysfunction, chronic lung disease, or questionable blood volume status should receive the benefits of Swan-Ganz catheter monitoring either before or immediately after the induction of anesthesia. As with any medical or surgical procedure, the benefits should be weighed against the potential hazards—the operator's ability and experience notwithstanding. Keep in mind that mortality and morbidity from inadequate or excessive volume replacement are far more common than are complications from invasive monitoring.[14]

Despite modern monitoring techniques, the urinary output level remains perhaps the most valuable guide to continued fluid therapy. Urinary output must be monitored in any lengthy operation where blood losses are expected to exceed 10 percent of the patient's blood volume. This monitoring is even more important for the patient in whom fluid balance and blood volume is unstable. Urinary output under these circumstances is the gauge against which the value of all other monitored physiological parameters are evaluated. The object of volume management is to maintain tissue perfusion and oxygenation. The CVP and PCWP may reveal to us how the heart and lungs are handling a given quantity of fluid but the urinary output level reveals the quality and quantity of the distribution of the cardiac output. The value of this information should not be underestimated because of the lack of sophistication of the technique. Fluids are administered during surgery to maintain a urinary output of near 1 ml/kg/hr. Oliguria, defined as 0.5 ml/kg/hr or less, or an unexpected diuresis is cause for reexamination and alteration in fluid therapy regardless of the data being received from the pressure monitors. However, the pressure monitors will usually reveal the trend toward hypovolemia or hypervolemia before it is revealed as a change in urine output. Thus, the combination of electronic monitor use and urinary output measurement is more valuable together than either is alone. The monitors allow one to keep "ahead" of the patient and the urinary output level will confirm or refute the ministrations of the anesthesiologist. The use of the Foley catheter is of further benefit during lengthy surgical procedures in that a distended bladder is a common and often unrecognized source of cardiac dysrhythmias and hypertension during surgery.

SPECIAL ANESTHETIC TECHNIQUES FOR BLOOD CONSERVATION

The increasing numbers and complexity of surgical procedures for trauma, radical cancer surgery, and cardiac surgery have resulted in an exponential increase in blood demands over the past decade. A proportional growth in population has not relieved this scarce national product. Less than 3 percent of the total population accounts for the blood donated annually. More than 5 percent of all patients receiving transfusions of homologous blood or blood products have some type of unfavorable reaction. This remains true despite the high standards maintained by modern blood banks.

Thus, the control of bleeding by improved surgical hemostasis and special anesthetic techniques reduces the need for multiple transfusions and the risks of transfusion complications. Several techniques have been developed within the past decade to reduce blood loss during surgery, which is of direct benefit to patients and the surgeon exclusive of the socioeconomic reasons for blood conservation.

Special anesthetic techniques for the prevention of blood loss include controlled hypotension, positioning, and autologous transfusion. The recent development of medical electronic monitoring has allowed the reexamination and refinement of hypotensive techniques as well as the development of several methods of autologous transfusion. Extensive experience has been gained in hypotensive anesthesia and autologous transfusions for open heart surgery, orthopedics, and neurosurgery. Hypotensive anesthesia has been commonly used for middle ear microsurgery in the United Kingdom. Only recently has the application of deliberate hypotension for this and other head and neck procedures been applied in the United States.[29]

Controlled Hypotension

Deliberate controlled hypotension was introduced in 1946 during an era when the risk of homologous blood transfusion was prodigious. As transfusion became safer in the 1950's, the popularity of hypotensive anesthesia decreased. The risks of hypotensive anesthesia, as it was then performed, became greater than the risks of blood transfusion. During the past 20 years the refinement of surgical techniques in all areas has made surgical results sufficiently reproducible that the surgical risk is often less than that of transfusion.

Hypotensive techniques have provided benefits in addition to blood conservation. Better surgical conditions are realized through better visualization. Orthopedic surgeons have used a localized form of hypotension with the use of tourniquets for just this purpose. Many would agree that the surgeon can see tumor margins better during hypotension, especially during head and neck dissections. Some centers report a significant reduction of surgical time. In addition, these techniques allow complex surgical procedures on patients with cross-matching problems as well as those whose religious beliefs prohibit transfusion.[18] Hypotensive anesthesia and autologous transfusion have been proven safe, effective, and easy to perform but proper patient selection is the pivot around which their reputation has gained favor. The use of these techniques is not to be taken casually and should not obscure the fact that surgical skill remains paramount in minimizing operative blood loss. Thus the need for hypotensive anesthesia during certain surgical procedures plus the availability of newer technology and drugs have spurred the resurgence in the use of hypotensive anesthesia.

Deliberate hypotension implies the purposeful lowering of a patient's blood pressure to systolic blood pressure levels of 65 to 70 mmHg (torr) or to a mean arterial pressure (MAP) of 55 to 60 mmHg. One might question why this might not be more appropriately termed deliberate shock. There is little doubt that the early attempts at this technique did produce shock. Better understanding of the principles of circulation has resulted in a very important distinction between shock and hypotension. Shock, from whatever the cause, is a syndrome complex in which hypotension is associated with the signs and symptoms of sympathetic hyperactivity. The neurohumoral response of vasoconstriction essential to survival in shock in the early stages makes shock, in time, a destructive force. The result is inadequate tissue perfusion of vital organs. There is persuasive evidence that the major component of the destructive pathophysiology of shock is due to sympathetic hyperactivity in the presence of untreated—relative or absolute—hypovolemia. Local tissue perfusion is clearly more important than absolute blood pressure. Hypotension combined with vasodilatation, blocking the compensatory vasoconstriction, produces more favorable conditions than hypotension accompanied by vasoconstriction.[18, 35, 39] If vascular resistance falls in proportion with the blood pressure, then local tissue perfusion will not be adversely affected, at least with mean arterial pressures down to 50 torr in normal healthy patients. Below this level, tissue perfusion will become pressure dependent. This explains in part why unintentional hypotension under anesthesia has been noted to produce fewer adverse effects than in unanesthetized patients. Sympathetic responses to the fall in blood pressure are blocked, and the reduction of tissue blood flow is less than when the vasoconstriction is present.

Controlled hypotension has been a most controversial subject in the past. Recent advances in our knowledge of circulatory hemodynamics and applied technology have led to a more rational application of these principles. Extensive studies on brain, heart, liver, and kidney function have been done with various types of controlled hypotension. These studies combined with published experiences with the technique indicate that few functional abnormalities occur when the hypotension is kept within safe limits.

The brain is the organ most sensitive to hypotension and brain damage is the most feared complication. The brain has a remarkable ability to maintain constant overall blood flow with perfusion pressures of 60 to 160 torr provided that normal ventilation and oxygenation is maintained. The perfusion pressure of the brain equals the MAP minus the venous pressure. Any situation that increases the venous pressure whether it is head down-tilt or an obstructed airway would reduce cerebral blood flow without a change in arterial pressure. Likewise, increased intracranial pressure limits cerebral perfusion and may represent a contraindication to induced hypotension. Notwithstanding the above considerations, if the MAP falls below 60 torr, cerebral autoregulation is compromised and the perfusion then becomes pressure dependent. The minimal permissible MAP is 50 torr. Rarely are pressure reductions of this magnitude

necessary to achieve a dry operative field. Cerebral aneurysm clipping is an exception to this rule but even then pressures lower than 50 torr are used only for very brief periods.

Coronary artery perfusion is determined principally by diastolic pressure. During induced hypotension, coronary blood flow may decrease, but the decrease in myocardial work and oxygen consumption as a result of the reduced afterload restores the balance between oxygen demand and supply in the absence of occlusive coronary artery disease. Renal and liver blood flow, though less well studied, also remain adequate when pressure is maintained at or above a mean of 60 torr. Preoperative evidence of coronary artery disease is a contraindication to elective induced hypotension (Table 6-7). In fact, evidence of com-

TABLE 6-7 CONTRAINDICATIONS TO CONTROLLED HYPOTENSION

Absolutes
Inexperienced anesthesiologist
Acute cardiovascular disease (unless used to reduce left ventricular afterload)
Reduced blood volume and/or gross anemia
Severe renal or hepatic disease
Leber optic atrophy, tobacco amblyopia, and vitamin B_{12} deficiency (nitroprusside)

Relative
Extremes of age
Coronary artery disease or congestive failure (except for afterload reduction)
Cerebral or peripheral vascular disease
Advanced pulmonary disease
Bronchospastic pulmonary disease (trimethaphan)
History of phlebitis or embolism
Symptomatic hypertension
Plasma cholinesterase deficiencies (trimethaphan)
Any contraindication for lumbar puncture if this technique is contemplated, i.e., bleeding diathesis, pernicious anemia
Glaucoma (with ganglionic blockers)

(Lawson, N. W., Thompson, D. S., Nelson, C. L., Flacke, J. W., and North, E. R. 1976. Sodium nitroprusside for supine total hip replacement. Anesthesia and Analgesia (Cleveland), 55: 654.)

promised blood flow to any critical organ obviates the use of deliberate hypotension. Organ perfusion becomes pressure dependent when the ability to autoregulate (i.e., arteriosclerosis) is lost. Thus, patients with coronary artery disease are in double jeopardy. Disaster is courted by either decreasing the MAP and oxygen supply or increasing the MAP, which increases oxygen demand.

METHODS

General anesthetics can alter sympathetic tone and can be used alone to produce hypotension. Halothane and enflurane have been used in selected patients with good results but the lowering of the blood pressure is primarily due to myocardial depression. Blood pressure may also be controlled by altering the resistance directly utilizing vasodilating drugs or indirectly with pharmacologic sympathectomy in addition to general anesthesia.

Temporary Sympathectomy. This technique can be used for head and neck procedures but has the disadvantage of poor control. A spinal or epidural anesthesia is given and then general anesthesia is administered. The operative site is elevated above the heart, and the patient positioned to allow venous pooling below the site of the block. This technique might predispose the patient to lower extremity thrombosis but might be useful when the drugs used for other techniques are contraindicated.

Ganglionic blockers are useful in producing hypotension. Pentolinium (Ansolysen) and trimethaphan (Arfonad) are the principal ganglionic blockers that have been used. Pentolinium is a long-acting agent whose primary disadvantage is poor controllability. Trimethaphan is a short-acting agent that can give good pressure control —if it works. Tachyphylaxis is a major problem with its use. The ganglionic blockade from either drug also produces fixed and dilated pupils during and following surgery, and hypoglycemia can be a problem. Bronchospastic disease is a contraindication to the use of either agent. These

drugs were the primary means of inducing hypotension before the application of direct acting vasodilators. Their use has been proven safe in properly selected patients.

Direct Acting Vasodilators. Recently, intravenous nitroglycerin has been introduced as a vasodilating agent for producing deliberate hypotension. Its action is primarily venodilatation when used for this purpose. Coronary arteries are also vasodilated, and this improves flow during induced hypotension in the absence of coronary artery disease. Blood pressure control is less reliable with this agent than with nitroprusside.

Sodium nitroprusside (Nipride) has been used in some centers since 1962 to produce deliberate hypotension. Nitroprusside is reported to produce a controlled hypotension that in contrast to other hypotensive techniques enhances cardiovascular dynamics. It is a potent antihypertensive which produces direct arteriolar vasodilatation independent of the autonomic nervous system. Nitroprusside produces predominantly arteriolar vasodilatation in contrast to nitroglycerin whose effect is predominantly venular. Blood pressure can be controlled easily, and little tachyphylaxis has been reported. This technique requires direct monitoring of arterial pressure and a calibrated drug pump for safest use. Given as a continuous infusion, pressure responses can occur within 2 minutes. The desired blood pressure level can be titrated by changes in the infusion rate. Should the pressure decline precipitously the infusion need only be discontinued and a rapid rise in pressure will ensue.

Nitroprusside appears to have no major side effects during short-term use. Prolonged use (> 24 hours) or high doses may cause accumulation of the nitroprusside metabolites thiocyanate and cyanide. The total dose of nitroprusside should not exceed 1.5 mg/kg. This maximum dose is very high for the usual patient. An occasional patient may develop resistance to nitroprusside in which case the infusion should be stopped and an alternate method of inducing hypotension should be used so as to avoid cyanide toxicity.[23] Another indication for discontinuing nitroprusside is the development of an unexplained metabolic acidosis, which must be considered cyanide toxicity until proven otherwise. The early effects of cyanide can be reversed by the intravenous administration of thiosulfate or hydroxocobalamin (vitamin B_{12A}). The administration of packed red cells may also be efficacious to serve as a fresh repository wherein cyanide can be converted to less harmful cyanmethemoglobin. Contraindications for the use of nitroprusside other than vascular disease include the presence of Leber optic atrophy, tobacco amblyopia, and vitamin B_{12} deficiency. All are indications that the metabolism necessary for the detoxification of cyanide has been altered. Even small amounts of nitroprusside in these cases may result in cyanide toxocity and accentuation of the disease.

A dry operative field during the course of surgery with hypotension should not foster complacency toward hemostasis. It is an absolute necessity with any hypotensive technique that the blood pressure be returned toward normal before skin closure is begun. If this is not done, postoperative hematoma may be a regular consequence.

Position

Regardless of the use of hypotensive anesthesia, a head-up posture is effective in reducing bleeding during head and neck surgery. In this position, venous and capillary pressures are reduced, affording some protection of cerebral perfusion during induced hypotension (cerebral blood flow = MAP − CVP). In addition, the amount of hypotensive drugs required to produce a given level of hypotension is reduced. The mean arterial blood pressure is reduced 2 mmHg for every inch that the operative site is above the heart. This is the effect of gravity operating against the column of blood being pumped to the brain from the heart. The reverse is true when the operative site is below the heart level. For example, neurosurgeons often place their patients in the full sitting position for posterior fossa craniotomies. The operative site may be as much as 18 inches above the heart. As a result, the intracranial MAP could be roughly 35 torr less than a cuff pressure would indicate, taken at the level of the heart. This pressure differential must be taken into account whenever the patient's position is other than supine. Radial artery cannulas are used during hypotensive anesthesia. It is then a simple matter to raise the transducer to the level of the operative site or the brain to get an accurate reflection of the perfusion pressure at the operative site. This counters the effect of gravity and is the pressure followed to produce a dry operative field—not the one at the heart level. This further assures that the organs below the operative site and certainly those below the heart (kidneys, liver) are receiving perfusion pressures approaching normotensive levels, whereas, only the operative site is hypotensive.

Autologous Transfusion

The use of autologous transfusion techniques is a developing area. These techniques have been of proven value in procedures that normally use high volumes of blood replacement such as open heart surgery, orthopedics, and trauma.

The following three types of autologous transfusion techniques are in use today:[8]

Preoperative blood collection, frozen storage, and reinfusion during or after surgery. Blood can be withdrawn many weeks before surgery and stored as frozen red cells. Studies indicate excellent patient tolerance of the withdrawal of 1 to 3 units over a period of time. Patients with preexisting transfusion incompatabilities should be considered candidates for this technique if preoperative time is available. The local transfusion hepatitis rate is another consideration.

Intraoperative phlebotomy with hemodilution. This technique has been used extensively for open heart surgery where two units of whole blood are removed during the procedure and the volume replaced with crystalloid (3:1). The blood is kept at room temperature and reinfused following hemostasis. The advantage here is that the patient is receiving his own whole fresh blood with intact clotting factors. This technique is likely of little value in head and neck cases, since the circulation is under less control than where cardiopulmonary bypass can be instantly instituted should the patient have an untoward effect from the blood withdrawal or crystalloid infusion.

Intraoperative shed blood salvage. This technique is being used to salvage blood by returning the blood from the surgical field to the circulation via a filter; however, the method is of limited value at the present time because the salvage may also include bile, bowel contents, sepsis, and particulate matter. Its successful use is reported primarily in trauma surgery where extensive blood salvage can be achieved. Intraoperative blood salvage during head and neck cancer surgery is not yet feasible as cancer cells from the operative site may also be reinfused. Current studies are focusing on better techniques to cleanse the salvaged blood; thus; it might become feasible in the future to employ blood salvage in cancer surgery.

These three methods of blood conservation are of limited value to the head and neck cancer surgeon and anesthesiologist but are mentioned as reference toward future developments.

AIR EMBOLUS

Venous air embolism should be anticipated in any head and neck case in which the patient is in a head-up position. The danger of air embolism is more likely when the CVP is low and the patient is breathing spontaneously. Air embolism is more closely associated with intracranial operations in the full sitting position. Its incidence is hard to assess in other operations on the head and neck though it has been reported.

Air embolism occurring with the patient in the sitting position is described as a catastrophic event associated with a mill-wheel murmur, circulatory collapse, and a high mortality. Newer monitors such as the Doppler chest piece have shown its occurrence to be more common than previously realized.[20] Patients undergoing surgical procedures in which air embolism is a real possibility should have a CVP catheter inserted so that its tip is located in the middle of the right atrium. CVP catheters are now marketed specifically for this purpose. The catheters serve as a wandering electrocardiograph electrode. During the insertion of the CVP, which may also be indicated for other purposes, the ECG is followed. When the p waves become biphasic and are larger in amplitude than the QRS, the catheter tip is located precisely in the midatrium. Studies of the incidence of air embolism with the Doppler and midatrial catheter have shown that a mill-wheel murmur is a late finding, as is cardiovascular collapse. Aspiration of air from the right atrium is diagnostic and therapeutic, and it can occasionally be detected before any other signs of air embolus appear.

Treatment of venous air emobolus in the absence of a midatrial CVP catheter consists of venous compression to retard air entry, discontinuation of nitrous oxide from the anesthetic circuit, elevation of the venous pressure at the wound by a sustained increase in airway pressure, and flooding of the wound with saline to detect the tear in the vessel. The judicious use of pressors that have a positive inotropic action may help disperse the air from the heart as well as support the circulation. Lidocaine may be required to treat ventricular arrhythmias.

The use of the left lateral Trendelenburg position can be effective treatment but is time consuming and difficult to achieve during surgery. The symptomatology of venous air embolism occurs because of blockage of right ventricular outflow by the air. Placing the patient in the left lateral Trendelenburg position will float the air away from the pulmonary valve and thus reestablish cardiac output. Systemic air embolism may also occur presenting other serious complications such as stroke. Approximately 20 percent of the normal population have a patent foramen ovale that is functionally closed but may open when the pulmonary artery pressure is elevated secondary to venous air embolus.[9] The result is the creation of a temporary right-to-left atrial shunt that will produce additional hypoxemia as well as allowing access of venous air to the systemic circulation. Obviously, prevention is better than treatment.

AIRWAY MANAGEMENT CONSIDERATIONS

One of the major advances in anesthesia and surgery has been the development of artificial airways. An artificial airway is defined as a tube inserted into the trachea that bypasses the upper airway and laryngeal structures as an integral part of the total airway. This means placing an endotracheal (oral or nasal) tube or performing a tracheostomy. The placement of an artificial airway is a serious step and definite criteria have been established to justify its use. These are the relief of airway obstruction, the protection of the airway, the facilitation of tracheal suctioning, and the facilitation of prolonged artificial ventilation. All four criteria are commonly met during the anesthetic management of head and neck cancer surgery.

Surgical difficulties on or around the upper airway are due to the anatomical complexities in a restricted field and the remarkable vascularity of the area. The surgeon requires unimpeded access to the area and a quiet and uncongested field. The anesthesiologist must provide for protection and patency of the airway at all times. In some instances the desire for operative space may clash with the need for a secure airway. The resolution of these conflicts requires the use of both skill and diplomacy to meet the fundamental requirements of the surgeon and anesthesiologist. Both parties should plan the airway management before surgery. The specific means by which the airway will be secured will be determined by

the surgical procedure, the patient's anatomy, the location of the tumor, the preexisting obstruction, and the need for continued ventilation after surgery.

The main difficulty in the anesthetic management of radical resection of the mandible, maxilla, or larynx is the establishment and maintenance of the airway. The larger proportion of emergencies that arise in relation to maintenance of the airway during anesthesia stem from failure both to recognize an airway problem before anesthesia and to anticipate its management. These problems can be described as involving three groups of patients. The first group consists of those patients with an unobstructed airway for whom introduction of an endotracheal tube is made difficult by anatomic or pathologic deformities. The second group are those patients who present with obvious and easily recognized obstruction; the problem then becomes a matter of planning the management of a recognized situation. The third group consists of patients in whom obstruction of the airway is not apparent and becomes evident only upon induction of anesthesia and relaxation of voluntary muscles. A large tongue or obesity are common causes of this difficulty.

Anatomic and functional abnormalities of the upper airway must be carefully evaluated. Patency of the nares is tested easily by alternate occlusion. Obvious nasal deformity and a history of obstruction warn of difficulties with nasotracheal intubation. Difficult laryngoscopy for intubation may be anticipated in individuals with deformities and fusion of the cervical spine; a short, thick neck; a receding lower jaw; prominent incisor teeth; a high arched palate; or a mouth that cannot be fully opened. Loose or prominent teeth should be noted before surgery as they may be lost or damaged during laryngoscopy. Following the preoperative examination, an airway management plan is formulated taking into account the surgeon's needs and the intended operation. For example, the surgeon may desire a nasotracheal tube during a maxillofacial dissection with the intention of doing a tracheostomy at the end of the operation. Examination of the patient might reveal that a nasotracheal intubation is not possible and an oral tube would be in the way. Thus, a tracheostomy may be performed at the start of the operation rather than an oral tube in order to remove the airway from the surgical field.

Nasal or oral endotracheal tubes may be inserted with the patient awake with local anesthesia and relaxation. In addition, nasal intubation can often be easily performed not only with the patient awake but without the need to visualize the vocal cords. The decision to perform an awake intubation is usually predicated on the presence of significant preoperative airway pathology or obstruction. The induction of anesthesia and relaxation are contraindicated for intubation if doubt exists about the ability to establish a patent airway. Patients presenting for laryngectomy epitomize the choices available for managing the airway. Indirect or direct laryngoscopy and radiologic studies of the neck provide information essential to the correct choice of airway management. Severe degrees of laryngeal obstruction from tumor require a preoperative tracheostomy under local anesthesia without benefit of an endotracheal tube. When the obstruction is less extreme, nasal or oral intubation can be performed with the patient awake under topical anesthesia. If the obstruction is only slight or absent, the intubation may be performed after administration of a short-acting barbiturate and a muscle relaxant. The dissemination of cancer cells is of concern when one intubates through an intralaryngeal tumor. If this is of concern to the surgeon, a tracheostomy may be performed under local anesthesia even though no airway obstruction exists.

Coiled wire endotracheal tubes (armored) are excellent for use in head and neck surgery. These tubes resist kinking even when bent at acute angles, which is an advantage over standard tubes. Because of their flexibility, they are the best tubes to use when working around the trachea or larynx and are ideally suited for laryngectomies.

The armored tubes may occasionally be difficult to insert because of their flexibility.

The development of the fiberoptic bronchoscope has been of great value in establishing the difficult oral or nasal airway.[28] This has alleviated problems where blind awake intubations or unprotected tracheostomies were necessary but undesirable. The glottic opening is identified through the scope, and the tube is then guided into the trachea over the scope. An adult fiberoptic bronchoscope cannot be used if a tube of 7.5 mm or less is indicated. Thus, a nasal intubation with this technique may not be indicated in the adult if the nares will not admit a larger tube. A pediatric scope can be used for tubes less than 7.5 mm to establish a temporary airway for controlled tracheostomy, or the bronchoscopic intubation can be performed orally.

Retrograde intubation can be performed in which a catheter is passed retrograde into the mouth or nose via a percutaneous cannulation through the cricothyroid membrane. The catheter is then threaded through the eye of the endotracheal tube and the tube then threaded into the trachea over the catheter. This technique has little application in head and neck surgery and is usually reserved for establishment of an emergency airway in trauma.

Tube Material

Current tube standards require that endotracheal tubes do not possess reactivity to animal tissues, allergenicity, or carcinogenicity. These standards require that plastics or rubber used for intratracheal airways be labeled with the symbol I.T. for "implantation tested" denoting that the material is nontoxic when implanted in rabbit muscle.[32, 33] Another symbol, Z-79, may be seen on airway devices. This stands for "Z-79 Committee for Anesthesia Equipment for the U.S.A. Standards Institute" indicating that the manufacturer has determined that the material used in the device is nontoxic to cell cultures. Any polymeric prosthetic device used today must carry one or both of these symbols to avoid liability in airway care.

Endotracheal and tracheostomy tubes are commonly made of Teflon, polyethylene, nylon, polyvinylchloride, or silicone. *Teflon* causes little tissue reaction and is easily sterilized by autoclaving without damage. Its prime disadvantage is rigidity and cost. *Polyethylene* is compatible with human tissue but is easily penetrated by general anesthetics, and autoclaving distorts the polymer. *Nylon* has been used for airways but is mentioned only to condemn the use of this material for airways. Nylon is degraded by moist heat, resulting in impurities that can become toxic to human tissue. These tubes are generally very rigid and are physically irritating. *Polyvinylchloride (PVC)* is the most widely used polymer for artificial airways, and today varying degrees of flexibility can be obtained by the use of nontoxic additives. Properly manufactured PVC tubes are nontoxic and possess the desired flexibility for use in surgery and postoperative care. These tubes are designed for disposal after use, since autoclaving will distort the PVC. They may be reused with ethylene oxide sterilization but must be throughly aerated and dried to avoid the formation of the toxic product ethylene glycol. *Silicone tubes,* which have the current disadvantage of high cost, are good prospects for use in the future as they are nontoxic, atraumatic to tissues, and can be autoclaved.

The Cuffed Tube

Artificial airways are used in surgical procedures and life-threatening conditions where the potential for harm seldom affects the decision to establish the airway. The immediate and specific complications of both the endotracheal tube and tracheostomy are well known. The late and postextubation complications of artificial airways are largely preventable and have in common the relatively recent use of the cuffed tube. Late complications are those occurring 24 to 48 hours after intubation. Postextubation complications are those occurring from 1 day to years following extubation. These complications include tracheal erosion, stenosis, dilatation, tracheoesophageal fistula, and erosion into the great vessels (Fig. 6-1). Patient factors that add to the incidence of cuff complications are airway sepsis, hypotension, and debilitation.

Stenosis at the tracheostomy site is excluded from the complications of cuffed tubes. Stomal site stenosis is unique to tra-

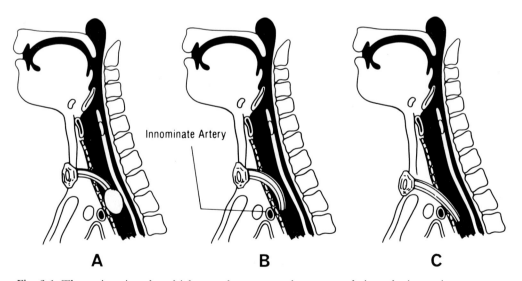

A **B** **C**

Fig. 6-1. Three situations by which a tracheostomy tube may erode into the innominate artery. (A) excessive cuff pressures, (B) short tube, and (C) low tracheostomy.

cheostomy where some degree of stenosis is inevitable. The incidence of stomal stenosis without cuffed tubes is less than 2 percent,[22] whereas the use of cuffed tubes increases the incidence of clinically evident stenosis to about 5 percent.[11] These data indicate that stomal stenosis will occur with or without the use of cuffed tubes. In contrast, stenosis resulting from cuffed tubes is usually found a few centimeters below the stoma in tracheostomies and at the corresponding cuff site with endotracheal tubes.

Tracheal stenosis following the use of cuffed tubes occurs more frequently than is generally appreciated. Clinical studies citing a 2 to 5 percent incidence of tracheal stenosis with cuffed tracheal tubes refer to the presentation of dyspnea, stridor, and recurrent pulmonary infection. Studies in which laminograms and bronchograms were used have demonstrated that stenosis can be found in up to 20 percent of those patients in whom cuffed tubes were required for mechanical ventilation.[6, 26] These discrepancies are accounted for not only by the method of study but by the fact that stenosis is seldom evident clinically in adults until more than 50 percent of the tracheal lumen is occluded. The incidence of symptomatic tracheal stenosis requiring surgical repair is approximately 0.5 to 2 percent in patients receiving ventilator support with cuffed tracheal tubes.[30]

The blood pressure at the arterial end of the adult tracheal wall capillaries is approximately 30 mmHg. The capillary venous pressure is 18 mmHg. These pressures are similar to airway pressures normally attained during positive-pressure ventilation. Thus, any cuff pressure which exceeds these pressures will interrupt mucosal blood flow. Cuff pressures in excess of 30 mmHg will result in ischemia whereas those less than 30 mmHg but greater than 18 mmHg will result in venous congestion. Pressures of greater than 5 mmHg on the mucosa will exceed lymphatic pressure and result in edema.

The tracheal tube cuff is a balloon. As air is injected into the cuff, the intra-cuff pressures rise slowly until the cuff contacts the tracheal wall. At this point any additional volume of air will cause a sharp rise in the cuff pressures.[4] Until recently, tracheal tubes incorporated cuffs of low residual volume. As a result the intra-cuff pressures required to achieve a seal often exceeded 300 mmHg. The area of tracheal contact is quite narrow, and small increments of air added to the cuff will cause exponential increases in the cuff-to-trachea pressure. Tracheal mucosal perfusion pressures will always be exceeded by virtue of the low residual volume of the cuff and produce distortion of the trachea as well as destruction of the mucosa. The use of low residual volume cuffs is disappearing but they are still commonly found in emergency rooms and on wards. They have no place in modern surgical or respiratory care as they can be tolerated only briefly before significant tracheal damage occurs.

Current cuff designs incorporate large residual volumes that allow the cuff to effect a seal while draping freely on the tracheal wall (Fig. 6-2). These cuffs will inflate to large volumes at essentially zero pressures and have proven successful in reducing cuff-site ischemia and resultant damage[5] (Fig. 6-3). The use of these low-pressure cuffs has not totally alleviated the problem of tracheal damage. Many cuffed tracheal tubes that are advertised as low-pressure cuffs do not reduce the pressures below the safe level of 25 torr. The floppy cuffs are easily torn, especially during nasal intubation, and can obstruct the airway if excessive volume is injected into the cuff (Fig. 6-4). The proper selection of the tube size is important to realize the benefits of the low-pressure cuff. If the selected tube is too small, the inflation pressure needed to effect a seal with the soft cuff will be excessive. Actual measurements of intra-cuff pressures are fraught with difficulties and only approximate the cuff-to-wall pressure. However, the actual cuff pressure of the high volume-low pressure cuffs will be near that measured. If a low-pressure cuff requires greater than 20 torr to achieve a seal,

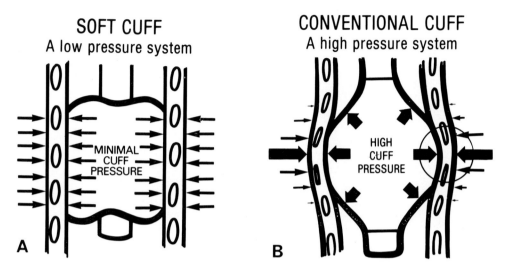

Fig. 6-2. A comparison of the method of seal between (A) the high volume-low pressure cuff and (B) the low volume-high pressure cuff. The low volume cuff effects a seal over a smaller surface area at very high pressure causing distortion of the trachea as well as ischemia.

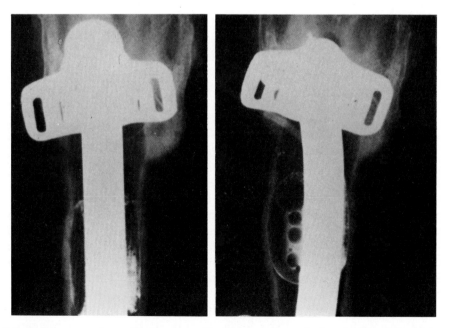

Fig. 6-3. X-rays were taken of both types of cuff using the no-leak technique. The high-pressure cuff (right) shows uneven inflation and tracheal distortion compared to the low-pressure cuff (left). The pressure at the time the leak ceased with the high-pressure cuff was 155 mmHg compared to 17 mmHg for the low-pressure cuff.

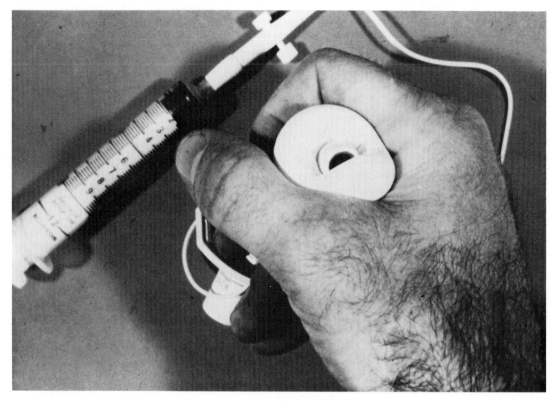

Fig. 6-4. High volume-low pressure cuffs can obstruct the airway if excessive volumes are used.

it means that the tube is too small and should be replaced.

Cuff Care

Proper inflation and deflation techniques of the cuffed tube are essential in the maintenance of the airway and avoidance of complications. Physiological necessity may require that the cuffs be used in a manner that is outside their envelope of safety. Experience in the care of the critically ill has demonstrated the advantages and limitations of both the cuffed endotracheal tube and tracheostomy.

Today over 90 percent of the patients receiving the benefits of mechanical ventilation for acute repiratory failure are in surgical intensive care units. The necessity for mechanical ventilation is the result of direct trauma, sepsis, or the combination of chronic lung disease coupled with a neces-

sary surgical procedure. Laryngectomy patients often fall into the latter category. Positive pressure ventilation requires a sealed airway mandating the use of the cuffed tube whether on an endotracheal tube or a tracheostomy. Several life-saving mechanical ventilation techniques include the use of positive end expired pressure (PEEP), continuous positive airway pressure (CPAP), and intermittent mandatory ventilation (IMV). These techniques require positive pressure ventilation and no-leak use of the cuffs. Most of the complications attributed to the use of cuffed tracheal tubes are found in patients who require mechanical ventilation.

Anticipated complications, however, must be viewed in relation to the benefits. Twenty years ago postextubation tracheal problems were rare, since most of the patients did not survive mechanical ventilation. This fact provides the proper perspective through which the problem of complications must be viewed. The possibility of tracheal stenosis is no contraindication to the use of cuffed tubes when indicated for proper airway management.

Two methods of cuff inflation may be used with the low-pressure cuffs. These are the minimal occlusion and the minimal leak techniques. Minimal occlusion means that only that volume of air necessary to stop the leak of air from around the cuff at the peak inspiratory pressure is used—and no more! This is attained by inflating the cuff while listening with a stethoscope over the trachea. The minimal leak technique, which is the safest method to use to avoid tracheal complications, is performed similarly to the minimal occlusion technique except that once the leak is sealed, the cuff is deflated just to the point that a small leak can be heard at peak inspiratory pressure. Cuff pressures are then measured to assure that they do not exceed 20 torr.

During head and neck surgery the no-leak method of cuff inflation is used to control ventilation and anesthesia as well as to prevent the aspiration of surgical debris. If the endotracheal tube or the tracheostomy tube is to remain in place after surgery, the cuff can then be totally deflated or reduced to minimal leak. Continued postoperative mechanical ventilation can be performed with the minimal leak cuff; however, the use of PEEP or CPAP will require the no-leak technique. The use of occluding cuffs in the postoperative period requires that cuff pressures be measured at least every 4 hours. Cuff pressures do not remain stable. Changes in the patient's temperature and the diffusion of gases, such as oxygen and nitrous oxide, into the cuff will alter cuff volumes. Oxygen may continue to diffuse into the cuff in the postoperative period whereas nitrous oxide will diffuse out at the conclusion of surgery. Pressures should be maintained or readjusted to keep the pressure below 20 torr. Five torr would be ideal if a seal can be maintained. The inflation of cuffs by injecting arbitrary volumes of air into the cuff is to be condemned and only invites needless complications.

"Trachea chasing" is a phenomenon common to patients receiving long-term positive pressure no-leak ventilation.[30] Cuffs that are inflated to seal during peak airway pressure will be overinflated during the exhalation phase when the tracheal lumen is reduced. This results in tracheal dilatation. Maintenance of no-leak ventilation then requires additional increments of cuff volume. Tracheal dilatation is rarely a problem in patients with no-leak cuffs who are breathing spontaneously, since intratracheal pressure changes are minimal. Severe degrees of tracheal dilatation may lead to esophageal compression and may contribute to the incidence of aspiration, dysphagia, and ulcerations caused by nasogastric tubes. Tracheal perforation may eventually occur (Fig. 6-5).

Periodic deflation of tracheal cuffs is not necessary if the inflating cuff pressures have been properly managed. Hourly deflation for 5 minutes is of less benefit than once believed. The original purpose of periodic deflation was to restore blood flow to the tracheal mucosa. There is no evidence to show that capillary blood flow is restored in less than 1 hour following deflation of the cuff from high occlusive pressures. Capillary mucosal blood flow is certainly not restored in the often prescribed 5 minutes. Patients who require controlled positive-pressure ventilation often do not tolerate deflation of the cuff. In addition, periodic inflation and deflation increases the possibility of careless inflation techniques and of possibly increasing cuff pressures and aspiration. Once the cuff is inflated using minimal occlusion or minimal leak the cuff is not routinely deflated. Proper cuff pressure management obviates the necessity for periodic deflation.

Certain safeguards must be taken whenever deflation of a tube cuff is necessary. The trachea must first be suctioned followed by suctioning of the pharynx above the cuff. The cuff may then be deflated followed by immediate tracheal suctioning to remove any secretions that may have

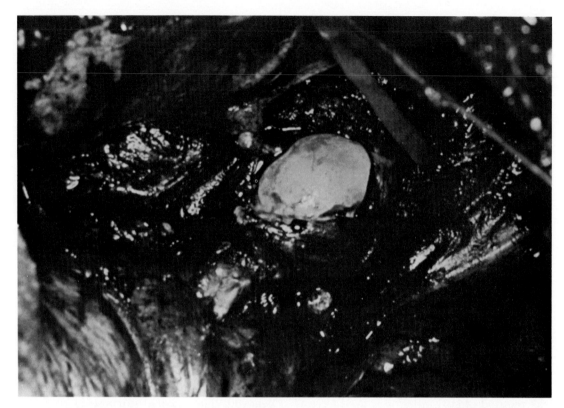

Fig. 6-5. This is an open thoracotomy looking toward the right medial apex. The cuff of an endotracheal tube has eroded through the trachea into the thorax. This complication was asymptomatic and was not suspected until the thoracotomy was performed. Routine x-rays did not reveal the erosion, since the uneven inflation of the cuff had eroded posteriorly and was not evident with an anteroposterior x-ray.

slipped past the tube when the cuff was deflated. Another maneuver is to apply positive pressure to the lungs while the cuff is being deflated to blow secretions back into the pharynx where they can be suctioned.

Humidification and Suctioning

The normal respiratory tract conditions and humidifies inspired air primarily in the upper airway. Nasal inspiration raises humidity to 80 to 90 percent at a temperature of 32° to 34°C; by contrast the humidity will be about 60 percent at a temperature of 21°C with mouth breathing. By the time it reaches the alveoli, inspired air is 100 percent humidified and the temperature is 37°C. If the upper airway is bypassed with an endotracheal tube, natural air and temperature conditioning mechanisms will be ineffective.

A patient with a tracheostomy, for example, has 10 percent less relative humidity and 6° to 7°C lower temperature than has a healthy person. Water is lost by evaporation from the lower respiratory tract because the upper airway has been bypassed.

Any gas, including room air, delivered to an artificial airway must be 100 percent humidified at body temperature. Failure to properly humidify the airway will result in dried secretions in the artificial airway and possible obstruction. In the past, this led to the frequent changing of artificial airways and the routine cleansing of inner cannulas of tracheostomy tubes every 3 to 4 hours. Humidification decreases this need, since crusting and obstruction of the airway is seldom encountered if the humidification equipment is functioning properly. With the use of humidification, there is no reason for routine changes in artificial airways; they should only be changed when there is a definite indication for a change. Unnecessary extubation and intubation should be avoided.

Humidification should be provided through a heated nebulizer. This humidification can be provided through any of the current mechanical ventilators for patients requiring postoperative ventilation. Patients who are breathing spontaneously through an artificial airway may be provided with heated humidification through a T-piece with a reservoir tubing on the exhalation end. This provides for a high flow system that allows complete control of temperature, humidity, and oxygen without adding resistance to the circuit. For those long-term patients in whom oxygen therapy is not essential, humidity may also be added to the airway via a tracheostomy mask.

Tracheal suctioning is necessary to remove viscous secretions in patients with artificial airways. Suction technique is one of the areas of greatest abuse in managing artificial airways. Hypoxia and atelectasis are immediate hazards as is the introduction of infection.[38] Suctioning techniques should be specifically written as part of the postoperative orders.

The choice of the suction catheter is as important as the suction technique. The catheters should have smooth molded ends with side holes to avoid damage to the tracheal mucosa. The catheters should have a proximal thumb-hole for control of the suction pressure, and the catheter size should be no larger than 2/3 of the internal diameter of the tube to be suctioned. If the catheter is larger, extreme negative pressures can be produced within the respiratory tract causing collapse of the lungs. Children are more susceptible to this disaster because of the variety of the size of their airways and because the casual attendant may not pay attention to this detail. High suction pressures will also cause the catheter to function as a curette denuding the tracheal mucosa during suctioning. Vacuum pressures in excess of −120 mmHg facilitate this process

but even proper vacuum levels of −80 to −120 mmHg do not entirely eliminate this process. Ring-tipped catheters have reduced the incidence of this type of injury. The relationship between suction damage to the trachea and tracheal infection remains unclear but it would seem obvious that less damage could only be better for the patient and a guard against infection.

The use of an artificial airway practically guarantees contamination of the airway but not necessarily infection. A gloved sterile technique should be used at all times. This technique includes the use of a sterile catheter and sterile rinsing solutions for the catheter. The catheter must never be reused. The incidence of complications and mucosal damage will be minimized using the following steps:

1. Suctioning should be preceded by several minutes of preoxygenation with 100 percent oxygen. This step will avoid arterial hypoxemia during the period of suctioning.

2. The catheter is inserted without vacuum (open thumb-hole) into the airway until the tip is at the desired suctioning level. Intermittent suctioning is then started rotating the catheter as it is removed. The intermittent suction and rotation minimizes mucosal damage and removes secretions more effectively. Suction time should never exceed 15 seconds. The total time from the start of suctioning until ventilation is reestablished should never exceed 20 seconds. These times will need to be shortened to 5 seconds for adults who are already hypoxic despite preoxygenation, for infants, and for children. Patients requiring frequent suctioning *must* be monitored with an electrocardiographic monitor. Many deaths often attributed to vagal reflexes have been reported during suctioning. Vagal reflexes may play a part in producing bradycardia during suctioning, but more often bradycardia or other arrhythmias are the result of hypoxia rather than some nebulous reflex. Any arrhythmia that develops during the suctioning is reason to immediately stop the suction and ventilate the patient with 100 percent oxygen.

3. After suctioning, the patient should be placed on 100 percent oxygen and given at least 5 deep breaths. Failure to hyperinflate the lungs with oxygen can result in prolonged hypoxia requiring up to 30 minutes before blood oxygenation has returned to the presuction level. Suctioning during this interval would lead to further hypoxia if the lungs are not hyperinflated after suctioning.

These three steps should be repeated until the airway appears clear. The tracheal catheter may then be used to clear oropharyngeal secretions but must never be reused in the trachea. These steps should be taken when one is taking culture specimens as well.

Extubation

The weaning of patients from ventilators should not be confused with weaning the patient from a tracheal tube. The indications for initiating or discontinuing mechanical ventilation will not be discussed; however, indications for extubation will be discussed assuming that mechanical ventilation has already been discontinued. Many patients who do not require mechanical ventilation may require an artificial airway for other reasons. These reasons are upper airway obstruction (i.e. edema), protection of the airway, and the need for suctioning and ventilation.

Generally, artificial airways can be removed when the cause for their placement is no longer present. If the airway was placed because of upper airway obstruction, the only sure way of testing whether or not the airway is needed is to extubate and watch for recurring signs of obstruction. Tubes that are placed for protection of the airway are more easily evaluated for extubation. This evaluation involves testing of the airway reflexes. Airway reflexes are obtunded from the top down, that is, pharyngeal, laryngeal, tracheal, and finally carinal. If the patient has a good swallowing mechanism (pharyngeal), it is likely that the laryngeal and carinal protective reflexes are

intact as well. The need for tracheal suctioning is dependent upon the patient's ability to cough. If the conscious patient has a vital capacity of 15 ml/kg and can sustain a negative inspiratory force of greater than 25 cm H_2O, it is reasonable to assume that airway hygiene can be achieved without an artificial airway or suctioning. Obviously the patient must be free of the need of mechanical ventilation before extubation. Once the decision is made to extubate, no one should remove an artificial airway who does not possess the skill to replace it.

Extubation should follow some basic steps:

1. Explain the procedure to the patient and elicit his cooperation.

2. Suction secretions from the trachea and then from the oral and nasal pharynx.

3. Increase the inspired oxygen concentration.

4. The tube should be removed at peak inspiration so that the patient can cough immediately upon removal. This may be accomplished by asking the patient to take a deep breath. At the very peak of inspiration the cuff is deflated and the tube rapidly removed. This may also be accomplished with a hand ventilator if the patient is uncooperative.

5. Supplemental humidified oxygen is administered immediately following extubation and the patient is observed for signs of obstruction. The patient is encouraged to cough and take deep breaths at this time. The patient is carefully watched until there is no doubt about his ability to function without the airway. Spare airways and equipment should remain at the bedside for a reasonable period of time following extubation.

Removal of the tracheostomy tube is not as pressing as that of the endotracheal tube. However, the indications for and technique of removing the tracheostomy tube are the same as those for removing an endotracheal tube. The tracheostomy imparts a greater degree of flexibility in extubation than does the endotracheal tube. The patients tolerate tracheostomy and are more easily evaluated for their ability to function without the tracheostomy by the use of a universal fenestrated tracheostomy tube. The fenestrated tube is one in which a window has been cut into the posterior of the outer cannula. When the tracheostomy is "corked," the patient can breathe around the tracheostomy tube and through the fenestration without having to remove the tube. The fenestrated tube allows the patient to speak but is not intended to be a long-term device. It is used primarily for testing the patient's ability to maintain the airway before actual extubation is performed. Following extubation of the tracheostomy the patient should be reassured that the stoma will close completely in about 48 hours. Epithelialization of the tract is rare unless tracheal infection is present.

In some cases tracheal buttons are used in the tracheostomy stoma following extubation. This may be done if future surgery is contemplated in which replacement of the tracheostomy tube may be necessary.

Proper management of the airway is a major factor in decreasing complications. There is little doubt that the variability in the standard of airway care across the country accounts for the disparity in published complication rates. Major factors contributing to airway complications are those factors that alone can cause problems: traumatic intubation, excessive cuff pressure, oversized tubes, improper tracheostomy procedure, duration of intubation, and toxic materials. Other predisposing factors include the age and sex of the patient.[30] The incidence of tracheostomy complications is much higher in children than in adults, and postintubation sore throat and granulomas are far more common in women than in men. This latter complication may be related to the frequent use of oversized tubes in women. Adjunctive factors in the development of complications relate to the patient's health. Hypoproteinemia, previous steroid therapy, or other factors related to poor healing will contribute to airway complications. All of these factors must be kept in mind whenever the complications of either endotracheal intubation or tracheostomy are discussed.

POSTANESTHETIC RECOVERY

The postanesthesia recovery room (PAR) holds an important place in the management of patients for head and neck surgery. It is a critical care area where the acute effects of surgery and anesthesia are observed and treated. During the immediate postanesthesia period, the patients are required to resume vital functions previously controlled by the anesthesiologist. Their ability to do this must be constantly monitored until it is safe to return them to the general nursing floors. Because of the magnitude of the operation or the presence of severe preexisting disease, some patients will be transferred to an intensive care unit directly from the operating room for extended observation or continued life support.

The need to describe objectively the physical condition of patients in the PAR has led to the development of a scoring system analogous to the Apgar score for newborns (Table 6-8). Five general categories consisting of activity, respiration, circulation, consciousness, and color are evaluated and scored 0, 1, or 2 on admission and periodically during the patient's stay. A score of 10 indicates a patient in the best possible condition. A total score of 7 or less is an indication for continued close monitoring.

Patients can present special problems during their PAR course. Some degree of hypothermia is usually present, which prolongs awakening time and increases the oxygen consumption on rewarming. The adequacy of intraoperative fluid management will become manifest as the intravascular volume equilibrates with the rest of the extracellular space. Incomplete fluid replacement will lead to progressive signs of hypovolemia; while vigorous hydration may lead to congestive heart failure in the mar-

TABLE 6-8 POSTANESTHETIC RECOVERY SCORE

Activity

Able to move 4 extremities voluntarily or
on command = 2
Able to move 2 extremities voluntarily or
on command = 1
Able to move 0 extremities voluntarily or
on command = 0

Respiration

Able to deep breathe and cough freely = 2
Dyspnea or limited breathing = 1
Apnea = 0

Circulation

Blood pressure ± 20% of preanesthetic level = 2
Blood pressure ± 20% to 50%
of preanesthetic level = 1
Blood pressure ± 50% of preanesthetic level = 0

Consciousness

Fully awake = 2
Arousable on calling = 1
Not responding = 0

Color

Pink = 2
Pale, dusky, blotchy, jaundiced, other = 1
Cyanotic = 0

(Modified from Aldrete, J. A., and Kroulik, D. 1970. A postanesthetic recovery score. Anesthesia and Analgesia (Cleveland), 49: 924.)

ginally compensated patient. Since head and neck cancer surgery usually involves manipulation or removal of structures in and around the airway, constant attention must be directed to the adequacy of ventilation and patency of the airway.

SUMMARY

From the preanesthetic assessment through the postanesthetic recovery phase, anesthesia for head and neck cancer surgery is a challenging and complicated area of anesthesia practice. Recognition of physiological derangements in these surgical patients and their adverse impact on the anesthetic has led to better preoperative preparation of these patients. Communication and planning by the surgeon and anesthesiologist avoid potential conflicts around a vital area where both must share the airway and adjacent structures. An understanding and agreement as to how the airway will be protected is of primary importance in assuring patient safety. An anesthetic plan which allows for any special needs of the proposed surgery and the patient must be formulated. Though important, the actual administration of a particular type of anesthetic assumes a secondary role to planning and intraoperative support of vital organs such as brain, heart, lungs, and kidneys. Meticulous attention to detail and alert monitoring of vital functions are required to prevent the development of life-threatening complications during surgery. The duration and degree of postoperative care must be anticipated and planned carefully.

REFERENCES

1. Aldrete, J. A., and Kroulik, D. 1970. A postanesthetic recovery score. Anesthesia and Analgesia (Cleveland), 49: 924.

2. Beecher, H. K., and Todd, D. P. 1954. A study of the deaths associated with anesthesia and surgery based on a study of 599,548 anesthetics in ten institutions 1948-1952, inclusive. Annals of Surgery, 140: 2.

3. Britt, B. A., Kwong, F. H., and Endrenyi, L. 1977. Management of malignant hyperthermia susceptible patients—a review. In Henschel, E. O., Ed.: Malignant Hyperthermia: Current Concepts. Appleton-Century-Crofts, New York, 63.

4. Carroll, R., Hedden, M., and Safar, P. 1969. Intratracheal cuffs: Performance characteristics. Anesthesiology, 31: 275.

5. Carroll, R. G., and Grenvik, A., 1973. A proper use of large diameter, large residual volume cuffs. Critical Care Medicine, 1: 153.

6. Cooper, J. D., and Grillo, H. C. 1969. The evolution of tracheal injury due to ventilatory assistance through cuffed tubes—a pathologic study. Annals of Surgery 169: 334.

7. Corrsen, G., and Sweet, R. B. 1967. Effects of halogenated anesthetic agents upon selectively starved cultured human liver cells. Anesthesia and Analgesia (Cleveland), 46: 575.

8. Couch, N. P., Laks, H., and Pilon, R. N. 1974. Autotransfusion in three variations. Archives of Surgery, 108: 121.

9. Daly, J. J. 1968. Venoarterial shunting in obstructive pulmonary disease. New England Journal of Medicine, 278: 952.

10. Dripps, R. D., Lamont, A., and Eckenhoff, J. E. 1961. The role of anesthesia in surgical mortality. JAMA, 178: 261.

11. Gibson, P. 1967. Actiology and repair of tracheal stenosis following tracheostomy and intermittent positive pressure breathing. Thorax, 25: 6.

12. Goldman, L., Caldera, D. L., Southwick, F. S., Nussbaum, S. R., Murray, B., O'Malley, T. A., Goroll, A. H., Caplan, C. H., Nolan, J., Burke, D. S., and Krogstad, D. 1978. Cardiac risk factors and complications in noncardiac surgery. Medicine (Baltimore), 57: 357.

13. Henschel, A., Mickelson, O., Taylor, H. L., and Keys, A. 1947. Plasma volume and thiocyanate space in famine edema and recovery. American Journal of Physiology, 150: 170.

14. Irvin, T. T., Hayter, C. J., Modgill, V. K., and Goligher, J. C. 1972. Clinical assessment of postoperative blood volume. Lancet, 2: 446.

15. James, P. M., and Myers, R. T. 1972. Central venous pressure monitoring: Misinterpretation, abuses, indications and a new technic. Annals of Surgery, 175: 693.

16. Jenkins, M. T., and Giesecke, A. H., Jr. 1974. Balanced salt solutions in clinical anesthesia. American Society of Anesthesiologists Refresher Courses, 2:9: 107.

17. Lappas, D., Lell, W. A., Gabel, J. C., Civetta, J. M., and Lowenstein, E. 1973. Indirect measurement of left-atrial pressure in surgical patients—pulmonary capillary wedge and pulmonary artery diastolic pressure compared with left atrial pressure. Anesthesiology, 38(4): 394.

18. Lawson, N. W., Thompson, D. S., Nelson, C. L., Flacke, J. W., and North, E. R. 1976. Sodium nitroprusside for supine total hip replacement. Anesthesia and Analgesia (Cleveland), 55: 654.

19. Lowenstein, E., and Bland, J. H. L. 1972. Anesthesia for cardiac surgery. In Norman, J. C., Ed.: Cardiac Surgery, 2nd edn. Appleton-Century-Crofts, New York, 75.

20. Martin, J. T. 1978. Positioning in Anesthesia and Surgery. W. B. Saunders, Philadelphia.

21. Mauney, F. M., Jr., Ebert, P. A., and Sabiston, D. C. 1970. Postoperative myocardial infarction: A study of predisposing factors, diagnosis and mortality in a high risk group of surgical patients. Annals of Surgery 172: 497.

22. Meade, J. W. 1961. Tracheostomy—its complications and their management. New England Journal of Medicine, 264: 587.

23. Michenfelder, J. D., and Tinker, J. H. 1977. Cyanide toxicity and thiosulfate protection during chronic administration of sodium nitroprusside in the dog—correlation with a human case. Anesthesiology, 47: 441.

24. Moster, J. W., Albano, P. C., Seniff, A., and Moore, R. H. 1968. Blood volume in patients with cancer. Anesthesia and Analgesia (Cleveland), 47(5): 643.

25. Nachlas, M. M., Abrams, S. J., and Goldberg, M. M. 1961. The influence of arteriosclerotic heart disease on surgical risk. American Journal of Surgery, 101: 447.

26. Pearson, F. G., Goldberg, M., and DaSilva, A. J. 1968. Tracheal stenosis complicating tracheostomy with cuffed tubes. Archives of Surgery, 97: 390.

27. Phillips, O. C., Frazier, T. M., Graff, T. D., and DeKornfeld, T. J. 1960. The Baltimore Anesthesia Study Commission. A review of 1024 postoperative deaths. JAMA, 174: 2015.

28. Raj, P. P., Forestner, J., Watson, T. D., Morris, R. E., and Jenkins, M. T. 1974. Technics for fiberoptic laryngoscopy in anesthesia. Anesthesia and Analgesia (Cleveland), 53: 708.

29. Schabery, S. J., Kely, J. F., Terry, B. C., Posner, M. A., and Anderson, E. F. 1976. Blood loss and hypotensive anesthesia in oral-facial corrective surgery. Journal of Oral Surgery, 34: 147.

30. Shapiro, B. A., Harrison, R. A., and Trout, C. A. 1975. Clinical Application of Respiratory Care. Year Book Medical Publishers, Chicago.

31. Skinner, J. F., and Pearce, M. L. 1964. Surgical risk in the cardiac patient. Journal of Chronic Diseases, 17: 57.

32. Spoerel, W. 1972. The unprotected airway. International Anesthesiology Clinics, 10: 1.

33. Stetson, J. B. 1970. Prolonged tracheal intubation for facilitation of tracheobronchial toilet and the treatment of atelectasis. International Anesthesiology Clinics, 8: 969.

34. Tarhan, S., Moffitt, E. A., Taylor, W. F., and Giuliani, E. R. 1972. Myocardial infarction after general anesthesia. JAMA, 220: 1451.

35. Taylor, T. H., Styles, M., and Lammins, A. J. 1970. Sodium nitroprusside as a hypotensive agent in general anesthetia. British Journal of Anaesthesia 42:   859.

36. Underwood, P. S., and Howland, W. S. 1966. Serial blood volume determinations associated with major cancer surgery. Anesthesia and Analgesia (Cleveland), 45:   797.

37. Underwood, P. S., Boyan, C. P., and Howland, W. S. 1966. Appraisal of RISA blood volume for clinical use: Anesthesia and Analgesia (Cleveland) 45:   1.

38. Urban, J. B., and Weitzner, S. W. 1969. Avoidance of hypoxemia during endotracheal suction. Anesthesiology, 31:   473.

39. Wildsmith, J. A. Q., Marshall, R. L., Jenkinson, J. L., MacRae, W. R., and Scott, D. B. 1973. Haemodynamic effect of sodium nitroprusside during nitrous oxide-halothane anesthesia. British Journal of Anaesthesia, 47:   71.

7 | General Principles of Radiation Therapy of Head and Neck Tumors

C. C. Wang, M.D.

GENERAL COMMENTS

Most of the malignant tumors originating in the mucous membranes of the aerodigestive tract are squamous cell carcinomas of varying malignant potential, ranging from in situ to poorly differentiated carcinoma. Tumors of the salivary glands, lymph nodes, bone, and soft tissue also occur in the head and neck regions. These tumors are less common although they are by no means less important in the practice of modern oncology. This chapter, however, is primarily concerned with the former—epithelial malignancies.

Squamous cell cancer of the head and neck region is a disease of middle and old age occurring especially in patients with a history of long-term cigarette smoking, alcoholism, and poor oral hygiene. It is a disease of mucosa and is often associated with multiple primary lesions, occurring either concurrently or sequentially; the incidence is as high as 15 to 20 percent. Men are more often affected, although the prevalance among women is rapidly increasing in the United States due to changes in the life style of American women.

The head and neck area is considered to be one of the most productive fields of cancer management in terms of cure rates. Many of these cancers can be readily seen, palpated, and evaluated and biopsied with relatively simple procedures. Because there is seldom a second chance to effect a cure, the choice of initial treatment must be the correct one, made after careful consideration of all the clinical features in each individual patient. This clearly requires that surgeons and radiation therapists know the strengths and weaknesses of their opposite disciplines and be thoroughly informed of the limitations of their chosen specialty. It is within the complimentary and cooperative efforts of this team that the welfare of the patient lies; this is particularly so for patients with advanced tumors.

Many good reference books related to the clinical, pathologic, and biologic aspects of this field are available; see the selected bibliography at the end of this chapter.

Carcinomas arising from the head and neck region are best described and discussed under their anatomical headings rather than under cell types. These regions include, among others, (1) oral cavity, (2) oropharynx, (3) hypopharynx, (4) larynx, (5) nasopharynx, (6) paranasal sinuses, and (7) salivary glands. In each of these locations, which often are subdivided into smaller areas, the tumor characteristics may be quite different. Each has its own natural history, separate mode of growth and spread, and different biologic behavior. The therapeutic management and results may differ greatly depending upon these factors.

In evaluating and reporting the therapeutic results in any malignant disease, whether treated by surgery or radiation therapy or combination of both, a commonly acceptable classification must be followed. For head and neck tumors, the

123

American Joint Committee for Cancer Staging and End Results Reporting (AJC) published a TNM staging system in 1977.[2] For tumors of the oral cavity and oropharynx, the T stage is determined primarily by the size of the lesion. For tumors of the nasopharynx, hypopharynx and larynx, the T stage is determined by the number of sites involved and the depth of invasion, which is reflected in the status of mobility of the involved structures in laryngeal and hypopharyngeal cancer or invasion of bone or nerves in nasopharyngeal cancer. For cervical nodal disease, the N stage is uniform throughout the head and neck region in that the size, number, and bilaterality of nodes are the determinant factors. Fixation of a particular node, however, is not taken into consideration at the present time. M stage is determined by clinical and radiographic findings. The AJC N and M staging is as follows:

N0—no clinically positive node.

N1—single clinically positive, homolateral node less than 3 cm in diameter.

N2a—single clinically positive, homolateral node 3 to 6 cm in diameter.

N2b—multiple clinically positive, homolateral nodes—none over 6 cm in diameter.

N3a—clinically positive homolateral node(s), at least one over 6 cm in diameter.

N3b—bilateral clinically positive nodes.

N3c—contralateral clinically positive node(s) only.

M0—no distant metastasis.

M1—distant metastasis present.

A variety of therapeutic measures are available for the management of carcinoma of the head and neck. These include surgical excision, radiation therapy, cryotherapy, laser excision, chemotherapy, immunotherapy and others. The choice of treatment modalities depends upon many factors such as (1) the site and extent of the primary lesion; (2) the likelihood of complete surgical resection; (3) the possibility of preservation of speech and/or swallowing mechanisms;

(4) the presence of bone and muscle involvement; (5) the presence of metastatic nodal disease; (6) the gross characteristics of tumor, i.e., exophytic-superficial vs endophytic-invasive; (7) the physical condition; (8) the social status and occupation of the patient; and (9) the experience and skill of both the surgeon and the radiation therapist.

At the present time, cryotherapy and laser excision is used in experienced hands primarily for superficial, accessible tumors with limited treatment success. Both chemotherapy and immunotherapy are used primarily for palliation or as adjuvant therapy, and their place in the curative management of carcinoma of the head and neck has yet to be established.

Surgery and radiotherapy are equally effective in eradicating limited cancers in the head and neck region. Each of these modalities has its own merits, indications, and limitations. Radiation therapy has the advantage of being able to control the disease in situ, thus avoiding sacrifice of a useful and necessary anatomic part as well as preserving speech and/or swallowing functions. Therefore, radiotherapy must be considered as the best "tissue and organ sparing procedure" available. On the other hand, for certain early lesions situated in less strategic locations, surgery can be carried out expediently and effectively without functional and cosmetic mutilation, and is therefore preferred.

In the management of advanced carcinomas, surgical failures are often due either to inability to excise microscopic tumor extension at the margin or to tumor seeding in the wound, both of which can result in local recurrence. Metastases via lymphatic or hematogenous routes are additional causes of treatment failure after surgery. The mechanisms of radiotherapeutic failures are different from those of surgery. The tumor core greater than 150 to 180 μm often contains hypoxic cells that are insensitive to radiation therapy. In contrast, the better oxygenated, well-nourished tumor cells at the tumor margins are more radioresponsive and are controllable by radiation. Local failure from radiation therapy therefore is central rather than marginal in nature. As with surgery, distant metastases through the lymphatic and hematogenous routes also constitute failures of local irradiation in a significant number of patients.

It is a well known fact in radiobiology that an approximate exponential relationship exists between the dose of ionizing radiation administered to a cell population and the surviving fraction of these cells. Experimental studies have demonstrated that relatively low doses will inactivate a vast number of cells in a tumor, i.e., D_{37} (dose to reduce survival cell population to the original 37 percent) ranges from 100 to 250 rads in most biologic systems. This is in keeping with the clinical observation that small microscopic aggregates of tumor cells, so-called subclinical disease, which cannot be palpated on physical examination and yet may be histopathologically detectable, can be controlled with a dose of 4,500 to 5,000 rads in 5 weeks in better than 90 percent of the cases.[17] However, for a large tumor, much higher doses such as 6,000 to 7,000 rads in 6 to 7 weeks are required for inactivation or eradication of the entire cell population to maximize the possibility of a lasting cure. For such advanced stage tumors, the radiation therapy is further handicapped by excessive tumor cell population as well as by the presence of a large number of hypoxic cells. In such situations, the radiation dose level must be increased significantly and sometimes beyond the limits of tolerance of the normal vasculoconnective tissues, thus making a lasting cure of such tumor impossible by radiation therapy.

Based on the mechanisms of treatment failures and the knowledge of modern radiobiologic techniques, the major strength of radiation therapy is therefore to eradicate the actively growing, well-oxygenated cells in the periphery of a tumor or the subclinical disease implanted in the wound or in the regional nodes. The strength of surgery on the other hand is to remove the centrally situated, radioresistant hypoxic tumor cells. For extensive tumors, which are rarely curable by either method alone, the logical approach at the present time is a combination of radiation therapy and surgery.

Attention must be paid to many important technical factors in the combined approach. The first of these is the dose and technique of administration of radiation therapy. It is beyond the scope of this chapter to describe various radiotherapeutic techniques for lesions arising from various sites of the head and neck. Certain generalizations, however, are warranted. It is clear that in expert hands radiation therapy with moderate doses of 4,000 to 4,500 rads administered over a period of 4 to 5 weeks can be delivered to any number of organ sites without significantly increasing postoperative morbidity and mortality. Even the magnitude of surgery remains unchanged and should include the original extent of the tumor. In higher radiation dosages, i.e., 6,000 to 6,500 rads over 6 to 7 weeks, which are cancerocidal in most epithelial tumors of the head and neck, the magnitude of surgery would have to be reduced in that only the residual disease should be removed.

High dose radical radiation therapy and radical resection invariably invites excessive, and at times, unacceptable postoperative morbidity and mortality. Timing of the operation is also most important. Clinical experience indicates that a dose of 4,000 to 4,500 rads delivered over a period of 4 to 5 weeks should be followed by an interval of about a month prior to surgery. If an operation is undertaken earlier, the operation is made technically more difficult because of mucosal edema, friability of tissues, and excessive bleeding in the operative field. On the other hand, a delay after radiation therapy beyond 8 to 10 weeks will frequently be accompanied by increasing fibrosis and postoperative complications.

During the past decade, two conceptual approaches to combined radiation therapy and surgery have emerged—preoperative and postoperative radiation therapy.

PREOPERATIVE RADIATION THERAPY

Conventional Preoperative Radiation Therapy

The aims of preoperative radiotherapy are to prevent marginal recurrences, to control subclinical disease in the primary site or in the nodes, and to convert technically inoperable tumors into operable ones. Theoretically, preoperative radiation therapy performed with the cancer cells in their maximum stage of oxygenation possesses a possible advantage over irradiation in the postoperative hypoxic condition.[28] A combination of preoperative irradiation and surgery has been found to decrease both local recurrence and the incidence of distant metastases.

The disadvantages of preoperative radiation therapy are that the exact tumor extent is obscured at the time of surgery, the surgery is delayed, and postoperative complications increase. The dosage employed in this conventional preoperative radiotherapy program is subcancerocidal consisting of 4,500 rads in 1 month. This is followed in 1 month by radical surgery encompassing all possible areas of disease as though radiation therapy had not been given. The program is applicable to medium-size or advanced tumors with poor radiotherapeutic or surgical cure rates including tumors of the oral cavity, such as the oral tongue, floor of the mouth, gum, hypopharynx, and larynx.

Cancerocidal Preoperative Radiotherapy or So-called Sequential Postradiation Resection

The radiation dosage used in this program is cancerocidal, i.e., 6,000 to 6,500 rads in 6 to 7 weeks delivered homogeneously to the primary site as well as to the first echelon lymph nodes. The treatment portal must be progressively reduced after 5,000 rads is achieved. Contrary to the conventional low dose preoperative program, radiation therapy is followed by limited surgical resection, and only the residual nidus of the primary lesion, mostly in the muscles or bone, is excised on the assumption that the peripheral, superficial disease has been controlled by high-dose radiation therapy. This approach is intended to avoid excessive functional and cosmetic mutilation by surgery and has been found useful in advanced lesions that arise from the retromolar trigone and faucil tonsil with involvement of the adjacent soft palate and base of tongue or gum. Following high-dose preoperative radiation therapy, radical surgery with intent to remove all involved areas according to the original extent of the lesion will most likely result in a high rate of postoperative complications, and is therefore ill-advised.

POSTOPERATIVE RADIATION THERAPY

The aims of postoperative radiation therapy are to eradicate residual disease at the resection margins and subclinical disease in the neck nodes or implanted in the wound. The procedure is usually carried out approximately 3 to 4 weeks after surgery when the wound is well healed. Generally, a dose of 5,500 rads in 6 weeks should not be exceeded if the surgery is radical in extent. On the other hand, if the surgery is primarily a debulking procedure, high-dose radiotherapy for gross residual disease must be given, i.e., 6,500 rads in 7 weeks through shrinking field technique to the area of known disease.

The decision for low-dose preoperative versus postoperative radiation therapy should be made on an individual basis that includes personal preference and experience. Although preoperative radiation therapy is often preferred at the Massachusetts General Hospital, there are, however, patients for whom postoperative radiation therapy—whether planned or unplanned—is definitely advised. These include the following: (1) Patients with extensive tumors of the larynx and hypopharynx in whom tracheostomy is required. In such circumstances, the infected larynx and tumor would be better removed prior to therapy so that radiation therapy can be carried out without the complications of pain, aspiration, and pulmonary infection, which are often present when laryngectomy is not done first. (2) Patients with extensive disease requiring laryngectomy, partial pharyngectomy, esophagectomy, and extensive reconstruction would be better treated by postoperative radiation therapy because of the belief that preoperative radiation therapy would add further difficulties to the already increased operative complications after such extensive surgery. (3) All patients with advanced T2, T3, and T4 lesions treated by primary excision who have questionable resection margins. (4) All patients with N2 and N3 nodes in the radical neck dissection specimens or N1 disease with disease extending outside the node capsule.

The management of metastatic nodes in the neck from a primary lesion arising from the head and neck region depends upon the size, the number of nodes, and the cell type and location of the primary lesion. Radiotherapy is highly curative for small metastatic nodes with primary tumors arising from Waldeyer's ring, i.e., nasopharynx, faucial tonsil, and base of tongue. Therefore, for such N1 and early N2 lesions, radiation should be given for cure and surgery should be reserved for salvage. For metastatic nodes with a primary lesion arising from the oral cavity and larynx in advanced stage, combined radiation therapy and surgery is the treatment of choice, i.e., radical neck dissection either preceded by or followed by radiation therapy.[21] A dose of 4,500 rads in 4 weeks as a preoperative procedure or 5,500 rads as a postoperative procedure should be planned. For inoperable metastatic nodes in the neck, high dose radiotherapy is necessary for local control. A dose of 7,500 or 8,000 rads over 7 to 8 weeks often is needed for N3 disease. This treatment program may result in painful fibrosis of the neck.

MODALITIES OF RADIATION THERAPY

Much emphasis is often placed on the equipment of radiation therapy; however, as in all medicine, the knowledge and skill of the therapist are the determinants of the success of a given treatment rather than the hardware. Nevertheless, the armamentarium of modern radiation therapy does make possible techniques previously unavailable, with a resultant improvement in cure rates and reduction of undesirable local side effects and complications.

The tools of radiation therapy used in the management of carcinoma of the head and neck are primarily megavoltage radiations, with energies at or above 1 million volts, and radioactive isotopes. These megavoltage radiation energies possess certain inherent physical advantages such as a skin sparing effect; an increase in depth dose, which is reflected by the fact that often a full course of curative radiation therapy can be given without causing radiation dermatitis; a sharp beam, which makes it possible to produce better beam collimation and to confine the irradiation to the individual lesions—thus minimizing unnecessary damage to the adjacent normal tissues and organs; and a bone sparing effect due to lesser differential absorption between soft tissue and bone, thus resulting in homogenous distribution of radiations throughout the irradiated volume.

Electromagnetic Radiations

The present day means of generating roentgen or gamma rays in the megavoltage range for the treatment of head and neck tumors are the telecobalt "bomb" and the linear accelerator. The former though technically not an x-ray machine is used in the same manner as and for all practical purposes is a megavoltage x-ray machine. The source of ionizing rays, in this case gamma rays having energies of 1.17 and 1.33 MeV, is several thousand curies of radioactive cobalt 60; the cobalt is housed in a shielded container, unfortunately called a bomb, with collimating devices and electrical circuits. It is a common and practical machine for clinical radiotherapy particularly for head and neck tumors and is available in most medical centers. Except for its relatively short half-life of 5.25 years, which may require frequent change of source in a busy department, there are certain technical advantages such as freedom from breakdown. The linear accelerator, commonly known as a linac or clinac, provides a compact source of x-rays in the range of 4 to 10 million volts. The heart of the device is a wave guide—a metal tube with a cross sectional geometry that permits it to conduct an electromagnetic wave or microwave frequency with high efficiency. An electron injected into an evacuated wave guide with sufficient velocity is caught up by the wave and carried along by it, gaining energy, and momentum from the wave. Either x-rays or electron beams can be produced. Linear accelerators have the advantage of high output (i.e., 200 to 1,000 rads per minute at isocenter) and compactness and have been found to be very popular in the major cancer centers.

Kilovoltage radiation, as generated by the 200 to 250 kV x-ray machines, may be used for transoral cone therapy or treatment of carcinoma of the lip. Otherwise, it has no place in the primary management of carcinoma of the head and neck. Most lesions treated by orthovoltage machines can be satisfactorily managed by low energy electron beam therapy.

Electron Beam

Energetic electrons can be generated by a linear accelerator or a betatron. Varying energies are used for radiation therapy of head and neck tumors including 6, 9, 12, 15, and 18 MeV or above. The characteristics of electron beams are rapid dose buildup and sharp fall-off beyond the specified energy applied; thus, the structures or organs im-

mediately beyond the treatment target receive relative protection. The principal areas of application suitable for 6 to 18 MeV electron beam therapy include lesions of the skin and lip, primary lesions of the head and neck located at 2 to 5 cm depth, parotid tumors, and metastatic cervical nodes. Frequently, electron beam therapy is given in conjunction with photon irradiation.

Radioactive Isotopes

Radioactive isotopes are important sources of gamma rays for the management of cancer of the head and neck and are primarily used interstitially either as a temporary or permanent implant. Radium 226, in the form of needles, was the isotope used most frequently in the past few decades. Because of its inherent hazards of radiation exposure to the radiation therapy staff, afterloading devices using angiocatheters with iridium 192 have been developed and extensively used in lieu of radium needles in clinical practice. Such implants are removed after delivering a prescribed radiation dosage to the tumor, usually requiring 2 to 3 days. Radon gas is a gaseous daughter product of radium and was used extensively in the past in the form of permanent, interstitially implanted seeds, but has been largely replaced by gold 198 or iodine 125 grains or others.

The modern practice of radiation therapy for head and neck tumors demands extreme technical sophistication. By using various treatment modalities and techniques (such as wedge filters and rotation) or a combination of photons and electrons, a maximum amount of radiation can be delivered to the tumor and yet a minimum to the adjacent normal tissues. Most of the irreparable radiation injuries of the bone and soft tissues, which were commonly seen in the past orthovoltage era, have decreased, and radical surgery often can be performed subsequently without significant postoperative complications.

TREATMENT PLANNING

After radiation therapy is elected, treatment should be carefully planned. In the modern practice of radiation therapy, the treatment planning is based on the nature, size and location of the tumor, the volume of the disease to be encompassed, the normal organ to be spared, and the intent of treatment—curative or palliative. Planning is carried out with the aid of a simulator and a dedicated computer prior to actual treatment. This procedural preparation for radiotherapy must be as thorough as is the preparation of a patient who is to undergo surgery. All work-ups should be completed, including evaluation of the extent of the primary lesion by inspection, palpation, and various diagnostic means such as radiographs (with or without contrast substance) and, when indicated, ultrasound and CT scans. This is mandatory in order to determine the exact tumor volume for optimum direction of the treatment beam. Since most of the lesions of the head and neck region are accessible for biopsy, a histologic confirmation of malignancy must be obtained prior to radiation therapy. A complete physical examination, including blood and urine studies and liver profile, for appraisal of patient's physical status is highly desirable. If anemia, weight loss, or electrolyte imbalance exists, these should be corrected because anemic and debilitated patients do not tolerate radiation therapy well.

THE INTENT OF RADIATION THERAPY

The intent of radiation therapy can be divided into three categories: curative, palliative, and adjunct to surgery.

Radical radiotherapy with intent to cure is not without morbidity and should be performed with both care and justification. In curative radiation therapy, the treatment course is usually prolonged and physically taxing; painful radiation reactions in the oropharyngeal mucosa may be quite severe resulting in dysphagia and impairment of nutrition. As a matter of fact, the discomfort suffered by the patient from curative radiation therapy is no less and is sometimes more than that of radical surgery. It is generally observed that elderly, debilitated patients and many alcoholics tolerate radical surgery procedures, i.e., partial glossectomy or total laryngectomy for advanced disease, far better than they tolerate a radical course of radiation therapy that extends for 6 to 7 weeks or that employs interstitial implant.

Extensive disease due to massive primary tumor or cervical metastases is rarely curable, and palliative radiotherapy for symptomatic relief should be the aim. Pain, bleeding, obstruction, and ulceration can be alleviated by radiation therapy; but unfortunately, for effective palliation for squamous cell carcinoma of the head and neck the dosage of radiation is generally quite high—approaching 5,000 rads or more in 6 weeks—if lasting effects are to be obtained. This palliative dose may produce symptomatic radiation reaction in the patient. Therefore, for the patients with far advanced but relatively asymptomatic lesions in a terminal stage, the best treatment is human kindness, morphine, and good nursing care.

In radiation therapy as in surgery, the first choice of treatment must be the correct one: there is seldom an equal chance later to cure the disease. If the lesion recurs after radiation therapy, it may have acquired resistance to irradiation because of impairment of local blood supply, increased fibrosis, and also formation of more radioresistant hypoxic cells, which is usually due to changes in the cellular component and other factors in or about the tumor. Consequently, in most instances when a full course of radiation therapy has been given, reirradiation with intent to cure is generally of little value and is less likely to be successful. Such recurrences should be treated by surgery if there is still a chance of cure. The exceptions to this rule, however, are nasopharyngeal cancer[41] and glottic cancer[33] where reirradiation has salvaged a few otherwise inoperable and incurable patients.

GENERAL GUIDELINES OF MANAGEMENT OF HEAD AND NECK CANCERS

Oral Cancer

Oral cancer is a relatively common malignancy of the head and neck and is predominately squamous cell carcinoma.[36] The TNM Staging System for Oral Cancer as recommended by the American Joint Committee in 1977[2] is as follows:

T1—tumor 2 cm or less in greatest diameter.

T2—tumor greater than 2 cm but not greater than 4 cm in greatest diameter.

T3—tumor greater than 4 cm in greatest diameter.

T4—massive tumor greater than 4 cm in diameter with invasion of bone, soft tissue, etc.

Pathologically, most of the carcinomas of the oral cavity are well- to moderately well-differentiated carcinomas. When the location of the lesions is further away from the lips and toward the oropharynx, as a general rule the tumors are less differentiated. Since squamous cell carcinomas represent mucosal abnormality, there are almost always some mucosal changes associated within the tumor and the lesions show some bleeding—the latter often after detailed examination and scraping with tongue depressors. Early mucosal lesions may appear as only a superficial granularity, as an indurated nodule, or as a shallow ulceration that may have minimal subjective symptoms. Advanced tumors often extend deeply into the underlying muscles or bone causing fixation and resulting in difficulty with speech and swallowing mechanisms. Metastases commonly occur to the ipsilateral subdigastric and upper jugular and midjugular nodes, although cross metastases to the opposite neck may also occur with lesions crossing the midline of the oral cavity. The incidence of regional lymph node metastases for the early lesions (T1) ranges from 10 to 20 percent; for the intermediate lesions (T2) 25 to 30 percent; and

advanced lesions (T3 and T4) 50 to 70 percent. Distant metastases below the clavicle are uncommon and occur late in the course of the disease.

The use of radiation therapy in the management of squamous cell carcinoma of the oral cavity, as is true for most squamous cell carcinomas of the head and neck, is based on the following principles:

1. Carcinomas of the head and neck are usually radioresponsive, and in early stages highly radiocurable.

2. The more differentiated the tumors, the less the radiation response.

3. Exophytic and well-oxygenated tumors are more radioresponsive than deeply infiltrative and hypoxic ones.

4. Squamous cell carcinomas when limited to the mucosa are highly radiocurable. Bone and muscle involvement adversely alters the radioresponsiveness of carcinomas and subsequently decreases their radiocurability.

5. Advanced cervical metastases, N2 and N3, are better treated by combined surgery and radiotherapy.

The treatment of carcinoma of the oral cavity is mostly by low megavoltage or cobalt 60 radiations with interplay of interstitial isotope implants. In general, external beam therapy is suitable for most lesions and in many instances is the procedure of choice.

The radiotherapy treatment program should include the primary and regional nodes, especially in patients who have cervical lymph node metastases. The irradiated volume is therefore large and often associated with some degree of radiation sequelae.

Interstitial isotope implant is only suitable for lesions situated in the anterior portion of the oral cavity such as the lip, floor of the mouth, tongue, and buccal mucosa. The irradiated volume of the implant is generally small but the radiation dosage is intense. The implant procedure requires skill, experience, and good judgment on the part of the radiation therapist, and is often used as a boost to the primary lesion. There are, however, inherent dosimetric difficulties in isotope implants in that inhomogeneity of dose distribution is invariably present and results in "hot" and "cold" spots. Interstitial implants are not suitable for lesions invading or adjacent to the jaw due to the risk of osteoradionecrosis or for lesions involving the tonsillar region or the base of the tongue.

Results of radiation therapy for carcinoma of the oral cavity are related to the size of the primary lesion and the presence or absence of metastatic nodes.[3, 4, 16] In early lesions (T1) the 3-year no evidence of disease (NED) rates should approach 75 to 80 percent and for intermediate lesions (T2) 50 to 60 percent. The radiotherapeutic results of advanced carcinomas (T3 and T4) are generally rather poor, approximating 10 to 20 percent. For the lesions without nodes, the 3-year NED rates range between 50 to 70 percent, while the presence of nodes reduces the cure rates from one-half to one-third.

From the standpoint of anatomic origin and method of management, cancer of the oral cavity can be further subdivided as follows: lip, oral tongue, floor of the mouth, retromolar trigone and anterior faucial pillar, buccal mucosa, gingival ridge, and palate. A brief discussion of each of these lesions is presented below.

LIP

Most of the squamous cell carcinomas of the lip are well-differentiated and are less than 1 cm in size. The AJC staging for lip carcinoma is as follows:[2]

T1—tumor less than 1 cm in size.

T2—tumor 1 to 3 cm in size.

T3—tumor greater than 3 cm in size.

T4—massive tumor with or without bone involvement.

As a rule, therapy is directed to the primary lesion if there are no palpable nodes. A small carcinoma of the lip can be dealt with expediently and successfully by V-excision, and the procedure will not result in cosmetic or functional deformity. Radiation therapy is best suited for superficial cancers involving more than one-third of the lip, for tumors which involve the oral commissure, for recurrent tumors after prior excision, or for patients who refuse surgery. Surgical excision is mandatory for radiation failures, for extensive cancers that involve the mandible, or for cancer associated with significant soft tissue destruction that will require major reconstruction after the lesion is controlled by radiation therapy. Since radiation therapy and surgery have each yielded extremely high cure rates for the small, limited cancers, i.e., 3-year NED rate of 90 percent, the selection of treatment modality must depend upon the cosmetic result that follows the treatment procedure. Radiation therapy for the superficial small tumor (T1) consists of low energy x-rays, such as 250 kV or low megavoltage electrons. For the extensive tumors (T2, T3) combined external beam therapy and interstitial isotope implant yields excellent cure rates and cosmetic results. For far advanced tumors, high energy or cobalt 60 radiation is used to include the primary and the metastatic nodes.

ORAL TONGUE

Squamous cell carcinoma of the oral tongue (anterior two-thirds of the tongue) invades underlying muscle early and tends to spread along the muscle planes with poorly defined margins. This tumor is difficult to manage by either radiation therapy or surgery alone because of the high incidence of local recurrence. Surgical resection is indicated for small cancers (T1 and T2) that can be expediently excised without resulting deformity and for tumors involving the tip of the tongue and for large infiltrative lesions (T3 or T4) that are associated with a great deal of muscle involvement.

Surgery is often used as a salvage procedure for recurrent lesions or residual disease following failure of radical radiation therapy. The superficial, exophytic T1 and T2 lesions without a great deal of muscle involvement are most amenable to radiation therapy and exhibit high local control and excellent cosmetic results. In certain moderately infiltrative lesions of less than 2 cm muscular invasion, a course of radiotherapy of 4,500 rads can be given first; this is followed by interstitial implant or "cone down" external beam therapy to 6,500 to 7,000 rads and surgery is used for salvage. For large, advanced, infiltrative T2, T3, and T4 lesions, a planned course of combined radiation therapy and surgery is the procedure of choice.

FLOOR OF THE MOUTH

Carcinoma of the floor of the mouth is commonly located in the anterior portion of the floor adjacent to Wharton's duct orifice. It may extend to the adjacent area of the tongue and gum and later invade the mandible.[9] When limited to the mucosa, it is highly curable by radiation therapy alone. Although bone involvement compromises treatment results, radiation therapy for such lesions is possible when bone is eroded but not infiltrated by tumor. In general, small lesions of the floor of the mouth are treated by external beam therapy or by combination of external beam and interstitial isotope implant. When preoperative radiation therapy of 4,500 rads is given prior to planned surgery, the margins of the tumor are tattooed prior to radiotherapy in order to define the extent of the surgery later required. Nodal metastases are associated with advanced disease and adversely affect the prognosis. For extensive carcinoma of the floor of the mouth with involvement of the mandible, the treatment of choice is preoperative radiotherapy of 4,500 rads in 5 weeks, which is followed by radical resection.

RETROMOLAR TRIGONE AND ANTERIOR FAUCIAL PILLAR

Squamous cell carcinomas arising from the retromolar trigone and anterior faucial pillar are generally under one heading for discussion and should not be confused with carcinoma of the tonsil. These lesions may spread to the adjacent soft and hard palate, gingiva, or adjacent buccal mucosa as well as to the tonsillar fossa, and inferiorly to the base of the tongue and floor of the mouth. Advanced lesions may extend to the pterygoid muscles resulting in trismus.

Most of these tumors are well-differentiated, and the superficial lesions can be treated successfully with external beam therapy. Primary radical surgery generally is attended by marked facial deformity and impairment of swallowing function and often results in a high incidence of marginal recurrence. Since these lesions tend to remain localized, salvage surgery is frequently efficacious to effect a lasting cure at the cost of cosmetic and functional multilation if radiation therapy fails to eradicate the entire lesion. The most common sites of failure after radiation therapy are the base of the tongue and the adjacent mandible that have been infiltrated by tumor. The residual disease after high dose radiotherapy is best managed by limited resection, i.e., nidusectomy. The large, infiltrative lesions, T3 and T4 with or without pterygoid invasion, are best treated by combination of high dose radiation therapy and composite resection.

BUCCAL MUCOSA

Carcinoma of the buccal mucosa is usually well-differentiated squamous cell carcinoma, frequently associated with areas of leukoplakia. Because the mucous membrane adheres closely to the muscle of the cheek, early invasion of the masseter muscle can occur and produce trismus. Once the deeper muscles are involved, there is an increased likelihood of cervical lymph node metastases. For early T1 and T2 lesions, radiotherapy has resulted in satisfactory control of the disease. If the buccogingival sulcus is not involved by the tumor, the best results of therapy have been achieved by combined external beam therapy and interstitial isotope implant. Unfortunately, the cure rates for extensive T3 and T4 lesions with deep muscular invasion are extremely poor with radiation therapy alone. Thus, en bloc excision of the primary lesion and its regional nodal metastases with preoperative or postoperative radiotherapy is the preferred procedure.

GINGIVAL RIDGE

Carcinoma of the gingival ridge usually arises in the posterior portion of the lower dental arch and is associated with leukoplakic changes. Since the mucous membrane adheres to the periosteum of the mandible, tumor arising from the gingival ridge is likely to invade underlying bone in its early stage of development. Most of these tumors are well-differentiated. Carcinoma of the maxillary gingiva is not an uncommon disease but should not be confused with tumors that originate from the maxillary sinus and secondarily extend to the gingiva. Radiography of the paranasal sinuses is helpful in differential diagnosis and also allows careful evaluation of the extent of the bony involvement. Treatment depends upon the extent of the lesion, degree of bony involvement, and the status of the cervical lymph nodes. Special note should be made of the smooth, erosive pressure defect that results from a slowly expanding tumor versus the moth-eaten type of bone destruction caused by tumor infiltration. The latter lesion cannot be successfully treated by radiation therapy, whereas the former can. The small T1 exophytic cancer without bone involvement can be well-managed by external beam therapy alone.[22] For advanced lesions that produce destruction of the mandible with or without metastases, radical surgery is preferred because partial mandibulectomy with radical neck dissection provides good survival rates.[8] Local spread of the disease along subperiosteal lymphatics is quite likely; for this reason, in advanced disease, radiation therapy is often given prior to or following resection in order to reduce the incidence of local recurrence.

PALATE

The palate is divided into the hard and soft palate. The hard palate is the most common site for occurrence of minor salivary gland tumors in the oral cavity. Squamous cell carcinomas arising from this site are quite rare and are usually ulcerative and generally invade the underlying bone. Early lesions without bone involvement can be treated satisfactorily by radiation therapy alone. Advanced, deeply infiltrative lesions of the hard palate with bone destruction are rarely curable by radiation therapy and are better treated by combined therapy. Malignant salivary gland tumors, as discussed on page 139, are traditionally treated by surgery and have recently been treated with increasing frequency by combination of surgery and postoperative radiation therapy. Some inoperable malignancies of the salivary glands in the oral cavity have been successfully controlled by high dose radiotherapy.

Most malignant tumors of the soft palate and uvula are well-differentiated squamous cell carcinomas and are included with oropharyngeal cancer by the AJC.[2] They are invariably ulcerated lesions with poorly defined borders and biologically and radiotherapeutically behave like carcinomas of the oral cavity; therefore, they are discussed herein. Surgical resection of such lesions is unsatisfactory and often results in marginal recurrences. Even when surgery is successful, impaired swallowing and speech often ensues unless prosthetic support is available. Because of the relatively superficial nature of most T1 and T2 lesions, good local control has been achieved by megavoltage radiation therapy.[18] For T3 and T4 lesions, often associated with regional nodal metastases, the results of radiotherapy are generally poor; such lesions, at the present time, are being considered inoperable and are treated by palliative radiotherapy, chemotherapy, or cryotherapy. If the lesion is still operable, combined radiotherapy and surgery should be carried out in hopes of improving the cure rate.

Oropharyngeal Cancer

The oropharyngeal lesions according to the American Joint Committee[2] include tumors arising from the faucial tonsil, base of the tongue, pharyngeal wall, and faucial arch. The faucial arch tumors, however, are included under the discussion of oral cavity tumors because of their similarity in terms of growth, spread, and prognosis to oral tumors. In contrast to carcinoma of the oral cavity, oropharyngeal carcinomas are generally poorly differentiated and include a special variant—so-called lymphoepithelioma. The staging for oropharyngeal carcinomas is the same as the staging for oral cancer. These lesions are characterized by high incidence of regional lymph node metastases, irrespective of the stage of the primary lesion, ranging between 50 and 75 percent at the time the diagnosis is made. Over half of the lesions with cervical metastases from the base of the tongue present with bilateral involvement.[26]

Radiation therapy for this disease is primarily external beam therapy either from a cobalt 60 unit or a low megavoltage linear accelerator. Technically, it is extremely difficult to obtain a satisfactory interstitial isotope implant in lesions situated in the base of the tongue or in the tonsillar fossa. Owing to the unusually high incidence of nodal metastases, radiation therapy commonly includes the primary tumor as well as the first echelon lymphatic areas in a continuous portal; this is so even in patients with clinically N0 necks. Radiotherapeutic results for carcinoma of the oropharynx were considered to be notoriously unfavorable. Recent studies at the Massachusetts General Hospital and Massachusetts Eye and Ear Infirmary (Wang, unpublished data) indicate that in tumors of similar size the local control for oropharyngeal cancer is comparable to that for carcinoma of the oral cavity. For early lesions (T1) the 3-year NED rates range from 75 to 85 percent and for intermediate lesions (T2) 50 to 60 percent. For extensive lesions (T3 and T4) the cure rate by radiotherapy is approximately 10 to 20 percent. Contrary to squamous cell carcinoma of the oral cavity, the presence of N1 nodal metastasis does not appear to affect the prognosis significantly, and many lesions with such early metastatic nodal dis-

ease can be controlled by radiotherapy alone without the necessity for neck dissection.

TONSIL

Squamous cell carcinoma of the faucial tonsil, as noted on page 132, is different from that which originates from the retromolar trigone and anterior tonsillar pillar. These lesions are prone to spread posteriorly to the lateral pharyngeal wall and the base of the tongue and superiorly to the soft palate.[29] Most of the carcinomas of the tonsil are radiosensitive and in early stages radiocurable. Therefore, for such early lesions, radiotherapy is the treatment of choice.[15, 18] Advanced tumors of the tonsil are best treated by combined therapies.[27] This includes high dose external beam therapy using a shrinking field technique to achieve a total dose of approximately 6,000 rads; this is followed by sequential surgery with removal of the residual disease commonly present in the base of the tongue or the adjacent mandible.[35] Any residual disease in the neck following high dose radiotherapy would be best dealt with by a neck dissection.

BASE OF TONGUE

This is the fixed portion or posterior third of the tongue starting anatomically from the circumvallate papillae posteriorly toward the epiglotticopharyngeal folds. In order to evaluate the extent of this disease, indirect laryngoscopy and digital palpation of the base of the tongue are necessary as a routine procedure. Xeroradiograms of the lateral base of the tongue may delineate the depth of the invasion of the tumor. Treatment of this disease is primarily by external beam therapy. Any residual disease following radiation therapy will be dealt with by limited surgery. Unfortunately, most of the primary cancers are so situated that appropriate surgery will have to include excision of tongue base and total laryngectomy for potential cure. For small lesions (T1 and T2),

3-year NED rates as high as 80 percent and 60 percent respectively can be achieved by radiation therapy alone.

PHARYNGEAL WALL

The pharyngeal wall includes the lateral and posterior walls and the posterior tonsillar pillar. Primary lesions arising from the posterior tonsillar pillar alone are extremely rare. Squamous cell carcinomas arising from these sites tend to be ulcerative and their exact extensions upward or downward are difficult to determine. Therefore, lateral soft tissue radiographs are essential to detect the extent of the tumor. Because of the location, surgery is unlikely to be successful due to a high frequency of marginal recurrences. These tumors are better treated by external beam therapy, which must include the entire pharynx from the nasopharyngeal vault down to the pyriform sinus.[34] Because of the proximity of the tumor to the spinal cord, care must be exercised to avoid excessive irradiation of the cord. Because of the high sensitivity of the oropharyngeal mucosa, patients generally experience rather severe, painful radiation reaction with impairment of nutritional status; therefore, radiation must be carried out with great caution. Any residual disease limited to the lateral pharyngeal wall after a course of radiotherapy occasionally may be dealt with by pharyngectomy, although cure rates generally are rather poor.[14]

Hypopharyngeal Cancer

Hypopharyngeal tumors include lesions arising from the pyriform sinus, the posterior pharyngeal wall, and the postcricoid area. The TNM staging system[2] is defined by tumor extension to the adjacent sites and by status of the mobility of the larynx if involved, and is as follows:

T1—tumor confined to site of origin.

T2—extension of tumor to adjacent region or site without fixation of hemilarynx.

T3—extension of tumor to adjacent region or site with fixation of hemilarynx.

T4—massive tumor invading bone or soft tissues of neck.

Owing to the lack of severe symptoms, carcinomas arising from these sites tend to be extensive, frequently with extensive cervical lymph node metastases that are often bilateral. Histologically, these tumors are moderately undifferentiated. These tumors tend to infiltrate to the adjacent structures with involvement of the underlying cartilage and musculature and have poorly defined borders. Treatment either by surgery or radiotherapy is unsatisfactory due to uncontrolled primary site and cervical lymph node metastases. Except in carcinoma of the posterior pharyngeal wall, combination of radiation therapy and surgery has been carried out for these tumors with improved results.

Carcinoma of the pyriform sinus is characterized by an extensive primary lesion and frequently by cervical nodal metastases. More than half of these patients when first seen present with T3 and T4 disease and two out of three patients present with cervical metastases. Distinction must be made between the lesions arising in the medial and lateral walls of the pyriform sinus and in the apical portion of the pyriform sinus. The tumor arising from the upper walls of the pyriform sinus tends to be exophytic and is curable by radiation therapy. The tumor arising from the apical portion of the pyriform sinus is often infiltrative and extensive with involvement of adjacent cartilage of the larynx or upper trachea and is therefore not likely to be radiocurable. Such a lesion would best be dealt with by a combination of radiotherapy and surgery. Primary radiotherapy is therefore not advisable. The overall 3-year NED rate for carcinoma of the hypopharynx is approximately 20 percent by radiotherapy. The control rates for patients with lesions arising from the pyriform sinus and the lateral pharyngeal wall are double with the use of combined treatment (radiotherapy and surgery) compared to the use of either modality alone.[43] The majority of the therapeutic failures are due to uncontrolled nodal disease in the neck, recurrence in the base of the tongue, tracheal stoma, and tumor extension into the cervical esophagus or into the base of the skull. A small number of patients die with distant metastases.

Laryngeal Cancer

Anatomically and therapeutically, the larynx can be divided into three separate portions—supraglottic, glottic, and subglottic. The supraglottic tumors include the lesions arising from the laryngeal surface and the rim of the epiglottis, the aryepiglottic fold, the arytenoid, the false cord, and the laryngeal ventricle. The glottic tumors originate from the vocal cord and anterior and posterior commissures. The subglottic lesions arise from the area approximately 1 cm inferior to the true cord down to the lower margin of the cricoid cartilage. The most common cancer of the larynx is squamous cell carcinoma of varying degree of malignant potential. This cancer is predominately a disease of the male in the fifth, sixth and seventh decades of life. The TNM staging system for laryngeal cancer as published in 1977[2] is as follows:

Supraglottis

T1—tumor confined to region of origin with normal mobility.

T2—tumor involving adjacent supraglottic site(s) or glottis without fixation.

T3—tumor limited to larynx with fixation and/or extension to involve postcricoid area, medial wall of the pyriform sinus, or preepiglottic space.

T4—massive tumor extending beyond the larynx to involve oropharynx, soft tissues of neck, or destruction of cricoid cartilage.

Glottis

T1—tumor confined to vocal cord(s) with normal mobility (including involvement of anterior or posterior commissures).

T2—supraglottic and/or subglottic extension of tumor with normal or impaired cord mobility.

T3—tumor confined to larynx with cord fixation.

T4—massive tumor with thyroid carti-

lage destruction and/or extension beyond the confines of the larynx.

Subglottis

T1—tumor confined to the subglottic region.

T2—tumor extension to vocal cords with normal or impaired cord mobility.

T3—tumor confined to larynx with cord fixation.

T4—massive tumor with cartilage destruction or extension beyond the confines of the larynx, or both.

GLOTTIS

The most common form of laryngeal cancer is well-differentiated squamous cell carcinoma of the vocal cords. Owing to its manifestation of disease by hoarseness of voice, glottic carcinoma is often discovered early, at which stage it is readily treatable and curable either by radiation therapy or surgery. When tumor is confined to the cord with normal mobility, the incidence of nodal metastases is extremely low and ranges from 0 to 2 percent. Therefore, the management of early glottic carcinoma does not include the management of cervical nodes.

Radiation therapy is preferred for T1 and T2 tumors with normal cord mobility.[20, 23] It not only provides excellent control of the disease, being in the neighborhood of approximately 90 percent 5-year NED, but also preserves a good, useful voice in approximately 95 percent of patients.[38] There is no doubt that a significant number of patients with laryngeal cancer in the early stage can be cured by primary surgery alone;[25] but total laryngectomy for early cancer should be condemned. Conservation surgery, such as laryngofissure with cordectomy or partial laryngectomy, by experienced physicians can control early glottic lesions in highly selected patients; but the functional results are inferior to those of radiation therapy because of the residual permanent hoarseness of voice following surgery. Salvage surgery is highly effective for radiation failures with few significant postoperative complications. For T2 lesions with impaired cord mobility, a trial course of radiotherapy is initially given. If the tumor shows good regression and/or return of normal cord mobility after a dose of 4,500 rads, radiation therapy may be continued to a curative dose level of about 6,500 rads and surgery is then reserved for salvage. The extensive T3 and T4 lesions with completely fixed cord are rarely curable by radiation therapy alone and are better treated by planned combination of radiotherapy and surgery. Lymph node metastases from laryngeal cancer indicate advanced disease and are managed by neck dissection and adjuvant radiation therapy.

SUPRAGLOTTIS

This ranks second to glottic carcinoma in incidence and is associated with a poorer prognosis. Usually the tumor is poorly differentiated squamous cell carcinoma. Owing to the abundant supply of lymphatics in this anatomic area, supraglottic carcinoma is characterized by a high incidence of lymph node metastases—reportedly as high as 50 percent. Because of frequent extension across the midline, bilateral cervical lymph node metastases are not uncommon and occur in 20 to 50 percent of supraglottic cancer patients; some series reported as high as 90 percent bilateral node metastases from the tumor arising from the base of the epiglottis, false cord, and ventricle. Treatment of this disease must therefore include management of the primary lesion as well as the lymph node metastases in the neck. The results of radiotherapy for supraglottic carcinoma are less satisfactory than for glottic carcinoma.[5, 19] The 5-year NED rates following radiation therapy vary depending upon the extent of the primary tumor and the status of the cervical nodes.[37] For a superficial, exophytic early lesion (T1 or T2), cure rate by radiotherapy alone is quite high, ranging from 70 to 90 percent; and therefore radiotherapy should be considered for such lesions. This is particularly true for the exophytic tumors arising from the tip of the epiglottis and free margins of the aryepiglottic fold. However, if the primary lesion is extensive and deeply ulcerative with fixation of the laryngeal structures and/or with cervical lymph node metastases (i.e., T3 N1 and T4 N1), the 5-year NED rates following radiotherapy are poor, approximately 20 to 25 percent. These advanced lesions are presently managed by the planned combined approach[30] (i.e., 4,500 rads in 5 weeks followed by total laryngectomy and comcomitant neck dissection) with considerably improved results.[43] Should the patient experience laryngeal stridor requiring emergency tracheostomy, it is recommended that the patient have primary surgery first, followed by postoperative radiotherapy to the entire neck, tracheal stoma, and upper mediastinum of approximately 5,500 rads in 5$\frac{1}{2}$ weeks. This should be carried out approximately 1 month after surgery.

SUBGLOTTIS

This is a rare tumor, constituting less than 1 percent of laryngeal cancers. Early tumors can be successfully dealt with by radiation therapy. Unfortunately, as most lesions are extensive and require tracheostomy, they are best dealt with by the combination of surgery and radiotherapy—with the latter administered either preoperatively or postoperatively.

Nasopharyngeal Cancer

Anatomically, the nasopharynx is considered to be a blind spot for routine clinical examination. Many metastatic carcinomas found in the cervical lymph nodes with an unknown primary cancer are from primary lesions arising in this area. Squamous cell carcinoma of the nasopharynx is a disease of the middle-aged and elderly and consists of various cell types including lymphoepithelioma, transitional cell carcinoma, and undifferentiated carcinoma. It is predominately a disease of the male and has a male to female ratio of 3:1. Asymptomatic mass in the neck, unilateral impairment of hearing with otitis media, nasal obstruction, epistaxis, and diplopia due to 6th cranial nerve involvement are the common manifestations of this disease and should arouse the suspicion of nasopharyngeal carcinoma. Evaluation of the extent of the lesion should include inspection and palpation of the lesion by direct or indirect nasopharyngoscopy and by digital examination. X-ray examinations include soft tissue films of the nasopharynx in the lateral projection and polytomes of the base of the skull in anteroposterior and lateral projections for evidence of bone destruction.

The AJC staging of carcinoma of the nasopharynx[2] is as follows:

T1—tumor involving one site, or a positive biopsy.

T2—tumor involving two sites.

T3—tumor extending to nasal cavity or oropharynx.

T4—massive tumor invading bone, cranial nerve, or soft tissues of the neck.

Owing to the rich lymphatic supply, carcinoma of the nasopharynx is known to have a high incidence of regional cervical lymph node metastases, ranging from 60 to 80 percent irrespective of T stage. Therefore, in the management of carcinoma of the nasopharynx, similar to carcinoma of the oropharynx and supraglottis, treatment must be directed both to the primary site and the neck even in cases of an N0 neck. Because of the rather inaccessible location of the tumor, primary surgery has no place in the curative management of this disease.[24] Because the nasopharynx is surrounded by many vital structures and organs, treatment of this disease by radiotherapy calls for careful techniques. High dose radiation is required for lasting control of the primary site. For small lesions (T1 and T2) without nodes, the radiotherapeutic results are reasonably satisfactory with a 5-year NED rate of better than 50 percent.[11, 39] Even among patients who have advanced disease with cranial nerve involvement, about one quarter may survive for 5 or more years, though some will still have disease.[42] Since these lesions tend to recur locally after external beam therapy, routine supplementary therapy with intracavitary cesium implant as part of the primary program for T1 and T2 lesions has reduced the incidence of local recurrence from 33 percent to less than 10 percent. Persistent nodal disease in the neck following radiotherapy should be dealt with by neck dissection, although the majority of the metastatic nodes can be controlled by radiotherapy alone.

Paranasal Sinus Cancer

Squamous cell carcinomas arising from the paranasal sinuses generally are relatively asymptomatic and early diagnosis can rarely be made. Most lesions, when first diagnosed, already present evidence of bone destruction. The maxillary and ethmoid sinuses are commonly involved. Tumor arising from the sphenoid or frontal sinuses alone are extremely rare. Detailed evaluation of this disease requires careful radiologic examination, including polytomes of paranasal sinuses in anteroposterior and lateral projections and occasionally CT scans.

The AJC staging for this tumor is as follows:[2]

T1—tumor confined to the antral mucosa of the infrastructure with no bone erosion or destruction.

T2—tumor confined to the suprastructure mucosa without bone destruction, or to infrastructure with destruction of medial or inferior bony walls only.

T3—more extensive tumor invading skin of cheek, orbit, antrum, ethmoid sinuses, pterygoid muscle.

T4—massive tumor with invasion of cribriform plate, posterior ethmoids, sphenoid, nasopharynx, pterygoid plates, or base of skull.

Treatment of this group of lesions, except for early mucosal carcinomas, is a combination of radiation therapy and surgery. Although most tumors are advanced lesions, the incidence of lymph node metastases is not high, being approximately 20 percent of all cases; therefore routine radical neck dissection or elective neck irradiation is not recommended in patients without nodes. The infected sinus must be drained before radiotherapy is given. In some instances, radical surgery is performed first and then followed 3 or 4 weeks later by postoperative radiotherapy of 6,000 rads in 6 weeks. For preoperative treatment, a dose of 5,000 rads in 5 weeks is generally well-tolerated and is followed by maxillectomy and ethmoidectomy in approximately 1 month. Further radiation may be given postoperatively to any area of residual disease with boost technique.

In spite of the advanced stage of the carcinomas of the paranasal sinuses, the therapeutic results following combined radiotherapy and surgery are still reasonably good.[13] Approximately one-third of the patients of the entire group can be cured. For the early lesions, better than one out of two patients enjoy freedom from disease for 5 or more years. Radical neck dissection is indicated only when the metastatic nodes in the neck become apparent.

Cancer of the Salivary Glands

Malignant tumors of the salivary glands are comprised of mucoepidermoid carcinoma, squamous cell carcinoma, acinic cell carcinoma, adenoid cystic carcinoma, adenocarcinoma, and others. The majority of tumors occur in the parotid salivary gland and a few in the oral cavity and oropharynx. The growth usually manifests as a painless swelling in the parotid region. The first therapeutic approach is surgical removal. Radiotherapy is indicated only for the following conditions: (1) inoperable lesions, (2) incomplete surgical removal with known residual disease and/or difficulty in clearance of the resection margin around the facial nerve, (3) tumor extension beyond the capsule found during histologic examination, (4) perineural involvement, (5) high grade malignant tumors, (6) cancers with one or more local recurrences after previous surgery, (7) for patients refusing surgery.

Generally a dose of 6,500 rads in 6½

weeks is given for lesions with known residual disease or of inoperable condition. For localized microscopic disease, a dose of 5,500 rads in 5½ weeks should be sufficient. This can be carried out by a combination of external beam therapy with electron beam boost or interstitial implant if accessible. Experience has shown that following radiotherapy of this magnitude, the local recurrence rate is less than 10 percent.

COMPLICATIONS OF RADIATION THERAPY

Since radiation affects both normal and abnormal tissue, certain effects of radiation therapy are expected, such as abnormal facial growth in children and epilation of irradiated areas. Long-term effects of radiation-induced malignancy, particularly in childhood, have been observed, but the incidence of such malignant transformation of irradiated tissue is extremely low and should not be seriously taken into consideration in the selection of radiation therapy for life-threatening malignant tumors.

Minor side effects such as xerostomia, loss of taste, and dental caries are relatively common following radiation therapy to the oropharynx and salivary glands; these effects can usually be managed by supportive measures in addition to careful oral and dental hygiene. Most of the unpleasant side effects relative to taste and dry mouth are temporary, although in some instances the effects may be long lasting. Although carious teeth should be extracted prior to radiation in order to minimize later infection of the alveolar bone and osteitis, most sound teeth can survive radiation therapy and need not be extracted if the radiation dosages are kept within the limits of tolerance of the mandible and a meticulous dental hygiene program such as prophylaxis and frequent fluoridation of teeth can be maintained after irradiation.

Major complications include soft tissue ulceration, orocutaneous fistulas, and osteoradionecrosis of the mandible and hard palate.[6, 12, 40] Invariably these are related to curative radiation but may be coincidental to unusually aggressive therapy or faulty treatment technique. Important factors in the occurrence of complications include the treatment modalities employed; the time-dose-fraction program, the size of the irradiated portals, and the magnitude of radiation dosages; the extent of the disease and its location; and the patient's age and nutritional status. The incidence is further exaggerated following combined radiation therapy and surgery due to an excessive impairment of local blood supply and secondary infection. This is particularly true when curative doses of radiation therapy are given first to tumors and then followed by radical excision. In such an environment, the postoperative morbidity and mortality could be exceptionally high and at times, unacceptable in the modern practice of oncology. Other uncommon radiotherapeutic complications are radiation-induced hypopituitarism, hypothyroidism, and cataract formation. All of these complications and unpleasant sequelae of treatment should be accepted as a risk in the management of extensive tumors, but may be minimized by observing careful radiotherapeutic and surgical techniques and principles. Radiation-induced transverse myelitis fortunately is extremely rare and should be avoided at all costs. Severe fibrosis may occur with entrapment of nerves resulting in neuropathies.

NEW RADIATION MODALITIES

It has been apparent for some time that surgery has reached its limit of applicability in the treatment of cancer of the head and neck. On the other hand, modern radiation therapy with high energy radiation from cobalt 60 machines or linear accelerators—with the aid of dedicated computers in treatment planning—has not significantly improved the therapeutic results, although the complication rates undoubtedly have been reduced considerably. Further improvement in cure rates by radiation therapy is much needed. Various new treatment modalities have emerged on the horizon and these are briefly summarized as follows:

Particulate Radiation

Heavy Charged Particles

Proton and alpha particles have been used for radiation therapy in the past few years. These heavy particles are generated from a cyclotron and can produce sharp beam margins deep in the body for specific high dose irradiation. When the heavy particles are slowed down in the tissues, they release their maximum ionizations shortly before stoppage, known as Bragg Peak phenomenon. By employing various thickness of absorber, the position of the Bragg Peak can be placed in a predetermined site. Also, by using a rotating wedge disc of the absorber, multiple Bragg Peaks can be spread within the desired width of volume of irradiation and thus form a so-called modulator beam. Although the relative biological effectiveness (RBE) is similar to x-rays, this form of radiation may improve dose distribution so that a high dose can be delivered to the target volume in the hope of increasing local tumor control and of decreasing radiation complications. This technique has been used for clinical radiation therapy in the head and neck region by radiation therapists at the Massachusetts General Hospital with the 160 MeV photons from the Harvard-MIT cyclotron.[32] At the present time, it is too soon to evaluate the therapeutic results.

High LET Radiation

Based on the biologic evidence, it is thought by some investigators that radiation therapy by means of x-rays or gamma rays has been hampered by the presence of hypoxic cells in advanced tumors. These hypoxic cells may be responsible for some of the local failures following irradiation. In order to overcome the problems of hypoxia, currently radiations with high LET have been employed for clinical trials. LET is a term designated as energy transfer per unit length of ionizing track. It is generally a useful and simple way to indicate the quality of different types of radiations. Cobalt 60 and 200 kV x-rays have low LET, while fast neutrons and heavy particles have high LET. Experimentally, the higher the LET the lesser the oxygen enhancement ratio (OER). Fast neutrons generated by the cyclotron have an intermediate OER of around 1.5 to 1.8 and yet maintain adequate penetration to treat deep seated tumors similarly to the cobalt 60 beam. In spite of various biologic advantages of fast neutrons over x-rays (such as low OER and lack of repair of sublethal or potentially lethal damage), a clinical randomized prospective trial for head and neck tumors did not show any improvement in survival rates, although local tumor control was definitely superior.[10] Scattered information thus far shows good control of parotid tumors and soft tissue sarcomas after neutron therapy. Further prospective trials are needed if the superiority of neutrons over x-rays in head and neck malignancies is to be confirmed.

Other particulate radiations such as pi-mesons, helium, carbon, and neon ions have been explored for clinical radiation therapy. No clinical data are available to indicate their usefulness.

Hyperbaric Oxygen Therapy

Hypoxic cell sensitizers have recently been introduced experimentally. These include metronidazole (marketed as Flagyl), RO-07-0582 (misonidazole), and others. Metronidazole sensitizer is only moderately efficient and fairly high concentrations are required to produce worthwhile radiosensitization for clinical use. Clinical trial use of RO-07-0582 has been carried out in the United States and abroad. The amount of drug administered is limited by the immediate symptoms such as anorexia, nausea, vomiting, and neuropathy. Because of its toxicity, the drug is limited to two treatments per week in conjunction with radiotherapy. Clearly, the hypoxic cell sensitizers are in their infancy and their efficacy has to be evaluated in due time.

Hyperthermia

Experimentally, it has been found hypoxic cells are more sensitive to elevated temperature than normally oxygenated cells.[31] When hyperthermia is combined with x-rays, the OER is reduced. Currently, local heating of the tumor can be given in conjunction with localized radiation therapy, although the problems of local heat delivery systems must be worked out satisfactorily. The results are sketchy and inconclusive and further work is needed if any significant progress is to be anticipated.

SUMMARY

Carcinomas of the head and neck are potentially curable malignant tumors. When the tumor is diagnosed and treated in its early stages (T1), the cure rate achieved either by radiation therapy or surgery is high. The choice of treatment modality is extremely complex and demands full knowledge of the biology of the tumors, advantages and disadvantages of various disciplines and treatment results, and sympathetic understanding on the part of the physician and the patient. The T2 tumors may perhaps be better treated by radiation therapy first, since satisfactory control of the disease can be achieved with preservation of normal function and anatomic part. Surgery can then be employed for radiation failures as a salvage procedure. Extensive disease—T3 and T4—is often associated with bone and muscle involvement in addition to cervical lymph node metastases and is better treated by combined modalities (i.e., radiation therapy and surgery) if the lesion is surgically resectable. If the lesions are obviously incurable by any means, palliative radiation therapy may offer some symptomatic relief. The management of cervical metastatic nodes depends upon the primary site and the size and number of nodes. The limited metastatic nodal disease (N1 and N2) from primary cancers arising from Waldeyer's ring can be satisfactorily controlled by radiation therapy alone, and the residual disease in the neck may be dealt with by salvage surgery. The large metastatic nodes (N2b, N3) from oral cavity, hypopharynx, and larynx are better treated by radical neck dissection with adjuvant radiation therapy. Chemotherapy is used as an adjuvant procedure or for palliation in incurable patients.

Although malignant tumors of the head and neck are considered to be among the most curable neoplasms, the therapeutic results for advanced carcinomas are still far from ideal. The need for early diagnosis and treatment cannot be too strongly emphasized. It is hoped that the newer treatment modalities such as heavy charged particulate and high LET radiations, radiation sensitizers, and hyperthermia with radiation therapy will one day come to fruition with further improvement in cure rates. Indeed, it is the full cooperation and efforts between the surgeons and radiation therapists that ultimately benefits the patients afflicted with this disease.

SELECTED BIBLIOGRAPHY

Ackerman, J. L., and del Regato, J. A. 1977. Cancer Diagnosis, Treatment and Prognosis. 5th edn. C. V. Mosby, St. Louis.

Buschke, F., and Parker, R. G. 1972. Radiation Therapy in Cancer Management. Grune & Stratton, New York.

Casarett, A. P. 1968. Radiation Biology. Prentice-Hall, Englewood Cliffs, NJ.

Fletcher, G. H. Ed. 1973. Textbook of Radiotherapy. 2nd edn. Lea & Febiger, Philadelphia.

Hall, 1978. Radiobiology for the Radiologist. 2nd edn. Harper & Row, Hagerstown, MD.

MacComb, W. S., and Fletcher, G. H. 1967. Cancer of the Head and Neck. Williams & Wilkins, Baltimore.

Moss, W. T., Brand, W. N., and Battifora, H. 1973. Radiation Oncology; Rationale, Technique, Results. 4th edn. C. V. Mosby, St. Louis.

Rubin, P., and Casarett, G. W. 1968. Clinical Radiation Pathology. 2 Vols. Saunders, Philadelphia.

REFERENCES

1. Adam, G. E. 1973. Chemical radiosensitization of hypoxic cells. British Medical Bulletin, 29: 48.

2. American Joint Committee for Cancer Staging and End Results Reporting. 1977. Manual for Staging of Cancer. American Joint Committee, Chicago.

3. Ash, Clifford L. 1962. Oral cancer: A twenty-five year study. Janeway lecture, 1961. American Journal of Roentgenology, 87:417.

4. Ballantyne, A. J., and Fletcher, G. H. 1965. Management of residual or recurrent cancer following radiation therapy for squamous cell carcinoma of the oropharynx. American Journal of Roentgenology,93: 29.

5. Bataini, J. P., Ennuyer, A., Poncet, P., and Ghossein, N. A. 1974. Treatment of supraglottic cancer by radical high dose radiotherapy. Cancer, 33: 1253.

6. Bedwinek, J. M., Shukovsky, L. J., Fletcher, G. H., and Daley, T. E. 1976. Osteonecrosis in patients treated with definitive radiotherapy for squamous cell carcinomas of the oral cavity and nasopharynx and oropharynx. Radiology, 119: 655.

7. Boone, M. L., Harle, T. S., Higholt, H. W., and Fletcher, G. H. 1968. Malignant disease of the paranasal sinuses and nasal cavity. Importance of precise localization of extent of disease. American Journal of Roentgenology. 102: 627.

8. Cady, B., and Catlin, D. 1969. Epidermoid carcinoma of the gum: A 20-year survey. Cancer, 23: 551.

9. Campos, J. L., Lampe, I., and Fayos, J. V. 1971. Radiotherapy of carcinoma of the floor of the mouth. Radiology, 99: 667.

10. Catterall, M., and Vonberg D. D.: 1974. Treatment of advanced tumours of head and neck with fast neutrons. British Medical Journal, 3: 137.

11. Chen, K. Y., and Fletcher, G. H. 1971. Malignant tumors of the nasopharynx. Radiogy, 99: 165.

12. Cheng, V. S. T., and Wang, C. C. 1974. Osteoradionecrosis of the mandible resulting from external megavoltage radiation therapy. Radiology, 112: 685.

13. Cheng, V. S. T., and Wang, C. C. 1977. Carcinomas of the paranasal sinuses: A study of sixty-six cases. Cancer, 40: 3038.

14. Cunningham, M. P., and Catlin, D. 1967. Cancer of the pharyngeal wall. Cancer, 20:1859.

15. Fayos, J. V., and Lampe, I. 1971. Radiation therapy of carcinoma of the tonsillar region. American Journal of Roentgenology, Radium Therapy, and Nuclear Medicine, 111: 85.

16. Fayos, J. V., and Lampe, I. 1972. Treatment of squamous cell carcinoma of the oral cavity. American Journal of Surgery, 124: 493.

17. Fletcher, G. H. 1972. Elective irradiation of subclinical disease in cancers of the head and neck. Cancer, 29: 1450.

18. Fletcher, G. H., and Lindberg, R. D. 1966. Squamous cell carcinomas of the tonsillar area and palatine arch. American Journal of Roentgenology, 96: 574.

19. Flynn, M. B., Jesse, R. H., and Lindberg, R. D. 1972. Surgery and irradiation in the treatment of squamous cell cancer of the supraglottic larynx. American Journal of Surgery, 124: 477.

20. Horiot, J. C., Fletcher, G. H., Ballantyne, A. J., and Lindberg, R. D. 1972. Analysis of failures in early vocal-cord cancer. Radiology, 103: 663.

21. Jesse, R. H., and Fletcher, G. H. 1977. Treatment of the neck in patients with squamous cell carcinoma of the head and neck. Cancer, 39 (2 suppl.): 868.

22. Lampe, I. 1955. Radiation therapy of cancer of the buccal mucosa and lower gingiva. American Journal of Roentgenology, 73: 628.

23. Lederman, M. 1971. Cancer of the larynx. I. Natural history in relation to treatment. British Journal of Radiology, 44: 569.

24. Lederman, M., and Mould, R. F. 1968. Radiation treatment of cancer of the pharynx: With special reference to telecobalt therapy. British Journal of Radiology, 41: 251.

25. Leroux-Robert, J. 1956. Indications for radical surgery, partial surgery, radiotherapy and combined surgery, and radiotherapy for cancer of the larynx and hypopharynx. Annals of Otology, Rhinology, and Laryngology, 65: 137.

26. Lindberg, R. 1972. Distribution of cervical lymph nodes metastases from squamous cell carcinoma of the upper respiratory and digestive tracts. Cancer, 29: 1446.

27. Perez, C. A., Lee, F. A., Ackerman, L. V., Ogura, J. H., and Powers, W. E. 1976. Nonrandomized comparison of preoperative irradiation and surgery versus irradiation alone in the management of carcinoma of the tonsil. American Journal of Roentgenology 126: 248.

28. Powers, W. E., and Palmer, L. A. 1968. Biological basis of preoperative radiation treatment. American Journal of Roentgenology, 102: 176.

29. Rider, W. D. 1962. Epithelial cancer of the tonsillar area. Radiology, 78: 760.

30. Silverstone, S. M., Goldman, J. L., and Ryan, J. R. 1970. Combined high dose radiation therapy and surgery of advanced cancer of the laryngopharynx. Frontiers of Radiation Therapy and Oncology, 5: 106.

31. Suit, H. D., and Shwayder, M.: 1974. Hyperthermia: Potential as an anti-tumor agent. Cancer, 34:122.

32. Suit, H. D., Goitein, M., Tepper, J. E., Verhey, L., Koehler, A. M., Schneider, R., and Gragoudas, E. 1977. Clinical experience and expectation with protons and heavy ions. International Journal of Radiation Oncology, Biology, Physics, 3:115.

33. Wang, C. C. 1967. Radical re-irradiation for carcinoma arising from the previously irradiated larynx. Laryngoscope, 77: 2189.

34. Wang, C. C. 1971. Radiotherapeutic management of carcinoma of the posterior pharyngeal wall. Cancer, 27: 894.

35. Wang, C. C. 1972. Management and prognosis of squamous-cell carcinoma of the tonsillar region. Radiology, 104: 667.

36. Wang, C. C. 1972. The role of radiation therapy in the treatment of carcinoma of the oral cavity. Otolaryngolic Clinics of North America, 5: 357.

37. Wang, C. C. 1973. Megavoltage radiation therapy for supraglottic carcinoma. Result of treatment. Radiology, 109: 183.

38. Wang, C. C. 1974. Treatment of glottic carcinoma by megavoltage radiation therapy and results. American Journal of Roentgenology, Radium Therapy, and Nuclear Medicine, 120: 157.

39. Wang, C. C. 1977. Treatment of carcinoma of the nasopharynx by irradiation. Ear, Nose, and Throat Journal. 56: 97.

40. Wang, C. C., and Doppke, K. 1976. Osteoradionecrosis of the temporal bone—Consideration of nominal standard dose. Inter-

national Journal of Radiation Oncology, Biology, Physics, 1:   881.

41. Wang, C. C., and Schulz, M. D. 1966. Management of locally recurrent carcinoma of the nasopharynx. Radiology, 86:   900.

42. Wang, C. C., Little, J. B., and Schulz, M. D. 1962. Cancer of the nasopharynx: Its clinical and radiotherapeutic considerations. Cancer, 15:   921.

43. Wang, C. C., Schulz, M. D., and Miller, D. 1972. Combined radiation therapy and surgery for carcinoma of the supraglottis and pyriform sinus. Laryngoscope, 82:1882.

8 | Dental Considerations in the Head and Neck Cancer Patient

Matthew J. Jackson, D.M.D., M.S.D.
James D. Billie, M.D., D.M.D.

INTRODUCTION

The current therapeutic approach toward head and neck cancer is a multifaceted regimen that may include surgery, chemotherapy, immunotherapy, radiotherapy, and dental therapy. The dental profession plays an important role in the care of the head and neck cancer patient. Many oral cancers are now discovered during routine thorough dental examinations. Proper preoperative, preirradiation, and prechemotherapy dental care can significantly decrease morbidity. For optimal patient care the participation of a general dentist, as well as an oral surgeon, maxillofacial prosthodontist, endodontist, or periodontist may be necessary.

The modern dentist's role is to evaluate and to treat systematically both the hard tissues (i.e., teeth and supporting structures) and the soft tissues of the oral cavity. He should be actively involved in the pretreatment, treatment, and posttreatment phases of cancer therapy. Dental expertise is particularly important in the care of patients who will require postoperative prosthetic devices, chemotherapy, or radiotherapy. Regardless of the anticipated modality of treatment of the primary lesion, it is essential to obtain pretreatment dental consultation if optimal oral health is to be maintained.

General Dental Considerations

Regardless of the anticipated treatment modalities, the general dental examination of the cancer patient is the same. Routine examination of the soft and hard tissues of the oral cavity is systematic. First, the mucosa in all areas is thoroughly inspected and palpated, and any abnormality is recorded. Any areas of anesthesia are also recorded. The extent of the tumor is ascertained by visualization and palpation. Next, a panoramic x-ray is take of both the edentulous and dentulous patient. This x-ray may reveal bone destruction by tumor, cysts, granulomas, abscesses, pathologic fractures, or other pathology of the mandible or maxilla. An occlusal x-ray often adds definition to lesions in the anterior regions of the mandible and maxilla. In dentulous patients, periapical and bite wing x-rays of all teeth may be obtained, as they add great definition to bony lesions near the tooth apices. Alveolar bone loss due to periodontal disease or tumor invasion is quantitated.

Each individual tooth is then inspected, utilizing appropriate dental instruments. Caries, erosion, and cementum exposure are evaluated. The periodontal or supporting structures are then evaluated; these include the gingiva and alveolar bone. Tooth mobility is recorded on a scale of zero to four. Alveolar bone loss is quantitated by bite wing x-rays. Pathologic periodontal pockets greater than 3 mm are measured with a periodontal probe and recorded. Vitality of all remaining teeth is evaluated by means of an electric pulp-testing device. The condition of existing fixed prostheses is noted. Partial or complete dentures, if present, are evalu-

145

ated for stability, condition, and fit. Finally, the interincisal opening is measured to ascertain the function of the temporomandibular joint, supporting structures, and muscles of mastication. The normal interincisal opening is approximately 45 mm.

The state of oral hygiene is then ascertained. All plaque and calculus are meticulously removed by means of appropriate curettes and dental pumice. The importance of excellent oral hygiene is stressed to the patient and family members. Home care should include frequent brushings using accepted techniques with a soft brush, daily flossing, and use of fluoride for certain patients. Time spent by the dentist or hygienist stressing the importance of proper oral hygiene is time well spent.

DENTAL THERAPY IN THE SURGICAL PATIENT

If the tumor will require only conservative soft-tissue excision with primary closure or local flap closure, dental therapy is limited to control of symptomatic teeth, routine fillings, and cleaning of teeth. This treatment could be readily completed in several days prior to surgery and is considered ideal if no other treatment modality is planned for tumor control.

If the tumor excision will result in an oral-antral or oral-nasal fistula or in velopharyngeal incompetence, a preoperative impression is taken for the construction of a surgical obturator. If the patient has a reasonable complement of teeth and segmental resection of the mandible will be included as part of the surgical treatment, preoperative dental impressions are taken for the construction of guiding planes, in case they may be needed. These protocols are discussed in detail in Chapter 9.

At the time of surgery, if segmental resection of the mandible is done, dentulous patients should be placed into intermaxillary fixation to stabilize the remaining mandibular segment.[20] Full arch bars are not necessary for this fixation. A short segmen-

tal arch bar with only three lugs on the bar usually will suffice. The segmental arch bar is applied, with twenty-four gauge wire, to the upper and lower first and second bicuspid region on the side opposite the surgery. Loose intermaxillary fixation is applied with elastics or wire simply to hold the mandible in the midline. The acid-etching bonded acrylic-type bracket may also be used for this limited intermaxillary fixation. Intermaxillary fixation is maintained continuously for 2 to 4 weeks except for inspection of the surgical site. Fixation at night should continue for another 4 to 8 weeks. In the fourth week, the patient is instructed to begin bite therapy by sitting in front of a mirror and practicing biting into centric occlusion. Leaving one elastic on often helps to guide the mandible into position at first. Next the patient is advanced to eating in front of a mirror, often with the help of one elastic band until the muscles of mastication are retrained to bite into a good occlusion; this may take 4 to 8 weeks or more. When the bite remains stable, the arch bars are removed. This sequence often can prevent a disabling malocclusion.

DENTAL THERAPY IN THE CHEMOTHERAPY PATIENT

The goal of dental therapy for the chemotherapy patient is to reduce morbidity and to avoid delay of chemotherapy treatments. Most cancer chemotherapy agents currently used for treatment of cancer of the head and neck region, as well as other regions of the body, have side effects on oral tissues. These effects vary with different agents as well as with dosage and are related to the cytotoxic, antimitotic, or photosensitization of the agents on mucosal tissues in general. Tissues with a high turnover rate—such as oral mucosa—which are subject to physical and chemical trauma are more likely to be affected by the chemotherapy agents. Intense mucositis and diffuse stomatitis often develop and may cause delay in chemotherapy administration. Due to decreased host resistance, normal bacterial, viral, and fungal flora of the oral cavity often become pathogens and may infect the injured mucosal tissues. For these reasons, dental therapy should be initiated before chemotherapy and followed through the entire course of chemotherapy.

Dental treatment at the prechemotherapy visit should include a thorough examination. Teeth which are beyond restoration should be extracted. Dental plaque and calculus must be removed, and the importance of strict oral hygiene for the duration of the chemotherapy treatment must be stressed. Periodontal disease should be corrected as well as possible by appropriate curettage or minor periodontal surgery. This is particularly important in areas where periodontal pockets of 5 mm or greater exist, since these pockets collect food debris and may be a focus for infection. If advanced generalized periodontal disease exists, it is best to extract the teeth in the involved areas prior to the initiation of chemotherapy. Adequate time, usually 7 to 10 days, should be allowed for healing of extraction sites.

Once chemotherapy is begun, dental therapy is directed at maintaining oral hygiene, decreasing mucositis effects, assisting the occasional patient who has xerostomia, and promoting adequate oral intake. Similar side effects occur with radiotherapy, and their treatment will be covered in the radiotherapy section.

Bleeding disorders involving the oral cavity sometimes occur with certain chemotherapy agents. These disorders may include eccymosis, petechiae, hematoma, or frank hemorrhage. The underlying cause is usually induced thrombocytopenia or disseminated intravascular coagulation. Oral care should include removal of local irritants. Systemic treatment of bleeding disorder may become necessary to control bleeding. Occasionally an arterial bleeder may develop in the gingiva. Local compression will usually control the bleeding and may be necessary in some cases. An alginate impression may also be useful for controlling bleeding. Topical thrombin or other agents, such as microfibrillar collagen, may be placed in the impression. The impression is then repositioned on the teeth so that the hemostatic agents will be held against the bleeding site. This procedure usually will stop the most difficult to control gingival bleeding site.

ORAL CARE OF THE IRRADIATED PATIENT

Radiotherapy may produce significant side effects. The objective of radiation therapy is to eradicate the tumor with doses of ionizing radiation adequate to destroy the tumor but able to be tolerated by the normal structures within the field of irradiation. However, tumoricidal doses of radiation will invariably cause some degree of transient or permanent damage to normal tissues.

The severity of this damage is directly related to the type of radiation and to the total dosage, fractionation, and duration of treatment. These problems may be eliminated or at least minimized by proper institution of preventive dental care. The effects of tumoricidal doses of ionizing radiation on oral tissues may be summarized as follows:

1. Xerostomia
2. Rampant decaying teeth ("radiation decay")
3. Early wearing of occlusal and incisal edges
4. Increased sensitivity of the teeth
5. Edema
6. Mucositis
7. Trismus
8. Loss of taste
9. Infection
10. Necrosis of soft and hard tissues.

Pretreatment Evaluation and Therapy

The oral side effects of radiation therapy are encountered when treatment is applied directly to oral or contiguous structures or both. Therefore, all patients receiving irradiation to the head and neck should be examined and treated by the dentist. During the initial oral examination, all necessary diagnostic aids should be employed to provide an adequate assessment of the hard and soft structures in the mouth. In addition, the dental "I.Q." of the patient must be evaluated in order to determine whether or not he will follow the necessary dental recommendations. Many of the patients have little understanding of oral care. All potential short-term and long-term sequelae are explained in an attempt to have the patient comprehend the severity of the problem. Appropriate dental treatment protocols are presented to the patient following this evaluation. Many of the patient's questions can be answered at this time, and the patient's mind can be set at ease.

After the dental protocol has been accepted by the patient, all procedures necessary to minimize or eliminate radiation sequelae are initiated. Any tooth that cannot be restored, whether due to periodontal disease, trauma, or caries, must be extracted prior to initiation of the treatment program.[3, 11, 20] If the patient is to have surgery before radiation therapy, those teeth that are to be extracted are removed and any necessary alveoloplasties are performed at the time of surgery. This usually provides adequate healing time and eliminates future anesthesia for the patient. However, if radiation therapy is to be given preoperatively or as the primary modality of treatment, the compromised teeth should be extracted and therapy to that area should not be started until adequate healing has occurred in order to prevent wound breakdown.[18, 20]

Those patients whose dentition is sound are instructed about proper oral hygiene and dental care. Fluoride carriers are constructed so that the patients may administer their own daily fluoride treatments at home. If a radiotherapy prosthesis is indicated, construction is initiated at this time.

The maintenance of as many sound teeth as possible is paramount, as the rehabilitation of the patient is greatly facilitated by the presence of teeth. These teeth will help the patient while chewing, as well as help to support such prostheses as resection appliances, obturators, and partial dentures.[27]

Immediate Dental Therapy

All symptomatic teeth must be managed, if possible, prior to beginning the treatment program in order to avoid difficulty during and after the treatment. Teeth that cannot be restored are extracted before therapy. Adequate healing cannot be obtained in less than 10 days following extraction. The more difficult the extraction, i.e., the more trauma involved, the longer the healing period will be. Impacted or ankylosed teeth may take 4 or more weeks to heal. Inadequate healing will invariably lead to soft and/or hard tissue necrosis.[18, 20, 27]

If the condemned teeth and their supporting bone are in the field of irradiation, or adjacent to it, it is imperative that alveoloplasties are performed at the time of the extractions. The aims of the alveoloplasty are to remove all loose spicules and sharp projections of bone, to provide an ideal edentulous ridge anatomy, and to permit the tissue to be closed primarily. This will prevent puncture or erosion of the bone through the gingival tissues and will prevent debris from entering into the sockets and delaying healing.[20] Those teeth that are not in the field of irradiation may be managed more conventionally.

If compromised teeth cannot be removed because of the rapidity of growth, size, or contiguity of tumor to the teeth, these teeth should not be considered for elective removal and alternative, conservative procedures should be instituted. However, all symptomatic teeth whether they need to be extracted or whether they are salvageable must be rendered asymptomatic as quickly as possible.[6]

DENTAL TREATMENT PROTOCOLS

Management of Short Term Sequelae

MUCOSITIS

Oral mucosa in the field of irradiation will develop a series of transient and permanent changes. The degree of mucositis is directly related to the total dose, the number of doses given, and the type of radiation. The chief complaints are pain, burning, and soreness, which usually occur during the first 2 weeks of therapy and last for several weeks after therapy has been completed. The tissue initially becomes edematous and hyperemic. This is followed by whitening, denudation, and ulceration of the mucosal surfaces. The injured mucosa is then covered by a fibrinous exudate (Fig. 8-1).

Medicaments such as viscous lidocaine, colloidal silver solutions, salt and soda rinses, Orabase, and peroxide rinses all have been used in controlling the problem. The objectives in the management of mucositis are to make the patient as comfortable as possible, to eliminate secondary infections, and to allow for the maintenance of proper nutrition. Salt may burn and should be discontinued when mucositis becomes painful.[22]

Eating will become a difficult chore. Coarse and highly seasoned foods are to be avoided. The use of topical viscous lidocaine swished in the mouth for several minutes before meals will anesthetize the irritated tissues and afford the patient more comfort in mastication and swallowing. Care must be

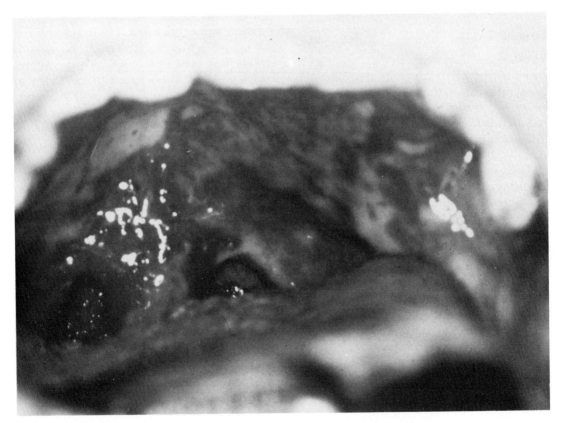

Fig. 8-1. Mucositis of the soft palate. The tissue is raw, edematous, and partially covered by a fibrinous exudate.

taken during the meal to avoid accidental aspiration of food and drink because of the abolishment of the gag reflex by the topical anesthetic.[6, 15]

Other topical medicaments may help the patient at rest or during eating; demulcents and antiseptics such as colloidal silver solutions have helped considerably.[22] Systemic analgesics may be of benefit in severe cases. However, it is impossible to totally eliminate the discomfort. Mucositis is a reversible situation; but the patient should know that although it is only a transient state, the tissue involved has become permanently compromised and will remain so even when the pain has subsided and the mucositis has healed. If the discomfort becomes severe and the nutritional status of the patient becomes compromised, a nasogastric tube should be inserted to ensure proper nutrition.

LOSS OF TASTE

The loss of taste (hypogeusia)[9] is experienced early in therapy at approximately 3,000 rads, due to the injury of the microvillae or the surfaces of the taste buds. This may be a transient problem; however, there could be some permanent taste loss at dosages of 6,000 rads or greater.[15] Partial sense of taste may return within 20 to 60 days following the completion of therapy, and should return fully within 2 to 4 months, if it is going to return.[6] The combination of loss of taste, mucositis, and xerostomia leads to a loss of appetite and of the desire to eat. This problem should be explained and the patient's nutritional intake and weight must be recorded in order to ensure proper monitoring.

Long Term Management Problems

XEROSTOMIA

Following irradiation of the major salivary glands there is a permanent quantitative and qualitative reduction of saliva. This se-

quela is related to the dose and duration of the ionizing radiation. Radiation-induced xerostomia is rapid in onset, pronounced, and usually irreversible. This in turn leads to a pronounced alteration of the oral environment. The watery or serous secretions are lost first. The residual salivary secretions after radiation-induced xerostomia are of the mucin type, which are thick, ropey, and tenacious. Patients complain of extreme dryness and difficulty in swallowing food. Changes in the intraoral soft tissues, such as cracking and bleeding, are common. This fragile, damaged tissue is extremely painful and distressing to the patient, especially when eating. Moistening or liquefying the food will facilitate eating and swallowing and help the patient to maintain an adequate nutritional intake.

Treatment of xerostomia is palliative.[15-18, 31] If the patient is made aware of the problems before onset, he will be more able to accommodate to them. The use of artificial saliva rinses may be prescribed. Numerous rinses have been developed with varying results, and Xero-Lube (First Texas Pharmaceutical) or Ora-Lube (Veteran's Administration Hospital, Houston, Texas) are now commercially available. The advantage of these medicaments is that their viscosity and electrolyte levels are similar to saliva.[32] Fluoride is added to enhance the mineralization capacity of the solution, which is high in calcium and phosphate. Other preparations can be employed with the objective of coating and lubricating the dry mucosa and of relieving the soft tissue symptoms.

DENTAL CARIES

With the onset of xerostomia, the inherent mechanical and chemical defenses against dental decay are greatly impaired. The saliva is no longer able to debride the teeth mechanically. Serous salivary secretions have been lost and what remains is a "stringy," thick, and tenacious mucinous secretion, which allows the accumulation of plaque and microorganisms on the teeth.

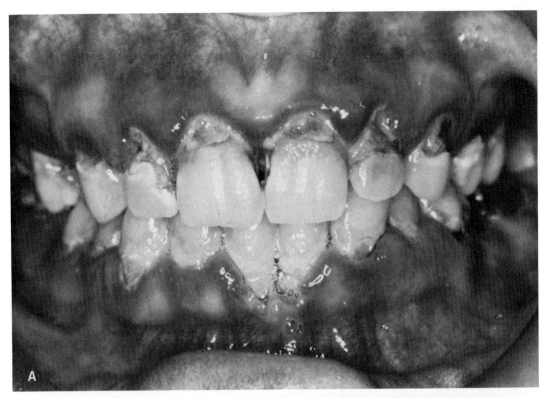

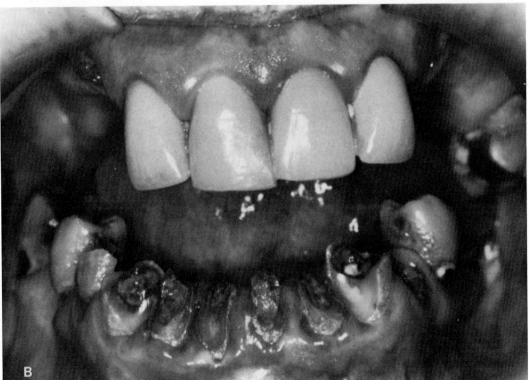

Fig. 8-2. (A) Rampant cervical decay involving virtually all teeth in the mouth; this developed 3 months after radiation therapy. Patient was not placed on prophylactic fluoride. (B) Amputation of the crowns of the lower incisor due to radiation decay.

Chemically, the saliva becomes more acidic and a highly cariogenic microflora and plaque appear. An increased number of yeast and *Streptococcus mutans* are noted. There is a drastic decrease in the protective salivary electrolytes and immunoproteins. Concurrent with the marked decrease of salivary flow is a change of diet from a detergent to a nondetergent type. This change of diet is a result of mucosal dryness and discomfort. All of these factors added together lead to a potentially enormous caries insult.[7, 25]

If the patient is not protected, the development of xerostomia will be followed by rampant dental decay involving virtually all teeth, no matter what the status of the dentition was prior to treatment (Figs. 8-2A and B). Radiation decay can be prevented by the daily use of fluoride and meticulous oral hygiene. Areas of demineralization will be remineralized and hardened by long-term fluoride use. Associated tooth sensitivity and occlusal and incisal wear will also be minimized by fluoride use.[6, 15, 18, 29, 32]

Various fluoride protocols have been devised for the irradiated patient. The one mentioned here is that developed at the M.D. Anderson Hospital and Tumor Institute.[11] It is a simple and inexpensive procedure and does not require much effort in addition to normal oral hygiene procedures. A 1 percent neutral sodium fluoride gel containing a disclosing agent is employed. The gel is placed into custom flexible carriers made on dental casts from impressions taken of the patient's dental arches (Fig. 8-3). The patient brushes and flosses his teeth following proper oral hygiene techniques. The carriers are then coated with the fluoride gel and placed over their respective dental arches (Fig. 8-4); they are left in place for only 5 minutes per day. The patient must use fluoride every day for the rest of his life.

Intimate fluoride contact of all tooth

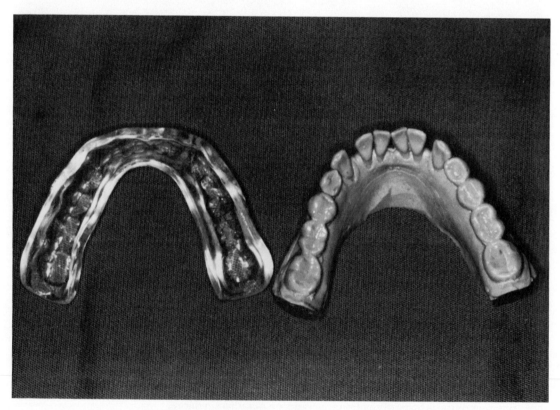

Fig. 8-3. Flexible fluoride carrier made to dental cast of patient's teeth.

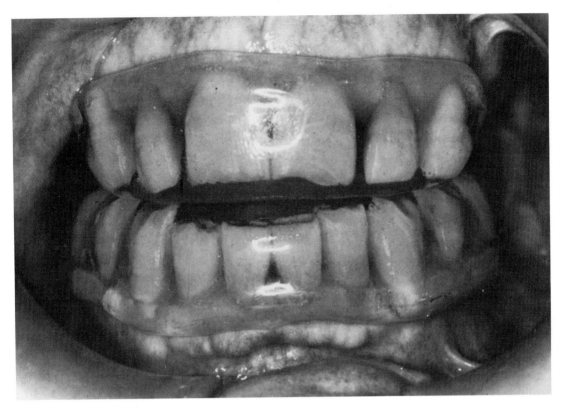

Fig. 8-4. Fluoride carriers in place in the patient's mouth.

surfaces is achieved by the use of the customized trays and by the pumping effect of clenching the teeth. After 5 minutes of contact, the carriers are removed and the gel is rinsed off. Those areas that have not been properly brushed or flossed appear red from the disclosing agent incorporated in the gel. The patient will then rebrush and floss those deficient areas. Fluoride applications may be increased as needed if demineralization is evident. A neutral fluoride gel and smooth and flexible carriers are used to minimize trauma to the fragile and sensitive oral mucosa.

SOFT AND HARD TISSUE NECROSIS

Therapeutic doses of irradiation to bone and soft tissue will cause the following basic physiological changes:

1. Impaired blood supply resulting in a decreased ability of the tissue to respond to injury.

2. Extracapillary fibrosis and decreased diffusion through the capillary wall.

3. Thickening of the basement membrane of the capillaries.

4. Arteriolar-capillary intimal hyalinosis.

5. Inhibition of both capillary sprouting and vascular remodeling.

6. Vessel occlusion, a decrease in the number of small vessels per area, and a compensatory dilatation of remaining capillaries—telangiectasia (Fig. 8-5).

7. Separation of periosteum or endosteum from the underlying bone resulting in denuded bone, which frequently dies from lack of blood supply.

8. Disturbance of the well-balanced process of destruction and reconstruction due to direct damage to the osteoblasts or osteocytes.[26]

The effects of radiation therapy on bone is due to injury to its cellular and vascular components. The end result is osteo-

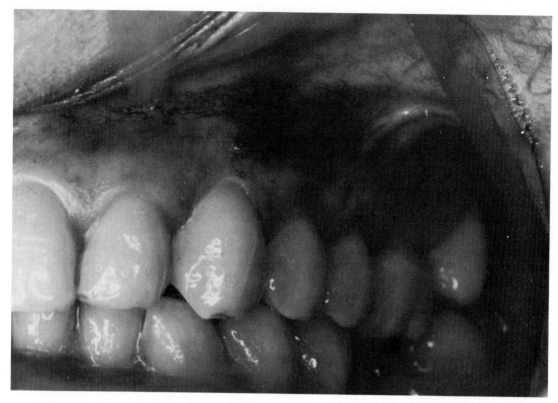

Fig. 8-5. Capillary engorgement (telangiectasia) of the buccal mucosa due to the effects of radiation.

porosis leading to osteonecrosis. This may occur under certain circumstances following high doses of radiation directly to these structures. However, radiation-induced osteitis or bone death is of little significance as long as the bone does not become infected or subject to great stress or trauma (Fig. 8-6). The prevention of radiation caries becomes paramount. If the decay process is allowed to proceed, microorganisms can easily traverse the dental tubules, enter the irradiated and compromised supporting osseous foundation, and lead to symptoms.

Necrotic soft-tissue ulcerations are painful, enlarge rapidly unless immediately treated, and are slow to heal; they can be the result of chemical, mechanical, or microbial insult. Early necrotic areas can be managed conservatively by irrigations with a mild solution of warm water mixed with salt and soda. For more severely affected areas, topical applications of a paste containing zinc

peroxide, carboxymethyl cellulose, and hydrogen peroxide or of a spray of 0.5 percent predisolone sodium phosphate with neomycin sulfate will be effective. These medicaments prevent further spreading of ulcerations and help to promote healing.

If the soft-tissue necrosis continues, the underlying devitalized bone will become exposed. Patients are most vulnerable to osteoradionecrosis within the first 2 years after therapy. Conservative management must first be attempted. Applications of zinc peroxide paste or 1 percent neomycin solutions are often adequate for stabilizing the problem. Additional procedures which will facilitate healing include gentle debridement of loose bone spicules, mild oral irrigations, and meticulous oral hygiene. Gross infection and severe pain will necessitate the use of systemic antibiotics and analgesics. Recently, hyperbaric oxygen therapy has been used in treating septic osteonecrosis. Only if

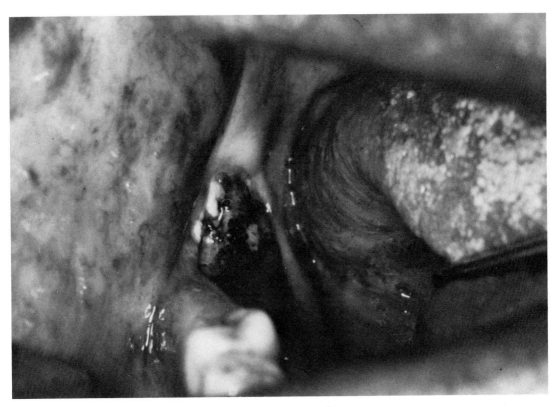

Fig. 8-6. Osteoradionecrosis of the mandible after placement of a removable partial denture immediately after therapy.

conservative methods have proven fruitless and the patient continues to have intractable pain, severe infection, and trismus, must surgical procedures then be employed to remove the necrotic areas; often, these procedures have severe debilitating results.[5, 11-15, 21, 24]

TRISMUS

Patients receiving radiation that directly affects the muscles of mastication or the temporomandibular joint (TMJ) may develop varying degrees of trismus.[6, 11, 15] This may be due to factors such as tonic spasms and fibrosis of the masticatory muscles, and/or fibrotic changes in the capsular elements of the TMJ. Trismus may occur during therapy or may in some cases not become apparent until 3 to 6 months after completion of radiotherapy. One must always be aware of possible tumor recurrence involving the muscles of mastication which can also lead to trismus.

Patients who are to receive high dosages of ionizing irradiation to the muscles of mastication or the TMJ, especially bilaterally, should be instructed about mouth-opening exercises in order to minimize muscle fibrosis and loss of interarch space. A simple exercise of opening the mouth as widely as possible 20 times, 3 to 4 times daily, should suffice.

For those patients who do develop frank trismus more definitive and intensive measures must be instituted. All possible conservative measures must be attempted before considering any surgical procedures to correct this problem. The degree of opening must be recorded and monitored at regular intervals. Intensive exercises and prostheses are utilized to regain the lost space. Appliances employing wedges, screws, springs, or elastics can be prescribed in an attempt to stretch the muscles and fibrotic contractures. (See Ch. 9 for more detail.)

RADIATION THERAPY PROSTHESES

The radiotherapist may need to use prosthetic devices to facilitate the treatment program. Any or all of the following can be devised and utilized: radiation stents, carriers, cone locators, tissue displacers, and shield appliances. In addition to optimizing the effects of head and neck irradiation, these devices can also prevent some of the sequelae.

A team approach requiring close collaboration between the prosthodontist and the radiotherapist is necessary to accomplish treatment goals. The radiotherapist must outline the area to be treated and the prosthodontist must analyze and explain to the therapist the limitations encountered in the construction of the device. The size and shape of the prosthesis depends on the fields of radiation planned for any given primary site. The desired amount of opening of the mouth likewise depends on the objectives of the prosthodontist and the therapist. The consequences of the prosthodontist's design can be assessed at the completion of therapy and thereafter. A sharply defined exudative mucositis is the best evidence that the geometry of the treatment has been reproduced at every period of irradiation. Posttreatment sequelae can often be predicted.

Some of the sequelae of radiation therapy can be severe and debilitating, even though the patient is free of disease. The objective is to eliminate or minimize the side effects of therapy. The use of therapy prostheses can be of great benefit in meeting these objectives. The need for treatment prostheses are as follows:

1. To outline and define fields of treatment.

2. To assist with the proper direction of the radiation beams.

3. To provide protection for contiguous normal tissues.

4. To displace the tongue, lips, or cheeks.

5. To serve as carriers for radium sources.

6. To facilitate patient set-up.

7. To permit duplication of the treatment arrangement.

8. To ensure accuracy of beam directions.

9. To simplify dosimetry in the tumor and in normal tissue.[14, 23]

The treatment program will achieve the goals of therapeutic success and minimal sequelae if the stent and/or shield meet the requirements listed above and the following common prosthetic considerations:

1. Comfort
2. Minimal weight
3. Stability
4. Accuracy
5. Self-retaining
6. Minimal adjustments
7. Breakage resistant
8. Easy to repair
9. Easy to clean
10. Allows the patient to breathe without much effort
11. Allows visualization of the tissues
12. Easy to place and remove.[28]

Types of Therapy Prostheses

TISSUE DISPLACERS

This type of device ensures that those tissues that need to be irradiated are positioned within the fields (e.g., tongue) and those tissues that are to be spared are correctly displaced (Figs. 8-7A and B). Variations in design are made according to the objectives of the therapy regimen (Fig. 8-8).

SHIELDS/TISSUE DISPLACERS

With the use of various types of radiation sources such as electron beam or orthovol-

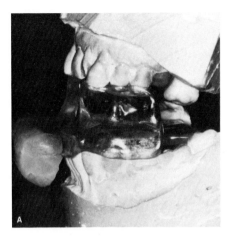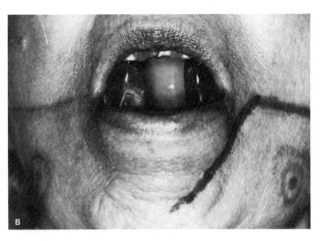

Fig. 8-7. (A) Tissue displacer in place on articulated casts of the patient. The prosthesis raises the maxilla and the lip out of the radiation field while the tongue platform with radiopaque ribbon secures the tongue into the field. (B) Stent in place in mouth. Note elevation of the maxilla and repositioning of the lower lip relative to field markings.

tage, shielding devices may be utilized to protect contiguous intraoral structures that need not be irradiated. Lead, or alloys of lead, of varying thicknesses may be embedded into the prosthesis to shield such structures as the tongue and gingiva (Tables 8-1 and 8-2). In addition to the shielding effect, there is usually a displacement of this tissue away from the radiation beam (Figs. 8-9A and B). This type of device will minimize radiation sequelae on normal structures that need not receive therapy. Close collaboration with the therapist is necessary to achieve realistic treatment goals.

CARRIERS

A carrier appliance is indicated when a radioactive source is administered by means of beads, capsules, or needles; usually radium or cesium 137 is the radiation source. The device is designed and constructed to place and hold the radiation source accurately and securely in the same position during each period of treatment (Figs. 8-10A–C). This provides accurate dosimetry to the tumor and to the adjacent marginal tissue and minimizes irradiation to normal structures that need not be exposed.

TABLE 8-1 MATERIAL THICKNESSES NEEDED TO STOP ELECTRONS

Electron Energy (MeV)	Lead or Cerrobend* (Lead-Alloy) Thickness (inches)†
6	$^1/_{16}$
9	$^1/_8$
12	$^3/_{16}$
15	$^1/_4$
18	$^5/_{16}$

*Metal Goods Corporation.
†Densities: Lead = 11.3 g/cm³, Cerrobend = 9.4 g/cm³.

TABLE 8-2 MATERIAL THICKNESSES NEEDED TO REDUCE X-RAY TRANSMISSION TO 5 PERCENT

Photon Energy	Lead or Cerrobend Thickness (inches)*
Cobalt 60 x-rays	2
4 MV x-rays	$2^1/_2$
10 MV x-rays	$2^3/_4$
25 MV x-rays	3

*Densities: Lead = 11.3 g/cm³, Cerrobend = 9.4 g/cm³.

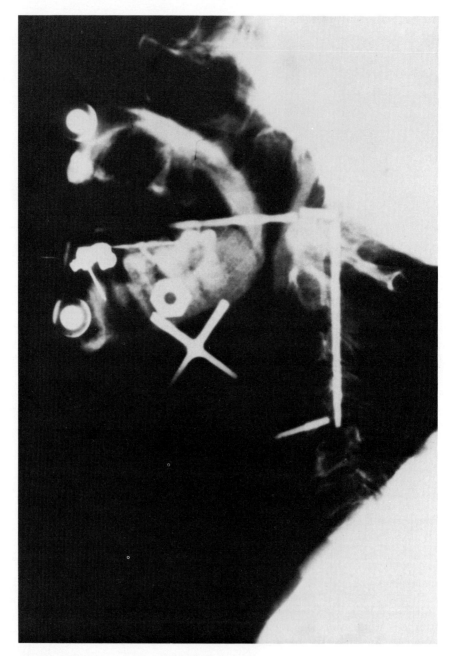

Fig. 8-8. Port film of the field of irradiation. Heavy line indicates radiation fields; lighter lines indicate the position of the lip and tongue. The lip and the maxilla are displaced out of the field while the tongue is depressed and secured within the field.

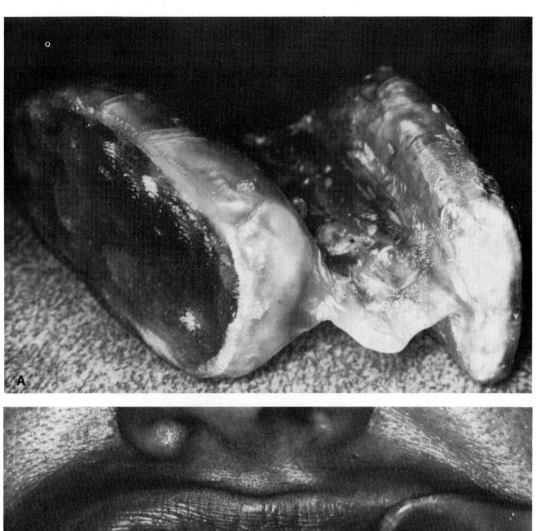

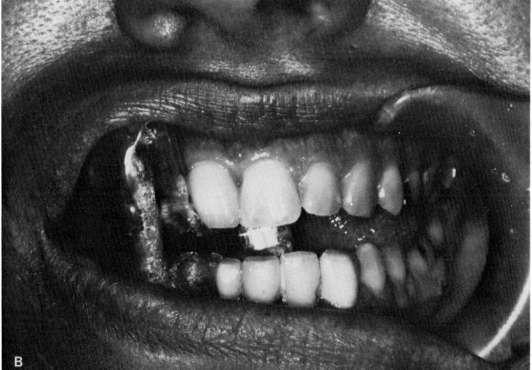

Fig. 8-9. (A) Stent of buccal and lingual lead alloy shields with occlusal index between. (B) Shield and tissue displacer in place. Note displacement of tongue and shielding of the buccal gingiva and tongue.

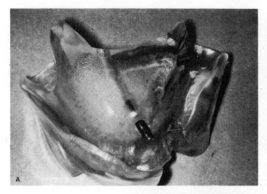
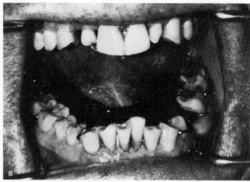
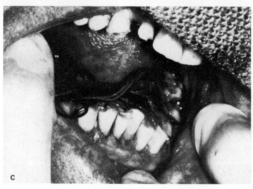

Fig. 8-10. (A) Appliance constructed to consistently receive and hold radiation source in place. (B) Prosthesis inserted covering the floor of mouth. (C) Radium needles held securely through prefabricated receptacles in the prosthesis of Figure 8-10B. (Courtesy of Dental Oncology, M. D. Anderson Hospital and Tumor Institute.)

CONE LOCATING DEVICE

This prosthesis positions the radiation beam precisely to the tumor (Fig. 8-11). An acrylic stent is custom fabricated to the intraoral cone, and a custom baseplate or occlusal index is attached to the acrylic cone. The cone locating device is inserted by the patient. The prosthesis positions the radiation beam accurately throughout the treatment and simplifies and improves intraoral radiotherapy technique (Fig. 8-12).

PROSTHODONTIC TREATMENT

The use of dentures or partial dentures over soft and hard tissue that has been irradiated is a controversial subject.[4, 10, 19, 28, 30] Patients, especially those who have worn prostheses before radiation therapy,[7] desire upon completion of therapy to immediately place their dentures back in the mouth for aesthetic and functional reasons. However, the indiscriminate use of a prosthesis in the oral cavity without proper knowledge of the new oral environment created by the radiation can be disastrous. A basic understanding of the anatomy and the effects of radiation on soft and hard tissues of the mouth is mandatory before any prosthetic intervention is contemplated.

The dentist must accumulate as much information as is possible from the patient, the radiotherapist, and the surgeon in order to fully evaluate the physical status of the oral cavity. Close consultation with the physician is necessary to determine the patient's general health and prognosis and the fields of radiation and the dosage the patient received.

The patient is questioned concerning previous denture experience, areas of sore-

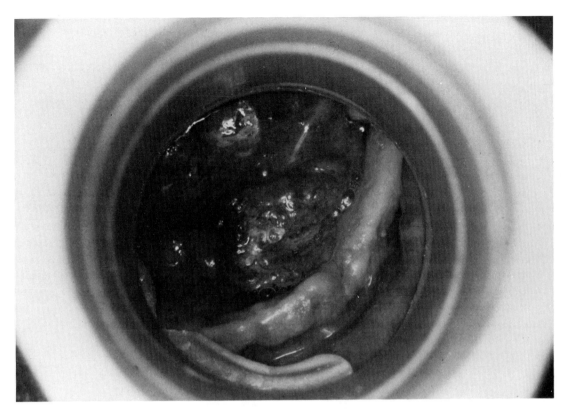

Fig. 8-11. Radiation cone secured by the stent.

ness, and ability to cope with the dryness. Oral habits such as drooling, clenching, or bruxing can be noted. The ability of the patient to cooperate in the treatment program should be assessed. The dentist must then perform a thorough and extensive examination of the remaining teeth, the soft tissue, and the ridge configuration. All data must be collected and analyzed before any prosthetic device is contemplated.

The radiotherapist will provide important information concerning how much of the mandible and the maxilla has been irradiated, what dosage and type of beam were used, whether or not the major salivary glands were within the fields, and whether the treatment was curative or palliative. Naturally, a thorough understanding of the patient's general health must be obtained. Problems such as malnutrition or alcoholism will adversely affect the denture foundation.

The status of the oral cavity following the completion of therapy is the most im-portant feature. Significant changes that predispose to tissue breakdown and infection occur within the radiation fields. Oral mucosa after radiation will demonstrate thinning, friability, and atrophy. The underlying connective tissue becomes fibrotic and avascular; bone will be devitalized.

The dentist must look for these signs and symptoms to provide himself with greater insight into the possibilities for success or failure of his prosthetic restoration. Areas of telangiectasia and scarring indicate tissue friability and potential areas of tissue breakdown. The severe dryness will result in the loss of the lubricating and retentive qualities of saliva necessary for denture comfort and retention. Tissue-bone undercuts, bony exostosis, knife-edge ridges, or any other bony impairment are areas of potential irritation and eventual tissue breakdown. In the final analysis, the dentist's mature clinical judgment and knowledge will determine whether a prosthesis can be constructed successfully. All necessary altera-

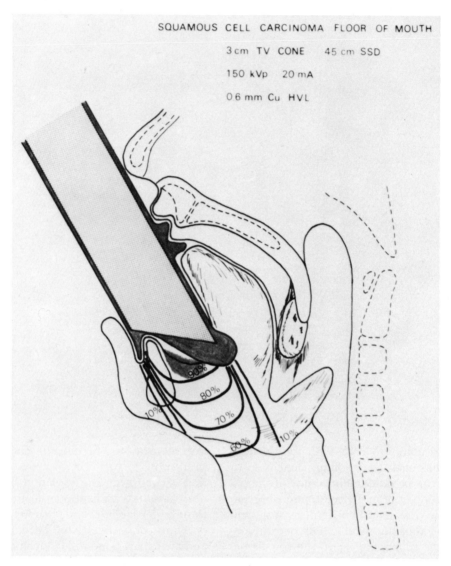

SQUAMOUS CELL CARCINOMA FLOOR OF MOUTH

3 cm TV CONE   45 cm SSD

150 kVp   20 mA

0.6 mm Cu HVL

Fig. 8-12. Dosimetry of the intraoral cone utilizing a cone locating stent for consistent placement.

tions must be designed into the prosthesis in order to accommodate for the irradiated foundation.

The placement of a prosthesis must depend upon the clinical findings within the patient's mouth. Patients who would be at severe risk are those who present with such telltale signs as telangiectasia, bony exostosis, thin friable tissue, and inflammation.

An adequate period of time following completion of therapy must be provided to allow the tissues to heal prior to wearing the denture. Some patients will be able to wear dentures comfortably several months after therapy. However, some patients with edematous and inflamed oral mucosa may need to be observed for long periods of time before dentures can be worn. There will be some patients who will never be able to tolerate a denture following treatment, even though they accepted dentures prior to treatment. For patients who did not accept dentures prior to therapy, there is little expectation that they will do so afterwards.

Technique of Construction

Sound prosthetic principles must always be followed to minimize the morbidity during the construction of the denture. All procedures should be atraumatic and nonirritating. A fully extended, nonpressure producing master impression is the first objective. Careful manipulation of the tissue and the impression can prevent problems. In reflex areas, such as the mucobuccal folds and the mylohyoid ridge, trays should not be overextended. The impression materials used should be nonirritating. Metallic oxide pastes are contraindicated because of their drying effect on the mucosa and because of the irritant effect of the eugenol. Plaster is rigid when set and generates heat; if used, special care must be taken to avoid abrading the soft tissues. Thermoplastics must be used with care. Low-fusing compounds are advisable to minimize trauma. Thiokol rubber bases, silicone bases, and irreversible hydrocolloids are recommended to prevent injury.

Maxillomandibular relationships may be accomplished by normal prosthetic procedures. A monoplane occlusal scheme is recommended using acrylic resin teeth. Proper horizontal and vertical buccal overlaps should be established to reduce lip, tongue, and cheek biting. The occlusion should be carefully established at the proper vertical dimension.

Variation may be used in selecting denture base materials, with some limitations. Heat-cured acrylic resins are most often employed. Care must be taken to avoid residual monomer after processing. Undercut areas must be adequately blocked out or relieved. Spicules or rough areas of acrylic resin on the finished prosthesis must be smoothed and polished. Silicone soft-liners may be used for minimizing trauma. However, the nonwettable properties of the silicones contribute to increased drag against the soft tissue and can be traumatic. This reduced wettability of the silicones takes on a greater significance on radiated and dry oral mucosa because the denture is no longer able to slip and slide as easily over the denture foundation during normal function. In addition, soft liners must be replaced more often and must be meticulously cared for.

Final insertion and postinsertion care of the prosthesis is very critical. All occlusal discrepancies are removed; areas of pressure are relieved. Pressure-indicating paste will locate potential sore spots so that adjustments can be made. Careful written and verbal instructions are given, describing how to care for and use the prostheses. The patient is told to remove the dentures at night or during one-third of the day. If areas of soreness or irritation develop, the dentures must be removed and the dentist contacted. The patient is seen every day for approximately 2 weeks. Thorough evaluation of any complaint of oral discomfort is mandatory; the patient must be seen and all necessary corrections made. When the patient is comfortable, a 3-month recall is sufficient. In the future, when a problem arises, the patient must be seen by the dentist for evaluation.

REFERENCES

1. Aramany, M. A., and Drane, J. B. 1972. Radiation displacement prostheses for dentulous patients. Journal of Prosthetic Dentistry, 27: 212.

2. Aramany, M. A., and Drane, J. B. 1972. Radiation protection prostheses for the edentulous patients. Journal of Prosthetic Dentistry, 27: 292.

3. Bedwinek, J. M., Shakovsky, L. J., Fletcher, G. H., and Daly, T. E. 1976. Osteonecrosis in patients treated with definitive radiotherapy for squamous cell carcinomas of the oral cavity and naso- and oropharynx. Radiology, 119: 665.

4. Beumer, J., III, Curtis, T. A., and Morrish, R. B., Jr. 1976. Radiation complications in edentulous patients. Journal of Prosthetic Dentistry, 36: 193.

5. Beaumer, J., III, Silverman, S., Jr., and Benak, S. B., Jr. 1972. Hard and soft tissue necroses following radiation therapy for oral cancer. Journal of Prosthetic Dentistry, 27: 640.

6. Braham, R. L. 1977. The role of dentistry in

the treatment of malignant disease. Journal of Preventive Dentistry, 4:   28.

7. Brown, L. R., Dreizen, S., Handler, S., and Johnston, D. A. 1975. Effects of radiation-induced xerostomia on human oral microflora. Journal of Dentistry Research, 54:   740.

8. Chalian, V. A., Drane, J. B., and Standish, S. M. 1971. Maxillofacial prosthetics: Multidisciplinary practice. Williams and Wilkins, Baltimore.

9. Conger, A. D. 1973. Loss and recovery of taste acuity in patients irradiated to the oral cavity. Radiation Research, 53:   338.

10. Curtis, T. A., Griffith, M. R., and Firtell, D. N. 1976. Complete denture prosthodontics for the radiation patient. Journal of Prosthetic Dentistry, 36:   66.

11. Daly, T. 1971. Management of dental problems in irradiated patients. The Radiological Society of North America, Refresher Course.

12. Daly, T. E., and Drane, J. B. 1972. Osteoradionecrosis of the jaws. Cancer Bulletin, 24:   86.

13. Daly, T. E., Drane, J. B., and MacComb, W. S. 1972. Management of problems of the teeth and jaw in patients undergoing irradiation. American Journal of Surgery, 124:   539.

14. Drane, J. B., and Guerra, L. L. 1972. Prosthetics and reconstruction. JAMA, 219:   351.

15. Dreizen, S., Daly, T. E., Drane, J. B., and Brown, L. 1977. Oral complications of cancer radiotherapy. Postgraduate Medicine, 61:   45.

16. Dykes, P., Harris, P., and Marston, A. 1960. Treatment of dry mouth. Lancet, 2:   1353.

17. Fine, L. 1975. Dental care of the radiated patient. Journal of Hospital Dental Practice, 9:   127.

18. Fletcher, G. H., Ed. 1975. Textbook of Radiotherapy. 2nd edn. Lea and Febiger, Philadelphia.

19. Griem, M. L., Robinson, J. E., and Barnhart, G. W. 1964. The use of a soft denture-base material in management of the post-radiation denture problem. Radiology, 82:   320.

20. Guralnick, W. C., Ed. 1968. Textbook of Oral Surgery. Little, Brown, Boston.

21. Guttenberg, S. A. 1974. Osteoradionecrosis of the jaw. American Journal of Surgery, 127:   326.

22. Jackson, M. J. 1976. Pilot investigation of neosilvol in the treatment of intraoral mucositis and infection in the irradiated patient. University of Texas Cancer System, M.D. Anderson Hospital and Tumor Institute.

23. Jackson, M. J. 1978. The radiotherapy stent—an adjuvant to therapy. Journal of Arkansas Medical Society, 75:   179.

24. King, E. R., Elzay, R. P., and Dettman, P. M. 1968. Effects of ionizing radiation in the human oral cavity and oropharynx: Results of a survey. Radiology, 91:   990.

25. Llory, H., Dammrun, A., Gioanni, M., and Frank, R. M. 1972. Some population changes in oral anaerobic microorganisms, *Streptococcus, mutans* and *yeasts* following irradiation of the salivary glands. Caries Research, 6:   298.

26. Moss, W. T., Brand, W. N., and Battifora, H. 1973. Radiation Oncology. 4th edn. C. V. Mosby, St. Louis.

27. Daly, T. E., and Drane, J. B. 1974. Dental care for irradiated patients. In M.D. Anderson Hospital, Ed. Neoplasia of Head and Neck. Year Book Medical Publishers, Chicago, 225.

28. Rahn, A. O., and Boucher, L. J. 1970. Maxillofacial Prosthetics; Principles and Concepts. W. B. Saunders, Philadelphia.

29. Rahn, A. O., and Drane, J. B. 1967. Dental aspects of the problems, care, and treatment of the irradiated oral cancer patient. Journal of the American Dental Association, 74:   957.

30. Rahn, A. O., Matalon, V., and Drane, J. B. 1968. Prosthetic evaluation of patients who have received irradiation to the head and neck regions. Journal of Prosthetic Dentistry, 19:   174.

31. Robinson, J. E. 1964. Dental management of the oral effects of radiotherapy. Journal of Prosthetic Dentistry, 14:   582.

32. Shannon, I. L., McCrary, B. R., and Starcke, E. N. 1977. A saliva substitute for use by xerostomic patients undergoing radiotherapy to the head and neck. Oral Surgery, Oral Medicine, Oral Pathology, 44:   656.

9 | Maxillofacial Prosthetic Rehabilitation

Mohamed A. Aramany, D.M.D., M.S.
Eugene N. Myers, M.D.

Radical surgery for cancer of the head and neck frequently requires extensive resection of orofacial structures leading to cosmetic, functional, and psychological impairment of the individual. Rehabilitation efforts must be planned and in some instances, initiated prior to the surgical intervention. The interaction between the prosthodontist and the surgeon begins during treatment planning stages. Effective communication is essential for the success of the rehabilitation and for the restoration of form and function to the affected organ. The goal of this joint effort is to sustain the patient's quality of life and to support the patient and his family psychologically throughout the ordeal of treatment.

Mutual understanding of the capabilities and limitations of both disciplines contributes greatly to the development of individualized and realistic treatment planning and results in a planned preservation of anatomic landmarks for improved prostheses retention and aesthetics. Preoperative consultation allows the surgeon, on the prosthodontist's recommendations, to retain, mobilize, or remove tissues, thus enabling the prosthodontist to construct the optimal prosthesis. Such planning is essential for both intraoral and extraoral defects.

The surgeon has become cognizant of the advisability of utilization of surgical prostheses in some situations and of the redundancy of their use in others. For example, an immediate surgical obturator is essential for maxillectomy patients, whereas a similar replacement is not effective for soft palate resection patients. Another example is the importance of preserving the tragus and external auditory meatus, whenever possible, in resection of the external ear, whereas preserving the ear lobe creates a problem in retention of a prosthetic ear.

The team effort at the University of Pittsburgh Health Center during the past 6 years has resulted in the initiation of a variety of protocols for dealing with different categories of patient problems. One of the most essential factors in achieving a meaningful team effort was the realization of the importance of having dental consultation prior to the institution of the treatment modalities. This was achieved by making dental consultation a routine part of the admission procedure for head and neck patients, thus enabling the dental evaluation to run concurrently with the medical evaluation.

Thorough dental examination, including radiographs, is carried out routinely. Dental impressions are made at this time if indicated. Oral hygiene protocol is mandatory in dentulous patients. Preservation and restoration of teeth usually provides a much better retained prosthesis. Patients with poor oral hygiene, rampant decay, or advanced periodontal disease may have surgery postponed so that these problems can be corrected. Healing of large intraoral wounds is improved by good oral hygiene. Dentulous patients who receive postoperative radiation therapy as a planned procedure or who have been previously radiated have fluoride treatments on a continuous basis.

Defects resulting from ablative surgical procedures produce varying degrees of disability, both functional and aesthetic. Utilizing the patient's own tissues for repair of these defects has many limitations, and the need for prosthetic restoration often arises. Surgical reconstructive techniques utilizing local or regional pedicle flaps and skin grafts are often an essential first step in the rehabilitation of the patient. Without adequate epithelial coverage, whether internal or external, it may be impossible to place a prosthesis. The extent of surgical excision and the type of reconstruction should be discussed preoperatively by the surgeon and the maxillofacial prosthodontist.

INTRAORAL PROSTHESES

Hard Palate Defects

Resection of the hard and soft palate and related structures results in a variety of anatomic and functional defects in the oral cavity and oropharynx. These defects are enormously inconvenient to the patient because of the loss of oronasal separation, which interferes substantially with the functions of swallowing and speaking.

Defects of the hard palate are less difficult to manage than those of the soft palate. The primary concern is that the opening in the hard palate be covered in order to restore oronasal separation. Since this is accomplished by replacement of a passive, rather than dynamic, anatomic unit, the important aspects to be considered are the location and the size of the defect and the retention and comfort of fit of the obturator. The problems in achieving adequate retention and comfort of fit are compounded in the presence of an edentulous maxilla, anterior maxillary defects leading to midfacial collapse, total hard palate resection, and previous radiation. Lack of patient acceptance of previous dentures also works against acceptance of the obturator.

PRESURGICAL CONSIDERATIONS

Patients who will have a resection of the palate should always be seen by the maxillofa-

cial prosthodontist well in advance of the surgical procedure. This is necessary so that impressions can be taken and the diagnostic cast can be made. The diagnostic cast is very important during the consultation phase between the surgeon and the maxillofacial prosthodontist. The structures to be resected during the ablative procedures are outlined on the cast by the surgeon. The prosthodontist may thereby be able to suggest modifications of the surgery that could be helpful in maximizing the effectiveness of the prosthesis. The efforts are directed toward preservation of structures that aid in support, retention, and stabilization of the prosthesis without compromising the ablative procedure.

SURGICAL CONSIDERATIONS

1. Preservation of as many anterior teeth on the side of the lesion as possible. The classical radical maxillectomy is usually done without regard for the preservation of the anterior teeth on the contralateral side, since the osteotomy through the midline to help to separate the specimen from its bony attachment is convenient and has been taught as the standard surgical treatment. Frequently the central and lateral incisors can be preserved, and in a few patients, the canine can be saved. This enables the prosthodontist to utilize cross-arch stabilization and indirect retention in the obturator design, thereby improving obturator stability.[4]

2. The bone cut should be made through the socket of the extracted anterior tooth closer to the segment to be removed, rather than next to the remaining tooth. This will preserve the alveolar bone adjacent to the tooth abutting the maxillary defect, thereby providing greater stability for this tooth. This tooth can be used safely in supporting the obturator (Fig. 9-1).

3. A local pedicle flap of mucosa from the hard palate of the maxilla to be resected is raised before making the bone cut on the palatal aspect of the maxilla. This is possible only if the tumor does not involve the palatal mucosa. The bone cut is made with an osteotome and the maxillectomy is completed.

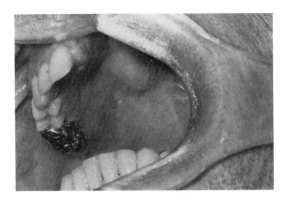

Fig. 9-1. The bone cut was made in the socket of the extracted tooth away from the central incisor to be preserved. A bony ridge is formed that adds to the stability of the central incisor. Gold crowns on maxillary molar teeth showing ledges on lingual surface to support metal framework. Note medial wall of the defect 9 months after palatal flap.

The palatal flap is reflected up onto the medial aspect of the defect and sutured to the nasal septum with through and through sutures, after a small area of the mucosa has been elevated from the inferior aspect of the nasal septum (Figs. 9-2A and B).

4. In the completely edentulous maxilla, preservation of bone anteriorly and/or posteriorly on the resection side improves the stability and retention of the obturator.

5. In edentulous patients, an undercut is created on the medial wall of the defect at the base of the nasal septum. This undercut is then covered with the palatal flap. Surveying of the dental cast is essential to avoid the presence of an antagonistic undercut on the buccal surface of the alveolar ridge on the nonresected side.

SURGICAL OBTURATOR

A surgical (immediate and temporary) obturator is always placed at the time of hard palate resection (Fig. 9-3). This maintains palatal integrity and reduces the postoperative morbidity. The patient is able to speak understandably immediately after surgery. He also retains the capability of oral feeding, thus eliminating the need for an indwelling nasogastric tube. The prosthesis also aids in healing, because it helps to hold the internal dressing against the skin graft. A better and cleaner environment is established for oral hygiene.

The design of the surgical obturator is arrived at by consultation between the surgeon and the prosthodontist and is recorded on a duplicate of the diagnostic cast. The teeth to be extracted are marked on the cast. On the palatal aspect of the same cast two lines are drawn, the first indicating the location of the bone cut and the second depicting the soft tissue flap that will eventually

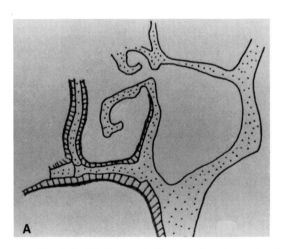

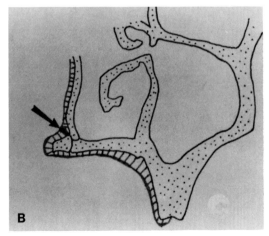

Fig. 9-2. (A) Coronal diagram showing palatal mucosa, nasal septum, and bone after the palatal mucosa is elevated and the bone cut is made during maxillectomy. (B) Palatal flap covers the bony margin and is sutured to the nasal septum.

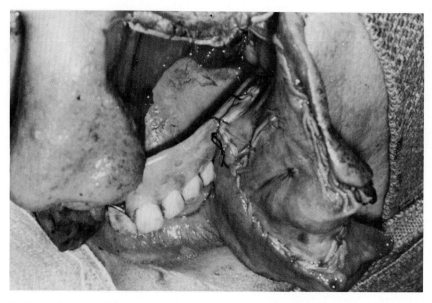

Fig. 9-3. After the maxillectomy, the split-thickness skin graft is inserted and the surgical obturator is sutured in place. The packing is applied before the skin closure is done.

cover the medial wall. These lines are transferred to the patient's tissues in the operating room at the time of the resection.

On the diagnostic cast, the prosthodontist removes the teeth designated for extraction. He plans the means of retention of the prosthesis by drilling holes in the buccal flange and/or adding wire clasps. Incorporating clasp retention whenever possible has proven essential for the eventual retention of the prosthesis during the transitional stage. In certain cases the surgical obturator is relined and used as a temporary obturator; if this is done anterior teeth are added to the prosthesis. In edentulous patients, the patient's denture may be modified and used as a surgical obturator instead of a new prosthesis being fabricated. In order to avoid future misunderstanding, the patient should be made aware that his denture will be altered. The surgical obturator is sterilized in Betadine (povidone-iodine) solution and is kept in a plastic container in the same solution until it is used in the operating room. We suture the surgical obturator in place after the skin graft has been sewn in and before the cavity is packed. This allows for more precise packing which helps

maximize the take of the skin graft. The facial wound is then closed.

TEMPORARY PROSTHESIS

Five to 7 days postoperatively the obturator is removed, the packing is taken out, and the defect is examined. The prosthodontist now has several options. He may elect to reline the surgical obturator with a resilient material, to modify the patient's denture to serve as a temporary obturator, or to construct a new prosthesis based on a new impression. The decision is dependent on various factors, such as extent of surgery, degree of recovery, condition of the local tissues, evaluation of the prosthesis, and, of course, patient attitude. The objectives are to make the prosthesis as retentive and as comfortable as possible, to eliminate leakage of fluids into the nasal cavity, and to restore normal speech. In order to achieve these objectives, the prosthesis must be adjusted frequently in the postsurgical period to accommodate the healing process. The resilient liners give the prosthodontist the opportunity to achieve his goals with the utmost patient comfort.

DEFINITIVE OBTURATOR

Obturators for acquired palatal defects are constructed for patients who are either completely or partially edentulous. The designs for these two types are completely different. When defects of the soft palate are also present, another dimension is added to the problem of prosthetic rehabilitation because then a dynamic anatomical structure must also be dealt with.

The obturator consists of two sections: a base prosthesis and a bulb portion. The base prosthesis is similar to a conventional prosthesis, whether it is a complete denture or a removable partial denture (Figs. 9-4, 9-5, and 9-6). A nasal extension section is added to occupy the defect area. This contributes to the effectiveness of the oronasal separation and improves the quality of speech. In the edentulous patient, the nasal extension also adds to the stability and retention of the obturator. The nasal extension is constructed either hollow or as a flange obturator[17] to decrease the weight of the prosthesis and to reduce the torque on the remaining teeth for better retention.

We have introduced a classification for partially edentulous patients based upon a review of 123 patients who required obturators.[3] This group was 67 percent male and 33 percent female. The location of the defect with respect to the remaining dentition

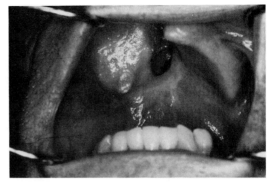

Fig. 9-5. Maxillary defect in edentulous patient. Note skin graft location and the scar bond formed at the junction of the mucosa of the cheek and the graft.

was used as a basis for the classification into six distinct groups (Fig. 9-7). Class sequence reflects the frequency of occurrence in the patient population. The metal framework for each class is designed differently to maximize the utilization of the remaining teeth and soft tissue structure within the limits of the physiological tolerance of these tissues. The different forces transmitted to the residual anatomic structures via the obturator are complex and include a variety of components: vertical dislodging force, occlusal vertical force, torque or rotational force, lateral force, and anteroposterior force. The weight of the obturator tends to exert a rotational stress on the abutment teeth due to

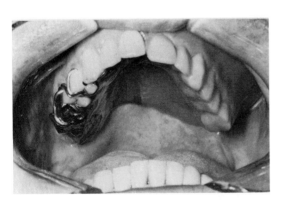

Fig. 9-4. The same surgical obturator (Fig. 9-3) in the patient's mouth. The cusp height on the defect side is flattened to reduce the stress on the remaining structures.

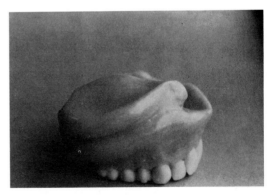

Fig. 9-6. The nasal extension of the obturator has a groove that accommodates the scar bond in the buccal wall of the defect. The extension is constructed as a hollow bulb.

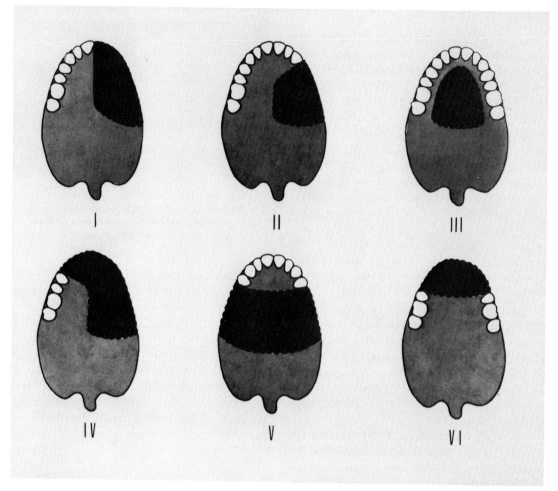

Fig. 9-7. Classification of maxillectomy patients based on relationship of the defect to the remaining teeth. (Aramany, M.A. 1978. Basic principles of obturator design for partially edentulous patients. Part I: Classification. Journal of Prosthetic Dentistry, 40:554.)

gravity. To counteract this effect, the obturator must be as light as possible, and the buccal flange must have a high vertical dimension to resist the dislodging force.

Stabilization of the obturator against lateral forces is effected by incorporating bracing components into the metal framework design and covering of the medial wall of the defect. This is particularly effective if the medial wall is covered with a palatal flap. Occlusal harmony and elimination of premature occlusal contacts adds greatly to the stability of the obturator. To prevent the obturator from displacement in an anteroposterior direction, the design should incorporate guiding planes to contact the proximal surfaces of the abutment teeth.

Preservation of as many teeth as possible helps in distribution of the occlusal load and adds to the stability of the obturator. The obturator design includes full palatal coverage to maximize obturator support and stability. The retention of the obturator in the partially edentulous patients can be improved greatly by utilizing the maximum number of teeth for retention through use of extracoronal clasps and indirect retention. The intracoronal retainers may be used in selected cases where the palatal defect is small and the remaining teeth are numerous with a good crown to root ratio. Maximum coverage of the remaining soft tissue is also advisable but the movable structure and low muscle attachment and frenulum must be avoided.

Before the construction of the definitive obturator, the oral hygiene of the patient is evaluated. All the restorative dental work must be completed. Frequently, the teeth selected to serve as abutment teeth are crowned with specially shaped gold restorations to accommodate the obturator's metal framework design. The crowns are shaped to provide support, retention, and stability for the obturator while placing minimum stress on the remaining teeth. Preserving the anterior teeth on the contralateral side converts a potential class I defect into a class II defect. Maintaining the incisor teeth enhances the cosmetic effect and increases the stability of the prosthesis through wide distribution of the occlusal forces occurring during mastication and swallowing. The metal framework will also include indirect retainers, which minimize the tendency of dislodgement of the prosthesis under gravity.

In edentulous patients where a classical maxillectomy has been performed, about 50 percent of the hard palate is maintained. The obturator should cover all available ridge and palatal structure. The nasal extension section is adapted to the buccal surface of the cheek, and the medial wall is adapted to the nasal septum. Covering the nasal septum with palatal mucosa improves the quality of the surface tissue and improves the success of the obturator. Surgical creation of a palatal shelf in the area of the nasal septum improves obturator retention.

The objective of these obturators is to effect oronasal separation. The functional demands, however, should be limited since obturators for the completely edentulous patient present a host of problems in retention, stability and functional proficiency. These problems occur in direct proportion to the extent of the palatal resection. In smaller defects created within the palatal structures, prosthetic replacement is successful. However, when the resection includes the major part of the hard palate the quality of the retention and the stability of the prosthesis is downgraded. In the latter cases, retention by "suspension" from undercuts located in the nasal defect is recommended using resilient denture base material. The patient's speech and swallowing will be improved,[5] but effective mastication of food is difficult to achieve.

Construction of functional complete denture for patients who have undergone maxillary resection is one of the most challenging problems in this field. Instability of these obturators frequently causes seepage of fluids in spite of the superior quality of speech. Fluids are forced into the nasal cavity during the act of swallowing when the tongue comes into contact with the soft palate. The fluids run along the medial side of the bulb and out through the nose. A bypass can be added to these obturators whereby most of the fluids passed to the nose can be redirected back to the oral cavity. Zaki's[19] technique of using an 8-gauge tubing that opens on the posterosuperior aspect of the bulb in a funnel shape and runs diagonally to open in the opposite bicuspid region orally has corrected this problem in most of the cases. Hence, the funnel portion of the tube is the lowest part of the top of the obturator; this will allow for easy collection of the fluids. The tortuous course of the tube helps to preserve the intraoral air pressure, so that the speech will not be affected.[19]

Cuspless teeth are used for the edentulous obturator, and teeth are set with no occlusal interference. The mandibular teeth are set to occlude with the maxillary teeth on the normal side, and they barely touch on the resected side of the oral cavity.

Denture adhesives have proved to be effective in improving the retention of edentulous obturators. The powder variety when used sparsely is better than denture creams.

We prefer that the patients attempt the use of the obturator without adhesives initially. Recommending adhesives should not be a substitute for utilizing sound basic principles of prosthesis construction.

Soft Palate Defects

Although loss of oronasal separation is also the primary consideration in resection of the soft palate, the prosthodontic rehabilitation of soft palate defects is more complex than is the rehabilitation of hard palate defects. The hard palate is a static structure and defects in it simply require coverage. However, the soft palate is a dynamic structure where mobility tends to act against prosthetic extension on the soft palate. The reduction of the size of the soft palate extension to prevent impingement upon the movable margins of the defect will lead to insufficient oronasal separation during functional activities. To understand the complexity of the problem of restoration of a soft palate defect, the mechanism of velopharyngeal closure will be reviewed.

Velopharyngeal Mechanism

In normal individuals, the muscles that are responsible for velopharyngeal closure include the superior constrictor, levator veli palatini, tensor veli palatini, palatopharyngeus, and salpingopharyngeus muscles. To accomplish velopharyngeal closure during the act of swallowing and in speech, the velum elevates and moves posteriorly, the posterior pharyngeal wall contracts and moves anteriorly, and both lateral pharyngeal walls move medially. This closure occurs at the level of the hard palate in the vicinity of the anterior tubercle of the atlas bone. Normal physiological movement is interrupted by ablative surgery as a result of removal of parts of the soft palate and/or pharyngeal walls and related structures. The muscle function of the soft palate is disrupted in a variety of ways depending on the site and size of the defect.

Prosthetic Treatment of Soft Palate

We do not use surgical obturators in conjunction with resection of soft palate tumors, a practice we use in hard palate resections. However, a base prosthesis, which is modified and inserted before the patient leaves the hospital, is designed and constructed. The temporary prosthesis is used by the patient during the hospital stay and is modified during the first few months. The final design of the prosthesis is then reproduced in the definitive obturator.

Attempts to cover the surgical defect in the soft palate, as is done with a defect in the hard palate, are not functionally adequate. The patient fails to recover normal speech and has the problem of escape of fluids through the nasal cavity. A different design for each category must be followed to give the patient a functionally adequate restoration. Three different prosthetic designs are used to restore the soft palate.[6, 8, 15]

Prosthesis for Total Soft Palate Resection. In this type of resection the soft palate, including all of its muscles, is totally removed. The function of the superior constrictor muscle of the pharynx remains intact. On eliciting the contraction of the superior constrictor muscle of the pharynx, there is a forward movement of the posterior wall and medial advancement of the lateral walls. This is similar to the unrepaired congenital cleft of the palate.[2]

A speech aid extending posteriorly from the base prosthesis into the pharyngeal region separates the oropharynx from the nasopharynx. The success of this prosthesis is dependent upon the action of the superior constrictor muscle of the pharynx separating the two cavities during speech and swallowing. In the rest position, there is a space around the pharyngeal part of the prosthesis to effect nasal breathing (Fig. 9-8 and 9-9). This type of prosthesis is similar to speech aids constructed for congenital cleft patients.[8]

Prosthesis for Median Palatal Defects. The resection may involve parts of the hard

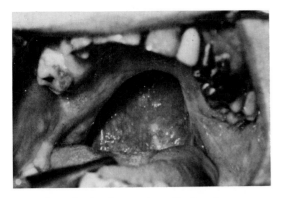

Fig. 9-8. Total resection of soft palate to treat a squamous cell carcinoma of the palate.

and soft palate. However, the levator palatini, tensor veli palatini, uvula, palatoglossus, and palatopharyngeus muscles are left functionally intact. While the normal physiological movement of the palate still takes place upon eliciting the velopharyngeal mechanism, the presence of the surgical defect will make this movement functionally inadequate. The anterior margin of the defect is not mobile, whereas the posterior aspect of the defect will move superiorly and posteriorly, increasing the size of the oronasal communication.

A velar extension from the base prosthesis passes through the soft palate defect, and in the rest position a space is present between the prosthesis and the posterior margin of the defect. The posterior extension of the prosthesis does not extend to the posterior or lateral pharyngeal wall. During speech or swallowing, the levator and tensor muscles contract and the margins of the defect elevate against the extension to separate the oropharynx from the nasopharynx. The size and shape of this extension is adjusted as healing and reorganization of the defect progresses.

Prosthesis for Lateral Soft Palate Defects. The resection of the tumor involves functional interruption of one-half of the paired muscles of the palate. The resection may be for a primary tumor. More often, however, this half of the soft palate unit is resected to provide adequate surgical margins for tu-

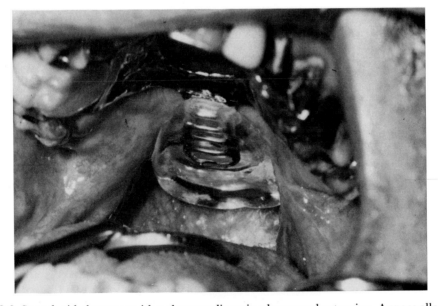

Fig. 9-9. Speech aid obturator with a clear acrylic resin pharyngeal extension. A space allowing nasal breathing exists around the pharyngeal extension during the rest position. When the pharyngeal muscles are activated, the pharyngeal lumen contracts around the acrylic extension leading to separation of the oropharynx from the nasopharynx.

mors of tonsil, retromolar trigone, and buccal mucosa. For instance, if the resection involves a lesion of the left side of the palate, the right levator, tensor, palatopharyngeus, palatoglossus, and uvula muscles remain intact. Since the palate is intended to function through a paired mechanism, the loss of one-half of the mechanism drastically alters the function of the palate during swallowing and speech. The soft palate tends to elevate more laterally toward the normal side and more superiorly, since there is no limiting action of the muscles on the other side.

A pharyngeal extension (retrovelar speech aid) from the base prosthesis passes through the defect and fills the potential space behind the remaining segment of the soft palate. Velopharyngeal closure is attained by the levator action of the remaining soft palate and the contraction of the pharyngeal muscles against the pharyngeal extension of the prosthesis. Some of the patients who have used the prosthesis for a period of time, may regain sufficient velopharyngeal closure so that they can get along without the prosthesis. A program of gradual reduction of the size of the pharyngeal extension is followed as the mechanism becomes effective. Although the exact mechanism is not known, it seems that either the presence of the pharyngeal extension of the prosthesis stimulates the muscle function or that some patients have the ability to spontaneously develop compensatory movements.

Patients with lateral soft palate defects are the most difficult to manage prosthetically. The more advanced tumors seen in this region tend to involve multiple anatomic sites. The more extensive resections required for tumor control produce more severe functional disability. The large regional pedicle flaps currently utilized for reconstruction provide static rather than dynamic replacement for the resected oropharyngeal musculature. This eliminates the pharyngeal component of velopharyngeal closure mechanism against the retrovelar speech aid. Many of these patients are edentulous, which makes adequate retention of these large prostheses difficult. Radiation therapy, applied to the oral cavity as part of the therapeutic program, may make wearing the prosthesis uncomfortable due to irritation of tissues.

Mandibular Resection

Resection of tumors involving the bone of the mandible and related soft tissue in the oral cavity may result in the loss of a section of the alveolar arch without loss of mandibular continuity. This is referred to as marginal resection. Resection of a segment of bone interrupts the continuity of the body or the ramus of the mandible. The muscular balance and the function of the stomatognathic system will be distributed in proportion to the extent of the surgically created defect.

TYPES OF MANDIBULAR RESECTION

Marginal Resection. Problems resulting from marginal resection of the mandible are treated much like those occurring in patients with severe atrophy of the alveolar ridges. Following resection, the loss of tissue may lead to obliteration of the vestibular depth, and in some cases the tongue may be sutured to the buccal mucosa, also obliterating the sulcus. Alveoplasty, with-or-without skin graft, may be used to improve the basal support of the mandibular denture. Although the bony continuity of the mandible is not affected, extending the mandibular denture over the surgical site is difficult unless the alveoloplasty is carried out.

Mandibular Dentures. Prostheses constructed for patients with marginal resection are designed to improve facial contour, to contain the saliva in the mouth, and to help in speech and mastication. If some of the mandibular teeth are still remaining, they are used for the retention, support, and stability of the denture. In the edentulous patient it is difficult to construct a prosthesis after mandibular resection.

Techniques of Alveoloplasty. The various methods of alveoloplasty to improve the denture-bearing area in the mandible are similar to those used for the maxillary arches. These techniques fall into three general classifications based upon the management of the exposed bony surfaces.[9]

The most ideal result is obtained by the technique of covering the bony surface with mucous membrane either through flaps or autogenous grafts. The thickness of the soft tissue, its ample blood supply, and its resiliency are thus preserved. Unfortunately, mucous membrane in the human body is not readily available for extensive grafting. A second possible technique, therefore, is to leave the exposed periosteum for secondary epithelization. This procedure is called *epithelization vestibuloplasty*. This is a rather slow process, and the quality of the resultant tissue is poor because of scarcity of subepithelial tissue.

Skin grafting is the third available technique and is used rather successfully. A serious disadvantage of alveolar-ridge skin graft alveoloplasty is the subsequent shrinkage of the graft and, hence, the loss of vestibular depth, the decrease in soft-tissue thickness, and the inelasticity of the skin graft as a denture-bearing surface. To overcome these disadvantages, the technique of skin grafting in the oral cavity has been subjected to repeated modifications. However, the basic principles underlying its use have remained essentially the same for the last half century. The technique was described by Esser in 1916[13] and was widely popularized by Obwegeser and MacIntosh.[14, 16] The most striking improvement was the utilization of the ring scar that develops on the buccal surface to engage a ledge created on the polished surface of the denture. The stent is constructed before surgery and inserted in the operating room before placing the gauze bolus. This procedure helps to preserve the depth of the vestibule, but this technique requires greater cooperation and a certain amount of dexterity on the part of the patient. The removal and insertion of the stent must be completely understood and mastered by the patient before he leaves the office after the denture-stent is inserted for the first time.

Staple Implant. Another alternative to increase the stability and retention of the lower denture in marginal resection of the mandible is the use of staple implants. A metal plate with projection is inserted through the inferior border of the mandible. The projection protrudes through the mucosa and is used to improve the retention of the lower denture.

Segmental Resections. The resection of a segment of the body or ramus of the mandible will lead to deviation of the remaining segments. The patient experiences difficulty in mastication because of the inability to maintain a centric relationship between the residual segments and the maxilla. The patient may suffer from continuous drooling and difficulty in speech especially if the tongue is involved. There is also a substantial cosmetic defect visible.

Atkinson and Shepherd[10] conducted a study on the changes that take place in the masticatory cycle following the resection of a large segment of the mandible compared with the normal movement of the mandible. They reported a lack of smoothness, a failure to return to centric occlusal position, and a pause between chewing cycles.

Mandibular Reconstruction

The ideal treatment for restoring the integrity of the mandible after segmental resection is by using an autogenous bone-graft. The grafting procedure is generally done as a secondary surgical procedure some months after tumor surgery. Attempts at immediate reconstruction may be complicated by the need for mobilization of distant tissue to ensure adequate coverage of the graft. Many times primary bone grafting fails due to local infection from contamination with saliva. In some patients a vestibuloplasty may be indicated after bone grafting and before the construction of a mandibular denture.

If bone grafting is not planned, the alternatives are:

Alloplastic material utilized as a temporary solution until future bone grafting is done. In some instances the alloplastic material is used as a definitive treatment for segmental resection. Varying degrees of success have been achieved with different implant materials such as acrylic resin, titanium, tantalum, and chrome cobalt alloys. The cast chrome cobalt mesh tubing as used by Hahn[13a] is a preferred approach to the restoration of a large mandibular defect. The material permits fibrous tissue to grow through its meshes and gives satisfactory results.

Reconstruction of mandibular defect by a combination of alloplastic materials and hemapoietic graft is another technique. Metal trays are filled with autogenous bone marrow grafts to effect repair of segmental defects of the mandible. Boyne[11] and other investigators have demonstrated the usefulness of autogenous bone marrow grafts in restoration of bony defects of the face. Tantalum trays of various sizes are filled with bone marrow grafts. This type of reconstruction creates a mandibular ridge form that is favorable in dimension for the reception and support of a prosthesis. Titanium mesh implants are used in a similar manner to restore mandibular defects. This metal is

easy to handle since it is prefabricated, can be adjusted in the operating room, and is easily autoclaved. Titanium screws and wires are used to attach the implant to the prepared bony abutments. The preformed titanium supportive metallic implant is illustrated in Figure 9-10.

Guiding flanges may be used in partially edentulous patients where at least a few sound teeth are present after partial resection of the mandible. A restoration can be constructed with a guiding flange. The guiding flange helps the patient achieve maxillomandibular occlusal contact and prevents deviation of the mandibular fragment. The patient is instructed to exercise the mandible following surgery to avoid scarring and permanent malalignment of the mandible. In some patients, the muscular adaptation seems to occur after a period of months so that the resection appliance is not needed. In these patients a sectional mandibular denture is constructed with 33° or 45° cusp teeth. The interdigitation of the teeth gives the patient positive guidance to intercuspal position.

A guiding flange is difficult to retain in completely edentulous patients. The lateral

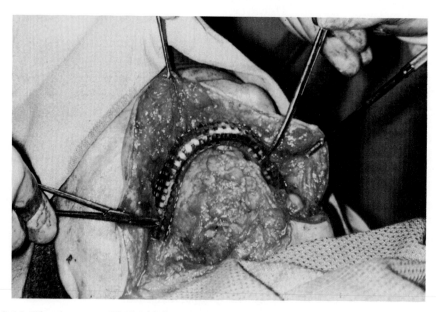

Fig. 9-10. Titanium tray filled with bone marrow to restore segmental resection of the mandible.

force on the upright flange causes dislodgment of the mandibular prosthesis.

Intermaxillary fixation may be utilized following segmental resection in edentulous patients. The mandible tends to deviate medially and superiorly so that the prosthodontist is faced with a problem when he tries to record the mandibular position in relationship to the maxillary arch.

The fixation of the mandibular segment to the maxillary arch immediately after the resection of the tumor helps to minimize the deviation resulting from postoperative scarring.[7] The immobilization of the fragment may be achieved by the insertion of modified Gunning splints constructed before the surgery.[1] The maxillary splint is fixed with intraosseous and circumzygomatic wiring. The mandibular splint is fixed with circummandibular wires. Elastics are used at night to maintain the relationship between the mandible and maxilla and are removed during the day to encourage early function of swallowing and speech. This program is maintained for a period of 7 weeks followed by an interim prosthesis, which is used until the definitive prosthesis is constructed.

The degree of mandibular deviation observed after the use of wiring in our patients was much less than the deviation observed in those patients who did not have intermaxillary fixation. By decreasing the deviation, a section of a complete denture when modified for mandibular-resection patients is likely to be accepted. When slight deviation occurs, the patient is fitted with a ramp on the maxillary denture that guides the mandibular segment, after the initial contact, into proper centric relations. In other cases, the denture may be made with a wide occlusal table or with two rows of teeth, or the teeth may be moved to the point where the mandible meets the maxilla without attempting to align the fragment.

Patient acceptance of the mandibular denture after extensive segmental resection is variable. The maxillary denture is easily accepted and helps to improve the patient's appearance and speech. Conventional lower dentures for mandibulectomy patients are usually rejected unless the remaining ridge is exceptionally good and the segmental resection is limited in nature. Functionally developed complete dentures rather than the conventional procedure proved to be more successful in some patients. The neutral zone concept of construction of complete denture is used. In this technique the neuromuscular mechanism dictates the location and shape of the restoration. The swallowing act is used to mold the impression material while recording the shape and extent of the fitting surface of the dentures and also the extent of the lower facial height. In essence, the impression of the ridges and the jaw relation records are made simultaneously. Intermaxillary fixation will alleviate the problem of deviation, but it is not as ideal as the restoration of the continuity of the mandible.

Dynamic Bite Opener

Limitation of mandibular movement may occur after surgery or radiation therapy due to fibrosis or to muscular rigidity. The physical limitation of mandibular opening in some patients interferes with proper oral hygiene practices and complicates the use of prostheses particularly during their insertion and removal. This limitation also complicates the impression procedure and other dental procedures.

The dynamic bite opener provides a gradual and intermittent force through the use of elastic traction to exercise the mandible. Initial separation of the arches is done by forcing tongue blades between the teeth to gain enough opening to insert the appliance.

The opener is composed of two U-shaped perforated metal plates with wire rods attached to the sides of each plate. Acrylic resin is applied on the perforated stent and inserted in the patient's mouth to record the imprints of the occlusal surfaces of the teeth.

The metal wires are contoured to provide loops to retain the elastic system in

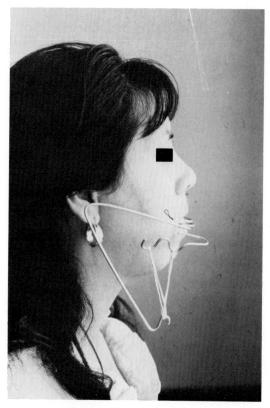

Fig. 9-11. Dynamic bite opener in place. Acrylic plate in the mouth with indentions of the teeth. The elastic bands exert downward force on the mandible.

order to transfer vertical opening force (Figure 9-11). The size and number of the elastic bands are varied until the patient feels downward pull on the mandible. He is then instructed to use the opener at short intervals throughout the day until he is capable of opening his mouth without assistance.

EXTRAORAL PROSTHESES

Facial appearance plays an important role in the life of the human being, as it is an important part of self-image and is the center of attention during social interaction. The resection of tumor involving part of the facial structures leads to facial disfigurement. Although the problem is primarily cosmetic it also has a great impact on the psychological well-being of the individual. Facial de-

fects predispose the patient to a state of depression and deprive him of daily social interactions.

Surgical reconstruction of facial defects by various flaps and grafting procedures has proven to be quite satisfactory in many instances. However, there are certain limitations imposed on the success of such procedures and the surgeon must realize the difficulties encountered in the attempts to surgically reconstruct the auricle, the impossibility of recreating the orbit after exenteration, and the problem of restoring extensive tissue loss with grafts. Compromise of the local blood supply due to radiation therapy or multiple surgical procedures resulting in dense local scarring adds to the complexity of the problem. Utilizing facial prostheses facilitates examination of the surgical site in follow-up visits.

The construction of a facial prosthesis that restores lifelike appearance requires an artistic and technical ability in addition to an understanding of the psychological implications to the patient. It is advisable to plan for the artificial restoration prior to the surgical procedure. Communication between the surgeon and the prosthodontist is essential in achieving a better looking and better fitting prosthesis.

Surgical Considerations

In general, a smaller defect lends itself to a better restoration; however, the margin of any facial defect should terminate at or be close to a natural anatomic landmark. This enables the prosthodontist to place the margins of the prosthesis within the natural skin folds. Bulky flaps or rudimentary tissue may interfere with positioning of the prosthesis. This is evident if the ear lobe or the ala of the nose are spared during the surgical procedure. This tissue may become distorted by scarring, consequently a prosthesis covering these structures will appear larger than the original.

In total resection of the auricle, preservation of a portion of the cartilage is helpful both for retention and for cosmetic reasons.

This cartilage must not be destroyed and has to be strategically located in order to conceal the margin of the prosthetic ear. Efforts should be directed toward preservation of the tragus and the external auditory canal, as this is essential if the anterior margins of the prosthetic ear are to be concealed (Figs. 9-12A and B). Preservation of cartilage is also important for proper orientation and is quite helpful for retention. This is an especially important consideration for patients who are visually handicapped.

In nasal resection, preservation of the upper lip is recommended to avoid the possibility of extending the inferior margin of the prosthesis on to the mobile part of the lip (Figs. 9-13A and B); if not avoided, then the seal between the prosthesis and the lip will be broken during function. In cases in which a portion of the upper lip is resected, the defect should be repaired with a local pedicle flap to provide adequate coverage and bulk, thus improving the appearance and retention of the prosthesis.

Residual tissue at the region of the ala interferes with proper shaping of the artificial nose. On the other hand, preservation of the nasal dorsum helps in retention and orientation of the nasal prosthesis. In orbital resection, the eyebrow helps in masking the superior margin of the prosthesis, and every effort should be made to preserve this structure The inferior margin of the defect should be located where the frame of the eye glasses will mask it.

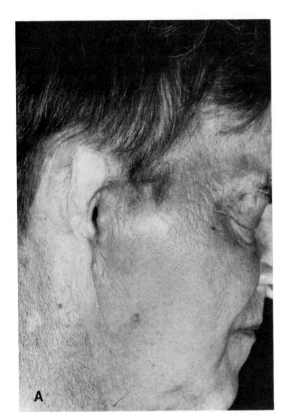
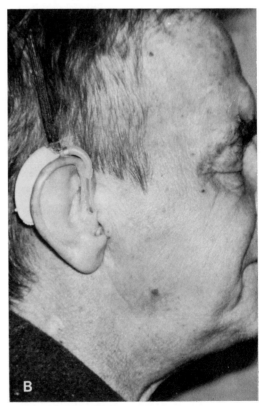

Fig. 9-12 (A) Resection of the ear preserving the tragus and external auditory meatus. A flap is rotated from the posterior margin to cover the inferior part of the surgical defect. This was planned to avoid placing the prosthesis on the skin that covers the angle of the mandible where it is mobile. The defect was covered with a skin graft. (B) The prosthesis was constructed and the patient's hearing aid was attached to it. (Fig. 9-12B courtesy of Mr. Ivo Zini, artist.)

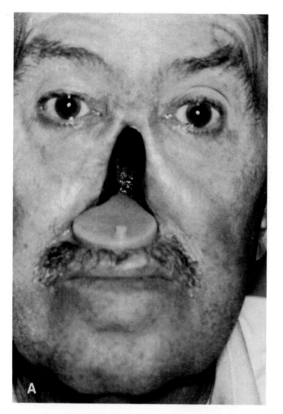
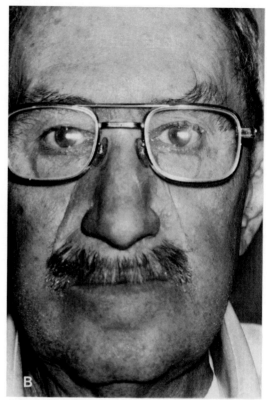

Fig. 9-13 (A) Resection of the nose and most of the hard palate. Intraoral prosthesis with a mushroom button for attachment of extraoral prosthesis in place. (Courtesy of Mark May, M.D.) (B) Intraoral and extraoral prosthesis are attached through the button and the button hole in extraoral prosthesis. The prosthesis has hair placed to blend with the natural mustache. (Courtesy of Mr. Ivo Zini, artist.)

Prosthetic Considerations

The protocol of prosthetic replacement begins with making a facial impression. If the disease process has not destroyed the affected organ, the cast is used to make an exact replica of that organ to be used after the resection. However, if the lesion has destroyed the anatomic configuration, the cast is used only as a guide in sculpting the replacement organ. Old photographs may be used as a guide. In some instances, a relative who bears a similarity to the patient is used as a model in order to achieve the most natural appearance possible for the facial replacement.

We prefer hand carving for all of our facial replacements because we have the advantage of an artist in residence. First, a fa-

cial moulage is made for patients who will undergo resection of facial structures. The cast is used to mark structures that must be removed for control of cancer and to outline proposed structures to be saved or removed for success of the prosthesis. Characterization of facial prostheses is achieved during the carving procedure by stippling the surface to duplicate skin pores and by incorporating surface texture and lines that blend naturally with the patient's own features.

Various plastic materials are used for the fabrication of facial prostheses. These materials may be grouped under two main categories: hard and resilient. Hard acrylic resin has been used in the past and is still used frequently when secretions pose a hygiene problem. The hard acrylic resin has less porosity and can be cleaned more easily than the resilient variety. Both materials can be colored intrinsically or by surface coloration. Hard acrylic resin, when the colors are incorporated during fabrication, retains the color for a longer period of time. It is dimensionally stable and gives a better fitting margin. However, it does not have the same pliability as normal human tissues and does not move with the soft tissue during function. Thus, its use is limited to smaller and nonmovable areas.

Resilient materials such as silicone, polyvinyl chloride (PVC) and polyurethane simulate the texture of the patient's tissues. The degree of this resiliency can be controlled during the fabrication process. These prostheses tend to change dimension after a period of use and the color tends to fade. The color stability varies from one material to the other and is dependent upon the amount of extrinsic coloring used after construction of the prosthesis. Environmental factors dictate the need for repainting the facial prosthesis. Exposure to the sun, application of cosmetics, hot climate, and exposure to chemicals all tend to shorten the life of the facial restorations. The quest for a durable facial material that is lifelike, will accept and retain color, and is easy to fabricate is being pursued by researchers in the field.

The facial prosthesis is processed in a custom-made mold, which can be made of dental stone, metal, or silicone material. Using silicone molds facilitates the construction of facial prostheses and reduces the time needed for completion of fabrication.

The technique for utilizing silicone molds has been developed and is advocated by our laboratory.[18, 20, 21] After carving the organ replacement, silicone 382 is applied to cover the carving and the area around it. The silicone is removed after vulcanization and a countermold is poured on the fitting surface to construct the second half of the mold.

Colors are incorporated into the facial material in patches. One patch for the basic color of the skin, a smaller patch mixed with red fibers for simulation of blood vessels, patches of brown pigments for blemishes, and patches of other characteristic colors found on individual patient's skin. To give the outer surfaces of the prosthesis a lifelike appearance, a clear coat is painted first, followed by an application of red fibers and brown areas as indicated by the patient's skin character. This is followed by the basic skin color. The balance of the mold is filled with material, the two parts of the mold are closed, and the prosthesis is cured. The surface is then touched up if needed. Chalian[12] uses heat vulcanizing silicone with metal molds, mixes the material with specific colors, then mills it in thin sheets before packing it into the mold. He relies mainly on an intrinsic coloring. The finished prosthesis is trimmed to remove any flash, proper adhesive is applied, and the prosthesis is secured in place on the patient's face.

In making orbital prostheses an acrylic resin eye is either painted to match the patient's normal eye, or a stock eye is selected and is adjusted to fit the tissue part of the prosthesis. This eye prosthesis is serviceable for many remakes, with replacement in the new prosthesis in the same manner as in the original prosthesis. The eye is always reoriented in correct alignment. It is important to have the same correction in both lenses of the eyeglasses so that each eye will be magnified to the same extent for a normal appearance (Figs. 9-14A and B). Prisms are used in patients to create the illusion of a proper alignment when the level of the defect side is different from that of the normal side.

Hair is incorporated during the processing of the facial prosthesis to blend in with the patient's hair around the ears and forehead or the patient's mustache. Techniques to incorporate the hair during fabrication of the prosthesis are far superior and more durable than attempts to use adhesives to secure it to a completed prosthesis. The hair is selected to match the patient's hair in color, type, and consistency.

We do not routinely attach facial prostheses to eyeglass frames, in order to

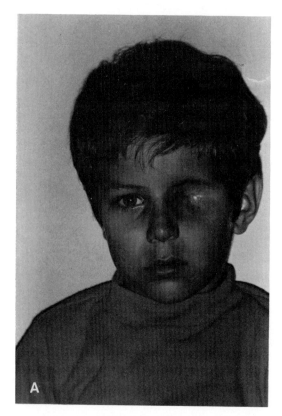
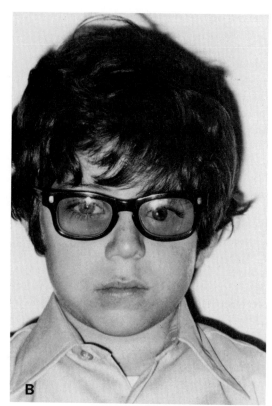

Fig. 9-14 (A) Eye defect following resection of rhabdomyosarcoma. (B) Eye prosthesis in place. Eye glasses, when slightly tinted, conceal the artificial look of the prosthesis. The glasses have the same magnification in both lenses.

avoid embarrassing situations when the patient needs to clean the lens of the normal seeing eye and inadvertently removes the glasses along with the entire prosthesis. However, we have fabricated such prostheses for retentive purposes in intraoral/extraoral large prostheses and for blind patients. Hearing aids may be attached to artificial prostheses and head bands are utilized for attachment of both the prosthesis and the hearing aid.

If the treatment plan calls for both intraoral and extraoral prostheses, the former should be completed before making the impression of the face for the extraoral prosthesis. The impression of the face is made with various elastic impression materials. Reversible hydrocolloid is the most commonly used material for this purpose. A cast is made in stone to which is added either clay or wax in preparation for carving the missing part. A metal mold is made if the facial prosthesis is to be constructed of PVC resin. Room-temperature vulcanizing silicone and heat-curing silicone materials and polyurethane may be fabricated in either stone or metal molds. The facial prosthesis is retained in place with various types of adhesives, creams, and tapes. Using these techniques, it is possible to restore almost any of the facial structures or combinations thereof.

The patient is taught how to apply and remove the facial prosthesis, is given verbal and written instruction in the care and cleaning of the prosthesis, and is instructed in the care of the defect area. In general, we recommend cleaning the prosthesis once a day by washing with pure soap and a soft brush. If the prosthesis includes an artificial eye, the eye is removed and washed, then oiled with mineral oil once a week. Proper instruction in the use of adhesive is discussed with the patient and family. The patient is warned against exposing the prosthesis to heat, flame, and chemicals and is instructed to avoid excessive exposure to sunlight.

SUMMARY

It is evident that construction of intraoral and extraoral prostheses that satisfy the patient's needs and restores function and lifelike appearance requires artistic and technical ingenuity. The task of the prosthodontist is greatly facilitated when he works within the framework of a team as an integral part of it. He examines the patient and has consultation with the various team members such as the surgeon, radiotherapist, chemotherapist, nurse oncologist, and speech pathologist before the initiation of treatment.

Early communication among team members, particularly between the surgeon and the prosthodontist, is essential to the success of the overall rehabilitation effort of head and neck cancer patients.

REFERENCES

1. Aramany, M. A. 1970. New trends in construction of splints. Journal of Prosthetic Dentistry, 23: 88.

2. Aramany, M. A. 1971. A history of prosthetic management of cleft palate: Paré to Suerson. Cleft Palate Journal, 8: 415.

3. Aramany, M. A. 1978. Basic principles of obturator design for partially edentulous patients. Part I: Classification. Journal of Prosthetic Dentistry, 40: 554.

4. Aramany, M. A. 1978. Basic principles of obturator design for partially edentulous patients. Part II: Design principles. Journal of Prosthetic Dentistry, 40: 656.

5. Aramany, M. A., and Drane, J. B. 1972. Effect of nasal extension sections on the voice quality of acquired cleft palate patients. Journal of Prosthetic Dentistry, 27: 194.

6. Aramany, M. A., and Matalon, V. 1970. Prosthetic management of post-surgical soft palate defects. Journal of Prosthetic Dentistry, 24: 304.

7. Aramany, M. A., and Myers, E. N. 1977. Intermaxillary fixation following mandibular resection. Journal of Prosthetic Dentistry, 37: 437.

8. Aramany, M. A., and Myers, E. N. 1978. Prosthetic reconstruction following resection of the hard and soft palate. Journal of Prosthetic Dentistry, 40: 174.

9. Aramany, M. A., Guerra, L. R., and Ballantyne, A. J. 1970. Skin grafting alveoloplasty following the resection of intraoral tumors. Journal of Prosthetic Dentistry, 24: 654.

10. Atkinson, H. F., and Shepherd, R. W. 1955. A preliminary report of investigations into mandibular movement. Australian Journal of Dentistry, 59: 267.

11. Boyne, P. J. 1969. Restoration of osseous defects in maxillofacial casualties. Journal of American Dental Association, 78: 767.

12. Chalian, V. A., Drane, J. B., and Standish, S. M. 1972. Maxillofacial Prosthetics: Multidisciplinary Practice. Williams and Wilkins, Baltimore.

13. Esser, J. F. 1917. Studies in plastic surgery of the face. I. Use of skin from the neck to replace face defects. II. Plastic operations about the mouth. III. Epidermic inlay. Annals of Surgery, 65: 297.

13a. Hahn, Y. W. and Corgill, M. D. 1969. Chrome cobalt mesh prosthesis. Oral Surgery, 27: 5.

14. MacIntosh, R. B., and Obwegeser, H. L. 1967. Preprosthetic surgery: A scheme for its effective employment. Journal of Oral Surgery, 25: 397.

15. Myers, E. N., and Aramany, M. A. 1977. Rehabilitation of the oral cavity following resection of the hard and soft palate. Transactions of the American Academy of Ophthalmology and Otolaryngology, 84: ORL-941.

16. Obwegeser, H. 1964. Surgical preparation of the maxilla for prosthetics. Journal of Oral Surgery, Anesthesia, and Hospital Dental Service, 22: 127.

17. Oral, K., Aramany, M. A., and McWilliams, B. J. 1979. Speech intelligibility with the buccal flange obturator. Journal of Prosthetic Dentistry, 41: 323.

18. Oral, K., Zini, I., and Aramany, M. A. 1978.

Construction of orbital prostheses using the silicone pattern technique. Journal of Prosthetic Dentistry, 40:   430.

19. Zaki, H. S. 1980. Modified bypass in maxillary hollow bulb obturator. Journal of Prosthetic Dentistry, 43:   320.

20. Zini, I., Krill, R. L., and Aramany, M. A.

1975. Direct wax method for fabrication of metallic facial molds. Journal of Prosthetic Dentistry, 33:   85.

21. Zini, I., Zaki, H. S., and Aramany, M. A. 1978. Universal simplified mold technique for construction of facial prostheses. Journal of Prosthetic Dentistry, 40:   56.

10 | Cancer of the Neck

James Y. Suen, M.D.
Stephen J. Wetmore, M.D.

INTRODUCTION

Cancer of the neck usually presents as a mass in the neck. The neck mass may represent a primary cancer originating from an anatomic structure within the neck or may represent a metastatic node from a primary in the upper aerodigestive tract, salivary glands, or skin of the face or scalp or from a primary below the clavicles. Neck masses should, therefore, be approached in an organized fashion. Most commonly the malignant neck mass will be a metastatic lymph node and the primary lesion can be identified by a careful head and neck examination. All too often a cervical node is removed for diagnostic reasons before an adequate search has been made for the primary lesion. This approach may result in an unnecessary procedure that can interfere with the definitive treatment and result in a decreased chance for cure. There are many controversial issues regarding cancer of the neck and this chapter represents our opinion. Some of the structures found in the neck, such as the salivary, thyroid, and parathyroid glands, will not be discussed in this section, since they are presented in separate chapters (see Ch. 20, 23, and 24).

ANATOMY

For purposes of this chapter the neck structures will include the muscles, nerves, vessels, submandibular glands, tail of the parotid gland, thyroid and parathyroid glands, and lymphatic system.

Cervical Triangles

Traditionally, the neck has been divided into two triangles, the *anterior cervical triangle* and the *posterior cervical triangle*. The anterior triangle is bounded by the midline of the neck, the anterior border of the sternocleidomastoid muscle, and the inferior border of the mandible. The posterior cervical triangle is bounded by the posterior border of the sternocleidomastoid muscle, the clavicle, and the anterior border of the trapezius muscle. This classical definition of the cervical triangles excludes the nodes deep to the sternocleidomastoid muscles from either major triangle; we feel these nodes should be included in the anterior cervical triangle.

The anterior cervical triangle can be subdivided into four lesser triangles (Fig. 10-1). The *submandibular triangle* is outlined by the inferior border of the mandible and the anterior and posterior borders of the digastric muscle. The *submental triangle* is outlined by the anterior belly of the digastric muscle, the hyoid bone, and the midline of the neck. The anterior triangle below the hyoid bone is divided by the omohyoid muscle into the *superior carotid triangle* and the *inferior triangle*.

The posterior cervical triangle can be divided into the *supraclavicular* or *omoclavicular triangle* and the *occipital triangle* by the

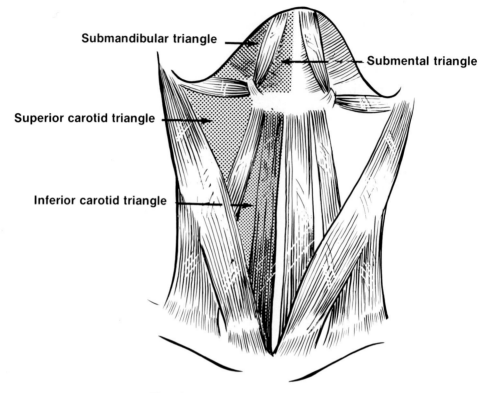

Fig. 10-1. Anterior cervical triangle.

posterior belly of the omohyoid muscle (Fig. 10-2).

Fascial Compartments

The superficial fascia and the deep cervical fascia divide the neck into several compartments (Fig. 10-3). The superficial fascia is the subcutaneous tissue of the neck and envelops the platysma. The deep cervical fascia consists of three layers: the superficial layer, which surrounds the sternocleidomastoid muscle, the strap muscles, and the trapezius; the pretracheal fascia, which is present along the anterior portion of the midline pharyngeal structures; and the prevertebral fascia, which encloses the vertebral column and its associated muscles. All three layers of deep cervical fascia join to form the carotid sheath. Knowledge of the fascial compartments is used clinically when performing a neck dissection. The nodal contents of the neck are theoretically contained within the superficial and deep layers of fascia and are, therefore, usually removed within their fascial envelopes.

Lymphatic System

Approximately 75 nodes are present on each side of the neck, most of which are in the deep jugular and spinal accessory chains (Fig. 10-4). The nodes most frequently involved in metastatic carcinoma are those in the deep jugular chain, which extends from the base of the skull to the clavicle. This deep jugular chain can be divided into superior, middle, and inferior groups. The other node groups are the submental, submandibular, superficial cervical, retropharyngeal, paratracheal, spinal accessory, anterior scalene, and supraclavicular.

The *superior deep jugular nodes* receive primary drainage from the soft palate, ton-

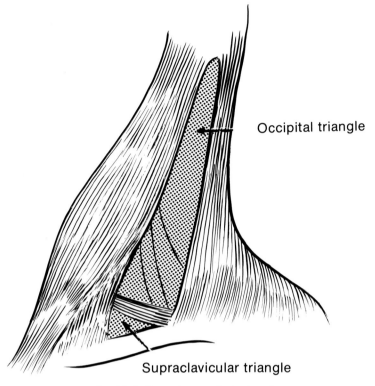

Occipital triangle

Supraclavicular triangle

Fig. 10-2. Posterior cervical triangle.

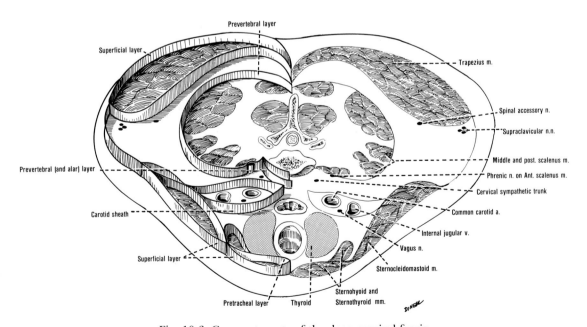

Fig. 10-3. Compartments of the deep cervical fascia.

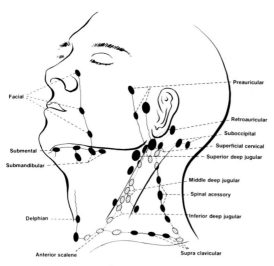

Fig. 10-4. Cervical lymphatic system.

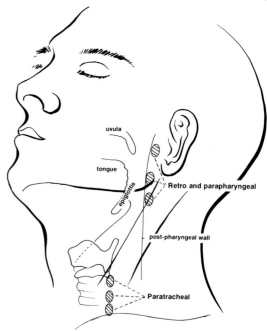

sils, tonsillar pillars, posterior oral tongue, base of the tongue, pyriform sinus, and supraglottic larynx. They receive secondary node drainage from the retropharyngeal, spinal accessory, parotid, superficial cervical, and submandibular nodes. The *middle deep jugular nodes* receive primary drainage from the supraglottic larynx, lower pyriform sinus, and posterior cricoid area. They receive secondary drainage from the superior deep jugular and lower retropharyngeal nodes. The *inferior deep jugular nodes* receive primary drainage from the thyroid, trachea, and cervical esophagus. They receive seondary drainage from the superior and middle jugular and paratracheal nodes.

The *submental nodes* receive drainage from the skin of the chin, the midportion of the lower lip, the tip of the tongue, the anterior oral cavity, and the nasal vestibule. The *submandibular nodes* receive drainage from the submental area, the lower nasal cavity, the upper lip, the lateral lower lip, the anterior oral cavity, and the skin of the midface. The submandibular nodes in turn drain into the superior deep jugular chain.

The *superficial cervical nodes* located along the external jugular vein receive drainage from the cutaneous lymphatics of the face, especially from around the parotid gland, retroauricular region, parotid nodes,

and occipital nodes. Melanomas of the skin and cancers of the parotid may drain into the superficial nodes.[3] These nodes then drain into the superior deep jugular chain. The *retropharyngeal nodes* receive drainage from the nasopharynx, posterior nasal cavity, paranasal sinuses, posterior oropharynx, and hypopharynx and drain into the deep jugular chain and to the upper spinal accessory nodes. The *paratracheal nodes* receive drainage from the lower larynx, hypopharynx, cervical esophagus, upper trachea, and the thyroid and in turn drain into the inferior deep jugular chain or superior mediastinal nodes.

The *spinal accessory nodes* are located along the spinal accessory nerves and receive drainage from the parietal and occipital regions of the scalp, the nape of the neck, and from the upper retropharyngeal and parapharyngeal nodes draining the nasopharynx, oropharynx, and paranasal sinuses. The upper spinal accessory nodes drain into the upper jugular nodes and into the lower spinal accessory nodes, which in turn drain into the supraclavicular nodes.

The *anterior scalene (Virchow's) nodes* receive drainage from the thoracic duct and are located at the junction of the thoracic duct and subclavian vein and usually are the site of metastasis from infraclavicular primary cancers. The *supraclavicular nodes* receive drainage from the spinal accessory nodes and from infraclavicular primary cancers.

The deep jugular chain drains into the jugular lymphatic trunk and empties on the left side into the thoracic duct and on the right side into the right lymphatic duct or directly into the venous system at the junction of the internal jugular and subclavian veins. The thoracic duct and right lymphatic duct also receive lymph drainage from the supraclavicular nodes.

DIFFERENTIAL DIAGNOSIS

When a mass in the neck is detected, one should consider the great variety of possible etiologies. Some neck masses turn out to be normal structures that are quite prominent in some patients. This can be best judged from experience gained after examining the necks of many patients.

The differential diagnosis should consider broad categories of diseases such as, neoplasms, infection, congenital anomalies, and miscellaneous conditions (Table 10-1).

PATIENT EVALUATION

The primary question is, of course, whether or not a neck mass represents a malignancy. Any neck mass suspected of being malignant should be approached in a rational, organized manner (Fig. 10-5), beginning with a pertinent history. Factors increasing the likelihood of malignancy include (1) age over 40 years; (2) excessive tobacco use, especially cigarettes; (3) excessive alcohol use; (4) nontender, enlarging mass; (5) obstructive symptoms of the airway; (6) hoarseness of over 3 weeks' duration; (7) persistent throat pain for more than 3 weeks; (8) nonhealing ulceration; (9) previous radiation exposure; and (10) history of cancer of the

TABLE 10-1. DIFFERENTIAL DIAGNOSIS OF A NECK MASS

I Neoplasms
  A. Benign
    1. Vascular—hemangioma, lymphangioma, arteriovenous malformation, aneurysms
    2. Chemodectoma
    3. Neural—neurofibroma, schwannoma
    4. Lipoma
    5. Fibroma
    6. Miscellaneous—fibromatosis
  B. Malignant
    1. Neck primary
      a. Lymphoma
      b. Sarcoma
      c. Thyroid carcinoma
      d. Salivary gland carcinoma
      e. Branchial cleft cyst carcinoma
      f. Thyroglossal duct cyst carcinoma
    2. Metastatic
      a. Head and neck primary—mucosal surfaces, skin, salivary glands, thyroid
      b. Infraclavicular primary—lung, kidney, prostate, gonads, stomach, breast
      c. Leukemias
II Infection
  A. Abscesses
  B. Cervical lymphadenitis
    1. Bacterial
    2. Granulomatous—tuberculosis, actinomycosis, sarcoidosis
    3. Viral—infectious mononucleosis
III Congenital
  A. Thyroglossal duct cyst
  B. Branchial cleft cyst
  C. Dermoid cyst
  D. Teratoma
IV Miscellaneous
  A. Zenker diverticulum
  B. External laryngocele
  C. Amyloidosis
V Normal Structures
  A. Hyoid
  B. Carotid bulb
  C. Transverse process of vertebrae
  D. Normal neck nodes (hyperplastic)

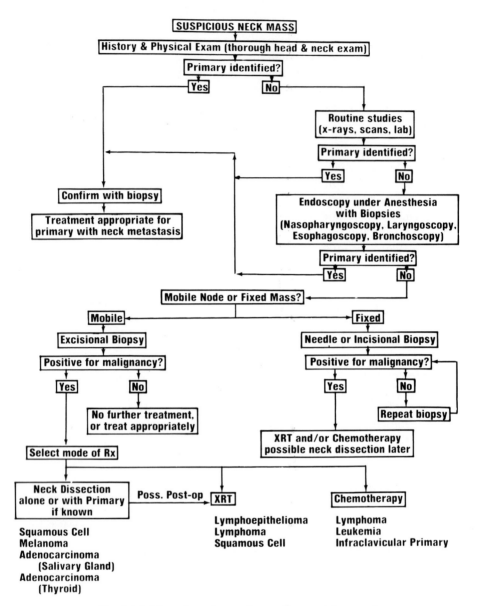

Fig. 10-5. Flow sheet for work-up of a suspicious node.

head and neck, especially of the skin or lip, that may have been locally controlled by excision several years previously and thought to be insignificant.

A complete examination of the head and neck must be performed. If the mass represents a cervical metastasis from a head and neck primary cancer, over 90 percent of the primaries can be found on this ex-amination. Lymphatic drainage is highly predictable and the location of the mass can direct the search. Lindberg[18] reviewed the records of 2,044 patients with previously untreated squamous cell carcinoma of the head and neck and described the incidence and topographic distribution of lymph node metastases on admission. The highest inci-dence of metastatic nodes from the oral cavity, oropharynx, supraglottic larynx, hypo-pharynx, and nasopharynx presented in the superior deep jugular chain.

A preauricular mass most commonly represents a primary tumor in the parotid or a metastasis from a primary cancer arising in the skin of the ipsilateral face, scalp, or ear (Fig. 10-6). Malignant nodes under the superior end of the sternocleidomastoid muscle and/or malignant superior-posterior cervical nodes would usually represent a primary cancer in the nasopharynx, posterior oropharynx, or maxillary sinus (Fig. 10-7). A submental node may represent a primary of the skin of the nose or lips or of the anterior floor of the mouth (Fig. 10-8). A submandibular triangle mass may represent a submandibular gland primary or a metastasis from a skin primary of the ipsilateral face or lips or from the oral cavity or paranasal sinuses (Fig. 10-9). Nodes in the superior deep jugular area may represent a primary of the posterior oral cavity, oropharynx, nasopharynx, hypopharynx, base of the tongue, or supraglottic larynx (Fig. 10-10).

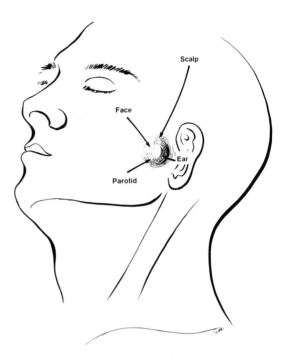

Fig. 10-6. Preauricular mass.

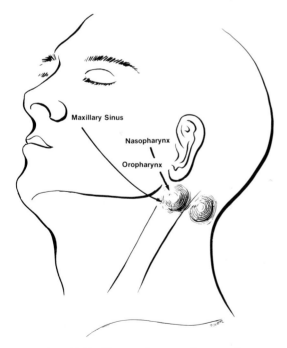

Fig. 10-7. Upper deep and posterior cervical nodes.

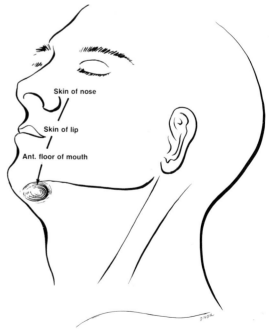

Fig. 10-8. Submental node.

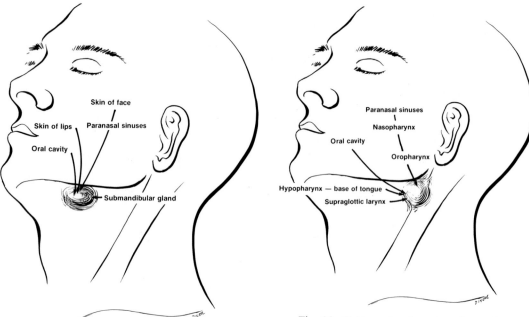

Fig. 10-9. Submandibular triangle mass.

Fig. 10-10. Superior deep jugular nodes (jugulodigastric).

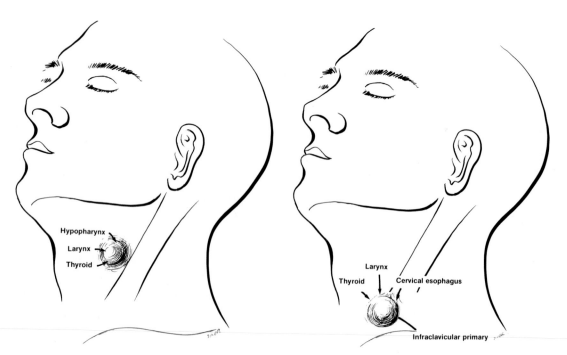

Fig. 10-11. Midjugular node.

Fig. 10-12. Lower jugular node.

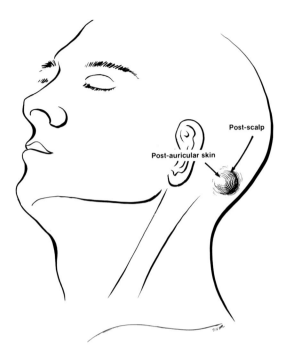

Fig. 10-13. Suboccipital node.

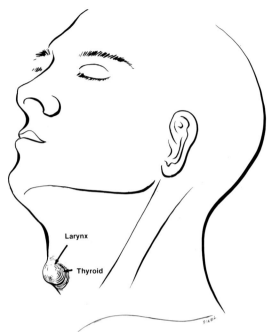

Fig. 10-14. Prelaryngeal (Delphian) node.

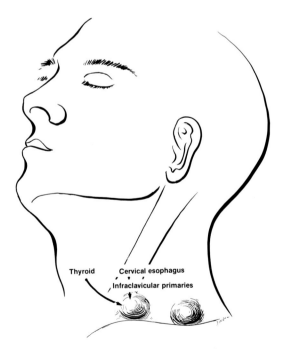

Fig. 10-15. Supraclavicular nodes.

A single midjugular mass would usually represent a laryngeal, hypopharyngeal, or thyroid primary (Fig. 10-11). A lower jugular mass most often represents a subglottic larynx, thyroid, cervical esophagus, or infraclavicular primary (Fig. 10-12).

Suboccipital nodes usually represent metastasis from a posterior scalp or auricle primary (Fig. 10-13). A prelaryngeal mass (Delphian node) would usually represent a primary from the thyroid or a laryngeal lesion with anterior commissure or subglottic extension (Fig. 10-14). Supraclavicular masses usually represent an infraclavicular primary or a cancer of the cervical esophagus or thyroid (Fig. 10-15).

Primary Identified

If a lesion suspected to be the primary is identified during the head and neck examination, a biopsy of the primary should be performed. If positive, then the neck mass should be considered metastatic node or nodes and the treatment will depend upon the site of the primary and the extent of the cervical metastasis.

No Primary Identified

If no primary is noted on examination, a reasonable search for the primary using other means should be undertaken. This should consist initially of a thorough review of the patient's history, including a review of systems, past history, family history, and occupational history, and a complete physical examination. Next, chest and sinus radiographs would be appropriate. A thyroid scan should also be considered in an effort to demonstrate a cold nodule. Other tests such as intravenous pyelography, upper gastrointestinal and barium enema x-rays, and liver and bone scans are not usually indicated for a patient without symptoms referable to these organs and are unnecessary expenses. Soft-tissue lateral x-rays of the neck, xeroradiograms, laryngograms, esophagrams, polytomograms, or computerized tomograms should be used primarily to determine the extent of disease once the cancer has been diagnosed. However, with an unknown primary, xeroradiograms of the lateral neck and an air-contrast esophagram may be helpful to suggest the primary site.

The next step, should the diagnosis remain obscure, would be a direct visual examination and palpation under general anesthesia to evaluate the nasopharynx, hypopharynx, larynx, esophagus, and tracheobronchial tree. Biopsies of all suspicious areas should be performed, and frozen sections requested. *Selected random* biopsies ("blind biopsies") can be done in areas of high probability based on the predictability of lymphatic drainage. Such areas include the nasopharynx, tonsils, and base of the tongue.

With careful physical examination and the above studies of a patient with a suspected metastatic neck node, the primary tumor site will be identified in nearly all cases. However, if the primary is still not identified, a biopsy of the neck mass can be performed. This may be done at the time of the examination under anesthesia. A neck dissection should be considered at the same operation if the node is positive for malignancy and is not a supraclavicular node. With a mass that is fixed to adjacent structures, a needle or incisional biopsy can be performed. If lymphoma is suspected, an excisional biopsy is indicated. Treatment of a fixed neck node is discussed later in this chapter.

With a mobile node, an excisional biopsy is preferred, taking care not to crush the node or tear the capsule. Placement of the incision for the biopsy should take into account future plans for the possibility of a neck dissection. Should the frozen section reveal a benign process, no further treatment may be necessary. If the pathologist is unsure and feels that permanent sections are necessary, it is more prudent to await the final pathologic interpretation. Should the node be interpreted as malignant on frozen section, treatment would depend upon the histology and the most likely primary origin.

Staging

CERVICAL NODE CLASSIFICATION (FIG. 10-16)

The following classification[1] of cervical lymph node metastasis is applicable to all malignant head and neck tumors. In evaluating the node the actual size of the nodal mass should be measured and allowances made for intervening soft tissue. Most masses over 3 cm in diameter are not single nodes but rather are confluent nodes or tumor that has extended outside of the node into the soft tissues of the neck. There are three stages of clinically positive nodes: N1, N2, and N3. The use of subgroups a, b, and c is recommended for more precise staging. Midline nodes are considered as homolateral nodes.

STAGING NECK NODES

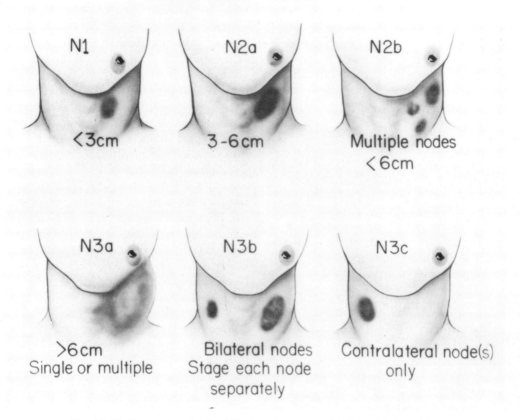

Fig. 10-16. Cervical node classification (courtesy of Michael Johns, M.D.).

NX   Nodes cannot be assessed.

N0   No clinically positive node.

N1   Single clinically positive homolateral node 3 cm or less in diameter.

N2   Single clinically positive homolateral node more than 3 cm but not more than 6 cm in diameter, or multiple clinically positive homolateral nodes none more than 6 cm in diameter.

N2a   Single clinically positive homolateral node more than 3 cm but not more than 6 cm in diameter.

N2b   Multiple clinically positive homolateral nodes none more than 6 cm in diameter.

N3   Massive homolateral node(s), bilateral nodes, or contralateral node(s).

N3a   Homolateral clinically positive node(s), at least one greater than 6 cm in diameter.

N3b   Bilateral clinically positive nodes (in this situation, each side of the neck should be staged separately; that is N3b; right, N2a; left, N1).

N3c   Only contralateral clinically positive node(s).

TREATMENT

Primary Cancers

Certain malignancies may arise from anatomic structures within the neck. These are the primary lymphomas and sarcomas, thyroid carcinomas, salivary gland (tail of parotid and submandibular) carcinomas, and the rare branchial cleft cyst carcinoma. Lymphomas, thyroid, and salivary gland carcinomas are discussed in other chapters in this book. Sarcomas and branchial cleft cyst carcinomas are quite rare and usually require wide resection and possibly a neck dissection, depending on the presence of clinically positive nodes.

Metastasis

The mode of treatment of cervical lymph nodes containing metastatic cancer will depend upon several factors. The major consideration is the site of the primary malignancy. The treatment varies depending upon whether the location of the primary cancer is in the head and neck region, the infraclavicular region, or unknown.

HEAD AND NECK PRIMARY

When the primary is identified in the head and neck, treatment must consider both the primary site and the metastatic node(s). The following recommendations are for squamous cell carcinomas and also adenocarcinomas of salivary gland origin. These recommendations are guidelines and cannot cover every possible situation.

With an *N1* neck, the most widely accepted treatment is a resection of the primary and a radical neck dissection, in continuity if possible. Postoperative irradiation (5,000-6,000 rads) is used if the primary is T4, sometimes with T3, and when pathology reveals more than one positive node. Other treatment modalities being used, although of unproven effectiveness, include a modified or regional neck dissection with postoperative irradiation, and irradiation alone.[19]

With an *N2a* or *N2b* neck, the most widely accepted treatment is a composite resection of the primary with a radical neck dissection, followed by postoperative irradiation. Preoperative irradiation is probably comparable in results to postoperative irradiation.

With an *N3a* or *N3b* neck, the most accepted treatment is a combination of irradiation and surgery if the nodes are resectable. If the nodes are fixed and felt to be unresectable, most patients are initially treated with irradiation in an attempt to "free up" the fixed mass. With bilaterally clinically positive nodes, which are still resectable, surgery usually consists of bilateral neck dissections. If bilateral dissections are performed during the same operation, we recommend doing a modified neck dissection on the least involved side, followed by irradiation. The rationale for this recommendation is based on the poor prognosis for patients with the extensive disease and the high morbidity and mortality for bilateral radical neck dissections. Some surgeons stage the radical neck dissections after preoperative irradiation. Another option would be no surgical treatment because of the poor prognosis.

There are certain exceptions to these guidelines. The accepted treatment for nasopharyngeal carcinoma with neck metastasis or any unresectable primary lesion is radiation therapy alone. Neck dissection is indicated for persistent neck disease only if the primary is controlled and there is no evidence of distant metastasis. When the primary site is in the posterior oropharyngeal or hypopharyngeal area, the neck dissection must include the retropharyngeal and parapharyngeal nodes, which are the first echelon nodes to be involved and may frequently be missed. These nodes should be palpated and removed if metastasis is present. If distant metastasis is noted, chemotherapy is probably the treatment of choice.

Adjuvant chemotherapy is being used in clinical trials in patients with Stage IV and with some Stage III malignancies in an effort to improve the cure rate, but this practice is still experimental as of now.

For further discussion see the chapters on specific primary sites.

INFRACLAVICULAR PRIMARY

An infraclavicular primary with neck metastasis will usually involve the supraclavicular and anterior scalene nodes. No surgical treatment of the neck is indicated in these cases. If treatment is to be administered, chemotherapy is employed for most infra-clavicular primaries with neck metastasis. Irradiation of the primary and its neck metastasis may be the treatment of choice for mediastinal and esophageal primaries.

UNKNOWN PRIMARY

The proper method of evaluating a suspicious neck mass is outlined in the section on Patient Evaluation. If a primary is not identified, then a needle or an open biopsy of the neck is indicated. The major question at this point is what to do if the node is positive for malignancy. The following treatment is recommended for the various cervical node situations depending upon the histology on frozen section.

A neck dissection should not be performed if the malignant diagnosis is lymphoma or lymphoepithelioma, because in this case radiation and/or chemotherapy would be the treatment of choice. With metastatic squamous cell carcinoma in the node, a neck dissection should be strongly considered, especially if other clinically positive nodes are noted on exploration. In this case, postoperative radiation therapy should be considered, covering all areas of potential primary origins (especially Waldeyer's ring) in the hope that the primary is small and radiation therapy will control it. Some surgeons, however, would not use radiation therapy and would follow the patient closely. Postoperative irradiation is mandatory after a neck dissection if the cancer has extended outside the node capsule, if multiple nodes are positive, or if lymphatic or nerve invasion is noted histologically.

If only one metastatic node is noted, some authorities feel that radiation therapy could be used to treat the neck without a neck dissection, including possible primary sites in the radiation portal in hopes of controlling microscopic disease.

A diagnosis of melanoma in the node should cause one to reexamine the likely primary sites in the skin, mucosa, and eyes.

Whether or not the primary is found in this instance, a neck dissection is the accepted treatment of choice.[3]

With a diagnosis of adenocarcinoma of salivary gland origin in the node, the treatment will depend on the possible primary and the location of the positive node. If the node is located in the submandibular triangle, the primary may be from the submandibular gland and the treatment would be a neck dissection. If the node is in the upper jugular chain, the primary could be from the parotid and the treatment would be a parotidectomy with a neck dissection.

An inferior or middle jugular, prelaryngeal, or a posterior cervical triangle node with adenocarcinoma may be from a thyroid primary. Thyroid carcinomas are not usually difficult to identify in a lymph node and the histology will direct attention to the thyroid gland.

Positive supraclavicular nodes or anterior scalene nodes usually represent metastasis from primaries below the clavicles. Nodes in these locations should be biopsied early if a primary in the head and neck region is not identified, since most of these positive nodes are from primaries outside of the head and neck.

Clinically Negative Neck

A controversy that is still unsettled is whether or not to do an elective neck dissection when the neck is clinically negative (no nodes palpable) after diagnosis of a primary cancer in the head and neck. At the present time no studies have definitively evaluated the worth of elective neck dissection.[15, 20, 22, 24, 27, 28, 30, 31, 33]

The primary argument for an elective neck dissection is that the incidence of occult nodes is quite high, especially with cancers arising in certain sites. Sako et al.,[27] in a study of 235 head and neck cancer patients, reported a 28 percent overall occult metastatic rate with 36 percent, 38 percent, and 55 percent rates for tonsil, oral tongue, and base of tongue, respectively. Other studies[6, 20, 23, 28, 30] have shown the presence of occult nodes in from 16 to 46 percent of their cases, with the higher figures generally occurring in the oral cavity and oropharynx. Other arguments for elective neck dissection are that allowing neck metastases to become clinically obvious before performing neck dissections may increase the incidence of distant metastases, and that the follow-up in patients with large necks may make early detection of cervical metastases difficult or impossible.

It seems rational that one would want to remove neck nodes that contain metastatic cancer. The problem is that the nodes containing microscopic deposits of cancer may not be clinically palpable. If elective neck dissections were performed routinely in every case, many unnecessary operations would be done. Some other arguments against the elective neck dissection include the significant morbidity from the shoulder-drop problem and some deformity of the neck that results from removing the sterno-cleidomastoid muscle; the indication, in some studies,[28] that a cure rate is no worse if one waits until the neck converts from N0 to N1; and the finding that radiation therapy may be effective for occult metastases.[9, 11, 14, 21, 25]

We feel that certain sites (oral cavity, pharyngeal and supraglottic larynx) with high risk of metastasis can be identified. If patients have a clinically negative neck but a large (T3 or T4) primary in one of these sites, each of which has greater than 25 percent chance of occult nodes, then an elective neck dissection would be indicated, especially if the neck would have to be entered to remove the primary. However, rather than a radical neck dissection, a modified neck dissection is recommended, preserving the 11th cranial nerve, sternocleidomastoid muscle, and jugular vein (see section on neck dissections). This removes some of the disadvantages of the radical neck dissection. This neck dissection also serves as a staging procedure for the neck, i.e., if two or more nodes are positive, then postoperative irradiation is indicated to help in local control.

Some studies[9, 11] appear to indicate that 5,000 rads or more of irradiation is effective in controlling occult metastases. These results would argue against the use of neck dissection and for the use of irradiation to control the neck disease.

Fixed Neck Mass

What is unresectable to one surgeon may be resectable to another. A fixed mass may be resectable depending upon the structure to which it is fixed.

Fixation to the mastoid process, paravertebral muscles, sternocleidomastoid muscle, larynx, or mandible does not alone imply unresectability. These masses may be resected in some cases but the decision whether or not to operate will require good judgment and experience. If all gross tumor can be removed, postoperative irradiation may be able to destroy the microscopic disease with a possibility for local control. With a fixed neck mass one must remember that the cure rate is extremely low. When trying to decide whether or not to do radical surgery and irradiation for local control only, one must weigh the morbidity and mortality of the treatment versus the morbidity and mortality of uncontrolled disease in the head and neck.

Masses fixed to the common or internal carotid artery, vertebrae, brachial plexus, or trachea are less likely to be resectable. In these cases it is not unusual to use irradiation first to see if the fixed mass will become "free," so that the mass can be removed surgically. Local control may be possible but cure is unlikely in these cases. If the mass remains fixed, then chemotherapy becomes the treatment of choice.

Recurrence in the Neck

Recurrence of cancer in the neck following what appeared to have been adequate treatment is a poor prognostic sign. When considering treatment one should know if the primary has recurred or persisted, or if this is metastasis from a second primary. Distant metastasis should also be ruled out.

Surgical resection would be indicated if the neck recurrence is still resectable and the primary is controlled. Major surgical resections should be done only after careful consideration, since the local control rate and cure rate with neck recurrence is extremely low.

If none has been given previously, radiation therapy can be used as the only treatment or with surgery if the recurrence is resectable. Chemotherapy can be selected if no further irradiation or surgery is indicated.

One should be very careful to look at the skin of the neck and upper chest for small subdermal metastases. When these occur, it is almost always after irradiation has been used. These subdermal metastases are easily missed and may appear as small benign-looking nodules (Figs. 10-17 A and B).

Surgery is rarely indicated, since these lesions are extremely difficult to control surgically. Methotrexate or other chemotherapy may be useful in treating these metastases.

Neck Dissections

In 1906 George Crile, Sr., described the classical radical neck dissection.[7] It has remained the primary operation for management of metastatic neck nodes for many years and is still considered by many authorities as the only operation for metastasis to the neck. The principle of the radical neck dissection continues to be valid; however, the indications are changing with the advent of other treatment modalities in conjunction with surgery.

RADICAL NECK DISSECTION

This operation was described by Crile as an en bloc dissection of all of the cervical lymphatic channels and glands draining a primary site of head and neck cancer. A description of the technique can be found in any atlas of head and neck surgery.

Rationale. When metastatic cancer cells have reached one group of nodes it is possible that a few cells have already involved

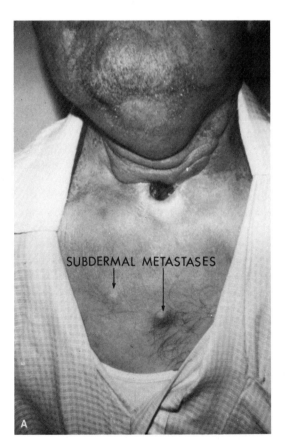

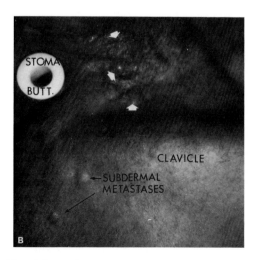

Fig. 10-17. (A & B) Two patients with subdermal metastases.

nonpalpable nodes in contiguous areas. Less than a radical neck dissection may risk leaving cancer cells behind, especially if surgery is the only treatment modality used.

Indications

1. With resection of a primary carcinoma of the head and neck when clinically positive cervical node(s) are present.

2. Regional metastases after the primary lesion has been controlled by surgery, irradiation, or a combination of these methods.

3. Clinically positive node(s) after previous irradiation to the neck.

4. Clinically positive node(s) when surgery is the only treatment.

5. Fixed neck mass that appears to become mobile following irradiation, or chemotherapy, or both.

6. High risk of occult nodes (procedure known as an "elective neck dissection").

7. Nodal involvement other than the first echelon group.

Contraindications

1. Uncontrolled cancer at the primary site.

2. Clinical or roentgenographic evidence of distant metastases.

3. Life expectancy of less than 6 weeks.

4. Fixed nodes unchanged by irradiation.

Advantages

1. Relative ease and straightforward nature of the operation.

2. Lower likelihood of leaving nodes behind.

Disadvantages

1. Trapezius muscle dysfunction with shoulder drop resulting in shoulder pain and limitation of motion.

2. Mild to moderate deformity of the neck.

3. Painful neuromas of the cervical plexus.

4. Increased facial swelling.

EXTENDED RADICAL NECK DISSECTION

This operation is a radical neck dissection plus dissection of adjacent node-bearing areas that are not included in the classical radical neck dissection but are, or may be, involved. These node-bearing areas include the suboccipital, parotid, retropharyngeal, paratracheal, and upper mediastinal areas.

The rationale for this procedure is that some head and neck primaries involve first echelon nodes that are not included in the classical radical neck dissection. These nodes would be the most likely to be involved and should be removed in addition to the ones removed with a radical neck dissection. The indications, contraindications, advantages, and disadvantages would be essentially the same as those for the radical neck dissection.

MODIFIED NECK DISSECTION (CONSERVATIVE OR FUNCTIONAL)

The modified neck dissection is essentially the same as a radical neck dissection except that the spinal accessory nerve, sternocleidomastoid muscle, internal jugular vein, and sometimes the cervical plexus nerves are preserved (Figs. 10-18 A and B). One or several of these structures could be included in the dissection and the procedure still be considered a modified neck dissection. The submental and/or submandibular triangles need not be included in the modified neck dissection if the chances for their involvement are small.

Rationale. Many of the pioneers in this speciality felt strongly that nothing less than a radical neck dissection should be performed. These feelings were expressed especially in earlier years when surgery was used as the primary, and frequently the only, modality of treatment. The availability of effective radiation treatment adds a different perspective to the management of neck nodes. Fletcher[9] has shown that microscopic disease can be controlled in many cases with a dose of 5,000 or more rads of radiation. Also, the probability of some nodal groups being involved with certain primaries is, predictably, low. For example, primary laryngeal carcinomas rarely metastasize to the submental, submandibular, or lower posterior cervical triangles[5, 29] and

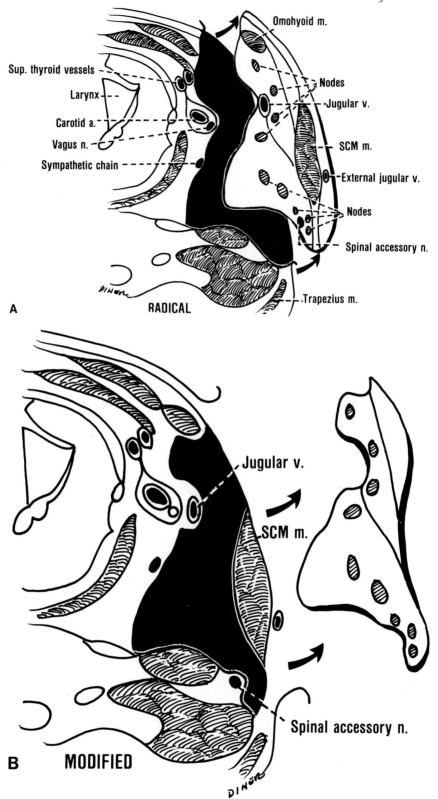

Fig. 10-18. (A) Structures removed with a radical neck dissection. (B) Structures removed with a modified neck dissection. SCM, sternocleidomastoid.

these areas would not necessarily require resection for control of neck disease. The fact that lymph drainage is highly predictable and irradiation is frequently used in combination with surgery makes modifications of the radical neck dissection more appealing. When selecting a modified neck dissection as treatment, one must be very careful to strictly adhere to the indications and contraindications as outlined below:

Indications

1. Clinically negative neck but significant (greater than 25 percent) risk of occult nodes; this is considered an "elective neck dissection." This situation would include this procedure on both sides of the neck with some midline primaries, such as in the base of the tongue and the supraglottic larynx. The modified neck dissection is usually performed in conjunction with resection of the primary.

2. Single node (<3 cm) when surgery is to be followed by irradiation, e.g., T3 or T4, N1M0 of oral cavity, oropharynx, or hypopharynx.

3. Differentiated thyroid carcinomas with neck metastasis.

4. If there are indications for bilateral neck dissections, a modified neck dissection saving the jugular vein and spinal accessory nerve on one side could be performed. These patients should receive postoperative irradiation.

Contraindications

1. Clinically positive nodes when surgery is the only treatment modality to be used.

2. Clinically positive nodes after irradiation has been given to the neck.

3. Clinically positive nodes after previous modified or regional neck dissection.

4. Melanoma with clinically positive nodes.

5. Inexperience of the surgeon.

Advantages

1. Avoidance of problems of shoulder drop, which occurs when the spinal accessory nerve is resected.

2. Lowered morbidity and mortality when performed on one side during bilateral neck dissections.

3. Greater protection or coverage for the carotid artery.

4. More tissue volume left for irradiation.

5. Value as a staging procedure in the N0 neck to determine the need for postoperative irradiation.

6. Avoidance of cosmetic deformity and permanent sensory deficit produced by radical neck dissection.

7. Fewer major complications with less chance for catastrophe.

8. Avoidance of painful neuromas if cervical plexus preserved.

9. Preservation of intracranial and facial venous drainage.

10. Possibility for conversion to a radical neck dissection if multiple clinically positive nodes are noted.

Disadvantages

1. Possible omission of occult positive nodes, especially the jugulodigastric and spinal accessory nodes.

2. Increased risk of cutting into positive nodes and seeding neck.

3. Increased risk of hematoma underneath the sternocleidomastoid muscle.

4. Increased difficulty and operative time over radical neck dissection.

5. Increased difficulty for a secondary radical neck dissection if nodes recur.

Technique of Modified Neck Dissection. A technique for the modified neck dissection was described by Bocca in 1967.[4] This technique originated with O. Suarez in Argentina. Over the past 25 years, Ballantyne from the M. D. Anderson Hospital and Tumor Institute developed his own technique, which differs slightly from that described by Bocca. The primary difference between these two techniques is that Bocca dissects the posterior cervical triangle contents behind the sternocleidomastoid muscle and then passes the contents anteriorly under the muscle with the fascial sheath, whereas Ballantyne dissects the posterior cervical contents from an anterior approach underneath the muscle. The anterior cervical triangle dissection is very similar with both techniques.

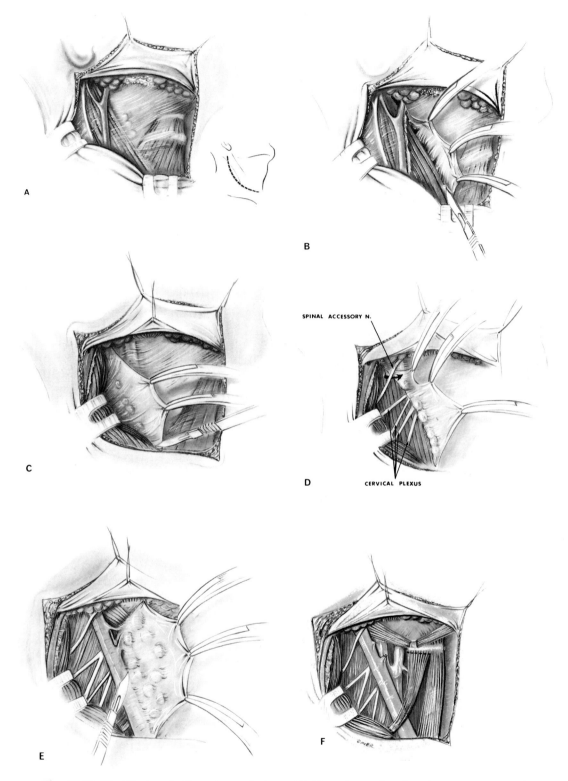

Fig. 10-19. Modified neck dissection technique. (A) Flap elevated and neck contents exposed. (B) Incision and elevation of the superficial fascia of the sternocleidomastoid muscle. (C) Fascia dissected from medial side of sternocleidomastoid muscle. (D) Cervical plexus nerves at posterior edge of sternocleidomastoid muscle. Tissue above spinal acessory nerve dissected out. (E) Dissecting tissue off of the jugular vein. (F) Neck anatomy of the modified neck dissection.

The operation described here is after the technique of Ballantyne and is the one we use. It requires the use of sharp knife dissection, constant traction and counter-traction, and extensive knowledge of the anatomy of the neck. It is usually done in conjunction with a primary resection.

First, a cervical flap is elevated to provide adequate exposure to the neck and primary (Fig. 10-19A). An incision is made into the superficial fascia of the sternocleidomastoid muscle along its entire length (Fig. 10-19B). With traction on the fascia, the superficial fascia is dissected anteriorly and then off the medial side of the sternocleidomastoid muscle (Fig. 10-19C) until the cervical plexus nerves are encountered at the posterior edge of the muscle (Fig. 10-19D). The sternocleidomastoid muscle must be retracted posteriorly during the dissection. The dissection can then include or exclude the cervical plexus nerves and is carried to the splenius capitus and levator scapulae muscles. Preserving the cervical plexus nerves makes the operation more difficult. Resecting the cervical plexus requires cutting the nerves at the posterior border of the sternocleidomastoid muscle and then again just after they exit from the vertebral foramina and give off branches to the phrenic nerve and the levator scapulae nerves.

During the dissection medial to the sternocleidomastoid muscle, the spinal accessory nerve is identified where it enters the muscle near the junction of the upper and middle one-third. The dissection should remove the tissue superior to the spinal accessory nerve and carry it under the nerve to be part of the posterior cervical contents being dissected (Fig. 10-19D).

After dissecting the posterior cervical contents and the tissues under the sternocleidomastoid muscle off the splenius capitus and levator scapulae muscles, the carotid sheath is encountered on its deep or posterior surface. This sheath is then dissected off the carotid artery, vagus nerve, and jugular vein from the deep side and over these structures and then anteriorly to the lateral pharynx, strap muscles, and the thyroid gland (Fig. 10-19E). The superior belly of the omohyoid muscle may be removed down to the tendon during the dissection or could be preserved. The rest of the dissection would be similar to the radical neck dissection depending on whether the submandibular and submental triangle contents were removed (Fig. 10-19F).

The dissection is difficult at the superior end; it requires dissection superiorly along the spinal accessory nerve to and over the jugular vein where the vein goes beneath the posterior belly of the digastric muscle. The digastric muscle must be retracted superiorly to be sure of removing the subdigastric nodes. The inferior part of the dissection removes the supraclavicular contents—with or without the superior belly of the omohyoid—over to the lower portion of the internal jugular vein, and then superiorly with the fascia of the strap muscles. The transverse cervical artery is usually preserved.

REGIONAL NECK DISSECTION (SELECTIVE OR PARTIAL)

A regional neck dissection, such as a submandibular triangle dissection and a jugulodigastric node dissection (Figs. 10-20A-D), or an interjugular node dissection with a wide field laryngectomy, removes a group or groups of nodes.

Rationale. The rationale for this operation is based upon the predictability of lymph node drainage and knowing the first and second echelon nodes most likely to be involved. It also is based on irradiation being effective for most subclinical disease. This operation is usually done in conjunction with resection of the primary. If the nodes removed in the regional neck dissection are negative, then further treatment to the neck may not be necessary. If one or more of the nodes is positive, then postoperative irradiation therapy would be indicated with reasonable chance for control of the neck.

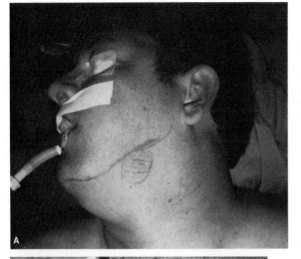

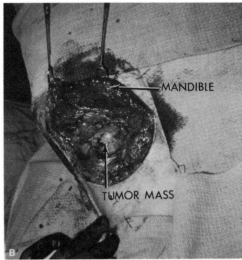

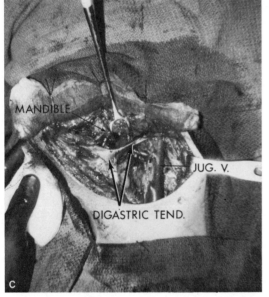

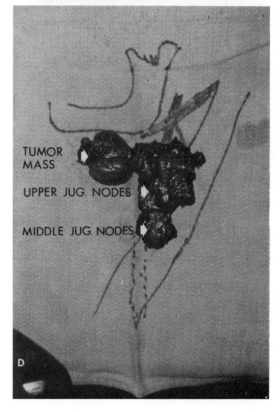

Fig. 10-20. Regional neck dissection (selective or partial). (A) Suspicious submandibular mass. (B) Submandibular and upper jugular area exposed. (C) Neck structures after regional neck dissection. (D) Regional neck dissection contents.

Indications

1. When resecting major salivary gland neoplasms suspected of being malignant and the neck is N0, the first and second echelon nodes may be removed in continuity as a regional node dissection.

2. When performing a wide field laryn-gectomy with an N0 neck, an interjugular node dissection is considered a regional node dissection.

3. When resecting a thyroid carcinoma with an N0 neck, an "anterior compartment dissection" is frequently performed and is considered a regional node dissection.

4. When removing a metastatic cervical node (N1) with an unknown primary, a regional neck dissection can be performed if irradiation is to be used postoperatively.

5. When a patient has received full course irradiation to the neck for an N1 or N2a node and the node does not completely regress, then a regional neck dissection may be indicated. This combination must be planned and the primary should be controlled.

Contraindications

1. Clinically positive nodes when surgery is the only treatment modality used.

2. Clinically positive nodes appearing after irradiation has been given to the neck.

3. Clinically positive nodes appearing after previous modified or regional neck dissection.

4. Melanoma with clinically positive nodes.

5. Multiple node involvement.

Advantages

1. The regional neck dissection can be used as a staging procedure when performed with resection of a primary cancer. If nodes are positive in the dissection, irradiation should be given postoperatively; if they are negative, then no further treatment may be necessary.

2. If combined with radiation therapy for the above indications, a radical neck dissection may be avoided with no increased risk of recurrence.

Disadvantages

1. Danger of missing some positive occult nodes if wrong group removed.

2. Difficulty of identifying "groups" of nodes.

Technique.   The technique requires that the surgeon be very familiar with the lymphatic drainage and node distribution. The procedure is performed primarily using knife dissection. A group.or groups of nodes can be removed as an en bloc dissection but these are not necessarily within fascial compartments.

INCISIONS

The arterial supply to the cervical skin[10, 16] runs primarily in a vertical direction, with one group consisting of tributaries of the facial artery, submental artery, superior thyroid artery, and sternocleidomastoid artery running from the upper neck inferiorly and the other group consisting of tributaries of the suprascapular artery, transverse cervical artery, and superficial clavicular artery running superiorly from the region of the lower neck (Fig. 10-21). Studies by Kambic[16] and Freeland[10] showed that the midneck was the least vascularized area of the neck and that poor anastomoses existed across the midline between the right and left sides of the neck.

The head and neck surgeon should be familiar with several versatile incisions so that he can manage a wide variety of extirpative and reconstruction procedures (Figs. 10-22 A-F). One should avoid an incision that has a trifurcation over the carotid artery.

The basic considerations for designing

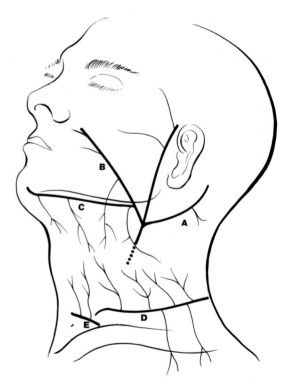

Fig. 10-21. Arterial blood supply to the cervical skin: A, Sternocleidomastoid branch of occipital artery; B, Facial artery; C, Submental branch of facial artery; D, Transverse cervical artery; E, Superficial clavicular artery.

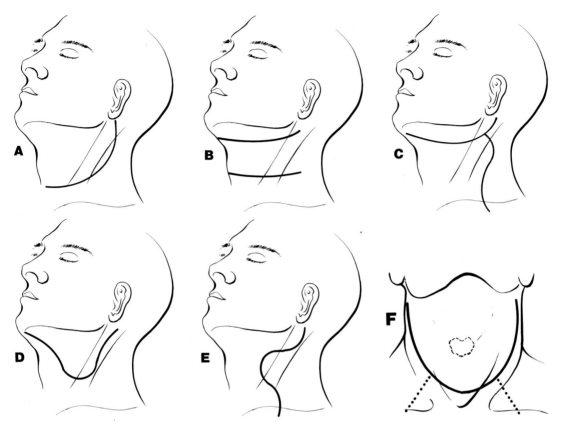

Fig. 10-22. Useful incisions for various neck operations: (A) utility flap; (B) McFee; (C) modified Schobinger; (D) unilateral apron; (E) "S" shaped flap; (F) apron or "U" flap.

an incision for neck surgery are the following:

1. Adequacy of exposure for resection of the primary and neck contents;

2. Safety of the flaps with regard to adequate circulation and coverage of carotid arteries, bone, and nerves;

3. Accommodation for reconstruction, e.g., flaps and implants; and

4. Cosmesis and function.

CAROTID INVOLVEMENT

Most surgeons consider fixation of a metastatic node to the carotid artery a criterion for unresectability, while a few will consider resecting the carotid and repairing it with an end-to-end anastomosis, vein graft, or synthetic graft. Whether or not the node is *fixed* to the carotid is primarily a judgmental decision.

Nodes that are larger than 5 to 6 cm usually indicate that the tumor has broken through the capsule and has begun to grow into adjacent structures. It is uncommon for a metastatic neck mass to become fixed to the carotid artery if no previous treatment has been administered. The mass may have infiltrated into the adventitia but can frequently be removed by dissection in a subadventitial plane. Signs of involvement of the carotid artery indicating unresectability include inability to move the mass (near the carotid) without moving the patient, Horner syndrome, vagus nerve involvement with a vocal cord paralysis, and ipsilateral carotid artery obstruction symptoms. In the absence of these signs and symptoms, the mass can probably be resected off of the carotid. The external carotid can usually be sacrificed without sequelae.

A carotid arteriogram is usually not helpful unless the surgeon is considering a carotid resection or ligation. In an older patient with a tortuous carotid artery, it may be possible to accomplish a segmental resection of the carotid with an end-to-end anastomosis. Ligation of the internal carotid artery is very hazardous in the older age group and frequently results in neurologic deficits, such as hemiparalysis or coma, or in death. Ligation of the common carotid is also hazardous but some blood could shunt from the external carotid artery to the internal branch thus creating less chance for cerebral injury.

If a tumor mass needs to be dissected from the muscular wall of the carotid artery, postoperative irradiation should be given. When dealing with a mass near the carotid artery after previous irradiation, it is much more difficult to determine unresectability. If a radical neck dissection is performed after previous irradiation, one must consider protection of the carotid artery with a dermal graft or muscle flap. A synthetic graft should not be used if the carotid is resected after irradiation or if the wound is contaminated, such as with a composite resection.

END RESULTS

The head and neck cancer literature is filled with statistics; the problem is finding meaningful data to help the physician base his treatment plan on a scientific foundation. The search for relevant data is complicated by a number of factors. First, different variations of the TNM classification system have been used over the last two decades, making comparison of data less accurate. Secondly, most studies are retrospective and contain the inherent problems of this type of study including incomplete data, nonrandom patient selection, and dissimilar control and treatment groups. Thirdly, data from different studies may be difficult to compare because of differing methods used to report this information. For example, survival data may be reported at 2 years, 3 years, or 5 years and may be the absolute survival at the interval or may be the determinant survival; the latter rate excludes cer-

tain patients such as those lost to follow-up or who died of other causes. In addition, the data may be expressed in terms of recurrence rate at different sites or conversely, the term "no evidence of disease" may be used to signify no recurrence at a particular site even though the patient may have died from his disease at other sites. With these factors in mind, we can examine some of the data in the recent literature.

Head and Neck Primary with Clinically Positive Nodes

Lee and Krause reported[17] 237 cases of therapeutic neck dissection for cancer of the oral cavity, oropharynx, hypopharynx, and larynx. The 5-year determinant survival rate (excluding patients with recurrence of the primary) for surgery alone was 60 percent. When the nodes were histologically positive, the 5-year determinant survival rate was 38 percent; when nodes were negative, the survival rate was 87 percent. The combined therapy group also had a 60 percent 5-year determinant survival rate.

Spiro et al.[32] reported a 30 percent 5-year determinant survival rate (excluding patients lost to follow-up or who died of other causes) for 328 patients with *solitary* nodes when nodes were histologically positive and a 63 percent 5-year determinant survival rate when nodes were histologically negative.

As a general rule, pathologically positive cervical nodes decrease the 5-year survival rate by 50 percent.

Head and Neck Primary with Clinically Negative Nodes

Controversy and conflicting data still cloud the therapy of the clinically negative neck. The critical question in the elective neck dissection controversy seems to be whether the neck dissection performed when lymph nodes are clinically positive will be less successful than the elective neck dissection performed when nodes are clinically negative but pathologically positive.

Shah and Tollefson[28] studied 141 patients with supraglottic carcinomas with N0 necks, 65 of whom underwent elective neck dissection. Twenty-two of the 65 patients (34 percent) had histologically positive nodes and this group had a 32 percent 5-year survival rate. Of the 76 patients who did not receive an initial radical neck dissection, 21 (28 percent) later developed neck metastases and subsequently underwent therapeutic radical neck dissection. This group of 21 patients had a 52 percent 5-year survival rate. These data do not appear to support elective neck dissection for patients with supraglottic carcinoma and a clinically negative neck; however, one must be careful in interpreting these figures because the patients who underwent elective neck dissection were not randomly selected but probably consisted largely of patients who had larger primary cancers with more chance for metastases. Therefore, one would expect a worse prognosis in patients in this study undergoing an elective neck dissection than in the group of patients who did not undergo one.

Spiro and Strong[31] studied patients undergoing a Commando procedure for oral cavity or oropharyngeal primaries. They compared the 27 percent 5-year determinant survival rate for 94 patients with clinically negative but pathologically positive necks with a 19 percent survival rate for 280 patients with both clinically and pathologically positive necks. Their study showed significantly better ($P < .06$) survival for patients undergoing elective neck dissection who were found to have pathologically positive necks compared to patients undergoing therapeutic neck dissection. These figures might seem to show the efficacy of elective neck dissection but the patients undergoing therapeutic neck dissection ranged from N1 to N3 and may have a higher tumor burden than those patients undergoing elective neck dissection.

Ogura et al.,[23] using a complicated probability model, reported a decrease in survival rate for patients with supraglottic carcinoma from 78 percent to 74 percent when occult nodes were allowed to become palpable before neck dissection. Using the same model for pyriform sinus carcinoma, they described a decrease in survival rate from 57 to 46 percent.

Although no definite conclusions about the efficacy of an elective neck dissection can be drawn from studies in the literature, most indicate improved survival for those having occult metastases who undergo an elective neck dissection versus those who undergo a therapeutic neck dissection for clinically positive nodes. Most of these studies report survival with treatment consisting of surgery alone. There seems to be plenty of proof that positive cervical nodes decrease the 5-year survival rate by 50 percent. A strong argument for an elective neck dissection would be its use as a staging procedure. Should occult positive nodes be found, postoperative radiation therapy should be used and this should improve the local control rate and cure rate. Some of the objections to the elective radical neck dissection could be overcome by using the modified neck dissection.

Unknown Primary

Jesse et al.[14] reported on 210 patients who received definitive treatment for neck metastases from an unknown primary. Only 3 of 26 patients with supraclavicular nodes were free of disease at 3 years. The remaining 184 patients had a 3-year absolute survival rate of 53 percent. The 3-year absolute survival rates were 57 percent, 48 percent, and 47 percent for surgery, radiation therapy, and combined therapy, respectively; the radiation therapy group had the greatest percent of patients with N3 necks. The 5-year absolute survival rate for all patients was 43 percent. Patients who later developed a primary lesion above the clavicle had a 31 percent chance of living 3 years, compared with a 58 percent chance for those patients whose primary remained occult.

Coker et al.[5] reported a 48 percent 5-

year determinant survival rate in 56 patients with neck nodes from an unknown primary who were treated with radiation, surgery, or combined therapy. The 5-year survival rate was 30 percent if the primary was found and 60 percent if it remained occult.

If, after an extensive search for a primary, none is found, the patient should be treated for cure, since survival of this type of patient is not as dismal as was once thought.

SUMMARY

A neck mass usually presents a diagnostic problem. The major concern is whether it may be a malignancy. Most of the malignant neck masses represent metastatic nodes from a head and neck primary, but they may be from an infraclavicular primary or sometimes an unknown primary. The evaluation should be done in an organized manner so that the diagnosis can be made without compromising the chance for cure.

What constitutes proper treatment may be controversial, but basically it involves surgery, or irradiation, or both in several possible combinations depending upon the situation. In view of modern techniques of irradiation and our knowledge of the predictable routes of lymphatic spread, one can argue for less than a radical neck dissection as adequate treatment of the neck.

The recurrence and survival statistics found in the literature seem confusing; therefore, only a few representative studies were presented. Patient survival does seem to be greatly influenced by the presence of histologically positive nodes in the neck.

Guidelines have been presented in this chapter in hopes of helping to organize a confusing, complicated subject in the reader's mind.

REFERENCES

1. American Joint Committee for Cancer Staging and End Results Reporting. 1979. Manual for Staging of Cancer, 1979. American Joint Committee, Chicago.

2. Ballantyne, A. J. 1967. Principles of surgical management of the pharyngeal walls. Cancer, 20: 663.

3. Ballantyne, A. J. 1976. Malignant melanoma of the head and neck region. In M. D. Anderson Hospital, Ed.: Neoplasms of the Skin and Malignant Melanoma. Year Book Medical Publishers, Chicago, 345.

4. Bocca, E., and Pagnataro, O. 1967. A conservative technique in radical neck dissection. Annals of Otology, Rhinology, and Laryngology, 76: 975.

5. Coker, D. D., Casterline, P. F., Chambers, R. G., and Jaques, D. A. 1977. Metastases to lymph nodes of the head and neck from an unknown primary site. American Journal of Surgery, 134: 517.

6. Conley, J. 1970. Lymph systems in the head and neck. In Conley, J., Ed.: Proceedings of the International Workshop on Cancer of the Head and Neck. Butterworth, Inc., Washington, 163.

7. Crile, G. 1906. Excision of cancer of the head and neck. Journal of American Medicine, 47: 1780.

8. Feldman, D. E., and Applebaum, E. L. 1977. The submandibular triangle in radical neck dissection. Archives of Otolaryngology, 103: 705.

9. Fletcher, G. H. 1972. Elective irradiation of subclinical disease in cancers of the head and neck. Cancer, 29: 1450.

10. Freeland, A. P., and Rogers, B. M. 1975. The vascular supply of the cervical skin with reference to incision planning. Laryngoscope, 85: 714.

11. Goffinet, D. R., Gilbert, E. H., Weller, S. A., and Bagshaw, M. A. 1975. Irradiation of clinically uninvolved cervical lymph nodes. Canadian Journal of Otolaryngology, 4: 927.

12. Jesse, R. H., and Fletcher, G. H. 1977. Treatment of the neck in patients with squamous cell carcinoma of the head and neck. Cancer, 39: 868.

13. Jesse, R. H., Ballantyne, A. J., and Larson, D. 1978. Radical or modified neck dissection: A therapeutic dilemma. American Journal of Surgery, 136: 516.

14. Jesse, R. H., Perez, C. A., and Fletcher, G. H. 1973. Cervical lymph node metastasis: Unknown primary cancer. Cancer, 31: 854.

15. Jesse, R. H., Barkley, H. T., Jr., Lindberg, R. D., and Fletcher, G. H. 1970. Cancer of the oral cavity. American Journal of Surgery, 120: 505.

16. Kambic, V., and Sirca, A. 1977. H incision-method of choice for radical neck dissection. Journal of Laryngology and Otology, 91: 383.

17. Lee, J. G., and Krause, C. J. 1975. Radical neck dissection: Elective, therapeutic, and secondary. Archives of Otolaryngology, 101: 656.

18. Lindberg, R. D. 1972. Distribution of cervical lymph node metastasis from squamous cell carcinoma of the upper respiratory and digestive tracts. Cancer, 29: 1446.

19. Lingeman, R. E., Helmus, C., Stephens, R., and Ulm, J. 1977. Neck dissection: Radical or conservative. Annals of Otology, Laryngology, and Rhinology, 86: 737.

20. Martis, C. S., and Karakasis, D. T. 1974. Prophylactic neck dissection in oral carcinomas. International Journal of Oral Surgery, 3: 293.

21. Million, R. R. 1974. Elective neck irradiation for TX N0 squamous carcinoma of the oral tongue and floor of the mouth. Cancer, 34: 149.

22. Nahum, A. M., Bone, R. C., and Davidson, T. M. 1976. The case for elective prophylactic neck dissection. Transactions of the American Academy of Ophthalmology and Otolaryngology, 82: 603.

23. Ogura, J. H., Biller, H. F., and Wette, R. 1971. Elective neck dissection for pharyngeal and laryngeal cancers. Annals of Otology, Rhinology, and Laryngology, 80: 646.

24. Reed, G. F., and Miller, W. A. 1970. Elective neck dissection. Laryngoscope, 80: 1292.

25. Rubin, P. 1971. Cancer of the head and neck, oral cavity: Neck nodes. JAMA, 217: 451.

26. Rufino, C. D., and MacComb, W. S. 1966. Bilateral neck dissections. Cancer, 19: 1503.

27. Sako, K., Pradier, R. N., Marchetta, F. C., and Pickren, J. W. 1964. Fallibility of palpation in the diagnosis of metastases to cervical nodes. Surgery, Gynecology and Obstetrics, 118: 989.

28. Shah, J. P., and Tollefsen, H. R. 1974. Epidermoid carcinoma of the supraglottic larynx. American Journal of Surgery, 128: 494.

29. Skolnick, E. M., Yee, K. F., Friedman, M., and Golden, T. A. 1976. The posterior triangle in radical neck surgery. Archives of Otolaryngology, 102: 1.

30. Southwick, H. W., Slaughter, D. P., and Trevino, E. T. 1960. Elective neck dissection for intraoral cancer. Archives of Surgery, 80: 45.

31. Spiro, R. H., and Strong, E. W. 1973. Epidermoid carcinoma of the oral cavity and oropharynx. Archives of Surgery, 107: 382.

32. Spiro, R. H., Alfonso, A. E., Farr, H. W., and Strong, E. W. 1974. Cervical node metastasis from epidermoid carcinoma of the oral cavity and oropharynx. American Journal of Surgery, 128: 562.

33. Staley, C. J., and Herzon, F. S. 1970. Elective neck dissection in carcinoma of the larynx. Surgical Clinics of North America, 50: 543.

11 | Cancer of the Skin

G. Thomas Jansen, M.D.
Kent C. Westbrook, M.D.

INTRODUCTION

Cancer of the skin is the most common form of malignant disease, and the skin of the head and neck is the site most frequently involved. However, the ease of early diagnosis and infrequency of metastatic spread usually provide an opportunity for cure at the time of treatment. Since exposure to sunlight is a predisposing factor, treatment must also stress prevention by avoidance of exposure, protection with appropriate sunscreens, and treatment of premalignant actinic keratosis. Therefore, patients at high risk because of fair skin, sun exposure, or occupation require repeated observations as the basis of a treatment program.

MacDonald has pointed out that lesions of the head and neck account for 90 percent of all skin cancers among white males and 85 percent among white females.[42] One-fourth of the patients with skin cancer have more than one lesion at the time of the first diagnosis. Approximately 60 percent of all cancers of the skin are basal cell type and 30 percent are squamous cell type. The other 10 percent are rare types. Half of all individuals, with the first diagnosis of skin cancer, are over 65 years of age at the time of this diagnosis.

Since the observation of Sir Percivall Pott in 1775 relating cancer of the scrotum in chimney sweeps to soot, other industrial exposures have been recognized. Exposure to pitch, tar or tar products, polycyclic aromatic hydrocarbons, and creosote are classic examples. Inorganic arsenic compounds still found in herbicides, pesticides, pharmaceutical products, and drinking water may increase the risk of skin cancer.

Unna in 1896 emphasized the relationship of sun exposure to skin cancer in his classic description of "sailor's skin."[63] The Celts have a susceptibility to skin cancer even in their homelands where limited ultraviolet light is available. The migrations of these people to the southwestern United States, Australia, and New Zealand has compounded the problem. Recent studies have shown that wind velocity and drying of the skin enhance ultraviolet injury.[53]

The clinician must recognize that epidermal cells and any cell type in the dermis or subcutaneous tissue can give rise to benign and malignant tumors. These cells differentiate into component parts of the skin including nerves, muscles, and circulating blood elements. Therefore, the complete clinical panorama is complex. Not only must the physician be aware of the clinical varieties, but he must also be knowledgeable of the microscopic variations. He cannot be content with reading the bottom line of the pathology report but must recognize the treatment implications of a basal cell carcinoma which has morphea elements or of a squamous cell carcinoma arising in actinically damaged skin. Correlations of the clinical pattern and histopathology influence the selection of treatment of skin cancer of the head and neck.

EPITHELIAL TUMORS

Basal Cell Carcinoma

CLINICAL VARIATIONS OF BASAL CELL CARCINOMA

Basal cell carcinoma is the most common type of skin cancer and presents an unusual number of clinical variations. The tumor may be flat and eczematous, with a tendency toward peripheral growth with no vertical invasion. A thread-like waxy border with atrophy and scarring may indicate this *superficial multicentric type* (Plate 11-1). Such lesions may be multiple and occur more often on the trunk and extremities than on the head and neck. *Nodular* lesions usually have a pinkish-red color because of the dilated vessels that course over the pearlescent tumor mass (Plate 11-2). These lesions are often about a centimeter in diameter. *Pigmented basal cell carcinoma* may resemble a pigmented nevus or a melanoma. At times, lesions ulcerate with a boring tendency that produces deep invasion and mutilation.

Perhaps the most deceptive clinical pattern is that of the *morphea* type (Plate 11-3). This lesion may be disregarded by the patient or the physician for long periods of time because it can be macular, whitish, and have indistinct margins. This type seems to have a special affinity for young women.

The *adenoid-cystic basal cell carcinoma* is a waxy, succulent lesion containing cysts filled with a gelatinous fluid. Genetic factors determine the *nevoid basal cell carcinoma syndrome*. In this syndrome, multiple basal cell carcinomas occur at a very early age on the head and neck associated with other developmental abnormalities.

The anatomic location of a lesion may give rise to a more aggressive behavior and may influence treatment. A basal cell carcinoma—of any morphologic type—occurring in embryonic fusion planes such as the preauricular and postauricular areas, the nasolabial fold, or the inner and outer canthus of the eye requires special consideration. Lesions of these areas invade into multiple tissue planes and have a higher rate of recurrence after any therapy.

Some types of basal cell carcinoma invade locally into cartilage, bone, nerves, and blood vessels. Subtle extensions beyond the clinically recognized margin result in a tendency for local recurrence. Although metastasis is extremely rare, this complication must be considered when lesions have recurred repeatedly or when treatment has been delayed for years.[31] In these instances, spread to the regional lymph nodes, lungs, or bones may occur.

MICROSCOPIC VARIATIONS OF BASAL CELL CARCINOMA

The most common histopathologic pattern of basal cell carcinoma is an anaplastic proliferation of basaloid cells in a solid mass extending into the papillary dermis. At the periphery, masses of columnar cells are arranged in palisades. The desmoplastic response may be minimal, but a dense lymphocytic inflammatory reaction will occur. Adenoidal interlacing strands of tumor cells may also form with or without cyst formation. The morphea type is characterized by small strands of disorganized anaplastic cells, an abundant desmoplastic response, and extensions along blood vessels, nerves, and periosteum.

TREATMENT OF EARLY BASAL CELL CARCINOMA

Multiple treatment modalities are available for basal cell carcinoma and the appropriate selection of lesions for each type of therapy is important.

Curettage Excision Combined with Electrosurgery. The most common form of treatment for basal cell carcinoma is curettage excision followed by electrodesiccation. A successful cure with preservation of function and cosmetic acceptability, as with any treatment, depends upon the skill of the operator and the proper selection of cases. In general, solid basal cell tumors less than 2 cm in diameter are selected for this treatment. Morphea lesions with a fibrous stroma cannot be curetted.

Following biopsy clarification and local anesthesia a small sharp dermal curette is used to remove the gelatinous basal cell lesion (Fig. 11-1). After primary curettage the entire base of the lesion is desiccated, curetted with a smaller curette, desiccated again, and curetted again. The feel of the curette

against firm tissue, at the base and all margins, is essential to ensure complete removal of the tumor and blend of the edges into the normal skin for a good cosmetic result. Healing occurs within several weeks with a flat white scar. The hypertrophic scar, usually present at the end of a month or two, flattens and is not a significant complication.

Scalpel Excision.   After appropriate local anesthesia, all accepted surgical techniques should be followed. The location and size of the tumor as well as the elasticity of the skin will determine the plan of removal. When primary closure is desired, wrinkle lines of the skin should be followed for the best cosmetic result. A margin of 3 to 5 mm beyond the visible or palpable borders is recommended, and the excised tissue should be submitted for pathologic verification of these margins. Primary closure can be done

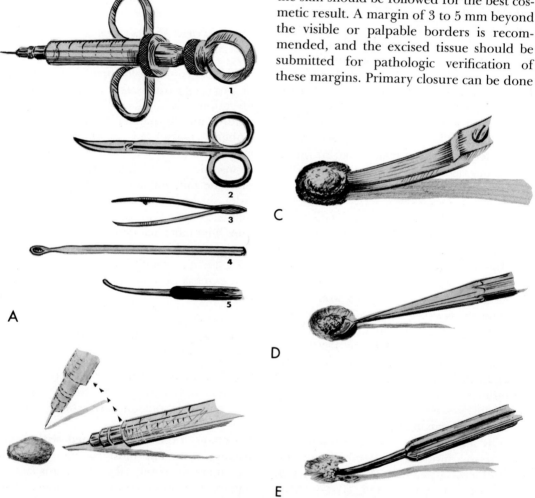

Fig. 11-1. (A) Curettage and electrodesiccation instruments suitable for many basal cell and squamous cell carcinomas: 1. anesthetic, 2. scissors, 3. forceps, 4. curette, and 5. electrode; (B) local anesthetic field block; (C) scissors biopsy; (D) curettage of tumor; (E) desiccation or fulguration of tumor.

in most areas if the excision is elliptical and has a length to width ratio of 4:1 (Fig. 11-2). Areas of fixed skin (scalp, occiput, forehead) and large lesions may require skin grafts or flap closure. Again, as with curettage, the cosmetic results correlate directly with the skill of the operator. An important rule to remember is that a cure at the time of primary treatment is more important than cosmetic considerations. Cosmetic reconstruction may be reserved for a period after initial healing when it has been determined that no residual tumor is present. Multiple frozen sections at the time of surgery may obviate this delay.

Radiation Therapy.   Lesions on the head and neck, because of the rich vascular bed, are especially amenable to radiation therapy. However, radiation therapy is more complex and protracted than other treatment methods and is reserved for patients in very poor health and for large lesions in difficult areas such as the eyelid, nose, or lip. If the tumor invades bone or cartilage, radiation therapy may be ineffective and may be followed by nonhealing or ulceration.

Careful evaluation of the size of the lesions as well as the depth of invasion should be determined. A 5 mm margin must be measured around the entire lesion, and the approximate depth of the lesion should be estimated. A depth dose chart indicates the appropriate quality of radiation to be used. In general, the quality of this superficial x-ray therapy is 80 to 100 kV with a half-value layer (HVL) of 0.7 to 1.6 mm aluminum. Although some therapists recommend a dosage as low as 3,500 rads, customary

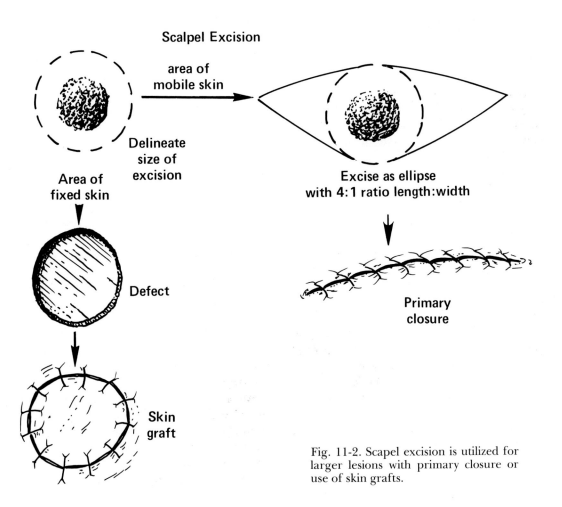

Fig. 11-2. Scapel excision is utilized for larger lesions with primary closure or use of skin grafts.

treatment of 4,500 to 5,000 rads fractionated over a three-week period is the more usual dosage.[34] Whenever possible, daily treatment appropriately fractionated over this period of time is desirable. Large doses of 500 to 900 rads per treatment can be given, but greater fractionation improves the cosmetic result with less chance of delayed radiation complication. Radium needles and plaques are still used by a few physicians who have years of experience with this modality. In general, radium offers no real advantage over radiation therapy in the treatment of most skin cancers. In special instances, more refined treatment techniques, such as the electron beam or linear accelerator, if available, can be used to handle difficult and complicated skin cancers of the head and neck. Shielding of surrounding structures including eyes, nose, and teeth is imperative.

Chemosurgery of Mohs.   The term chemosurgery may seem confusing. In this context, it refers to the method of microscopically controlled excision of cancer as developed by Mohs.[51] The unexcelled effectiveness of this treatment especially for tumors involving the nasolabial fold, ocular canthi, and circumauricular areas has produced wide acceptance. Complete microscopic surveillance of the excised tissue is accomplished by layer after layer excision with frozen section examination of the undersurface of each segment removed.

The classic technique relies upon chemical fixation in situ following application of zinc chloride paste. Four to 24 hours after application of the zinc chloride, carefully oriented segments of tissue 1 to 3 mm thick are removed from the entire tumor base, inverted, and examined by frozen section (Fig. 11-3). The excision level is in the fixed tissue just superficial to the underlying viable tissue so no pain or bleeding occurs. Some pain results at the time of fixative penetration. As each piece of tissue is removed, a diagram is made showing the specimen location in relationship to anatomic landmarks. This permits the operator to determine the exact location of any remaining

cancer, to mark it on the diagram, and to reexcise additional tissue after further chemical fixation. Once a clear base is obtained microscopically, the excised area can be permitted to heal by secondary intention or can be closed surgically. A modification of this classic technique—the *fresh tissue technique*—is more widely used at this time. It differs from the fixed technique in that zinc chloride fixation is omitted and local anesthesia is utilized. Sequential layer excision with microscopic control is performed in the usual way. This fresh technique is more rapid and less painful. For cancers of moderate extent, it offers sufficient microscopic control.

Cryosurgery.   Cryosurgery has been an accepted mode of treatment for benign lesions since the turn of the century. Availability of liquid nitrogen, advancements in cryobiology, and improvement of cryosurgical units have led to its acceptance in the treatment of selected cancers. Generally, basal cell carcinomas with clinically definable margins and depth may be treated with cryosurgery. A thermocouple is inserted into the base of the tumor to insure freezing to $-30°C$ (Fig. 11-4). Margins of the lesion are marked and a cryospray is used to freeze 5 mm beyond the extent of the tumor. The area is permitted to thaw, and the thaw time is recorded. It should be at least 60 seconds. The lesion is refrozen in similar fashion, and once again the thaw time is recorded.

Long-term cure rates seem to justify the acceptance of cryosurgery for appropriately selected lesions. Relatively small tumors of the eyelid, nose, or ear are especially amenable to cryosurgical treatment with minimal scarring. Some authorities feel that lesions in the scalp or nasolabial fold have an increased recurrence rate with cryosurgical treatment and should be managed by other techniques.[68]

Topical Chemotherapy.   Cytotoxic agents are effective in the treatment of premalignant skin lesions as well as in the treatment of selected basal cell carcinomas. A number of compounds, including colchicine, methotrexate, and nitrogen mustard have been

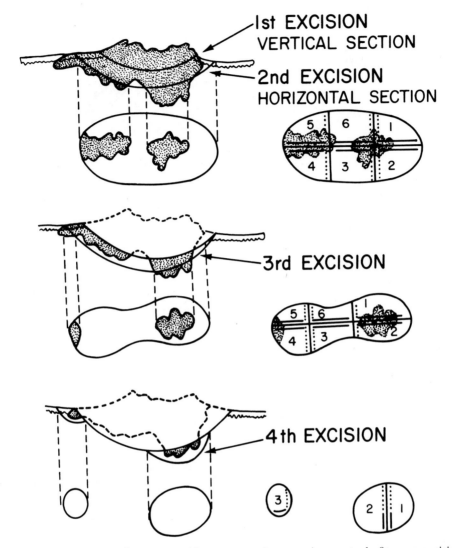

1st EXCISION
VERTICAL SECTION

2nd EXCISION
HORIZONTAL SECTION

3rd EXCISION

4th EXCISION

Fig. 11-3. Mohs chemosurgery provides accurate tissue section control of tumor excision.

tried; but 5-fluorouracil in propylene glycol or an ointment base is the topical chemotherapeutic agent of choice.[32] A trial of topical 5-fluorouracil is justified in selected superficial erythematous basal cell carcinomas. A 1 to 5 percent preparation is applied twice daily for 4 weeks. A brisk inflammatory reaction and erosive change in the skin should be noted. Careful observation is essential, and retreatment should be attempted if a recurrence is noted. Since the cure rate is less predictable than that of more traditional modes of therapy, topical chemotherapy for infiltrative lesions should be reserved for special instances when patient factors prohibit standard treatments.

TREATMENT OF ADVANCED BASAL CELL CARCINOMA

Appropriate primary treatment of basal cell carcinoma of the head and neck is attended by at least a 90 percent cure rate. However, occasionally there are advanced lesions that present special treatment problems. Today, fewer patients delay treatment because of complacency, ignorance, or fear of

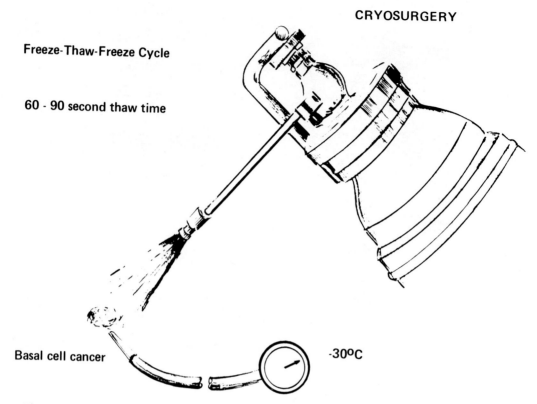

CRYOSURGERY

Freeze-Thaw-Freeze Cycle

60 - 90 second thaw time

Basal cell cancer

-30°C

Fig. 11-4. Cryosurgery requires accurate temperature control plus freezing of a margin of normal tissue.

cancer. Therefore, most advanced lesions are seen after failure of initial treatment.

A multidisciplinary approach is valuable in treatment selection for advanced lesions. Open and candid discussion among trained professional colleagues will usually lead to the best treatment selection. If a treatment modality has failed, it is usually wise to change to another modality. This decision, however, must be modified by the availability of various physician skills. Each treatment modality has an inherent weakness, and success will depend upon the experience and skill of those doing the treatment.

Curettage excision with electrosurgery, cryosurgery, or topical chemotherapy are not ordinarily appropriate for advanced or recurrent lesions. Chemosurgery of Mohs using the fixed tissue technique can be skillfully used for lesions even in the external auditory canal, the orbit, or the nasolabial

fold, or for aggressive basal cell carcinomas of the scalp. Periosteal involvement can be defined and excised. Linear extension of the recurrent tumor along blood vessels and nerves can be followed.

Radiotherapy is frequently applicable for large lesions. In some locations, surgical excision or chemosurgery excision of advanced lesions may produce extensive deformity whereas appropriately fractionated radiation therapy may produce minimal tissue loss.[62] Radiation therapy may be utilized for advanced untreated lesions when they are large, in difficult areas, and not fixed to bone. It is not recommended if tumor is fixed to cartilage or bone. For recurrent lesions, radiation therapy is selected for multifocal recurrence, morphea basal cell carcinoma, or lesions with vague margins. Bone or cartilage involvement is usually a contraindication for radiation therapy.

Many advanced basal cell carcinomas,

either primary or recurrent, require radical surgical excision. Surgical ablation is usually recommended for patients with previous radiotherapy, for bone or cartilage involvement, or for discrete lesions that can be handled more readily with surgery than with radiation therapy.

Surgical management of advanced basal cell carcinoma requires meticulous attention to surgical technique in order to prevent failure. For lesions with a distinct border, a surgical margin of 1 cm may be adequate. Lesions in which the border cannot be accurately delineated require wider resection margins. The deep margin should be as wide as the lateral margins. However, this may be quite difficult to obtain.

Cartilage or bone invasion creates special problems. Full-thickness excision of involved cartilage is required. The extent of any bone involvement dictates the surgery needed. Removal of the periosteum may be adequate when actual invasion is absent. This technique, however, results in a tissue defect that cannot be closed with a split-thickness skin graft. Closure will require local flap rotation or delayed skin grafting after removal of bone and development of a granulating bed. Penetration into the bone may require resection of the outer table or full-thickness of the bone. If only the outer table is resected, this can usually be reconstructed with the use of a rotational flap or of a secondary split-thickness skin graft. Full-thickness resection of the skull necessitates large flap closure. Occasionally, a combination of surgery and postoperative radiotherapy is necessary. If the surgical procedure fails to yield free margins, such combined treatment is indicated.

Definitive surgery for advanced basal cell carcinoma is designed to cure the cancer, maintain function, and provide a satisfactory cosmetic result. However, one should not let cosmetic factors compromise adequate cancer surgery. Immediate reconstruction is sometimes necessary and requires free margins on frozen section evaluation. Delay of reconstruction may be preferable to ensure that recurrent disease is not going to develop. If massive ablation without reconstruction is necessary, adequate rehabilitation may frequently be accomplished with a prosthesis. Prostheses can provide satisfactory coverage of large facial defects on either a temporary or a permanent basis.

Squamous Cell Carcinoma

Squamous cell carcinoma of the skin of the head and neck is exceeded in incidence only by basal cell carcinoma. Most of the tumors occur on areas exposed to sunlight. The most significant observation the clinician can make when dealing with squamous cell carcinoma is to determine whether the lesion is arising from an area of actinic keratosis with solar degeneration or arising denovo. This distinction is important for treatment planning, since squamous cell carcinomas arising in actinic keratoses are less agressive and have an excellent prognosis. Differentiation may at times be determined clinically, although in certain instances it may be necessary to rely on the pathologist for the determination.

CLINICAL VARIATIONS OF SQUAMOUS CELL CARCINOMA

As with basal cell carcinoma, multiple variations will occur in the clinical presentation. The typical squamous cell carcinoma is usually ulcerative and infiltrates adjacent tissues (Plate 11-4). An *actinic keratosis* may slowly progress into a *cutaneous horn*. A papillomatous proliferation with indistinct solid infiltrating margins and a slowly forming ulcerated center may occur. This raw, crusted lesion will bleed easily. In general, a persisting lesion that bleeds must be presumed malignant and warrants a biopsy. At other times squamous cell carcinoma will show limited tendency for vertical growth but will spread in superficial fashion with an eczematous change. This usually represents a *squamous cell carcinoma in situ* (either Bowen disease or a Bowenoid solar keratosis).

MICROSCOPIC VARIATIONS OF SQUAMOUS CELL CARCINOMA

The physician must understand the clinical variations of squamous cell carcinoma and the correlations with the microscopic patterns in order to select the best plan of management. The therapist must know what the pathologist's ability is to distinguish squamous cell carcinoma arising in actinic change from that arising in solar change. In solar keratosis with squamous cell carcinoma, the dermal-epidermal membrane is disrupted at one or more sites and atypical squamous cells extend into the papillary dermis with or without pearl formation.[40] This invasion may be superficial, intermediate, or deep. The pathologist can use special staining techniques to diagnose squamous cell carcinoma arising in actinic degenerative change. With few exceptions, squamous cell lesions of this type do not behave in an aggressive manner and lack the ability to metastasize and can be treated with conservative methods. However, in about 6 percent of such lesions, acantholytic dyskeratotic cells will be noted (Fig. 11-5). This acantholysis usually occurs in very old patients in lesions located on or about the ear. When this acantholytic change invades the dermis, the lesion assumes the feature of an *adenoid squamous cell carcinoma*. These lesions are more aggressive and about 3 percent of patients with lesions larger than 2 cm will have deep invasion and metastasis. Hence, recognition and aggressive therapy is important.[24]

Denovo squamous cell carcinoma may occur on both sun-damaged or covered skin. These lesions show hyperkeratosis, spotty parakeratosis, irregular acanthosis, and ulceration. Special stains may assist the pathologist in determining whether actinic change is present or not. At least 8 percent of patients with denovo squamous cell carcinoma will develop regional or distant metastases or both.[25]

Another microscopic variant of squa-

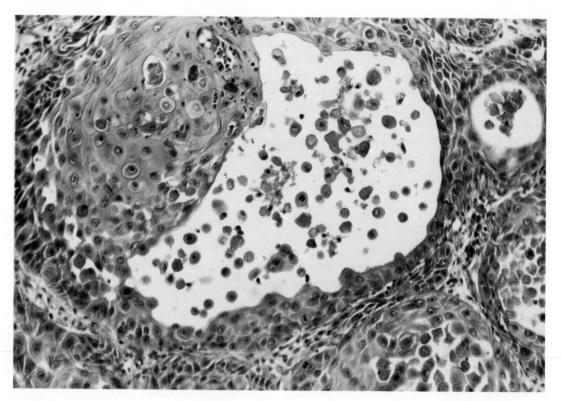

Fig. 11-5. High power view of adenoidal squamous cell carcinoma with acantholytic changes.

mous cell carcinoma of the head and neck is the *spindle cell carcinoma*. This lesion usually occurs at the site of chronic trauma. Chronic radiodermatitis or a burn scar would be a characteristic location for such a lesion. The squamous cells take on a spindle configuration with enlongated nuclei and a swirling pattern. At times the anaplasia may be great enough to resemble a sarcoma or an amelanotic melanoma. If the biopsy specimen does not reveal distinct connections with the epidermis, a final decision that this represents squamous cell carcinoma may be difficult. Spindle cell tumors are aggressive and may occur at multiple foci in the scarred tissue. Treatment should include removal of the specific lesion plus prophylactic surgical removal of the entire scar.

TREATMENT OF EARLY SQUAMOUS CELL CARCINOMA

Electrosurgery was once considered inappropriate in the treatment of squamous cell carcinoma. However, appreciation of the clinical significance of this lesion arising in sun-damaged skin has led to its use in appropriately selected tumors. Electrosurgery is especially useful in relatively small lesions that have developed in actinically damaged skin (Fig. 11-1). Large lesions and those squamous cell carcinomas that arise denovo should be treated by other techniques.

Surgical excision and primary closure under local anesthesia is ideal for many early squamous cell carcinomas. It is particularly appropriate for lesions in areas of movable skin where an excellent cosmetic result can be obtained. It is more difficult and less applicable for those lesions located where multiple tissue planes intersect such as the nasolabial, periocular, preauricular, and postauricular areas.

Squamous cell carcinoma of the skin can certainly be controlled with radiation therapy. However, such treatment usually necessitates multiple visits and is not ideal for early lesions which can be treated with simpler techniques. Topical chemotherapy requires prolonged application with unpredictable results. Therefore, topical 5-fluo-

rourical is reserved for unusual patients, e.g., nursing home patients that cannot be available for other treatment techniques.

In summary, early squamous cell carcinoma of the skin may be treated very similarly to basal cell carcinoma of the skin. However, one must recognize and appropriately handle the more aggressive forms.

TREATMENT OF ADVANCED SQUAMOUS CELL CARCINOMA

It is hoped that squamous cell carcinoma will be detected early and adequate primary treatment will be given to prevent development of advanced lesions. Occasionally, patients neglect lesions until they are far advanced and then present themselves for treatment. Also, even following superb treatment by skilled physicians, certain lesions will persist or metastasize. The greater aggressiveness of denovo, adenoidal, and spindle cell carcinoma produces serious clinical problems.

Treatment of advanced squamous cell carcinoma involves many of the principles outlined for the treatment of basal cell carcinoma. However, in addition to management of the primary lesion, consideration must be given to management of regional nodes. The primary lesion, in advanced squamous cell carcinoma, may be treated by Mohs chemosurgery, radiation therapy, or surgical ablation. Mohs chemosurgery, as outlined previously, gives excellent results in skilled hands. However, application of this technique is limited by the relative lack of skilled therapists and also by its somewhat cumbersome application.

Control of advanced untreated squamous cell carcinoma is usually possible with radiotherapy if the lesion does not involve bone or cartilage. Adequate radiation therapy requires careful delineation of tumor margins, wide field therapy, and protracted treatment over at least 5 weeks. Radiotherapy is also used in patients with previous surgical excision and recurrent disease with indistinct margins or with perineural invasion. Rarely should more than one course of radiotherapy be attempted.

Surgical resection of advanced squamous cell carcinoma requires wide lateral margins (1 to 2 cm) and adequate deep excision. Bone and cartilage must be removed if involved. Either frozen section or permanent section evaluation of all margins is necessary. However, one must remember that free margins do not guarantee that the disease has been eliminated.

Reconstruction after surgical ablation may consist simply of split-thickness skin grafting and observation of the area. If portions of the skull have been excised, more elaborate reconstruction techniques are necessary. One must either use a local or regional flap or delayed skin grafting.

Metastasis to regional lymph nodes may occur with both early and advanced squamous cell carcinoma. The metastatic pattern is heavily influenced by the location of the primary cancer. Squamous cell carcinoma involving the scalp, forehead, temple, and auricle may metastasize to the paraparotid or intraparotid lymph nodes as well as to the deep cervical lymph node system. Such cancer located elsewhere on the skin of the head or neck generally metastasizes to the deep cervical nodes only.

Regional lymph node metastasis may become apparent some years after treatment of the primary cancer. Patients may present with a mass in the parotid or cervical region without an obvious primary cancer, and unless questioned specifically they may not even mention treatment of a skin cancer in the past.

Since the incidence of nodal metastasis from squamous cell carcinoma of the skin is quite low, radical neck dissection is usually not indicated at the time of resection of the primary if the neck is clinically negative. However, patients with a clinically positive neck require radical neck dissection if the primary is controlled or controllable. If control of the primary cancer cannot be determined with certainty, then the site of the primary cancer should be excised at the time of radical neck dissection.

Patients with metastasis to the parotid area with or without evidence of cervical lymph node involvement should have total or subtotal parotidectomy in continuity with neck dissection. If the metastasis is in the inferior portion of the gland or in the upper neck, the lower division of the facial nerve should be sacrificed and the gland inferior to the upper division resected. If the metastasis involves the entire gland, then the entire facial nerve must be excised along with the parotid tissue. If the mass is large and deeply situated, the masseter muscle must be taken as a deep margin of resection.

If the facial nerve has been sacrificed, an attempt at reanimation should be made by utilizing a free nerve graft from the cervical plexus, if uninvolved with tumor, or by using hypoglossal-facial anastomosis. In some cases the parotid mass will have been biopsied and the skin may be fixed to the mass. Such scars or involved skin must be excised. If primary closure cannot be accomplished, the area should be resurfaced—preferably with local or regional flaps or, if necessary, skin grafting. Radiation therapy should be considered following radical neck dissection with or without parotidectomy so as to maximize regional control. Radiation therapy is particularly important if more than one node is positive, if a single involved node is larger than 2.5 cm, if the tumor replaces the entire node, if there is evidence of capsular invasion or extracapsular spread, or if there is invasion of nerves, vessels, or lymphatics.

Other Epithelial Carcinomas

METATYPICAL CANCER

A dilemma in classification exists in some tumors of epithelial origin that have a microscopic pattern combining characteristics of both basal and squamous cell carcinoma. These intermediate lesions may have no particular clinical pattern and have been called *basosquamous cell carcinomas*. The World Health Organization has proposed the designation of metatypical carcinoma of the skin. Metatypical carcinoma has biologic characteristics similar to those of basal cell carcinoma and management is essentially the same.

KERATOACANTHOMA

Pseudomalignancy, which represents transitional lesions between benign and malignant disease, can occur in any organ system. The keratoacanthoma is an example of such a lesion that has been recognized since the early 1950's. Keratoacanthoma occurs most often in males, occasionally has a history of preceding trauma, and grows to 1 or 2 cm in a few weeks.[22] The lesion initially may be a tense, smooth, rounded papule or nodule (Fig. 11-6). As the tumor evolves, the center becomes umbilicated and covered with a scale. Removal of this central keratinous material will reveal a crater filled with horny material or reveal a rough wart-like surface. Histologically, the lesion looks like a well-differentiated squamous cell carcinoma (Fig. 11-7). Biologically, however, these lesions may undergo spontaneous resolution leaving a depressed scar, especially if the hyperkeratotic center is removed.

Keratoacanthoma occurs most often on the head, neck, arms, and hands; those occuring on the vermillion margin of the lip tend to increase in size for longer than 2 months and to take a year to involute spontaneously. Destructive lesions on the nose and eyelids pose a real problem for the clinician and pathologist in determining a benign rather than a malignant course. It is imperative that an adequate biopsy, including the paracentral area of the lesion, be submitted to the pathologist. The clinical impression of keratoacanthoma, with rapid

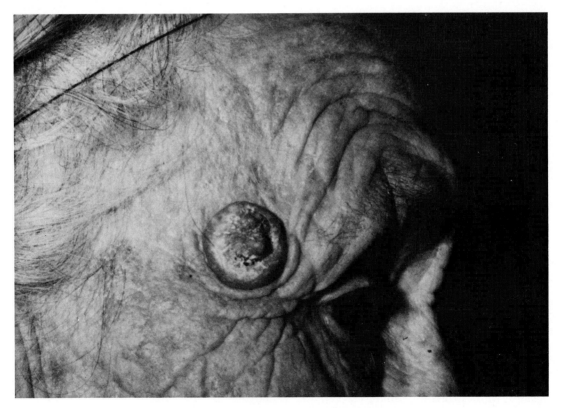

Fig. 11-6. Clinical appearance of keratoacanthoma.

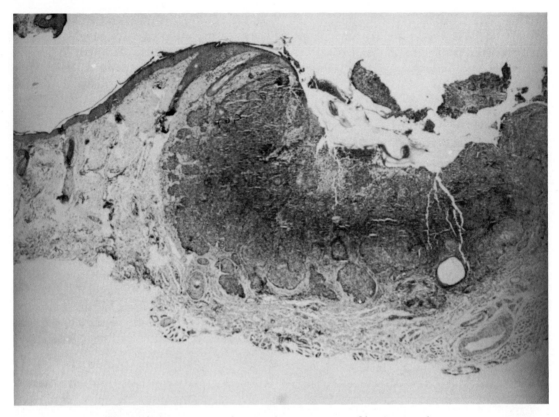

Fig. 11-7. Low power microscopic appearance of keratoacanthoma.

growth in a short period of time, should be documented as well. Ultrastructural studies have implied a viral origin for keratoacanthoma.[54]

Unfortunately, the exact nature of this pseudomalignancy and its benign or malignant potential has become less distinct with time. Usually, keratoacanthoma is treated by simple surgical excision. Recurrences following removal average about 5 percent but are more common for keratoacanthomas surrounding the lips or nose.[55] Recurrence following removal usually produces a similar lesion. Retreatment with wider excision is recommended. Transition of the microscopic pattern toward squamous cell carcinoma may be noted. Conversion of a keratoacanthoma into a squamous cell carcinoma is still controversial. Lever feels such lesions were probably squamous cell carcinoma from the time of origin.[40] Intralesional injection with 5-fluorouracil has be-

come an accepted mode of therapy for selected cases.

ORAL FLORID PAPILLOMATOSIS

This tumor also falls into the zone of questionable malignancy. It involves primarily the oral mucosa but may extend onto the skin of the head and neck. This rare and unusual problem begins as wart-like lesions on the oral mucosa, the lips, or the vermillion.[67] Rather than a self-limited course, the lesions become proliferative, cauliflower-like in appearance, and continue to recur after excision, electrosurgery, or cryosurgery.[56] An ability to change into squamous cell carcinoma has led to the opinion that this tumor represents a type of verrucous carcinoma from the time of onset. Counterparts of this chronic proliferative process are considered to be the giant condyloma acuminata of Buschke and Loewenstein seen in the genital area and the fungating low grade carcinomas of the cuniculatum type seen on the foot or hand.

Appropriate treatment for the proliferative process must certainly be individualized to the agressiveness of the specific case. Destruction with surgery, electrosurgery, or cryosurgery are the preferred methods of treatment. However, in complicated cases, chemotherapy with methotrexate or bleomycin may be indicated.[33]

CARCINOMA OF SKIN APPENDAGES

Carcinoma of sebaceous glands, eccrine sweat glands, and apocrine glands may occur on the head and neck area. Carcinoma of sebaceous gland origin is the most significant of these and occurs most frequently on the eyelids as a malignant alteration in the meibomian gland. No characteristic clinical picture may be present, but a nodular, ulcerated verrucous growth is perhaps the most common appearance. Widespread aggressive metastatic disease is often seen when sebaceous carcinoma originates on the eyelid. Similar lesions may occur elsewhere on the face but are less aggressive. Pathologically, it is necessary to distinguish sebaceous carcinomas from sebaceous epitheliomas. The sebaceous epithelioma represents a basal cell carcinoma with sebaceous gland differentiation. The sebaceous carcinoma has no basal cell component. The irregular lobules show great variation in size, consist of undifferentiated cells, and contain distinct sebaceous cells with foamy cytoplasm in the center.[40]

Carcinoma of eccrine sweat glands and apocrine glands can occur on the head and neck, since both glandular structures are present. No specific clinical configuration is known and diagnosis follows appropriate pathologic interpretation. Both of these lesions are locally invasive and tend not to metastasize. The pathologist may, however, have difficulty in deciding whether these are primary lesions or represent metastatic disease from other glandular sites. Extramammary Paget disease as a variation of apocrine carcinoma can occur as an eczematous process in the external auditory canal or the orbital skin.

Treatment of these malignant appendage tumors includes the techniques noted for basal or squamous cell carcinoma, but usually the tumors are excised surgically. Sebaceous carcinoma of the eyelid should be noted for its more aggressive nature and tendency for local metastasis.

NONEPITHELIAL TUMORS

Tumors of Vessels

Primary malignant tumors of vessels in the head and neck are rather rare and include *malignant angioendothelioma, Kaposi sarcoma,* and *hemangiopericytoma.* Of these, the malignant angioendothelioma has a predilection for the scalp and face of elderly persons. The lesions of lymphatic origin appear usually as a dusky, colorless thickening of the skin, while those of blood vessel origin have a purplish-blue color. The most common location is the skin on the face or the scalp with a slow centrifugal spread with the result that even the skin of the neck may be involved. Metastases to the cervical lymph nodes or hematogenous spread to the lungs, liver, and elsewhere can occur, but a more common course is that of slowly progressive destruction.

Kaposi sarcoma is usually characterized by purplish-red or dark-brown plaques and nodules in the skin. The lesions most often occur on the extremities, but the disease may be generalized and include visceral lesions and lymph node involvement. The disease is slowly progressive, and local control of the involved sites with radiation therapy is considered to be the treatment of choice. Low dose superficial radiation therapy to a total of 900 rads (which may be repeated if necessary) has been the classic treatment schedule, although more aggressive, deeper therapy with a cobalt source has proved to be of more lasting benefit.[30]

Hemangiopericytoma is rarely found on the head and neck. Recognition depends upon appropriate histologic examination. The skin, subcutaneous tissue, or musculoskeletal tissue may be involved. Occasionally, lesions are noted in the oral cavity. Hemangiopericytomas of the skin are less apt to be metastatic than those arising in internal organs.[23] These metastases may be to lymph nodes, lungs, or other areas.

A rare benign vascular lesion may be mistaken for the malignant vascular tumor. This unique *angiolymphoid hyperplasia* with associated eosinophilia occurs most often on the head and neck of young adults. While these purplish red lesions may occur anywhere, they are most often noted around the ear. They begin as small plaque-like infiltrates but may reach a size of 5 to 10 cm. The characteristic vascular proliferation with associated tissue eosinophilia and the relatively young age of the patient help to distinguish this benign lesion from malignant angioendothelioma.

All of these vascular tumors are treated by surgical excision with the exception of Kaposi sarcoma. Extent of the excision depends upon the nature, size, and location of the tumor. Occasionally, local radiotherapy or systemic chemotherapy are indicated.

Tumors of Nerves

Malignant tumors of the nerves of the skin and subcutaneous tissue of the head and neck are uncommon. When they occur, they usually represent malignant degeneration in a neurofibroma of Von Recklinghausen disease. When a neurofibroma becomes malignant it produces an anaplastic fibrosarcomatous pattern. Treatment of malignant tumors of nerve origin usually involves radical surgical excision.

Miscellaneous Tumors

Tumors of muscle origin, either smooth or striated, are usually in the subcutaneous tissue on the head and neck. Liposarcomas are rare. Fibrosarcomas can occur but they must be separated from the more important *atypical fibroxanthoma*. This fibroxanthoma is a benign lesion, which is fairly common and can be mistaken for a true malignancy because of its histologic picture. It usually appears as a nodule on sun-exposed areas on the head and neck of elderly persons and may occur in areas of irradiation. The lesion may either grow slowly or very rapidly. At times the epidermis is intact on the smooth glistening nodule, and at other times an ulcer may be present. These lesions are usually less than 2 cm in diameter. Microscopically, the lesion is characterized by an unusual, aggressive infiltrate extending into the subcutaneous fat; pleomorphic elongated cells with hyperchromatic nuclei; bizzare multinucleated atypical giant cells; and frequent mitoses. The pathologist must separate this lesion from dermatofibrosarcoma or fibrosarcoma, which usually gain origin from the deeper subcutaneous layer and fascial tissue. Simple excision of the atypical fibroxanthoma is adequate treatment.

Metastatic carcinoma to the skin or subcutaneous tissue of the head and neck can occur. There is nothing specific in the clinical appearance. However, the lesions are usually subcutaneous, infiltrated, and firm and vary in color from the normal skin. The scalp is a common site for metastatic lesions especially for the kidney, breast, and prostate. The pathologist will sometimes be able to determine the primary site. At times, malignancies of skin appendage origin can be taken for metastatic disease.

Mycosis fungoides (a cutaneous form of lymphoma), lymphomas, and leukemic infiltrates can occur on the skin of the head and neck. Again, there is nothing specific in the clinical appearance and the clinician will have to depend upon the microscopic examination for diagnosis of these tumors. These tumors involve multiple body sites, and treatment must be directed toward the generalized process as well as toward the specific lesions on the skin of the head and neck.

MALIGNANT MELANOMA

Incidence and Etiology

INCIDENCE

The incidence of malignant melanoma has increased dramatically in recent years. Data from various geographic locations have documented an increase in incidence of about 50 percent from 1956 to 1970 accompanied by an increase in mortality.[20] While the population of Queensland, Australia increased by 52 percent between 1950 and 1970, the number of melanoma cases increased 370 percent.[16] At the Columbia Presbyterian Medical Center in New York City, the average number of melanoma cases increased from 10 to 26 per year from 1947 to 1973. Similarly, the incidence of melanoma doubled between 1950 and 1970 in the state of New York and increased four-fold in Connecticut between 1935 and 1970. The number of recorded deaths from melanoma in New York City increased from approximately 90 per year in 1950 to about 165 per year in 1970, although the size of the population remained stable. No significant change in the anatomic location of the melanomas occurred.[14]

In summary, the incidence of melanoma throughout the world has approximately doubled in the last 20 years. This trend has existed for at least 35 to 40 years. With this increased incidence, interest in the possible etiology of melanomas has mounted.

HEREDITY

In 1962, the occurrence of cutaneous melanoma in a father and two of his three children was reported.[12] Based on a study of melanoma patients including one kindred with melanoma in 15 individuals, Anderson, Smith, and McBride concluded that hereditary melanoma was not sex-linked, appeared at an early age, and was often multiple.[3, 4] In Queensland, it is believed that approximately 10 percent of the causation

of melanoma is due to heredity.[65] While no definite hereditary pattern can be established in most patients with melanoma, heredity certainly determines skin pigmentation. Increased skin pigmentation provides protection against melanoma.[38]

A form of multiple pigmented nevi with frequent occurrence of melanoma has been described (B-K nevus syndrome). Malignant melanoma in these patients is almost certainly familial.[26]

EFFECT OF SUNLIGHT

Various observations incriminate exposure to sunlight as an etiologic factor in melanoma. The mortality from melanoma increases as one approaches the equator where greater sunlight exposure occurs.[16, 35, 45] Elwood and Lee studied melanoma development related to the skin surface area of various anatomic sites. Areas with significant incidence of melanoma were in sun-exposed regions and included the face, leg, neck, and arm in woman and the face, ear, neck, and back in men.[20]

The correlation between melanoma and sunlight exposure is not simple. The anatomic distribution of melanoma is different from that of squamous cell carcinoma, which is more clearly related to sun exposure. Squamous cell carcinomas occur primarily on the head, neck, forearm, and dorsum of the hand, while melanomas occur over the entire body; some in areas never exposed to sunlight. Further, if the development of melanomas were directly correlated with sunlight exposure, there should be an increased incidence with age and multiple primary melanomas in elderly patients. This is not the case.[16, 37, 45] In summary, there appears to be a relationship between sun exposure and development of melanoma in some patient populations. It is difficult, however, to correlate development of a specific melanoma with sunlight exposure.

NEVI

The origin of melanomas from preexisting nevi (moles), while at one time widely accepted, has been challenged by Clark.[13] It is proposed that a mole is simply a site where relatively normal melanocytes are concentrated and is not a definite precursor of malenoma. However, although the causal relationship is unclear, at least 30 percent of melanomas appear to arise in the melanocytes of a mole.[17, 26]

OTHER FACTORS

Many patients incriminate trauma as a factor in the development of their melanomas, but there is no clear evidence for this relationship. Comparison of a group of patients who have cutaneous melanoma with a group of patients who have basal cell carcinoma seemed to indicate that trauma was related to the development of cutaneous melanoma.[20] Most authors, however, reject the idea that trauma is important.[16, 36, 38]

Melanomas are very rare in childhood, develop occasionally in adolescence, are fairly frequent in middle age, and continue to develop into old age. Melanoma is more common in females, suggesting a hormonal relationship. The high incidence, however, is primarily in melanomas of the lower legs and may be related to sun exposure. The relationship of melanoma to pregnancy is unclear. There have been isolated case reports indicating that pregnancy stimulated melanomas.[38]

Clinical Presentation

Approximately 20 percent of all melanomas occur in the head and neck areas.[16] The majority present as cutaneous lesions manifested by a change in a preexisting pigmented lesion or by the development of a new pigmented lesion. The lesions may be amelanotic and appear pinkish or white. Mucosal melanomas occur in the upper aerodigestive tracts. Occasionally metastatic melanoma to cervical nodes is seen without an obvious primary tumor.

Any change in a pigmented lesion or mole may be significant. Specifically, any of the following should arouse suspicion: (1) increased size; (2) change in configuration; (3) change in color with either increased or decreased pigment; (4) change in surface with a previously smooth surface becoming rough, irregular, scaly, or ulcerative; (5) occurrence of any serous or bloody drainage; (6) development of satellite lesions; and (7) any change in sensation especially the occurrence of itching or tingling.[17]

The differentiation of melanoma from various benign lesions can be difficult. In younger persons, nevi in various stages of evolution (junctional, compound, intradermal) are frequently seen. Less common lesions such as the Spitz nevus and the blue nevus may be difficult to differentiate from melanoma clinically. Older patients frequently present with pigmented lesions of a benign nature including seborrheic keratosis, senile hemangiomas, and cherry-red hemangiomas. In general, the physical features of a melanoma can be summarized in one word—irregular—irregular color, irregular shape, and irregular surface. Any pigmented lesion with these irregularities must be suspected of being a melanoma.[49]

The diagnosis of melanoma must be made histologically. A few patients may be treated on the basis of clinical assessment, but patients should have a histologic diagnosis before definitive therapy. Small lesions with any suspicious characteristics should be excised under local block anesthesia with narrow margins (2 mm) and the underlying fascia should be left intact. Large lesions may be biopsied by an incisional technique. If the biopsy proves to be malignant, a definitive operation should be done within a week. Incisional biopsy followed by a delayed surgical procedure does not alter the prognosis for melanoma.[21] However, an excisional biopsy should be done if this is technically feasible.

In hospitals in which a large number of melanoma patients are treated, frozen section evaluation is often used. Patients with a clinically suspicious lesion are anesthetized, the lesion is excised, and frozen section examination is performed. Definitive diagnosis and treatment are based upon the frozen section. At the Princess Alexandra Hospital in Queensland, frozen section evaluation was 98.8 percent accurate in 316 patients with melanoma.[41]

Mucosal melanomas account for less than 10 percent of the melanomas arising in the head and neck region. The lesions usually occur in the oral cavity or nasal cavity. Oral cavity melanomas are often pigmented and are either flat or raised. They may be fairly large by the time of diagnosis. Nasal cavity melanomas present with nasal obstruction or epistaxis. Examination shows an abnormally pigmented, exophytic mass, which may be ulcerated.[57, 60]

Metastatic melanoma may present with no primary site detectable. The metastatic lesion may appear as lymphadenopathy or as a subcutaneous mass or as distant metastasis. Cervical node metastasis probably originates in a primary lesion of the head and neck. Of 71 male patients with metastatic melanoma and no known primary lesion, 41 presented with node metastasis, 10 of which were cervical nodes. These metastases probably developed from primary lesions that had undergone spontaneous regression.[5]

Pathology

Recently, the heterogenous group of tumors previously labeled "malignant melanoma" has been divided into morphologic types and further characterized by depth of invasion. Mehnert and Heard classified melanomas into in situ, superficial, intradermal, and subcutaneous depending upon depth of penetration. Deeper lesions had a poorer prognosis than the superficial ones.[47]

The clearest delineation of melanoma types has come from Clark, Bernardino, and Mihm who separated cutaneous melanomas into three types: lentigo maligna melanoma (MM), superficial spreading melanoma (SSM), and nodular melanoma (NM).[13, 48] The types are delineated by clinical and histologic features. In addition to

these three invasive forms of melanoma, a noninvasive (or in situ) lesion, lentigo maligna (LM), is seen in the head and neck.

LENTIGO MALIGNA

Lentigo maligna (circumscribed precancerous melanosis of Dubreuilh or melanotic freckle of Hutchison) is a noninvasive lesion occurring primarily on the face of elderly patients. It may remain noninvasive for years but enlarges by centrifugal growth. Lentigo maligna is usually a flat, tan lesion with an irregular border and areas of lighter pigmentation (Plate 11-5). Histologically, there is an increased number of atypical melanocytes in the epidermal basal cell layer often adjacent to relatively normal melanocytes. Nests of these atypical melanocytes may be seen. No melanocytes are present in the dermis[6] (Fig. 11-8).

LENTIGO MALIGNA MELANOMA

Invasive melanoma may develop in lentigo maligna and is termed lentigo maligna melanoma. This malignant degeneration is heralded by the development of raised brown or black nodules within previous flat, tan or brown areas. Lentigo maligna melanoma is characterized by a completely irregular outline and a flat surface with only small areas of elevation and is usually brown in color (Plate 11-6). The intraepithelial changes seen in lentigo maligna are still present in lentigo maligna melanoma. However, invasion into the dermis is also present. The invasive component is similar to that seen in other forms of invasive melanoma except that there is a greater number of spindle cells[19] (Fig. 11-9).

Electron microscopy confirms the presence of normal and atypical melanocytes within the basal layer of the epidermis. Some cells have nuclei that are quite large with a narrowed perikaryon. Additionally, nuclear membrane abnormalities may be present. Cytoplasmic features are usually relatively normal.[13]

Lentigo Maligna

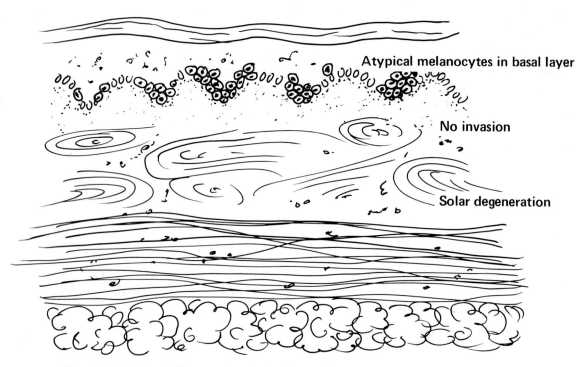

Atypical melanocytes in basal layer

No invasion

Solar degeneration

Fig. 11-8. Lentigo maligna (melanotic freckle of Hutchinson) is in situ melanoma and histologically consists of malignant cells confined to the epidermis.

Lentigo Maligna Melanoma

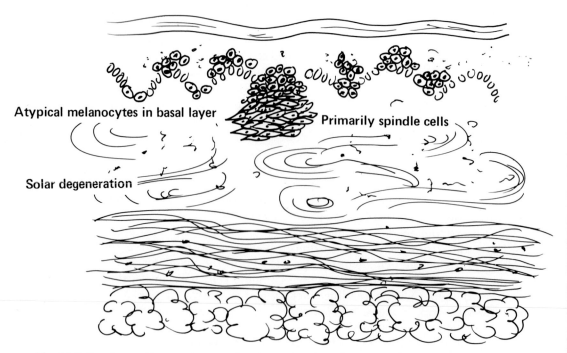

Atypical melanocytes in basal layer

Primarily spindle cells

Solar degeneration

Fig. 11-9. Lentigo maligna melanoma develops when invasion occurs in a lentigo maligna.

SUPERFICIAL SPREADING MELANOMA

Superficial spreading melanoma may occur anywhere on the body and affects primarily patients of middle age. The lesion is basically circular with a defect on one side giving an arc or bean shape. The surface is usually elevated above the surrounding skin and is frequently scaly. The lesions have a haphazard combination of all colors including brown, tan, gray, black, pink, blue, and white. Areas of spontaneous regression are common (Plate 11-7).

Superficial spreading melanoma is characterized by large epithelioid cells (Fig. 11-10) These cells occur in nests and as an intraepidermal component at least three rete pegs away from the area of invasion. This intraepidermal component is the radial growth phase of SSM. The cells are uniform in appearance but definitely abnormal. They are primarily epithelioid and have relatively uniform nuclei and an abundance of dusty cytoplasm. The vertical growth phase of superficial melanoma consists of malignant cells that invade into the dermis for a variable distance. Frequently, there are clusters of cells that vary in appearance from one cluster to another. A lymphocytic infiltration is fairly common around these invasive cells. Electron microscopy demonstrates that the intraepidermal cells have cytoplasm filled with melanosomes that are abnormal and lack the cross linkage seen in normal melanosomes.[13, 19]

NODULAR MELANOMA

Nodular melanoma (NM) is the least common of the three forms of invasive melanoma, has various clinical appearances, and occurs over the entire body; this melanoma usually has a uniform appearance and color throughout its area. It is always palpable but surface characteristics vary from lesion to lesion. Some are spherical and resemble a blueberry under the skin; others appear as an elevated, irregular black plaque; and still

Superficial Spreading Melanoma

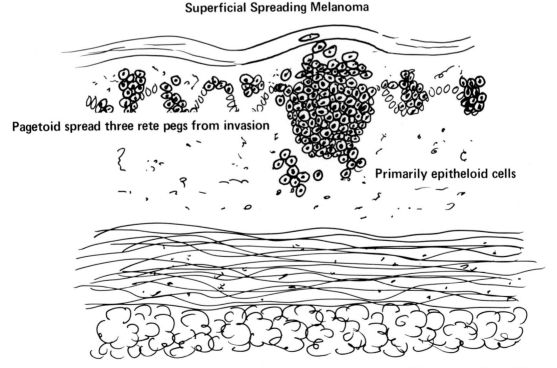

Pagetoid spread three rete pegs from invasion

Primarily epithelioid cells

Fig. 11-10. Superficial spreading melanoma is characterized by radial growth (Pagetoid spread) and vertical growth (invasion).

others present as a nodular mass with ulceration (Plate 11-8).

Histologically, the entire lesion is invasive and there is no intraepidermal component without underlying invasion (Fig. 11-11) Generally, nodular melanomas invade deeper than do lentigo maligna melanomas or superficial spreading melanomas. Epithelioid cells predominate and may be pigmented or amelanotic.[19]

Evaluation of Invasion

Recent correlation between the depth of invasion and the metastatic potential and ultimate prognosis of melanoma has been established.[8, 13, 46-48] Two classification systems related to the depth of invasion have evolved. The first, Clark's levels of invasion,

relates the depth of invasion to normal histologic skin structures (Fig. 11-12). Clark levels are as follows: level I, tumor confined above the basement membrane; level II, tumor extending into the papillary layer of the dermis; level III, tumor through the papillary dermis and accumulated at the junction of the papillary and reticular dermis; level IV, tumor invading into the reticular dermis; and level V, tumor invading into the subcutaneous fat. The risk of dying of melanoma has been correlated with the level of invasion and is about 0 percent for level I, 10 percent for level II, 25 percent for level III, 50 percent for level IV, and 90 percent for level V.[13, 48]

The second method of quantitating the depth of invasion involves a direct measurement of the thickness of the melanoma as

Nodular Melanoma

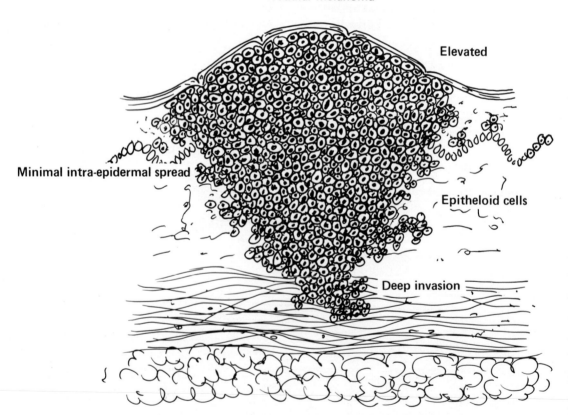

Fig. 11-11. Nodular melanoma usually appears as uniform malignant cells with deep invasion and little intraepithelial spread.

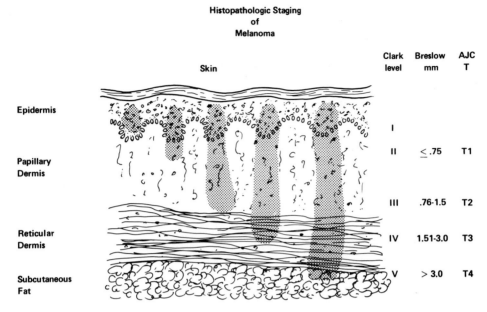

Fig. 11-12. The Clark and Breslow classifications are both utilized in the American Joint Committee staging system.

described by Breslow (Fig. 11-12). The maximal thickness of the lesion from the skin surface to the deepest point of invasion is determined by direct micrometer measurement. Lesions are divided into thin (.75 mm or less), intermediate (.76 to 1.5 mm), and thick (greater than 1.5 mm). The prognosis decreases as the thickness of the lesion increases. Breslow stressed the significance of cross sectional area of the lesion with regard to the prognosis and found that larger lesions had a worse prognosis.[8]

These concepts concerning melanoma types and depth of invasion have only recently been applied to malignant melanoma of the head and neck. In 119 patients with head and neck melanoma seen at the Sloan-Kettering Memorial Hospital in New York, 23 had lentigo maligna melanoma, 37 had superficial spreading melanoma, and 59 had nodular melanoma. Lentigo maligna melanoma occurs almost exclusively as a head and neck lesion, but it is less common than either superficial spreading or nodular melanomas. Lentigo maligna melanoma had a peak incidence in the seventh decade, a male to female ratio of 1:3, and usually occurred on the cheek. The other two types occurred in all age groups, involved various anatomic areas, and had a male to female ratio greater than 2:1. Nodular melanomas were most invasive (level IV or V), and lentigo maligna melanomas were least invasive (level II).[18] At the University of California at Los Angeles, 69 patients with head and neck melanomas were reviewed. Lesions were generally distributed over the entire skin surface. Survival was better for superficially invasive lesions but pathologic involvement of the regional lymph nodes was the most important determinant of prognosis.[61]

Clinical Staging

The American Joint Committee has combined the various pathologic aspects of melanoma into a staging system. Four stages are defined utilizing the T (tumor), N (node), and M (distant metastasis) system[1] (Table 11-1). Stage I disease is localized to the primary site and is either IA (thin) or IB (thick). Stage II has regional spread either as satellites, intransit metastasis, or movable

TABLE 11-1 AMERICAN JOINT COMMITTEE STAGING

T = Primary Tumor
    T0 No evidence of primary
    T1 Level II and/or less than .75 mm
    T2 Level III and/or .76 to 1.5 mm
    T3 Level IV and/or 1.51 to 3.0 mm
    T4 Level V and/or greater than 3.0 mm
    T1 to T4 may be modified by:
        a. Satellite(s) within 2 cm of primary
        b. Satellites more than 2 cm from primary and/or intransit metastasis toward primary drainage

N = Nodal Involvement
    N0   No node involvement
    N1a First station node involvement, small movable
    N1b First station node involvement, massive or fixed
    N2a Contralateral, bilateral, or secondary node involvement, movable, small
    N2b Contralateral, bilateral, or secondary node involvement, massive or fixed

M = Distant Metastasis
    M0   No known distant metastasis
    M1a Skin, subcutaneous tissue, or distant lymph node metastasis
    M1b Visceral metastasis

Stage Grouping

Stage	TNM Description	Clinical
IA	Any T1 or T2, N0, M0	Localized, thin
IB	Any T3 or T4, N0, M0	Localized, thick
II	Any T, N1a, M0	Regional spread—satellites, intransits, or movable nodes
	Any Ta or Tb, N0 or N1a, M0	
III	Any T, N1b or N2a or N2b, M0	Extensive node metastasis
IV	Any T, N, M1a or M1b	Distant spread

regional nodes. Stage III is characterized by advanced nodal metastasis either as large fixed nodes, contralateral nodes, or second level nodes. Stage IV disease includes all patients with distant metastasis.

Clinical assessment includes both physical examination and laboratory evaluation. Physical examination includes a careful description and measurement of the primary lesion, a search for satellite lesions, and palpation of regional lymph nodes. Regional lymph node palpation is about 75 percent accurate in predicting the presence of metastasis. Remainder of the physical examination is directed toward the common metastatic sites: liver, lung, brain, and bone. The extent of laboratory evaluation necessary is controversial. Certainly, routine stud-

ies (chest x-ray, complete blood count, urinalysis, liver function tests, and screening chemistries) are indicated. However, nuclear scans (brain, liver, and bone) are not recommended unless there is clinical evidence of metastasis. Scans are useful in experimental protocols but do not help in routine management of melanoma patients who do not have evidence of metastasis.

Management

PRIMARY LESION MANAGEMENT

Surgical excision is the appropriate treatment of melanoma. Radiation therapy, chemotherapy, and cryosurgery play no role in the treatment of primary lesions. Surgical management includes "adequate resection" with reconstruction of the defect. Traditional adequate resection includes a 5 cm margin around the tumor plus the underlying fascia. Such a margin is frequently inappropriate for head and neck lesions. The extent of excision should be based on the pathologic characteristics, the size, and the location of the tumor.[6] Lentigo maligna melanoma need not be excised as widely as spreading or nodular melanoma. Breslow and Macht reviewed the optimal size of resection for thin (less than 0.75 mm) melanomas. The resection margin varied from 0.1 to 5.5 cm, and 32 percent of the patients had a margin less than 1 cm. No patient developed local recurrence or metastasis.[11] Small lesions do not require as wide a margin as do larger lesions. In the head and neck, location may limit the extent of resection. A melanoma between the eyes cannot be resected as widely as one located on the scalp. In general, small thin lesions may be resected with narrow margins (1 to 2 cm). Larger tumors, deeply invasive lesions, and lesions with satellites must be resected with wide margins (2 to 5 cm).

Closure of the defect may be accomplished primarily or with a skin graft. If adequate skin is available, the lesion is excised with an ellipse and primary closure performed. Many lesions of the head and neck will require a skin graft. This is especially true of those located where the skin is fixed to bone or cartilage such as the nose, forehead, and scalp.[29] A thick split-thickness skin graft (.018 to .020 inch) from the upper chest provides good cosmetic matching for the face. Scalp lesions are usually covered with a skin graft from the leg. There is no difference between local, regional, and systemic control in patients with primary closure compared to those with a skin graft.[2]

MANAGEMENT OF CLINICALLY POSITIVE NODES

When nodes are clinically positive but resectable and there is no evidence of distant metastasis, regional lymph node dissection is indicated if the primary lesion is controlled. In planning an operation the surgeon must consider the lymphatic drainage of the involved site and modify or extend a classical neck dissection as indicated. The dissection may need to include occipital nodes, parotid nodes, postauricular nodes, and others[6] (Fig. 11-13). The addition of radiotherapy to radical node dissection in patients with pathologically positive nodes does not affect survival or the disease-free interval.[15]

MANAGEMENT OF CLINICALLY NEGATIVE NODES

The management of patients with clinically negative nodes is controversial. The classic argument for elective or prophylactic node dissection is as follows: (1) clinical evaluation of nodes is inaccurate; (2) pathologic examination of elective node dissections will reveal metastatic disease in 25 percent of patients; (3) removal of these nonpalpable positive nodes will give better results than waiting until they become palpable. Retrospective studies support the use of an elective neck dissection.[27, 59]

Recently, the Clark and Breslow classifications have been used to predict which patients should have elective node dissections. Lesions that are level II or III (Clark) and less than 1.5 mm thick (Breslow) rarely metastasize to lymph nodes. Proponents of elective node dissection suggest that patients with deeper lesions (level IV or V or thicker than 1.5 mm) should undergo elective node dissection. Retrospective studies seem to validate this concept.[9, 29, 61, 66]

There are no published prospective randomized studies regarding the use of elective node dissection for melanoma of the head and neck. Recently, two such trials of extremity melanomas have been performed. The World Health Organization Melanoma Group studied patients with invasive melanomas of the leg. Patients with clinical stage I (localized) melanoma were prospectively randomized; 267 patients re-

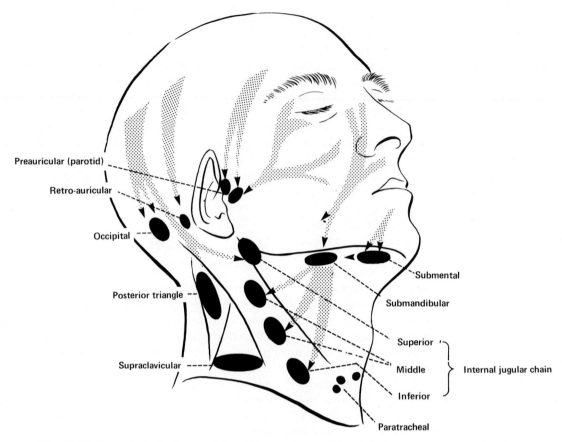

Preauricular (parotid)

Retro-auricular

Occipital

Posterior triangle

Supraclavicular

Submental

Submandibular

Superior

Middle   Internal jugular chain

Inferior

Paratracheal

Fig. 11-13. Lymphatic drainage of the skin must be considered in the management of patients with skin cancer of the head and neck.

ceived excision plus immediate node dissection while 286 received excision and delayed node dissection if metastasis developed. There was no difference in survival between the two groups regardless of how the data were analyzed (according to sex, site, maximum diameter, or thickness).[64] A similar trial performed at the Mayo Clinic randomized patients with clinical stage I melanomas into three treatment groups: no lymphadenectomy, delayed (2 to 4 months after primary excision) lymphadenectomy, or immediate lymphadenectomy. Patients were excluded with midline lesions, head and neck lesions, lesions situated directly over nodes, or level I or II lesions. Of 173 patients studied, 110 had elective node dissections. Only 7 of the 110 patients had histologically positive nodes. The authors concluded that there was "no significant benefit to the patient from immediate or delayed elective lymphadenectomy."[58] While both of these studies exclude head and neck lesions, neither demonstrates any improvement in survival with elective node dissection for stage I melanoma.

Currently, management of patients with melanoma of the head and neck and clinically negative nodes varies from surgeon to surgeon. Many perform elective node dissections on patients who meet the following criteria: (1) Invasion to level IV or V or over 1.5 mm thick, (2) predictable lymphatic drainage, (3) good general medical condition, and (4) no evidence of distant metastasis. Other surgeons simply treat the primary lesion, instruct patients in self-examination of nodes, institute regular follow-up,

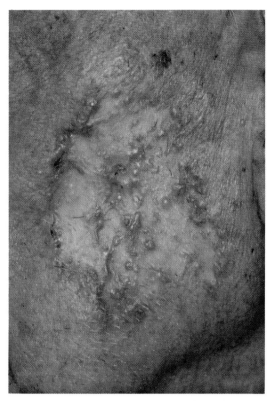

Plate 11-1. Superficial multicentric basal cell carcinoma.

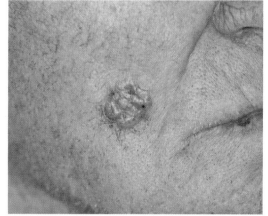

Plate 11-2. Nodular basal cell carcinoma.

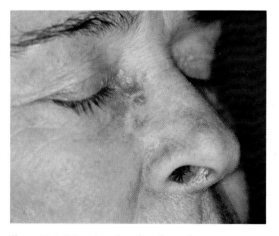

Plate 11-3. Morphea basal cell carcinoma.

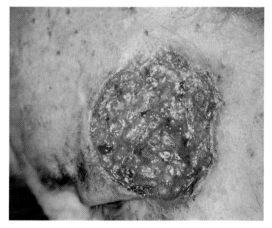

Plate 11-4. Squamous cell carcinoma.

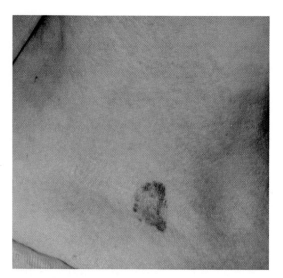

Plate 11-5. Lentigo maligna (melanotic freckle of Hutchinson).

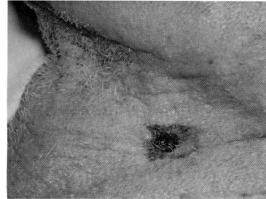

Plate 11-6. Lentigo maligna melanoma.

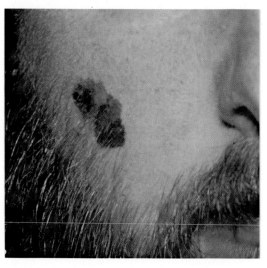

Plate 11-7. Superficial spreading melanoma.

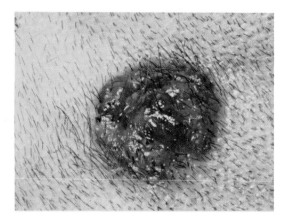

Plate 11-8. Nodular melanoma.

and do a therapeutic node dissection if nodes become positive. Breslow reviewed this question and concluded "as for the role of elective node dissection in the treatment of cutaneous melanoma, the literature prior to 1977 . . . is worthless".[10]

To date it has not been proved that elective node dissection is beneficial. Certainly node dissection is not indicated for minimally invasive lesions or for lesions with unpredictable drainage (as in midline structures). Further studies may clarify what patients, if any, with clinically negative nodes will be benefited by elective node dissection.

ADJUVANT THERAPY

About 50 percent of the patients with melanoma will eventually succumb to their disease. This means that many patients initially felt to have curable disease die from metastatic melanoma. Utilizing clinical and histologic evaluation, a group of patients with a high risk of recurrent disease may be selected. Patients who have a greater than 50 percent chance of developing recurrent disease include the following: (1) patients with a clinically localized lesion (stage I) that is greater than 1.5 mm thick or is of level IV or V invasion, or (2) patients with histologically positive nodes.

Since high risk patients can be identified, the use of adjuvant chemotherapy or immunotherapy may be warranted. It is well-documented that 20 percent of patients with advanced melanoma will respond to chemotherapy. Selected advanced lesions will respond to immunotherapy. Since some advanced lesions respond to chemotherapy and immunotherapy, it is logical to assume that minimal residual disease in high risk patients should respond.

Numerous investigators have utilized chemotherapy, immunotherapy, and chemoimmunotherapy as an adjuvant to surgery. Adjuvant chemotherapy protocols are usually based on dimethyl triezeno imidazole carboxamide (DTIC). The nitrosoureas (BCNU, CCNU, methyl-CCNU) have been added or substituted in some regimens. Reviews summarizing all reported adjuvant studies have been published. Results are conflicting, with several studies suggesting that adjuvant chemotherapy may prolong the tumor-free interval and others finding no effect.[39, 46]

Adjuvant immunotherapy has primarily taken the form of nonspecific immunostimulation with bacillus Calmette-Guerin (BCG). Specific immunotherapy has only been tried in limited experiments. Again, results are not consistent. Most studies using prospective randomized protocols have not shown a statistically significant improvement with adjuvant immunotherapy. However, trials with historical controls have suggested an improvement with adjuvant treatment.[39, 44]

Chemoimmunotherapy has also been tried in some trials usually with a combination of DTIC and BCG. Again, no clear-cut beneficial effect has been demonstrated.[39, 44]

Randomized clinical trials have shown no clear benefit from the adjuvant use of chemotherapy, immunotherapy, or chemoimmunotherapy. Improvement of adjuvant treatment must probably await the development of new drugs or immunotherapy agents of increased effectiveness.

LOCALLY RECURRENT DISEASE

Melanoma of the head and neck may recur in the primary site, as satellites around the primary site, or as regional node metastasis. Local recurrence is usually associated with systemic disease. However, local treatment should be undertaken in an effort to achieve local control. Uncontrolled disease in the head and neck area is a serious medical and social problem.

Surgical excision, intralesional immunotherapy, or radiotherapy may be used to treat local disease. Occasionally, radical excision of local or satellite recurrence followed by skin grafting may achieve control.[6] Regional node recurrence in a previously undissected area dictates an appropriate neck dissection. Nodes that develop in an area of previous dissection may occasionally be excised with hopes of local control, but this excision is usually doomed to failure.

Numerous groups have reported on the injection of BCG into dermal metastasis. About 66 percent of injected nodules undergo regression, with 22 percent of patients experiencing regression of some of the uninjected nodules and 27 percent of patients who had intralesional injections going into complete remission.[39, 43, 52] Intralesional injection of dermal metastasis of the head and neck is worthwhile in selected patients.

Radiation therapy is not a primary treatment modality for melanoma. Significant palliation, however, can be obtained with irradiation of recurrent disease. Treatment of skin, subcutaneous, and lymph node metastasis with radiotherapy utilizing 600 rads or more once or twice weekly resulted in a complete or partial regression in 29 of 33 lesions.[28]

In summary, the treatment of recurrent disease confined to the head and neck may utilize one of several modalities. Localized recurrence or nodal metastasis is usually treated with surgical excision. Diffuse dermal metastasis is best treated with intralesional BCG. Recurrence not suitable for surgery or immunotherapy should be treated with radiotherapy.

MANAGEMENT OF DISSEMINATED MELANOMA

About half of all patients with melanoma eventually develop widespread disease. Sites commonly involved include the lung, liver, brain, skin, bone, and gastrointestinal tract. Systemic chemotherapy is the only treatment available for these patients.

Many drugs have been used as single agents against melanoma. The most effective single agent is DTIC, which has a response rate of about 20 percent. Approximately 5 percent of patients obtain complete remission for a long period of time. The nitrosourea derivatives (BCNU, CCNU, methyl-CCNU) yield a slightly lower response rate.

Because of the relatively low response rate to single agents, combination chemotherapy has been attempted. Most combination regimens have included DTIC plus other agents. The superiority of combination regimens over DTIC alone is still questionable. Therefore, advanced disseminated melanoma is treated with DTIC alone or in combination with nitrosoureas.[7, 19, 39]

Prognosis of Melanoma of the Head and Neck

The prognosis of melanoma is determined primarily by the location, histopathologic microstaging, clinical stage, and pathologic status of the regional nodes. In general, melanoma of the head and neck has an intermediate prognosis, whereas trunk lesions have a worse prognosis and extremity lesions have a better prognosis.[17] Utilizing the Clark level classification, patients with level II lesions have about a 90 percent probability of a 5-year survival, while those with level V lesions have a 10 percent probability of a 5-year survival. Level II and III lesions are intermediate in prognosis. Melanoma arising in lentigo maligna has the best prognosis and nodular melanoma has the worst prognosis.

Probably, the single most important determinant of prognosis is the pathologic status of the regional lymph nodes. If they are positive, approximately 10 percent of patients survive 5 years. If the regional lymph nodes are negative, approximately 90 percent of patients survive 5 years.[29]

The prognosis of melanoma has improved significantly in the last 20 years. In Australia, information from the Queensland melanoma group documents a better survival than in other areas around the world. This is ascribed to excellent public and professional education. Melanoma is very common in Australia and suspicious lesions are biopsied early. This experience seems to point out the need for better education of the public and physicians if the survival of melanoma patients is to improve.[17]

SUMMARY

Cancer of the skin of the head and neck is very common. Basal cell carcinoma is the most common histologic type and is curable in about 95 percent of patients. Electrodessication and curettage is used for small discrete lesions, surgical excision for larger tumors in accessible locations, and chemosurgery or radiotherapy for lesions that are not discrete or are located in difficult locations. Early squamous cell carcinoma arising in sun-damaged skin is managed in a similar fashion. Aggressive squamous cell carcinoma, morphea basal cell carcinoma, and recurrent lesions may require radical surgery, chemosurgery, or radiation therapy.

Melanoma presents several different clinical and histologic patterns. The type, location, and clinical stage dictate the indicated therapy. While survival of melanoma has improved in recent years, further advances will depend on either earlier diagnosis or better adjuvant therapy.

REFERENCES

1. American Joint Committee for Cancer Staging and End Results Reporting, 1977. Manual for Staging of Cancer. American Joint Committee, Chicago.
2. Ames, F. C., Sugarbaker, E. V., and Ballantyne, A. J. 1976. Analysis of survival and disease control in stage I melanoma of the head and neck. American Journal of Surgery, 132: 484.
3. Anderson, D. E. 1971. Clinical characteristics of the genetic variety of cutaneous melanoma in man. Cancer, 28: 721.
4. Anderson, D. E., Smith, J. L., and McBride, C. M. 1967. Hereditary aspects of malignant melanoma. JAMA, 200: 741.
5. Baab, G. H., and McBride, C. M. 1975. Malignant melanoma—The patient with an unknown site of primary origin. Archives of Surgery, 110: 896.
6. Ballantyne, A. J. 1976. Malignant melanoma of the head and neck region. In Anderson Hospital, Ed.: Neoplasms of the Skin and Malignant Melanoma. Year Book Medical Publishers, Chicago, 345.
7. Bellet, R. E., Mastrangelo, M. J., Berd, D., and Lustbader, E. 1979. Chemotherapy of metastatic malignant melanoma. In Clark, W. H., Goldman, L. I., and Mastrangelo, M. J., Eds.: Human Malignant Melanoma. Grune & Stratton, New York, 325.
8. Breslow, A., 1970. Thickness, cross-sectional areas and depth of invasion in the prognosis of cutaneous melanoma. Annals of Surgery, 172: 902.
9. Breslow, A., 1975. Tumor thickness, level of invasion and node dissection in stage I cutaneous melanoma. Annals of Surgery, 182: 572.
10. Breslow, A., 1978. The surgical treatment of stage I cutaneous melanoma. Cancer Treatment Reviews, 5: 195.
11. Breslow, A., and Macht, S. D., 1977. Optimal size of resection margin for thin cutaneous melanoma. Surgery, Gynecology, and Obstetrics, 145: 691.
12. Cawley, E. P., Kruse, W. T., and Pinkus, H. K. 1952. Genetic aspects of malignant melanoma. Archives of Dermatology and Syphilology, 65: 440.
13. Clark, W. H., Jr., From, L., Bernardino, E. A., and Mihm, M. C. 1969. The histogenesis and biologic behavior of primary human malignant melanomas of the skin. Cancer Research, 29: 705.
14. Cosman, B., Heddle, S. B., and Crikelair, G. F. 1976. The increasing incidence of melanoma. Plastic and Reconstructive Surgery, 57: 50.
15. Creagan, E. T., Cupps, R. E., Ivins, J. C., Pritchard, D. J., Sim, F. H., Soule, E. H., Soule, E. H., and O'Fallon, J. R. 1978. Adjuvant radiation therapy for regional nodal metastases from malignant melanoma: A randomized prospective study. Cancer, 42: 2206.
16. Davis, N. C., 1976. Cutaneous melanoma. The Queensland experience. Current Problems in Surgery, 13: 1.
17. Davis, N. C., McLeod, R., Beardmore, G. L., Little, J. H., Quinn, R. L., and Holt, J. 1976. Primary cutaneous melanoma: A report from the Queensland melanoma project. CA. A Cancer Journal for Clinicians. 26: 80.
18. Donnellan, M. J., Seemayer, T., Huvos, A. G., Mike, V., and Strong, E. W. 1972. Clinicopathologic study of cutaneous melanoma of the head and neck. American Journal of Surgery, 124: 450.
19. Elder, D. E., Ainsworth, A. M., and Clark, W. H. 1979. The surgical pathology of cutaneous malignant melanoma. In Clark, W. H., Goldman, L. I., and Mastrangelo, M. J., Eds.: Human Malignant Melanoma. Grune & Stratton, New York, 55.
20. Elwood, J. M., and Lee, J. A. H. 1975. Re-

cent data on the epdemiology of malignant melanoma. Seminars in Oncology, 2:   149.

21. Epstein, E., Bragg, K., and Linden, G. 1969. Biopsy and prognosis of malignant melanoma. JAMA, 208:   1369.

22. Finley, A.G. 1954. Kerato-acanthoma. Australian Journal of Dermatology, 2:   144.

23. Forrester, J. S., and Houston, R. A. 1951. Hemangiopericytoma with metastases. Report of a case with autopsy. Archives of Pathology, 51:   651.

24. Graham, J. H., 1976. Selected precancerous skin and mucocutaneous lesions. In Anderson Hospital, Ed.: Neoplasms of the Skin and Malignant Melanoma. Year Book Publishers, Chicago, 69.

25. Graham, J. H., and Helwig, E. B. 1977. Cutaneous premalignant lesions. In Montagna, W., and Dobson, R. L., Eds.: Advances in Biology of the Skin. Vol. 7. Carcinogenesis. Permagon Press, New York, 277.

26. Green, M. H., and Fraumeni, J. F. 1979. The hereditary variant of malignant melanoma. In Clark, W. H., Goldman, L. I., and Mastrangelo, M. J., Eds.: Human Malignant Melanoma. Grune & Stratton, New York, 139.

27. Gumport, S. L., and Harris, M. N. 1974. Results of regional lymph node dissection for melanoma. Annals of Surgery, 179:   105.

28. Habermalz, H. J., and Fischer, J. J. 1976. Radiation therapy of malignant melanoma: Experience with high individual treatment doses. Cancer, 38:2258.

29. Harris, M. N., Roses, D. F., Culliford, A. T., and Gumport, S. L. 1975. Melanoma of the head and neck. Annals of Surgery, 182:   86.

30. Holecek, M. J., and Harwood, A. R. 1978. Radiotherapy of Kaposis sarcoma. Cancer, 41:   1733.

31. Jackson, R., and Adams, R. H. 1973. Horrifying basal cell carcinoma: A study of 33 cases and a comparison with 435 non-horror cases and a report on four metastatic cases. Journal of Surgical Oncology 5:   431.

32. Jansen, G. T., Dillaha, C. J., and Honeycutt, W. M. 1967. Bowenoid conditions of the skin: Treatment with topical 5-fluorouracil. Southern Medical Journal, 60:   185.

33. Kanee, B. 1969. Oral florid papillomatosis complicated by verrucous squamous carcinoma. Treatment with methotrexate. Archives of Dermatology, 99:   196.

34. Kopf, A. W. 1971. Therapy of basal cell carcinoma. In Fitzpatrick, T. B., Arndt, K. A.: Clark, W. H., Eisen, A. Z., Van Scott, E. J., and Vaughan, J. H., Eds.: Dermatology in General Medicine. McGraw-Hill, New York, 472.

35. Lancaster, H. O. 1956. Some geographical aspects of the mortality from melanoma in Europeans. Medical Journal of Australia, 1:   1082.

36. Lea, A. J. 1965. Malignant melanoma of the skin: The relationship to trauma. Annals of the Royal College of Surgeons of England, 37:   169.

37. Lee, J. A., and Yongchaiyadha, S. 1971. Incidence of and mortality from malignant melanoma by anatomical site. Journal of the National Cancer Institute, 47:   253.

38. Lee, J. A. 1975. Current evidence about the causes of malignant melanoma. Progress in Clinical Cancer, 6:   151.

39. Lejeune, F. J., and DeWasch, G. 1978. Malignant melanoma. In Staquet, M. J., Ed.: Randomized Trials in Cancer: A Critical Review by Sites. Raven Press, New York, 339.

40. Lever, W. F., and Schaumburg-Lever, G. 1975. Histopathology of the Skin. 5th edn. J.B. Lippincott, Philadelphia.

41. Little, J. H., and Davis, N. C. 1974. Frozen section diagnosis of suspected malignant melanoma of the skin. Cancer, 34:   1163.

42. MacDonald, E. J. 1976. Epidemiology of skin cancer. In Anderson Hospital, Ed.: Neoplasms of the Skin and Malignant Melanoma. Yearbook Publishers, Chicago, 27.

43. Mastrangelo, M. J., Bellet, R. E., and Berd, D. 1979. Immunology and immunotherapy of human cutaneous malignant melanoma. In Clark, W. H., Goldman, L. I., and Mastrangelo, M. J., Eds.: Human Malignant Melanoma. Grune & Stratton, New York, 355.

44. Mastrangelo, M. J., Bellet, R. E., and Berd, D. 1979. Postsurgical adjuvant therapy. In Clark, W. H., Goldman, L. I., and Mastrangelo, M. J., Eds.: Human Malignant Melanoma. Grune & Stratton, New York, 309.

45. MacDonald, E. J., Johnson, M. S., and Murphy, A. 1971. Regional patterns in morbidity from melanoma in Texas, 1944–1966. Cancer Bulletin, 23:   51.

46. McGovern, V. J. 1970. The classification of melanoma and its relationship with prognosis. Pathology, 2:   85.

47. Mehnert, J. H., and Heard, J. L. 1965. Staging of malignant melanomas by depth of invasion. American Journal of Surgery, 110:   168.

48. Mihm, M. C., Jr., Clark, W. H., Jr., and From, L. 1971. The clinical diagnosis, classification, and histogenetic concepts of the early stages of cutaneous malignant melanomas. New England Journal of Medicine, 284: 1078.

49. Mihm, M. C., Jr., Fitzpatrick, T. B., Lane Brown, M. M., Raker, J. W., Malt, R. A., and Kaiser, J. S. 1973. Early detection of primary cutaneous malignant melanoma. A color atlas. New England Journal of Medicine, 289: 989.

50. Milton, G. W. 1977. Malignant Melanoma of the Skin and Mucous Membrane. Churchill Livingstone, Edinburgh.

51. Mohs, F. E. 1978. Chemosurgery: Microscopically controlled surgery for skin cancer—past, present and future. Journal of Dermatologic Surgery and Oncology, 4: 41.

52. Morton, D. L., Eilber, F. R., Malmgren, R. A., and Wood, W. C. 1970. Immunological factors which influence response to immunotherapy in malignant melanoma. Surgery, 68: 158.

53. Owens, D. W., Knox, J. M., Hudson, H. T. and Troll, M. S. 1975. Influence of humidity on ultraviolet injury. Journal of Investigative Dermatology, 64: 250.

54. Prutkin, L. 1967. An ultrastructure study of experimental keratoacanthoma. Journal of Investigative Dermatology, 48: 326.

55. Rook, A., Kexdel-Vegas, R., and Young, J. A. 1967. Recurrences in keratoacanthoma. Medicina Cutanea, 11: 17.

56. Samitz, M. H., Ackerman, A. B., and Lantis, L. R. 1967. Squamous cell carcinoma arising at the site of oral florid papillomatosis. Archives of Dermatology, 96: 286.

57. Shah, J. P., Huvos, A. G., and Strong, E. W. 1977. Mucosal melanomas of the head and neck. American Journal of Surgery, 134: 531.

58. Sim, F. H., Taylor, W. F., Ivins, J. C., Pritchard, D. J., and Soule, E. H. 1978. A prospective randomized study of the efficacy of routine elective lymphadenectomy in management of malignant melanoma: Preliminary results. Cancer, 41: 948.

59. Simons, J. N. 1972. Malignant melanoma of the head and neck. American Journal of Surgery, 124: 485.

60. Snow, G. B., Van Der Esch, E. P., and VanSlooten, E. A. 1978. Mucosal melanomas of the head and neck. Head & Neck Surgery, 1: 24.

61. Storm, F. K., III, Eilber, F. R., Morton, D. L., and Clark, W. H., Jr. 1978. Malignant melanoma of the head and neck. Head & Neck Surgery, 1: 123.

62. Tapley, N. D. 1976. Radiotherapy for basal and squamous cell carcinoma of the skin. In Anderson Hospital, Ed.: Neoplasms of the Skin and Malignant Melanoma. Year Book Medical Publisher, Chicago, 155.

63. Unna, P. G., The Histopathology of the Diseases of the Skin. Macmillan, New York.

64. Veronesi, U., Adamus, J., Bandiera, D. C., Brennhovd, I. O., Caceres, E., Cascinelli, N., Claudio, F., Ikonopisov, R. L., Javorskj, V. V., Kirov, S., Kulakowski, A., Lacour, Jr., Lejeune, F., Mechl, Z., Morabito, A., Rode, I., Sergeev, S., VanSlooten, E., Szczygiel, K., Trapeznikov, N. N., and Wagner, R. I., 1977. Inefficacy of immediate node dissection in stage I melanoma of the limbs. New England Journal of Medicine, 297: 627.

65. Wallace, D. C., Exton, L. A., and McLeod, G. R. 1971. Genetic factor in malignant melanoma. Cancer, 27: 1262.

66. Wanebo, H. J., Fortner, J. G., Woodruff, J., MacLean, B., and Binkowski, E. 1975. Selection of the optimum surgical treatment of stage I melanoma by depth of microinvasion: Use of the combined microstage technique (Clark-Breslow). Annals of Surgery, 182: 302.

67. Wechsler, H. L., and Fisher, E. R. 1962. Oral florid papillomatosis. Clinical, pathological, and electron microscopic observations. Archives of Dermatology, 86: 480.

68. Zacarian, S. A. 1977. Cryosurgery for Cancer of the Skin. In Zacarian, S. A., Ed. Cryosurgical Advances in Dermatology and Tumors of the Head and Neck. Charles C Thomas, Springfield, Ill., 68.

12 | Cancer of the Nasal Cavity and Paranasal Sinuses

George A. Sisson, M.D.
Stephen P. Becker, M.D.

INTRODUCTION

Cancer of the paranasal sinuses is so rare that individual surgeons see very few cases in a lifetime of practice unless special interest dictates their attention and study or some coincidental personal experience compels a sustained interest.

The latter was such the case for me (G.A.S.) when in 1960 my senior medical partner—a Professor of Otolaryngology at Upstate Medical Center, Syracuse—developed a cancer of the left maxillary sinus that was difficult to diagnose and to which, after five years, he succumbed at age 61. As a result, early in my practice this rare condition consumed much of my time, creating great frustration with humility.

ANATOMY

Nasal Fossa

If we are to treat tumors of the nasal fossa or paranasal sinuses surgically, the complex anatomy must be well understood by the surgeon. This anatomy is only learned by dedication and repetition.[12]

The nasal fossa begins at the pyriform aperture and consists of paired cavities divided from each other by the nasal septum. The cavities are triangular in shape being wide inferiorly and narrow superiorly. The anterior openings of the nasal cavities are the external nares, while posteriorly the nasal cavities are connected to the nasopharynx by the posterior choanae.

The interior of the nasal fossa is composed of a medial wall formed by the nasal septum, a lateral wall, roof, and floor. The septum is composed of the quadralateral cartilage anteriorly and the perpendicular plate of the ethmoid and the vomer posteriorly. The roof of the nasal fossa is formed by the cribriform plate, which separates the nasal cavity from the anterior cranial fossa. The floor of the nasal fossa is formed by the palatine process of the maxillary bones and the palatine bone and separates the nasal fossa from the oral cavity.

Projecting from the lateral nasal wall are three and sometimes four structures called turbinates (Fig. 12-1). These structures increase the functional surface of the nasal fossa. The inferior turbinate is a separate bone, while the middle and superior and, in cases where it is present, the supreme turbinate are part of the ethmoid bone. Each turbinate has a meatus beneath and lateral to it named for that turbinate. The inferior meatus consists of rather thin bone and contains the ostium of the nasolacrimal duct. The middle meatus is largely membranous and contains the ostia of the maxillary and anterior ethmoid sinus (Fig. 12-1).

The nasal fossa is lined by mucous membrane attached to the periosteum and perichondrium. This mucous membrane is pseudostratified ciliated columnar epithelium (respiratory membrane) containing

242

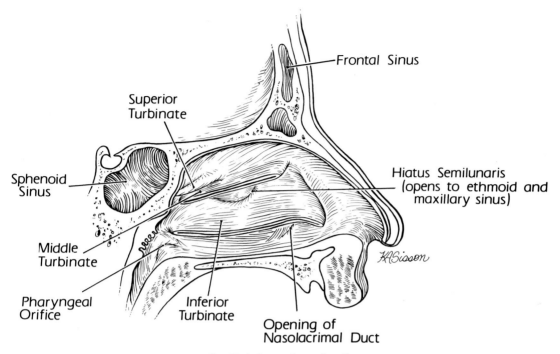

Fig. 12-1. Lateral nasal wall.

mucous and serous glands and is quite vascular. A limited area of the roof and superior aspect of the septum and lateral wall of the nasal fossa is lined by olfactory mucous membrane. It is a nonciliated epithelium and contains the olfactory nerve fibers, which pass through the cribiform plate from the anterior cranial fossa.

The mucosa of the nasal fossa is innervated by the anterior ethmoidal and maxillary nerves. The blood supply is derived from the branches of the sphenopalatine artery, the anterior and posterior ethmoid arteries, and the facial artery. Autonomic innervation comes by way of the greater superficial petrosal nerve. The important relationships of the nasal cavity are to the paranasal sinuses as discussed, the anterior cranial fossa superiorly, the oral cavity inferiorly, and the nasopharynx posteriorly.

Paranasal Sinuses

The paranasal sinuses begin their development as invaginations from the mucosa of the nasal fossa during the third and fourth

fetal months, with the maxillary and ethmoid air cells being present at birth.

MAXILLARY SINUS

The maxillary sinuses (maxillary antrum) are located in the body of the maxilla and are paired and usually symmetrical. The anterior wall is the facial surface of this sinus whereas the posterior wall relates to the infratemporal space and the pterygopalatine fossa. The floor of the antrum is the alveolar process of the maxilla and the roof of the antrum forms the major portion of the floor of the orbit (Fig. 12-2). The medial wall forms a portion of the lateral wall of the nasal fossa. The important relationships of the maxillary sinuses are, therefore, to the soft tissues of the face anteriorly, the orbit superiorly, and the teeth and oral cavity inferiorly.

The maxillary sinus is lined by a respiratory epithelium continuous with the nasal fossa and drains into the nasal fossa through its natural ostium in the middle meatus. The innervation and blood supply of the maxil-

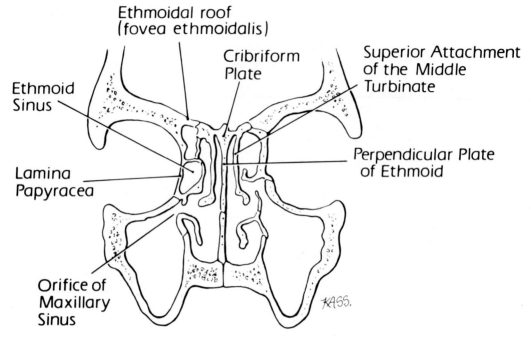

Fig. 12-2. Coronal section of maxillary and ethmoid sinus.

lary sinus comes by way of branches derived from the posterior-superior alveolar, infraorbital, and anterior-superior alveolar nerves and arteries.

ETHMOID SINUS

Three to eighteen air cells occupying each ethmoid sinus are formed by invaginations of nasal mucosa into the ethmoid bone. The anterior group of cells drain into the middle meatus, and the posterior group of cells drain into the sphenoethmoidal recess.

The roof of the ethmoid sinus (fovea ethmoidalis) along with the cribriform plate (the roof of the nasal cavity) form a portion of the floor of the anterior cranial fossa. The floor of the ethmoid labyrinth is separated from the supermedial aspect of the maxillary antrum by a thin plate of bone. The lateral wall of the ethmoid sinus is formed by the lamina papyracea, or paper plate, which as the name implies is extremely thin bone. The lacrimal bone just anterior to the lamina papyracea is also quite thin and makes up the anterior part of

the wall between the ethmoid sinus and the orbit. The medial wall of the ethmoid sinus is the middle meatus and turbinate.

The ethmoid air cells are lined by a respiratory epithelium continuous with the nasal fossa. The arterial supply is from the posterior nasal branches of the sphenopalatine artery as well as the anterior and posterior ethmoid arteries. The venous drainage is into the ophthalmic vein and the pterygoid plexus. Innervation is through the anterior and posterior ethmoidal branches, the first division of the trigeminal nerve. The important relationships of the ethmoid sinus are the maxillary sinus inferiorly, the nasal fossa medially, the orbit laterally, the optic nerve posteriorly, and the anterior cranial fossa superiorly (Fig. 12-2).

FRONTAL SINUS

The frontal sinuses are paired, often asymmetrical outgrowths of ethmoid air cells. They are separated by a partition called the interfrontal septum. The frontal sinus is lined by a respiratory epithelium continuous with the nasal fossa. The sinus drains through the nasofrontal duct into the middle meatus.

The blood supply is from branches of the supraorbital artery and the venous drainage to the supraorbital and superior ophthalmic veins. Nerve supply to the frontal sinus is derived from the supraorbital nerve.

The important relationships of the frontal sinus are with the soft tissues of the forehead anteriorly, the anterior cranial fossa posteriorly, and the orbit inferiorly.

SPHENOID SINUS

The sphenoid sinus is formed by the invagination of nasal mucosa into the sphenoid bone. The sinuses are generally paired and asymmetrical. They are lined with respiratory epithelium and drain into the sphenoethmoidal recess from the ostium in the anterior wall of each sinus. The blood supply is by way of branches of the sphenopalatine and posterior ethmoid arteries. The innervation is by way of the sphenopalatine ganglion and posterior ethmoidal nerves.

The important relationships of the sphenoid sinus are the nasal fossa anteriorly, the optic nerve and the cavernous sinus laterally, and the pituitary gland and anterior cranial fossa superiorly.

Lymphatics

The skin of the nose and vestibule drain primarily into the submandibular nodes. The mucosa of the nose is divided into an olfactory and a respiratory area. A rich lymphatic capillary network lines this mucosa. The respiratory area, which includes the middle and inferior turbinates, septum, and superior aspect of the floor of the nose, drains posteriorly in a horizontal fashion towards the nasopharynx (Fig. 12-3A). The lymphatic capillary networks converge on an area just anterior to the eustachian orifice on the lateral wall of the nasopharynx (pretubal plexus) (Fig. 12-3B). A posterior collecting channel from the pretubal plexus ends in the lateral pharyngeal lymph nodes near the base of the skull. From this point, lateral collecting channels terminate in the subdigastric nodes of the internal jugular chain.[13]

The lymphatic network of the olfactory region is in close contact with the perineural spaces of the penetrating olfactory nerves. The subarachnoid space follows the olfactory nerve fibers to a submucosal position

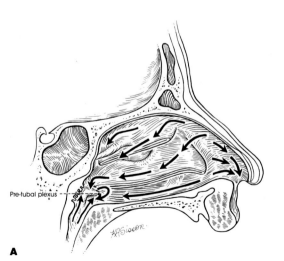

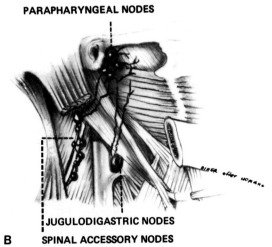

Fig. 12-3. (A) Lymphatic drainage of turbinates. (B) Lymphatic drainage from the retropharyngeal and parapharyngeal nodes. (Fig. 12-3B is modified from Fletcher, G. H., Healey, J. E., Jr., McGraw, J. P., and Million, R. R. 1967. Nasopharynx. In MacComb, W. S., and Fletcher, G. H., Eds. Cancer of the Head and Neck. © (1967) The Williams & Wilkins Co., Baltimore, 152.)

and it is thought that the submucosal lymphatic network in this area exists on both sides of the cribriform plate. The collecting trunks of the olfactory area along with the mucosa adjacent to it are directed posteriorly to terminate in the lateral retropharyngeal nodes.[13]

The ethmoid and maxillary sinuses are lined by a lymphatic capillary network that connects with the network of the nasal fossa. These lymphatics drain into the lateral retropharyngeal and/or the subdigastric nodes. The frontal and sphenoid sinuses also connect with the lymphatics of the nasal fossa and drain in a similar manner.

ETIOLOGY

The origin of cancer of the nose and sinuses is poorly understood. There is, however, thought to be an increased incidence of these malignancies in patients with a history of chronic sinusitis and protracted nasal polyposis.[8]

Of particular interest is an epidemiologic study published in the British Medical Journal in 1968.[1] This report offered strong evidence that woodworkers in the Buckinghamshire furniture industry were found to be at risk with respect to adenocarcinoma of the nasal cavity (particularly the turbinates) and ethmoid sinuses. The maxillary sinus was not a site of origin. There was a 500-fold increased risk in these workers. Machinists and cabinet workers were afflicted almost exclusively and had the greatest exposure to wood dust, which was the substance implicated as being carcinogenic. Carpenters and polishers had very little exposure to wood dust and only rarely contracted the disease.

Barton's excellent article[2] "Nickel Carcinogensis of the Respiratory Tract," which was the topic of the 1976 Schall Lecture at Harvard University, details the role of nickel as a carcinogen in cancer of the nose and paranasal sinuses. This relationship was first noted in a report of ten cases of squamous cell carcinoma, originating in the ethmoid sinuses, which had developed in 1921 and 1922 among nickel workers at a refinery in Wales where the so-called carbonyl process was employed. Changes in the process and the institution of methods of protection virtually eliminated this hazard among the nickel workers.

Such cancer has also been noted among the nickel workers in Canada, Russia, Germany, Japan, and Norway. In Norway, cancer of the nose and paranasal sinuses occurred at 28 times the expected rate in workers in a certain nickel works.[2] A program was instituted to modify the refining process and to protect the workers and monitor them with regular physical and x-ray examinations and blood and urine tests for nickel. This program appears to have resulted in a trend toward a gradual lowering of the rate of respiratory tract cancer.

Other workers for whom an occupational relation in cases of nasal or paranasal sinus cancer has been reported include boot makers, makers of mustard gas and isopropanol, and "luminizers" who were exposed to ionizing radiation while using radium paint on watch dials.

CLASSIFICATION

Tumors of the nose and paranasal sinuses can be classified as benign, intermediate, malignant, and tumor-like disease (Table 12-1).[27] Malignant tumors of the nose and paranasal sinuses make up 0.5 percent of all body tumors and 3 percent of all tumors of the upper respiratory tract. Fifty-nine percent involve the maxillary sinuses, 24 percent the nasal cavities, 16 percent the ethmoid sinuses, and less than 1 percent involve either the sphenoid or frontal sinuses. When considering the paranasal sinuses alone, 77 percent of malignancies arise in the maxillary sinuses, 22 percent in the ethmoid sinuses, and less than 1 percent in the sphenoid and frontal sinuses.

TABLE 12-1. TUMORS OF THE NOSE
AND PARANASAL SINUSES

I. Benign
  A. Soft tissue
    1. Epithelial
      a. Papilloma
        (1) Squamous cell
        (2) Epithelial
      b. Adenoma
      c. Dermoid
      d. Nevus
      e. Mixed tumor
      f. Oncocytoma
    2. Connective tissue
      a. Nasal glioma
      b. Myxoma
      c. Meningioma
      d. Fibroma
      e. Hemangioma
      f. Lymphangioma
      g. Chondroma
      h. Ganglioneuroma
      i. Neurilemmoma
      j. Lipoma
      k. Hamartoma

  B. Osseous
    1. Primary osseous (nonodontogenic)
      a. Osteoma
      b. Exostoses (torus)
      c. Osteoid osteoma
      d. Giant cell lesions
        (1) Giant cell reparative granuloma
        (2) Giant cell tumor
        (3) Osteitis fibrosa cystica
        (4) Cherubism
      e. Cysts
        (1) Median fissural
        (2) Simple unicameral
        (3) Aneurysmal bone
    2. Odontogenic
      a. Epithelial
        (1) Cysts
          (a) Dentigerous
          (b) Radicular
        (2) Ameloblastoma (adamantinoma)
        (3) Pindborg (calcifying epithelial odontogenic tumor)
        (4) Adenoblastoma
        (5) Ameloblastic fibroma
      b. Mesodermal
        (1) Myxoma
        (2) Fibroma
          (a) Odontogenic
          (b) Cementifying
        (3) Dentinoma
        (4) Cementoma
      c. Mixed (epithelial and mesodermal)
        (1) Ameloblastic fibroma
        (2) Ameloblastic odontoma
        (3) Ameloblastic hemangioma
        (4) Ameloblastic neurilemmoma
        (5) Odontoma

II. Intermediate
  A. Soft Tissue
    1. Epithelial
      a. Inverting papilloma
      b. Basal cell
      c. Ameloblastoma
      d. Leukoplakia
    2. Connective tissue
      a. Angiofibroma
      b. Esthesioneuroblastoma
      c. Chordoma
      d. Plasmacytoma
      e. Rathke's pouch tumors
        (1) Craniopharyngioma
        (2) Intracranial cysts
    3. Fibro-osseous
      a. Ossifying fibroma
      b. Fibrous osteoma
      c. Fibrous dysplasia
      d. Desmoplastic fibroma

III. Malignant
  A. Soft tissue
    1. Epithelial
      a. Carcinoma in situ
      b. Squamous cell carcinoma
      c. Adenocarcinoma
      d. "Spindle cell" carcinoma
      e. Undifferentiated carcinoma
      f. Lymphoepithelial carcinoma
      g. Malignant melanoma
      h. Minor salivary gland tumors
        (1) Malignant mixed
        (2) Adenoid cystic carcinoma (cylindroma)
        (3) Mucoepidermoid
      i. Metastatic carcinoma
    2. Connective tissue
      a. Wegner granulomatosis (malignant histiocytoma, lethal midline granuloma)

TABLE 12-1—CONTINUED

      b. Rhabdomyosarcoma
          (1) Embryonal (sarcoma botryoides)
          (2) Alveolar
          (3) Pleomorphic
      c. Fibrosarcoma
      d. Angiosarcoma
      e. Lymphosarcoma
      f. Reticulum cell sarcoma
      g. Myxosarcoma
      h. Chondrosarcoma
   3. Osseous
      a. Osteogenic sarcoma
      b. Ewing sarcoma
      c. Malignant giant cell tumor

IV. Tumor-like lesions
   A. Mucocele
   B. Pyocele
   C. Pyogenic granuloma
   D. Granuloma gravidarum
   E. Rhinoscleroma
   F. Nasal polyp
   G. Sarcoidosis
   H. Amyloidosis
   I. Infections
      1. Tuberculosis
      2. Syphilis
      3. Fungal
         a. Actinomycosis
         b. Blastomycosis
         c. Rhinosporidiosis
         d. Coccidioidomycosis
         e. Aspergillosis
         f. Candida
         g. Mucormycosis

(Adapted from Sisson, G. A., and Goldstein, J. C. 1973. Tumors of the nose, paranasal sinuses and nasopharynx. In Paparella, M. M., and Shumrick, D. A., Eds.: Otolaryngology, Vol. III: Head and Neck. W. B. Saunders, Philadelphia, 123.)

Squamous cell carcinoma is the predominant malignant tumor type, being present in 80 percent of the patients studied. In general, well-differentiated squamous cell carcinomas appear to arise in the anterior nasal cavity and antrum; the more undifferentiated tumors arise in the posterior ethmoid cells and posterior nasal cavity. These carcinomas spread by local extension with few nodal metastases even at late stages of the disease. Most of the information available in the literature having to do with lymphatic spread and treatment according to the biologic behavior of carcinoma of the paranasal sinuses is based upon the experience with squamous cell carcinoma.

Marchetta et al.[20] in 1969, in their series of 119 cases, noted that by the time the diagnosis of cancer was made, there was in every patient extension beyond the confines of the maxillary antrum to the orbit, nasal cavity, oral cavity, or skin of the cheek. It should not be surprising then that the 5-year cure rate runs about 25 percent,[3] usually due to late diagnosis.

The grading of these tumors from well differentiated to undifferentiated often shows a peculiar shift in the same patient when followed over a long period of time. What starts out as a well-differentiated lesion may, when seen as a recurrence, be graded as poorly differentiated. The reverse is seldom true.

Included with the undifferentiated tumors are lymphoepitheliomas. The lymphoepithelioma most frequently occurs in the nasopharynx and is a poorly differentiated epithelial cancer with a predominant lymphoid stroma. When it occurs in the posterior nasal cavity it behaves in a similar fashion producing characteristic early metastases to the spinal accessory and upper deep jugular nodes and is usually sensitive to radiation therapy. The survival rate is approximately 30 percent.

The association of inverting papilloma with squamous cell carcinoma must be recognized.[32] The inverting papilloma causes unilateral nasal obstruction and occurs most often in males aged 50 to 70. The anatomic site of origin is the lateral nasal wall and ethmoid sinus. This neoplasm has a tendency for early recurrence and in 10 to 15 percent of cases is associated with invasive squamous cell carcinoma at some time within the course of the disease. Wide local resection of the entire lateral nasal wall including the ethmoid sinus is required for cure. Serial and sometimes subserial sections of the entire specimen are necessary, since areas of malignancy can coexist with areas of benign papilloma. Some mitotic activity in the basal layers is acceptable, but where there is marked increase in mitosis or atypia of the cells, serial sections should be sought. Recurrent lesions should likewise be treated with suspicion of malignant potential even if the initial lesion was benign.

Malignant melanomas comprise about 1 percent of nasal and paranasal sinus cancers. Melanomas manifest local multicentricity known as satellitosis and metastasize early by vascular and lymphatic pathways. When detected in the nose, a polypoid growth pattern is seen. Slate gray, blue, or black color is present in 45 percent of intranasal cases. Results of treatment were reviewed in 1973 by Freedman et al.[9] When studied according to site of origin, patients with intranasal melanoma (44 percent 5-year survival rate) were found to have a better prognosis than those with melanoma arising in the paranasal sinuses (none alive at 5 years).

In those patients with melanoma whose primary treatment was surgical resection the 5-year survival rate was 61.3 percent as compared to 34.2 percent for those treated with radiation either before or after surgery.[9] No patient treated primarily by radiation survived 5 years. Death is most often due to local recurrence or distant metastases. Regional nodal metastases are not as important in this entity as in other head and neck malignancies.[31] Radical local surgery with extensive removal of mucosa may help to prevent local recurrence because of the multicentric nature of the mucosal lesions. Survival data indicate a constant risk of death by melanoma no matter how long after treatment the patient lives, in contrast to other lesions in which there is a marked drop in the risk of death after the patient survives 1 or 2 years. The response of mucosal melanoma to chemotherapy is poor as compared to some of the encouraging results with skin lesions. Immunotherapy has recently been advocated for patients with advanced lesions as well as for those with distant metastasis.

Adenocarcinomas make up 10 to 14 percent of all nasal and paranasal sinus malignancies. Included in this group are the adenoid cystic carcinomas. This group of tumors is thought to arise in the minor salivary glands of the hard palate and then to penetrate to the nasal cavity and maxillary antrum. Conley and Dingman[5] have shown that these tumors can spread intracranially along nerve trunks and manifest their presence many years after initial resection. Recent evidence shows that surgery is the only type of treatment associated with control of disease. However, when dealing with adenoid cystic carcinoma, many surgeons include postoperative radiotherapy as an adjunct in hopes of sterilizing areas of perineural spread. Adenocarcinomas (other than cylindromas) are most often seen in the ethmoid and maxillary sinuses where they demonstrate three growth patterns—sessile, papillary, and alveolar mucoid. When these lesions exhibit a papillary pattern, they have a similarity to carcinoma of the colon.[3] Metastases from adenocarcinoma are infrequent. The mechanism of spread is by invasion and destruction of the adjacent soft tissue and bone. Even with radical surgery and adjunctive radiation therapy, the survival rate is only 20 percent over 5 years.

Cancers of mesodermal origin constitute 5 percent of malignant tumors of the nose and paranasal sinuses. These include ameloblastomas, fibrosarcomas, chondrosarcomas, osteogenic sarcomas, plasmacytomas, rhabdomyosarcomas, and lymphomas. Fibrosarcomas, chondrosarcomas, and osteogenic sarcomas are treated in a similar fashion to other sinus and nasal malignancies even though the sarcomas are more difficult, and in most cases, impossible to control. In our experience of five cases of chondrosarcoma, all responded to irradiation in varying degrees.

Rhabdomyosarcomas are aggressive tumors most often occurring in children and the elderly. Children with embryonal rhabdomyosarcomas have a survival rate of 20 to 35 percent but some encouraging results have been obtained more recently, the results of which were reported in 1974 by the Memorial Sloan-Kettering Cancer Center in New York.[6a] These investigators used surgical extirpation of all the tumor or as much of it as possible followed by chemotherapy and irradiation (4,500 to 7,000 rads). Chemotherapy consisted of cycles of sequential administration of dactinomycin, Adriamycin, vincristine, and cyclophosphamide. Patients with Stage I through Stage IV disease were treated. Of the 29 patients treated, 24 (82 percent) continued to survive with no evidence of disease for periods ranging from 4 to 42 months.

Patients with extramedullary plasmacytomas, when solitary lesions, have a 5-year survival rate of 50 to 60 percent. Treatment is with radiation therapy and surgery.

Various types of extranodal non-Hodgkins lymphoma may arise in the paranasal sinuses (see Ch. 26 for more details).

Neurogenic tumors comprise less than 1 percent of sinus and nasal tumors. The two major types encountered are the olfactory neuroblastoma (esthesioneuroepithelioma) and malignant schwannomas. The olfactory neuroblastoma arises from the olfactory bulb high in the nasal fossa but can be also encountered in the maxillary and ethmoid sinuses and nasal floor. The primary mode of therapy is wide surgical excision and radiotherapy with the 5-year survival rate at 50 percent. Recurrences may often occur much later than the 5-year period and distant metastases are not rare, occurring most frequently in the cervical lymph nodes, lungs, and long bones.[30]

Metastases to the nose and paranasal sinuses from other primaries make up about 1 percent of malignancies found in this area. The most frequent is renal cell carcinoma. Others are undifferentiated tumors from lung, breast, prostate, and pancreas. The overall prognosis in these situations is extremely poor; therefore, it is important to determine the site of the origin of the primary cancer before considering debilitating therapy for sinus malignancies.

Special Characteristics of Nasal Cavity Tumors

The nasal cavity and paranasal sinuses are intimately related in this complex anatomic area. Malignant tumors in this area overgrow natural boundaries and usually involve two or more anatomic sites by the time the diagnosis is made. When we classify the site of origin of tumors in this area, we find that more adenocarcinomas arise in the nasal fossa and ethmoid than in the maxilla. Lymphomas occur as often in the nasal cavity as in the maxilla, while melanomas are found in equal numbers in the nasal cavity and the ethmoids.[18]

It is rare for a malignancy to arise as a primary within the nasal cavity but when it does occur, it is more common in males and 15 percent of the patients give a past history of chronic sinusitis or polyposis. Squamous cell carcinoma is the most frequent cancer and usually arises as a polypoid or papillary lesion from the lateral nasal wall.[3]

The well-differentiated low grade squamous cell carcinoma found in the area of the columella and nasal ala has been referred to as the "nose pickers' " cancer. This lesion arises in the area of the septum at the mucocutaneous junction or laterally in the nasal vestibule. The nasal vestibule includes the area inside the opening of the nose encircled by the crura of the lower lateral cartilage and is lined with skin. Tumors arising in this site present with symptoms such as local soreness or burning. These cancers metastasize rarely but when they do it is to lymph nodes in the submandibular region adjacent to the facial artery and vein.[7] Nasal fossa malignancies are best treated by wide local surgical resecton. If nodes are palpated, then a neck dissection is indicated followed by postoperative irradiation.

Tumors arising on the nasal septum are more aggressive than those arising laterally in the vestibule. While wide local resection is again the preferred treatment, the surgeon must be certain that the posterior and superior margins of the resection are clear of disease because recurrences are common. Neck dissections are indicated for palpable metastatic lymph node deposits. Postoperative radiotherapy has also been found to be useful in selected cases.[3]

The esthesioneuroblastoma arises from the olfactory bulb in the roof of the nasal cavity. Lesions arising in this area can grow to immense size, causing deviation of the nasal bone, and may fill almost the entire nasal cavity prior to detection. These tumors may also involve the ethmoid and maxillary sinuses. The extent of any of these intranasal lesions often cannot be determined until surgical exploration at the time of biopsy and staging.

Tumors involving the posterior part of the nasal cavity have a pattern of lymphatic spread similar to that of the antral-ethmoid complex, and occasionally the retropharyngeal and upper deep jugular nodes are involved and palpable.

PATIENT EVALUATION

Signs and Symptoms

The most ominous symptoms of tumors arising from the nose are nasal obstruction and bleeding. Obstruction is usually relatively long-standing. Unfortunately, nasal obstruction and bleeding are also symptoms of chronic inflammatory disease, so that oftentimes these symptoms are not given the full consideration that they warrant. It is very difficult indeed on the basis of the symptoms of obstruction and nasal bleeding to know whether a tumor is primary in the nasal fossa or arises in the paranasal sinuses with extension to the nasal fossa.

Other symptoms include pain localized to the area of the nose or paranasal sinuses. Pain in the upper teeth may represent invasion of tumor into the alveolar nerve. Lateral nasal swelling may result from infiltration of the overlying bone or infiltration of the skin by a tumor arising primarily in the nasal fossa, maxillary antrum, or ethmoid sinus. Frontal headache may be due to direct extension to the anterior fossa by way of the cribriform plate. Headache and facial pain may also be due to secondary infection of the paranasal sinuses due to obstruction of the natural ostium of the sinus by intranasal tumor.

The most common symptom of tumor in the maxillary-ethmoid complex is unilateral nasal bleeding or atypical facial or gum pain. This may be a straightforward event such as persistent or recurrent mild epistaxis or may be subtle such as the patient seeing specks of blood, mixed with mucus, on the handkerchief after he blows his nose. The pain may be intermittent and lancinating or a constant dull ache, like a toothache. Unilateral nasal obstruction due to growth of tumor from the sinuses into the nasal cavity is also quite common. Patients with cancer of the maxillary sinus in late stages often present with a mass overlying the antrum due to extension of tumor through the bony anterior wall. In such cases, a mass will be palpable obliterating the gingivobuccal sulcus. The overlying skin may also be infiltrated and have a reddened appearance as with inflammation. There may be numbness in the area of the distribution of the infraorbital nerve, due to destruction of the nerve in its canal or in the soft tissues. Numbness of the teeth due to direct infiltration of the anterior-superior and/or posterior-superior alveolar nerves may also occur (Fig. 12-4). Infiltration of these nerves may result in retrograde perineural spread of tumor into the middle cranial fossa.

The patient may present with a mass in the maxillary alveolus or the palate itself due to growth of the tumor inferiorly. Some patients complain of a feeling that their dentures are not fitting well, while others complain of ulceration of the palate or antral-oral fistula. Posterior extension of these tumors may invade and destroy the pterygoid plate or the internal pterygoid muscle

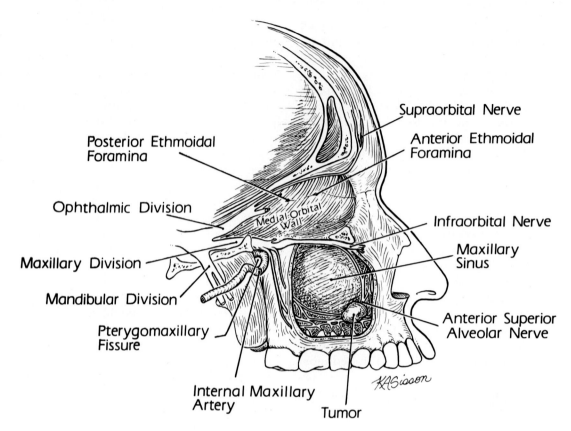

Fig. 12-4. Relationship of nerves to maxillary sinus.

causing trismus (Fig. 12-5) and, occasionally, middle ear effusion secondary to functional obstruction of the eustachian tube. Direct invasion of the infraorbital canal and nerve may result in numbness of the face and may be the pathway for intracranial extension through the foramen rotundum into the middle cranial fossa. Invasion of the sphenopalatine nerve may result in anesthesia of the palate. Posterior extension may involve the mucosa of the nasopharynx, and this involvement renders the patient technically inoperable.

Superior extension of cancer from the sinus into the orbit may produce proptosis, resulting in diplopia caused by displacement of the eye.

Tumors arising in the ethmoid sinuses also may present with unilateral nasal obstruction and bleeding. In the more advanced stages of the disease, invasion through the fovea ethmoidalis into the anterior cranial fossa with symptoms of headache or increased intracranial pressure may occur. Downward and lateral displacement of the eye due to invasion through the lamina papyracea to the orbit may also occur. Occasionally, there may be invasion of the skin of the medial canthus with fungation of the tumor through this area.

Symptoms referable to the frontal sinus are usually unilateral nasal bleeding, pain in the frontal area, an obvious mass in the frontal area, and headache from local causes as well as from involvement of the anterior cranial fossa. Proptosis due to invasion of the orbit and displacement of the orbital contents may result in diplopia. Since mucoceles are more common in the frontal sinuses than malignancies and cause similar signs and symptoms, this condition must be excluded early in the differential diagnosis.

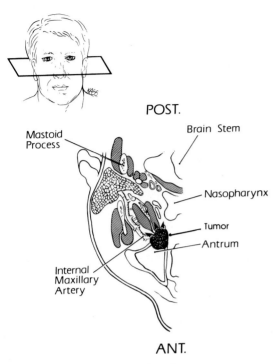

POST.

Mastoid Process

Brain Stem

Nasopharynx

Tumor

Antrum

Internal Maxillary Artery

ANT.

Fig. 12-5. Relationship of pterygomaxillary space to maxillary sinus.

Symptoms referable to the sphenoid are deep boring retro-ocular pain, proptosis, headache, blindness due to optic nerve destruction, and cranial nerve paralyses due to involvement of the cavernous sinus.

Physical Examination

Thorough inspection of the nasal cavity is essential. This requires adequate light, a nasal speculum, and suction. Suction of these friable and infected tumors often produces bleeding, which, though brisk at times, does not necessarily indicate that the tumor is vascular. Only rarely may one determine from the speculum examination the exact site of origin.

The nasopharynx must also be examined either by way of an indirect mirror or direct examination with the fiberoptic nasopharyngoscope. This examination is most important, since infiltration of the mucosa of the nasopharynx is a contraindication to surgery. The oral cavity must also be exam-

ined in order to ascertain whether there is trismus or whether frank tumor is present. When palpation of the canine fossa reveals a mass or softening of the underlying bone, this indicates that the anterior wall of the antrum has been invaded and partially destroyed by neoplasm. The function of the cranial nerves must also be evaluated, with particular attention to the 5th cranial nerve. The soft tissues of the face should be examined in order to ascertain whether a mass is present and if so, whether the skin is fixed by infiltration. The eyes must be examined to ascertain whether there is displacement or fixation of the globe. The neck must be thoroughly palpated to determine the presence or absence of nodes. In our experience with over 150 cases, only 10 percent metastasized to the cervical lymph nodes.

Patterns of Spread

Both benign and malignant lesions arising either in the nasal cavity or the paranasal sinuses may encroach upon surrounding structures at some time in their stage of development. Local spread will depend upon the primary site of origin. Tumors arising in the *infrastructure of the maxillary sinus* may spread inferiorly into the alveolar process or the gingivobuccal sulcus, or they may spread into the soft tissues of the cheek below the zygoma causing pain or anesthesia due to involvement of the maxillary divisions of the trigeminal nerve. They may extend medially into the nasal cavity or hard palate, sometimes with swelling of the nasolabial fold but infrequently with pain. Rarely will these tumors spread posteriorly to involve the pterygoid plates.

Tumors arising in the *suprastructure of the maxillary sinus* may spread anterolaterally into the zygoma, causing trigeminal pain, or posterolaterally into the infratemporal fossa and may cause trismus. Tumor may spread superiorly and medially into the ethmoid sinuses and cribriform plate. Early orbital involvement with eye deviation and proptosis is not uncommon and gives these tumors a poor prognosis. Epiphora is frequent due to blockage of the nasolacrimal duct. Posteriorly, the tumor may extend into the pterygoid space, sphenoid sinuses, or base of the skull. Spread into the pterygoid space may involve the trigeminal nerve. Absent or decreased corneal reflex is usually due to involvement of the sphenopalatine ganglion.

Ethmoid sinus tumors may spread inferolaterally into the antrum through the ethmoidomaxillary plate or laterally into the orbit. Medial spread will involve turbinates and even the septum. Posterior spread usually involves the sphenoid sinus, nasopharynx, or base of the skull. Superior extension may involve the frontal sinus, cribriform plate, or the anterior cranial fossa.

Frontal sinus tumors may spread anteriorly producing a mass in the forehead often with secondary infection or inferiorly into the ethmoid sinuses and orbit. Posterior extension will involve the dura and even the frontal lobes. If these tumors extend medially, the other frontal sinus will be involved.

Sphenoid sinus tumors may spread inferiorly into the nasopharynx, which makes them difficult to differentiate from primary nasopharyngeal cancer. Superior extension will involve the middle cranial fossa, and lateral extension will involve the superior orbital fissure. The posterior ethmoid cells and nasal cavity will be involved with anterior extension. Medial extension will involve the other sphenoid.

The routes of lymphatic flow from the nose and paranasal sinuses are major pathways of metastatic dissemination of carcinoma involving this region. The direction of spread depends on the site of involvement. Expanding lesions of the paranasal sinuses often involve the deep structures of the orbit and may invade the deep dermal lid lymphatics and the tarsal plexus of lymphatics. These drain to collecting trunks in the medial and lateral canthi. The medial collecting trunks follow the facial vein into the prevascular or postvascular nodes of the submandibular group. The lateral collecting area drains to the periglandular parotid nodes.[13]

Lesions of the maxillary sinus that penetrate and involve the buccal or gingival aspect of the mucosa may drain through the lymphatics to the submandibular nodes. However, if the lingual aspect of the gingival or the palatal mucosa is involved, tumor cells flow to the retropharyngeal and, thence, to the upper deep jugular nodes.[13] While this posterior spread has been taught and mentioned in the literature for many years, our experience has revealed a palpable mass or node in the retropharyngeal space in only 3 percent of cases.

As already noted, malignant tumors of the paranasal sinuses spread by an embolic phenomenon through the lymphatics to the regional areas but may also be disseminated through hematogenous spread to distant sites such as the liver, brain, lungs, and spine. We have observed spread to all of these distant metastatic sites, although such spread is rare. Certain types of tumor, such as adenoid cystic carcinoma, spread by perineural invasion. Melanoma, the unpredictable cancer, almost always spreads to distant sites by hematogenous pathways.

The signs and symptoms produced by tumors are, then, not only directly related to variabilities of the specific tumors but also to the anatomic relationships of the adjacent structures to the nose and paranasal sinuses.

Defining Extent of Disease

Defining the site and extent of the disease is important for formulating a treatment plan, predicting prognosis, and reporting results of treatment. Two noninvasive radiologic studies can assist in defining the extent of disease, computerized tomography (CT scanning) and polytomography.

It must be emphasized that these tests are not pathognomonic of sinus cancer, as false negatives as high as 30 percent were encountered in our series and have been reported by others. An exploratory antrostomy is the only certain test to determine if and where the cancer is present in the sinuses. It is the only sure way the extent may be staged.

Bone destruction on x-ray examination is the finding most indicative of squamous cell carcinoma of the antrum. Polytomography of these areas further outlines the areas of bone destruction, such as that occurring in the nasoantral wall, orbit, or clivus.

It should be remembered that a tumor can obstruct a sinus ostium and cause opacification by secretions, thus creating a false impression of malignant involvement. Computerized tomography is of value in outlining tumors and in differentiating a soft-tissue mass in a sinus from a fluid-filled sinus. CT scanning is better than polytomography for visualizing the limits of a soft-tissue mass and may be equal to it in outlining bone destruction.[15] CT scans are well suited to the delineation of tumor invasion of the orbital and retro-orbital areas, and orbital displacement may be readily demonstrated (Figs. 12-6A and B). It is also useful for assessment of intracranial extension in the area of the base of the skull, i.e., cribriform plate, ethmoid roof, planum sphenoidale, or pituitary fossa.[15] Patients with known esthesioneuroblastoma or ethmoid

carcinoma should be studied for intracranial extension, as this is a part of the biologic behavior of these tumors. Demonstration of intracranial extension may not be successful in tumors that have the same density as the surrounding brain tissue. If the tumor is avascular, contrast enhancement will not improve tumor detection. CT scanning also improves the outlining of nasopharyngeal masses.[15] While most sinus malignancies are avascular, preoperative angiography is used when the lesion is suspected to be vascular, is possibly invading or bound to a major vascular structure, or is likely to be an angiofibroma of the nasopharynx extending into the nose or sinuses.

Biopsy

All malignant tumors of the nose and paranasal sinuses must be biopsied and submitted for a histopathologic examination before diagnosis and treatment are possible.

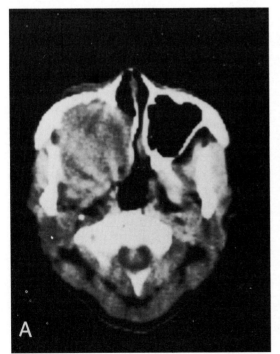 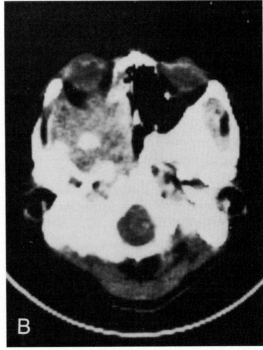

Fig. 12-6. (A) CT scan through the maxillary sinuses demonstrating extensive sarcoma with bone destruction of the left antrum. (B) Same tumor demonstrating involvement of orbit, ethmoids, and base of skull on the left side.

This is of enormous importance because many of the signs, symptoms, and radiographic findings are the same in both benign and malignant disease. A good example is a mucocele of the frontal sinus causing x-ray evidence of bone destruction.

BIOPSY OF NASAL LESION

A tissue mass presenting in the nasal cavity may be primary in that location, may be an expression of tumor growth from any one of the paranasal sinuses, or, in rare instances, may prove to be from a distant origin, such as from hypernephroma in the kidney. Biopsy in the nasal cavity may be performed under local anesthesia utilizing both topical and local infiltration. The addition of adrenalin to the local anesthetic will help to reduce bleeding in this vascular area. A good light source, suction, and trained assistance facilitate the procedure.

Generous amounts of tissue should be taken, especially from the interior of the mass because many of these tumors are inflamed and necrotic on their periphery. In addition, different areas of the cancer may vary in histologic features, especially tumors of minor salivary gland origin. Since many of the tissues in this area provide difficulty in diagnosis even under the best of circumstances, care should be taken not to crush the tissue as crushing may create artifacts. Packing may be necessary at the completion of the procedure to control bleeding.

EXPLORATION AND BIOPSY OF THE MAXILLARY ANTRUM (A MINI-CALDWELL-LUC OPERATION)

If the suspicion of carcinoma of the maxillary antrum arises, the radiographs are equivocal, and no abnormal tissue is present in the nasal cavity, then an exploratory antrostomy should be performed. This procedure may be performed under local anesthesia with an incision in the inferior portion of the canine fossa. This incision permits removal of the biopsy site at the time of a definitive surgery. The anterior wall of the sinus is removed in order to visualize its interior. If preoperative irradiation is to be considered, a nasoantral window assists in drainage of the necrotic antral contents during radiation.

BIOPSY OR EXPLORATION OF THE ETHMOID FOR DIAGNOSIS

If no abnormal tissue is present in the nasal cavity but the index of suspicion is high, an ethmoidectomy may be necessary for biopsy. Several techniques are available and will be described in some detail. An intranasal ethmoidectomy approach for biopsy can be performed. The anterior tip of the middle turbinate is removed by scissors and snare and the anterior ethmoid cells and bulla are entered. It is important to palpate the roof of the ethmoid, which is at the level of the superior attachment of the middle turbinate. Tissue can then be removed for biopsy. Caution should be utilized when biopsying in the posterior ethmoid cells because of the proximity of the optic nerve. The lateral wall (lamina papyracea) must also be respected in order to avoid injury to the orbital contents.

Some surgeons prefer to biopsy via the external ethmoidectomy approach because they believe it is a safer technique. This is carried out through an incision in the area of the medial canthus. The incision is taken down to bone. The medial canthal ligament is detached and the lacrimal sac displaced from the lacrimal groove. The periorbita is then separated from the bone. The frontoethmoidal suture is identified at its origin at the superior aspect of the lacrimal bone. The anterior and posterior ethmoidal arteries are identified and preserved as landmarks. This is extremely important because in most cases the roof of the ethmoid and, therefore, the cranial cavity will be at or just above this landmark.

The ethmoid sinus may then be entered through the thin bone of the lacrimal fossa and lamina papyracea. Often these bones will have been destroyed by the pathologic process in the ethmoid. Tissue may then be removed for biopsy purposes. At the time of exploration, if the surgeon feels that this lesion may be benign, all tissue should be removed from the ethmoid labyrinth. This may be done with the use of an operating microscope. By cautiously following the roof of the ethmoid posteriorly, the sphenoid sinus may also be identified and entered for exploration and biopsy.

Our preference for biopsy is via the intranasal route because an external route might well lead to unnecessary local manipulation and spread of the cancer.

EXPLORATION AND BIOPSY OF THE SPHENOID SINUS

The sphenoid sinus may be approached through either a transantroethmoid or transseptal route. The transseptal view gives better exposure of the roof of the sphenoid and the transantroethmoid view affords a better exposure of the posterior wall of the sinus.

The transseptal approach is begun by elevating the mucoperichondrium off the left side of the cartilaginous portion of the nasal septum. The septum is divided caudally just anterior to the perpendicular plate of the ethmoid and vomer and then detached inferiorly from the crest of the maxilla and nasal spine. The mucoperiosteum is elevated from both sides of the posterior bony nasal septum. A sublabial incision is then started by incising the mucosa in the canine fossa. The periosteum is elevated exposing the pyriform aperture and nasal spine. A rim of bone is removed from the pyriform aperture and the nasal spine is lowered. A hypophysectomy speculum is inserted and the bony nasal septum removed up to the rostrum of the sphenoid sinus. For orientation, a cross table lateral radiograph of the sphenoid sinus may be obtained by using a C-arm image intensifier. The rostrum and a portion of the anterior wall of the sphenoid sinus is removed with a sphenoid punch. The interior of the sphenoid sinus can then be examined and biopsied.

BIOPSY OR EXPLORATION OF THE FRONTAL SINUS FOR DIAGNOSIS

This approach is quite similar to the trephine operation used for acute frontal sinusitis. An incision should be made in the supermedial aspect of the medial canthus along the floor of the frontal sinus. It is placed posterior to the supraorbital ridge and should be approximately 2 cm in length. A scalpel is used to carry the dissection directly down to the periosteum. The periosteum is elevated with a small periosteal elevator, and the sinus is entered by drilling through the bone with a cutting burr. Delicate curettes and cup forceps can then be used to remove portions of suspicious tissue for biopsy.[21]

TABLE 12-2 SISSON'S 1963 CLASSIFICATIONS OF TUMOR STAGING FOR MAXILLARY SINUS CANCER

T1a	Invasion anterior wall
T1b	Invasion nasoantral wall
T1c	Invasion anteromedial palate (Fig. 12-7)
T2a	Invasion lateral wall not involving muscle
T2b	Invasion superior wall not involving orbit (Fig. 12-8)
T3a	Invasion pterygoid muscle
T3b	Invasion orbit
T3c	Invasion anterior ethmoid cells but not cribriform plate
T3d	Invasion anterior wall with skin involvement (Fig. 12-9)
T4a	Invasion cribriform plate
T4b	Invasion pterygomaxillary fossa
T4c	Extension to nasal fossa or contralateral antrum
T4d	Invasion pterygoid plates
T4e	Invasion posterior ethmoid cells
T4f	Extension to ethmoid—sphenoid recess or sphenoid sinus (Fig. 12-10)

N and M classification as with other neoplasms.

(Adapted from Sisson, G. A., Johnson, N. E., and Amiri, C. S. 1963. Cancer of the maxillary sinus: Clinical classification and management. Annals of Otology, Rhinology and Laryngology, 72:1050.)

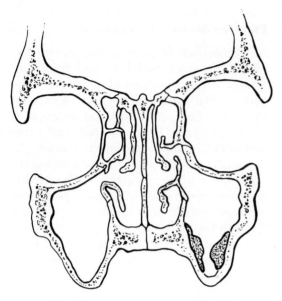

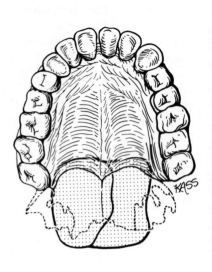

Fig. 12-7. T1 antral carcinoma.

CLASSIFICATION

It is evident that proper staging enables the surgeon to apply therapy in a systematic and effective manner. It also helps to predict prognosis and permit comparison of treatment regimens. The senior author in 1963, using Ohngren's lines as guides, attempted to apply the basics of the TNM system to the sinuses, which had not heretofore been included in a TNM system of staging[28] (Table 12-2).

Ohngren,[23] who first classified sinus tumors over 40 years ago, described an imaginary line that divided the superior ana-

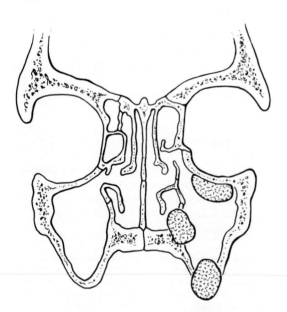

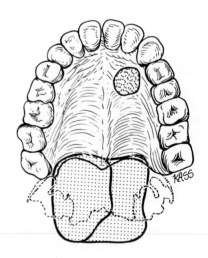

Fig. 12-8. T2 antral carcinoma.

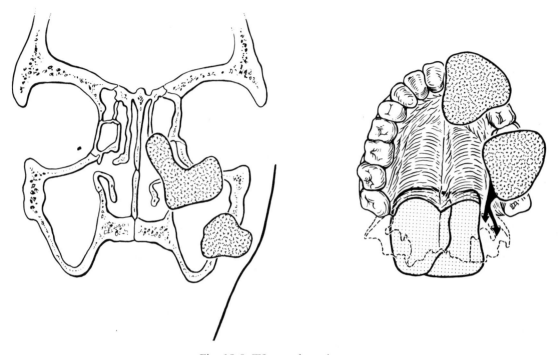

Fig. 12-9. T3 antral carcinoma.

tomic portions of the paranasal sinuses from the inferior. The line extended from the medial canthus of the eye to the angle of the mandible and divided the maxillary sinus into an anterior-inferior and posterior-superior portion. This has been referred to as Ohngren's line. He then made a gross correlation that if tumor were posterior-superior the prognosis was poor.

Not until 1978 was a TNM system adopted by the Joint Committee on Staging and essentially it was an improved revision of the 1963 Sisson TNM system (Table 12-3).

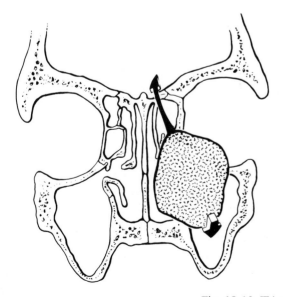

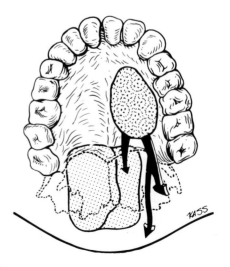

Fig. 12-10. T4 antral carcinoma.

TABLE 12-3 TNM CLASSIFICATION OF MAXILLARY SINUS CANCER, AJC 1978

Primary Tumor (T)

TX   Tumor that cannot be assessed by rules

T0   No evidence of primary tumor

T1   Tumor confined to the antral mucosa of the infrastructure with no bone erosion or destruction

T2   Tumor confined to the suprastructure mucosa without bone destruction of medial or inferior
bony walls only

T3   More extensive tumor invading skin of cheek, orbit, anterior ethmoid sinuses, or pterygoid muscle

T4   Massive tumor with invasion of cribriform plate, posterior ethmoids, sphenoid nasopharynx, pterygoid
plates, or base of skull

Nodal Involvement (N)

NX   Nodes cannot be assessed

N0   No clinically positive node

N1   Single clinically positive homolateral node 3 cm or less in diameter

N2   Single clinically positive homolateral node more than 3 cm but not more than 6 cm in diameter

   N2a   Single clinically positive homolateral node more than 3 cm but not more than 6 cm in diameter

   N2b   Multiple clinically positive homolateral nodes, none more than 6 cm in diameter

N3   Massive homolateral node(s), bilateral nodes, or contralateral node(s)

   N3a   Clinically positive homolateral node(s), one more than 6 cm in diameter

   N3b   Bilateral clinically positive nodes (in this situation, each side of the neck should be staged separately;
that is, N3b; right, N2a; left, N1)

   N3c   Contralateral clinically positive node(s) only

Distant Metastasis (M)

MX   Not assessed

M0   No (known) distant metastasis

M1   Distant metastasis present

Stage Group

Stage I   T1N0M0

Stage II   T2N0M0

Stage III   T3N0M0

            T1 or T2 or T3 with N1M0

Stage IV   T4N0M0 or T4N1M0

            Any T with N2 or N3 and with M0

            Any T with any N and with M1

(Adapted from American Joint Committee for Cancer Staging and End Results Reporting. 1978. Manual for Staging of Cancer. American Joint Committee, Chicago.)

TREATMENT

Malignant Neoplasms of the Maxillary Sinus and Antraethmoid Complex Cancer

HISTORICAL ASPECTS

Lizars, in 1826, was the first to report the successful resection of the upper jaw and sinus. In 1888, Parsons reported the destruction of a tumor in the sinuses by the use of cautery. With the introduction of radiotherapy, surgeons from 1910 until about 1925 began to combine irradiation with electrosurgery. From 1925 to 1940, there were a number of reports on the use of electrodessication and radium implantation combined with surgery. From 1945 until 1955, there was a reawakening of interest in radical surgery, which usually included a total maxillectomy and exenteration of the orbit. Orthovoltage irradiation was given in cases where disease was left behind.

At the present time there is no standard treatment endorsed by all surgeons. More recent reports stress the importance of individualizing each case and of developing a treatment after consideration of the histology, location, extent (stage) of the tumor, and various patient factors.

RADIATION

Many radiotherapists no longer believe that preoperative radiation therapy seals off the lymphatics by creating fibrosis so that tumor cells become "locked up." There is good radiobiologic evidence that radiation therapy before surgery has lethal or sublethal biologic effects on the tumor cell itself.[22] Theoretically, previously irradiated tumor cells left behind after surgery demonstrate a decreased propensity for mitotic activity. This is referred to as a "mitotic link death." It is also believed that cells in the periphery are more sensitive to irradiation than those in the core of the tumor because the center is more anoxic due to a decreased blood supply. Although it is not entirely accepted at this time, we postulate that because of a more compact tumor bed after preoperative radiation a less radical operation with a decrease in metastatic potential can be offered.

These same radiotherapists feel that the disadvantage of preoperative radiation is the difficulty in determining how much of the radiographic changes are due to secondary infection from obstruction of ostia rather than to actual tumor invasion. Proponents of postoperative radiation also state that they can delineate the exact extent of involvement of the cancer during surgery and remove the anoxic, necrotic portions prior to irradiation.

SURGERY

At one time, we performed extensive radical surgery for all cases of antral carcinoma that were considered resectable and followed this by intracavity radium or orthovoltage external beam radiation. In 1963, the results for 54 cases were carefully reviewed by Sisson, Johnson, and Amiri.[28] A determinant 5-year cure rate of 22 percent was reported. The concept of less radical surgery, *where it applies to orbital preservation,* does not significantly decrease survival rates when larger doses of preoperative radiation are added. The concept of exenteration of the orbital contents where there is invasion and destruction of only the orbital floor and rim is questioned. It is the inferior rim of the orbit with the periosteum or the invaded structure that needs to be resected and not the orbital contents. Clearly, gross invasion of the orbit with extension to the orbital fat and extraocular musculature requires exenteration of the orbital contents.

Since 1963 our therapeutic approach has continued to be greatly altered by treating antral carcinomas with preoperative cobalt 60 radiation therapy. While the cure rate has not been significantly improved, it is no lower than it was in 1963 and the number of orbital exenterations has been greatly reduced (fewer than 25 percent in the last 65 cases).

The data for the last 12 years at Northwestern University were recently reviewed. We have continued to increase the number of cases in which the orbital contents were preserved without detrimental effects. From a total of 52 cases, 35 patients with nasal and antral cancer had a follow-up of 3 or more years. Preoperative radiation and postoperative chemotherapy were applied frequently in all 52 cases. Planned combined radiation was used in over 90 percent of cases. The overall survival rate demonstrated 26 percent free of disease at 3 or more years. Looking more specifically at the large tumors, the T3 lesion patients had a 33 percent disease-free rate and 16 percent of the T4 lesion patients showed no evidence of disease at 3 years or more. Fifty-three percent of patients with T3 lesions and 74 percent of those with T4 lesions were dead of disease at 3 or more years. No patients with positive cervical nodes or distant metastasis at the time of staging survived.

CHEMOTHERAPY

Regional infusion chemotherapy may, in spite of earlier shortcomings, have a place in the treatment of advanced squamous cell carcinoma of the maxillary antrum. Goepfert, Jesse, and Lindberg in 1973 reported the results of 26 patients with advanced cancer of the paranasal sinuses and nasal cavity who were treated by intra-arterial infusion of chemotherapy and external radiotherapy from 1963 to 1970.[11] Five-fluorouracil (6 mg/kg/day) was administered into the external carotid artery for 2 weeks. External radiotherapy was started on the second day of infusion and was continued for 6 to 7 weeks at the rate of 1,000 rads per week. At the end of the first 2 weeks the catheters were removed. Only one patient in this group had had any previous therapy.

The disease was staged according to the 1963 classification by Sisson et al.[28] Accordingly, there were 15 T4 cases and 8 T3 cases. Twenty-three of the 26 patients (22 with squamous carcinoma and 1 with adenocarcinoma) completed the treatment according to the protocol. Eleven of the 23 patients who completed their treatment had no local recurrence from 24 months to 84 months (median 44 months). Nine of these 11 patients were still alive and free of cancer at the time of the report. Two of the 11 patients died at 50 and 63 months, respectively, of unrelated causes. The absolute survival at 2 and 5 years for these 23 patients was 48 percent and 26 percent respectively. Only two patients required a maxillary resection and in one of them it was secondary to radionecrosis of soft tissue and bone.

Everts and Thomas reported in 1979[6] the use of regional intra-arterial infusion of bleomycin and methotrexate in eight cases of T4 and T3 antral lesions. This was followed by radiation therapy, 5,500 to 6,500 rads, and then surgery. No evidence of residual tumor was found in the surgical spec-

imen in four of eight patients, and one of the other four patients only had a microscopic focus. Four of eight patients were free of disease at 20 months. While these figures were encouraging, no conclusions can be drawn because of inadequate follow-up.

There is no conclusive data available as to the effect of systemic chemotherapy for cancer of the paranasal sinuses. Many of the protocols apparently have been abandoned for reasons not known to us at this time. The figures for intra-arterial use are encouraging in suggesting that perhaps these tumors might respond to the proper combination of chemotherapeutic agents.

When we use chemotherapy, we use high dose methotrexate with leucovorin rescue for Stage IV disease. We have not, however, been consistent in our application of this modality.

PRESENT POLICY OF TREATMENT OF MAXILLARY SINUS CANCER

We do not believe combining preoperative chemotherapy with irradiation adds anything to patient survival. For an aggressive definitive treatment of any malignant tumor three factors are important: the histologic diagnosis, the site and extent of disease, and the general condition of the patient. With thorough knowledge of the above factors a rational plan of management can then be formulated.

The current management program for carcinoma of the antrum on the Head and Neck Service at Northwestern University is based upon a total experience of over 150 cases. Our present policy includes the following:

1. Exploratory antrostomy is performed on all cases in order to stage the disease.

2. T1 and T2 lesions are treated by either subtotal or radical maxillectomy at the time of exploration if the diagnosis can be firmly established, or within several days of the exploration after permanent sections are reported. Adjuvant high dose methotrexate chemotherapy or postoperative ir-

radiation are usually not added except in "selected cases." Selected case implies a particular individual problem that makes us believe that the location or the biology of the tumor warrants additional therapy. This is a clinical judgment related to experience and hard guidelines cannot be dictated.

3. T1 and T2 lesions also receive postoperative irradiation when margins of resection are in question or when recurrent disease is evident.

4. T3 and T4 lesions are debulked at the time of an exploratory antrostomy. The medial (nasoantral) wall of the antrum is removed to facilitate evacuation and drainage of necrotic tumor during radiotherapy.

5. T3 and T4 tumors receive 6,000 rads of cobalt 60 irradiation over a period of 4 to 6 weeks. Four to 5 weeks following completion of irradiation, an exploratory antrostomy is again performed to ascertain the amount of residual tumor. While ablative surgery, particularly in T4 cases, usually includes radical maxillectomy with orbital exenteration, T3 cases, after irradiation, will often demonstrate complete resolution of tumor obviating the need for orbital exenteration. It is mandatory with T3 and T4 tumors that the osseous borders of the maxillary and ethmoid sinuses be completely removed with the entire floor of the orbit. The orbital contents are suspended by using a strip of temporalis fascia as a sling or by using a folded dermal graft. Adjuvant chemotherapy is given in selected cases.

6. For massive T3 or T4 lesions demonstrating invasion of the anterior cranial fossa or with extension into the sphenoethmoid recess or sphenoid sinus, radical excisional surgery should be undertaken only after judiciously reviewing the results of the preoperative radiation. Often it is necessary to perform a combined craniofacial procedure for these cases. Should this procedure be considered, first the neurosurgeon performs anterior craniotomy to determine whether or not the tumor is resectable. If after inspection of the dura overlying the fovea ethmoidalis and cribriform plate no tumor is visualized, a partial or complete maxillectomy with or without an orbital exenteration is performed. This can result in long-term palliation and in some cases, cure.[29] We have performed over 25 of these procedures for T4 Stage IV sinus cancer. The procedure is somewhat technically complicated and is successful only when there is close cooperation with a competent neurosurgical team.

7. For all N1 and N2 lesions the neck is included in the preoperative irradiation and later is treated surgically by unilateral or bilateral neck dissection, which may be performed at the time of maxillary resection.

Having described a treatment protocol for patients with localized primary disease in the maxillary antrum with or without regional lymph node metastasis, it is also important to recognize that there are groups of patients who, when seen initially, have contraindications for curative treatment. Those patients who refuse treatment require our understanding, sympathy, and supportive care. Those patients who have spread of their disease into the nasopharynx are technically inoperable because there is no possibility of resecting the anatomic structures involved in this area. Patients who have demonstrable distant metastases or unresectable regional metastases should also be disqualified from the treatment program. Patients with invasion of the base of the skull, except in the area of the cribriform plate and fovea ethmoidalis, which may be resectable, have a poor chance for cure.

Patients with unresectable or otherwise incurable disease can benefit from such procedures as palliative decompression, debulking, and drainage through a large antrostomy. Palliative doses of radiation therapy and chemotherapy used in combination with cryosurgery are all helpful in reducing discomfort.

Lateral Rhinotomy—Initial Exposure. A lateral rhinotomy is a procedure used to provide the necessary exposure so that the boundaries of the tumor can be defined (Figs. 12-11 A–C). This is the initial step prior to most subtotal maxillectomies,

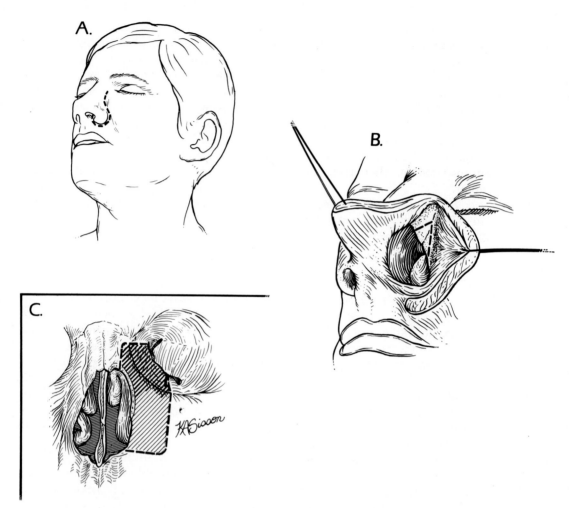

Fig. 12-11. (A) Lateral rhinotomy incision. (B) Nasal bone removal. (C) Antral bone removal.

radical maxillectomies, and radical maxillectomies combined with orbital exenteration. The orbital contents and globe are a part of the surgical field and the cornea must be protected by suturing the eyelids together.

This approach when combined with a maxillectomy is begun with an orbital incision running along the lower lid about 3 mm from the edge of the tarsal plate. This incision then continues inferiorly in the nasofacial crease, follows the ala to the base of the columella, and is continued into the philtrum without splitting the upper lip, unless there is no other way to obtain adequate exposure.

A flap is developed by periosteal elevation exposing the anterior surface of the

maxilla, the inferior aspect of the orbit, the frontal process of the maxilla, and a portion of the nasal bone. The lateral rhinotomy is completed by lateral osteotomy with, in some cases, an anterior-superior division of the nasal septum. The nose is retracted towards the side opposite the lesion. It is often necessary to remove the cartilage of the nasal septum to facilitate evaluation of the tumor boundaries. This maneuver is made in an area far removed from the growth. Bone is removed from the lateral wall of the pyriform aperture and a section of the nasal bone resected for better exposure of the nasal cavity (Fig. 12-11C).

The periosteum is elevated from the medial and inferior walls of the orbit. If one is able to free the periosteum easily without encountering tumor, orbital exenteration should not be necessary. Frozen-section control is important. If one finds the periosteum involved with tumor and there is no gross invasion of the orbital contents, the eye can still be saved. The periosteum and tumor are left attached to the specimen.

If the lesion is primarily located in the ethmoid and the extent of the disease in the antrum has not been surveyed, then an antrostomy is performed through the canine fossa to explore the maxillary sinus and to decide which portions of the maxilla are involved by the cancer.

Radical Maxillectomy. Most T1 and T2 antral lesions will be treated adequately by this procedure. By following the technique outlined for the lateral rhinotomy, exposure is achieved and the limits of the disease defined. After the incisions (Fig. 12-12A), the flap of facial skin and periosteum is raised further laterally, exposing the entire anterior surface of the maxilla. Exposure of the anterolateral portion of the zygomatic process of the frontal bone, the

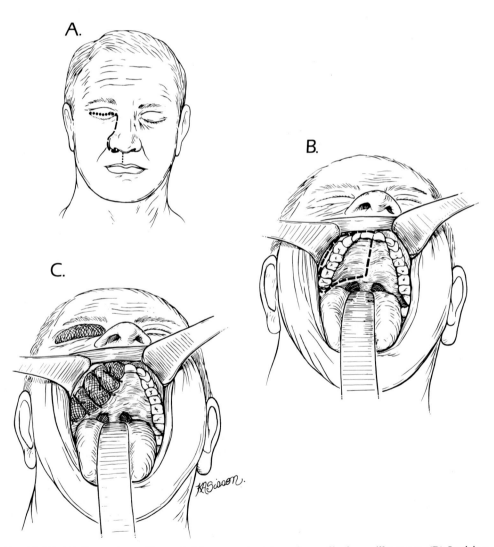

Fig. 12-12. (A) Extension of lateral rhinotomy incisions for radical maxillectomy. (B) Incision used to spare soft palate. (C) Gauze packing sewn in place.

frontal process of the maxilla, and the medial and inferior walls of the orbit is required. When the periosteum and overlying soft tissue are reflected off the bone strict attention is paid to any area where tumor may have penetrated the bone and involved the periosteum, muscle, or skin. If the periosteum and soft tissue are invaded, then they are removed en bloc with the bone. The incision is continued, encompassing the involved area (Fig. 12-12B) but leaving a margin of soft palate.

The decision regarding preservation of the eye will have been made as noted previously. If orbital exenteration is indicated, the incision in the lower lid must be extended around the medial and latheral canthi and then just above the tarsal plate in the upper lid (Fig. 12-12A). The palpebral skin is elevated superiorly exposing the orbicularis oculi muscle. The periosteum along the superior orbital rim is incised and the orbital periosteum reflected off the roof and the medial and lateral aspect of the orbit. The orbital contents are then retracted inferiorly to permit ligation and transection of the ethmoid and ophthalmic vessels. The orbital contents are removed in-continuity with the roof of the maxillary sinus. If the eye is not to be included in the resection, the periosteum is elevated from the orbital floor and lamina papyracea and the ethmoidal arteries are ligated and transected as they penetrate their corresponding foramina.

An incision is made in the palate, and the mucoperiosteum is elevated. If the floor of the maxilla is to be removed, the musculature of the soft palate is then separated from the hard palate at their junction.

If a previous oroantrotomy incision (exploration and biopsy) is present, the incision along the alveolus of the maxilla (buccogingival incision) is made superior to this site so that the previous incision can be included in the specimen. The buccogingival incision begins in the midline and joins the midline incisions in the philtrum and palate. It is then carried posteriorly around the maxillary alveolar tuberosity to the midline of the

palate. This frees the buccal flap from its last attachment to the maxilla.

Following the elevation of the soft tissue from the underlying bony framework bone cuts are performed without cutting through tumor tissue. The extent of the bone resection is individually modified according to the extent of the tumor. The first bone cut is an osteotomy just below the frontoethmoid suture or on a level passing just inferior to the anterior and posterior ethmoid foramina (Fig. 12-13A). Anteriorly, this cut passes through the frontal process of the maxilla. The bone of this strong anterior buttress is most easily transsected with a Stryker saw. When the orbital contents are saved, care must be taken to avoid damaging the optic nerve. Therefore, the posterior extent of the horizontal ethmoid osteotomy stops at the level of the posterior ethmoidal artery and a vertical cut is made carefully to provide a fracture line at the posterior aspect of the labyrinth. Laterally, a Stryker or a Gigli saw is used to transect the frontal and temporal (zygomatic arch) projections of the zygoma. The hard palate is easily transsected with a Gigli saw inserted intranasally and grasped at the posterior margin of the hard palate by way of the oral cavity. The last bone cut is at the base of pterygoid process (Fig. 12-13B); however, prior to this manuever, all other areas of transsected bone should be examined with an osteotome to be sure of the detachment of the specimen at these sites. This should be the last osteotomy, since this last bone cut is a deep cut in the area of the potentially bloody pterygoid plexus. If the internal maxillary artery has not been visualized and ligated up to this point, it will bleed and must be secured. This step is facilitated by rotating the maxillary block medially to gain better exposure of the vessel. Any remaining soft-tissue attachments are cut and the specimen removed from the field.

Any remaining ethmoid sinus fragments are meticulously removed with ethmoid forceps and the ipsilateral frontal sinus floor is likewise removed. This allows

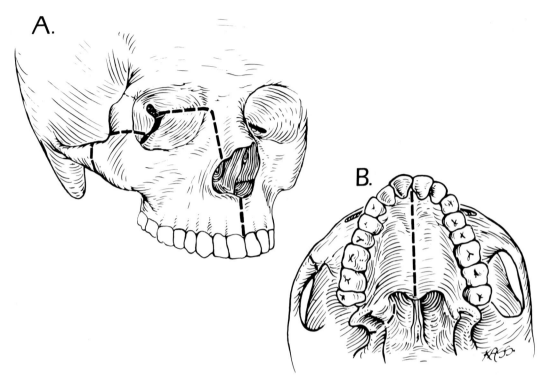

Fig. 12-13. (A and B) Bone cuts for radical maxillectomy and orbital removal.

for better drainage of the sinus as well as adds to the margins of the resection. If the patient is edentulous or all teeth are missing on the remaining maxilla, the lower one-third of the septum can be removed in order to create an undercut to facilitate retention of the upper dental prosthesis.

All bleeding vessels are clamped and ligated or cauterized. Careful hemostasis is required before proceeding to the reconstructive phase of the operation.

When disease is located in the inferior portion of the maxilla and involves only the hard palate or alveolar process, a subtotal maxillectomy may be possible (Fig. 12-14). The resection can be further modified to accommodate lesions of the nose invading the ethmoid complex and the common wall between the nasal cavity and the maxilla. Through a lateral rhinotomy incision, the ethmoid complex and medial aspect of the maxilla including the lateral nasal wall are removed as a block.[25] This may be combined

with a craniofacial resection to resect the cribriform plate and ethmoid roof. A piecemeal resection is thus avoided and facial contour is preserved.

This limited approach has its greatest applicability for lesions such as adenocarcinoma of the ethmoid, lesions of the lateral nasal wall, olfactory esthesioneuroblastoma, and chondrosarcoma. Squamous cell carcinoma of the antrum requires maxillectomy due to its invasiveness in multiple scattered sheets and nests. The more superior, posterior, and medial the disease, the more lethal the potential. Overt superior extension of an antral lesion into the orbital cavity or extension laterally into the orbit from the ethmoid lesion will often require orbital exenteration or a combined cranial-facial resection. Superior medial extension into the orbital apex or posterior extension into the pterygoids may signal invasion of the base of the skull. The latter problems may herald an unresectable situation.

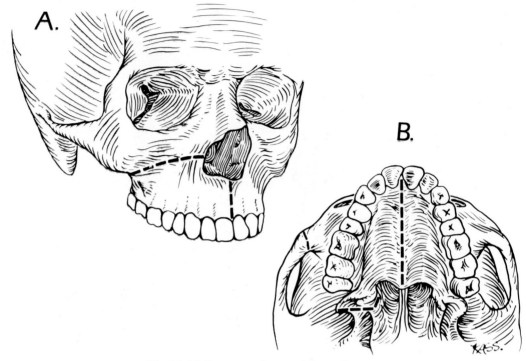

Fig. 12-14. Bone cuts for partial maxillectomy.

An extensive cavity remains following radical maxillectomy with or without orbital exenteration. No matter what the extent of the resection, the cavity that is left should be easily available for postoperative inspection and cleansing. Bone and soft tissue surrounding the opening into the cavity are removed so that inspection of all areas of the maxillectomy cavity will be a simple office procedure. The sinuses surrounding the cavity (frontal and sphenoid) must be opened widely so that a postoperative recurrence is not hidden. This also helps to eliminate confusion between recurrent disease and granulation tissue, as such confusion can be fostered by an inflamed irregular segment of mucosa that may present at the orifice of a residual infected ethmoid cell or remaining intact sphenoid sinus.

Reconstruction of the Defect.   The raw surfaces of the entire cavity are lined with a split-thickness or dermal skin graft taken from the anterior thigh. The graft should be between 0.016 and 0.020 inches thick. If the eye is retained, a fascial sling is em-

ployed on the undersurface of the orbit before it, too, is grafted. The skin graft is sewn in place with an absorbable suture and covered with a layer of Gelfoam. The bony cavity is packed with a continuous strip of gauze impregnated with antibiotic ointment (Fig. 12-12C). This provides hemostasis and holds the skin graft in place. A soft Silastic sponge is cut to fit the lower half of the cavity and is then inserted into the palatal defect.

If skin from the cheek was resected with the specimen, the defect may be reconstructed with a forehead pedicle flap (Fig. 12-15) or a sternomastoid myocutaneous flap (Fig. 12-16) and a split-thickness graft used to line the inner surface of either flap. Heavy preoperative radiation to the head and neck may require advancement of a tubed pedicle flap from a distant site (Fig. 12-17). In institutions where the services of a maxillofacial prosthodontist are readily available a temporary surgical obturator is constructed and placed in the cavity immediately. This enables the patient to take liq-

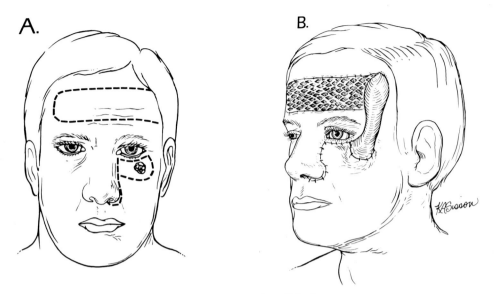

Fig. 12-15. Forehead pedicle flap.

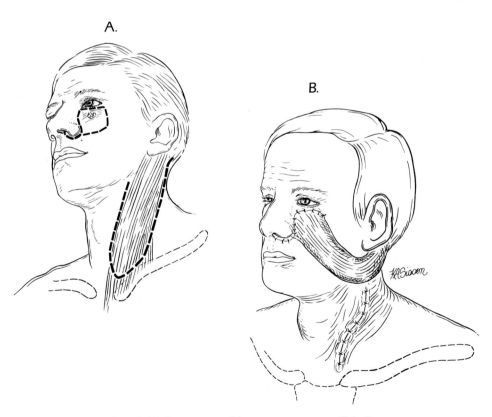

Fig. 12-16. Sternomastoid myocutaneous pedicle flap.

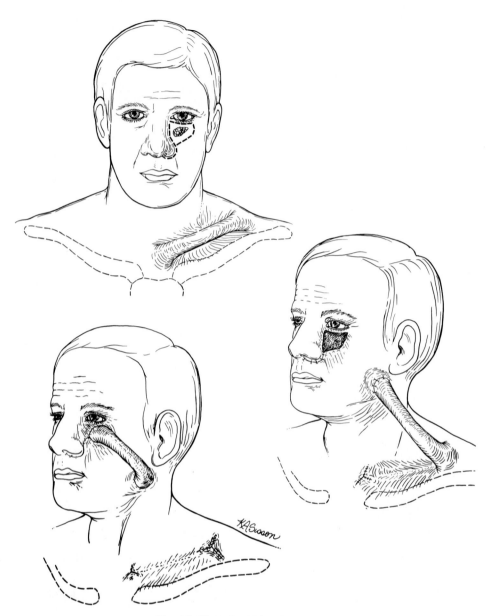

Fig. 12-17. Tubed bipedicle flap.

uids and soft foods immediately postoperatively until a permanent prosthesis can be constructed by the prosthodontist. (For more detail on obturators and facial prosthetics, see Ch. 9.) In our experience the Silastic sponge works as well as a temporary surgical obturator and is less costly. Finally, the nasofacial and palpebral incisions are approximated with a 4-0 chromic or other absorbable suture for the subcutaneous tissue and with a 5-0 and 6-0 nylon suture for the skin. The packing is carefully removed 7 to 10 days postoperatively.

Craniofacial Resection.   Malecki[19] reported on a combined craniofacial approach for neoplasms of the ethmoid sinus extending into the cribriform area.

We have been performing this procedure on selected cases during the past 18 years and find it valuable in the management of advanced antroethmoid cancer.[29] A well-organized, experienced neurosurgical-otolaryngologic team that works comfortably together can safely offer this operation to the patient with advanced cancer who has only minimal penetration of the floor of the anterior fossa (Fig. 12-18). This approach may also be combined with an exenteration of the orbit and total maxillectomy when indicated.

The patient is prepared for frontal craniotomy and a facial approach to the nose and paranasal sinuses. The hip and thigh are prepared for an iliac-crest graft, a split-thickness graft, or a dermal graft. Frontal craniotomy is performed, and the frontal lobes are retracted to expose the base of the anterior cranial fossa (Figs. 12-19 and 12-20). As the dura and frontal lobes are reflected off the floor of the cranial vault, exposure is enhanced by releasing cerebrospinal fluid through a previously placed subarachnoid catheter. Resectability is determined at this point. If the tumor extends through the bone of the cribriform plate, the lesion may still be resected by leaving the overlying dura attached to the specimen.[16] Contraindications to further surgery are the following:

1. Extension of the neoplasm superiorly through the dura and into the frontal lobes.

2. Posterior extension of the tumor beyond the cribriform plate or beyond the roof of the ethmoid complex to a point where there would be excessive traction on the optic nerve.

3. Tumor involving both optic nerves.

4. In most cases, lateral extension outside the boundaries of the fovea ethmoidalis and into the region of the superior orbital fissure.

After estimation of the superior extent of the tumor, involvement of the orbital

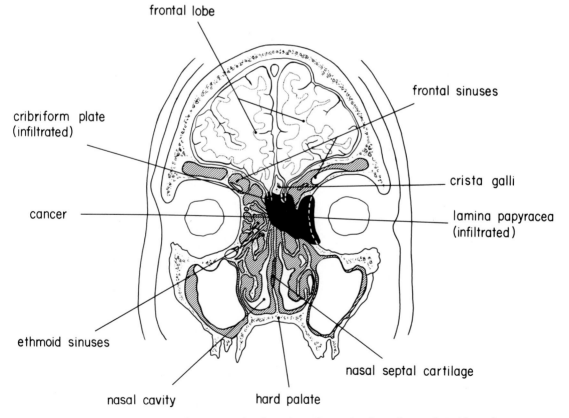

Fig. 12-18. Coronal section demonstrating invasion of anterior fossa from ethmoid carcinoma.

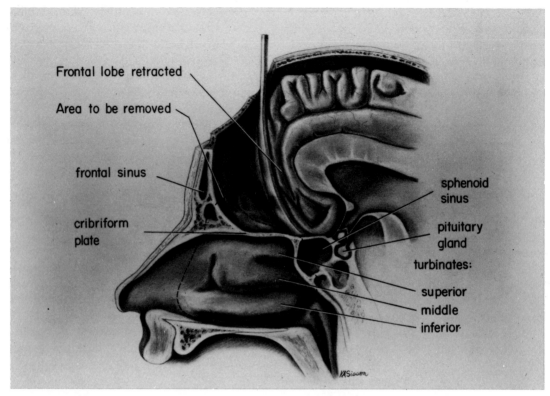

Fig. 12-19. Floor of anterior cranial fossa exposed by retraction of frontal lobes.

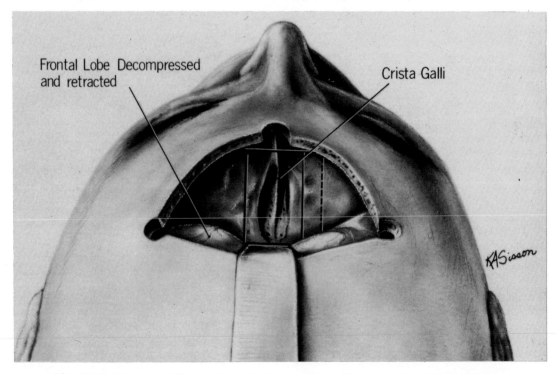

Fig. 12-20. Exposure of floor of anterior fossa enhanced by retraction of frontal lobes.

contents is determined and the size of the lesion is assessed. The facial approach is begun with a modified Weber-Fergusson incision (Fig. 12-12A). A single limb incision is used in the orbit running along the lower lid 3 mm from the edge of the tarsal plate. The incision continues inferiorly in the nasalfacial crease and follows around the ala into the philtrum without splitting the upper lip. The remainder of the procedure, since it entails an exploration of the orbit and evaluation of the need to remove the eye, is carried out as described under lateral rhinotomy.

After the boundaries of the tumor are assessed, bone-cutting instruments are used to excise the block of involved bone and a margin of normal tissue from its attachments. The placement of these bone cuts varies with the extent of the neoplasm (Fig. 12-21). A partial or total maxillectomy, with or without an orbital exenteration, is performed in conjunction with removal of the ethmoid complex.

Osteotomies are used to mobilize both sides of the cribriform plate and fovea ethmoidalis. Cuts along the lateral aspect of the roof of the ethmoid sinus are matched with those of the frontoethmoid suture made during the facial approach (Fig. 12-20). The ethmoid complex on the side opposite the tumor is removed. The posterior wall of the frontal sinus is included in the resection. If necessary, the anterior portion of the roof of the sphenoid sinus is removed (Fig. 12-19).

After the tumor is mobilized, it is grasped inferiorly while pressure is exerted through the cranial defect on the block of bone. Remaining attachments are cut and the specimen is delivered inferiorly through the facial defect.[16] Hemostasis is obtained after the specimen is removed. Clips are placed on the terminal branches of the internal maxillary arteries. Electrocautery, bone wax, and firm packing also can be used if necessary.

Several methods are available for repair of the cribriform defect (Figs. 12-22 and 12-23). Fascia lata and direct suturing are used to mend dural tears and serve as the superior layer of a three-layered repair. A middle supporting layer of iliac-crest bone, septal cartilage, or posterior lamina of frontal bone provides rigidity to prevent dehiscence of anterior cranial contents into the nasal fossa. The inferior layer forms part of the lining of the common nasal and maxillectomy cavity and may consist of a rotated septal pedicle flap (selected cases), a free dermal graft, or a split-thickness skin graft. Some dural tears are more easily repaired by working through the facial defect.

The facial cavity is lined with splitthickness skin grafts. Packing is inserted that will be removed in 7 to 10 days and replaced by a fresh pack, which is left in place for another week. The incision in the area of the eyelids is closed, but the lateral rhinotomy segment is left open on selected cases to serve as an observation portal during the postoperative period. This allows easy manipulation of packing, better control in case of sudden hemorrhage, and easier repair of cerebrospinal fluid leaks. Once the cavity is healed, usually within 2 months, this defect is repaired. Closure of the incision in the philtrum and lower nasal alar region is completed at the time of the primary surgery. The craniotomy is closed conventionally.

Operative Approach—Frontal Sinus. The posterior wall of the fronal sinus forms part of the floor and anterior wall of the anterior cranial fossa. A malignant tumor in this area would therefore require a combined craniofacial resection. The neurosurgeon first performs a craniotomy and evaluates possible invasion of the dura or frontal lobe. Involvement of the olfactory tracts and the optic nerve is then assessed. With high grade adenocarcinoma or squamous cell carcinoma, bilateral optic nerve invasion should be considered a sign of unresectability. Extensive involvement of the frontal lobe carries the same outlook. If extensive posterior invasion is not present, then the facial approach is initiated. The same steps as indicated under the craniofacial approach are utilized. The orbital periosteum including the superior and medial

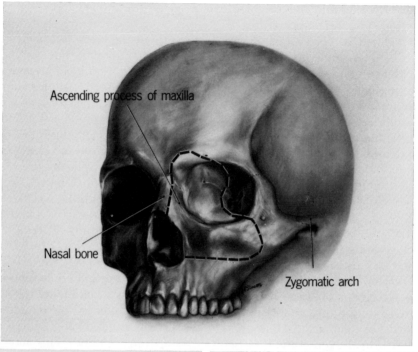

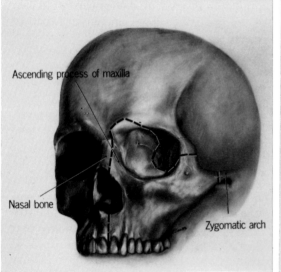

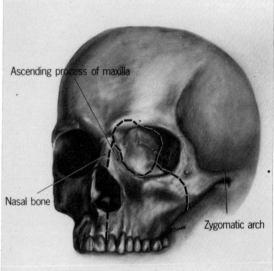

Fig. 12-21. Osteotomies for craniofacial resection.

aspect of the orbit is incised and reflected. The need to remove the eye is determined, and a lateral rhinotomy is employed to evaluate ethmoid extension. Osteotomies are performed to create a facial block of tissue that will include, at the least, part of the inferior portion of the frontal bone, superci-

liary arch, orbital roof and medial wall, glabella (if necessary), and ethmoid complex. Radiation should be administered in a planned combined program.

Operative Approach—Sphenoid Sinus. For malignant tumors of the sphenoid sinus. surgery can provide a correct diagnosis

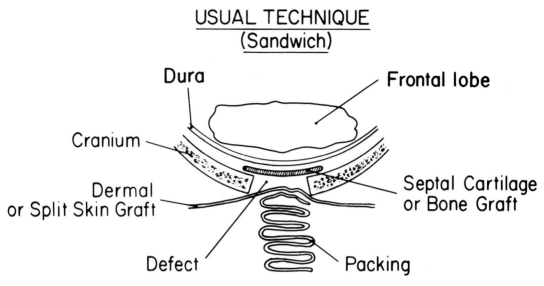

Fig. 12-22. Usual technique for repair of cribriform defect.

and decompression but not a block resection. Sphenoid sinus tumors, particularly those with a superior or lateral extension, are not totally resectable due to the complex anatomic boundaries and vital structures that surround the sinus. The approach for a biopsy has been discussed.

Decompression can be obtained by a transseptal, transpalatal, or transantral ethmoid approach. After making an inverted "U" incision in the posterior hard palate the mucoperiosteum is elevated from the hard palate and the mucosa elevated from the soft palate. The posterior aspect of the hard palate and nasal septum and the medial aspect of the ethmoid sinus complex, including both middle turbinates, are removed. This provides visualization for the resection of the anterior and inferior walls of the sphenoid sinus for drainage and decompression. All tumor that can be visualized is removed.

The defect is left open, and the patient is fitted with a prosthesis to facilitate postoperative speaking and swallowing and to provide easy observation and cleaning of the cavity.

Recently some encouraging results with

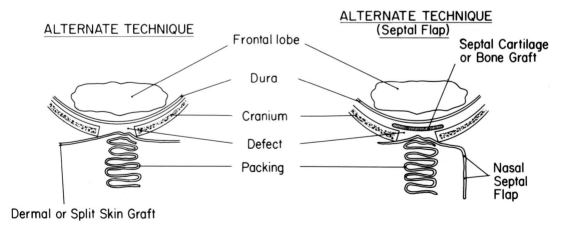

Fig. 12-23. Alternate techniques for repair of cribriform defect.

the slower-growing lesions (chondrosarcomas and adenoid cystic carcinomas) have been obtained using the air drill and diamond burr to remove the lesion from around the optic nerves. Palliation has been improved by this technique.

Complications of Surgery. *Hemorrhage.* This may be immediate and is usually accompanied by marked edema of the cheek and obvious bleeding. The patient should be returned to the operating room and the pack removed. Specific bleeding sites should be searched for and ligated. A fresh, tight pack is then inserted. Most significant bleeding comes from the internal maxillary artery; therefore, we recommend self-locking clips be placed on the terminal branches of this vessel at the time of surgery. Delayed hemorrhage at 2 to 3 weeks after surgery was a problem in the early development of craniofacial resections, and the above manuever has been effective in controlling this difficulty.

Infection. Infection may occur due to the contamination by secretions from the nose, oropharynx, and paranasal sinuses, even though all of our patients are placed on postoperative antibiotic prophylaxis. Those patients with infection should all be placed on parenteral antibiotics specific for pathogens cultured from the wound. The problem of infection can be especially acute in postoperative craniofacial resection. The sequelae, if uncontrolled, might be meningitis and/or brain abscess. Daily packing changes with aggressive debridement of infected radionecrotic bone are required before healing can be complete. Most of our patients have received preoperative or postoperative radiation in excess of 6,500 rads. In our series there were no major postoperative infective complications in patients who were irradiated postoperatively. If a planned combined treatment program is employed for a patient undergoing craniofacial resection, postoperative radiation is preferred but not always practical if one hopes to spare the eye. Because of this, when the eye is in jeopardy, we give preoperative irradiation and accept the inci-

dence of osteoradionecrosis as a complication. This contrasts with our approach to radical maxillectomy, for which we recommend preoperative radiation.

Cerebrospinal Fluid Leak. No prolonged cerebrospinal fluid leak occurred in patients undergoing craniofacial resection perhaps because of the three-layered repair of the defect in the skull base. We have changed our technique of repair in recent years and it differs from those previously described in that we now use a supporting layer of autogenous bone graft or cartilage (Figs. 12-22 and 12-23). The craniofacial approach in itself provides good exposure for the reconstruction of the floor of the anterior cranial fossa. None of our patients became comatose after surgery, and there were no instances of subdural abscess or hematoma. One patient developed meningitis 6 days postoperatively but responded promptly to antibiotics.

PROGNOSIS AND END RESULTS

The correlation between the TNM system and prognosis is evident. The more advanced the TNM staging, the poorer the prognosis.

From 1963 to 1967, at Upstate Medical Center, State University of New York at Syracuse, the senior author (G.A.S.) applied the system to prospective cases and found similar results.[26] It clearly reflected how early diagnosis results in better prognosis. Using the same TNM system, others have analyzed cases and reported the same conclusions.[14]

The results of treatment in the series of Jackson et al.[14] of patients with malignant neoplasms of the nasal cavity and paranasal sinuses demonstrated that in patients with antral carcinoma the local recurrence rate was 44 percent, while in other sites it was 50 percent. It is noteworthy that most patients in this series presented with advanced disease and that patients with residual disease after treatment were counted as recurrences. The figures on local recurrence still remain impressive. Distant metastases developed in 30 percent of those with antral lesions and 35 percent of those with nonantral lesions. No distinct pattern or site of predilection for local recurrence of antral or nonantral cancer was noted. Jackson et al.[14] analyzed their 67 patients using the Sisson classification and reported their 5-year statistics (Table 12-4). Survival rates based on modes of therapy showed the best survival with preoperative radiotherapy and surgery (43 percent) or surgery alone (59 percent).

A series of 50 patients reported by Schecter and Ogura in 1972[24] showed that failure to control the primary lesion was the major problem. On close analysis the treatment failures related to local recurrence (19 patients) were associated with positive margins (6/19), extensive pterygoid invasion (5/19), positive ethmoid currettings (2/19), extensive orbital invasion (1/19), or poor cellular differentiation (3/19), with no reason for recurrence in 2 of the 19 patients. The patients with local recurrence and positive margins were all treated prior to 1961. Since that time larger doses of preoperative radiation therapy and a more radical technique for maxillectomy have been used. The later, more aggressive techniques have resulted in a decrease in local recurrence associated with positive margins.

Those cases with cervical nodes are pre-destined for a poor prognosis. Schecter and Ogura[24] reported that of 7 patients with carcinoma of the maxilla presenting with positive cervical nodes, none were free of disease at 1 year. Of 13 patients who developed cervical nodes after treatment, only 1 was alive at 2 years. Jackson et al.[14] reviewed a series of 115 patients with cancer of the paranasal sinuses. They found cervical nodes clinically enlarged in 9 percent of maxillary sinus patients but not in any of the patients with tumor primary in other sites. Moss et al.[22] and other radiotherapists are proponents of radiation of the clinically negative neck, but most surgeons, ourselves included, do not advocate this approach. Certainly, the preoperative ports should include the retropharyngeal and pterygomaxillary areas.

The following table (Table 12-5) from a 1970 study by Gallagher and Boles[10] shows the biologic behavior of this tumor. Surgery consisted of radical maxillectomy, and radiation therapy was in the range of 6,900 to 7,100 rads. Note the poor survival rate in those T2 and T3 tumors treated with radiation alone. This is no place for the attitude of "radiate and watch."

TABLE 12-4 ANALYSIS OF 67 PATIENTS BY THE SISSON CLASSIFICATION

Tumor Classification	Number of Patients	5-Year Survival Rate (%)
T1N0M0	3	100
T2N0M0	11	30
T3N0M0	21	53
T3N1M0	3	33
T3N2M0	2	0
T4N0M0	26	13
T4N2M0	1	0

(Adapted from Jackson, R. T., Fitz-Hugh, G. S., and Constable, W. C. 1977. Malignant neoplasms of the nasal cavities and paranasal sinuses: A retrospective study. Laryngoscope, 87: 726.)

TABLE 12-5 FIVE-YEAR ABSOLUTE SURVIVAL RATES BY TUMOR STAGE AND TREATMENT TYPE FOR SQUAMOUS CELL CARCINOMA OF THE MAXILLARY ANTRUM WITHOUT RECURRENCE

Treatment	Survivors/No. of Patients				Overall by Treatment (Percent)
	T1	T2	T3	T4	
No Treatment	—	—	0/5	0/2	0
Surgery	1/1	2/2	1/5	—	50
Radiation	—	2/8	3/16	0/7	16
Combined	—	1/2	5/6	0/2	60
Overall by Stage (Percent)	100	42	33	0	

(Adapted from Gallagher, R. M., and Boles, R. 1970. Symposium: Treatment of malignancies of paranasal sinuses. Carcinoma of the maxillary antrum. Laryngoscope, 80: 924.)

SUMMARY

Malignant tumors in the nasal cavity and paranasal sinuses are hidden within secluded bony cavities and tortuous recesses. The symptoms and signs from these lesions mimic those of benign inflammatory disease (nasal obstruction and sinusitis) or degenerative disease (epistaxis, atypical facial pain). The diagnosis is therefore obtained only by maintaining a high degree of suspicion and aggressive surgical exploration. By the time the tumor is discovered it often has extended to destroy the bony walls of adjacent sinuses or to involve the orbit or base of the skull. Adequate surgery, therefore, requires wide-field en bloc regional resection of the tumor and attached structures. There has been a recent trend toward preservation of the orbital contents. Form and function have been improved without adversely affecting survival rates. The more frequent application of the craniofacial resection has improved the survival rates of the patients with T4 lesions invading the floor of the anterior cranial fossa. Planned combined surgery and irradiation is a standard part of the treatment of all but the smallest lesions. Radiation alone in order to save the patient from a procedure that causes a cosmetic deformity results in residual submucosal islands of tumor and most often a disastrous final outcome.

Further advances leading to improved survival rates will depend on early diagnosis and adequate intensive initial treatment. We must look to the research laboratory of the chemotherapist and immunologist as well as to the inventiveness that fosters new surgical techniques to advance the treatment of one of the most severe afflictions of mankind.

REFERENCES

1. Acheson, E. D., Dowdell, R. N., Hadfield, E., and Macbeth, R. G. 1968. Nasal cancer in woodcutters in the furniture industry. British Medical Journal, 1: 587.

2. Barton, R. T. 1977. Nickel carcinogenesis of the respiratory tract. Journal of Otolaryngology 6: 412.

3. Batsakis, J. G. 1975. Tumors of the Head and Neck: Clinical and Pathological Considerations. Williams and Wilkins, Baltimore.

4. Brownson, R. J., and Ogura, J. H. 1971. Primary carcinomas of the frontal sinus. Laryngoscope, 81: 71.

5. Conley, J., and Dingman, D. L. 1974. Adenoid cystic carcinoma in the head and neck (cylindroma). Archives of Otolaryngology, 100: 81.

6. Everts, E. C., and Thomas, R. 1979. Advanced squamous cell carcinoma of the maxillary antrum. Presented at the April, 1979, meeting of the American Society for Head and Neck Surgery, Boston.

6a. Exelby, P. R. 1974. Management of embryonal rhabdomyosarcoma in children. Surgical Clinics of North America, 54: 849.

7. Fletcher, G. H., and MacComb, W. S. 1967. Cancer of the Head and Neck. Williams and Wilkins, Baltimore.

8. Frazell, E. L., and Lewis, J. S. 1963. Cancer of the nasal cavity and accessory sinuses. A report of the management of 416 patients. Cancer, 16: 1293.

9. Freedman, H. M., Desanto, L. W., Devine, K. D., and Weiland, L. H. 1973. Malignant melanoma of the nasal cavity and paranasal sinuses. Archives of Otolaryngology, 97: 322.

10. Gallagher, T. M., and Boles, R. 1970. Symposium: Treatment of malignancies of paranasal sinuses. Carcinoma of the maxillary antrum. Laryngoscope, 80: 924.

11. Goepfert, H., Jesse, R. H., and Lindberg, R. D. 1973. Arterial infusion and radiation therapy in the treatment of advanced cancer of the nasal cavity and paranasal sinuses. American Journal of Surgery, 126: 464.

12. Goss, C. M., De. 1959. Gray's Anatomy. 27th edn. Lea and Febiger, Philadelphia.

13. Haagensen, C. D., Feimd, C. R., Herter, F. P., Slanetz, C. A., Jr., and Weinberg, J. A. 1972. The Lymphatics in Cancer. W. B. Saunders, Philadelphia.

14. Jackson, R. T., Fitz-Hugh, G. S., and Constable, W. C. 1977. Malignant neoplasms of the nasal cavities and paranasal sinuses: A retrospective study. Laryngoscope, 87: 726.

15. Jing, B-S., Goepfert, H., and Close, L. G. 1978. Computerized tomography of paranasal sinus neoplasms. Laryngoscope, 88: 1485.

16. Ketcham, A. S., Chretien, P. B., VanBuren, J. M. Hoye, R. C., Beazley, R. M., and Herdt, J. R. 1973. The ethmoid sinuses: A re-evaluation of surgical resection. American Journal of Surgery, 126: 469.

17. Larsson, L. G., and Martensson, G. 1954. Carcinoma of the paranasal sinuses and the nasal cavities: A clinical study of 379 cases treated at Rudiumhement and the Otolaryngologic Department of Karolinski Sujkhuset, 1940–1950. Acta Radiologica, 42: 149.

18. Lewis, J. S., and Castro, E. B. 1972. Cancer of the nasal cavity and paranasal sinuses. Journal of Laryngology and Otology, 86: 255.

19. Malecki, J. 1959. New trends in frontal sinus surgery. Acta Oto-Laryngologica, 50: 137.

20. Marchetta, F. C., Sako, K., Mattick, W. L., and Stinziano, G. D. 1969. Squamous cell carcinoma of the maxillary antrum, American Journal of Surgery, 118: 805.

21. Montgomery, W. W. 1971. Surgery of the Upper Respiratory System. Vol 1. Lea and Febiger, Philadelphia.

22. Moss, W. T., Brand, W. N., and Battifora, H. 1973. Radiation Oncology: Rationale, Technique and Results. 4th edn. C. V. Mosby, St. Louis.

23. Ohngren, L. G. 1933. Malignant tumours of the maxillo-ethmoidal region. Acta Oto-Laryngologica, suppl., 19: 1.

24. Schechter, G. L., and Ogura, J. H. 1972. Maxillary sinus and malignancy. Laryngoscope, 82: 796.

25. Sessions, R. B., and Larson, D. L. 1977. En bloc ethmoidectomy and medial maxillectomy. Archives of Otolaryngology, 103: 195.

26. Sisson, G. A. 1970. Symposium—Paranasal Sinuses. Laryngoscope, 80: 945.

27. Sisson, G. A., and Goldstein, J. C. 1973. Tumors of the nose, paranasal sinuses, and nasopharynx. In Paparella, M. M., and Shumrick, D. A., Eds.: Otolaryngology, Vol. III: Head and Neck. W. B. Saunders, Philadelphia, 123.

28. Sisson, G. A., Johnson, N. E., and Amiri, C. S. 1963. Cancer of the maxillary sinus: Clinical classification and management. Annals of Otology, Rhinology and Laryngology, 72: 1050.

29. Sisson, G. A., Bytell, D. E., Becker, S. P., and Ruge, D. V. 1976. Carcinoma of paranasal sinuses and cranial-facial resection. Journal of Laryngology and Otology, 90: 59.

30. Skolnik, E. M., Massari, F. S., and Tenta, L. T. 1966. Olfactory neuroepithelioma. Review of the world literature and presentation of two cases. Archives of Otolaryngology, 84: 644.

31. Snow, G. B., Van der Esch, E. P., and Von Slooten, E. A. 1978. Mucosal melanomas of the head and neck. Head and Neck Surgery, 1: 24.

32. Vrabec, D. P. 1975. The inverted Schneiderian papilloma: A clinical and pathological study. Laryngoscope, 85: 186.

13 | Cancer of the Lip

Shan Ray Baker, M.D.
Charles J. Krause, M.D.

ANATOMY

The lips are the anterior boundary of the oral cavity and are formed embryologically by the union of mesenchyme from five facial processes. Two lateral maxillary processes fuse with a centrally located frontonasal process to form the upper lip. Two mandibular processes meet in the midline to form the lower lip.[47]

The musculature of the lips derives from the second branchial arch, which later migrates to the facial processes. The orbicularis oris is the sphincter of the mouth lying within the lip and encircling the oral aperture. This muscle extends upward almost to the columella of the nose and downward to the mental crease. The muscle fibers decussate in the midline of the mouth and occasionally form a raphe in the lower lip.[47]

A point near the corner of the mouth is considered as the point of origin of the orbicularis oris (Fig. 13-1) and marks where five muscles of facial expression converge, blending their muscle fibers: the levator anguli oris arises from the face of the maxilla; the zygomaticus major arises from the bone of the same name; the risorius arises from the parotid fascia and is joined by the posterior fibers of the platysma; and the depressor anguli oris arises from the oblique line of the mandible.

Three muscles arise from the inferior orbital margin and insert into the upper lip. They are the levator labii superioris, levator labii superioris alae nasi, and zygomaticus

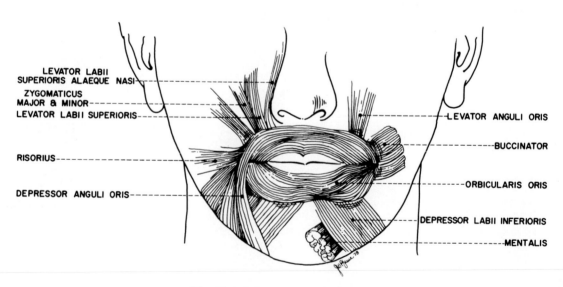

LEVATOR LABII
SUPERIORIS ALAEQUE NASI

ZYGOMATICUS
MAJOR & MINOR

LEVATOR LABII SUPERIORIS

RISORIUS

DEPRESSOR ANGULI ORIS

LEVATOR ANGULI ORIS

BUCCINATOR

ORBICULARIS ORIS

DEPRESSOR LABII INFERIORIS

MENTALIS

Fig. 13-1. Musculature of the lips.

minor. The second and third muscles are mere slips.

The depressor labii arises from the oblique line of the mandible and inserts into the midportion of the lower lip. Its medial border decussates with that of its fellow above the mental crease leaving a triangular space below the crease. This space is occupied by the mentalis muscle, which arises from the incisive fossa of the mandible to attach widely to the skin of the chin.

The buccinator is considered a muscle of the cheek. However, it extends from the superior constrictor of the pharynx and blends with fibers of the orbicularis oris in the upper and lower lips. Some fibers decussate behind the angle of the mouth: the upper fibers passing into the lower lip and the lower fibers into the upper lip.

The sensory innervation of the lip is supplied by the second and third division of the trigeminal nerve (Fig. 13-2). The infraorbital branch of the maxillary nerve (V^2) supplies sensation to a major portion of the skin and mucous membrane of the upper lip. The oral commissure area is supplied by the buccal branch of the mandibular nerve (V^3). Portions of this nerve pierce the buccinator muscle to supply the mucous membrane of the commissure. The mental branch of the mandibular nerve emerges through the mental foramen to supply the skin and mucous membrane of the lower lip.

The facial or seventh cranial nerve is the nerve of the second branchial arch and thus the motor nerve to the muscles of the lip. The buccal branch of the facial nerve is superficial to the masseter muscle but runs

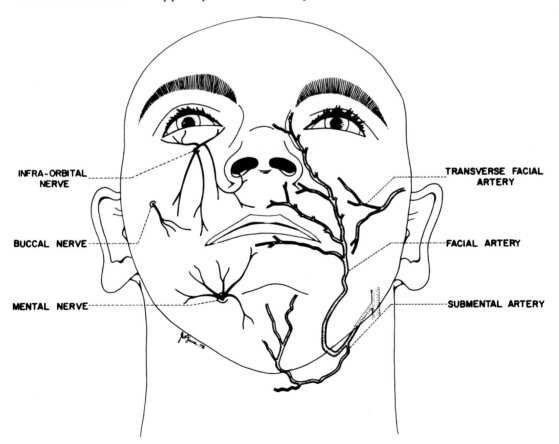

Fig. 13-2. Sensory innervation and blood supply of the lips.

in the same direction as the buccal branch of the trigeminal nerve to supply the upper lip musculature. It is aided in part by zygomatic branches of the facial nerve. The mandibular branch assisted by a portion of the cervical branch of the facial nerve innervates the muscles of the lower lip.

The buccinator-orbicularis complex is concerned with oral competence and its primary action is sphincteric. It is innervated in a segmental fashion permitting individual portions to contract separately. The muscles of facial expression that surround the orbicularis oris in a radial fashion are also innervated by the seventh nerve. These muscles act as synergist or antagonist singly or in concert to fix or retract a portion of the lip.[22]

The major blood supply of the lip is from branches of the facial artery (Fig. 13-2). This artery gives off a small submental artery to the lower lip and continues forward passing approximately 1.5 cm from the angle of the mouth, where it gives rise to the inferior and superior labial arteries. These vessels together with those of the opposite side encircle the mouth between the orbicularis oris and the submucosa of the lip. The transverse facial artery may supply portions of the lateral aspect of the upper and lower lip. The lip also receives small branches from the internal maxillary artery; these branches accompany the branches of the trigeminal nerve.

The anterior facial vein runs posterior to the facial artery and gives off branches corresponding to the artery providing venous drainage of the lip. This vein makes important connections with the pterygoid

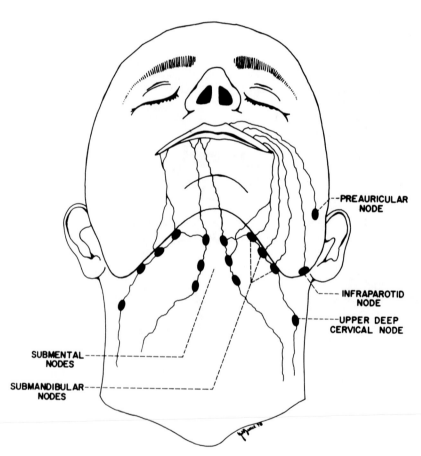

Fig. 13-3. Lymphatic drainage of the lips.

PREAURICULAR NODE

INFRAPAROTID NODE

UPPER DEEP CERVICAL NODE

SUBMENTAL NODES

SUBMANDIBULAR NODES

plexus through the deep facial vein, with the cavernous sinus through the superior ophthalmic vein, and with the frontal diploic veins through the supraorbital vein. The anterior jugular vein also aids in venous drainage of the lower lip and of the mental area in the midline. The transverse facial vein and deep facial vein parallel the buccal artery and drain the commissure and upper lip.

The lymphatic drainage of the lip has been well described by Most[34] and Rouviere[38] (Fig. 13-3). The upper and lower lips have a cutaneous and a mucosal system of lymphatics, both of which take origin from a fine capillary network in the vermilion border. The network in the lower lip usually combines to form one medial and two lateral main collecting trunks; the latter are located one on each side of the midline. The medial trunk drains the inner one-third, the lateral trunks drain the outer two-thirds of each half of the lower lip. The medial trunk drains to submental lymph nodes. The lateral trunks drain into submandibular triangle lymph nodes. Submandibular lymph nodes are segregated in relationship to the submandibular gland and the facial artery and vein. Preglandular lymph nodes are located anterior to the submandibular gland. Prevascular and postvascular lymph nodes are located anterior and posterior to the facial vessels respectively.

Numerous anastomoses from the lymphatic vessels of the two halves of the lip are present near the midline and account for the bilateral metastases from tumors that are located near to or across the midline. Collecting lymphatic trunks have been shown to enter the mental foramen in 22 percent of patients.[48] The upper lip lymphatic network forms three to five main collecting trunks, which drain to preauricular, infraparotid, submandibular triangle, and submental lymph nodes. In the upper lip, only a few of the cutaneous lymph trunks empty into contralateral nodes. No crossing of the midline has been documented for the mucosal lymphatics of the upper lip. Efferent lymphatic channels from nodes located in the submental, submandibular triangle, and periparotid areas drain into the lymph nodes of the upper and occasionally the middle deep cervical lymphatic chain.

ETIOLOGY

The incidence of carcinoma of the lip in the United States is 1.8 per 100,000 population.[45] The lip is the most common site of cancer of the oral cavity.[3, 26, 54] All reported series of carcinoma of the lip show that the disease occurs most frequently on the lower lip of elderly males (Table 13-1). The male to female ratio is 79:1 for the lower lip and 5:1 for the upper lip.[27]

Carcinoma of the lip is most commonly observed in the white male smoker who has a fair or ruddy complexion, light hair, and blue or gray eyes. The disease occurs primarily in males of the sixth decade. The av-

TABLE 13-1. CARCINOMA OF THE LIP

Study	Number of Patients	Males (%)	Females (%)	Mean Age (yr) or Largest Incidence Decade	Upper Lip (%)	Lower Lip (%)
Burkell[9]	534	98.6	1.4	59.6	2.6	97
Cross et al.[13]	563	98.0	2.0	62.0	3.4	88.3
Jørgensen et al.[23]	869	97.2	2.8	6th	1.8	98.2
Molnar et al.[33]	2,373	89.8	10.2	5th	6.9	93.1
Ward and Hendrick[48]	259	96.9	3.1	6th	7.7	92.3

erage age of onset is between 59 to 62 years of age, though it is not limited to that period. Cases have been reported as early as the second and third decades of life.[25]

On the lower lip, cancer is most frequently found to originate on the exposed vermilion border, just outside the line of contact with the upper lip. Tumor most often arises at a point approximately halfway between the midline and the commissure, occurring there in 85 percent of the cases.[3] Tumors arising from the commissure comprise less than 1 percent of reported cases.[25, 53] When tumors occur on the upper lip they frequently arise near the midline and account for 1.8 to 7.7 percent of all lip cancer.[23, 48]

More than one third of the patients with carcinoma of the lip have outdoor occupations.[9, 29, 30, 33] Prolonged exposure to sunlight has been implied as a major etiologic factor. Damaging effects of solar exposure are found in most patients with lip carcinoma regardless of their ages. Loss of elastic fibers, atrophy of fat and glandular elements, and hyperkeratosis with atypical cells are common features. The lower lip receives considerable solar radiation under normal sunlight conditions, while the upper lip is by comparison shaded. This is probably the reason for the infrequent occurrences of carcinoma involving the upper lip.[9, 13, 23] The lip is susceptible to actinic change because it lacks a pigment layer for protection. The black race has pigment in the lip, which may explain the rare occurrence of carcinoma of the lip in this portion of the population. Lip cancer is 10 times more common in whites than in non-whites.[6]

Early literature suggested tobacco in the form of pipe smoking as a possible etiologic agent for carcinoma of the lip.[7, 14, 33] The high temperatures generated within the stem from the smoke may cause irritation sufficient to induce carcinomatous degeneration. Moderate to heavy cigarette smoking is now more frequently observed among lip cancer patients than is pipe smoking.

An association of carcinoma of the lip and a positive Wasserman reaction or clinical signs of syphilis had been implied in earlier patient series. Such an occurrence had been reported to be as high as 20 percent in some studies. Recent papers, however, indicate that not more than 2 percent of patients with carcinoma of the lip have syphilis, and it is now believed that syphilis plays no significant part in the development of lip cancer.[9, 48]

Poor dental hygiene may play an etiologic role in cancer of the lip. In nearly all series reported, fewer than 15 percent of patients have what is considered to be good oral and dental hygiene.[13, 30] Poor fitting dentures, sharp jagged teeth, and chronically infected gingiva may cause persistent irritation of the lips.

Chronic alcoholism may be another factor in the development of carcinoma of the lip. Although the association of excessive alcoholism with carcinoma of the oral cavity has long been recognized, Molnar, Ronay, and Tapolcsany found that 47 percent of 2,623 patients with carcinoma of the lip were habitual alcohol consumers.[33]

Recently, carcinoma of the lip has been found to be associated with chronic immunosuppression. Berger et al. reported a case of epidermoid carcinoma of the lip in a 27-year-old male and in a 17-year-old female.[4] Both patients had previous renal transplantation and were receiving immunosuppressant drugs. Immunologic systems may provide a "surveillance" function by which neoplastic cells are identified and either destroyed or restricted. Immunosuppressive therapy may prevent this system from recognizing tumor-specific antigens located on the surface of the neoplastic cell, thus increasing the risk of neoplasia.

CLASSIFICATION

The vast majority of neoplasms of the lip are squamous cell carcinoma. Occasionally, a basal cell carcinoma will extend from the skin of the lip onto the labial surface. When basal cell carcinoma involves the lip, it is twice as common on the upper lip as the lower lip, and is the most common form of cancer to involve the upper lip.[12, 51] The remainder of the malignant epithelial neoplasms of the lip are of minor salivary gland origin, predominately adenoid cystic carcinoma, adenocarcinoma, or mucoepidermoid carcinoma.[11, 19]

Three morphologic types of squamous cell carcinoma of the lip are seen: exophytic, ulcerative, and verrucous. The exophytic type is slightly more common than the ulcerative type. Verrucous carcinoma rarely occurs on the lips.[3] The exophytic form grows superficially and tends to metastasize late. It begins as an area of thickened epithelium that eventually extends lateral and deep into the substance of the lip, forming a disc-like base. This base is usually only a few millimeters under the epithelium. The lesion becomes heaped up and may extend a centimeter or more above the surface of the lip. Deep narrow crypts and crevices form within the substance of the tumor and secondary infection supervenes. This form of tumor may reach a size of 6 to 7 cm with very little local destruction of tissue. The superficial portions of the tumor, however, eventually become necrotic and frank ulceration usually occurs when the lesion has reached the size of 1 cm. The ulcer becomes covered by a reddish-brown or black crust, which when removed reveals an easily bleeding grayish-red or deep red granular surface. Exophytic carcinomas gradually become deeply infiltrative in more advanced cases and lose their papillomatous character.

The ulcerative type of squamous cell carcinoma of the lip begins like the exophytic type, as an epithelial thickening or blister. However, in the early stages the tumor is minimally elevated above adjacent tissues. Ulceration occurs earlier than in the exophytic type, and the lesion may be ulcerated from the beginning (Fig. 13-4). The tumor is usually round or oval and tends to bleed more readily than the exophytic type. In addition, the ulcerative type manifests a relatively greater tendency for rapid infiltration

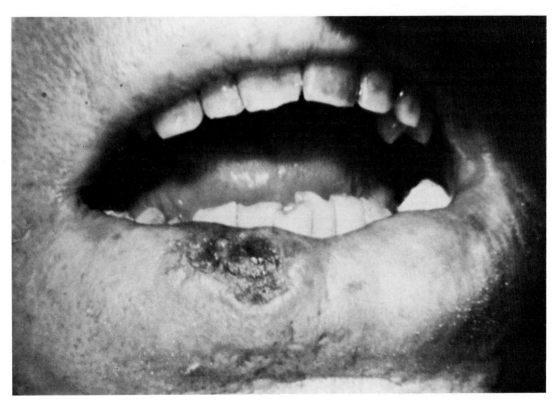

Fig. 13-4. Ulcerative squamous cell carcinoma of the lower lip. The ulcer has a disc-like base.

and invasion (Fig. 13-5) and is usually of a higher histologic grade than the exophytic type. Because of its infiltrative growth, secondary bacterial infection occurs more frequently.

The distance between the surface epithelium of the lip and the orbicularis oris is only about 2 mm, because of the very thin layer of submucosal tissue that is present. As the ulcerative squamous cell carcinoma continues to grow, it fixes the skin and deeply invades into the substance of the lip. Muscle involvement is therefore an early finding with this form of lip carcinoma. Unlike skin cancer, which is considered to be infiltrative when tumor involves musculature, it is not possible to make muscle invasion the basis for classification in cancer of the lip.

Verrucous carcinomas of the lip are rare. These tumors may grow to considerable size by lateral spread, but they do not deeply invade the lip substance. The neoplasm usually evolves in an indolent fashion in areas of leukoplakia. It has the appearance of a piled-up growth with a papillary surface. Histologic examination demonstrates hyperplastic, well-differentiated squamous cell carcinoma in finger-like extensions. Cellular atypism and mitoses are rare.

Broders, in 1920, established a microscopic grading of carcinoma of the lip. A slight revision was later made, and for the most part, this system is used today in assessing cancer of the lip (Table 13-2).[8] Broders' classification was based on cellular differentiation. It is well established that the poorer the differentiation of carcinoma of the lip, the greater the incidence of metas-

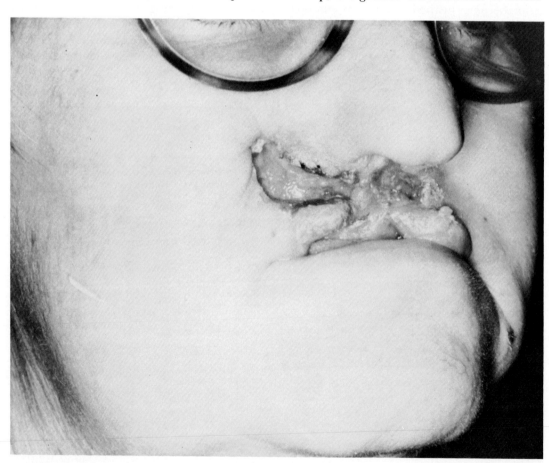

Fig. 13-5. Ulcerative squamous cell carcinoma of the upper lip with extensive invasion into the cheek and nasal areas.

TABLE 13-2. BRODERS' CLASSIFICATION FOR CARCINOMA OF THE LIP[8]

Grade of Malignancy	Cellular Differentiation Expressed in Percent of the Total Cellular Elements
I	near 75 to 100
II	50 to 75
III	25 to 50
IV	0 to 25

tasis and the worse the prognosis for survival.[2, 7, 8, 20, 27] In 537 cases of cancer of the lip reported by Broders, no metastases were present in grade I neoplasms whereas all grade IV neoplasms demonstrated metastases.[8]

Approximately 85 percent of squamous cell carcinomas of the lip are well differentiated and fall into grade I or II of Broders' classification.[3, 12, 27] Only 5 percent are poorly differentiated tumors and spindle-cell variants.[2] Poorly differentiated carcinoma and spindle-cell variants are much more aggressive in their growth pattern. They spread along neural pathways and metastasize early to cervical lymphatics.

In addition to grade of differentiation, metastases are also closely related to size of the neoplasm, the location on the lip, and the involvement of the mandible. Nearly all studies indicate increased incidence of metastases with increasing size of tumor. A partial explanation for this is that larger lesions tend to be less differentiated. Carcinomas of the upper lip and of the commissure grow more rapidly, ulcerate sooner, and metastasize earlier than lower lip cancer. Lesions larger than 2 cm or involving the upper lip or extending to the lateral commissure thus have a poorer prognosis.[13] Mandibular involvement with tumor also offers a poor prognosis and a high incidence of regional metastases. Early bone involvement suggests a more aggressive tumor. Creely and Peterson found only a 33 percent three-year survival rate in those patients with mandibular involvement.[12]

Clinically apparent cervical lymph node metastases are present in fewer than 10 percent of patients presenting with squamous cell carcinoma of the lower lip and slightly more frequently among patients with upper lip carcinoma.[9, 14, 20, 23, 27, 43, 54] Approximately 20 percent of clinically apparent cervical lesions involving the commissure present with clinical metastases on initial examination.[27] Subsequent development of cervical metastases following treatment of the primary neoplasm ranges from 5 to 15 percent.[14, 23, 30, 32, 54] Most metastases present within 2 years following treatment of the primary tumor. The likelihood of their occurrence increases with increased duration and size of the tumor at presentation. The risk of developing metastases also increases with repeated local recurrences.

As a rule, metastases occur later in the course of the disease with lip cancer than with lesions found in other sites within the oral cavity, and further dissemination also tends to occur later. Cervical metastases from both the upper and lower lip generally progress in an orderly fashion. From tumors occurring in the midportion of the lower lip, the submental nodes are more commonly involved first, while from tumors of the lateral portion of the lip, the submandibular triangle nodes are most frequently involved. Subsequent metastases develop in the upper deep cervical nodes and later in the middle and lower deep cervical nodes. Contralateral or bilateral metastases may develop when the primary lesion is near to or crosses the midline of the lip. Metastatic spread from upper lip carcinoma tends to occur first to the preauricular or infraparotid lymph nodes.[30] Spread then occurs more rapidly to the submandibular triangle nodes and to the upper and middle nodes of the jugular chain that is seen with lower lip lesions.

Most metastases that develop subsequent to initial treatment of upper or lower lip carcinoma follow the same progression: first, the submandibular triangle and submental lymph nodes and then to the deep cervical lymphatic chain.[39] Until advanced stages, metastatic disease from carcinoma of the lip tends to remain above the level of the clavicle. General dissemination eventually occurs to viscera in 15 percent of patients dying of lip carcinoma.[30] In such instances, regional cervical metastases have been present for prolonged periods of time.

Several different criteria for classifying carcinoma of the lip have been defined by various authors in reporting their series of cases. The TNM system for the oral cavity has not included the lip because of the significant difference in biologic activity of lip cancer as compared to oral cavity cancer. Articles in the recent literature have staged carcinoma of the lip according to the Union Internationale Contre le Cancer (UICC) at the meeting in Geneva in 1974 (Table 13-3).[21] This classification places emphasis on infiltration in addition to size, since both features correlate with tumor behavior and prognosis. For example, a tumor may be less than 2 cm in its greatest dimension and still be classified as T3 if it is deeply infiltrative. The recent Task Force for Head and Neck Sites suggested a T classification that is different from that used in other head and neck malignancies as well as from the UICC classification (Table 13-4).[42] Clinical staging of lymph nodes is the same for carcinoma of the lip as for carcinoma of all other areas of the head and neck (Table 13-5).

TABLE 13-3. CLASSIFICATION OF CARCINOMA OF THE LIP ACCORDING TO THE UNION INTERNATIONALE CONTRE LE CANCER GENEVA 1974[21]

T1S	Preinvasive carcinoma (carcinoma in situ)
T0	No evidence of primary tumor
T1	Tumor measuring 2 cm or less in largest dimension and strictly superficial or exophytic
T2	Tumor measuring 2 cm or less in largest dimension with minimal infiltration in depth
T3	Tumor measuring more than 2 cm in largest dimension or one with deep infiltration irrespective of size
T4	Tumor involving bone

TABLE 13-4. CLASSIFICATION OF CARCINOMA OF THE LIP ACCORDING TO THE TASK FORCE FOR HEAD AND NECK SITES 1976[42]

T1S	Carcinoma in situ
T1	Tumor smaller than 1 cm in its largest dimension
T2	Tumor between 1 and 3 cm in size
T3	Tumor larger than 3 cm
T4	Deep invasion of bone and muscle

TABLE 13-5. CLINICAL STAGING OF CERVICAL METASTASES FOR CARCINOMA OF THE LIP[42]

N0	No lymph nodes palpable
N1	Single homolateral node less than 3 cm
N2	Single homolateral node 3 to 6 cm or multiple homolateral nodes up to 6 cm
N3	Homolateral node greater than 6 cm or bilateral, or contralateral only
	When bilateral nodes are present, each neck should be classified separately

Many different stage-groupings for carcinoma of the lip have been offered by investigators reporting retrospective patient studies. There has been no uniformity in such staging. Stage-grouping of cancer of the lip has not as yet been established by either the Task Force for Head and Neck Sites or the Union Internationale Contre le Cancer. At present, lip carcinoma should be classified according to the TNM extent of disease classification.

PATIENT EVALUATION

Carcinoma of the lip tends to have a protracted clinical course. In its early stages it usually demonstrates relatively indolent behavior and frequently the only early symptom is the presence of a blister or induration arising in an area of leukoplakia. A history of recurrent lip crusting that bleeds readily on removal of the crust is characteristic of this lesion. Such crusting may exist for many years before evidence of infiltration develops. This indolent behavior tends to lull the physician and patient into a false sense of security. It is uncommon for carcinoma to arise de novo from an entirely normal-appearing lower lip.

Clinically, it is easy to recognize carcinoma of the lip. Its superficial location makes the tumor easily accessible to inspection and palpation. The appearance is in general so typical that a mistake in diagnosis is uncommon. Fortunately, most lip carcinomas remain localized for an extended period of time as an exophytic or ulcerative growth that slowly increases in size. Tissue destruction by the neoplasm is not prominent. Although the diagnosis of carcinoma is easily made on a clinical basis, it must be confirmed by biopsy.

In more advanced stages, extension of the tumor into the skin of the lip is seen. Secondary infection and necrosis develop. The lesion becomes surrounded by erythema, and a purulent exudate forms in the ulcerated center of a tender, swollen tumor mass. Only when infection is present are pain and tenderness prominent features. As the tumor enlarges, involvement of the mandible may occur and erosion of bone becomes demonstrable on roentgenograms. The patient must be closely examined for hypesthesia in the distribution of the mental nerve. Even in the absence of cortical bone destruction, the tumor may grow along the mental nerve into the medullary portion of the mandible and may even extend as far as the cranial cavity.[40] Involvement of the mental nerve may be by perineural invasion or by direct extension from mandibular involvement with the tumor. In patients who are edentulous and have undergone considerable alveolar bone resorption, the mental nerve is in a more superficial location and is more vulnerable to tumor invasion.

Lymphadenopathy is seen more frequently in carcinomas larger than 2 cm than in smaller carcinomas. Metastases develop first in the submandibular and submental triangles. Subsequent metastases appear in the upper and middle cervical chain. Only in very late stages do distant metastases develop. Visceral metastases are very uncommon even in postmortem inspection of patients who died of lip cancer.

Approximately 3 percent of patients will develop metastases very early in the course of disease when the primary lesion is 1 cm or less in size.[30] This usually indicates a very aggressive biologic behavior. Not all lymphadenopathy, however, represents metastases. Infection of the tumor or poor oral hygiene may cause the regional adenopathy. Lymph nodes larger than 2 cm are rarely inflammatory, however, and most often represent metastatic disease. Metastatic nodes are much more firm to palpation compared to inflammatory nodes.

The distinction of carcinoma from benign lip lesions is seldom difficult. Hyperkeratosis and cheilitis frequently occur alone or concurrent with lip cancer. Leukoplakia in association with carcinoma of the lip has been reported in from 2 to 75 percent of cases.[20, 30, 41] Leukoplakia is a clinical term denoting a white plaque, which may possess varying degrees of histologic differentiation from hyperkeratosis through carcinoma in situ to invasive carcinoma. The frequency with which malignant changes occur in leukoplakia of the lip is unknown but may approach 30 percent.[52] Carcinoma of the lip tends to be more indurated than benign lesions and has a more discrete margin. If secondary infection is severe the borders may be less distinct.

Cheilitis may be associated with chronic dermatitis and eczema or with prolonged exposure to sunlight. It is characterized by scaling of the vermilion border, inflammation and exudate, crusting extending to the skin of the lip, and fissuring of the commissure. Cheilitis is a frequent precursor of lip cancer especially in patients having had prolonged exposure to actinic rays. It is necessary to follow its course closely so that an early malignancy is not overlooked. In suspicious cases, histologic examination is mandatory.

There are a number of benign and malignant neoplasms that may occasionally be confused with squamous cell carcinoma of the lip. Malignant melanomas are rare within the vermilion portion of the lip but may occur in the skin. Such tumors usually arise in a melanotic area and often display distinct pigmentation giving the growth a bluish-black color. These lesions demonstrate less tendency for necrotic ulceration than do squamous cell carcinomas. Sarcomas of the lip are also rare and may be difficult to distinguish from carcinomas. Microscopic examination is required.

Benign and malignant tumors of minor salivary gland origin are rare in the lip. These tumors develop within the depths of the lip substance without any connection with the mucous membrane. Because they are covered with mucosa and do not appear on the vermilion surface, they may be confused with fibromas, lipomas, and retention cysts of the lip. Myoblastomas have also been reported to occur in the lip but remain beneath the mucosa.[14]

Granuloma pyogenicum, keratoacanthoma and papillomas are commonly confused with lip cancer, because they are exophytic and occur on the vermilion border or adjacent skin. Granuloma pyogenicum has a bluish-red tint and rises above the vermilion epithelium like a cupola. It bleeds copiously when manipulated and has a softer consistency than cancer.

Benign papillomas of the lip are more exophytic for their size than are carcinomas and tend to be pedunculated. Because the base of the papilloma is situated chiefly in the epithelium of the lip, there is minimal induration of the lip substance.

Keratoacanthoma (molluscum sebaceum) can occur on the cutaneous aspect of the lip and give the appearance of a squamous cell carcinoma. These lesions are usually circular in shape with a central crater and may demonstrate rapid growth. They have a tendency to regress spontaneously, but concern about malignancy should not be relaxed until growth has ceased and there are signs of involution. Histologically, they are well circumscribed and have a central keratinizing core.

The lips may be the site of an extragenital chancre, which can present diagnostic difficulties. The history of a rapidly developing ulcerated firm lesion with evidence of spirochetes on darkfield examination should establish the diagnosis of syphilis. Acute tuberculous ulcers can occur on the buccal mucosa of the lips and are associated with an active pulmonary focus. Lupus vulgaris does not occur primarily on the vermilion but may extend to the area from adjacent skin. Leprosy, sarcoidosis, and Crohn disease are other causes of granulomatous cheilitis and must occasionally be differentiated from carcinoma of the lip.

Biopsy of the lip is mandatory prior to treatment, because hyperkeratosis, cheilitis, keratoacanthoma and other benign lesions can be confused with carcinoma of the lip. An elliptic incision encompassing a portion of the lesion as well as adjacent normal-appearing tissue is achieved under local anesthesia. The biopsy specimen should be sufficiently deep to assess the invasiveness of the tumor. Biopsy in the center of ulcerative or exophytic tumors may reveal keratin or necrotic debris and show no evidence of malignancy.

TREATMENT

Radiation Therapy

Radiotherapeutic treatment of carcinoma of the lip may consist of interstitial, contact, or external radiation therapy. Interstitial and contact applications of radium were once the standard technique of radiologic treatment. Surface or contact applications of radiation may be effective for early lip carcinoma that does not demonstrate deep invasion of more than 3 mm; however, deeply infiltrating tumors are more effectively treated by external therapy or by a combinaton of surface and interstitial needle application.

Accurate spacing of interstitial seeds or needles is not a simple procedure and overlapping of the radiation points creates problems of uneven distribution of the irradiation. Tumor dose computation is difficult with contact radium application. In addition, there is the additional disadvantage of frequent exposure of the therapist to radium. An average of six to eight applications are usually necessary for treatment. For these reasons and others, contact and interstitial radiotherapy has largely given way to external roentgen therapy, which is more versatile and controllable.

Low voltage roentgen radiation (100 kV) has produced satisfactory results for small shallow lesions less than 1.5 cm in diameter. A total dose is given of 3,000 to 4,500 rads (measured in air) in divided doses over 1 to 4 weeks of therapy. Higher energy (200 kV) with good filtration is preferable for tumors larger than 1.5 cm in diameter. These large lesions require a much larger field. A total dose of 4,500 to 6,000 rads (measured in air) is delivered in fractions over a 4 to 6 week period.

More recently, electron beam irradiation in the order of 7 to 18 MeV has been used for treating carcinoma of the lip.[46] The advantage of 7, 9, or 11 MeV electron beams over conventional voltage radiation therapy is the additional depth of penetration. The electron beam results in 80 to 100 percent of delivered energy at a depth of 2 cm with 7 MeV and of 3 cm with 11 MeV. An added advantage of this form of irradiation is the rapid fall off in dose beyond those depths. Thus, the mandible receives very little irradiation in treating most lip carcinomas. Very small lip cancers subjected to electron beam irradiation may be treated with 2,000 rads delivered in 2 weeks or less. Large deeply infiltrating tumors are treated with 7,000 to 8,000 rads in fractions over 6 to 7 weeks.

Regardless of the form of radiotherapy used, care must be taken to protect uninvolved tissue by the use of a cutout lead contact. This will limit the beam to the desired area, and confine the side effects of radio-mucositis and radiodermatitis to a minimal area of the lip. Permanent increased sensitivity of the treated area to thermal and actinic stimuli is present. This is a disadvantage of radiation therapy for patients having occupations requiring long periods of time in the sun.

Surgical Treatment

Early carcinomas of the lip may be treated successfully by either surgery or irradiation, and the results are cosmetically acceptable with both methods. In advanced lesions, surgery or a combination of surgery and irradiation are preferred. Primary surgery offers the advantages of eradication of disease, pathologic survey of margins, and reconstruction of the defect in a single procedure. Surgical procedures to reconstruct the lip after excision of tumor may be classified as follows: those limited to the remaining lip segment; those that borrow tissue from the opposite lip; those that utilize adjacent cheek tissue; and those that utilize distant flaps.[24]

PRIMARY CLOSURE OPERATIONS

A V-shaped excision is the simplest form of surgical treatment for lip carcinoma. A full-thickness wedge-shaped excision of the tumor with a margin of at least 0.5 cm of normal-appearing tissue beyond the recognized limits of the tumor can be performed under local anesthesia. Modifications of the V excision have been advocated, changing it to an S-plasty or Z-plasty to create a step-like closure. Any of these techniques (the V, S, or Z) offer an acceptable scar. The incision should not extend beyond the mental crease, however, since to do so results in an unsightly pointed chin. If tumors require excision of more than one half the entire width of the lip, a V-excision should be combined with some form of cheiloplasty.

When leukoplakia is present in association with a small invasive carcinoma, V-excision should be combined with vermilionectomy (Fig. 13-6).[17, 35, 44] Vermilionectomy,

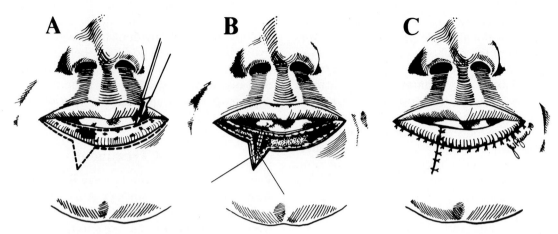

Fig. 13-6. Vermilionectomy combined with a V-excision of the lower lip. This technique can be used when leukoplakia is present in association with a small invasive carcinoma of the lip.

or "lip shave," may be used for superficial lesions confined to the mucous membrane and for treatment of multicentric areas of carcinoma in situ. Reconstruction of the vermilion is performed by advancing mucous membrane flaps from the oral cavity.

LIP AUGMENTATION PROCEDURES

Reconstruction of the lower lip should occur immediately after surgical resection of carcinoma. Local flaps are preferable because of close skin color and texture match and the availability of mucous membrane. Vertical defects no larger than one half of the width of the lower lip are best closed using a full-thickness flap pedicled on the vermilion border of the opposite lip, containing a labial artery (Fig. 13-7). Estlander's original operation was devised for closure of lower lip defects near the commissure of the mouth.[16] Since its original description the operation has been modified in many ways to accommodate surgical defects anywhere in the lower lip.

Defects may similarly be reconstructed in accordance with the techniques described

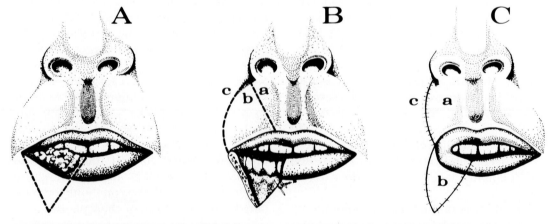

Fig. 13-7. Estlander type of pedicled flap for reconstruction of a lower lip defect. Incisions should follow the nasolabial crease so that the subsequent scar will fall within natural skin lines.

by Abbe.[1] The Estlander and Abbe flaps (lip-switch flaps) should be reconstructed so that the height of the flap equals the height of the defect. The width of the flap should be one half that of the resected segment so that the two lips are reduced in width proportionately. The pedicle should be made narrow to facilitate rotation, but care must be taken not to injure the labial artery. The secondary defect should be closed in three layers. Accurate approximation of the vermilion border of the flap with that of the defect prevents a notched appearance. If the pedicle of the flap crosses the oral stoma (Abbe flap) it should be severed in 2 to 3 weeks. A Z-plasty often facilitates good ap-

proximation of vermilion borders at the time of pedicle severance.

ADJACENT CHEEK FLAPS

Advancement of the remaining lip segments after resection of tumor may allow reconstruction of the lip. Defects of the midportion of the upper lip are closed by the method of Dieffenbach and Webster in which a crescent of perialar cheek skin is excised to allow for advancement of the lip segments medially.[49] If the wound closure is too tight, an Abbe flap may be added in the midline (Fig. 13-8).

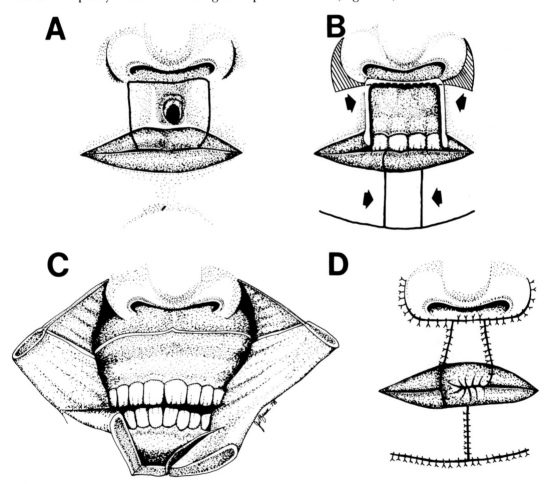

Fig. 13-8. Advancement of remaining lip segments after resection of a tumor of the upper lip. Perialar cheek skin excisions allow advancement of the lip segments, and an Abbe flap from the lower lip prevents excessive tension on wound closure.

Midline lower lip defects may similarly be closed by full-thickness advancement flaps as described by Burow,[10] Bernard,[5] May,[31] and Webster et al.[49] These techniques require excision of the tumor of the lower lip as a wedge-shaped or square segment (Fig. 13-9). Excisions of additional triangles in the nasolabial region are performed to allow advancement of the cheek flaps. The triangular excisions should follow the lines of the nasolabial crease and should include only skin and subcutaneous tissues. The underlying muscle is mobilized to form a new commissure. The mucous membrane is separated from the muscle and turned outward to provide a vermilion border. Incisions are made in the gingivobuccal sulcus as far back as the last molar tooth if necessary to allow proper approximation of the remaining lip segments without tension.

When lower or upper lip defects are not too large, nasolabial transposition flaps may be used. A full-thickness flap is incised in the area of the nasolabial crease based on the facial artery inferiorly. The flap is transposed into the lip defect and sutured in three layers. Mucosa from the flap is advanced to create a vermilion. Defects as large as three-fourths of the lip width may be reconstructed by such a technique.

DISTANT FLAP OPERATIONS

In very large defects of the upper or lower lip if flaps from adjacent areas are not applicable or sufficient, a distant flap must be used. Excision of the lower lip, chin, and middle section of the mandible for carcinoma often requires such flaps for closure. The deltopectoral (Bakamjian) flap is perhaps the most commonly used. Such a flap may be lined with a skin graft or turned on itself to supply the inner lining of the reconstructed lip.

The temporal based forehead flap may be used for upper lip reconstruction; it may be lined with a split-thickness skin graft or mucosal graft from the oral cavity if necessary. In males, hair-bearing scalp may be incorporated to provide hair growth to camouflage surgical scars.

Postoperative Care

Wound care following surgical resection of lip carcinoma should include keeping the

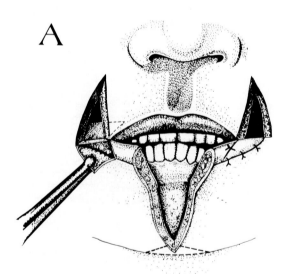
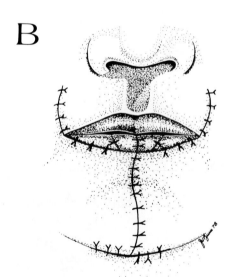

Fig. 13-9. Large resection of lower lip tumors require full-thickness cheek advancement. The excisions include only skin and subcutaneous tissues. The underlying muscle is mobilized to form a new commissure. The mucous membrane is separated from the muscle and turned outward to provide a vermilion border.

suture line clean and dry. Dressings are not necessary for local flaps or if primary closure of the surgical defect has been accomplished. Sutures may be removed between the fifth and seventh day postoperatively unless the patient has had previous irradiation. An antibiotic ointment may be applied to the suture line, but systemic antibiotics are not necessary. Should wound infection supervene, it should be treated by appropriate antibiotics and local wound care.

Postoperative feeding in patients who have had surgery of the lip should be restricted to liquids for the first 48 hours followed by a soft diet for 4 to 5 days. Soft foods require less biting and chewing and thus less movement of the lips. Patients with pedicle flaps crossing the oral stoma, as in the Abbe flap, must be maintained on a semiliquid diet until division of the pedicle takes place.

Postoperative complications include lip ectropion, disruption of the vermilion, and microstomia. The first two complications can be minimized by not allowing suture lines to come under tension and by careful approximation of vermilion margins. Microstomia can be prevented by liberal use of local and regional flaps. Commissure distortion occurs following operations involving this region. Lip-switch operations at the commissure often require secondary commissuroplasty to prevent distortion and microstomia.

Complications following radiotherapeutic treatment of lip carcinoma include dermatitis and chronic ulceration with cicatrical scarring of the lip. An anatomic defect is left following radiation therapy of advanced lesions if tissue destruction has occurred. Radiation osteomyelitis may be seen in large lesions if the radiation fields include the mandible.

Treatment of Lymph Node Metastases

In the opinion of most authors the treatment of cervical metastases is a surgical problem.[9, 15, 23, 27, 36, 54] Although cervical metastases may be treated with interstitial radium or external roentgen therapy, these treatments are less successful than surgery. Radiotherapeutic control of clinically involved cervical nodes from lip carcinoma is successful in approximately 35 percent of cases if nodes are palpable at the time of initial presentation. Subsequent development of cervical metastases that occurs after the initial lip lesion has been treated can be controlled by radiotherapy in 16 percent of cases.[27] Surgical treatment of cervical metastases offers a five-year control rate of 50 percent. In patients with nodes developing after initial therapy, treatment by operation is about as successful as for patients operated on for nodes found on admission. Information is not available concerning the efficacy of combined radiotherapy and surgery for the treatment of cervical metastases from lip carcinoma. Presumably, combined therapy might allow greater control of neck metastases in cases in which metastatic nodes are large, multiple, or bilateral.

Although metastases are usually confined to the submandibular and submental triangle areas for extended periods of time before extension to the deep cervical lymph nodes occurs, supraomohyoid dissection is not recommended. Such an operation offers a higher recurrence rate than a complete neck dissection. When the tumor invades or approaches the midline, however, the therapeutic neck dissection on the affected side should include a prophylactic contralateral suprahyoid dissection. The presence of bilateral metastases calls for bilateral neck dissections.

Prophylactic neck dissection for occult metastatic disease is not indicated for two reasons. First, the percentage of patients who subsequently develop cervical metastases following treatment of their primary lesions is less than 10 percent (Table 13-6).[18, 36, 37] Second, the cure rate for therapeutic neck dissection compares favorably with the cure rate in patients undergoing a prophylactic neck dissection for confirmed occult metastases.[15, 27] The small group that will eventually develop metastases thus have

TABLE 13-6. INCIDENCE OF SUBSEQUENT
METASTASES: PATIENTS WITHOUT EVIDENCE OF
METASTASES ON ADMISSION

Study	Total Patients	Subsequent Metastases	Percent
Martin et al.[30]	313	27	8.6
Richards[37]	275	11	4.0
del Regato and Sala[36]	498	39	7.8
Jørgensen et al.[23]	869	45	5.2
Burkell[9]	534	16	3.0
Gladstone and Kerr[18]	519	47	9.1
Modlin[32]	156	15	9.6

a fair chance of survival with adequate surgical treatment. Prophylactic neck dissection may be advised, however, for large undifferentiated tumors that involve the oral commissure and the upper lip.

RESULTS

The prognosis for cure in carcinoma of the lip varies, depending upon the extent of disease at the time of initial examination. Lesions less than 2 cm in diameter that involve the lower lip enjoy an excellent prognosis. The cure rates for T1 and T2 lesions without evidence of cervical node metastases are generally greater than 90 percent for surgery or radiation therapy. If the lip cancer population is considered as a total group (Table 13-7), the average 5-year absolute and determinate survival without evidence of disease is found to be approximately 65 and 80 percent respectively in the combined series of 10,230 patients. Treatment in these series consisted of irradiation, surgery, and combinations of the two.

It is remarkable how similar the survival rates are for carcinoma of the lip treated with radiation therapy or surgery. Molnar et al. reported a determinate 5-year survival of 86 percent in patients treated primarily by irradiation.[33] Bernier and

Clark, in a large series of lip cancer patients treated mainly by surgery, noted a 5-year determinate survival of 82 percent.[6] In a comparison study of patients with lip carcinoma treated with surgery versus radiation therapy, Ashley et al. reported that of 106 surgically treated patients, 87 percent were free of tumor through 5 years.[2] Forty-three patients were treated initially with radiation therapy and 77 percent survived 5 years without recurrence. While half of the radiation therapy recurrences developed in the lip, most of the recurrences after surgery developed in the neck. Sixty percent of the postirradiation recurrences were salvaged by subsequent operations.

The incidence of recurrent disease increases and the cure rate drops significantly in large cancers of the lip.[13, 23, 27, 36, 48] Jørgensen et al. reported that persistent or recurrent disease occurred in 7.4 percent of tumors measuring more than 2 cm in diameter or having deep infiltration.[23] Ward and Hendrick demonstrated a 5-year cure rate of 95 percent for lesions under 1 cm in diameter.[48] Curability fell to 59 percent for lesions 2 to 3 cm in diameter and to 41 percent for tumors larger than 3 cm in diameter. Gladstone and Kerr reported a cure rate of 92 percent for tumors smaller than 2 cm and 86 percent for lesions larger than 2 cm.[18]

TABLE 13-7. FIVE YEAR SURVIVAL OF PATIENTS WTH LIP
CARCINOMA

Study	Total Number of Patients	5-Year Survival (%) Determinate*	Absolute
Burkell[9]	534	89.5	79.8
Gladstone and Kerr[18]	519	82.4	65.1
Schreiner and Christy[41]	636	74.4	58.9
Wookey et al.[54]	1,128	85.1	58.4
Ebenius[14]	749	79.4	67.5
Molnar et al.[33]	2,066	86.0	75.7
Cross et al.[13]	563	58.5	49.9
Jørgensen et al.[23]	869	96.7	84.4
MacKay and Sellers[27]	3,166	89.0	65.0
	10,230	X̄ 82.3	X̄ 67.2

*Determinate: Subtracting those cases who died from intercurrent disease without evidence of cancer or those who have been lost to follow-up evaluation.

The relationship of histologic grade to recurrence and curability has been stressed by many investigators.[13, 48] Grade I carcinomas are less likely either to recur or to metastasize than are tumors of higher pathologic grades. Ward and Hendrick showed a 3-year cure rate of 95.4 percent for grade I carcinomas of the lip but only 45.5 and 38.3 percent respectively for grades III and IV.[48] Cross et al. demonstrated a 3-year cure rate of 75.5 percent for grade I and 48.5 percent for grade III lip carcinoma.[13] In this series the occurrence of regional lymph node metastases as well as the rate of recurrence was directly proportional to the grade of the malignancy of the primary neoplasm. Interestingly, the investigators demonstrated that the cure rate for patients with regional metastases was directly related to the pathologic grading of the tumor as well. The highest percentage of cures was obtained in the group of patients having the lowest histologic grade tumor.

Cancer control in patients with cervical metastases is considerably more difficult. The overall curability of patients with carcinoma of the lip and regional node metastases approaches 50 percent (Table 13-8). The poorest results are obtained when cervical node metastases are fixed to the deep structures of the neck or when there is radiographic evidence of mandibular involvement.

A statistical review of 3,166 patients with confirmed squamous cell carcinoma of the lip demonstrated that when regional lymph nodes were not involved on admission, the primary lesion was controlled in 85 percent of the cases by the initial treatment.[27] An additional 8 percent were controlled by subsequent treatment when recurrence developed. Of the patients presenting with lymph node involvement on admission, however, the primary lesion was controlled in 68 percent of the cases by the initial treatment and in an additional 7 percent by subsequent treatment. Initial treatment of the neck disease was not as good. Control of cervical metastases was obtained in only 58 percent of cases. Subsequent treatment of neck recurrence was successful in a mere 1 percent of cases. For patients with nodes developing after the initial treatment of the primary, control was obtained

TABLE 13-8. FIVE-YEAR SURVIVAL OF PATIENTS WITH LIP
CARCINOMA AND CONFIRMED REGIONAL METASTASES
(THERAPEUTIC NECK DISSECTION)

Study	Total Number of Patients	5-Year Survival (%) (Absolute)
Modlin[32]	25	52.0
Mahoney[28]	45	46.7
Cross et al.[13]	39	35.9
Jørgensen et al.[23]	27	55.5

in 35 percent of cases and subsequent treatment of recurrent neck disease was successful in 4 percent of cases.

Investigators of carcinoma of the lip have consistently observed poorer results in patients who have had previous treatment of their cancer.[13, 18, 36] Gladstone and Kerr showed a 90 percent 3-year determinate survival for patients treated initially, and a 70 percent survival for previously treated patients.[18] Cross et al. demonstrated a 78.7 percent 5-year cure rate for primary cases versus 34.6 percent for cases treated secondarily.[13] This finding is not surprising, since secondarily treated tumors have failed initial therapy and often are more advanced lesions and are of a higher histologic grade.

A few investigators have used combined therapy for large tumors of the lip with regional metastases, but the number of patients reported is small. Ward and Hendrick reported on 39 patients treated with combined radiotherapy and surgery.[48] A 3-year survival rate of 58 percent and a 5-year survival rate of 51 percent were recorded. Cross et al. reported almost identical figures on 36 cases treated with combined therapy.[13] A 3-year cure was noted in 58.3 percent of cases and a 5-year cure in 51.6 percent.

Malignant tumors of the upper lip account for 1.8 to 7.7 percent of all carcinomas of the lip. There is a greater proportion of women with cancer of the upper lip than with cancer of the lower lip. The male to female ratio of patients with upper lip cancer approaches 5:1.[27] Malignant neoplasms of the upper lip have a worse prognosis than those of the lower lip because they grow more rapidly and metastasize earlier. Metastases may be widespread throughout the preauricular nodes and cervical chain at the time of initial treatment. The 5-year survival rate for upper lip cancer is 50 to 60 percent (Table 13-9).

Both lips or the commissure are involved with carcinoma in 1 to 2 percent of cases.[6, 27] Multicentric lesions occur in approximately the same percent of cases. The prognosis for commissure lesions is not as good as for carcinomas located elsewhere on the lips. Recurrences are frequently seen. Commissure tumors behave similarly to tumors involving the buccal mucous membrane and have similar cure rates. Cross et al. reported only a 34 percent 5-year survival rate for 42 patients with oral commissure carcinoma.[13]

TABLE 13-9. FIVE-YEAR SURVIVAL OF
PATIENTS WITH UPPER LIP
CARCINOMA

Study	Total Number of Patients	5-Year Survival (Absolute)
Martin et al.[30]	21	41.0*
Eckert and Petry[15]	18	50.0
Molnar et al.[33]	154	57.8
Schreiner and Christy[41]	22	40.9

*Five-year determinate survival.

REFERENCES

1. Abbe, R. 1898. A new plastic operation for the relief of deformity due to double hare-lip. Medical Records, 53: 477.

2. Ashley, F. L., McConnell, D. V., Machida, R., Sterling, H. E., Galloway, D., and Grazer, F. 1965. Carcinoma of the lip: A comparision of five year results after irradiation and surgical therapy. American Journal of Surgery, 110: 549.

3. Batsakis, J. G., 1974. Tumors of the Head and Neck. Clinical and Pathological Considerations. Williams and Wilkins, Baltimore.

4. Berger, H. M., Goldman, R., Gonick, H. C., and Waisman, J. 1971. Epidermoid carcinoma of the lip after renal transplantation: Report of two cases. Archives of Internal Medicine, 128: 609.

5. Bernard, C. 1853. Cancer de la levre inferieure opéré par un procédé nouveau. Bulletin et memoirs. de la Société de Chirugie, 3: 357.

6. Bernier, J. L., and Clark, M. L. 1951. Squamous cell carcinoma of the lip: A critical statistical and morphological analysis of 835 cases. Military Surgeon, 109: 379.

7. Broders, A. C. 1920. Squamous cell epithelioma of the lip: A study of five hundred and thirty-seven cases. JAMA, 74: 656.

8. Broders, A. C. 1941. The microscopic grading of cancer. Surgical Clinics of North America, 21: 947.

9. Burkell, C. C. 1950. Cancer of the lip. Canadian Medical Association Journal, 62: 28.

10. Burow, C. A. 1855. Beschreibung einer Neuen Transplantations-Methode (Methode der Seitlichen Dreiecke) zum Wiederersatz Verlorengegangener Theile des Gesichts. Nauck, Berlin.

11. Byers, R. M., Boddie, A., and Luna, M. A. 1977. Malignant salivary gland neoplasms of the lip. American Journal of Surgery, 134: 528.

12. Creely, J. J., Jr., and Peterson, H. D. 1974. Carcinoma of the lip. Southern Medical Journal, 67: 779.

13. Cross, J. E., Guralnick, E., and Daland, E. M., 1948. Carcinoma of the Lip: A review of 563 case records of carcinoma of the lip at the Pondville Hospital. Surgery, Gynecology and Obstetrics, 87: 153.

14. Ebenius, B. 1943. Cancer of the lip. Acta Radiologica. Supplementum (Stockholm), 48: 1.

15. Eckert, C. T., and Petry, J. L 1944. Carcinoma of the lip. Surgical Clinics of North America, 24: 1064.

16. Estlander, J. A. 1872. Eine Methode aus der einen Lippe Substanzverluste der Anderen zu Ersetzen. Archiv Für Klinische Chirurgie. 14: 622.

17. Gaisford, J. C., Ed. 1969. Symposium on Cancer of the Head and Neck: Total Treatment and Reconstructive Rehabilitation. Vol. 2. C. V. Mosby, St. Louis.

18. Gladstone, W. S., and Kerr, H. D. 1958. Epidermoid carcinoma of the lower lip: Results of radiation therapy of the local lesions. American Journal of Roentgenology, 79: 101.

19. Heidelberger, K. P., McClatchey, K., Batsakis, J. G., and Van Wieren, C. R. 1977. Primary adenocarcinoma of the lip. Journal of Oral Surgery, 35: 67.

20. Hendricks, J. L., Mendelson, B. C., and Woods, J. E. 1977. Invasive carcinoma of the lower lip. Surgical Clinics of North America, 57: 837.

21. International Union Against Cancer, 1974. TNM Classification of Malignant Tumors. 2nd edn. Imprimerie G. de Buren S. A., Geneva.

22. Jabaley, M. E., Clement, R. L., and Orcutt, T. W. 1977. Myocutaneous flaps in lip reconstruction. Applications of the Karapandizic principle. Plastic and Reconstructive Surgery, 59: 680.

23. Jørgensen, K., Elbrond, O., and Andersen, A. P. 1973, Carcinoma of the lip: A series of 869 cases. Acta Radiologica, 12: 177.

24. Kazanjian, H., and Converse, J. M. 1959. The Surgical Treatment of Facial Injuries. 2nd edn. Williams and Wilkins, Baltimore.

25. Longenecker, C. G., and Ryan, R. F. 1965. Cancer of the lip in a large charity hospital. Southern Medical Journal, 58: 1459.

26. MacComb, W. S., and Fletcher, G. H. 1967. Cancer of the Head and Neck. Williams and Wilkins, Baltimore.

27. MacKay, E. N., and Sellers, A. H. 1964. A statistical review of carcinoma of the lip. Canadian Medical Association Journal, 90: 670.

28. Mahoney, L. J. 1969. Resection of cervical lymph nodes in cancer of the lip: Results in 123 patients. Canadian Journal of Surgery, 12: 40.

29. Marshall, K. A., and Edgerton, M. T. 1977. Indications for neck dissection in carcinoma of the lip. American Journal of Surgery, 133: 216.

30. Martin, H., MacComb, W. S., and Blady, J. V. 1941, Cancer of the lip. Annals of Surgery, 114: 226.

31. May, H. 1960. Reconstructive and Reparative Surgery. 2nd edn. F. A. Davis, Philadelphia.

32. Modlin, J. 1950. Neck dissections in cancer of the lower lip: Five-year results in 179 patients. Surgery 28: 404.

33. Molnar, L., Ronay P., and Tapolcsanyi, L. 1974. Carcinoma of the lip: Analysis of the material of 25 years. Oncology, 29: 101.

34. Most, A. 1906. Die Topographie des Lymphgefässaparates des Kopfes und des Halses in ihrer Bedeutung für die Chirurgie. Verlag von August Hirschwald, Berlin.

35. Paletta, X., Coldwater, K., and Booth, F. 1957. The treatment of leukoplakia, and carcinoma in situ of the lower lip. Annals of Surgery, 145: 74.

36. Regato, del, J. A. and Sala, J. M. 1959. The treatment of carcinoma of the lip. Radiology, 73: 839.

37. Richards, G. E. 1936. The radiological treatment of cancer 1929–1936, IV. Carcinoma of the lips. Canadian Medical Association Journal, 35: 490.

38. Rouviere, H. 1938. Anatomy of the Human Lymphatic System. Edwards Brothers, Ann Arbor.

39. Sack, J. G., and Ford, C. N. 1978. Metastatic squamous cell carcinoma of the lip. Archives of Otolaryngology, 104: 282.

40. Schmidseder, R., and Dick, H. 1977. Spread of epidermoid carcinoma of the lip along the inferior alveolar nerve. Oral Surgery, Oral Medicine, Oral Pathology, 43: 517.

41. Schreiner, B. F., and Christy, C. J. 1942. Results of irradiation treatment of cancer of the lip: Analysis of 636 cases from 1926–1936. Radiology, 39: 293.

42. Schulz, M.D., Ketcham, A. S., Sellers, A. H., and Vaage, M. 1976. Staging cancer of the lip. In American Joint Committee for Cancer Staging and End-Results Reporting Ed.: Manual for Staging of Cancer, 1976. American Joint Committee, Chicago.

43. Sharp, G. S., Williams, H. F., and Pugh, R. E. Jr. 1950. Irradiation as the preferred treatment of cancer of the lip. JAMA, 142: 698.

44. Spira, M., and Hardy, S. B. 1964. Vermilionectomy: Review of cases with variations in technique. Plastic and Reconstructive Surgery, 33: 39.

45. Szpak, C. A., Stone, M. J., and Frenkel. 1977. Some observations concerning the demographic and geographic incidence of carcinoma of the lip and buccal cavity. Cancer, 40: 343.

46. Tapley, N., and Fletcher, G. H. 1973. Applications of the electron beam in the treatment of cancer of the skin and lips. Radiology, 109: 423.

47. Villoria, J. M. F. 1975. A study of the development of the orbicularis oris muscle. Plastic and Recontructive Surgery, 55: 205.

48. Ward, G. E., and Hendrick, J. W. 1950. Results of treatment of carcinoma of the lip. Surgery, 27: 321.

49. Webster, J. P. 1955. Crescentic peri-alar cheek excision for upper lip flap advancement with a short history of upper lip repair. Plastic and Reconstructive Surgery, 16: 434.

50. Weitzner, S. 1975. Basal-cell carcinoma of the vermilion mucosa and skin of the lip. Oral Surgery, Oral Medicine, Oral Pathology, 39: 634.

52. West, T. L. 1962. Epidermoid carcinoma of the gingiva following long-standing leukoplakia. Oral Surgery, Oral Medicine, Oral Pathology, 15: 701.

53. Wilson, J. S. P., and Kemble, J. V. H. 1972. Cancer of the lip at risk. British Journal of Oral Surgery, 9: 186.

54. Wookey, H., Ash, C., Welsh, W. K., and Mustard, R. A. 1951. The treatment of oral cancer by a combination of radiotherapy and surgery. Annals of Surgery, 134: 529.

14 | Cancer of the Oral Cavity

Elliot W. Strong, M.D.
Ronald H. Spiro, M.D.

INTRODUCTION

According to current American Cancer Society estimates, the oral cavity gives rise to 5 percent of all cancers in men and 2 percent of all cancers in women. Unfortunately, these low incidences are counterbalanced by the needless misery of many of the afflicted patients and the frustration of those who treat them. Relatively few primary care physicians perform an adequate oral examination, which should include digital palpation of any suspicious areas. Even fewer are trained to recognize early oral cancer. Inasmuch as symptoms may be minimal or absent when an oral cancer is small, this means that diagnosis and treatment are too often delayed until the cancer is large or cervical lymph node metastasis is apparent.

ANATOMY

The oral cavity is the portal of entry to the aerodigestive tract, which extends from the lips anteriorly to the faucial arch posteriorly. The latter, including the palatine tonsils, the tonsillar pillar and the soft palate, is considered a part of the oropharynx. For convenience, the oral cavity has been divided into the following sites (Fig. 14-1):

Lip. The lips form the anterior boundary of the oral vestibule, commencing at the junction with the facial skin (vermilion border). Designation as lip in origin implies that a tumor has arisen from that portion of the vermilion surface that comes into contact with the opposite lip.

Buccal or cheek mucosa. The mucous membrane covering the inner surface of the cheeks and lips extends from the line of attachment of the upper and lower alveolar ridges to the point of contact of the lips.

Bordered above and below by the gingivobuccal sulci, the buccal mucosa forms the lateral wall of the oral vestibule and terminates posteriorly at the junction with the mucous membrane overlying the ascending ramus of the mandible (retromolar trigone) and anterior tonsillar pillar.

Gums (gingivae). The gingivae surround the teeth and cover the upper and lower alveolar ridges from the line of attachment laterally in the gingivobuccal sulci to the junction with the floor of the mouth and palate mucosa medially. The lower gingiva terminates at the last molar tooth, where it is contiguous with the mucous membrane overlying the anterior border of the ascending ramus of the mandible (retromolar trigone).

Retromolar trigone (retromolar gingiva). When the upper and lower jaws are in occlusion, there is communication bilaterally between the vestibule and the oral cavity proper through a space bordered by the molar teeth and the retromolar gingiva. This triangular-shaped area of mucous membrane is attached to the anterior surface of the ascending ramus of the mandible. The base of this triangle starts just posterior to the last molar tooth, and the apex terminates adjacent to the maxillary tuberosity. Laterally, this area is contiguous with the cheek mucosa that overlies the anterior tonsillar pillars.

301

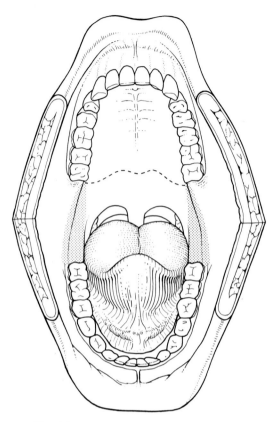

Fig. 14-1. The oral cavity extends from the vermilion border of the lips to the posterior margin of the hard palate and the junction of the glossopalatine folds with the tongue. Shading indicates the retromolar areas. The soft palate and the base of the tongue are oropharyngeal structures.

Hard palate. This forms the roof of the oral cavity and consists of the mucous membrane overlying the palatine process of the maxilla from the inner aspect of the superior alveolar ridge to the junction with the soft palate posteriorly.

Oral tongue (anterior two-thirds). The line of the circumvallate papillae defines the junction between the mobile, oral portion of the tongue and the base, or posterior one third, which is considered an oropharyngeal structure. The oral tongue is divided into the following topographic areas: tip, dorsum, lateral borders, and undersurface. Sometimes called the ventral aspect, the un-

dersurface of each side of the tongue communicates anteriorly at the attachment of the lingual frenum.

Floor of the mouth. This is the crescent shaped area between the lower gingiva and the undersurface of the tongue. Posteriorly, the mucosa blends with that overlying the base of the anterior tonsillar pillar; anteriorly, it is divided in half by the lingual frenum. Immediately adjacent to the frenum on either side is the mucosal elevation marking the termination of each submaxilary duct (plica sublingualis).

Lymphatic drainage. The structures of the oral vestibule drain by a submucosal capillary lymphatic plexus into the tributaries that terminate in submental and submandibular lymph nodes. The same is true for the mucosa that covers the lateral aspect of the upper and lower alveolar ridges. Lymphatics from the hard palate or lingual gingival mucosa may lead to upper deep jugular or submandibular lymph nodes.

Lymphatic networks are especially profuse in the tongue in the submucosal layer as well as within muscle. Superficial and deep tributaries drain directly from the anterior portion of the tongue into submental lymph nodes. Lymphatics from the lateral aspect either drain into the ipsilateral submandibular or deep jugular lymph nodes. The lymphatic channels of the central and posterior areas of the tongue have access to deep jugular lymph nodes in both sides of the neck. From the anterior floor of the mouth, lymphatics communicate with nodes in the submandibular triangle, whereas those from the posterior floor of the mouth lead to the upper deep jugular chain of lymph nodes.

ETIOLOGY

Several epidemiologic studies have documented that the incidence of oral cancer varies greatly throughout the world.[25] In the United States less than 5 percent of all carcinomas arise in the oral cavity[17] compared with a peak incidence of 50 percent reported in parts of India.[81] Although the etiology of oral carcinoma remains unknown, the observed variation seems directly related to certain cultural and environmental factors.

Tobacco

The incidence of oral squamous cancer is directly related to the use of tobacco in any form. In the United States, the relative risk in men and women who smoke increases with the amount smoked and the duration of the habit.[105] In recent years the dramatic increase in cigarette consumption by women has reduced the male predominance for this disease significantly.[83] Among cigarette smokers, the incidence of oral carcinoma has been estimated at six times that observed in the nonsmoking population.[83]

Another report concerning patients "cured" of an oral cavity cancer indicates that 40 percent of those who continued to smoke developed a second cancer in tobacco-contact tissues, compared to 6 percent of those who stopped smoking.[63] Moreover, 5-year survival rates are significantly higher in nonsmokers than in smokers. [63, 83]

Crude and processed tobacco is smoked in various ways in much of the world, including an unusual custom called reverse smoking. In parts of India, Sardinia, Venezuela, and Panama, where the burning end of the cigarette is inserted into the mouth, the incidence of hard palate cancer appears to be significantly increased.[52, 73]

The habit of holding raw tobacco against the mucous membrane in one area of the mouth is responsible for a verrucous variant called "snuff dipper's" carcinoma, which typically involves the cheek mucosa.[94] In India and other parts of Southeast Asia, the extremely high incidence of oral carcinoma can be related to a similar habit using a compound of dried and cured tobacco leaf, powdered betel nut, and betel leaves coated with slaked lime.[52, 81] The portion of the oral cavity affected by cancer corresponds to the area in which the quid is kept.

Alcohol

The relationship of alcohol consumption, particularly hard liquor, to squamous carcinoma has long been appreciated.[45, 103] In heavy drinkers, cancer of the upper aerodigestive tract occurs with almost six times the frequency observed in nondrinkers.[41]

Whether alcohol acts as a direct irritant or merely reflects underlying nutritional deficiencies has not been determined, but there is evidence that the incidence of oral cancer in those who use both tobacco and alcohol excessively may be as much as 15 times greater than in those who neither smoke nor drink.[74] One retrospective study of patients with tongue cancer confirms that the chronic alcohol and tobacco users more often die from the original tumor, a second primary tumor, or intercurrent disease than do those with tongue cancer who never use tobacco or alcohol.[40]

Exposure to Sunlight

In certain sunbelt areas of the United States, notably Texas, the lower lip is the oral site most often involved with squamous carcinoma.[96] Apparently, repeated ultraviolet exposure over several decades may cause the mucosa of the lower lip to undergo atrophic changes that may develop into carcinoma. This concept has recently been challenged by a study that showed poor correlation between the incidence of skin and lip cancer in the same areas and a disparity in the incidence of lip cancer between survey populations situated at the same geographic latitude.[96]

Other Factors

The role of metabolic and dietary deficiencies in the etiology of oral squamous carcinoma has long been suspected, but remains unproved. Degenerative mucosal changes occur in riboflavin deficient diets, and this may explain part of the relationship between alcoholism and oral cancer.[104] The high incidence of oral, as well as hypopharyngeal, squamous carcinoma in Scandinavian women seems related to the prevalence of Plummer-Vinson syndrome, in which iron deficiency is responsible for severe atrophic and ulcerative mucosal changes as well as anemia.[106]

Poor oral hygiene, mechanical irritation from sharp teeth or dentures, and specific infectious agents have been implicated as possible causes of oral cancer. Aside from older reports of squamous carcinoma of the tongue associated with the atrophic glossitis of tertiary syphillis, the relationship of these factors is most likely coincidental. Heavy users of alcohol and tobacco often have poor oral hygiene or show evidence of dental neglect.

PATHOLOGY

More than 90 percent of malignant oral tumors are squamous carcinomas arising directly from the lining membrane. Most of the remainder are "minor salivary gland" carcinomas indistinguishable histologically from similar neoplasms occurring in the major or paired salivary glands. These minor salivary tumors originate in mucous glands that lubricate the epithelium of the upper aerodigestive tract and are found most often in the palate, cheek mucosa, and lips (Table 14-1).

On rare occasion, lymphoma, melanoma, or sarcoma can arise in the oral cavity. Metastatic carcinoma is even more unusual. Our discussion will hereafter be limited to the diagnosis and treatment of the patient who has oral *squamous* carcinoma.

Premalignant Lesions

Under normal circumstances, healthy oral epithelial cells progress towards the surface and desquamate without appreciable keratin accumulation. The presence of a white patch—which clinicians call "leukoplakia"—indicates several possibilities. The superficial mucosal layer (stratum corneum) may be thickened (hyperkeratosis), the propor-

TABLE 14-1. ORAL CARCINOMA—MEMORIAL HOSPITAL, NEW YORK CITY (1966–1974)

Location	Total Number of Patients	Squamous Carcinoma— Number (%)	Minor Salivary Carcinoma— Number	Lymphoma— Number	Melanoma— Number	Sarcoma— Number
Tongue (anterior 2/3)	312	309 (99)	2	0	0	1
Floor of the mouth	290	284 (98)	4	0	0	2
Gingiva	185	172 (93)	5	3	5	0
Cheek mucosa	147	123 (84)	17	2	3	2
Lip	118	107 (91)	11	0	0	0
Hard palate	68	33 (48)	29	3	1	2
Total	1120	1028	68	8*	9	7†
%	100	91.6	6.1	0.8	0.8	0.7

*4 Histiocytic lymphoma, 4 lymphosarcoma.
†Includes embryonal rhabdomyosarcoma 2 patients; spindle cell sarcoma 2 patients; fibrosarcoma 1 patient; hemangiosarcoma 1 patient; and myxoliposarcoma 1 patient.

tion of nucleated cells may be increased near the surface (parakeratosis), and the basal layer (stratum granulosum) may show accentuation with elongation of the rete ridges into the submucosa (acanthosis).

All of the foregoing changes are harmless and stand in contrast to premalignant "leukoplakia," which on microscopic examinations show abnormal cell orientation, proliferation, and staining characteristic. The stratum corneum may be hyperkeratotic or thin, and differentiation from carcinoma in situ may be difficult. Not only is there a significant risk that carcinoma may develop in such dysplastic areas, but these mucosal alterations may mask a carcinoma or may be associated with invasive carcinoma in other areas.

Oral "leukoplakia" is most common in older individuals. Accurate prediction of the histology is seldom possible by gross appearance alone, and a biopsy will usually be required. In one review of 332 biopsies taken from areas of leukoplakia, the diagnosis was carcinoma in situ in 6 (1.8 percent) and invasive squamous carcinoma in 27 (8.1 percent).[98] Relatively few white lesions prove to be malignant, and it is not unusual for potentially malignant areas to be erythematous, rather than white (erythroplasia)[60, 77, 78] (Fig. 14-2).

Gross Appearance

Superficially invasive cancer may be indistinguishable clinically from certain types of leukoplakia or erythroplasia, but the typical oral squamous carcinoma is an obvious ulcerated lesion with a greyish shaggy base. Extending laterally from the margin of this ulcer, as well as deeply into the underlying tissue, is induration of variable extent. The tumor may protrude above the surface of the adjacent normal mucous membrane

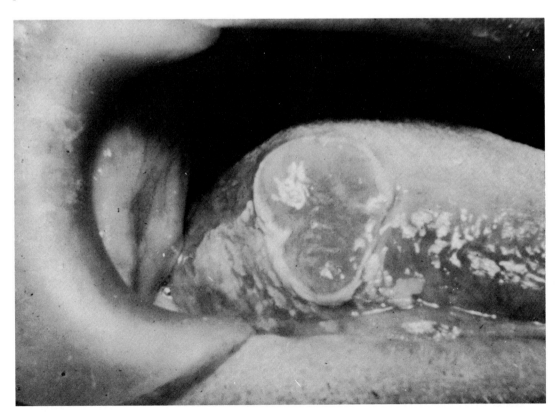

Fig. 14-2. Typical squamous carcinoma of the lateral border of the tongue with adjacent leukoplakia.

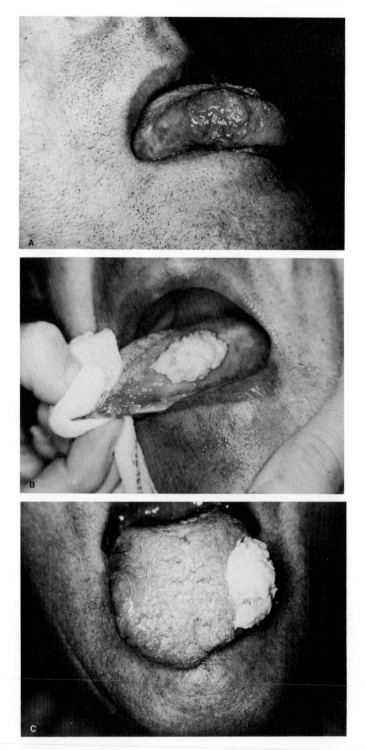

Fig. 14-3. (A) Endophytic and (B) exophytic tongue carcinomas on the right and left side, respectively, in the same patient. (C) Anterior view of both lesions.

(exophytic), infiltrate deeply with minimal projection above the surface (endophytic), or, not infrequently, show combinations of both growth patterns (Figs. 14-3 A–C).

At times, ulceration may be inconspicuous and the principle finding is a firm mass covered with abnormal-appearing mucosa. Some lesions may present as plaque-like elevations with the epithelium replaced by a velvety or granular erythematous membrane and almost no induration.

The term *verrucous carcinoma* refers to certain exophytic tumors that are heaped above the surface and have a papillary, micronodular, or mamillated appearance. Similar appearing lesions occur in the larynx, nasal cavity, and elsewhere.[44] These tumors may be reddish-white or white in color and usually carry a more favorable prognosis than do the more common ulcerated cancers because of the tendency to

lateral, rather than deep extension[7,30] (Fig. 14-4).

Microscopic Appearance

Many pathologists subclassify oral squamous carcinoma according to histologic criteria formulated years ago by Broders.[13] The presence of epithelial pearls and keratinization with minimal pleomorphism and few mitoses indicates that a tumor is of low histologic grade. High grade tumors are characterized by cellular and nuclear pleomorphism and negligible keratinization.

We feel that the value of histologic grading is likely to remain limited even if standardized criteria are accepted by all. Most patients have tumors that are intermediate in grade, and delineation of the few with high or low grade tumors may prove difficult if a small biopsy is not represen-

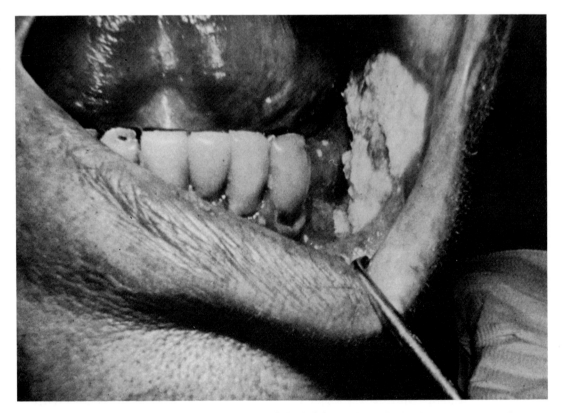

Fig. 14-4. Verrucous squamous carcinoma of the left lower buccal (cheek) mucosa extending into the gingivobuccal sulcus.

tative or if interpretation differs between pathologists. Moreover, even if high grade lesions have a faster growth rate and greater propensity for metastasis, our experience suggests that the prognosis for any patient depends much more on the extent of the tumor at the time of initial therapy than its microscopic appearance.

Regional Metastasis

Primary squamous carcinomas of the oral cavity have a well-demonstrated propensity for spread through lymphatic channels to the lymph nodes of the cervical region. For convenience, the nodes can be divided into levels according to their anatomic location. We have customarily designated the sub-mandibular area as level I.

Upper, middle, and lower jugular nodes are considered levels II, III, and IV, respectively, and the posterior triangle is level V (Fig. 14-5).

Depending upon the site of the oral tumor, certain patterns of metastatic involvement are evident. Lesions in the lip, anterior cheek mucosa, floor of the mouth, and adjacent anterior gingiva typically metastasize to level I initially. Level II is more often first involved in patients with tongue, posterior gingiva, or retromolar carcinoma. When multiple cervical nodes are involved, there is usually a progression from higher to lower node levels. Metastasis to submental or supraclavicular nodes (level V) is unusual from a primary in the oral cavity, as is involvement of a low jugular lymph node in the absence of nodal disease higher in the neck.

About one-third of our patients with a squamous carcinoma arising in the tongue, floor of the mouth, gingivae, or cheek mucosa have clinical evidence of cervical metastasis when first seen. The incidence is usually directly related to the size of the primary; extensive nodal disease with a small or inapparent primary tumor—as seen in some patients who have a pharyngeal lesion—is unusual in those with oral

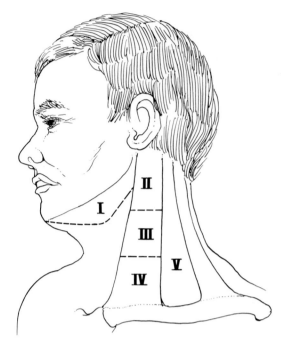

Fig. 14-5. A useful system for describing the levels of cervical lymph node metastasis from an oral primary is illustrated. Level I indicates submandibular nodes, whereas, levels II, III, and IV refer to upper, middle and lower jugular nodes, respectively. The posterior triangle nodes are considered level V.

cancers. The lower incidence of cervical metastasis in patients with hard palate or lip cancer may relate to the less extensive lymphatic network in the immobile palate mucosa or the fact that most lip cancers are relatively small and well differentiated when first seen.

The presence of an enlarged lymph node proven histologically positive is an ominous finding in any patient who has an oral squamous carcinoma.[88] Survival rates in such patients will be about half of those achieved in patients whose disease is confined to the site of origin. When nodal involvement is multiple, and extends low in the neck, or when tumor erodes through the node capsule into the soft tissues of the neck, relatively few patients are "cured" regardless of the treatment employed.[80]

Distant Metastasis

Characteristic of oral squamous cancer is the tendency for the tumor to remain localized to the primary site and regional lymph nodes until relatively late in the course of the disease. Clinical estimates of the incidence of distant spread from a primary tumor anywhere in the upper aerodigestive tract vary from 5 to 24 percent, and the incidence is as high as 47 percent in some autopsy series.[61]

Tumor involvement of distant sites is usually associated with recurrent or persistent disease above the clavicles. Lungs and bone are the sites most often involved, and the reported incidence of distant metastases from oral primaries seems to be significantly less than that observed in patients who have a tumor arising in the pharynx. Preliminary data suggest that distant metastasis occurs with significantly increased frequency in patients who receive postoperative irradiation.[61]

Multiple Primaries

Fifteen to twenty percent of patients treated for oral cancer may have one or more cancers in other sites. In our experience, at least half of these tumors involve the upper aerodigestive tract. They may occur synchronously or metachronously.

CLINICAL STAGING

In order to discuss treatment alternatives and compare results, patients with malignant tumors are grouped according to histologic diagnosis, the site of origin, and the extent of the lesion. Staging offers the clinician a succinct, standardized language that categorizes the extent of a tumor.

According to the currently accepted TNM staging system,[53] an oral primary is designated T1 if it is 2 cm or less in size and T2 if more than 2 but not more than 4 cm. T3 refers to a lesion which exceeds 4 cm,

and T4 describes a massive, deeply invasive tumor.

Neck node status (N) depends upon the presence or absence of lymph node enlargement, whether the enlargement is solitary or multiple, and the estimated size of the largest node in either side of the neck. The current T and N classification is summarized in Table 14-2.

By adding M0 or M1 to indicate the absence or presence of distant metastases, three TNM categories are derived. Using these variables, the extent of disease is defined by one of four stages (Fig. 14-6). In patients with oral cancer, this staging is entirely clinical and is restricted to previously untreated patients.

TABLE 14-2. TNM STAGING SYSTEM FOR ORAL SQUAMOUS CANCER[53]

Primary Tumor (T)

T1	Greatest diameter of primary tumor less than 2 cm.
T2	Greatest diameter of primary tumor 2 to 4 cm.
T3	Greatest diameter of primary tumor more than 4 cm.
T4	Massive tumor greater than 4 cm with deep invasion to involve antrum, pterygoid muscles, root of tongue, or skin of neck.

Cervical Nodal Involvement (N)

N1	Single clinically positive homolateral node less than 3 cm.
N2a	Single clinically positive homolateral node 3 to 6 cm.
N2b	Multiple clinically positive homolateral nodes, none over 6 cm in diameter.
N3a	Clinically positive homolateral node(s), one over 6 cm.
N3b	Bilateral clinically positive nodes (each side staged separately).
N3c	Contralateral clinically positive node(s) only.

Distant Metastasis (M)

M0	No (known) distant metastasis.
M1	Distant metastasis present.

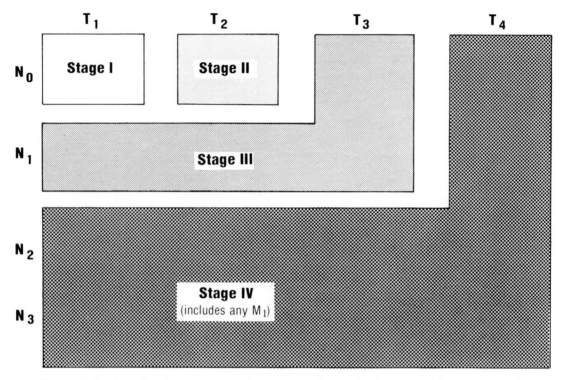

Fig. 14-6. Staging of oral squamous carcinoma according to the American Joint Committee.[53]

Few will question the value of clinical staging as a concept, but every staging system has limitations that must be appreciated. Although oral primaries are usually accessible for measurement, tumor size can be grossly underestimated if the extent of the ulceration rather than the induration is measured. Furthermore, clinical estimates of primary tumor size are two dimensional and do not consider the depth of infiltration. This means that a 4.5 cm lesion that may show only superficial infiltration will be designated T3, whereas a 2 by 2 cm tumor that infiltrates to the same depth—and carries a more ominous prognosis—may be listed as T1.

Accurate assessment of cervical metastases can also be troublesome. Not only will estimates of node size vary between examiners—particularly if the patient has a short, muscular neck—but about 10 to 20 percent of palpable node enlargement will prove to be inflammatory, rather than neoplastic. The presence of multiple, as op-

posed to solitary, enlargement seems to be a reliable guide, possibly because discrepancy between clinical and histologic findings is unusual when more than one node is enlarged.[92] The current N system deliberately excludes fixation as a criterion because it is almost impossible to define in reproducible, clinical terms.

It is important to remember that staging systems are subject to revision and modification. For this reason, TNM designations should supplement, but never replace an accurate description of the size, shape, position, consistency, and mobility of a primary oral tumor and its metastases.

SELECTION OF THERAPY

The choice of therapy for a patient who has an oral squamous carcinoma is most influenced by the location of the primary tumor and its extent. Either irradiation or surgery yields effective control of a small lesion that is confined to the site of origin (stage I), but local excision may often be easier for the patient (Fig. 14-7). A small, anterior tumor can even be excised under local anesthesia if necessary. The surgical defect is either sutured primarily, grafted, or allowed to heal by secondary intention and functional impairment is rarely a problem.

Although exophytic or undifferentiated tumors are likely to be radiosensitive, results comparable to those reported after excision may require a combination of external and interstitial irradiation. For the elderly or debilitated patient, this may entail many outpatient treatment sessions as well as hospitalization and general anesthesia.

Radiotherapy offers an obvious advantage for the patient whose oral lesion is small but posteriorly situated, ill defined in extent, or otherwise inaccessible for excision through the open mouth. In this situation, the risk of irradiation damage to bone or adjacent normal soft tissue must be weighed against the functional and cosmetic sequelae of a more extensive operation. The training and experience of the responsible clinician will understandably affect this decision.

For patients who have a more extensive

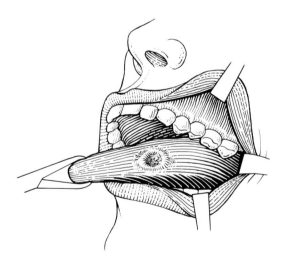

Fig. 14-7. Small cancers situated anteriorly, such as this tongue lesion, can often be easily excised through the open mouth (peroral approach).

oral carcinoma (stages II and III), experience suggests that treatment modalities should probably be combined in hopes of reducing local recurrence and improving survival rates. In a prospective, randomized study some years ago, preoperative radiation totaling 2,000 rads in five treatment sessions significantly reduced neck recurrence but had no impact on "cure."[95] Retrospective reports from other hospitals using higher dosage preoperative irradiation have shown improved results in patients with pharyngeal and supraglottic laryngeal primaries.[8, 15, 33]

Despite the theoretic advantages of irradiation before surgery, postoperative teletherapy seems just as effective and is preferred by most surgeons. Wound healing problems tend to increase as preoperative doses exceed 4,000 rads; whereas, postoperative irradiation can usually be carried to 4,000 to 6,000 rads with minimal additional morbidity.[39] Currently, we give postoperative irradiation to selected patients who either have bulky primary tumor (T3 or T4), extensive nodal metastases (N2 or N3), or unfavorable pathologic findings such as involved margins or jugular vein invasion. When indicated, we prefer to start postoperative irradiation as soon as the wound has healed.

Peroral excision is often not feasible in the patient who has a very extensive oral carcinoma. When the lesion is too large or is situated too far posteriorly, a cheek flap approach is usually required (Fig. 14-8). If the mandible is directly invaded by tumor, segmental resection is indicated. A marginal mandibulectomy, which preserves jaw continuity, may provide an adequate margin around a tumor that approaches but does not involve the bone (Fig. 14-9). On occasion, the mandible may be divided and rewired in the midline when the jaw is uninvolved, but access is a problem (Fig. 14-10). Portions of the maxilla may have to be resected when the primary tumor arises in the hard palate or upper gingiva, or when a lesion in the cheek mucosa or retromolar area involves the upper jaw by contiguity (Fig.

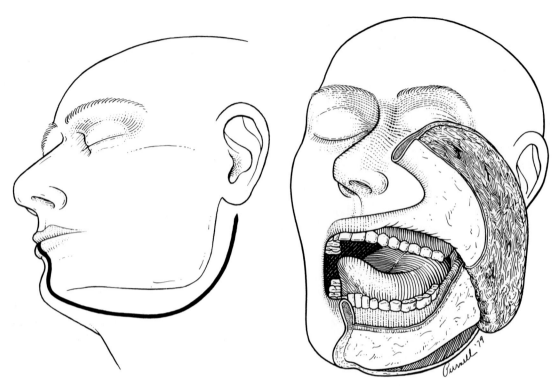

Fig. 14-8. When the cancer is larger and more posteriorly situated, the lower lip can be divided in the midline and a cheek flap elevated in order to provide better access (cheek flap approach).

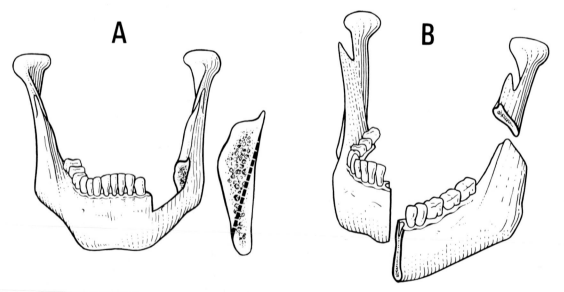

Fig. 14-9. Mandible resection may be either (A) marginal or (B) segmental. Marginal mandibulectomy is most appropriate when the tumor approaches, but does not involve, bone and can be performed through the open mouth for anterior lesions. When the mandible is involved with cancer, segmental mandibulectomy is best performed through a cheek flap approach.

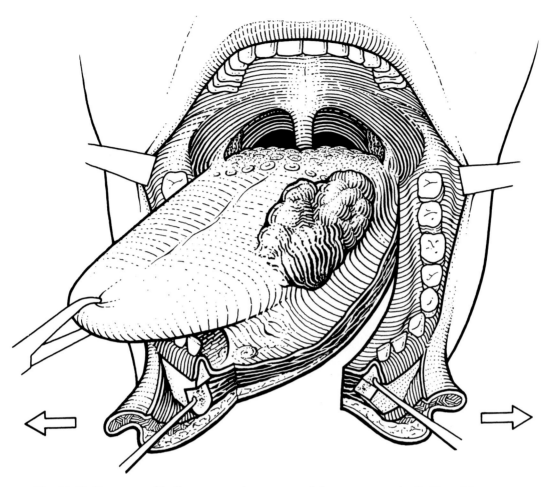

Fig. 14-10. Exposure of bulky or posterior cancers of the tongue can be facilitated by a mandibulotomy approach. The mandible is divided through the symphysis and rewired to preserve appearance and function.

14-11). When excision through the open mouth is not possible, the upper lip is divided and a Weber-Fergusson approach is used (Fig. 14-12).

Although some therapists claim that small metastatic deposits can be controlled by radiotherapy, [76, 102] radical neck dissection has traditionally been considered an essential part of the initial treatment for any patient who has clinical evidence of cervical lymph node involvement. Despite recent suggestions that this operation can be modified,[10] we prefer the classical, unmodified operation.[59] Treatment failure in the neck occurs in almost 50 percent of those who have node involvement, if treated with rad-

ical neck dissection alone[26] Our concern is that a modified procedure will result in an even further reduced cure rate. The lymphadenectomy is performed in continuity with the oral excision when feasible (combined resection, composite resection, or "Commando" operation), but this does not appear to be essential.[90]

In the absence of clinically apparent cervical node metastasis (N0), neck dissection may be indicated on an elective basis. When a cheek flap approach is required for resection of a sizable oral primary, the neck must be entered. In this situation we proceed with a neck dissection in most N0 patients. About one-third already have micro-

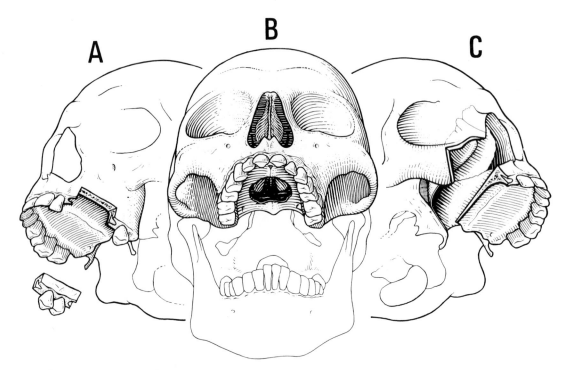

Fig. 14-11. (A) Maxillary alveolectomy or (B) partial palatectomy can often be performed through the open mouth in conjunction with the excision of small primary cancers of the palate or upper gingiva. (C) Subtotal maxillectomy for larger cancers usually requires an upper cheek-flap approach (Weber-Fergusson).

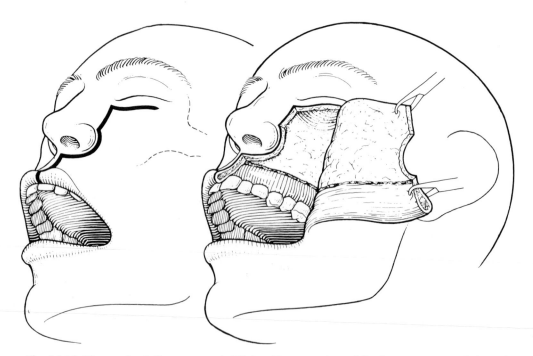

Fig. 14-12. Upper cheek-flap approach (Weber-Fergusson) used for larger cancers of the palate or upper gingiva. The infraorbital portion of the incision can be extended as far laterally as necessary.

metastases, and neck dissection is likely to be more tedious if deferred until the metastases are obvious. Elective neck dissection should also be considered when the patient has a muscular neck which is difficult to evaluate, the patient is unable or unlikely to return for regular follow-up visits, and the probability of subsequent node involvement seems particularly high.

Recent experience with elective neck irradiation for patients who have oropharyngeal primaries has indicated a significant decrease in anticipated metastases and no appreciable morbidity after 5,000 to 5,500 rads.[29] Prospective, randomized studies are needed before it can be safely assumed that occult neck metastases in the patient who has an oral cancer can be as effectively controlled by irradiation as by lymphadenectomy.

The role of chemotherapy remains to be defined. Several drugs appear to have significant antitumor effect in patients with squamous carcinoma arising in the upper aerodigestive tract. Cis-diamino-dichloro-platinum (cis-platinum), methotrexate, and bleomycin—alone, in combination, and/or in conjunction with external irradiation —have yielded partial response rates (PR of at least 50 percent regression) approaching 70 percent in patients with locally advanced, unresectable previously untreated tumor.[9, 46, 71, 101] Unfortunately, the duration of response has usually been measured in months.

Based on this limited, but encouraging experience, there has been much interest in adjunctive chemotherapy given preoperatively to patients who have a resectable tumor. As with preoperative irradiation, the extent of the operation is based on the initial evaluation even if significant tumor shrinkage occurs. As of this writing, few conclusions can be drawn. The use of chemotherapy as the first treatment modality does not appear to increase the morbidity of subsequent surgery or irradiation or both, but definitive treatment may be delayed if significant drug complications occur.

CANCER OF THE TONGUE

Presentation

Before the seventeenth century there are few references to cancer of the tongue in the medical literature. This has intrigued many investigators, including Martin,[54] who pointed out that cancer of the tongue was not necessarily a rare entity. Diagnostic confusion was obvious in eighteenth-century reports of operations on lingual tumors. In fact, the distinction between malignant, benign, and especially inflammatory lesions such as gummas was not clarified until Virchow's time in the midnineteenth century. Nevertheless, it seems likely that cancer of the tongue was rather uncommon more than two centuries ago considering that the peak incidence presently is in the sixth and seventh decades of life (median about 60 years) and the average life expectancy in eighteenth-century Europe was only about 40 years of age. Moreover, several significant etiologic factors such as tobacco, distilled spirits, and syphilis had only first appeared in the fifteenth and sixteenth centuries.

Currently there is a lack of awareness that cancer of the tongue can occasionally afflict the young. About 1 percent of patients are less than 30 years of age, and rare occurrence in early adolescence has been reported.[14] The proportion of women treated for cancer of the tongue in our hospital has steadily increased from 13 percent in the 1930's to more than 26 percent in a more recent report 30 years later.[31, 58, 91] This undoubtedly reflects the increasing consumption of alcohol and cigarettes by women during the same period.

Most cancers of the tongue arise in the oral portion or anterior two-thirds, but the proportion arising in the base of the tongue, the area posterior to the circumvallate papillae, has increased from 25 percent to almost 50 percent recently in our hospital. Most squamous cancers involve the lateral borders or ventral aspect of the tongue; involvement of the dorsum is uncommon and midline lesions are quite rare.

In its early stages, cancer of the tongue is often asymptomatic. Unless pain supervenes, which is a surprisingly uncommon occurrence, the cancer may often attain a size of several centimeters before the patient becomes aware of discomfort. Growth can be so gradual and discomfort so minimal that medical advice is not sought until an enlarged cervical lymph node becomes apparent. Pain radiating to the ear, slurring of speech, difficulty in swallowing, and bleeding are ominous late symptoms.

Patient Evaluation

Cancer of the tongue arises most often as an indurated, nontender ulcer in the lateral border of the middle-third of the tongue. As the cancer enlarges, the margin becomes granular and elevated, the ulceration spreads laterally, and infiltration into the underlying musculature increases. On occasion, ulceration may be inconspicuous or even absent, but palpation invariably confirms that the lesion is larger than it appears on inspection.

Extension of the tumor into the adjacent floor of the mouth or into the tonsillar pillars is not unusual. With a massive primary (T4), involvement of the base of the tongue, floor of the mouth, and mandible may be so extensive that the exact site of origin cannot be ascertained. Restriction of tongue movement is common in this situation and indicates considerable deep infiltration of the tongue musculature.

Most patients with cancer of the oral tongue have a primary that is staged as T2 (2.1 to 4 cm) when first seen. The proportion with T1 lesions has remained relatively constant in our hospital (about 20 percent), and massive tumors fortunately are seen less often.

Metastasis to cervical lymph nodes is clinically apparent initially in about 30 percent of patients who have a primary cancer of the oral tongue, in contrast with more than 60 percent in those with lesions in the base of the tongue. Submandibular or upper jugular lymph nodes (levels I and II) are most often involved. Bilateral metastases may be present when the tumor involves the midline of the tongue. In patients with locally advanced disease, it may be difficult at times to distinguish between cervical metastasis and extensive, deeply infiltrating tumor that invades the upper neck.

Selection of Treatment

Radiation and surgery each have a major role in the treatment of tongue cancer, but there has been varying preference for one modality over the other for much of this century. Martin's[54] admonition in 1940 seems entirely appropriate today: "It is unfortunate that the current medical literature should still contain reports attempting to prove the superiority of one method alone—either radiation or surgical therapy—in the treatment of this disease . . . Any such partisan attitude is entirely out of place in the management of so serious a problem as lingual cancer."

For the patient who has a T1 lesion, either partial glossectomy or irradiation is highly effective therapy, but surgery offers the advantage of simplicity (Fig. 14-7). The smaller the tumor and the more anterior its location, the easier is the surgical excision. Restricted tongue mobility and slurring of speech are usually minimal following this procedure.

Lower voltage irradiation given through a peroral lead cone shield was extensively used in the past and is still preferred by some radiotherapists,[28] but for small tongue tumors many radiotherapists currently express a strong preference for the implantation of radioactive sources directly into the tumors.[11, 75] Radium needles have been most often used for this interstitial therapy (brachytherapy), but other radioactive substances such as radon seeds, gold 198 seeds, cobalt or cesium needles, tantalum 182 wires, and irridium 192 have also been employed.

Implantation of the tongue is an exacting technique, which is best performed under general anesthesia by an experienced radiotherapist. A tracheostomy may be required until tongue swelling subsides. It is possible to deliver a high dose (as much as 10,000 rads) uniformly throughout the tumor, sparing the adjacent normal tissues. Persistent, painful soft tissue ulceration and mandibular osteoradionecrosis are complications occasionally seen but usually heal with time. Afterloading techniques, in which sources are later inserted into previously implanted, hollow nylon tubes, may offer more precise dosimetry while reducing radiation exposure to the therapist.[69]

When a primary cancer of the tongue is larger and more deeply infiltrative (T2), partial glossectomy remains feasible, but resection through the open mouth is not always possible. Occasionally, the lower lip must be divided in the midline and a cheek flap reflected in order to provide adequate exposure for resection. If irradiation is selected in this situation, a course of external irradiation is often delivered to the primary tumor and the ipsilateral neck before the implant is performed. If enlarged lymph nodes indicate a strong likelihood of metastasis, radical neck dissection is indicated. Most radiotherapists recommend neck dissection rather than attempting to control obvious nodal involvement by irradiation alone.

The indications for treating the neck of the patient with cancer of the tongue who has no evidence of cervical metastasis(N0) remains controversial. Our experience indicates that more than 40 percent of patients with T2N0 lesions treated by partial glossectomy alone will develop nodal involvement subsequently; and the incidence approaches 70 percent for those with T3N0 tumors. With few exceptions, radical neck dissection should be part of the initial surgical treatment of any patient who has a T3 lesion and is recommended for selected patients who have T2N0 lesions.[89] Experience in some radiotherapy centers suggests that comparable results may be achieved by "elective" irradiation of the neck.[1, 62]

Control of a bulky tongue primary (T3 or T4) is difficult to achieve by surgery or irradiation alone, and the current trend is to use both modalities in combination. Tumors of this size usually invade adjacent tissues and encroach upon the mandible; cervical metastases are usually palpable. Adequate surgery may involve segmental mandibulectomy in addition to a radical neck dissection. The resultant disability is directly related to the extent of the tongue and jaw resection and may be significantly reduced by appropriate reconstruction.

In our hospital, postoperative teletherapy to the tongue and ipsilateral neck commences as soon as the wound is healed and is usually carried to at least 5,000 rads. Preoperative chemotherapy has been added to the therapeutic program for selected patients who have stage IV disease in the hope that the combination of all three modalities may enhance resectability and prolong survival.

Results

In a report from our hospital in 1962, the five year cure rate for 843 patients treated for carcinoma of the oral tongue was 40.7 percent.[31] By 1974, this had increased to 49.1 percent in a survey of 236 patients treated after treatment preference had shifted almost exclusively to surgery.[91] A comparable cure rate of 45 percent has been reported for patients treated predominantly with irradiation.[47]

Any study suggesting the superiority of one modality must be analyzed with care. As a rule, the choice of therapy has not been randomized and different results are predictable, if, for example, the patients with small anterior lesions have surgery and those with large posterior tumors receive irradiation.[99] Moreover, comparison of results achieved in patients treated in different hospitals is seldom valid, for one or more of the following reasons: data may be given for multiple oral sites rather than a single site, different clinical staging criteria are used, a selected, rather than a total experience is presented, or different statistical reporting methods are used.

Despite these obstacles, it seems clear that about 90 percent of early cancers (T1) can be controlled locally either by partial glossectomy[89, 100] or by interstitial irradiation.[19, 69] Although preference has been expressed for surgery *and* irradiation for the patient who has a large tumor or cervical metastases, there is no evidence as yet that results are significantly improved, nor is there agreement as to how the two modalities should best be combined. Answers to these questions are unlikely until prospective, randomized studies are organized by cooperating hospitals.

The prognosis for patients with cancer of the oral tongue depends upon the size of the primary tumor and the presence or absence of involved cervical lymph nodes. Our 5-year cure rate varied from 69.2 percent in patients with stage I disease to 52.7 and 36.6 percent in those with stage II and stage III lesions, respectively.[91] Gradual improvement in overall cure rate can be anticipated as the proportion of favorable cases increase. Fortunately, relatively few patients present with stage IV oral tongue tumors. Salvage of such patients is unusual regardless of the treatment employed.

CANCER OF THE FLOOR OF THE MOUTH

Presentation

Carcinoma occurs in the floor of the mouth with a frequency approaching that seen in the tongue and, similar to cancer of the tongue, is a disease of the sixth and seventh decades (median about 60 years). In the past it was unusual to find a cancer of the floor of the mouth in a woman. In more recent reports, the male-female ratio has dropped to between three and four to one.[32, 36]

In searching for causative factors, it would seem that the floor of the mouth is less susceptible to chronic irritation and dental trauma than is the tongue. The work of Moore and Catlin[64] suggests that the high incidence of cancer in this dependent site may reflect greater exposure to ingested food and salivary secretions. Although specific data are lacking, our experience indicates that a history of excessive alcohol consumption can be elicited from all but a few of these patients.

The typical cancer arises anteriorly, often in relation to one or both submandibular gland ducts. Early cancers are seldom symptomatic. The patient may be unaware of a swelling until the tumor is several cm in size, by which time discomfort or pain is usually noted. A mass in one or both submandibular triangles is suggestive of either cervical node metastasis or enlargement of the submandibular gland due to obstruction of Wharton's duct by the tumor, or both.

Patient Evaluation

In its earliest stage, squamous carcinoma in the floor of the mouth is typically superficial and erythematous. The mucosa may be slightly ulcerated or may present as a granular plaque-like elevation. The periphery of the tumor may be ill defined; deep red areas may be interspersed with patches of leukoplakia, and multifocal origin is not unusual.

As the cancer enlarges, ulceration becomes more prominent and there is lateral spread to involve the ventral aspect of the tongue and the adjacent lingual gingiva. In several reported series[23, 36, 42, 82] the tumor was localized to the floor of the mouth in less than half of the patients. It is essential that the extent of deep infiltration be ascertained by careful bimanual palpation. One or both submaxillary ducts may be obstructed by tumor infiltration. If patients have extensive lesions, the tongue may be tethered due to invasion of its musculature. The tumor may also involve the retromolar trigone, tonsillar pillar, or may even cross the gingiva to infiltrate the cheek mucosa.

We consider radiographs unreliable in the detection of minimal mandibular involvement and believe that this assessment is best made on clinical grounds. If the tumor is not freely movable with respect to the lingual surface of the mandible, this may only mean that periosteum is involved. The dense cortical bone of the mandible serves as an effective barrier to tumor invasion; however, obvious bone exposure or extensive infiltration through the muscular support of the floor of the mouth with involvement of submental skin usually indicates extensive osseous involvement.

The incidence of lymph node involvement at the time of initial presentation varies from 39 to 63 percent of patients.[6, 23, 36, 42] Stage I tumors are encountered in about 20 percent of patients; almost one-half of patients have stage III or IV disease. A mass in the submandibular triangle may be difficult to evaluate. Needle aspiration or excisional biopsy may be necessary in order to establish the presence of metastatic carcinoma; preferably the latter should be deferred until the surgeon and the patient are both prepared for appropriate, definitive treatment.

Selection of Treatment

Small cancers confined to the floor of the mouth can be treated effectively either by surgery or irradiation. When the cancer is superficial and situated anteriorly, local excision is simple and is usually more convenient for the patient. The surgical defect can either be sutured, resurfaced with a skin graft, or left open to heal by secondary intention, all with minimal dysfunction (Figs. 14-13 A-D). If the transected submandibular duct can be identified, reimplantation posteriorly may reduce the likelihood of stenosis and postoperative enlargement of the submandibular gland due to duct obstruction. Comparable local control rates have been achieved with irradiation, when a combination of external irradiation and interstitial implantation was used.[19, 69]

The surgical approach to large cancers that are still localized to the floor of the mouth is determined by the extent of deep infiltration and the proximity to the mandible. Peroral wide local excision is appropriate if the tumor is relatively superficial. This can be accomplished in conjunction with resection of the alveolar process or inner table of the adjacent mandible (i.e. marginal mandibulectomy) if the cancer encroaches upon or seems adherent to the periosteum (Fig. 14-9).

Extension to contiguous tongue, gingiva, and mandible is usual when patients have a large cancer (T3 or T4) and occurs earlier in the course of the disease when the tumor is laterally situated. Adequate exposure for resection is best achieved using a cheek-flap approach (or occasionally a visor-flap approach for anterior lesions) (Figs. 14-8 and 14-14). The involved mandible may require segmental resection.

The cosmetic deformity and functional disability associated with segmental resection of the mandible is significant and increases in proportion to the amount of mandible (and especially mandibular arch) that is removed. For the patient with a bulky tumor that invades the mandible, irradiation may offer an alternative to such deforming surgery; but the prospect of local control is small and the risk of irradiation damage to the mandible is high. Recently, the impact of radical surgery on the patient who has an extensive tumor has been decreased by a trend towards preservation of mandibular continuity by aggressive marginal resection in the presence of superficial bone involvement[34] and by refinements in reconstructive techniques.

In the absence of enlarged cervical lymph nodes (N0), several options are available. If peroral excision of the primary tumor proves feasible, it may be preferable to defer treatment of the neck and to follow the patient closely. Persistent postoperative swelling of one or both submandibular glands may create a problem in trying to determine whether this is due to surgical trauma to the ducts or represents metastases to the submandibular lymph nodes. This dilemma must occasionally be resolved by biopsy. Elective neck dissection may be appropriate when a cheek flap approach is required for excision of a larger primary

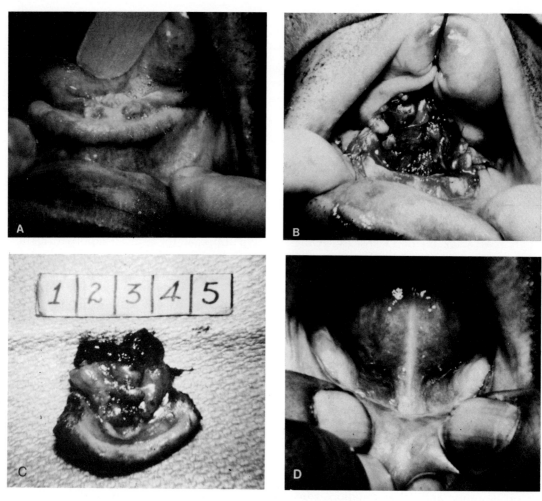

Fig. 14-13. Squamous carcinoma of (A) the floor of the mouth (B) resected with marginal mandibulectomy. (C) Resected specimen. (D) Appearance 3 months later. Wound was left open to heal by secondary intention, rather than grafted or sutured primarily. (Spiro, R.H., and Strong, E.W. 1976. Mouth cancer, a surgical perspective. Clinical Bulletin of the Memorial Sloan-Kettering Cancer Center, 6:6.)

cancer because the neck has been entered and the likelihood of occult nodal involvement is higher with the large tumors. Elective neck irradiation is preferred for such lesions in some treatment centers.

We believe that radical neck dissection is indicated for any patient who has clinical evidence of metastasis. Many patients have tumors that approach or cross the midline, and nodal involvement in both sides of the neck is not unusual. Our preference is to stage bilateral neck dissections whenever possible, inasmuch as the morbidity and mortality of simultaneous bilateral radical neck dissection is high.[65] Simultaneous bilat-

eral dissection may occasionally be required if tumor-bearing tissue must be transected in order to stage the operations. Considering the small prospect of tumor control by single modality therapy when neck metastases are extensive (N2 and N3) or the primary lesion is massive (T4), there is much interest currently in combined therapy.

Results

Cure rates approaching 90 to 70 percent respectively can be achieved in groups of patients with stage I and II lesions when either surgery or a combination of external

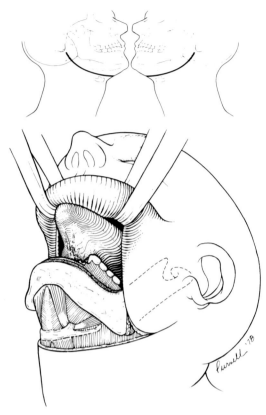

Fig. 14-14. In the visor flap approach, the skin of the entire chin is elevated off of the mandible in order to provide access to anteriorly situated oral cancers.

and interstitial irradiation is used. Salvage rates for those patients who have stage III or IV disease leave much to be desired. A combination of surgery and irradiation is thought to offer the best prospect for control, but thus far there is insufficient statistically valid evidence to support this view. Overall cure rates are about 50 percent, with at least some of the improvement explained by the fact that in recent years fewer patients have presented with far advanced cancers that are suitable for palliative therapy only.

CANCER OF THE GINGIVA

Presentation

Cancer of the gingiva (gum, alveolar ridge) is most unusual before the age of 50, and men are afflicted two to three times more often than women.[16, 66] In a large series reported by Cady and Catlin[16] 80 percent of the lesions occurred in the lower gingiva and 60 percent involved the area posterior to the bicuspid teeth. According to current classifications, some of the latter patients probably had cancers that were retromolar, rather than gingival in origin.

Tobacco usage by patients with cancer of the gingiva was carefully evaluated in the Cady and Catlin study.[16] Ninety-four percent of the men were smokers, compared to only 48 percent of the women; and the proportion of men who were cigar or pipe smokers (34 percent) was significantly higher than that observed in the general population. The authors emphasized the potential for multiple lesions in the patient with gingival cancer by pointing out that at least 17 percent of patients treated successfully for the first primary lesion later developed another cancer in the oral cavity.

The patient typically has a history of pain or ulceration and usually has sought professional advice within a few months of the occurrence of these symptoms. In the absence of pain or bleeding, delay in diagnosis is more common, and the inability to wear a previously well-fitting denture may be the only symptom. Most individuals initially consult a dentist for these symptoms. Not infrequently, the gingival changes are assumed to be inflammatory and appropriate therapy is delayed by extraction of teeth or other useless measures.

Patient Evaluation

The papillary ulcer of early cancer of the gingiva usually arises on the apex of the gingiva and less often on the buccal or lingual aspect. The mucous membrane and the underlying dense fibrous tissue provide only a 1 or 2 mm covering over the alveolar process of the maxillae and mandible. The periosteum, however, tends to form a barrier; and thus, initial tumor spread is usually lateral into the cheek, hard palate, or floor of the mouth. If a tooth is extracted, however, access is then provided for rapid, deep invasion of bone by way of the socket. Once the dense cortical bone of the mandible is penetrated and the underlying cancellous bone or neurovascular tissues are involved, the cancer may extend proximally or distally well beyond what is anticipated by radiographic or clinical examination. Radiographic findings must therefore always be interpreted with caution. Histologic examination may prove negative despite the impression that bone is involved radiographically, and about one-third of patients without x-ray evidence of bone destruction may have histologic evidence of involvement.

Martin[55], in his study of cancer of the gingiva at Memorial Hospital, found that only 10 percent of patients had a cancer less than 2 cm in size. The cancer had produced obvious bone destruction in 35 percent and extended beyond the gingivae into neighboring structures in 90 percent of patients. Clinically positive lymph nodes were found on admission in 35 percent of patients with cancer of the gingiva. More recently in the same hospital,[16] 23 percent had cancers that were 2 cm or less in size, but the proportion with bone involvement, extension beyond the gingiva, and clinically involved lymph nodes on admission remained about the same.

Nodal metastasis occurs with slightly greater frequency in patients with cancer of the lower gingiva as compared to upper gingiva, with the submandibular lymph nodes usually involved first. Metastasis to upper jugular (subdigastric) lymph nodes is seen more often in the patients who have lesions arising in the upper gingiva.

Selection of Therapy

Peroral local excision in conjunction with marginal resection of the mandible is easily accomplished in patients with a small cancer localized to the gingival mucosa (T1N0) and situated anteriorly. When a cancer of the lower gingiva is large or obviously invades the mandible and other adjacent tissues, a cheek flap approach and segmental resection of the mandible will usually be required. For bulky lesions arising in the upper gingiva, a partial maxillectomy is performed through a Weber-Fergusson incision (Fig. 14-12).

Radical neck dissection is indicated when enlarged nodes are present and may be appropriate electively when a clinically negative neck is entered during a cheek flap approach to a large primary of the lower gingiva.

External irradiation or teletherapy directed through a peroral cone may be administered to patients with cancers localized to the gingiva. In those patients with large cancers, the risk of bone exposure and osteoradionecrosis increases in proportion to the extent of osseous involvement. As with other sites in the oral cavity, a combination of surgery and irradiation is preferred when the primary tumor is extensive or cervical metastases are evident.

Results

Determinate 5-year cure rates for all treated patients increased from 35 to 64 percent during the 20-year period reviewed by Cady and Catlin[16] as preference shifted from irradiation to surgery. The survival rate increased to more than 80 percent for the group of patients with localized disease. Although the incidence of cervical metastasis remained unchanged, the proportion with only level I involvement increased. The salvage rate for the latter group of patients rose to 54 percent, compared to 35 percent for the group with involvement of nodes at other levels.

In the M.D. Anderson Hospital experience[48] with 101 determinant patients who had cancers of the lower gingiva, 48 percent remained alive and free of cancer during the period of evaluation. When these patients were grouped according to the extent of the tumor, the salvage rate was 78 percent for stage I, 64 percent for stage II, 35 percent for stage III, and 15 percent for stage IV. Surgical results seemed clearly superior to those achieved by radiotherapy alone. There are insufficient data[48, 66] to support the contention that the combination of surgery and radiotherapy is more effective for patients with advanced disease.

Retromolar Trigone

The term *retromolar* has long been used by clinicians who recognized that certain oral cancers that involve the posterior lower gingiva, cheek mucosa, floor of the mouth, or the anterior tonsillar pillar may overlap any or all of these contiguous sites. In fact, it is most unusual for an oral cancer to be confined within the limits of the retromolar trigone as defined above. The mucosa of the retromolar trigone blends imperceptibly with that of the anterior tonsillar pillar, as well as with that of the adjacent posterior lower gingival mucosa when molar teeth are missing.

For this reason, at Memorial Sloan-Kettering Cancer Center (Memorial Hospital) most posterior and lateral oral cancers are classified according to the predominant site of involvement (gingiva, floor of the mouth, cheek mucosa, or anterior tonsillar pillar) and are rarely listed as retromolar in origin. The characteristic features of cancers that involve these sites are described in the appropriate section.

CANCER OF THE CHEEK (BUCCAL) MUCOSA

Presentation

In the United States, cancer rarely arises in the cheek mucosa of persons less than 40 years of age. The median age is generally well into the seventh decade. Such cancers occur in men about three times as frequently as in women.[22, 67] Reports from India show that in India the incidence of cancer of the cheek mucosa is second only to that of the tongue.[68] Indian patients tend to be younger and women are more often afflicted.[84] These differences seem directly related to indigenous tobacco chewing habits, also a factor in patients from the southern United States who develop "snuff-dipper's" cancer.[94]

Observing that most cancers appear to arise opposite the point where the teeth meet (occlusal line), Martin[57] assumed that trauma from sharp or broken teeth or from ill-fitting dentures was the most important causative factor. As with other oral sites, more recent studies[22, 67] implicate alcohol and cigarette consumption.

Despite the ease with which the tongue can detect a roughening or ulceration on the surface of the cheek mucosa, the small lesion is often ignored. In O'Brien and Catlin's review of 248 patients,[67] the mean duration of symptoms was 7 to 12 months. Small lesions arising in the cheek mucosa are seldom symptomatic. Pain, local infection, and trismus usually indicate extensive and sometimes unresectable disease.

Patient Evaluation

Carcinoma of the cheek mucosa usually begins as a small, ulcerated, indurated mass that may or may not protrude above the surface. Ordinarily, lesions arise in the central and posterior portion of the cheek lining, but in tobacco chewing patients the lower sulcus is typically involved in the area where the quid is retained. Growth patterns may vary considerably, with many lesions—particularly in tobacco chewing patients—having the papillary appearance of relatively superficial verrucous carcinoma (Fig. 14-4). In contrast, other patients may have deeply infiltrating tumors that penetrate through to involve the skin. If the lesion arises posteriorly, there may be early infiltration of the retromolar mucosa and underlying pterygoid musculature with pain and trismus. As the cancer enlarges, lateral spread into the upper or lower jaw, oral commissure, or lips may ensue. The occasional patient who has avoided treatment may finally seek attention because a foul, through-and-through cheek defect has made it impossible to eat (Figs. 14-15A and B).

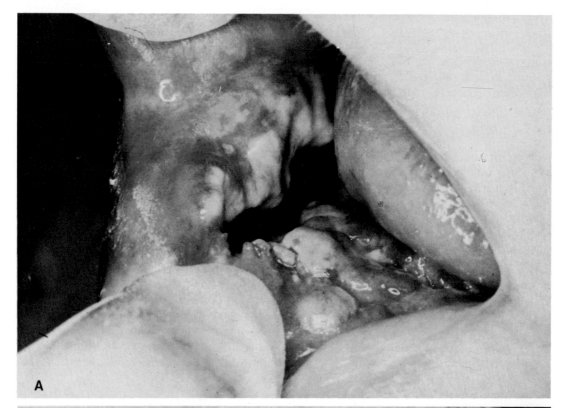

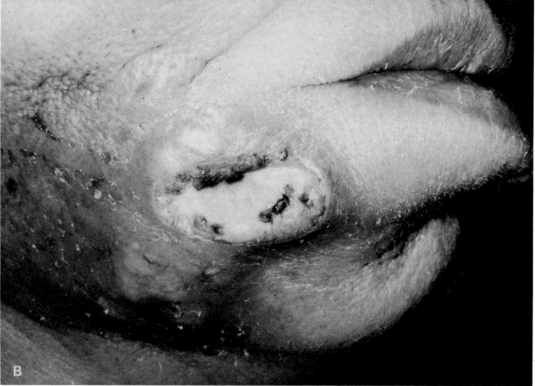

Fig. 14-15. (A) Locally advanced squamous carcinoma of the cheek mucosa with (B) extensive invasion and destruction of the overlying skin.

Surprisingly, the proportion of patients with disease confined to the cheek mucosa was one-third in Martin's report in 1935[57] as well as in O'Brien and Catlin's study[67] thirty years later. A more recent review by Conley and Sadoyama[22] lists 11 percent and 26 percent as having stage I and stage II lesions, respectively.

Clinically positive cervical lymph nodes are evident initially in 37 to 44 percent[22, 67] of patients, and the incidence may be slightly higher when the lesion is situated posteriorly.[68] Regional lymph node involvement is often confined to the submandibular triangle, but metastasis directly to the internal jugular chain is not unusual when the lesions arise posteriorly. The overall incidence of cervical metastasis approaches 50 percent including those patients who develop nodal involvement subsequent to treatment.

Selection of Therapy

Small cancers localized to the cheek are easily and effectively treated by wide excision or by irradiation. The surgical defect may be sutured primarily or a skin graft applied. When larger tumors infiltrate deeply towards skin or laterally into the upper or lower jaw or pterygoid musculature, local control is more difficult to achieve using irradiation alone. A more extensive, full-thickness resection of the cheek or even a composite resection may be required.

Until relatively recently, enthusiasm for radical extirpation of advanced cancers of the cheek mucosa was tempered by concern about incapacitating functional and cosmetic sequelae. Reconstruction of large cheek defects and restoration of oral competence can now be accomplished with a variety of innovative techniques[2, 22] and is best initiated at the same time as the resection.

Radical neck dissection is performed when nodes are present and may also be indicated electively when the neck must be entered to resect a large primary cancer. Postoperative irradiation is often recommended for those patients who have had a resection of stage III or IV disease as well as for those patients with positive margins on histologic examination of the surgical specimen.

Results

MacComb and Fletcher have reported a 5-year cure rate of 70 percent for 115 patients, 75 (65 percent) of whom had T1 or T2 lesions localized to the cheek mucosa.[47] Salvage was 92, 86, 65, and 15 percent for groups of patients with stage I through IV disease, respectively. Except for patients with stage IV lesions, results seemed better for the 60 percent who received irradiation rather than surgery. Part of the difference may be explained by the fact that surgery was preferred for patients with more advanced lesions, which invaded the mandible or maxilla.

The 5-year cure rate was 51 percent in O'Brien and Catlin's study[67] including 21 percent who required additional treatment for local recurrence. All but 5 percent were treated surgically. Of those patients with N0 disease, 56 percent were salvaged. Only 23 percent remained alive and well when cervical lymph nodes were involved.

Conley and Sadoyama[22] reported that 12 of 20 determinant patients (60 percent) who had surgery and 9 of 17 patients (53 percent) who had irradiation remained alive and well 5 years later. Only 5 of 31 patients (16 percent) treated with irradiation *and* surgery were salvaged. Local recurrence occurred in 40 percent of their patients, and the overall cure was 38 percent. The poor results seen in patients who received combined therapy should come as no surprise. Salvage rates invariably depend more on the stage of a tumor than its treatment, and combined therapy was usually reserved for those who had the most extensive cancers.

CANCER OF THE PALATE

Presentation

The hard palate, more so than any other site in the oral cavity, gives rise to tumors of varied histologic appearance. In fact, only about one-half of hard palate lesions prove to be epidermoid carcinoma. Useful clinical information about hard palate cancer is limited either because tumors of different histology have been grouped together or because published reports make no distinction between cancers arising in the hard palate, soft palate, or upper gingiva (alveolar ridge). In a study of 123 patients by Ratzer, et al.,[72] more than 80 percent were men and the tumor occurred most often in the seventh decade.

Chronic irritation seems an unlikely causative factor in palate carcinoma, although leukoplakia or areas of mucosal atrophy are often associated.[56] The correlation with alcohol and tobacco consumption is less impressive when compared to other sites within the oral cavity, with the exception of the high incidence of palate cancer seen in certain parts of India.[73]

Median duration of symptoms is usually several months. Pain or swallowing difficulty may occasionally be reported by patients who have small tumors in the soft palate, but painless irregularity of the mucous membrane is usually the only symptom in hard palate carcinoma until late in the course of the disease. Some patients may seek medical attention only because an upper denture no longer fits properly.

Patient Evaluation

The first sign of cancer of the hard palate is usually a superficial, granular ulcer with rolled, elevated edges. Initially, growth tends to be exophytic and despite close proximity to the periosteum, invasion of bone does not usually occur until the tumor is sizeable. The cancer on initial presentation appears to be localized to the mucosa of the hard palate in about half of the patients.[72] Suspected invasion of the underlying palatal bone, the maxillary antrum, or the nasal cavity should be assessed by appropriate radiographs or by computerized axial tomography (CT).

In the more advanced cases, bone de-

struction and invasion of the floor of the maxillary antrum or nasal cavity may be so extensive as to suggest that the tumor originates from these sites rather than from the hard palate. Lateral extension into the gingivae, lip or cheek mucosa, soft palate, or pterygoid area is common in this setting and is usually associated with pain and difficulty in swallowing. The incidence of cervical lymph node metastasis on initial presentation (16 percent) is less than half that recorded for patients with soft palate lesions (37 percent).[72] The lymph nodes in the submandibular triangle and upper jugular chain are most often involved.

Selection of Therapy

At Memorial Hospital, there has been strong preference for surgery in the treatment of cancer of the hard palate. Radioresponsiveness appears to be less than that seen in patients with the cancer primary in the soft palate, and the dosage may be limited by the proximity of the underlying bone in order to minimize the risk of bone exposure and necrosis. Irradiation may be appropriate for selected small cancers that do not invade bone. Dysfunction is thought to be less in such cases, and surgical salvage is still possible if radiation fails.

Small cancers that include a portion of the underlying bone can be resected through the open mouth. Larger cancers usually require a partial maxillectomy through a Weber-Fergusson approach (Fig. 14-12). Not infrequently, extension to the maxillary antrum, nasal cavity, or pterygomaxillary space may not be appreciated until the time of surgery but should be anticipated if preoperative assessment has been adequate. Sizeable antral defects are usually skin-grafted, and the communication between the oral cavity and the antrum and nasal cavity is closed by a specially fabricated dental prosthesis (see Ch. 9). The latter can be wired in place at the time of the resection, to facilitate oral alimentation postoperatively.

The occasional patient who presents initially with cervical node metastasis is treated with a radical neck dissection at the same time as the excision of the primary cancer. As with other sites in the oral cavity, current preference calls for irradiation in addition to surgery in patients who have larger cancers, invasion of bone, or obvious regional metastases.

Results

Determinant 5-year cure was achieved in 31 percent of patients treated by surgery at Memorial Hospital,[72] whereas, the 3-year cure was 40 percent in another treatment center where radiotherapy alone or irradiation and surgery in combination were preferred.[43] Results are not comparable because the latter report includes upper gingival and soft palate cancers, but excludes patients whose lesions could not be staged.

The salvage rate varies from 56 to 86 percent for patients whose primary cancer is less than 3 cm in size. Ratzer et al.[72] reported that only 8 percent of patients who had positive nodes on admission remained alive and well. Konrad et al.[43] have suggested that their salvage of 5 of 14 patients (36 percent) with Nl disease may reflect the beneficial effect of irradiation when added to surgery.

NONEPIDERMOID CANCER

Nonepidermoid cancers comprise less than 10 percent of the cancers arising in the oral cavity. Although they seldom occur in the tongue on the floor of the mouth (1 or 2 percent), more than half of the cancers arising in the hard palate prove to be other than epidermoid carcinoma (Table 14-1). Most of these are minor salivary in origin, but melanoma, lymphoma, and various types of sarcoma may also occur. Metastatic deposits from distant sites are rarely seen in the oral cavity, and if seen are usually in association with widely disseminated disease.

Minor Salivary Gland Tumors

Submucosal mucous glands (minor salivary glands), which lubricate the lining epithelium of the upper aerodigestive tract, may give rise to neoplasms histologically identical to these seen in the major, or paired, salivary glands. In our experience,[93] more than 85 percent of minor salivary tumors are malignant and adenoid cystic carcinoma is the tumor most often encountered (Table 14-3). About 70 percent of all minor salivary tumors arise in the oral cavity and more than half involve the palate. Benign lesions—almost always pleomorphic

TABLE 14-3. ORAL MINOR SALIVARY GLAND TUMORS

Type of Tumor	Palate	Tongue	Cheek, Lips	Gums	Floor of Mouth	Total
Benign	41	2	9	0	0	52
Adenoid cystic	65	27	13	11	5	121
Adenocarcinoma, solid and other	43	12	19	6	8	88
Mucoepidermoid	21	10	8	9	4	52
Malignant mixed	7	1	0	2	0	10
Oat cell	4	2	0	0	0	6
Acinic	0	0	0	1	0	1
Total	181	54	49	29	17	330

(Spiro, R. H., Koss, L. G., Hajdu, S. I., and Strong, E. W. 1973. Tumors of minor salivary origin, a clinicopathologic study of 492 cases. Cancer 31:117.)

adenomas (benign mixed tumors)—typically occur in the palate or cheek mucosa and are most unusual in other sites. The median age of our patients with this type of cancer is in the sixth decade and both sexes are equally represented.

Minor salivary gland tumors originating in the oral cavity characteristically present as an asymptomatic swelling beneath intact mucous membrane (Fig. 14-16). Ulceration may occasionally be present usually as a result of denture or other trauma. Pain is reported with greater frequency by those who prove to have malignant tumors, but neither symptomatology nor appearance is of assistance in predicting the histology. Although the duration of symptoms is usually measured in months, many years may elapse before some patients seek medical attention. We have encountered a few patients who had an asymptomatic swelling—later proved to be malignant—that had been present for more than 20 years.

Definitive treatment is surgical. Conservative local excision may be feasible through the open mouth for patients who have small cancers arising in the buccal mucosa, lips, or tongue. More often, as for cancers of the palate or gingiva, en bloc excision including underlying bone is indicated. A partial maxillectomy may be required in the case of large cancers involving the palate. Radical neck dissection is usually reserved for those who present with clinically positive cervical nodes (less than 15 percent of patients). Elective neck dissection may be indicated for a few patients who require a cheek flap approach in order to resect a bulky cancer of the tongue, floor of the mouth, or lower gingiva but is otherwise avoided, since the overall incidence of cervical metastasis is less than 25 percent.

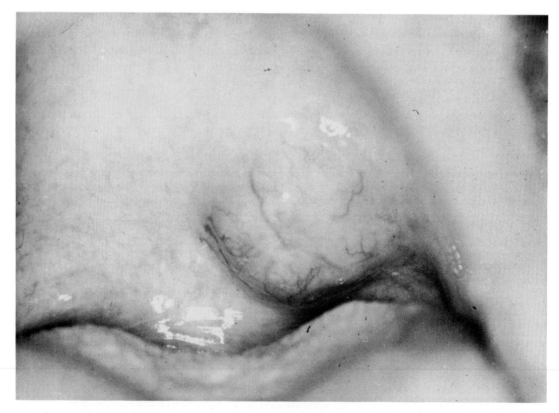

Fig. 14-16. Typical appearance of a minor salivary tumor arising beneath the intact mucosa of the palate. The lesion proved to be an adenoid cystic carcinoma.

Conventional 5-year cure rates may be misleading as it can take decades of observation to appreciate the indolent, yet lethal course in some patients, particularly those with adenoid cystic carcinoma. About 40 percent of our patients with malignant minor salivary neoplasms of the oral cavity remain alive and well for 10 years after treatment. This is a significantly better salvage rate than that which we have observed for patients who have minor salivary tumors in less accessible sites.

Some cancers of minor salivary gland origin, notably adenoid cystic carcinoma, appear to be radioresponsive but rarely radiocurable. For this reason, there is currently much interest in the use of adjunctive teletherapy after appropriate surgery for patients who have unfavorable lesions. Anecdotal responses to chemotherapy have been described, but we are not yet aware of a single agent or drug combination that can produce a significant objective response rate in patients with malignant minor salivary neoplasms.

Mucosal Melanoma

Fewer than 10 percent of melanomas of the head and neck arise in mucosa, and 25 to 50 percent of mucosal melanomas involve the oral cavity.[21, 79] The occurrence of these tumors is unusual in patients younger than 30 years. The peak incidence is in the sixth and seventh decades. Although the sex incidence is about equal in patients with skin melanomas, mucosal melanomas occur about twice as often in men.

Oral pigmentation in black individuals is very common, but benign, pigmented mucosal lesions are rare in whites. Therefore, any pigmented oral lesion in a white patient must be viewed with concern. Many mucosal melanomas arising in the palate or buccal

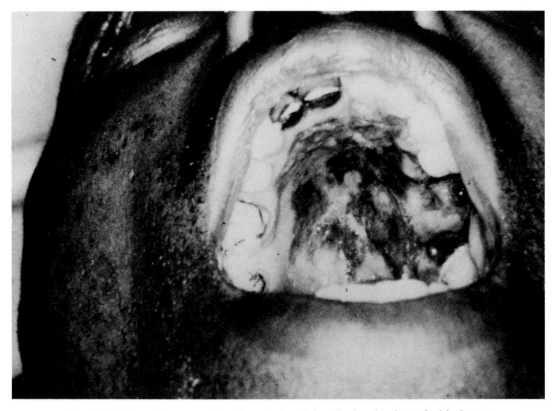

Fig. 14-17. Extensive mucosal melanoma involving the hard palate of a black man.

mucosa are smooth, flat, and may have a lacy pattern of brown or brownish-grey pigmentation that looks deceptively benign (Fig. 14-17). Despite the fact that these tumors are prone to extensive local spread as a consequence of submucosal lymphatic permeation, the incidence of cervical lymph node metastasis is appreciably less than that recorded for skin melanoma.

Treatment usually consists of radical excision. Radiation alone has little to offer, but electrodesiccation has been suggested for certain patients who have extensive, but superficial lesions.[21] Elective radical neck dissection is seldom appropriate for patients with oral melanoma.

Only 10 to 15 percent of patients remain alive and well 5 years after curative surgery; almost all of the remainder succumb with local recurrence. Various drug combinations occasionally yield transient responses in patients who have unresectable disease or distant metastasis.

SURGICAL RECONSTRUCTION

Most radical operations for oral cancer produce significant changes in the patient's function and appearance. Slurring of speech and swallowing impairment is in proportion to the amount of tongue resected and the extent to which the mobility of the remaining tongue is reduced by its use in repair of the surgical defect. Drooling may result if the lips cannot be approximated after resection or if the natural reservoir provided by the floor of the mouth and lower gingivobuccal sulcus is removed. Facial contour is altered and much of the ability to chew solid food may be lost when segmental resection of the mandible is performed. The disability after excision of the arch of the mandible is particularly distressing to both the patient and the surgeon. As a rule, the severity of the functional and cosmetic problems is directly related to the extent of the ablative surgery. When indicated, reconstruction is usually best accomplished at the time of resection.

With the recent increased interest in immediate reconstruction, there has been a flurry of reports advocating specific techniques. Overriding concern with the "how?" of reconstruction has sometimes obscured the more important question: "which patient?" A complex primary reconstruction may not only fail to achieve desired functional and cosmetic goals, but may also add significantly to postoperative morbidity if flap necrosis, sepsis, or other complications occur. The fact is that for many patients very satisfactory rehabilitation can be accomplished merely by skillful approximation of the tissues that remain after resection.

Adequate advance planning is essential, whether one surgeon is to be responsible or a joint effort is contemplated using an ablative and a reconstructive team. In addition to the anticipated disability based upon the extent of the operation proposed, other factors must also be considered. Aggressive rehabilitation is essential for a young, productively employed individual, but may be less important for an elderly retiree. Patient motivation and expectation are also important factors to consider. Finally, the likelihood of increased operating time and greater blood loss make the surgeon decide against immediate reconstruction for certain poor risk patients.

In the past, reconstruction was usually deferred if patients had extensive disease and a very poor prognosis. Actually, the importance of reconstruction increases as the prospect for cure by a radical operation decreases. Restoration of speech and swallowing is crucial to the quality of survival when surgery is likely to be palliative at best. Flap necrosis, planned fistulae, and other problems after reconstruction may seriously interfere with planned postoperative irradiation or other adjunctive therapy.

Some techniques we have found useful for oral reconstruction will be briefly described. A detailed review of this complex subject is beyond the scope of this presentation. The reader is referred to Chapter 27 and other sources,[20, 51] for additional information.

Moderate-Sized Defects

Defects involving mobile tissues such as the tongue or the buccal mucosa are in some cases easily closed by advancement and primary suturing. In contrast, a mucosal gap in the hard palate cannot be sutured, and primary closure of a sizeable wound in the floor of the mouth usually tethers the tongue. Appearance and function will be most satisfactory if the latter wounds are allowed to heal by secondary intention, even if some bone has been exposed (Fig. 14-13); alternatively, a split-thickness skin graft can be used for epithelial coverage in some cases.[37]

Another useful method for repair of posterior defects in the retromolar area, cheek, palate, or floor of the mouth involves the posteriorly based tongue flap[18] (Fig. 14-18). The versatility of this flap depends upon the size and location of the defect, and its reliability is much reduced if the oral cavity has previously been irradiated. Moreover, large tongue flaps may significantly reduce tongue mobility.

Larger Defects

The skin of the neck is convenient and useful for resurfacing sizeable defects in the tongue and floor of the mouth.[4] Although the blood supply of superiorly based cervical flaps is randomly derived, these flaps are reasonably reliable in well-nourished patients. Cervical skin flaps should be avoided in hirsute men with a low beard line or when there has been irradiation to the neck. Either a small flap can be introduced into the mouth through a planned fistula, closing the neck primarily with the remaining skin, or almost the entire ipsilateral neck skin can be fashioned into a large flap. In the latter case, a second, medially

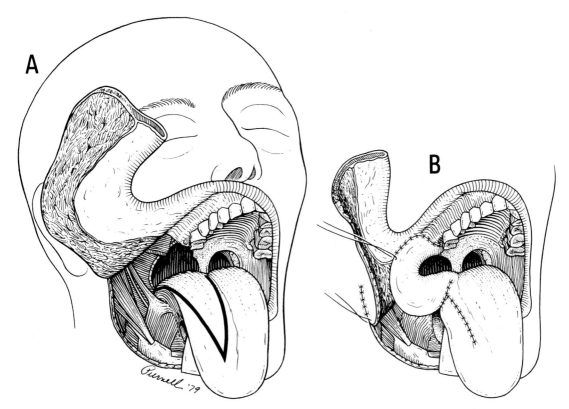

Fig. 14-18. (A and B) Mucosa and a small portion of the underlying musculature of the tongue elevated and rotated as a flap to resurface a defect remaining after resection of a cancer of the retromolar trigone.

medially based deltopectoral flap is used to resurface the neck[27] (Figs. 14-19, 14-20 and 14-21). The smaller flap provides adequate tissue to reconstruct the floor of the mouth with minimal restriction of tongue movement. The larger cervical-apron flap can replace sizeable resected portions of the tongue and facilitate articulation and swallowing (Figs. 14-22A–F).

Other useful techniques include the forehead flap[38, 50] or the deltopectoral flap,[3, 5] both of which can be introduced directly into the oral cavity. Full-thickness cheek and lip defects pose a particularly challenging problem, which can be solved by modifications of single flaps or by the use of one flap for lining and a second flap for external coverage (Fig. 14-23). The use of myocutaneous flaps has recently been described.[49, 70] Our early experience with these flaps has been encouraging.

Reconstruction of the Mandible

Although much has been written about reconstruction of the mandible, we find it appropriate for relatively few patients. Mandibular deviation and loss of facial contour associated with resection of a portion of the body of the mandible varies greatly from patient to patient. Most patients find their appearance to be more acceptable than anticipated (Fig. 14-24). The desired goal of successful jaw reconstruction is the ability to retain a lower denture and to chew solid

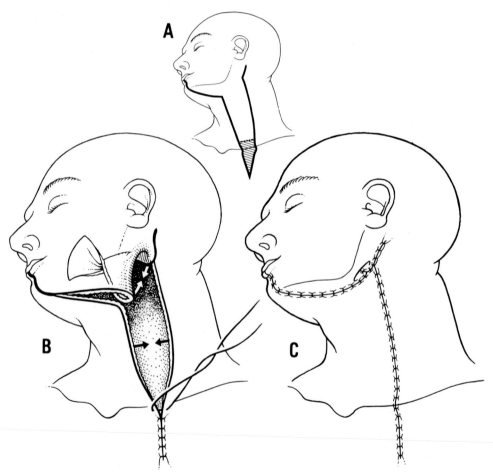

Fig. 14-19. (A) Cervical-apron flap used to repair moderate-sized oral defects; the distal third of the flap (shaded portion) is discarded. (B) The neck incision can be closed primarily. (C) A second procedure is necessary to close the planned orocutaneous fistula.

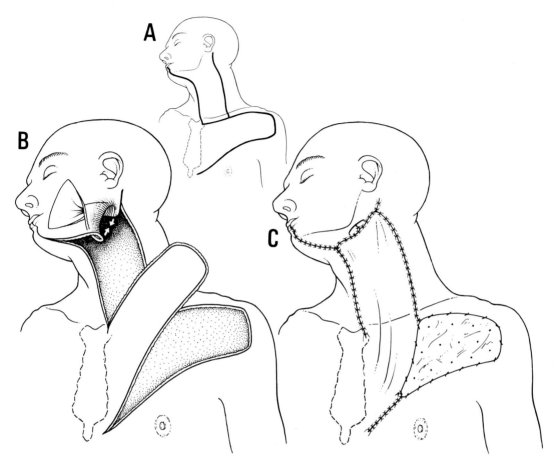

Fig. 14-20. (A) Incision for a large cervical flap, which can be used to repair sizeable oral defects. (B) A median-based deltopectoral flap is used to resurface the neck. (C) The raw area on the chest wall is grafted, and the planned orocutaneous fistula is closed about 4 weeks later.

foods. When the patient learns that this is not often achieved, there may be reluctance to proceed for cosmetic reasons alone. Mandibular deviation may be treated successfully in many patients by using various bite appliances (see Ch. 9).

Even with careful patient selection, however, success is not likely unless certain principles are observed. There is general agreement that mandible reconstruction is more likely to be successful when performed as a clean, second stage procedure than when attempted in a contaminated field immediately after the tumor resection. Even more important is the need for adequate oral lining. When indicated this is provided by a skin flap transposed into the mouth at the initial operation. Aside from restricting the movement of the

tongue, inadequate lining greatly increases the risk that intraoral soft tissue breakdown over the reconstruction may lead to sepsis and failure.

Available techniques include the use of a piece of autologous bone (preferably from the iliac crest),[86] prefabricated alloplastic prostheses (most often stainless steel or titanium),[35, 97] or a tray that is filled with autologous bone particles.[12] Autologous bone segments are subject to some resorption and are less than satisfactory for defects in the mandibular arch. Porosity seems to be an important consideration when alloplastic materials are used. Without the fixation afforded by ingrowth of fibrous tissue, movement usually leads to bone resorption where the applicance is attached and eventual loss of fixation.

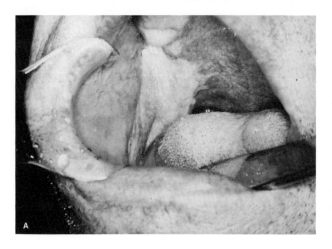

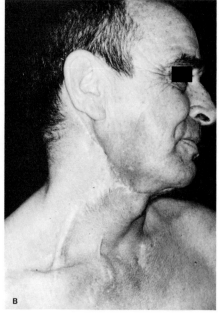

Fig. 14-21. (A) Cervical-apron flap of the type illustrated in Figure 14-19A has been used to repair an oral defect after resection of a retromolar primary. (B) Appearance of the neck after staged closure of the planned orocutaneous fistula.

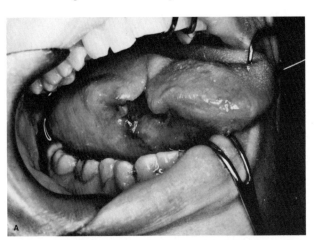

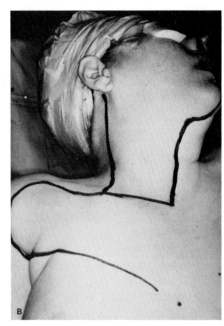

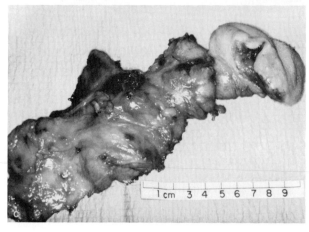

Fig. 14-22. (A) Massive squamous carcinoma of the oral tongue. (B) Incision outlining a large cervical-apron flap for reconstruction of the tongue and a deltopectoral flap for resurfacing of the neck as illustrated in Figure 14-20. (C) Most of the oral tongue removed in-continuity with the contents of the right side of the neck through a mandible splitting approach.

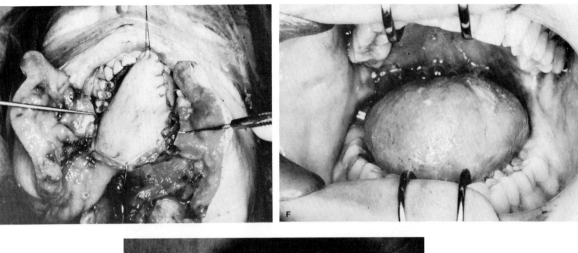

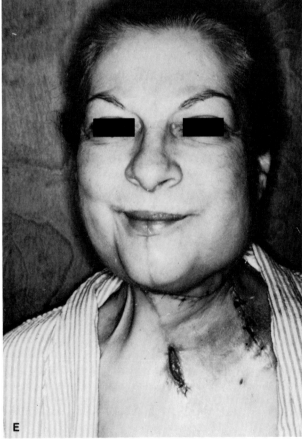

Fig. 14-22 continued. (D) Access provided by the mandibulotomy approach is illustrated. The cervical skin-flap is sutured to the remaining tongue. (E) Appearance of the patient $3^{1}/_{2}$ months after her initial surgery and one week after contralateral radical neck dissection. (F) Appearance of the reconstructed tongue $3^{1}/_{2}$ months after resection.

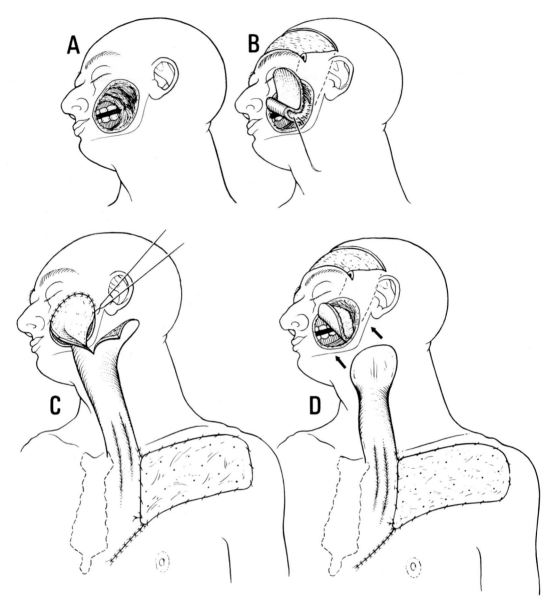

Fig. 14-23. Several useful techniques for repair of (A) a through-and-through cheek defect are illustrated. (B) A forehead flap can be turned back upon itself for lining and external coverage. In (C) a median based deltopectoral flap is split distally to provide lining as well as skin coverage. (D) Lining and external coverage can also be fashioned separately from forehead and deltopectoral flaps. Each of these techniques requires secondary revision for watertight closure.

COMPLICATIONS

Aside from failure to control cancer in the oral cavity, either surgery or irradiation may have many other undesired consequences. Suture line disruption, tissue necrosis, hemorrhage, or sepsis can occur after any surgical procedure in the contaminated oral environment. These problems can be minimized by good technique and appropriate prophylactic antibiotic coverage and seldom cause serious difficulty unless an external fistula develops.

Potentially serious complications more

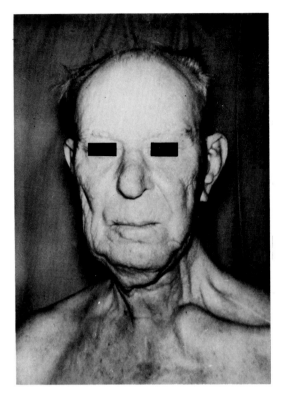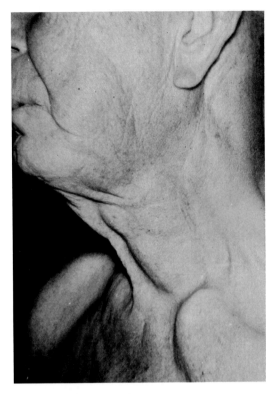

Fig. 14-24. Appearance of a patient 5 years after a composite or "Commando" operation for resection of a tongue cancer. Cosmetic and functional results after hemimandibulectomy can be very satisfactory without plastic reconstruction.

often relate to the neck dissection performed in conjunction with the oral excision. Any significant loss of skin-flap coverage or mucosal lining that exposes the carotid artery or its major branches may lead to exsanguinating hemorrhage. Tissue necrosis and sepsis are the usual precipitating factors and occur more frequently in previously irradiated patients. Carotid catastrophe is seen most often in the patient whose infected neck wound communicates with the oral cavity or pharynx. Careful placement of skin incisions in the neck can reduce the chance of carotid exposure and is particularly important for the patient who has been irradiated. Dermal grafts or muscle flaps can be used to protect the carotid vessels when healing problems are anticipated.[85]

Operative mortality depends significantly upon the extent of the operation performed and may vary from near zero for those who have a local excision of a small oral primary to more than 15 percent for the exceptional patients who require a radical, en bloc resection with simultaneous, bilateral radical neck dissection. Many patients with cancer of the oral cavity are elderly and have respiratory, gastrointestinal, and other problems aggravated by chronic alcohol and tobacco abuse. When postoperative death occurs, it is more often related to these systemic ailments rather than to wound breakdown.[88]

SUMMARY

Oral cancer remains a challenge and a frustration to the clinician. If treated when the tumor is small and localized, almost 70 percent of oral cancer patients can be "cured." Therapeutic approaches to "early" oral cancer may differ, but the results are often gratifying and cosmetic and functional sequelae are usually minimal. These results contrast greatly with those for patients who have advanced oral cancers. Despite radical treatment and the use of different modalities in combination, survival rates are low and the morbidity is high. Hopefully, new developments in immunotherapy, chemotherapy, and radiation therapy will improve the outlook. Meanwhile, the increased risk of oral cancer for those who smoke or drink excessively deserves more emphasis. Primary care physicians need more training in order to detect oral cancer in its earliest stages.

REFERENCES

1. Bagshaw, M. A., and Thompson, R. W. 1971. Elective irradiation of the neck in patients with primary carcinoma of the head and neck. JAMA, 217:   456.

2. Bakamjian, V. Y. 1974. The surgical management of cancers of the cheek. Journal of Surgical Oncology, 6:   255.

3. Bakamjian, V. Y. 1975. The deltopectoral flap. In Grabb, W. C., and Myers, M. B., Eds.: Skin Flaps. Little Brown, Boston, 225.

4. Bakamjian, V. Y., and Littlewood, M. 1964. Cervical skin flaps for intraoral and pharyngeal repair following cancer surgery. British Journal of Plastic Surgery, 17:   191.

5. Bakamjian, V. Y., Long, M., and Rigg, B. 1971. Experience with the medially based deltopectoral flap in reconstructive surgery of the head and neck. British Journal of Plastic Surgery, 24:   174.

6. Ballard, B. R., Suess, G. R., Pickren, J. W., Greene, G. W., Jr., and Shedd, D. P. 1978. Squamous cell carcinoma of the floor of the mouth. Oral Surgery, Oral Medicine, Oral Pathology, 45:   568.

7. Batsakis, J. G. 1974. Tumors of the Head and Neck: Clinical and Pathological Considerations. Williams and Wilkins, Baltimore.

8. Biller, H. F., Ogura, J. H., Davis, W. H., and Power, W. E. 1969. Planned preoperative irradiation for carcinoma of the larynx and laryngopharynx treated by total and partial laryngectomy. Laryngoscope, 79:   1387.

9. Blum, R. H., Carter, S., and Agre, K. 1973.

A clinical review of bleomycin, a new antineoplastic agent. Cancer, 31:   903.

10. Bocca, E., and Pignataro, O. 1967. A conservation technique in radical neck dissection. Annals of Otology, Rhinology and Laryngology, 76:   975.

11. Botstein, C., Silver, C., and Ariaratnam, L. 1976. Treatment of carcinoma of the oral tongue by radium needle implantation. American Journal of Surgery, 132:   523.

12. Boyne, P. J., and Zarem, H. 1976. Osseous reconstruction of the resected mandible. American Journal of Surgery, 132:   49.

13. Broders, A. C. 1926. Carcinoma, grading and practical application. Archives of Pathology and Laboratory Medicine, 2:   376.

14. Byers, R. M. 1975. Squamous carcinoma of the oral tongue in patients less than thirty years of age. American Journal of Surgery, 130:   475.

15. Cachin, Y., and Eschwege, F. 1975. Combination of radiotherapy and surgery in the treatment of head and neck cancers. Cancer Treatment Reviews, 2:   178.

16. Cady, B., and Catlin, D. 1969. Epidermoid carcinoma of the gum. Cancer, 23:   551.

17. Cancer Facts and Figures. 1978. American Cancer Society, New York.

18. Chambers, R. G., Jacques, D. A., and Mahoney, W. D. 1969. Tongue flaps for intraoral reconstruction. American Journal of Surgery, 118:   783.

19. Chu, A., and Fletcher, G. H. 1973. Incidence and causes of failures to control by irradiation the primary lesions in squamous cell carcinoma of the anterior two thirds of the tongue and floor of mouth. American Journal of Roentgenology, 117:   502.

20. Conley, J., and Dickinson, J. T., Eds. 1972. Plastic and Reconstructive Surgery of the Face and Neck. Vol. 2. Grune and Stratton, New York.

21. Conley, J. C., and Pack, G. T. 1974. Melanoma of the mucous membranes of the head and neck. Archives of Otolaryngology, 99:   315.

22. Conley, J. and Sadoyama, J. A. 1973. Squamous cell cancer of the buccal mucosa. Archives of Otolaryngology, 94:   330.

23. Correa, J. N., Bosch, A., and Marcial, V. A. 1967. Carcinoma of the floor of the mouth: Review of clinical factors and results of treatment. American Journal of Roentgenology, 94:   302.

24. Daly, T. E., Drane, J. B., and MacComb,

W. S. 1972. Management of problems of the teeth and jaw in patients undergoing irradiation. American Journal of Surgery, 124: 539.

25. Ezzatollah, M. (Mahboubi, E.) 1977. The epidemiology of oral cavity, pharyngeal and esophageal cancer outside of North America and Western Europe. Cancer, 40: 1879.

26. Farr, H. W., and Arthur, K. 1972. Epidermoid carcinoma of the mouth and pharynx. Journal of Laryngology and Otology, 86: 243.

27. Farr, H. W., Spiro, R. H., and Shah, J. P. 1976. Immediate repair of the commando defect by cervical and pectoral flaps. American Journal of Surgery, 132: 533.

28. Fayos, J. V., and Lampe, I. 1969. Peroral irradiation of carcinoma of the oral tongue. Radiology, 93: 387.

29. Fletcher, G. H. 1972. Elective irradiation of subclinical disease in cancers of the head and neck. Cancer, 29: 1450.

30. Fonts, E. A., Greenlaw, R. H., Rush, B. F., and Rovin, S. 1969. Verrucous squamous cell carcinoma of the oral cavity. Cancer, 23: 152.

31. Frazell, E. L., and Lucas, J. C., Jr. 1962. Cancer of the tongue, report of the management of 1554 patients. Cancer, 15: 1085.

32. Fu, K. K., Lichter, A., and Galante, M. 1976. Carcinoma of the floor of the mouth, an analysis of treatment results and causes of failures. International Journal of Radiation Oncology, Biology, Physics, 1: 829.

33. Goldman, J. L., and Friedman, W. H. 1969. High dose preoperative irradiation in cancer of the larynx. Otolaryngologic Clinics of North America, 2: 473.

34. Guillamondegui, O. M., and Jesse, R. H. 1976. Surgical treatment of advanced carcinoma of the floor of the mouth. American Journal of Roentgenology, 126: 1256.

35. Hagh, G. W., and Corgill, D. A. 1969. Chrome cobalt mesh mandibular prosthesis. Journal of Oral Surgery, 27: 5.

36. Harold, C. C. 1971. Management of cancer of the floor of the mouth. American Journal of Surgery, 122: 487.

37. Helsper, J. T., and Fister, H. W. 1967. Use of skin grafts in the mouth in the management of oral cancer. American Journal of Surgery, 114: 596.

38. Hoopes, J. E., and Edgerton, M. T. 1966.

Immediate forehead flap repair in resection for oropharyngeal cancer. American Journal of Surgery, 112: 527.

39. Jesse, R. H., and Lindberg, R. D. 1975. The efficacy of combining radiation therapy with a surgical procedure in patients with cervical metastasis from squamous cancer of the oropharynx and hypopharynx. Cancer, 35: 1163.

40. Johnston, W. D., and Ballantyne, A. J. 1977. Prognostic effect of tobacco and alcohol use in patients with oral tongue cancer. American Journal of Surgery, 134: 444.

41. Kissin, B. Kaley, M. M., Su, W. H., and Lerner, R. 1973. Head and neck cancer in alcoholics, the relationship to drinking, smoking and dietary patterns. JAMA, 224: 1174.

42. Kolson, H., Spiro, R. H., Roswit, B., and Lawson, W. 1971. Epidermoid carcinoma of the floor of the mouth. Archives of Otolaryngology, 93: 280.

43. Konrad, H. R., Canalis, R. F., and Calcaterra, T. C. 1978. Epidermoid carcinoma of the palate. Archives of Otolaryngology, 104: 208.

44. Kraus, F. T., and Perez-Mesa, C. 1966. Verrucous carcinoma. Cancer, 19: 26.

45. Lowenfels, A. B. 1974. Alcohol and cancer. New York State Journal of Medicine, 74: 56.

46. Lane, M., Moore, J. E., III, Levin, H., and Smith, F. E. 1968. Methotrexate therapy for squamous cell carcinomas of the head and neck. JAMA, 204: 561.

47. MacComb, W. S., and Fletcher, G. H. 1967. Cancer of the Head and Neck. Williams and Wilkins, Baltimore, p. 122.

48. MacComb, W. S., and Fletcher, G. H. 1967. Cancer of the Head and Neck. Williams and Wilkins, Baltimore, p. 147.

49. McCraw, J., Dibbell, D. G., and Carraway, J. H. 1977. Clinical definition of independent myocutaneous vascular territories. Plastic and Reconstructive Surgery, 60: 341.

50. McGregor, I. A. 1963. The temporal flap in intraoral cancer: Its use in repairing the post-excisional defect. British Journal of Plastic Surgery, 16: 318.

51. McGregor, I. A. 1977. Reconstruction following excision of intraoral and mandibular tumors. In Converse, J. M., Ed., Reconstructive Plastic Surgery. Vol. 5. W. B. Saunders, Philadelphia, 2642.

52. Mahboubi, E. 1977. The epidemiology of oral cavity, pharyngeal and esophageal cancer outside of North America and Western Europe. Cancer, 40: 1879.

53. Manual for Staging of Cancer, 1977. American Joint Committee for Cancer Staging and End Results Reporting, Chicago.

54. Martin, H. E. 1940. The history of lingual cancer. American Journal of Surgery, 48: 703.

55. Martin, H. E. 1941. Cancer of the gums (gingivae). American Journal of Surgery, 54: 765.

56. Martin, H. E. 1942. Tumors of the palate (benign and malignant). Archives of Surgery, 44: 599.

57. Martin, H. E., and Pflueger, O. H. 1935. Cancer of the cheek (buccal mucosa). Archives of Surgery, 30: 731.

58. Martin, H. E., Munster, H. and Sugarbaker, E. D. 1940. Cancer of the tongue. Archives of Surgery, 41: 888.

59. Martin, H. E., DelValle, B., Ehrlich, H., and Cahan, W. G. 1951. Neck dissection. Cancer, 4: 441.

60. Mashberg, A., Morrissey, J. B., and Garfinkel, L. 1973. A study of the appearance of early asymptomatic oral squamous cell carcinoma. Cancer, 32: 1436.

61. Merino, O. R., Lindberg, R. D., and Fletcher, G. H. 1977. An analysis of distant metastases from squamous cell carcinoma of the upper respiratory and digestive tracts. Cancer, 40: 145.

62. Million, R. R. 1971. Elective neck irradiation for $T_X N_0$ squamous carcinoma of the oral tongue and floor of the mouth. Cancer, 34: 149.

63. Moore, C. 1971. Cigarette smoking and cancer of the mouth, pharynx and larynx. JAMA, 218: 553.

64. Moore, C., and Catlin, D. 1967. Anatomic origins and locations of oral cancer. American Journal of Surgery, 114: 510.

65. Moore, O. S., and Frazell, E. L. 1964. Simultaneous bilateral neck dissection. Experience with 151 patients. American Journal of Surgery, 107: 565.

66. Nathanson, A., Jacobsson, P. A., and Wersäll, J. 1973. Prognosis of squamous cell carcinoma of the gums. Acta Otolaryngologica, 75: 301.

67. O'Brien, P. H., and Catlin, D. 1965. Cancer of the cheek (mucosa). Cancer, 18: 1392.

68. Paymaster, J. C. 1956. Cancer of the buccal mucosa. Cancer, 9: 431.

69. Pierquin, B., Chassagne, D., Baillet, F., and Castro, J. 1971. The place of implantation in tongue and floor of mouth cancer. JAMA, 215: 961.

70. Quillen, C. G., Shearlin, J. C., Jr., and Georgiade, N. G. 1978. Use of the latissimus dorsi myocutaneous island flap for reconstruction in the head and neck area: Case report. Plastic and Reconstructive Surgery, 62: 113.

71. Randolph, V. L., Callejo, A., Spiro, R. H., Shah, J., Strong, E. W., Huvos, A. H., and Wittes, R. E. 1978. Combination therapy of advanced head and neck cancer, induction of remissions with diammedichloroplatinum (II), bleomycin and radiation therapy. Cancer, 41: 460.

72. Ratzer, E. R., Schweitzer, R. J., and Frazell, E. L. 1970. Epidermoid carcinoma of the palate. American Journal of Surgery, 119: 294.

73. Reddy, C. C. R. M. 1974. Carcinoma of hard palate in India in relation to reverse smoking of chuttas. Journal of the National Cancer Institute, 53: 615.

74. Rothman, K., and Keller, A. 1972. The effect of joint exposure to alcohol and tobacco on risk of cancer of the mouth and pharynx. Journal of Chronic Diseases, 25: 711.

75. Saxena, V. S. 1970. Cancer of the tongue: Local control of the primary. Cancer, 26: 788.

76. Schneider, J. J., Fletcher, G. H., and Barkley, H. T. 1975. Control by irradiation alone of nonfixed clinically positive lymph nodes from squamous cell carcinoma of the oral cavity, oropharynx, supraglottic larynx and hypopharynx. American Journal of Roentgenology, 123: 42.

77. Shafer, W. G., and Waldron, C. A. 1961. A clinical and histopathological study of oral leukoplakia. Surgery, Gynecology and Obstetrics, 112: 411.

78. Shafer, W. G., and Waldron, C. A. 1975. Erythroplakia of the oral cavity. Cancer, 36: 1021.

79. Shah, J. P., Huvos, A. G., and Strong, E. W. 1977. Mucosal melanomas of the head and neck. American Journal of Surgery, 134: 531.

80. Shah, J. P., Cendon, R. A., Farr, H. W., and Strong, E. W. 1976. Carcinoma of the oral cavity, factors affecting treatment failure at the primary site and neck. American Journal of Surgery, 132: 504.

81. Shanta, V., and Frishnamurthi, S. 1959. A

study of aetiological factors in oral squamous cell carcinoma. British Journal of Cancer, 13: 381.

82. Shedd, D. P., VonEssen, C. F., Connelly, R. R., and Eisenberg, H. 1968, Cancer of the floor of the mouth in Connecticut, 1935–1959. Cancer, 21: 97.

83. Silverman, S., and Griffith, M. 1972. Smoking characteristics of patients with oral carcinoma and the risk for second oral primary carcinoma. Journal of the American Dental Association, 85: 637.

84. Singh, A. D., and VonEssen, C. F. 1966. Buccal mucosa cancer in south India, etiologic and clinical aspects. American Journal of Roentgenology, 96: 6.

85. Smithdeal, C. D., Corso, P. F., and Strong, E. W. 1974. Dermis grafts for carotid artery protection: yes or no? A ten year experience. American Journal of Surgery, 128: 484.

86. Snow, G. B., Kruisbrink, J. J., and Van-Slooten, E. A. 1976. Reconstruction after mandibulectomy for cancer. Archives of Otolaryngology, 102: 207.

87. Southwick, H. W. 1977. Radiation-associated head and neck tumors. American Journal of Surgery, 134: 438.

88. Spiro, R. H., and Frazell, E. L. 1968. Evaluation of the radical surgical treatment of advanced cancer of the mouth. American Journal of Surgery, 116: 571.

89. Spiro, R. H., and Strong, E. W. 1971. Epidermoid carcinoma of the mobile tongue, treatment by partial glossectomy alone. American Journal of Surgery, 122: 707.

90. Spiro, R. H., and Strong, E. W. 1973. Discontinuous partial glossectomy and radical neck dissection in selected patients with epidermoid carcinoma of the mobile tongue. American Journal of Surgery, 126: 544.

91. Spiro, R. H., and Strong, E. W. 1974. Surgical treatment of cancer of the tongue. Surgical Clinics of North America, 54: 759.

92. Spiro, R. H., Alfonso, A. E., Farr, H. W., and Strong, E. W. 1974. Cervical node metastasis from epidermoid carcinoma of the oral cavity and oropharynx, a critical assessment of current staging. American Journal of Surgery, 128: 562.

93. Spiro, R. H., Koss, L. G., Hajdu, S. I., and Strong, E. W. 1973. Tumors of minor salivary origin, a clinicopathologic study of 492 cases. Cancer, 31: 117.

94. Stecker, R. H., Devine, K. D., and Harrison, E. G. 1964. Verrucous "snuff dippers" carcinoma of the oral cavity. JAMA, 189: 838.

95. Strong, E. W. 1969. Preoperative radiation and radical neck dissection. Surgical Clinics of North America, 49: 271.

96. Szpak, C. A., Stone, M. J., and Frenkel, E. P. 1977. Some observations concerning the demographic and geographic incidence of carcinoma of the lip and buccal cavity. Cancer, 40: 343.

97. Terz, J. J., Beal, E. S., King, R. E., and Lawrence, W., Jr. 1974. Primary reconstruction of the mandible with a wire mesh prosthesis. Surgery, Gynecology and Obstetrics, 139: 198.

98. Waldron, C. A., and Shafer, W. G. 1975. Leukoplakia revisited, a clinicopathologic study of 3256 oral leukoplakias. Cancer, 36: 1386.

99. Wawro, W. N., Babcock, A., and Ellison, L. 1970. Cancer of the tongue. American Journal of Surgery, 119: 455.

100. Whitehurst, J. O., and Droulias, C. A. 1977. Surgical treatment of squamous cell carcinoma of the oral tongue, factors influencing survival. Archives of Otolaryngology, 103: 212.

101. Wittes, R. E., Cvitkovic, E., Shah, J., Gerold, F., and Strong, E. W. 1977. Cis-diamminedichloroplatinum (II) (DDP) in the treatment of epidermoid carcinoma of the head and neck. Cancer Treatment Reports, 61: 359.

102. Wizenberg, M. J., Bloedorn, F. G., Weiner, S., and Gracia, J. 1972. Treatment of lymph node metastases in head and neck cancer, a radiotherapeutic approach. Cancer, 29: 1455.

103. Wynder, E. L. 1971. Etiological aspects of squamous cancers of the head and neck. JAMA, 215: 452.

104. Wynder, E. L., and Klein, U. E. 1965. The possible role of riboflavin deficiency in epithelial neoplasia. Cancer, 18: 167.

105. Wynder, E. L., and Stellman, S. D. 1977. Comparative epidemiology of tobacco related cancers. Cancer Research, 37: 4608.

106. Wynder, E. L., Hultberg, S., Jacobsson, F., and Bross, I. J. 1957. Environmental factors in cancer of the upper alimentary tract, a Swedish study with special reference to Plummer-Vinson (Patterson-Kelly) syndrome. Cancer, 10: 470.

15 | Cancer of the Oropharynx

Donald A. Shumrick, M.D.
Jack L. Gluckman, M.D.

INTRODUCTION

Cancer of the oral cavity, pharynx, and larynx is increasing in frequency. At a time when certain cancers, e.g., stomach and uterus, are showing a decline in incidence, quite the reverse appears to be occurring for cancer involving the upper aerodigestive tract. Not only is there an absolute increase in the number of cases being diagnosed, but there appears to be a change in incidence with regard to both age and sex. This condition used to be most commonly diagnosed in the 60 to 70 year age group, however, today cases in the fourth and fifth decades are not uncommon. In addition, with a changing life-style, especially in women, and most particularly with regard to alcohol and tobacco abuse, the male-to-female ratio has changed from 10:1 to today's figure of 4:1.

Tumors may, of course, arise from anywhere within the oropharynx, however, by far the most common site of origin is the palatine arch, including the tonsil and retromolar trigone. Approximately, 4,000 new cases of cancer of the oropharynx are diagnosed every year in the United States[8a] (Third National Cancer Survey, 1969–1971). Unfortunately, even in the best of hands, between 40 and 50 percent of these cancers have a fatal outcome for a wide variety of reasons, e.g., late presentation with advanced disease, the presence of multiple primary carcinomas and general ill health due to old age and chronic alcohol and tobacco abuse.

342

ANATOMY

For clinical purposes the oropharynx can be regarded as consisting of the oropharynx proper and the palatine arch. The oropharynx is continuous anteriorly with the oral cavity through the oropharyngeal isthmus. It communicates with the nasopharynx above and with the hypopharynx below (Fig. 15-1).

The palatine arch includes the soft palate, the anterior tonsillar pillar, and the retromolar trigone. While the retromolar trigone is actually located within the oral cavity, it blends medially with the anterior tonsillar pillar; lesions in this area behave in a similar fashion to those arising in the oropharynx. The retromolar trigone is a triangular area that covers the anterior aspect of the ramus of the mandible posterior to the third molar tooth (Fig. 15-2).

The roof of the oropharynx is formed anteriorly by the pharyngeal portion of the soft palate, but is posteriorly incomplete and communicates with the nasopharynx via the nasopharyngeal isthmus. This isthmus is bounded anteriorly by the uvula and free margin of the soft palate. The lateral and posterior boundaries are formed by some of the fibers of the palatopharyngeus muscle, which encircles the pharynx inside the superior constrictor and forms a ridge against which the soft palate impinges when elevated by the levator palati (Passavant's ridge). Other fibers of the palatopharyngeus form the posterior tonsillar pillar (Figure 15-3).

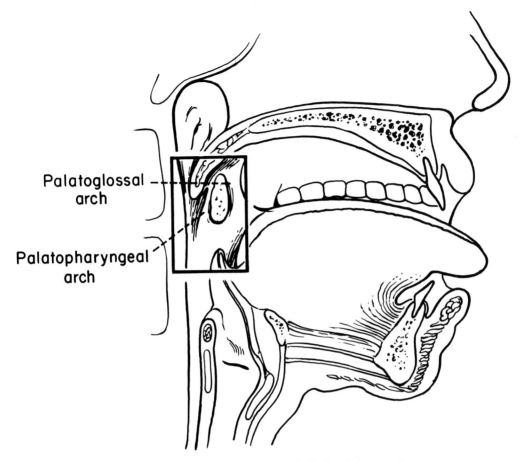

Fig. 15-1. Diagram depicting the anatomic limits of the oropharynx.

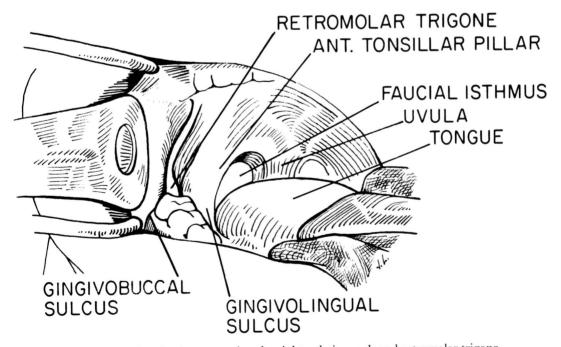

RETROMOLAR TRIGONE
ANT. TONSILLAR PILLAR

FAUCIAL ISTHMUS
UVULA
TONGUE

GINGIVOBUCCAL
SULCUS

GINGIVOLINGUAL
SULCUS

Fig. 15-2. Oral cavity demonstrating the right palatine arch and retromolar trigone.

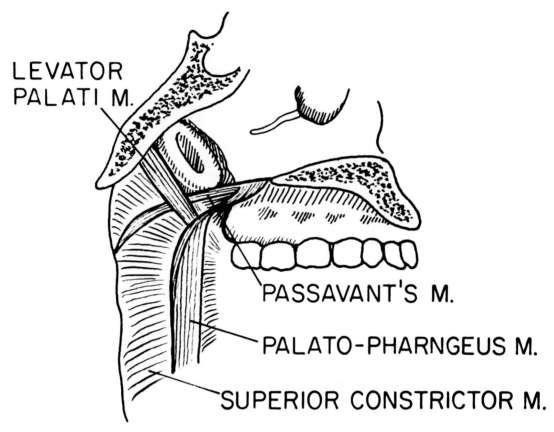

LEVATOR
PALATI M.

PASSAVANT'S M.

PALATO-PHARNGEUS M.

SUPERIOR CONSTRICTOR M.

Fig. 15-3. The palatopharyngeus muscle. Note how some of the fibers form Passavant's ridge and the rest the posterior tonsillar pillar.

The anterior boundary of the oropharynx consists of the base of the tongue and the oropharyngeal isthmus opening into the oral cavity. This isthmus is bounded by the soft palate above, the anterior tonsillar pillars laterally, and the dorsum of the tongue at the circumvallate papillae below. The mucosa of the base of the tongue is extremely irregular, due to the underlying lingual tonsil, which varies considerably in size. A midline mucosal fold, the glossoepiglottic fold, connects the base of the tongue to the epiglottis. The pharyngoepiglottic fold extends from the lateral margins of the epiglottis to the lateral pharyngeal walls on both sides. The pharyngoepiglottic folds separate the oropharynx from the hypopharynx. The area bounded by the epiglottis, base of the tongue, and pharyngoepiglottic folds is known as the valleculae.

The limits of the lateral walls of the oropharynx are formed by the anterior and posterior tonsillar pillars, which are mucosal folds overlying the palatoglossus and palatopharyngeus muscles. The tonsillar fossa occupies the space between these two pillars. Deep to this space, the lateral wall consists of the superior constrictor and upper fibers of the middle constrictor, with contributions to the lateral wall by the palatoglossus, palatopharyngeus, salpingopharyngeus, and stylopharyngeus muscles. Between the base of the tonsillar fossa laterally and the base of the tongue medially lies the tonsillolingual sulcus, which forms part of the lateral food passage.

The faucial tonsil is a mass of lymphoid tissue that fills the tonsillar fossa. The free surface varies considerably in appearance and consists of a large number of narrow crypts (tonsillar crypts). The normal tonsil varies in size at different periods of life and, therefore, at times may bulge into the pharynx and later may be sessile and limited to the tonsillar fossa. The deep surface is covered by a fibrous tissue capsule to which fibers of the palatoglossus and palatopharyngeus are attached. The major blood supply to the tonsil is derived from the tonsillar branch of the facial artery. Other branches are from the ascending pharyngeal and the dorsalis linguae arteries, as well as from the palatine branches of the internal maxillary and the facial arteries. The peritonsillar veins emerge from the deep surface of the tonsil and, after piercing the inferior constrictor, terminate in the common facial vein and pharyngeal plexus.

The posterior wall of the oropharynx is related to the second and third cervical vertebrae.

Inferiorly, the boundary between the oropharynx and hypopharynx is formed by the upper border of the epiglottis anteriorly and the pharyngoepiglottic folds laterally.

Parapharyngeal Space

Knowledge of the anatomy of this space is essential to the understanding of the signs and symptoms produced by direct tumor extension into this area (Fig. 15-4). This space is divided into a prestyloid and poststyloid space by the styloid process and the three muscles arising from it, i.e., stylohyoid, stylopharyngeus, and styloglossus. The prestyloid space is bounded medially by the buccopharyngeal fascia overlying the superior constrictor muscles and laterally by the medial pterygoid muscle. The glossopharyngeal nerve lies within this space and enters the pharynx between the superior

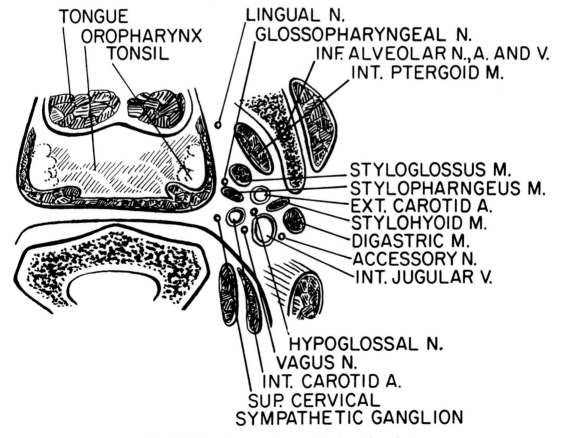

Fig. 15-4. Parapharyngeal space (horizontal section).

and middle constrictor muscles. This nerve supplies the motor branches to the pharyngeal musculature and the sensory branches to the oropharynx. The lingual nerve, which is a branch of the mandibular division of the trigeminal nerve, also runs through the prestyloid space; it supplies the mucous membrane of the floor of the mouth and the anterior two-thirds of the tongue. Between the medial pterygoid and the mandible lies the poststyloid space, through which the inferior alveolar nerve and internal maxillary artery run. Not only can tumors cause signs and symptoms due to direct involvement of these nerves, but tumor can extend up to the base of the skull by perineural extension.

Lymphatic Drainage

The most important primary drainage site from the oropharynx is the jugulodigastric (tonsillar) node. Also of importance are the retropharyngeal and parapharyngeal nodes, which drain the pharyngeal portion of the soft palate, lateral and posterior oropharyngeal walls, and base of the tongue (Fig. 15-5). These nodes lie in the retropharyngeal and parapharyngeal space and are closely related to the last four cranial nerves, the internal jugular vein, and the internal carotid artery at the base of the skull. The most superior lateral node is known as the node of Rouviere. The efferent channels from these nodes pass to the jugulodigastric and posterior cervical group. The area of the retromolar trigone can drain directly into the submaxillary node. Bilateral metastases are possible in midline lesions.

Pharyngeal Phase of Deglutition

To better understand the sequelae of disease and surgery in this area, a brief description of the pharyngeal phase of deglutition is useful.

In the voluntary act of swallowing, the bolus of food is forced by the tongue through the oropharyngeal isthmus into the pharynx. Once this has occurred the palatoglossus muscle contracts, thereby reducing the size of the oropharyngeal isthmus and preventing reflux of the food into the mouth. The larynx is elevated against the epiglottis, which in turn is pushed backwards and downwards by the movement of the base of the tongue. The nature of the bolus now determines its subsequent progress. If fluid or semifluid, the thrust of the tongue is sufficient to project it into the esophagus. If, however, it is solid, the pharyngeal muscles contract and propel the food into the esophagus.

Any process interfering with the musculature can result in dysphagia, aspiration, or reflux by incompetent nasopharyngeal and oropharyngeal sphincters.

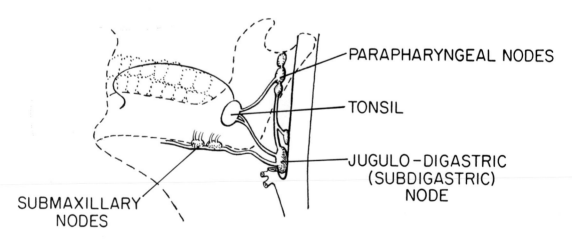

Fig. 15-5. Lymphatic drainage of oropharynx.

ETIOLOGY

The anatomy of the upper aerodigestive tract renders it extremely vulnerable to a wide variety of exogenous carcinogens. A carcinogen by definition is an agent that is capable of initiating the development of cancer, with the effects being manifest after a considerable time delay. This carcinogenic effect is heightened by cocarcinogens.

Carcinogens

In man, numerous chemical and ionizing carcinogens have been demonstrated to be active in the upper aerodigestive tract. The aromatic hydrocarbons of tobacco are probably the most important, regardless of whether the tobacco is snuffed, chewed, or smoked. These hydrocarbons are weakly carcinogenic and require a large total dose to have any effect. The smaller the dose, the longer the required exposure. Controversy exists as to whether cessation of smoking will avoid the formation of further carcinoma. There does appear to be evidence that the possibility of further cancer development is considerably decreased. but not completely eliminated.[20]

Ionizing radiation treatment for benign problems in the head and neck area, e.g., adenoid hypertrophy and acne, has been implicated as a cause of carcinoma. There also appears to be an increased incidence of carcinoma for those who were exposed to the atomic bomb in Japan and to atomic tests in the Pacific Islands.

Cocarcinogens (Promoting Factors)

Other factors, known as cocarcinogens, obviously play a part in carcinogenesis; however, these factors are less easily identifiable.

1. *Alcohol:* Alcohol and tobacco abuse are commonly found together in patients seen with carcinoma of the oropharynx;[12] and alcohol appears to have a synergistic effect with tobacco.[24] The incidence of oropharyngeal cancer is far greater among alcoholics than among the general popula-

tion.[12] The exact carcinogenic mechanism through which alcohol acts is obscure, but may be related to many possibilities, such as local mucosal irritation, associated malnutrition seen in alcoholism, or a possible alteration in the hormonal balance or the status of the patient's natural immunity because of the effect on the liver.[30]

2. *Local mucosal irritation,* which may be due to chronic infection, poor oral hygiene, or ill-fitting dentures.

3. *Nutrition:* Malnutrition, frequently seen in alcoholics, may well be a factor. Mucosal atrophy and hyperkeratosis have been demonstrated in cases of riboflavin deficiency. Certainly, there is a high incidence of pharyngeal cancer, particularly in the postcricoid area and esophagus, in the Plummer-Vinson syndrome, which is associated with iron deficiencies. Carcinogens among food additives have also been implicated.

4. *Immunity:* Impaired immunity may play an important, but as yet unexplained role. It has been well-documented that patients who are immunosuppressed, e.g., because of organ transplants, show a much higher incidence of cancer.

5. *Saliva reservoirs:* Saliva may act as a medium for the carcinogen, and this would explain the predominance of lesions on the saliva-dependent portions of the oral cavity and oropharynx, i.e., floor of the mouth and base of the tongue. The carcinogen in the saliva would remain in prolonged contact with the mucosa in these areas.[18]

Multiple etiologic factors seem to be involved in most of the patients with cancer of the oropharynx. In 1944, Willis[34] stated that when carcinogenic stimuli are in contact with epithelial tissue, all of the epithelia in that area are affected similarly, but not necessarily equally. Neoplasia, therefore, is more likely to commence when the stimuli have been maximal, and neoplastic response may occur later in adjacent tissue that was exposed to the same carcinogens. This "condemned mucosa" or "field cancerization" theory certainly applies to the upper aerodigestive tract and explains the high incidence—12.5 percent in our experience—of synchronous multiple primaries that are diagnosed if carefully looked for.

PATHOLOGY

Benign, as well as malignant, tumors are found in the oropharynx. A classification of these lesions is presented in Table 15-1.

Benign

EPITHELIAL

Papilloma. This common pedunculated, fimbriated lesion may arise on the tonsil, fauces, or palate and may be single or multiple. It has a fibrovascular cord. Papillomas are usually asymptomatic and discovered in-

TABLE 15-1. TUMORS OF THE
OROPHARYNX

Benign

    Epithelial

        Papilloma
        Adenoma and pleomorphic adenoma
        Mucous cyst

    Mesenchymal

        Fibroma
        Lipoma
        Hemangioma
        Neuroma

Malignant

        Squamous cell carcinoma, including
          lymphoepithelioma
        Adenocarcinoma
        Lymphoma
        Sarcoma

Parapharyngeal tumors

        Parotid
        Neurogenic (e.g. neurolemmoma)
        Vascular (e.g. chemodectoma, aneurysm,
          arteriovenous malformation)

---

cidentally by the patient, dentist, or physician; in rare instances, they may be large enough to cause an irritating sensation. Papillomas can be excised under local anesthesia for diagnostic and therapeutic purposes.

Simple Adenoma and Pleomorphic Adenoma present as a small mucosal covered mass. They are rare with the most common site being the hard palate; appearance on the soft palate seldom occurs. Treatment is surgical excision.

Mucous Cysts. The importance of these common lesions is that they should be differentiated from other submucosal tumors. Treatment consists of simple incision and drainage.

MESENCHYMAL

Lipomas and Fibromas rarely occur; they may be pedunculated or submucosal.

Hemangiomas can occur in the palate, tonsil, and posterior and lateral walls of the oropharynx, or can be situated entirely in the parapharyngeal space. Angiography is useful in aiding diagnosis and evaluating the extent of the lesion. If lesions increase in size or become symptomatic, e.g., bleeding or dysphagia, they should be excised after preoperative embolization, if feasible.

Malignant

Squamous Cell Carcinomas constitute the most common group of malignancies found in the oropharynx and in general are more biologically aggressive and more undifferentiated than squamous cell carcinomas of the oral cavity. The current concept regarding lymphoepithelioma is that it represents a poorly differentiated squamous carcinoma. Clinically it behaves somewhat differently from most squamous cell carcinomas, with the former having a propensity to early nodal and distant metastases. Histologically, lymphoepitheliomas consist of nests of epithelial cells with lymphocytes scattered between the cells. These tumors are, however, truly epithelial in nature with the lymphocytes not actively participating in the genesis of the tumor. Histologic variations of the tumor may closely resemble a lymphoma.

Adenocarcinomas usually arise from minor salivary glands and present in the palate, faucial regions, or base of the tongue as an ulcerated or a mucosa-covered mass. These tumors have a lethal behavior with a propensity for regional and distant metastases. Aggressive surgical excision is the treatment of choice. Adenocarcinomas are associated with a high local recurrence rate.

Lymphomas. Hodgkin and non-Hodgkin lymphomas occur in the tonsil and base of the tongue in adults and occasionally in children. They can present as a unilateral enlargement of the tonsil with or without ulceration or can simulate a peritonsillar abscess. Association with enlarged cervical nodes may also exist. Tonsillectomy may be necessary for most accurate histologic diagnosis. Appropriate tests for staging of the disease must be carried out prior to instituting a definitive radiotherapeutic and/or chemotherapeutic regimen (see Ch. 26).

Sarcomas. Rhabdomyosarcoma of the pterygoid muscles may present as a parapharyngeal mass.

Parapharyngeal Tumors

Osteomas and chondromas arising from the anterior surface of the cervical vertebrae may present as a bulge in the posterior oropharynx. Neurogenic tumors, chemodectomas and aneurysms, and tumors arising from the deep lobe of the parotid should be considered in the differential diagnosis of parapharyngeal lesions. These tumors may distort the lateral pharyngeal walls and mimic tumors arising from the oropharynx proper.

METHODS OF SPREAD

As discussed on page 342, the oropharynx can be divided into a number of distinct regions anatomically. In practice, however, it is impossible (except in very early cases) to determine the exact site of origin of these lesions, as the limits of these anatomic boundaries are not respected by the cancer and when the cancer is first seen several sites are frequently involved. It is, therefore, preferable to regard the posterior oral cavity and oropharynx as a mucosal field that includes several anatomic structures with a common lymphatic drainage. The similarity and prognosis of cancers in this region supports this view. It is because the posterior oral cavity and oropharynx are regarded as a mucosal field that the retromolar trigone lesions are included in this group by some authors.

Overall, cancers of the oropharynx are more aggressive and less differentiated than those of the oral cavity. Clinically they can be divided into four types: superficial spreading, exophytic, ulcerative, and infiltrative. The first two types are usually found in areas of condemned mucosa, particularly on the palatine arch. They are rarely associated with metastasis. The latter two types, however, have a marked tendency to regional metastasis, i.e., 50 percent from the tonsil and 70 percent from the base of the tongue.[7] Because of the rich network of lymphatics there is a tendency towards bilateral and contralateral metastases. It is of interest that the retropharyngeal nodes are the most direct drainage site, but are not as frequently involved as the superior deep cervical nodes.[7]

CARCINOMA OF THE TONSIL AND TONSILLAR FOSSA

These lesions are the most common of all cancers arising in the oropharynx. They can be exophytic and spread superficially, but are more commonly ulcerative and infiltrative, with only the tip of the iceberg being evident on clinical examination. They spread directly to involve the palatine arch, base of the tongue, pharyngeal walls, and hypopharynx. Extension along the periosteum of the mandible with invasion of the pterygoid muscle and masseter can occur, resulting in pain and trismus. The lesions can also involve the mandible and maxilla directly. In addition, direct extension into the floor of the mouth can occur with subsequent extension to the submaxillary space. By penetrating the superior constrictor and invading the parapharyngeal space, the lingual, hypoglossal, glossopharyngeal and inferior alveolar nerves can become involved. The base of the skull can be invaded by direct extension or perineural spread along the above nerves. Fifty percent of cases have cervical metastasis at the time of initial presentation.[25]

CARCINOMA OF THE PALATINE ARCH

The palatine arch, i.e., the soft palate and the anterior faucial pillars, is regarded as the junctional area between the oral cavity and the oropharynx. Lesions in this area tend to behave more like oral cavity lesions —they tend to be superficial and better differentiated and to remain localized for longer periods of time than others in the oropharynx. There is often associated widespread erythroplasia. In many instances the early lesions may present as areas of erosion in diffuse erythroplasia, resulting in difficulty in delineating the extent of the tumor. As the lesions extend more laterally and become more deeply infiltrative, they tend to behave more like pharyngeal lesions with an increased tendency to cervical metastases. Tumors of the palatine arch may present early by causing pain and interfering with the oropharyngeal sphincter. Occasionally, the patient may notice a lesion in the mirror. Contiguous structures can be involved by direct extension as described for carcinoma of the tonsil.

CARCINOMA OF THE POSTERIOR AND LATERAL PHARYNGEAL WALLS

Because of the lack of symptoms associated with lesions presenting in this area, they are usually diagnosed late and by this time the lesion has attained a considerable size. Submucosal spread can occur to regional oropharyngeal structures, i.e., soft palate, ton-sil, tongue, or to the nasopharynx or hypopharynx. Only rarely, however, does deep posterior infiltration, with involvement of the anterior spinal ligament, occur. Parapharyngeal involvement can occur. Sixty-six percent of cases will eventually have cervical metastasis.[8] Extremely poor prognosis is related to the late presentation and frequent metastasis.

CARCINOMA OF THE POSTERIOR THIRD OF THE TONGUE

The posterior third of the tongue is frequently involved secondarily by large tumors arising elsewhere in the oropharynx or in the supraglottic larynx. Lesions can, however, arise primarily in this area. There appears to be a particularly high incidence of base of tongue cancers in India and in patients with Plummer-Vinson syndrome.[3] Because of the site of origin, they are relatively asymptomatic until late and unfortunately may be missed even when large, as the lesion may be mistaken for the lingual tonsils. All too frequently, the first sign of disease is the presence of cervical metastasis with the primary lesion not being visible on indirect laryngoscopy and only detected on palpation. Lesions tend to be deeply infiltrative and to take the line of least resistance, which is spreading to the intrinsic lingual musculature with direct spread to the preepiglottic space and root of tongue occurring (Fig. 15-6). The lesions may spread to involve other oropharyngeal structures and even the larynx and hypopharynx. Seventy percent of cases show cervical metastases, either unilateral or bilateral, when lesions are first diagnosed, and distant metastases can occur.

Lymphatic Spread

Due to the late diagnosis, most oropharyngeal lesions are seen at an advanced stage. Sixty percent of patients have clinically positive nodes on the initial examination; this percentage varies according to the location of the primary lesion. In addition, another 10 to 20 percent of patients have clinically

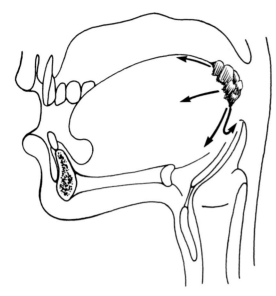

Fig. 15-6. Carcinoma of the base of the tongue—routes of spread.

negative but histologically positive nodes. This is of great prognostic importance, as the presence of clinically positive nodes will decrease the 5-year survival rate by 50 percent for those with lesions of the base of the tongue. Histologically-proven metastasis in palpable nodes decreases the survival by a further 25 percent.[3]

The superior jugular nodes (jugulodigastric or subdigastric) are usually the first echelon of nodes to be involved. If a carcinoma is situated in the anterior oropharynx, the next most common nodal group involved is that of the submaxillary triangle nodes and the middle jugular nodes. If a lesion is situated posteriorly, the retropharyngeal nodes are more likely to be involved with a greater incidence of contralateral and multiple cervical metastases.

The presence of retropharyngeal lymph nodes is well documented; however, their involvement by carcinoma is seen primarily in lesions of the posterior nasopharynx, oropharynx, and hypopharynx. They are found in the areolar tissue behind the musculature of the pharynx and consist of two groups: a lateral group (node of Rouviere), which lies near the base of the skull in close relationship to the internal carotid

artery, the last four cranial nerves, the sympathetic chain, and the internal jugular vein; and a medial group, which lies more inferiorly and is closely related to the pharyngeal musculature.

The efferent pathways are to nodes in the deep lobe of the parotid, to upper jugular nodes, and to posterior triangle nodes.

Ballantyne in 1964[1] found metastases to retropharyngeal nodes in 44 percent of cases of cancer of the pharyngeal walls. Involvement of these nodes has a significant effect on the prognosis of the patient because they are frequently not included in the dissection. Surgery for cancer in this area should, therefore, include active dissection of these nodes with resection where necessary. The nodes are identified by retracting the pharynx and dissecting the tissue medial to the carotid artery at the base of the skull.

A clinical syndrome has been described in patients with enlarged metastatic retropharyngeal lymph nodes; it is characterized by pain in the ipsilateral neck and head with radiation to the eye and is often associated with stiffness of the neck.[1]

Distant Metastasis

As newer therapeutic methods enable us to gain better local control of the disease, the patients succumb later to distant metastasis. An increased incidence of distant metastasis appears to be related to the following factors: the site of the tumor, e.g., the posterior third of the tongue and posterior pharyngeal wall; the nodal staging; and the recurrence of tumor.

PATIENT EVALUATION

Undoubtedly the most important reason for the poor prognosis associated with cancer of the oropharynx is failure of early recognition of the disease. Patients are usually asymptomatic in the early stages. Even when they do become symptomatic, the vast majority are treated conservatively for a considerable period of time because of misdiagnosis before the condition is recognized. It is essential that greater physician awareness of lesions in this area be promoted, in order to ensure earlier diagnosis. The average time interval between the first presenting symptom and diagnosis is 6 months.

Symptoms

The most common symptom is a persistent, usually unilateral, sore throat that has proven refractory to various conservative measures. This symptom may be associated with referred otalgia. The nerve pathway ascends the glossopharyngeal nerve to the petrosal ganglion, then with the tympanic nerve (Jacobson's nerve) to the tympanic cavity. A vague irritation of the throat associated with a persistent desire to clear the throat occurs occasionally. Change in the quality of speech to the so-called hot potato speech may be associated with lesions of the base of the tongue. The patient may frequently present because of a lump in the neck. Odynophagia, dysphagia, or trismus occur in large lesions. Bleeding may occur from lesions of the base of the tongue and must be differentiated from hemoptysis. The patient invariably complains of weight loss.

Examination

It is important not to confine the examination to the head and neck but to perform a general physical examination. The patient's nutritional status must be evaluated. The physical age is as important as the chronologic age. The presence and severity of associated diseases, such as cardiovascular and pulmonary, may influence the therapeutic approach in the individual. Also of importance is assessment of the mental status; the patient's knowledge that he has cancer and the fear of radical therapy may cause profound depression.

A complete head an neck examination should be performed, including indirect lar-

yngoscopy and nasopharyngoscopy to assess the extent of the primary lesion and, of course, to exclude a second malignancy. The usual finding is a definite mass or an ulcerative lesion. The lingual tonsils may mask a lesion of the posterior third of the tongue; thus, this area of the tongue should always be palpated as a routine part of the examination and if any asymmetry is noted a malignant lesion should be suspected. Having the patient protrude his tongue for the degree of fixation will provide information regarding involvement of the root of the tongue. The state of dentition should be assessed so that carious teeth may be repaired. The appropriate cranial nerves should be tested. Trismus may be present because of involvement of the medial pterygoid muscle and would indicate an extensive infiltrative lesion. The neck must be examined in detail for evidence of metastases or direct extension of tumor.

Special Studies

In addition to the routine workup, a radiograph or xeroradiograph of the mandible should be obtained to ascertain whether the bone is involved and to assess the teeth if present. If indicated, tomography of the base of the skull and of the sinuses should be obtained. All cases should be evaluated by a prosthodontist preoperatively for advice regarding the use of prostheses or dentures. If a lesion is large or there is evidence of extensive cervical metastasis, a screening metastatic workup including a chest x-ray, full blood count, and a liver profile, is performed. Further tests, such as bone, liver, spleen, and brain scans should be done if the index of suspicion of distant metastasis is high.

Examination Under Anesthesia

Panendoscopy, i.e., laryngoscopy, bronchoscopy, and esophagoscopy, as well as direct examination of the oropharynx and mirror examination of the nasopharynx should be performed under anesthesia on all cases of cancer of the upper aerodigestive tract, irrespective of their size or situation or amenability to evaluation under local anesthesia. The reasons for this examination are that it is easier to accurately assess the tumor under general anesthesia; it allows adequate tattooing of the lesion where indicated and it enhances the possibility of diagnosing an unsuspected second synchronously developing primary tumor.

Tattooing

If planned preoperative radiotherapy is to be used or if salvage surgery at a later stage is a possibility, the margins of the proposed resection should be outlined prior to the commencement of radiation.[2] Unless tattooed, the response of the tumor to irradiation may make recognition of adequate margins difficult, no matter how carefully the margins have been documented. This may result in ablative surgery being performed too conservatively because the shrinkage of the tumor may lull the surgeon into a false sense of security. The aim at surgery is to remove the same amount of tissue as if no prior radiation had been given.

The tattooing technique consists of making puncture marks with a size 18 needle dipped in India ink. These are made 1 cm apart, approximately 2 cm around the palpable margin of the tumor, and not just around the visible ulceration. Care is taken to restrict the injection of ink to the full thickness of the mucosa only. Deeper staining results in excessive staining of the tissues and will not mark discretely, thereby making identification of the mark more difficult at a later stage. In the case of cancer of the base of the tongue or vallecula, the needle may be introduced through a laryngoscope.

Biopsies are taken after the lesion has been tattooed. Careful documentation should be kept of the tumor and a tumor registry data sheet completed.

Use of Toluidine Blue

In selected cases, particularly where a lesion has developed in "condemned mucosa," there may be lesions that are not obvious to the naked eye. In order to aid assessment, in vivo staining with toluidine blue 0.2 percent can be used.[29] The suspicious area should be blotted dry and if necessary, acetic acid can be used to remove the excess mucus. The dye is then swabbed onto the area and after a short period of time irrigated off with saline. The stain is selectively taken up by nucleic acids and deposited in intercellular spaces. The greater the atypism, the greater is the nucleic acid-cytoplasm ratio and the further apart are the cells; therefore, the dye uptake will be greater. Areas of atypism are stained deep violet. Because the stain penetrates no deeper than four or five layers, submucosal disease cannot be detected. While this is a useful aid, the inexperienced observer may have great difficulty with interpretation.

Staging

After careful examination the cancer should be staged. In reviewing the literature, there appears to be an even distribution between the two major TNM classifications and this may lead to confusion in assessing results. The international system (UICC) and the American Joint Committee (1956) classify according to site, while the new American Joint Committee (1975) classifies according to size. While both types of classifications are given (see Table 15-2), it is recommended that the newer classification be adopted to ensure uniformity for future comparison of results.

TREATMENT

At the present time, there is no therapeutic regimen that offers a clearly superior survival rate over other methods. Indeed, this lack of significant advantage of one method

TABLE 15-2. DEFINITION OF T CATEGORIES OF THE OROPHARYNX
(LOCATION AND EXTENT OF PRIMARY TUMOR)

Based on AJC Subcommittee 1965

Anatomic Description

Posterior Wall	*Lateral Wall*	*Anterior Wall*
Extends from free borders of the soft palate to the tip of the epiglottis	Includes the tonsillar pillars, the tonsillar fossa and contents	Consists of the lingual surface of the epiglottis, and the folds of mucosa which bound the vallecula

T1—Tumor limited to one site of the oropharynx

T1—Tumor limited to the posterior wall	T1—Tumor limited to the lateral wall	T1—Tumor limited to the anterior surface of the epiglottis or to the folds of mucosa bounding vallecula

T2—Tumor Extending into two sites of the oropharynx

T2—Tumor of the posterior wall extending onto a lateral wall	T2—Tumor of the lateral wall extending into the posterior wall or anteriorly into the pharyngoepiglottic fold or the glossoepiglottic fold	T2—Tumor of the anterior surface of the epiglottis, with extension into the lateral wall of the oropharynx

T3—Tumor extending beyond the oropharynx

T3—Tumor of the posterior wall extending into prevertebral fascia or laterally into soft tissues of neck by direct extension	T3—Tumor of the lateral wall extending laterally by direct extension into soft tissues of neck, or posteriorly into prevertebral fascia, or anteriorly into base of tongue, or into pyriform sinus	T3—Tumor of the anterior surface of epiglottis, with extension into base of tongue, into larynx, into pyriform sinus, or into soft tissues of the neck

Based on Revisions Recommended by AJC Subcommittee 1975

Primary tumor

T1S—Carcinoma in situ
T1—Lesion 2 cm or less in greatest diameter
T2—Lesions greater than 2 cm but not exceeding 4 cm in greatest diameter
T3—Lesion greater than 4 cm in greatest diameter
T4—Lesions greater than 4 cm with invasion of bone, soft tissues of the neck, or root of tongue

---

over another has led to constant change in approach in an attempt to obtain both maximal results and less morbidity. The selection of treatment for a specific lesion in an individual depends on the following factors:

1. The staging of neoplasm, i.e., large lesions require radical treatment, which results in significant morbidity and disfigurement.

2. The presence of associated systemic disease; this may prohibit major surgical resection.

3. The psychological attitude of the patient. Many patients will refuse to undergo

mutilating surgery under any circumstances.

4. Attitude of the relatives. Too frequently relatives with the best intentions refuse to allow the patient to undergo radical treatment.

5. Philosophy and experience of physician. The outlook and experience of the physican, either radiotherapist or surgeon, is important in dictating the type of treatment, particularly in cases of advanced lesions.

6. The facilities that are available. The presence or absence of an experienced surgeon or radiotherapist will affect the approach to the patient. In addition, lack of supportive facilities and professionals, e.g., intensive care, nursing, and paramedical personnel, must also be taken into consideration. There is no doubt that ideally these cases should be managed in major institutions having sufficient support facilities to handle the complications that invariably occur when many cases are treated.

The current available modes of therapy are surgery, radiation, combined radiation and surgery, chemotherapy, and palliative therapy.

For many years oropharyngeal cancers were regarded as exceptionally radiosensitive and radiotherapy alone was regarded as the treatment of choice. This may suffice for early lesions; however, in some areas (for example, the base of tongue) radiotherapy alone gives a dismal 5-year survival rate, varying from 10 to 26 percent depending on the stage of the disease.[33] Combination therapy (surgery *and* radiation) is increasingly being utilized in an attempt to improve these figures. The poor prognosis seems related to the lack of early diagnosis, inaccessibility of the area to examination, and early cervical metastases. These factors result in advanced disease at the time of diagnosis. In general, the T1 and T2 lesions can be treated with surgery or radiation, whereas the T3 and T4 lesions should be treated with combined therapy.

Surgery

METHODS OF APPROACH

Major surgery in the oropharynx should only be performed by a surgeon well trained in this field who has a team experienced in the postoperative management of these patients. In addition, a surgical pathologist is essential in order to ensure satisfactory margins of resection by means of frozen section at the time of surgery. There are a number of methods of approach to the lesion depending on the site or sites involved, size of the lesion, cervical involvement, and experience of the surgeon.

Intraoral Resection. The obvious advantage of this technique compared to the composite resection is the minimal morbidity. The intraoral resection should be used primarily for small lesions in the oropharynx, excluding the base of the tongue. Lesions of the palatine arch and posterior oropharyngeal wall are particularly amenable to this approach. After resection, the margins of the defect must be evaluated by frozen section and a wider excision performed if indicated.

Some of the surgical defects may be allowed to granulate in, while others may be closed primarily after undermining the surrounding mucosa. Usually, however, the area must be grafted using a split skin graft. The graft may be stented into position, but this usually necessitates a tracheostomy to prevent upper airway obstruction. A more practical approach has been to employ the "quilting technique" to fix the graft into position.[15] This technique immobilizes the graft by suturing it to the underlying musculature at 1 cm intervals. This usually obviates the need for a stent and tracheostomy.

Resection via Mandibular Osteotomy (Fig. 15-7). For years the standard operation for cancer of the posterior oropharynx has been a composite resection of the primary lesion and hemimandible, together with a radical neck dissection (the Commando, or

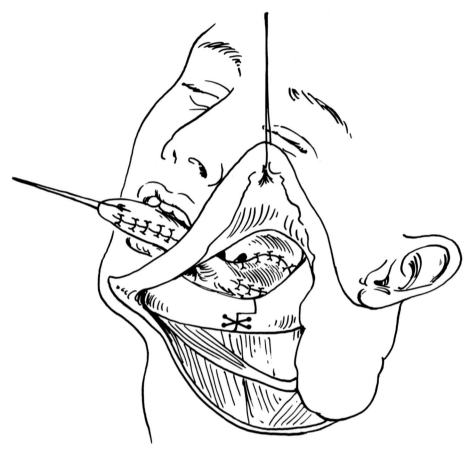

Fig. 15-7. The technique of lateral osteotomy and laterally based tongue flap for reconstruction.

jaw-neck, operation). While there is little argument as to the need for excision of the primary tumor and the neck dissection, the importance of removing the hemimandible as part of the dissection is now being questioned.

The rationale for removal of the adjacent mandible has been to allow both easier access to the tumor and ease of primary closure. In addition, it was felt that complete tumor removal required mandibular resection to remove the periosteal lymphatic involvement. This, however, has been refuted, as microscopic involvement of the periosteum or mandible has not been demonstrated when grossly normal tissue is interposed between the tumor and the mandible.[17] Therefore, in an attempt to preserve the mandible the technique of lateral oste-

otomy as first described by Trotter 50 years ago has been reintroduced.[10] The absolute contraindication to the use of this method is involvement of the mandible or periosteum. If involvement is noted at the time of surgery, the procedure can easily be converted to a composite resection.

This osteotomy is performed in a step fashion and wired at the end of the procedure. If postradiotherapeutic surgical salvage is to be performed this technique should not be used, because the risk of osteoradionecrosis and nonunion of the osteotomy is high. The use of the mandibular osteotomy following planned preoperative radiotherapy may also be complicated by this problem.

Median Translingual Pharyngotomy (Median Labiomandibular Glossotomy) (Fig.

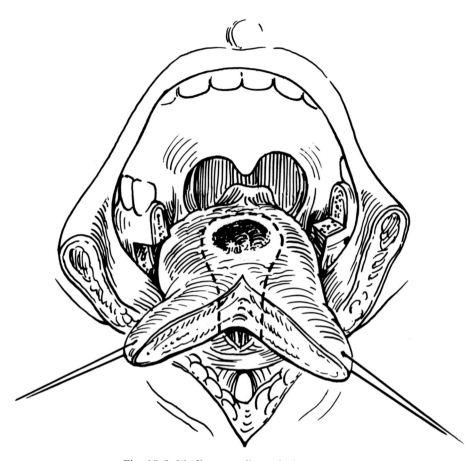

Fig. 15-8. Median translingual pharyngotomy.

15-8). This technique has been used in a limited way to approach cancers situated at the base of the tongue, posterior pharyngeal wall, and epiglottis (Fig. 15-9). It was originally devised by Trotter in 1929 and consists of splitting the lower lip, mandible, and tongue in the midline. Dissection of the tongue is continued posteriorly until the lesion is sufficiently exposed so that it can be resected with a wide margin of normal tissue. There is usually a need for a skin graft when posterior pharyngeal wall lesions have been excised, whereas primary closure is usually possible with base of the tongue lesions. This approach produces minimal cosmetic and functional deformity, although a temporary tracheostomy will be necessary. Wiring of the mandible, together with intermaxillary fixation, is recommended. The median translingual pharyngotomy is not suitable for concomitant neck dissection.

Lateral Pharyngotomy (With or Without Mandibular Osteotomy (Fig. 15-10). This operation is an excellent approach to the posterior pharyngeal wall, but also gives access to tumors arising from the tip of the epiglottis and posterior third of the tongue. It may be combined with a lateral mandibular osteotomy for improved access and with a neck dissection.

Transhyoid Pharyngotomy. The transhyoid pharyngotomy (Fig. 15-11) is an excellent approach to lesions involving the tip of the epiglottis, posterior pharyngeal wall, or base of the tongue. A horizontal incision is made above or below the hyoid and the pharynx entered in the vallecula. Care must be taken to avoid injury to the hypoglossal nerves, lingual arteries, and superior laryngeal nerves. Since the vallecula is entered

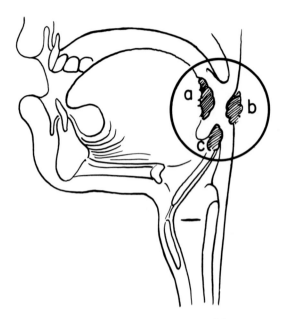

Fig. 15-9. Sites of tumors accessible to resection by the median translingual pharyngotomy, the lateral pharyngotomy, or the transhyoid approach: a, base of the tongue; b, posterior pharyngeal wall; c, epiglottis.

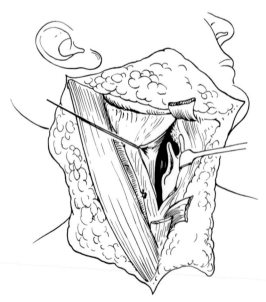

Fig. 15-10. Lateral pharyngotomy. This may be combined with a lateral osteotomy to obtain better exposure.

blindly, there is a danger of compromising the lines of resection. The resultant defect is closed primarily; such closure results in a good cosmetic result and excellent speech and swallowing rehabilitation. A temporary tracheostomy is necessary.

Midline Osteotomy With Mandibular Swing.   Another approach to the base of the tongue is via a midline osteotomy and splaying of the mandible laterally. The base of the tongue is approached by an incision along the lateral floor of the mouth; the incision stays close to the lingual aspect of the mandible but leaves a cuff of mucosa on the mandible to aid later reconstruction. The lesion is then excised, and the defect reconstructed primarily or by using regional flaps. Occasionally there may be difficulty swinging the mandible laterally and exposure may be compromised.

Discontinuous Intraoral and Cervical Approach.   Occasionally certain oropharyngeal lesions may be treated by discontinuous intraoral resection and neck dissection, e.g., small pharyngeal wall or palatine arch lesions. Traditionally, in-continuity neck dissection together with the primary lesion has been regarded as essential to the success of the operation; however, many surgeons no longer regard en bloc dissection as being necessary.[10] Careful patient selection is essential if this approach is to be used.

Composite Resection (Jaw-neck, or Commando, procedure).   This technique, consisting of a neck dissection, partial mandibulectomy, and in-continuity excision of the oropharyngeal lesion, has been regarded for years as the cornerstone for management of cancer of the oropharynx. It is without doubt the method of choice for extensive lesions and lesions with obvious involvement of the mandible, and certainly in postirradiation salvage surgery. The technique can be performed as the primary modality or combined with radiation therapy. While it is an extensive radical procedure, in most cases it is associated with an acceptable cosmetic result and adequate rehabilitation with regard to deglutition and speech.

Patients who are to undergo composite

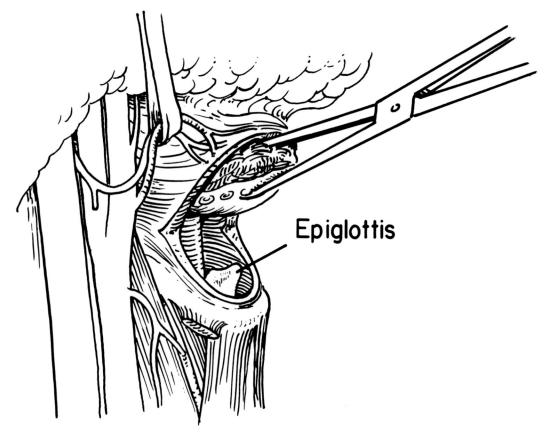

Fig. 15-11. Transhyoid pharyngotomy.

resection may have been subjected to planned preoperative irradiation followed by a 4 to 6 week recuperation period. Full details of the resection are adequately described in most surgical atlases, and only the highlights of this technique will be discussed here.

A tracheostomy is indicated and can be performed at the beginning or end of the procedure. In planning the incision, it must be remembered that the patients may have had previous radiation (planned preoperative or unplanned full course) and should complications occur, the carotid artery would be vulnerable. Many incisions have been described but the following are most commonly used in our department.

The *modified Frazier incision* has a curved horizontal component stretching from the mastoid to the opposite submandibular triangle and crossing the midline at the level of the hyoid bone; an S-shaped vertical component extends down to the clavicle (Fig. 15-12). This incision is by far the easiest to work with, but poses a potential threat in that the vertical component of the incision is often adjacent to the common carotid artery. Should wound separation and retraction of flaps occur in the postoperative period, the carotid may be vulnerable to drying and possible rupture. Therefore, the vertical component should be placed as far posterior as possible. In our experience, a lip-splitting incision is rarely indicated.

The *McFee incision* consists of parallel horizontal incisions resulting in a bipedicled flap. The advantage of this incision is that carotid coverage is ensured. Occasionally, difficulty is encountered with the midneck dissection under the flap.

A standard radical neck dissection is then performed with the neck dissection

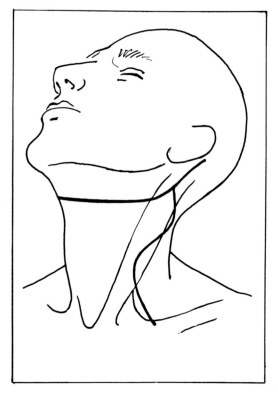

Fig. 15-12. Modified Frazier incision.

performed just below the sigmoid notch, or the condyle can be divided just below the temporomandibular joint. The temporomandibular joint can be disarticulated if necessary to obtain an adequate margin of excision.

A heavy scissors is used intraorally to deepen the mucosal cuts on the soft palate through the nasopharynx and to continue the dissection along the mucosal incisions. The latter is continued around to the lateral gingivobuccal sulcus at the site of the anterior osteotomy. The posterior segment of the mandible is then splayed outward exposing the full extent of the tumor, which can now be easily resected via the external approach by following the previously performed mucosal cuts.

The pterygoid musculature is divided at the end, as dissection in this area is often accompanied by profuse bleeding from the internal maxillary artery. The secret of removal is adequate exposure and for the surgeon to have an exact three-dimensional concept of the extent of the proposed excision. Figure 15-14 demonstrates the resultant defect.

At this stage all margins of the defect should be checked by means of frozen section to ensure that no residual tumor remains. The cut end of the body of the mandible is rongeured to prevent the sharp edge from eroding through the skin. The defect is then reconstructed, either primarily or using alternative methods described below. After reconstruction and closure of the pharynx and oral cavity, a dermal skin graft is routinely placed over the upper end of the common carotid artery, its bifurcation, and its proximal portions of the internal and external carotid arteries to protect them should they become exposed. Large hemovacs are used for postoperative drainage.

In an uncomplicated case, the postoperative management is relatively simple, with the tracheostomy being removed at 7 days and the nasogastric tube the following day. There may be difficulty with deglutition and aspiration initially, but the patient quickly

being pedicled at the angle and posterior third of the body of the mandible. At this stage, it is important to ensure that the neck dissection is completely free from the carotid system. The mouth is opened, and the proposed margin of excision (previously tattooed) is infiltrated with 1:100,000 epinephrine and the mucosal cuts are made (Fig. 15-13). A spinal needle is then passed from the oral cavity at the site of the anterior tattoo mark so that it is seen external to the mandible and will mark the proposed anterior osteotomy. If no tattooing has been done, then the needle is passed anteriorly through the mucosa at a safe margin into the neck.

Attention is then turned once again to the neck, and the periosteum is incised along the lower aspect of the body of the mandible. The periosteum is carefully elevated superiorly exposing the area of the mandible to be excised. Using a Gigli or Stryker saw, the anterior osteotomy is then performed. A superior osteotomy can be

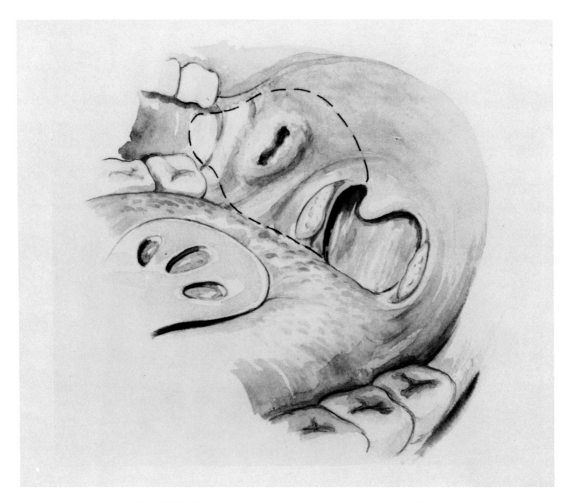

Fig. 15-13. Composite resection: proposed area of excision.

learns to overcome this. Antibiotics are used prophylactically in the perioperative period.

Indications for Associated Laryngectomy. Squamous cell cancer of the posterior third of the tongue usually extends inferiorly to involve the supraglottic larynx and the pre-epiglottic space. In these cases a decision has to be made as to whether total or supraglottic laryngectomy should be performed in combination with the glossectomy.[13, 22, 33] A number of factors need to be taken into account in this decision-making process, i.e., general status of the patient, age, the respiratory reserve, extent of tumor, the amount of tongue that needs to be removed, and the residual function.

In general, in a young healthy patient, if less than half of the base of the tongue is removed leaving at least one hypoglossal nerve intact, a supraglottic laryngectomy together with a cricopharyngeal myotomy can usually be successfully performed without aspiration problems. If, however, a large portion of the base of the tongue needs to be excised, and/or both hypoglossal nerves sacrificed, there is no place for conservative procedures and total laryngectomy should be performed in order to prevent severe postoperative aspiration and swallowing problems.

For the poor risk patient, it may be advisable to perform a total laryngectomy even if a partial laryngectomy is technically feasible.

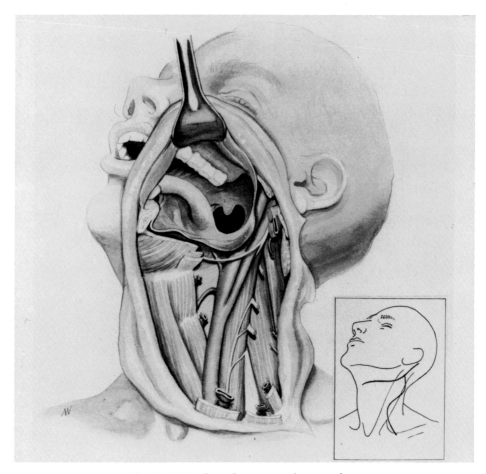

Fig. 15-14. Defect after composite resection.

RECONSTRUCTION

While almost all defects can technically be closed primarily, this may well compromise the future rehabilitation of the patient and, therefore, an alternative plan should always be available in case primary closure does not appear appropriate. Particularly following a composite resection, a poorly conceived primary closure may cause considerable distortion of the position of the remaining mandible and shortening and restriction of the tongue resulting in difficulty with speech, mastication, and deglutition. In an irradiated field a primary closure should not be attempted if there is tension on the suture line, as primary closure under this condition may result in breakdown of the closure site and fistula formation.

Primary Closure.   Following a composite resection, primary closure is usually possible. The procedure consists of a three-layered closure that results in the tongue being tethered in the region of the lateral pharyngeal wall (Fig. 15-15). This method is undoubtedly the quickest and easiest, but the advantages should be weighed against the disadvantages for each case. This type of closure after extensive resection usually markedly downgrades the patient's ability to swallow and speak. With time and exercise, some mobility of the tongue may be regained, and a tongue release with skin graft can be performed at a later stage to obtain more mobility. If healthy teeth are present, intermaxillary fixation or a bite plane can be used to ensure adequate position of the mandible. Lesions on the posterior pharyn-

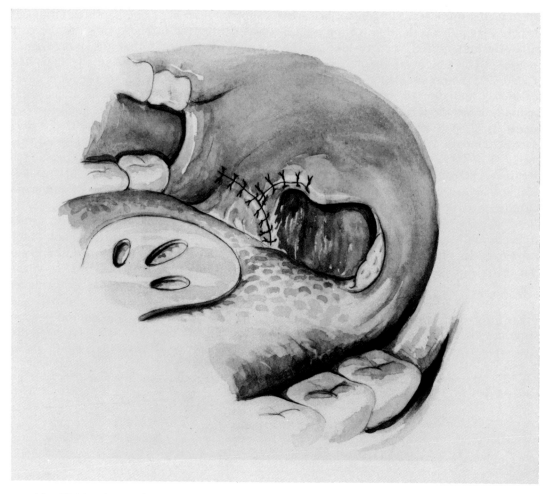

Fig. 15-15. Primary closure of composite resection. Note trifurcation formed. In this diagram only a small portion of the angle of the mandible has been removed.

geal wall or palatine arch can be closed primarily by undermining the surrounding mucosa or can be allowed to granulate in.

Free-skin Graft or Dermal Graft. These grafts are extremely useful in closing defects of the posterior pharyngeal wall and can be maintained in position by means of stenting with the quilting technique. The use of these grafts is once again coming into vogue for reconstruction following a composite resection and a large pouch of dermis or split skin is utilized to cover the defect. Although the free-skin and dermal grafts do not appear to be saliva-tight and do tend to shrink, the protagonists of this technique claim that if carefully performed this graft-ing gives as satisfactory a result as use of regional or local flaps.

Local Flaps. The use of a tongue flap where feasible is an excellent alternative to the above technique. The advantages of tongue flaps are the availability of a good blood supply, which usually ensures viability; that the external appearance is not altered; and that 50 percent of the tongue can be utilized without compromising mastication or deglutition. Articulation is usually unaffected but may occasionally be altered. The continuity of the ipsilateral lingual artery is not essential for flap survival.

Numerous tongue flaps are available for reconstruction; however, the easiest and the one that supplies the largest surface area is based laterally on the floor of the mouth after the tongue has been divided in the midline. The tongue is then filleted, unrolled, and then rotated 180° into the surgical defect and sutured into place. The remaining portion of the tongue is closed upon itself. A posteromedially based flap can be similarly utilized (Figs. 15-16 and 15-17).

Regional Flaps. The advantages of regional flaps are that they enable adequate closure without tension and without the need of viable nonirradiated healthy tissue to be brought in to facilitate healing. The forehead flap is the most reliable, with alternatives including the deltopectoral and nape of neck flap.

When the forehead flap is to be used, every effort must be made to preserve the superficial temporal artery during the neck dissection so as to ensure an adequate blood supply to the flap. The flap is carefully elevated from the forehead down to the pericranium, ensuring that the postauricular vessels are incorporated in the flap. The flap is then rotated into the oral cavity through a separate incision 2 cm below the zygoma. Care must be taken to ensure that the incision is large enough so that it does not constrict the flap. The flap is used to close the defect in the oropharynx and is tubed above the defect. A split-thickness skin graft is then placed over the donor site (Fig. 15-18, 1–3).

Another possible route is to bring the flap under the zygoma, with resection of the zygomatic arch being performed to prevent constriction of the flap. In 2 to 3 weeks the base of the flap is contricted by a tourniquet to determine the viability of the flap and then as a second stage, the unused portion is severed and returned to the forehead defect (Fig. 15-18, 4). If the flap is brought in

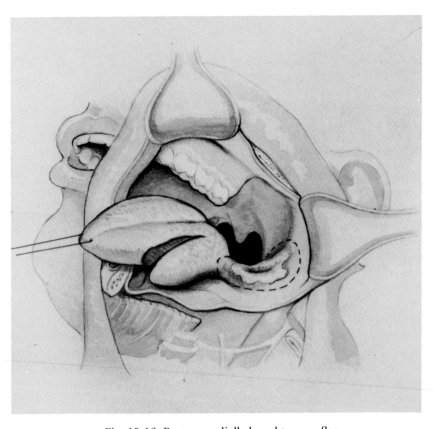

Fig. 15-16. Posteromedially based tongue flap.

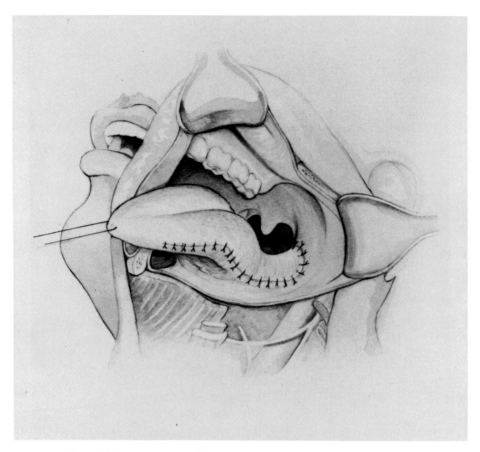

Fig. 15-17. Posteromedially based tongue flap placed into position.

under the zygoma, the second stage may be complicated by difficulty in separating the flap from the surrounding tissue. The major disadvantages of this flap are that it results in a marked cosmetic deformity at the donor site that is difficult to camouflage adequately and that it requires two stages.

The versatile deltopectoral flap also can be used to reconstruct a large defect in this area. This flap is tunnelled under the neck flaps and sutured into position with the pedicle inversely tubed; the tubing creates a controlled pharyngostome that is closed as a second stage.

CONTROLLED PHARYNGOSTOME

The use of a controlled pharyngostome should be considered for poor risk patients and for late salvage after irradiation, i.e.,

any situation where danger of fistula formation is great. The creation of a temporary controlled pharyngostome is useful because it decreases the tension in primary closures and acts as a controlled salivary fistula. Construction is easily accomplished by using a modified Frazier or McFee incision and suturing the edges of the skin flaps to the margins of the mucosal defect. As soon as adequate healing has occurred, the pharyngostome can be closed by using regional flaps.

COMPLICATIONS OF SURGERY

The complications encountered in head and neck surgery are considered in more detail in Chapter 28. Wound breakdown and orocutaneous fistula are not uncommon complications in major oropharyngeal surgery

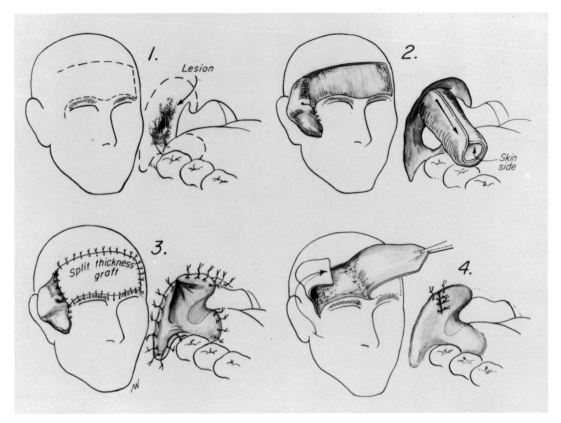

Fig. 15-18. Forehead flap: (1) Flap outlined. (2) Incision made 2 cm below zygoma. Flap delivered into oropharynx. (3) Split-thickness skin graft placed on donor site. Flap sewn into defect. (4) After 2 to 3 weeks unused portion of flap returned to donor site. Incision in buccal mucosa and skin sutured.

because of the extent of the extirpative surgery, poor nutrition, and previous radiation therapy. Carotid rupture can result, although the incidence of this life-threatening situation has in our experience decreased considerably because of the prophylactic use of dermal graft over the carotid system. Facial nerve palsy due to over vigorous retraction of the superior flap has been seen, and osteitis of the end of the mandible occurs rarely. Postsurgical velopharyngeal incompetence and distortion of the mandible can result in deglutition, mastication, and speech difficulties.

Radiation

This subject is dealt with in more detail elsewhere in this book (see Ch. 7); however, a few words are indicated for completeness. As surgical techniques have advanced considerably in the past decade, so too have radiotherapeutic techniques. As in surgery, the results of radiation vary according to the skill and experience of the radiotherapist and to his available facilities. The results of using only radiation in the treatment of stage I and II lesions of the oropharynx are comparable to those obtained from using surgery. Usage entails delivery of a dose of 6,000 to 7,000 rads to the cancer and to both sides of the neck. However, as the staging increases, the efficiency of using only radiotherapy declines and the use of planned combined therapy appears to offer the best chance for cure.[5, 32]

Radiation, therefore, may be used effectively in the following situations: for small limited cancers; where no experienced head and neck surgeons are available; as part of planned combined therapy; if the patient is physically unable to undergo extensive surgery; if the patient refuses surgery; and finally, to offer palliation for extremely advanced tumors. Radiation should not be indiscriminately used with the idea of salvaging the patient later by surgery should the first line of therapy not be successful. The success rate with surgical salvage is extremely poor, and of course, the surgery after irradiation is associated with a high morbidity. Radiation itself may be associated with complications and unpleasant sequelae, such as xerostomia, loss of taste, osteoradionecrosis, mucosal ulceration, pharyngeal necrosis with fistula formation, and hemorrhage.

Combination Surgery and Radiation Therapy

The concept of combined therapy for cancer of the tonsil was first proposed nearly 50 years ago; however, only in the past 15 years has it been carried out in a planned fashion. The rationale for its use is based on the following observations regarding surgery and radiotherapy: The main reason for surgical failure is that following surgery viable tumor cells remain in the patient either as a result of dissemination of tumor cells during the operation, unrecognized peripheral projection of malignant cells, or undetected lymphatic or hematogenous metastases. The reasons for radiation failure are peripheral projection of the tumor outside the treatment field, the presence of anoxic cells in the center of the neoplasm being relatively unaffected, or the presence of undetected distant metastases. Therefore, planned combined radiation and surgery should be able to minimize the source of the failure in each method.

While it is strongly suggestive that combined therapy offers the best prognosis, there remain some unresolved points. There have as yet been no properly controlled trials that support this argument. In addition, the dosage of radiation to be used is unresolved, and while it is believed by some that 1,000 to 2,000 rads is adequate, others prefer a higher dosage. The problem is to choose the dosage of radiation that will increase the cure rate but will not cause a prohibitive increase in the postoperative morbidity. The question of preoperative or postoperative irradiation is still unresolved, with each method having its own advantages and disadvantages.

It is our opinion that a regimen of planned preoperative radiation consisting of 4,500 to 5,000 rads to the tumor and both sides of the neck followed by a 4-week delay before radical surgery is performed is the best method of approach for larger lesions with or without cervical metastases.[16, 23] It is important to emphasize the word planned, as the timing and dosage of the radiation, the rest period, and the timing of surgery are vital to the success of this regimen. During the waiting period, there is an opportunity to consider the various other aspects of the overall management—such as nutritional and medical problems, which can be corrected on an elective basis. Dental care and assessment by the prosthodontist should, of course, be done prior to irradiation.

Chemotherapy

In recent years renewed interest has been shown in the use of chemotherapeutic agents alone or as an adjunct to both surgery and radiation for treatment of head and neck cancer. Reliable data from trials using these drugs have been limited due to the small number of patients in most studies and the multiplicity of prognostic factors involved, e.g., prior therapy and nutritional status.[6] Nevertheless, several studies have reported significant regression of advanced primary tumors with the use of chemotherapy.[4, 11] Whether adjunct chemotherapy will aid in the control of disease when subclinical tumor dissemination is likely to be present is as yet unanswered (see Ch. 29 for more detail).

Palliative Therapy

The management of a patient who is incurable, either because of late presentation or failed therapy, is a tremendous challenge to the physician. Every attempt should be made to alleviate suffering and to allow the patient to spend his last days with some dignity. The use of radiation or chemotherapy to obtain tumor shrinkage or alleviate pain should be considered. Tracheotomy, esophagostomy, or gastrostomy may be indicated. Placement in an institution, even for short periods to relieve the burden on relatives and friends, may be necessary. The patient's medication, e.g., analgesics, must be constantly reevaluated to ensure that pain is controlled.

REHABILITATION

For too long, the act of excising the carcinoma—no matter how extensive the procedure—in order to cure the patient was regarded as the goal for both the surgeon and the patient. In recent years, however, greater emphasis has been placed on the total rehabilitation of the patient, which has been successfully accomplished in many instances. Probably the most important factor for such success is the motivation of the patient. Without the patient wanting to be rehabilitated, the surgeon and the paramedical team are helpless. Total rehabilitation is the function of a team of professionals, with the surgeon playing a lesser role. Speech therapists, physical therapists, social workers, occupational therapists, and prosthodontists together with the patient's immediate family are all vital members of this team. A number of factors have to be considered.

Cosmetic appearance. Although a composite resection is undoubtedly a mutilating procedure, the end result—particularly if only a small portion of the mandible is removed—is usually acceptable, provided a forehead flap has not been used. The scars in the neck can be covered with scarves, and for women the hair may be styled to cover the defect. In males a beard may be grown. A lateral osteotomy with preservation of the mandible is, of course, more acceptable cosmetically.

Speech. There is no doubt that dysarthria results in those patients who have had a large amount of tongue removed. The best treatment is prevention by ensuring that the tongue is not tethered too high or too low during primary closure or by interposing flaps or grafts to provide more mobility when indicated.

Once this situation has occurred, however, the problem can be improved by dividing the scar tissue and placing a generous split-thickness skin graft to release the tongue. This is usually successful. A speech therapist is invaluable in aiding these patients. Another cause of speech problems is a velopharyngeal incompetence because of removal of much of the soft palate. This can be helped or corrected by means of a speech appliance. (See Ch. 9 for more detail.)

Deglutition. When a large portion of the tongue has been removed and the remaining tongue tethered, the posterior propulsion of food into the hypopharynx becomes awkward. The bolus is propelled down the surgical defect on the operated side and from there is funnelled directly into the larynx due to a frequently partially obliterated pyriform sinus. This results in aspiration problems with all its sequelae of repeated lower respiratory tract infections, fear of eating, and debility. Most patients can be trained to correct this problem by avoiding some liquids initially and concentrating on a blenderized diet. A further cause of problems in deglutition is the velopharyngeal incompetence with reflux of food through the nose. This can be helped by use of the speech appliance.

Mastication. Particularly in those patients who have had a partial mandibulectomy performed, the mandible is frequently deviated by scarring, which results in interference with mastication. Two devices employed to correct this are the maxillary guide plane and the mandibular flange prosthesis (see Ch. 9). The maxillary guide plane is a plastic ramp that extends the occlusal surfaces of the posterior teeth on the functional side towards the midline. The teeth of the remaining mandible make contact on the plane and are guided into occlusion by the ramp.

The mandibular flange prosthesis is used in dentulous cases. Metal frameworks are fitted to both maxillary and mandibular arches and the flange built up vertically from the buccal aspect of the lower teeth; the buccal aspect extends into the maxillary buccal sulcus where it rests against the bar extending from the maxillary framework. As the patient opens and closes his mouth, the flange prevents any horizontal deviation of the mandible. These prostheses are removed at a later stage. Exercises to maintain proper occlusion are helpful.

Rehabilitation may be hampered by the xerostomia frequently seen following preoperative irradiation and if the cranial nerves, such as the hypoglossal nerve, are damaged.

Psychosocial functioning. Too often, with the physician's attention zeroing in on the patient's physical adjustments, insufficient attention is devoted to the tremendous psychological adjustments the patient has to make. The emotional status of the patient in the postoperative period is important. He is frequently depressed and this interferes with his motivation for physical rehabilitation. An experienced and understanding nursing and paramedical staff are, therefore, important in aiding the patient to overcome this problem.

There may, in addition, be a change in the patient's relationship with his immediate family because of the fear of being rejected by them. Adequate family counseling is vital. The patient must learn to accept his situation and make the necessary alterations in his lifestyle to compensate for his particular disability.

END RESULTS

Comparisons of survival rates for cancer of the oropharynx are extremely difficult because of the changing methods of classification and the difference in interpretation of the material. For this reason, controversy still exists as to the relative advantages and disadvantages of one form of therapy over another. It is our opinion that a single modality treatment, be it radiation or surgery, may well be adequate for very early lesions and that for these lesions the possible benefits of combined therapy may be negated by increased morbidity and even by mortality. However, the larger lesions and those with cervical lymph node metastases appear to do better with combined therapy, and in our experience a regimen of planned preoperative radiation followed by definitive surgery appears to offer improved results without a significantly increased morbidity.

Base of tongue lesions, unfortunately, are usually diagnosed late and have an overall poor prognosis varying from 10 to 42 percent.[13, 19, 27, 33] If, however, they are seen early and aggressive therapy is instituted, these figures may be improved: a high of 63 percent 5-year survival rate has been reported for stage II lesions[28] (see Table 15-3).

A considerable discrepancy is noted in the reported results for patients with cancer of the tonsil and tonsillar fossa,[14, 16, 21, 26, 31] but with aggressive therapy the prognosis is not as dismal as might be expected. Five-year survival rates can vary from 63 percent

TABLE 15-3. FIVE-YEAR SURVIVAL FOR CANCER OF THE OROPHARYNX[28]

Location	Stage I (percent) ⟶	Stage IV (percent)
Tonsil & tonsillar fossa	63	21
Base of tongue	42 to 63	10 to 21
Palatine arch & pharyngeal wall	77	20

for stage I tumors to 21 percent for stage IV tumors.[14] An overall 2-year survival rate of 59 percent can be expected for patients undergoing planned combined therapy.

In the best hands, cancer of the palatine arch and pharyngeal walls can be expected to yield from a 77 percent 5-year survival rate for stage I lesions to a 20 percent rate for stage IV lesions.[15]

Of interest is an analysis of why therapy fails. Inability to eradicate the cancer at the primary site, with local recurrence, is the most important cause of failure. This invariably occurs within 2 years and is related to the size of the tumor and to tongue involvement. The next most common cause of failure is recurrence occurring in the neck; this is related to the degree of initial nodal disease.

Nine and one-half percent of patients develop distant metastases;[14] these are more likely to occur if there was evidence of cervical metastases at the initial presentation. In addition, a small percentage of patients die because of the treatment itself.

Of those patients who survive, the chances of developing another primary cancer are high (37 percent)[14] and thus, this possibility will also affect the prognosis.

In conclusion, it appears that as more aggressive local and regional treatment becomes successful in controlling the local disease, a greater number of patients will survive only to become victims of distant metastases and second primaries at a later date.

REFERENCES

1. Ballantyne, A. J. 1964. Significance of retropharyngeal nodes in cancer of the head and neck. American Journal of Surgery, 108: 500.

2. Baluyot, S. T., and Shumrick, D. A. 1972. Pre-irradiation tattooing. Archives of Otolaryngology, 96: 151.

3. Batsakis, J. G. 1975. Tumors of the Head and Neck: Clinical and Pathological Considerations. Williams & Wilkins, Baltimore.

4. Blum, R. H., Carter, S. K., and Agre, K. 1973. A clinical review of Bleomycin—A new antineoplastic agent. Cancer, 31: 903.

5. Cardinale, F., and Fischer, J. J. 1977. Radiation therapy of carcinoma of the tonsil. Cancer, 39: 604.

6. Carter, S. K. 1977. The chemotherapy of head and neck cancer. Seminars in Oncology, 4: 413.

7. Conley, J. 1970. Concepts of Head and Neck Surgery. Georg Thieme, Stuttgart.

8. Cunningham, M. P., and Catlin, D. 1967. Cancer of the pharyngeal wall. Cancer, 20: 1859.

8a. Cutler, S. J., and Young, J. L., Eds. 1975. Third National Cancer Survey: Incidence Data (Monograph 41). National Cancer Institute, Bethesda, MD.

9. DeSanto, L. W. 1977. Cancer of the posterior oral cavity. Surgical Clinics of North America, 57: 597.

10. DeSanto, L. W., Whicker, J. H., and Devine, K. D. 1975. Mandibular osteotomy and lingual flaps: Use in patients with cancer of the tonsil area and tongue base. Archives of Otolaryngology, 101: 652.

11. Goldberg, N. S., Chretien, P. B., and Elias, E. G. 1977. Preoperative high dose Methotrexate—A well tolerated regimen in head and neck cancer. Proceedings of the American Association for Cancer Research and American Society of Clinical Oncologists, 18: 292.

12. Hakulinen, T., Lehtimaki, L., Lehtonen, M., and Teppo. L. 1974. Cancer morbidity among two male cohorts with increased alcohol consumption in Finland. Journal of the National Cancer Institute, 52: 1711.

13. Harrold, C. C. 1967. Surgical treatment of cancer of the base of tongue. American Journal of Surgery, 114: 493.

14. Jesse, R. H., and Sugarbaker, E. V. 1976. Squamous cell carcinoma of the oropharynx: Why we fail. American Journal of Surgery, 132: 435.

15. McGregor, I. A., and McGrouther, D. A. 1978. Skin-graft reconstruction in carcinoma of the tongue. Head & Neck Surgery, 1: 47.

16. Maltz, R., Shumrick, D. A., Aron, B. S., and Weichert, K. A., 1974. Carconoma of the tonsil: Results of combined therapy. Laryngoscope, 84: 2172.

17. Marchetta, F. C., Sako, K., and Badillo, J. 1964. Periosteal lymphatics of the mandible and intraoral carcinoma. American Journal of Surgery, 108: 505.

18. Mashberg, A, and Meyers, H. 1976. Anatomical site and size of 222 early asymptomatic oral squamous cell carcinomas: A con-

tinuing prospective study of oral cancer. II Cancer, 37: 2149.

19. Montana, G. S., Hellman, S., Von Essen, C. F., and Kligerman, M. M. 1969. Carcinoma of the tongue and floor of the mouth: Results of radiotherapy. Cancer, 23: 1284.

20. Moore, C. 1971. Cigarette smoking and cancer of the mouth, pharynx and larynx. JAMA, 218: 553.

21. Perez, C. A., Mill, W. B., Ogura, J. H., and Powers W. E., 1970. Carcinoma of the tonsil: Sequential comparision of four treatment modalities. Radiology, 94: 649.

22. Rappaport, I., Shramek, J., and Brummett, S. 1967. Functional aspects of cancer of the base of tongue. American Journal of Surgery 114: 489.

23. Rolander, T. L., Everts, E. C., and Shumrick, D. A. 1971. Carcinoma of the tonsil: A planned combined therapy approach. Laryngoscope, 81: 1199.

24. Rothman, K., and Keller, A. 1972. The effect of joint exposure to alcohol and tobacco on the risk of cancer of the mouth and pharynx. Journal of Chronic Diseases, 25: 711.

25. Scanlon, P. W., Gee, V. R., Erich, B. B., Williams, H. L., and Woolner, L. B. 1958. Carcinoma of the palatine tonsil. American Journal of Roentgenology, Radium Therapy, and Nuclear Medicine, 80: 781.

26. Shumrick, D. A., and Quenelle, D. J. 1979. Malignant disease of the tonsillar region, retromolar trigone and buccal mucosa. Otolaryngologic Clinics of North America, 12: 115.

27. Skolnik, E. M., and Saberman, M. N. 1969. Cancer of the tongue. Otolaryngologic Clinics of North America, 2: 603.

28. Strong, E. W. 1979. Carcinoma of the tongue. Otolaryngologic Clinics of North America, 12: 107.

29. Strong, M. S., Vaughan, C. W., and Incze, J. S. 1968. Toluidine blue in the management of carcinoma of the oral cavity. Archives of Otolaryngology, 87: 527.

30. Vaughan, C. W. 1972. Carcinogenesis in the oral cavity. Otolaryngologic Clinics of North America, 5: 291.

31. Wang, C. C. 1972. Mangement and prognosis of squamous-cell carcinoma of the tonsillar region. Radiology, 104: 667.

32. Weller, S. A., Goffinet, D. R., Goode, R. L., and Bagshaw, M. A., 1976. Carcinoma of the oropharynx; results of megavoltage radiation therapy in 305 patients. American Journal of Roentgenology, Radium Therapy, and Nuclear Medicine, 126: 236.

33. Whicker, J. H., DeSanto, L. W., and Devine, K. D. 1972. Surgical treatment of squamous cell carcinoma of the base of the tongue. Laryngoscope, 82: 1853.

34. Willis, R. A. 1944. The modes of origin of tumors: Solitary localized squamous cell growths of skin. Cancer Research, 4: 630.

16 | Cancer of the Nasopharynx

George Choa, M.D.

INTRODUCTION

Cancer of the nasopharynx is synonymous with squamous cell carcinoma affecting the nasopharynx. There are at least three unusual features of this disease, one of which is the uneven distribution among ethnic groups. While uncommon among most white and black groups, it is among the most common malignant diseases affecting the Cantonese people (people from Kwangtung province in China) (Fig. 16-1). As a result of population movements in the last century, pockets of Cantonese people may be found in most parts of the world. Clinicians should have a working knowledge of the management of nasopharyngeal cancer (NPC), since the disease also affects these immigrant Cantonese.

Secondly, the management of this disease is also somewhat unusual when contrasted with that of other cancers in the head and neck area, in that radiation plays a dominant role in the treatment program and surgery plays a relatively minor role. Marked improvement in techniques of radiation therapy has increased the survival rate of this once invariably fatal cancer.

The third unusual feature of this disease is that the many and variously presenting symptoms of NPC are not directly referrable to the nasopharynx itself, but to its anatomic relationships. Awareness of the importance of the symptoms of epistaxis, middle ear effusion, masses of the neck, and various neurologic signs with no apparent primary source should direct the physician's attention to the nasopharynx. Earlier diagnosis, thus stimulated, may further improve the cure rate.

ANATOMY

Boundaries

The nasopharynx lies behind the nasal cavities and above the soft palate and is roughly cuboidal in shape (Fig. 16-2).

Anteriorly, it communicates freely with the nasal cavities on each side of the free edge of the nasal septum.

Roof. The sphenoid bone and the basiocciput make up the roof of the nasopharynx as far posteriorly as the pharyngeal tubercle. The upper portion of the posterior wall lies in front of the anterior arch of the atlas. A collection of lymphoid tissue, the nasopharyngeal tonsil (adenoids), is found embedded in the mucous membrane.

Posterior Wall. The roof curves gently into the posterior wall, which extends from the pharyngeal tubercle to the level of the soft palate. It is formed mainly by the atlas and its related ligaments and muscles.

Lateral Wall. The lateral wall is clinically the most important in the study of NPC. The eustachian tube opening into the lateral wall forms a prominent and important landmark. Between the cartilaginous, mobile medial end of the eustachian tube (torus) and the posterior wall is the lateral pharyngeal recess (fossa of Rosenmüller) (Fig. 16-3).

The Fossa of Rosenmüller

The fossa of Rosenmüller or lateral pharyngeal recess is a lateral extension of the nasopharynx lying above and behind the medial end of the eustachian tube (torus) (Fig. 16-3). It is variable in size and is

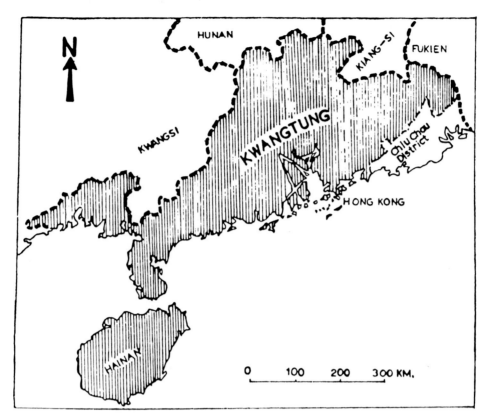

Fig. 16-1. Map of Kwangtung, China. (Ho, H. C. 1967. Nasopharyngeal carcinoma in Hong Kong. In Muir, C. S., and Shanmugaratan, K., Eds.: Cancer of the Nasopharynx. Munksgaard, Copenhagen, 58.)

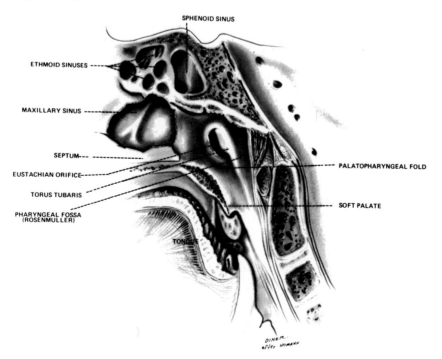

Fig. 16-2. Midsagittal section of the nasopharynx, showing the related structures. (Modified from Fletcher, G. H., Healey, J. E., Jr., McGraw J. P., and Million, R. R. 1967. Nasopharynx. In MacComb, W. S., and Fletcher, G. H., Eds.: Cancer of the Head and Neck. © (1967) The Williams and Wilkins Co., Baltimore, 152.)

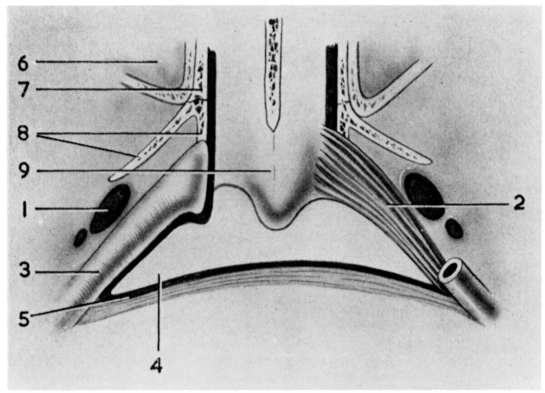

Fig. 16-3. The fossa of Rosenmüller seen from above (after Prentiss) 1, foramen ovale; 2, levator palatini muscle; 3, eustachian tube; 4, fossa of Rosenmüller; 5, internal lamina of the pharyngeal fascia; 6, antrum; 7, palatine bone; 8, internal and external pterygoid; 9, soft palate. (From Lederman, M. 1961. Cancer of the Nasopharynx: Its Natural History and Treatment. Courtesy of Charles C Thomas, Publisher, Springfield, Il.)

scarcely visible in an infant. By adult life, especially among the Southern Chinese, it is cleft-like and may be as deep as 1.5 cm. Fibrous trabeculae are often seen to traverse the entrance to the recess, making visualization difficult. Its apex reaches the anterior margin of the carotid canal and its base opens into the nasopharynx at a point below the foramen lacerum medially. The fossa is related to the internal carotid artery both at the apex and at the base, the former where the artery enters the petrous portion of the temporal bone and the latter where the artery passes from the petrous portion of the temporal bone to the interior of the skull. The interior wall of the fossa is formed by a delicate mucosa covering the eustachian tube and levator palatini muscle, and the posterior wall is formed by the mucosa covering the dense pharyngobasilar fascia from the upper border of the superior constrictor

to the base of the skull in the region of the sinus of Morgagni. The mandibular division of the 5th nerve lying in the parapharyngeal space is anterolateral to the apex of the fossa and is separated from it by fascia, the eustachian tube, and the tensor palatini muscle.

Histology

The histology of the nasopharynx epithelium in adults is significant in the study of the pathology of NPC. In infancy, the nature of the epithelium is respiratory (columnar ciliated). From 12 years of age, metaplasia can be observed to occur with a change to squamous epithelium. In adults, most of the epithelium has undergone squamous metaplasia, with only islands of respiratory epithelium remaining[1, 2] (Fig. 16-4). Some transitional epithelium may also be present.

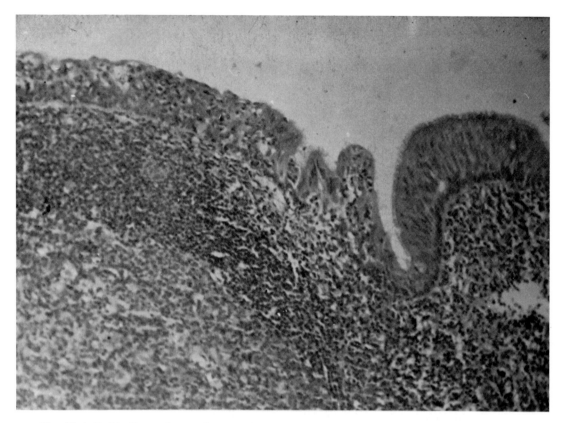

Fig. 16-4. Epithelium of nasopharynx showing ciliated epithelium (on right) and squamous epithelium (on left). The picture also shows marked inflammatory change and cellular infiltration.

Teoh[51] has shown that carcinoma in situ develops in this metaplastic epithelium.

Nerve Supply

All muscles of the soft palate except the tensor veli palatini are supplied by the pharyngeal plexus. The motor fibers are mainly derived from the 11th cranial nerve motor root. They are carried by the vagus and distributed by the pharyngeal branch of the vagus. The tensor veli palatini muscle is innervated by the mandibular division of the 5th cranial nerve through the otic ganglion (phylogenetically a muscle of mastication).

Blood Supply

The blood supply of the pharynx is derived from the ascending pharyngeal artery, the ascending palatine branches of the facial artery, and the greater palatine branch of the maxillary artery. In addition, small twigs are derived from the dorsalis lingual artery, the tonsillar artery, and the artery of the pterygoid canal.

Venous Drainage

According to Batson[4] the veins are arranged in two well-defined plexuses—an internal submucous and an external pharyngeal—with numerous communicating branches. The submucous plexus drains definite areas of the mucous membrane. In addition this plexus forms, in several places, an extensive network found on the posterior wall of the pharynx and around the entrance to the larynx. These networks communicate with the veins of the dorsum of the tongue, the superior laryngeal veins, the esophageal veins, and with the external pharyngeal plexus. The latter drains to the internal jugular and the anterior facial veins. The pharyngeal plexus is also closely connected to the cavernous sinus through emissary veins.

Lymphatic Drainage

There is a rich lymphatic capillary plexus throughout the nasopharynx. The efferent vessels usually drain into ipsilateral nodes but frequently cross the midline and drain to the contralateral side. The first echelon of nodes to be involved in NPC is the lateral retropharyngeal nodes; the uppermost one is known as the node of Rouviere.[45] These nodes lie deep in the upper neck and cannot be palpated (Fig. 16-5).

The jugulodigastric nodes and the deep nodes of the posterior triangle (spinal accessory nodes) are the other primary nodes (Fig. 16-5) that become involved in NPC. The cancer may spread to these nodes through efferent vessels from the retropharyngeal nodes or directly from the nasopharynx. Further extension may involve the nodes of the posterior triangle and the jugular nodes.

ETIOLOGY AND EPIDEMIOLOGY

The following factors may be related to the etiology of cancer of the nasopharynx and will herein be discussed: (1) race; (2) household carcinogens; (3) heredity; (4) environment; (5) chronic sepsis; (6) anthropology; (7) virus; (8) genetics; (9) occupation and socioeconomic level; and (10) other medical factors.

One or more factors are frequently found in patients with NPC. How much, however, they are actually responsible for in the development of the disease remains uncertain. From present knowledge, there is more than one factor involved in each case.

Race

In Hong Kong the racial factor stands out prominently, because natives of the Kwangtung province are affected almost exclusively (Fig. 16-1). In 30 years, I have seen only one white patient with the disease even though Hong Kong has a white population of over 100,000. It has been shown by various researchers[39] that in Southeast Asian

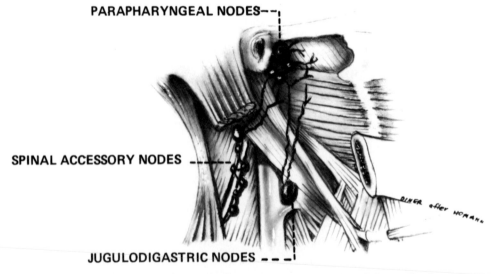

Fig. 16-5. Major lymphatic drainage of the nasopharynx. (Modified from Fletcher, G. H., Healey, J. E., Jr., McGraw, J. P., and Million, R. R. 1967. Nasopharynx. In MacComb, W. S., and Fletcher, G. H., Eds.: Cancer of the Head and Neck. © (1967) The Williams and Wilkins Co., Baltimore, 152.)

countries, with very few exceptions, it is still the Chinese and the mixed races with Chinese parentage who are affected with NPC.[3, 9, 21, 27, 37] The crude annual morbidity in Hong Kong is 124 per million, nearly 25 times that estimated by Godfredsen[15] for Denmark and Sweden.

Household Carcinogens

It has been suggested that deposits from cooking fumes and smoke carry carcinogens and that these deposits could be a factor in the etiology of NPC.[49] The studies of Ho[21, 27] do not support this theory. He has shown that boat dwellers in Hong Kong, who living on their fishing boats can easily avoid the smoke from cooking and incense used in worship, have a higher incidence of NPC than does the land population of Hong Kong. Furthermore, Buddhist monks, exposed to incense all day and every day, are very rarely seen with the disease. This observation is supported by my own experience.

Clifford,[7] working in Kenya, has contrary views. He believes that smoke from burning exotic wood (for example, eucalyptus and wattle) as fuel in poorly ventilated huts may play a part in causing the disease. Specimens of soot from the roof of these huts have been examined at the Memorial Sloan-Kettering Institute in New York and were, on analysis, found to contain significant quantities of benzopyrene, benzanthracene, benzofluoranthesen, and other polynuclear aromatic hydrocarbons. The Bantu and the Nilo-Hamitic tribes living in high altitudes often suffer from vasomotor rhinitis with a thick mucoid discharge. Clifford believes that this discharge could be the vehicle of inhaled carcinogens but somehow only the nasopharynx is susceptible. These tribesmen live in small, poorly-ventilated huts that have an open fire burning inside all day, for both cooking purposes and warmth. The incidence of the disease among these people is higher than among those living in low lands, where there are well-ventilated homes and cooking is done

outdoors. Another form of vasomotor rhinitis—one characterized by sneezing bouts and a clear, watery discharge—seems to "protect" a person from NPC.

Heredity

There have been only a few families on record in which more than one sibling has suffered from the disease. Ho[22] found a significantly higher frequency of NPC in close blood relatives of NPC patients.

Environment

This is probably an important factor. Zippin et al.[57] investigated the place of birth of 31 Chinese males in the University of California, the majority of whom were natives of the southern Kwangtung province of China. He found that the observed to expected ratio (OE) by age group was eight times higher for Chinese in the 55 years and under age group who were born outside the United States than for those of the same age group who were born in the United States. Ho[27] is of the opinion that diet is an important factor in the development of NPC in the Chinese and especially can have an effect on Chinese babies who live on boats. These babies and young children have in their diet salted fish (which contain nitrosamine—a potent carcinogen) and a low vitamin C intake, both of which may well be factors in the causation of NPC. Vitamin C is able to block the nitrosification of amines, which are derived from the digestion of proteins in the stomach and upper intestines.

Chronic Infection

Chronic nasal catarrh and maxillary sinusitis are extremely common in Hong Kong. Such irritations could cause metaplasia and may eventually cause carcinoma in situ. Some investigators, however, are of the opinion that metaplasia is not essential for the development of a squamous carcinoma in the nasopharynx because there are areas in the nasopharynx where the epithelium is transitional. Furthermore, squamous carcinoma can develop from the basement layer of the ciliated columnar epithelium normally present in the nasopharynx.[23]

Anthropology

Because of a possible difference in the configuration of the Southern Chinese skull compared with that of Northern Chinese, it is postulated that this difference facilitates the deposit of nasal discharge in the nasopharynx. Proetz,[41, 42] in his studies on air currents through the nose, showed that soot tends to deposit beyond the bend of a glass tube and that if an air current is forced through a constricted portion, the soot deposits beyond the constriction. Following this principle, one may conjecture that inhaled carcinogens tend to be deposited on the posterior pharyngeal wall or to find their way into the pharyngeal recess by forcible sniffing (a common Chinese habit).

Virus

Ho and his associates[26] have made an in-depth study into the relationship between the Epstein-Barr virus (EBV) and NPC. They are of the opinion that the association of the virus with NPC is now firmly established. Old et al.[40] had demonstrated the presence of precipitating antibodies to EBV-related antigens in sera from patients with the cancer. This discovery was followed by the demonstration that NPC patients in widely separated parts of the world had higher geometric mean titers (GMT) of antibodies to EB viral capsid antigen (VCA) than members of control groups made up of patients with other head and neck cancers and normal subjects had.[11–13, 17, 19, 34] The GMT of antibodies to VCA increases with advancing clinical stage of the disease.[14, 18, 19, 22] De-Thé et al.[14] demonstrated that VCA titers for NPC correlated with titers of antibodies to three other EBV-specific antigens: early antigen (EA), nuclear antigen (EMNA), and soluble antigen (CF/S). Henle et al.[18] showed that in NPC

antibodies to the diffuse component of the EBV-induced EA were not usually demonstrable in stage I of the disease, but from stage II onwards there was an increasingly higher titer. Thus, it would seem that the various EBV antibodies are related to the total tumor burden.

It is particularly interesting that VCA-specific IgA antibodies were rarely present in normal individuals but were almost invariably present in high titer patients with NPC. Therefore, it has been suggested that the absence of these antibodies in a patient with clinical features suggestive of NPC may be used to exclude the diagnosis of NPC.

Genetics

Clifford[8] believes that in Kenya, persons with blood Group A are "protected" or at less risk of NPC than are persons of other blood groups. In contrast, Ho[22] failed to find any significant difference between the blood group distribution (A/O and B/O) in 1,000 consecutive Chinese NPC patients and in controls.

Occupation and Socioeconomic Level

Neither in Singapore[47] nor in Hong Kong[22] has the risk of the disease been found to be related to occupation or social status.

Other Medical Factors

No convincing evidence has been reported to associate the risk of NPC with malnutrition, avitaminosis, hormonal imbalance, chronic upper respiratory infection, or vasomotor rhinitis.[22] However, I believe that chronic upper respiratory infection may predispose to NPC by causing squamous metaplasia. Vasomotor rhinitis may present in two forms. In one form, the main symptom is nasal obstruction associated with a postnasal drip, which is generally mucoid in nature. The second form is characterized by sneezing bouts especially in the mornings and is associated with a profuse watery discharge with or without obstruction (a form of physical allergy). In the course of many years, I have noted that patients suffering from the latter—the "wet" form of vasomotor rhinitis—seldom develop NPC. No exact explanation can be given, but it is possible that the excessive watery nasal discharge may be responsible for cleansing the nasopharynx of any carcinogen that may be lodged there by inhalation.

CLASSIFICATION

Rare benign conditions encountered in the nasopharynx are tuberculosis, angiofibroma, and benign cysts. An extensive carotid body tumor may present with a bulging into the oropharynx by displacing the tonsil medially and be confused with an infiltrating NPC.

The differential diagnosis of angiofibroma and cysts presents no difficulty. Patients with tuberculosis complain of blood-stained sputum, and on examination, features not unlike an ulcerated carcinoma are seen. Other features noted in tuberculosis are a generalized epipharyngitis, a nodular appearance, or a lesion that is almost indistinguishable from infected and ulcerated adenoids. Biopsy is necessary to confirm the diagnosis. Tuberculous epipharyngitis as an isolated lesion is rare, and adequate chemotherapy should serve to cure this disease. Cervical lymphadenopathy is not necessarily a feature of tuberculous epipharyngitis. Tuberculous cervical lymphadenopathy without epipharyngeal ulceration is much more common. Here again, a diagnosis can only be made by a lymph node biopsy after malignancy of the head and neck areas is excluded. Tuberculous nodes are frequently diffuse, discrete, and bilateral, involving mainly the posterior triangle. A node with metastatic carcinoma from the nasopharynx is painless as a rule and appears first with the enlargement of the upper posterior cervical triangle group of lymph nodes, rarely, if ever, below the level of the sixth cervical vertebra.

According to the "Histological Typing of Upper Respiratory Tract Tumours" published by the World Health Organization, Geneva in 1978,[48] the following classifications for malignant tumors of the nasopharynx have been adopted:

1. Nasopharyngeal carcinoma—(a.) squamous cell carcinoma (keratinizing squamous cell carcinoma); (b.) nonkeratinizing carcinoma; and (c.) undifferentiated carcinoma (undifferentiated carcinoma of nasopharyngeal type)
2. Adenocarcinoma
3. Adenoid cystic carcinoma
4. Others

Teoh[51] studied necropsy material of nasopharyngeal carcinomas from 31 Chinese patients from the standpoint of structure, histogenesis, and behavior. He found that the histologic features of nasopharyngeal carcinomas (and their metastases) may show marked structural variations, even in the same tumor, or particular features may pre-

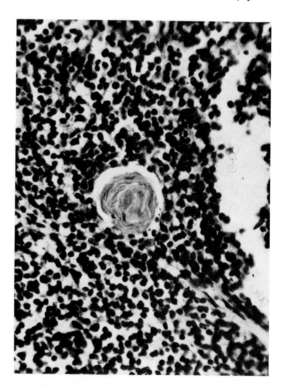

Fig. 16-6. Small, rounded tumor cells with a keratinized focus in the primary growth.

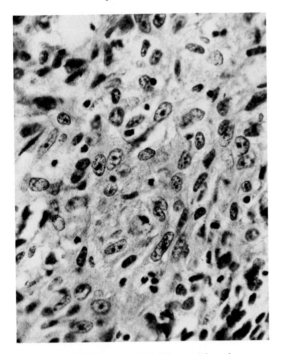

Fig. 16-7. Large cells with ovoid vesicular nuclei and prominent nucleoli in primary growth.

dominate. Frank epidermoid features, such as prickle cells and keratin, may be present (Fig. 16-6) or glycogen-containing clear cells (Fig. 16-7) and even transitional cell patterns may be noted. The term *lymphoepithelial carcinoma* is used to describe nonkeratinizing and undifferentiated nasopharyngeal carcinomas that have numerous lymphocytes found among the tumor cells[43, 46] (Figs. 16-8 and 16-9). The close admixture of lymphocytes and tumor cells is the main reason for the name lymphoepithelioma. Lymphocytes are only incidental components of these cancers. Electron microscopic study of these cancers reveals the presence of keratin fibrils.[50]

It has been established[51] that nasopharyngeal carcinoma arises from the stratified squamous epithelium of the nasopharynx. From a personal series of over 500 cases studied, as well as from reviewing other studies published from Hong Kong, I have found that the vast majority of cases are

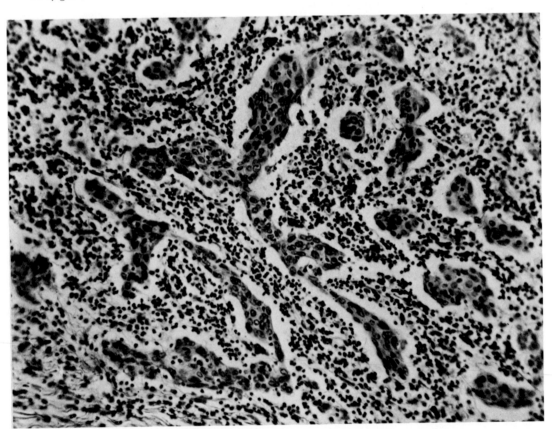

Fig. 16-8. Previously irradiated primary growth with heavy stromal infiltration of lymphocytes and plasma cells.

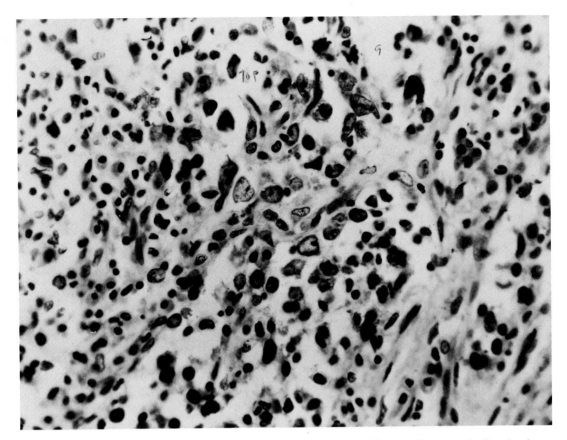

Fig. 16-9. Large irregular cells with vesicular nuclei, some with prominent nucleoli, mixed with lymphocytes and plasma cells in the primary growth.

poorly differentiated (anaplastic) epidermoid carcinomas.

Other types of malignant tumors are rarely encountered. These include adenocarcinoma, adenoid cystic carcinoma, melanoma, lymphomas, chordoma, and plasmacytoma,[24] and in children, embryonal rhabdomyosarcoma.

ROUTES OF SPREAD

Nasopharyngeal carcinoma can spread by direct infiltration or by metastasis (the latter in two-thirds of cases), or by both routes. Direct infiltration may or may not involve the cranial nerves. If these nerves are not involved, spread by direct infiltration may be within the nasopharynx (early) or beyond the nasopharynx.

Direct Infiltration

Direct infiltration to the basiocciput and middle cranial fossa is common[52] (Figs. 16-10 and 16-11 and Table 16-1).

In general, the infiltrative type of lesion eventually results in cranial nerve palsies. The most common nerves involved are the 5th, 6th, 9th, 10th, 11th, and 12th. The 3rd and 4th nerves can only be involved by direct invasion of the orbit or by involvement of the cavernous sinus. The sympathetic chain may also be involved.

In late cases, tumor tissue can extend beyond the confines of the nasopharynx and in the presence of sepsis, the internal carotid artery can rupture, giving rise to fatal hemorrhage. The carotid artery can also be damaged by radiotherapy, resulting in the thinning of its wall and subsequent rup-

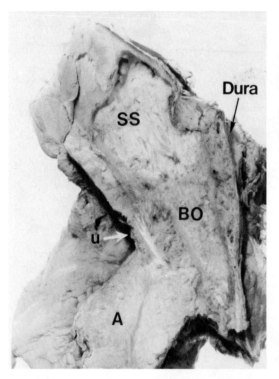

Fig. 16-10. Direct tumor infiltration. SS, sphenoid sinus; BO, basiocciput; U, ulcerated area in nasopharynx; A, atlas.

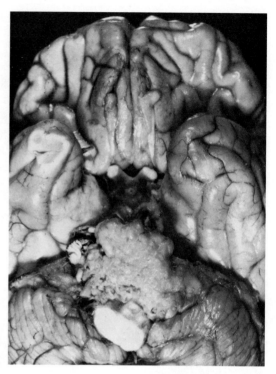

Fig. 16-11. Infiltration to the base of the brain.

TABLE 16-1. EPIDERMOID CARCINOMA OF NASOPHARYNX: FREQUENCY OF DIRECT INVASION (183 POSTMORTEMS)

	Number of cases	%
Basi-occiput bone	85	46
Cranial fossae	70	38

(Teoh, T. B. 1971. The pathologist and the surgical pathology of head and neck tumours. Journal of the Royal College of Surgeons of Edinburgh, 16:117.)

ture[52] (Fig. 16-12). Cancer cells can also penetrate the wall of the large veins, and thus result in generalized dissemination[52] (Fig. 16-13).

Metastasis

Early in the disease, the retropharyngeal nodes are probably the first to be involved, followed by the upper posterior triangle nodes. It is often the enlargement of the cervical lymph nodes that brings a patient to see a doctor. The nodes initially noted to be involved are the upper posterior cervical group located at the apex of the posterior triangle or just below the angle of the jaw (Fig. 16-14). Bilateral cervical node involvement is common. Late in the disease, lymph nodes as far as the inguinal group may be involved. Generalized lymphadenopathy has been seen and mistaken for a lymphoma. No metastasis to the brain has ever been recorded although infiltration into the cranium through the foramina at the base of the skull is well known (Fig. 16-11).

Teoh[51] studied the sex, age, and metastatic patterns in 31 cases of epidermoid carcinoma of the nasopharynx (necropsy findings) (Table 16-2). Metastases were present in cervical lymph nodes in 27 cases, other lymph nodes in 4, lungs in 6, liver in 12, bones in 4, and other sites in 4 cases. In five of the cases with lung metastases, these appeared only as small subpleural plaques; in

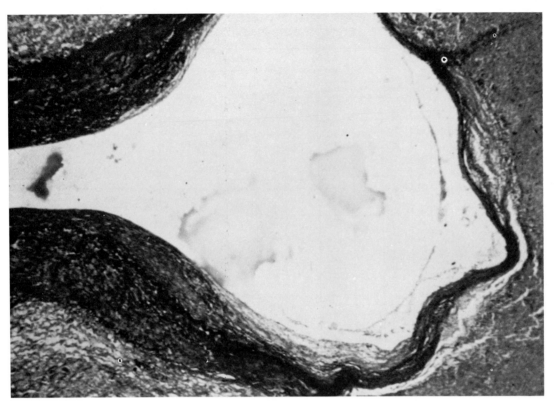

Fig. 16-12. Thinning of the arterial wall (on right) after radiotherapy.

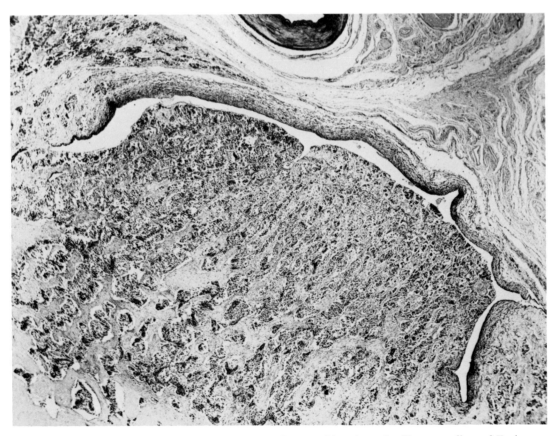

Fig. 16-13. Invasion of lumen from one side of internal jugular vein. Hematoxylin and Eosin and Weigert's elastic tissue stain. (Magnification × 15.)

TABLE 16-2. SEX, AGE AND METASTASES IN 31 CASES OF EPIDERMOID CARCINOMA OF NASOPHARYNX

Case	Sex	Age	Cervical lymph-glands		Cervical veins invaded	Other lymph-glands	Lung	Liver	Bone	Other sites
			L.	R.						
1	M	49	++	++	+	—	—	+++	—	—
2	M	37	+++	++	+	—	—	+	Skull (+) Ribs (+++)	—
3	F	32	—	—	—	—	—	—	—	—
4	F	54	—	+	—	—	—	—	—	—
5	M	55	++	++	—	—	—	—	—	—
6	M	54	+++	—	+	—	—	+	—	Extrapleural L. costovertebral angle (+)
7	M	28	+++	+++	—	—	++	++	Skull (+)	—
8	F	34	++	+	+	+	—	+++	—	Dura mater (+) Larynx (+)
9	F	46	—	+++	—	—	—	—	—	—
10	M	38	++	++	+	+	++	+++	—	—
11	F	51	++	+	—	—	—	—	—	—
12	F	30	—	+	—	—	—	—	—	—
13	M	28	++	++	—	+	++	—	—	Kidneys (+++) Dura mater (+++)
14	F	46	+	++	—	—	—	—	—	—
15	M	53	—	—	—	—	—	—	—	—
16	M	36	++	+	—	—	—	—	—	—
17	M	50	—	—	—	—	—	—	—	—
18	M	20	—	+	—	—	—	—	—	—
19	F	26	+	+++	+	—	—	+	—	—
20	M	53	—	—	—	—	—	—	—	—
21	M	50	+	—	+	—	—	+++	Ribs (++) Vertebræ (++) Skull (+)	—
22	F	48	+	—	—	—	—	+	—	—
23	M	40	+++	+++	+	—	—	+++	—	—
24	M	37	+	+++	+	—	—	+	—	R. adrenal (+)
25	M	40	++	+++	+	+	+	++	—	—
26	M	47	++	+	—	—	—	—	—	—
27	M	35	—	++	—	—	—	—	—	—
28	M	46	++	+	—	—	+	—	Ribs (++) Vertebrae (+) Skull (+)	—
29	F	18	++	+++	+	—	+	—	—	—
30	F	59	++	++	—	—	—	—	—	—
31	M	35	+++	+++	—	—	—	—	—	—

+, ++ or +++ indicates number or size of metastases.

(Teoh, T. B. 1957. Epidermoid carcinoma of the nasopharynx among Chinese: A study of 31 necropsies. Journal of Pathology and Bacteriology, 73: 451.)

TABLE 16-3. EPIDERMOID CARCINOMA OF NASOPHARYNX FREQUENCY AND SITE OF METASTASES (183 POSTMORTEMS)

	Number of Cases	%
Cervical lymph nodes	128	70
Liver	90	49
Bones	89	49
Lung	70	38
Spleen	18	10

(Teoh, T. B. 1971. The pathologist and the surgical pathology of head and neck tumours. Journal of the Royal College of Surgeons of Edinburgh, 16:117.)

the sixth case, tumor nodules were present in the parenchyma of the lung. All four cases with bone metastases showed bone destruction. In addition, Teoh[52] reviewed the frequency and site of metastases of nasopharyngeal carcinoma in postmortem examinations of 183 patients with NPC (Table 16-3).

PATIENT EVALUATION

Clinical Features

History. In order of frequency, the most common presenting symptoms in my experience[6] are bleeding, enlarged cervical

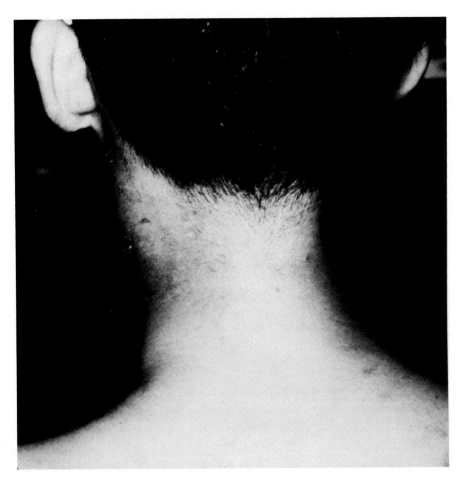

Fig. 16-14. Enlarged upper posterior cervical node. Classical position as seen from behind.

nodes, ear symptoms, and nasal obstruction. Less frequent presenting complaints are headache, diplopia, facial numbness and hypesthesia, trismus, ptosis, and hoarseness. The average time elapsed between the appearance of the first symptom and the first consultation is about 6 months, but this varies from weeks to years.

Age. NPC occurs at a younger age than do most solid cancers. In a personal series of over 500 cases, I found that the peak incidence was 44 years of age in both sexes, with the youngest patient being 18 and the oldest 76. The age specific incidence rates in a series published by Ho[21] revealed that the peak rate was in the 40 to 44-year-old age group in males and the 60 to 64-year group in females. The youngest patients recorded

have been 4[33] and 4.5 years[10] of age. In Hong Kong, the youngest patient seen has been 13 years of age.[21] In whites, the peak age is higher; for example, the peak incidence rate in Godfredsen's Scandinavian series of 454 patients was found to be in the 55 to 59-year-old age group for all cases.[15]

Sex. The male to female ratio is two or three to one in Hong Kong and this ratio is universally true, except in a Scandinavian series, in which there was a female preponderance in the 65 to 69-year-old age group.

Symptoms and Signs

Bleeding. Profuse epistaxis is an infrequent presenting symptom of NPC; however, blood in the postnasal drip is a very significant finding for the early diagnosis of the disease. Though bleeding is synonymous with ulceration, ulcers may be so small as to be easily missed by clinical examinations. Swabbing with cotton wool often reveals blood when ulceration is present in suspicious areas.

Cervical adenopathy. The nodes first involved are probably the retropharyngeal nodes. As they are not palpable, a clinical diagnosis of stage I (disease confined to the nasopharynx) is often not a diagnosis of pathologic stage I. The most common palpable node is deep to the upper fourth of the sternomastoid muscle, at the apex of the posterior triangle, and is pathognomonic of NPC (Fig. 16-15). Any affected nodes below the level of the cricoid cartilage (C6), if the first to be affected, are not likely to be caused by NPC. The involved nodes are, as a rule, painless.

The metastatic nodes are usually solitary at first but with the passage of time may enlarge and become multiple. They are at first firm and mobile but later become hard and matted together and later still, without treatment, malignant cells may erupt through the capsule of a node and spread directly into surrounding tissues with fixation to skin or underlying structures (Fig. 16-16). At this stage, the skin may become ulcerated (Fig. 16-17). In Hong Kong, because many patients still consult herbalists, this ulcerative process is enhanced by the application of herbs.

Metastases to lymph nodes outside of the neck are occasionally seen and may be mistaken for a lymphoma. Involvement of preauricular nodes is rare and may be mistaken for a parotid tumor (Fig. 16-18). However, in order for cancer cells from the nasopharynx to reach these nodes, the prestyloid space must be traversed and thus, additional complications such as facial paralysis would be evident. Nodes can appear initially on the side of the neck contralateral

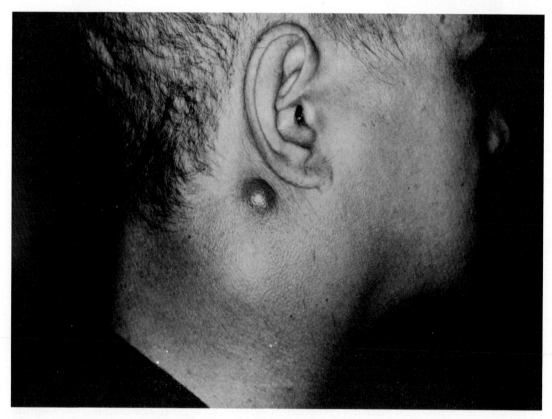

Fig. 16-15. Classical position of upper posterior cervical node involvement.

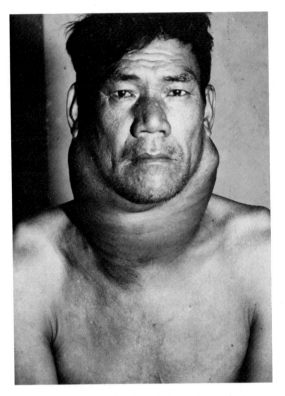

Fig. 16-16. Massive bilateral cervical node involvement.

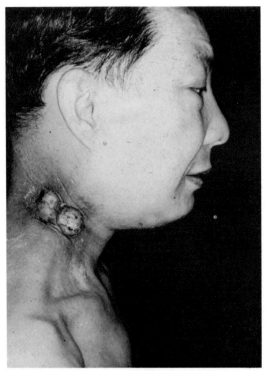

Fig. 16-17. Nodal involvement with fixation and ulceration of the skin.

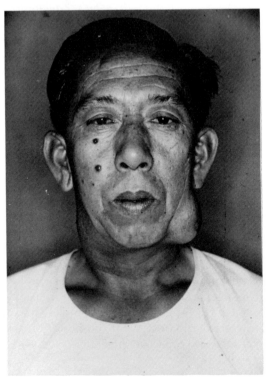

Fig. 16-18. Atypical site of metastasis.

to the side of the primary lesion, an important point to remember when doing a biopsy.

Hearing loss. Conductive deafness due to middle ear effusion is often the first symptom of NPC. The blockage may be due to infection in the nasopharynx, paralysis of the tensor veli palatini muscles, obstruction of the torus by the tumor, or actual invasion of the tubal orifice. Adults with recent onset of unilateral or bilateral conductive hearing loss due to middle ear effusion should be suspected of having NPC. This is especially true in patients without history of prior ear problems, antecedent upper respiratory infections, or barotrauma.

Invasion of the middle ear is extremely rare (one case in my series). Chronic otitis media is a common complication of long-standing disease and sometimes needs operative treatment. If surgery follows radiotherapy, healing is poor (Fig. 16-19).

Nasal obstruction. Nasal obstruction is not present unless the tumor is large, thus

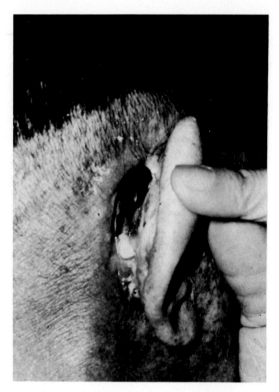

Fig. 16-19. Breakdown of postauricular incision in a previously irradiated patient.

blocking the choana, or has actually infiltrated the nasal cavity.

Headache and facial pain. The trigeminal nerve (especially the second division) is the nerve most commonly involved, and involvement gives rise to temporal headache, facial pains, and hypesthesia of the face. The loss of the corneal reflex may be the first sign of the trigeminal, or indeed any, cranial nerve involvement. The headache of NPC may further be due to involvement of the meninges. At this late stage, the pain is boring, severe, and indistinguishable from that of meningitis.

The 6th nerve paralysis has not been a prominent finding in my own series, but other authorities agree that it is the second most frequency involved cranial nerve[24, 33] (Fig. 16-20).

Diminished lacrimation, which is sometimes obvious, is due to the involvement of the nerve to the pterygoid canal (7th nerve).

Headache, diplopia, facial numbness,

trismus, ptosis, and hoarseness are all indicative of tumor spread outside the confines of the nasopharynx.

Other disease entities may be associated with NPC and include the following:

Endocrine changes. Cushing syndrome[5] has been observed in advanced disease. This is, of course, not a feature peculiar to NPC but can occur with other carcinoma.

Dermatomyositis. In Hong Kong, the most common cause of symptomatic dermatomyositis is NPC.

Pseudomyasthenia gravis. Also known as Eaton-Lambert syndrome, pseudomyasthenia gravis has also been reported.

Physical Examination

NASOPHARYNGEAL INSTRUMENTS

Instruments used in the physical examination are as follows (Fig. 16-21):

Postnasal mirror. This instrument is ideal because one can scan the whole of the postnasal space with it, including the superior surface of the soft palate. Ideally, the face of the mirror should be slightly rotated to the left as one holds the mirror and the angle between the mirror surface and the handle should be slightly reduced. The handle of the mirror should be touching the left angle of the patient's mouth (for a right-handed examiner) so that the hand is completely out of the way, allowing maximum illumination (Fig. 16-22).

Lack's angled tongue depressor. This is most helpful. A straight blade depressor is difficult to handle, particularly when the patient is nervous and cannot relax the tongue (Fig. 16-22).

The Yankauer speculum only allows the lateral wall of the nasopharynx and part of the roof and posterior wall to be seen. The choanae, especially the superior margins, cannot be visualized. It is, however, useful for taking a biopsy from the posterior and lateral walls, especially the latter (Figs. 16-23 and 16-24).

Swab test. Cotton on a carrier is used to swab the nasopharynx and the choanal

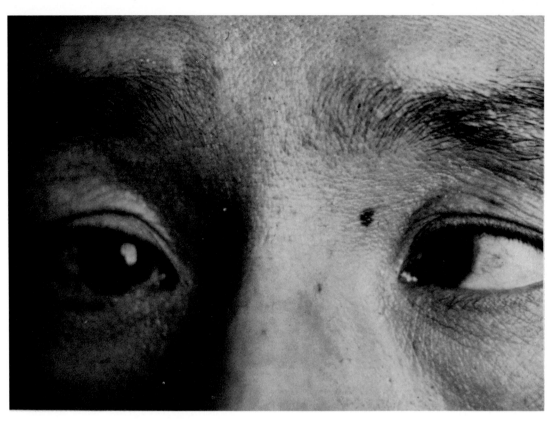

Fig. 16-20. Sixth nerve palsy of left eye.

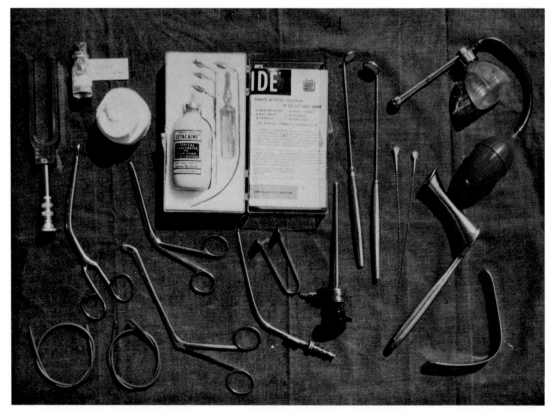

Fig. 16-21. Instruments used to examine the nasopharynx.

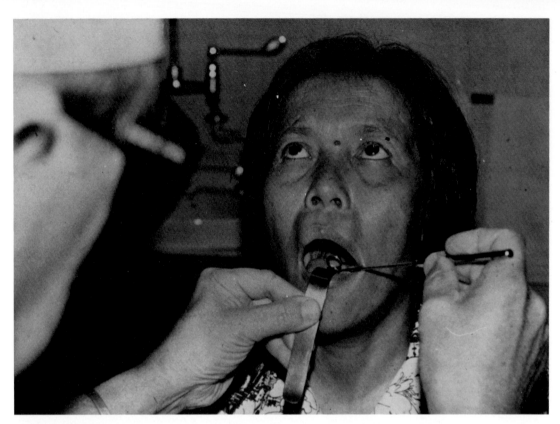

Fig. 16-22. Indirect nasopharyngeal examination using a Lack's tongue depressor and post-nasal mirror.

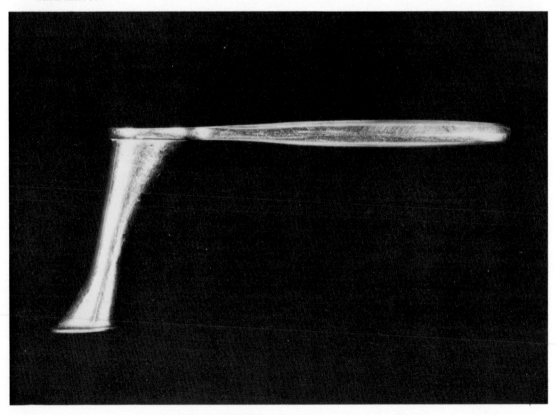

Fig. 16-23. The Yankauer speculum.

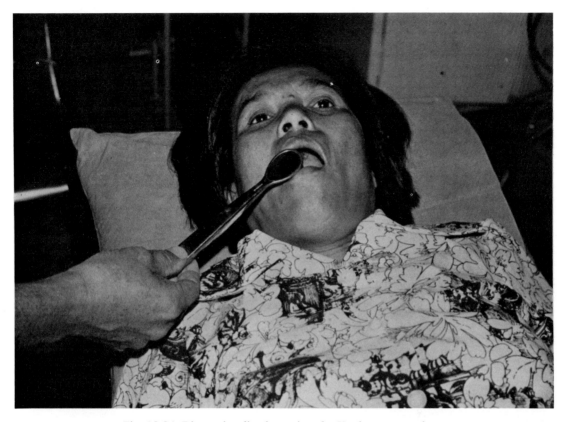

Fig. 16-24. Direct visualization using the Yankauer speculum.

area. If the cotton is blood-stained, ulceration can be assumed to be present.

The nasopharyngoscope is particularly useful in detecting small lesions and superficial ulcerations (because it gives a magnified view) and in visualizing the floor of the lateral pharyngeal recess when mirror examination has not been clear. However, the depth of the recess may not be visible in the Oriental because of its slit-like form. In addition, many patients are found to have bands traversing the entrance to the recess, making visualization even more difficult. This instrument, in addition to its examination function, is also used to guide a biopsy forceps accurately to a diseased site. To use the nasopharyngoscope, the nasal fossae and the nasopharynx should first be anesthetized with a topical anesthetic. The instrument is indispensable when trismus is present.

A routine ENT examination, with special attention to the nasopharynx, should be made. If posterior cervical nodes are involved, all superficial lymph node bearing areas of the body should be examined. Lymph nodes as far as the inguinal region may be enlarged in disseminated NPC.

The nasopharynx may be examined by either indirect or direct techniques. The instrument for indirect technique is the mirror, as it allows the examiner to scan the whole of the nasopharynx including the superior surface of the soft palate (Fig. 16-25).

Direct visualization of the nasopharynx can be achieved by either the Yankauer speculum (Fig. 16-24) or a nasopharyngoscope. The relative merits of these two instruments have already been mentioned. In some patients, it is not possible to do a satisfactory examination even with topical anesthesia because of an excessive gag reflex. This problem can be overcome by the use of the nasopharyngoscope. Should the exam-

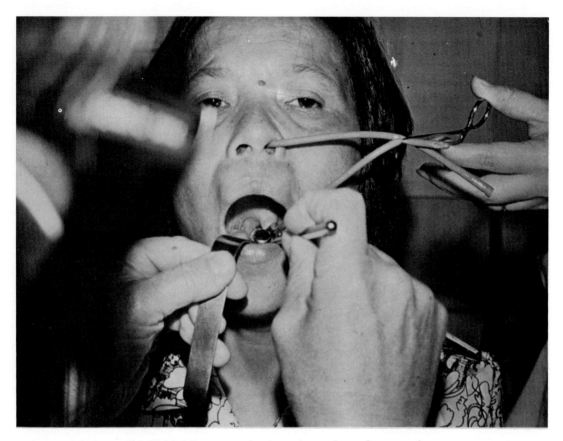

Fig. 16-25. Mirror examination using catheter for retraction.

iner be inexperienced in the use of this instrument, then a general anesthetic would be required. Under general anesthesia, the postnasal space can be examined by either a mirror or a Yankauer speculum. The soft palate can be retracted with a catheter to expose the nasopharynx for visualization with a mirror (Fig. 16-25). Palpation of the nasopharynx often provides additional information.

NECK EXAMINATION

The patient's neck including the trapezius area should be inspected down to the level of the clavicles. Careful palpation should be carried out to detect enlargement of the various groups of cervical nodes. In the case of NPC, one should concentrate on the upper jugular group and the nodes at the apex of the posterior triangle. In early cases, it may not be easy to detect a lymph node deep to the sternomastoid muscle. The two sides of the neck should be compared. A fullness would be noted on the side with early metastasis, as would a loss of the sternomastoid-mandibular groove. Metastatic nodes in the neck from NPC are, as a rule, painless and when present in large numbers, tend to be matted together.

CRANIAL NERVE EXAMINATION

The cranial nerve most commonly involved is the trigeminal. In early stages the patient would complain of paresthesia of the mid or lower face, and in more advanced disease, anesthesia supervenes. The corneal reflex is commonly lost. Involvement of the 7th nerve (in the pterygoid canal) with a diminution of lacrimation on the affected side can occur. Loss of lacrimation can be tested very easily by inserting a small piece of thin filter paper between the conjunctiva and the eyeball so that two-thirds of the paper overhangs the lower lid (Schirmer test). The nasal mucosa of the tested side is then stimulated either by the inhalation of something pungent or by swabbing it with a piece of cotton-wool on a stick (direct irritation).

The next group of cranial nerves commonly involved are the last four: 9th, 10th, 11th, and 12th. They should be checked in every case for diminution of function.

The 3rd and 4th nerves are involved only when advanced disease has infiltrated the orbit or has entered the anterior cranial fossa or the cavernous sinus. At this advanced stage, the 6th nerve—in addition to others—is usually also involved. Oftener than not, a patient with 6th nerve palsy consults an ophthalmologist because of double vision. In my experience. the 6th nerve involvement is not common (Fig. 16-20).

The level of function of the trapezius must be ascertained to rule out involvement of the accessory nerves. Again, the two sides should be compared. The involved side is then usually obvious to the examiner.

The above mentioned cranial nerves may be involved individually or in combination (Figs. 16-26 and 16-27).

When there is massive involvement of cervical nodes, or direct invasion from the nasopharynx encroaching onto the carotid sheath and cervical vertebrae, the sympathetic trunk becomes involved.

Clinical Findings

Ulcerations, nodular elevations, or a smooth bulging of the roof, posterior wall, or the lateral wall extending down to the oropharynx have been observed. The first sign of ulceration may be the presence of blood-tinged sputum. Blood clots are highly sug-

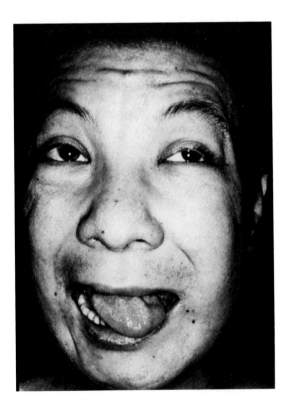

Fig. 16-26. Paralysis of the hypoglossal and sympathetic nerves. Note ptosis of left eyelid and deviation of tongue.

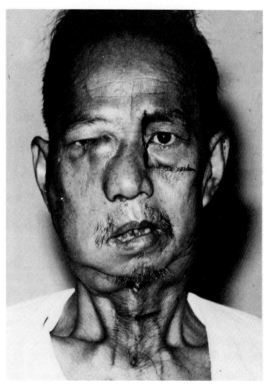

Fig. 16-27. Involvement of the nasal fossa, antrum, orbit, and bilateral neck with paralysis of 5th, 7th, and sympathetic nerve (ptosis) on right side.

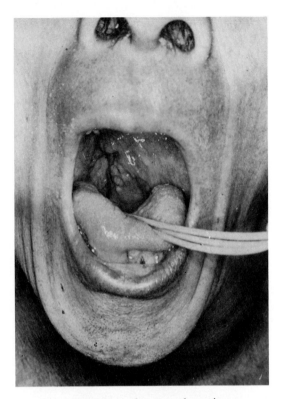

Fig. 16-28. Nasopharyngeal carcinoma extending into the oropharynx displacing the soft palate and tonsil and immobilizing them.

gestive of an ulcerated growth. Fungating growths occupying the fossa of Rosenmüller, the roof, and posterior or lateral walls are easily visible.

Large growths have been seen to occupy the whole of the nasopharynx, with extension into the nasal fossae, and may even be visible in the oropharynx, displacing the soft palate downwards and immobilizing it (Fig. 16-28). Infiltrative tumor tissue on the eustachian cushions (which form the anterior wall of the fossa of Rosenmüller) and in the fossa of Rosenmüller can escape detection. Comparison of the two sides should be made. The presence of edema, thickness, or nodularity in the eustachian cushions (torus) should be checked.

Radiology (for Extent of Disease)

Supporting evidence may be provided by radiology. Radiographs of the skull, i.e.,

lateral, submento-occipito-mental, occipito-maxillary (25° occipitofrontal) and soft tissue lateral (xerogram) views, are of value. These views give the following information: soft tissue swelling in the prevertebral space, obliteration of the lateral pharyngeal recess, and/or bony erosion.

Further radiographs of the skeleton may be required. Bone scans are obtained if any significant bone pain is present. A chest x-ray is taken as a routine to rule out pulmonary tuberculosis and to detect metastasis if present.

Computerized tomography (CT) is not routinely done for suspected intracranial spread. It is an expensive procedure that will help delineate the tumor but does not affect the treatment plan significantly. Figures 16-29 A, B, and C show a CT scan of one patient.

Biopsy Procedures

If no lesion is clearly visible in the nasopharynx but symptoms and signs arouse a high index of suspicion, a biopsy of both the fossa of Rosenmüller and the adjacent posterior wall and roof should be done. One should concentrate on the side where enlarged neck nodes or evidence of cranial nerve palsy is present, keeping in mind that a primary lesion may be present on the side opposite the enlarged cervical nodes. A single negative biopsy is of no significance. Biopsies may need to be performed multiple times if there are signs of the disease.

BIOPSY TECHNIQUES

Blind Techniques. The nasal cavity is anesthetized by the use of a topical anesthetic solution on ribbon gauze; the gauze is left in place for at least 20 minutes. The nasopharynx is also anesthetized by a topical local anesthetic (Cetacaine or tetracaine). Biopsy of the growth itself is painless but if the nasopharyngeal mucosa or deeper tissue is required for tissue examination, pain may occur requiring an infiltration

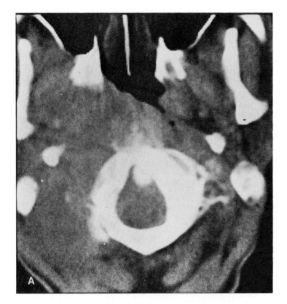
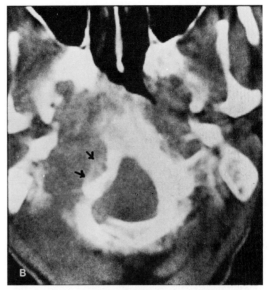

Fig. 16-29. (A), (B), and (C) Computerized tomography demonstrating a tumor mass of the right nasopharynx, extending into the retropterygoid fossa and destroying adjacent bone.

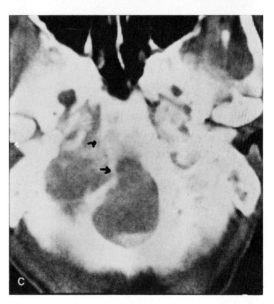

anesthetic. A Tilley-Henkel type of forceps is then introduced through the nasal fossa that is on the side of the suspected lesion (Figs. 16-30 A and B). A large tumor can be easily felt by the forceps and a biopsy specimen is taken. Bleeding is rarely severe in a biopsy procedure.

Forceps and Mirror Technique. The tumor is identified by means of a mirror. The biopsy forceps is then guided into position by the examiner with the help of the mirror. This is the ideal technique and the one most frequently practiced. Topical anesthesia is required. Retraction of the soft palate is sometimes necessary; this is done by passing a small catheter from the nose to the mouth, with the two ends held in place by a pair of forceps (Fig. 16-25).

Forceps and Yankauer speculum. When a small growth is confined to the fossa of Rosenmüller, forceps introduced through the nasal fossa would not reach it unless they are angled at the tip, but forceps with an angled tip cannot pass through the nasal fossa with ease. Therefore biopsy, utilizing forceps passed through the Yankauer speculum under direct vision, is desirable. The Yankauer speculum must be passed through the mouth, beneath the soft palate, and into the nasopharynx. When the patient is too nervous or the gag reflex persists in spite of topical anesthesia, this procedure has to be done under general anesthesia.

Forceps and nasopharyngoscope. This is a good technique. The forceps can be guided into position through the nasal fossa while the operator looks through the scope. It is indispensable when trismus is present.

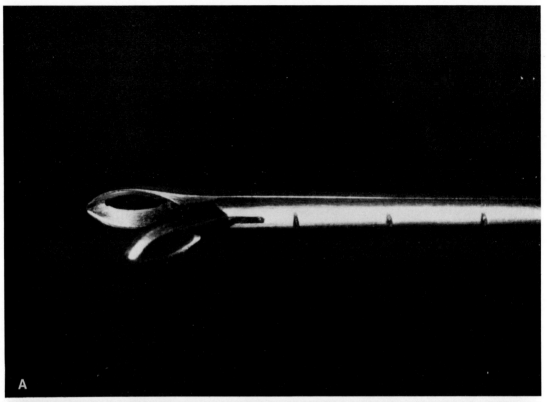

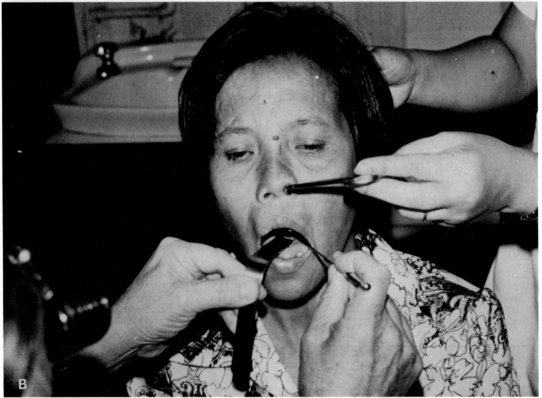

Fig. 16-30. (A) Tip of biopsy forceps. (B) Biopsy forceps guided into place by a postnasal mirror.

WHERE TO TAKE A BIOPSY

As a general policy, the side of presenting symptoms is first biopsied, that is, the side with either cranial nerve involvement or cervical nodes metastasis. In almost all cases, a positive biopsy will be obtained on the side of presenting symptoms. On the rare occasions when the first biopsy is negative, then the rest of the postnasal space is explored with multiple specimens taken from the posterior wall, roof, and the fossa of Rosenmüller of the opposite side.

A lymph node biopsy is done only when an exhaustive study of the nasopharynx and other relevant areas is negative. Removal of a node as a primary diagnostic procedure should rarely be done, for the following reasons:

1. It is unnecessary in 99 percent of patients;

2. A positive pathologic report often does not indicate the primary site of malignancy;

3. The tumor-bearing area in the node may be missed because a complicating disease such as tuberculosis is evident instead;

4. Removal of a painless node gives the patient a false sense of security and he may then default on follow-up; and

5. It has been reported that in patients who have had a neck node biopsy prior to treatment the chance of cure is reduced and they have a poorer long-term survival.[36, 38]

In Hong Kong, if the patient is a Southern Chinese with a positive cervical node and no primary tumor identified, a full course of radiotherapy is given after ruling out all other possible malignancies in the head and neck areas, thus assuming that the patient has NPC.

Staging

The tumor, node, metastases (TNM) system of describing the extent of a malignant tumor according to the extent of its primary tumor, the extent of involvement of the regional lymph nodes, and the presence or absence of clinically demonstrable metastases was recommended by the International Union Against Cancer (UICC) in 1962 and revised in 1974. The T stages in the UICC classification[54] are:

T Primary tumor

T1S Preinvasive carcinoma (carcinoma in situ)

T0 No evidence of primary tumor

T1 Tumor limited to one region

T2 Tumor extending into two regions

T3 Tumor extending beyond the nasopharynx without bone involvement

T4 Tumor extending beyond the nasopharynx with bone involvement, including the cartilaginous portion of the eustachian tube

Ho feels that this separation of tumors confined to the nasopharynx into T1 and T2 is not practical. In some patients, examination of the nasopharynx is notoriously difficult and it is not always possible to ascertain the limits of the tumor (T) within the nasopharynx. Furthermore, a tumor may occur submucosally making it difficult to evaluate its extent. The diagnosis of such cases is established only by biopsy, which, however, does not give an indication of the extent of tumor. The difference between T3 and T4 in the UICC classification is the presence or absence of bone involvement, but no mention is made of the involvement of cranial nerves which may occur without demonstrable bone involvement. Since the tumor must have already entered the cranial cavity before it could invade a cranial nerve, nerve involvement carries with it an even graver prognosis than mere involvement of a bone, especially when involvement occurs below the base of the skull. For these reasons, Ho has adopted the following T staging:

T Primary tumor

T1 Tumor confined to the nasopharynx (space behind the choanal orifices and nasal septum and above the posterior margin of the soft palate in the resting position)

T2 Tumor extended to the nasal fossa, oropharynx, or adjacent muscles or nerves below the base of the skull

T3 Tumor extended beyond T2 limits and subclassified as follows:

T3a Bone involvement below the base of the skull (floor of the sphenoid sinus is included in this category)

T3b Involvement of the base of the skull

T3c Involvement of cranial nerve(s)

T3d Involvement of the orbits, laryngopharynx (hypopharynx), or infratemporal fossa

Ho's experience has shown that, within the T3 group, T3a is associated with the best prognosis and T3d the poorest.

The UICC nodal or N staging was designed primarily to guide surgical treatment (block dissection) and to indicate prognosis when surgery is the main form of treatment. For instance, N1 involvement (homolateral mobile node or nodes) would require at least a block dissection on one side, N2 (contralateral or bilateral node or nodes) would require bilateral block dissections, and N3 (fixed node or nodes) would probably not be dissectable; hence, this staging is considered to carry with it the worst prognosis irrespective of the level of involvement.

However, in 1974, the UICC[54] recognized that the level of involvement of cervical lymph nodes has a bearing on both treatment and prognosis and recommended that such involvement should always be recorded; but they felt that it was not possible at the time to incorporate these levels in the N classification.

Since nasopharyngeal carcinomas are treated mainly by radiation therapy (RT), the staging of NPC nodal involvement should be based on the results of RT and not on the results of surgical treatment of other head and neck cancers. Furthermore, as the sequence of nodal involvement in NPC is usually from above downward and nodal fixation presents no problem in RT, the N involvement should, therefore, be staged according to the level of involvement, because the latter has been shown to determine the prognosis regardless of the mobility of the nodes or the laterality of involvement (Table 16-4). The staging in this

TABLE 16-4. FIVE-YEAR RESULTS OF NASOPHARYNGEAL CARCINOMA PATIENTS WITH T1 OR T2 TUMORS BY LEVEL OF NODAL INVOLVEMENT REGARDLESS OF MOBILITY OR LATERALITY OF THE NODES, 1965–1967

Level	Alive	Probability and Significance	Relapse Free	Probability and Significance
N1	55/102 (53.9%)	N1 vs N2 $\chi^2 = 14.99$ $P < 0.0001$ S.	49/102 (48.0%)	N1 vs N2 $\chi^2 = 12.40$ $P < 0.0004$ S.
N2	56/183 (30.6%)	N2 vs N3 $\chi^2 = 12.89$ $P < 0.0003$ S.	50/183 (27.3%)	N2 vs N3 $\chi^2 = 21.21$ $P < 0.000004$ S.
N3	23/161 (14.3%)		13/161 (8.1%)	

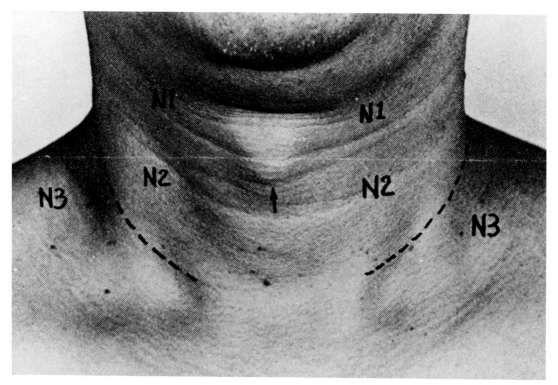

Fig. 16-31. Front view of neck showing the N levels. Skin crease dividing N1 and N2 is arrowed. (Reprinted with permission from International Journal of Radiation: Oncology, Biology, Physics, 4:181, Ho, H. C., An epidemiologic and clinical study of nasopharyngeal carcinoma. Copyright 1978, Pergamon Press, Ltd.)

table is according to Ho's 1970[22] classification, which gives the N and group TNM stage classifications as follows:

N Regional lymph nodes (Figs. 16-31 and 16-32)

N0 None palpable (nodes thought to be benign excluded)

N1 Node(s) wholly in the upper cervical level bounded below by the skin crease extending laterally and backward from or just below the thyroid notch (laryngeal eminence)

N2 Node(s) palpable between the crease and the supraclavicular fossa, the upper limit being a line joining the upper margin of the sternal end of the clavicle and the apex of an angle formed by the lateral surface of the neck and the superior margin of the trapezius.

N3 Node(s) palpable in the supra-clavicular fossa and/or skin involvement in the form of carcinoma *en cuirasse* or satellite nodules above the clavicles

Grouped TNM staging

I Tumor confined to the nasopharyngeal mucosa

II Tumor extended to nasal fossa, oropharynx, or adjacent muscles or to nerves below the base of the skull (T2), and/or N1 involvement

III Tumor, extended beyond T2 limits, or bone involvement (T3), and/or N2 involvement

IV N3 involvement, irrespective of the primary tumor

V Hematogenous metastasis and/or involvement of skin or lymph node(s) below the clavicles (M)

The above stage classification has evolved from the successive analyses of

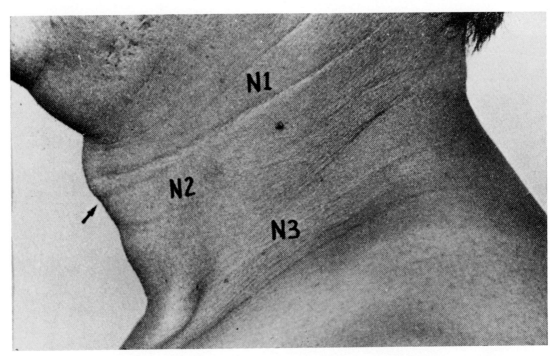

Fig. 16-32. Side view of Figure 16-31. (Reprinted with permission from International Journal of Radiation: Oncology, Biology, Physics, 4:181, Ho, H. C., An epidemiologic and clinical study of nasopharyngeal carcinoma. Copyright 1978, Pergamon Press, Ltd.)

treatment results obtained in Ho's institute since 1965.

TREATMENT

Radiotherapy

The mainstay of treatment for NPC is radiotherapy. The anatomical structures included in the portals covering the primary lesion are determined by the clinical and radiographic evidence of involvement of specific contiguous structures. When the cancer involves the nasopharynx proper, included in the treatment of the primary are most of the posterior part of the nasal cavity, the posterior ethmoid cells, and the sphenoid sinus. When there are known extensions beyond the nasopharynx, the fields are modified to include them.

The lymphatics of the neck and parapharyngeal spaces are usually irradiated in continuity with the primary tumor regardless of whether palpable nodes are present (Fig. 16-33). The rationale is to control microscopic disease in the cervical nodes in the clinically negative neck.

Generally, the dosage of irradiation to the primary tumor is between 6,500 to 7,500 rads over $6^{1}/_{2}$ to $7^{1}/_{2}$ weeks. The nasopharynx and neck are usually treated to 5,000 rads, then boosts to 6,500 to 7,500 rads are given to areas that contain gross tumor using smaller fields (Figs. 16-34 A and B).

VALUE OF PROPHYLACTIC IRRADIATION OF CERVICAL LYMPH NODES

In 1971, Ho initiated a randomized clinical trial to test the value of prophylactic irradiation of cervical nodes in NPC patients with T1, T2, or T3 tumors. One group (Group A) was given prophylactic irradiation and the other (Group B) was not given irradiation until the nodes became palpable. For those treated in 1971, 5-year results are now

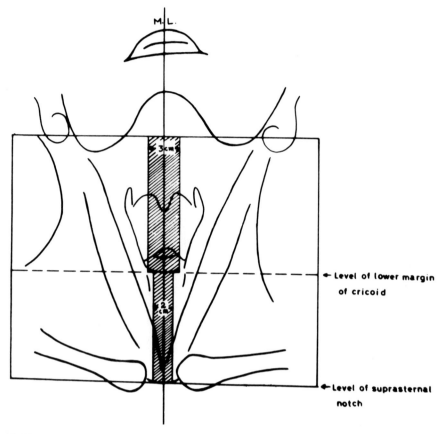

Fig. 16-33. Anterior cervical field. For prophylactic irradiation the inferior margin is at the level of the lower cricoid margin. With nodal involvement it is at the suprasternal notch. (Reprinted with permission from International Journal of Radiation: Oncology, Biology, Physics, 4:181, Ho, H. C., An epidemiologic and clinical study of nasopharyngeal carcinoma. Copyright 1978, Pergamon Press, Ltd.)

available, and for those treated in 1972 only 4-year results are available. Only the results of stage I (T1N0) cases have been analyzed and will be reported here (Table 16-5).

The patients in the two groups were treated by the same technique and with the same dosage scheme. The technique and dosage scheme for patients treated in 1971 were different from those for patients treated in 1972. In 1971 the mean tumor dose to the nasopharynx was 420 rads twice a week until 5,040 rads total were given (1,855–1,860 roentgens equivalent therapeutic [ret]). In 1972 the dose fraction was reduced to 400 rads and the total to 4,800 rads (1,767–1,722 ret). In 1971 the dose to the cervical nodes on both sides of the neck above the level of the lower margin of the cricoid cartilage (reckoned at 90 percent isodose level through an anterior cervical field with the larynx and spinal cord shielded) was 580 rads weekly for 7 weeks to 4,060 rads (1,687 ret), but this was reduced in 1972 to 560 rads weekly for 7 weeks to 3,920 rads (1,629 ret) to avoid undue fibrosis.

All patients in the two groups had what might be described as nonkeratinizing squamous carcinoma, which includes undifferentiated, anaplastic, and poorly differentiated variants. In fact, of 404 NPC patients registered in 1971 at Queen Elizabeth Hospital, 395 or 97.8 percent had nonkeratinizing squamous carcinoma. Of the remaining nine, only one patient had well-differentiated squamous carcinoma and the rest had what was described in the biopsy reports as

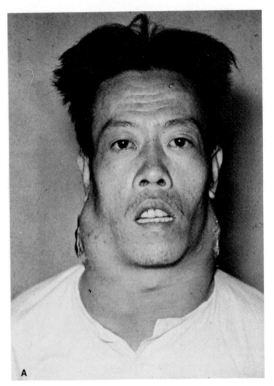
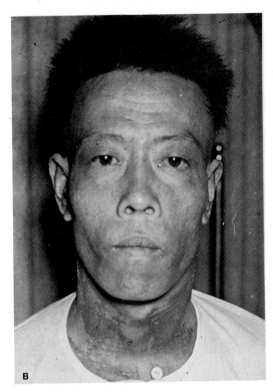

Fig. 16-34. (A) Before radiotherapy. Massive bilateral neck disease with partial ulceration. (B) After radiotherapy.

moderately differentiated squamous carcinoma.

Only one patient—a member of Group B—was lost to follow-up, but he was well without evidence of disease when last seen after the first year. Because his subsequent condition was not known, he was excluded from the analysis.

Table 16-5 shows the results of the trial for the two groups, and Table 16-6 for those patients aged 40 years or over. All the patients tolerated the treatment well. The mucosal reactions were surprisingly mild, and no patients developed radiation neuropathy. Soft tissue fibrosis in the neck was either minimal or not detectable when the weekly dose was reduced to 560 rads at 90 percent isodose level.

There were five patients in Group B who following radiation therapy to the nasopharyngeal region developed palpable nodes in the neck, unaccompanied by a recurrence of the primary tumor. After they had irradiation of the cervical nodes, four of them remained well without evidence of disease. The remaining one later developed pulmonary and liver metastases, but 4 years after his initial therapy he was alive with no evidence of residual disease in the neck. Consequently, no patients in Group B had simple nodal relapse.

These data indicate that prophylactic irradiation for stage I cancer of the nasopharynx is not essential and that cervical node disease can be controlled when it becomes clinically evident. One must be cautious with more advanced primary tumors because the likelihood of subsequent cervical disease is extremely high and prophylactic irradiation would be warranted.

FAILURE OF TREATMENT

According to Ho,[22] failure may be due to the following reasons:

1. *The failure of existing methods of radio-*

TABLE 16-5. STAGE I WITH AND WITHOUT PROPHYLACTIC
CERVICAL NODAL IRRADIATION OBSERVED FOR 4 TO 5 YEARS

| | Cases(%) Prophylactic Irradiation | | | |
	With (Group A)	Without (Group B)	Probability	Significance
Alive	25/34(74)	23/32(72)	$\chi^2 = 0.023$ $P = 0.88$	N.S.
No evidence of disease	22/34(65)	22/23(69)	$\chi^2 = 0.121$ $P = 0.73$	N.S.
Cause of death				
Primary tumor	5	6		
Metastases	0	1		
Intercurrent disease	4	2		
Relapse				
Primary	4	4		
Node	1	0		
Primary & node	3	6		

therapy to eradicate or control the primary tumor; radiotherapy appears to be ineffective in about one-third of cases, even when the disease appears to be still confined to the nasopharynx.

2. *The presence of cranial spread* with the brain posing a limit to the dose of radiation that could be given without risking fatal or incapacitating radiation neuropathy. Ho has not encountered a single proven case of hematogenous brain metastasis from NPC, although metastases in bone and other viscera are common. The brain is not immune to spread from an adjacent meningeal metastasis or to a direct spread from the primary tumor through the base of the skull. In the case of the latter, there is always far more pressure-softening and necrosis than tumor infiltration.

3. *Uncontrolled cervical nodal metastases.* This is the least important reason for treatment failure now that the radiotherapist has at his disposal megavoltage x-rays or gamma rays from kCi telecobalt units and high energy electrons, all of which have enabled him to deliver a cancericidal dose to the cervical nodes without risking radiation myelopathy.

4. *Distant metastases.*

For patients with recurrent disease of the nasopharynx only, reirradiation—utilizing an implant with a radiation source

TABLE 16-6. STAGE I PATIENTS AGED ≥ 40 YEARS WITH
AND WITHOUT PROPHYLACTIC CERVICAL NODAL
IRRADIATION OBSERVED FOR 4 TO 5 YEARS

| | Cases (%) Prophylactic Irradiation | | | |
	With (Group A)	Without (Group B)	Probability	Significance
Alive	12/21(57)	13/19(68)	$\chi^2 = 0.541$ $P = 0.462$	N.S.
No evidence of disease	11/21(52)	12/19(63)	$\chi^2 = 0.474$ $P = 0.491$	N.S.

—to another 5,000 rads or more may be helpful and occasionally curative.

Surgery

Surgery is seldom indicated for cancer of the nasopharynx except for adenoid cystic, rhabdomyosarcomas, and chordomas. Occasionally a palatal fenestration procedure or a neck dissection may be indicated.

PALATAL FENESTRATION

Palatal fenestration may take the form of either a subtotal maxillectomy with the removal of half of the hard palate in order to allow intracavitary irradiation for a residual neoplasm in the maxillary antrum, or a temporary or permanent opening in the palate for exploring the nasopharynx or to allow intracavitary irradiation.

A temporary opening may be indicated when conservative methods of biopsy have failed to give a positive result. I seldom use a temporary opening; however, there are clinics in Europe that use it almost routinely.

The indications for a permanent opening are (1) when there is residual cancer in the epipharynx when radiotherapy has failed, and further radiation needs to be given, usually in the form of caecium 137 sources or electron beam therapy; (2) to control sepsis, especially when there is bone destruction and osteomyelitis, which is usually foul-smelling; and (3) to facilitate inspection and biopsy of the nasopharynx.

The technique for a temporary fenestration is illustrated in Figures 16-35 A–D.

Prior to creating a permanent fenestration, the patient should be seen by the maxillofacial prosthodontist so that an impression of the palate can be made in order to create a prosthesis to cover the defect for eating and speaking (Figs. 16-36 and 16-37).

NECK DISSECTION

In Hong Kong, no en bloc dissection is done for neck nodes from NPC. This policy has been adopted for the following reasons:

First, because radiotherapy must remain the mainstay of treatment for NPC, prophylactic neck dissection is not justified before the appearance of nodal involvement, as metastasis sometimes takes place on the side contralateral to the primary lesions. Furthermore, it is the experience of Ho[27] that prophylactic irradiation of lymph nodes does not improve the long-term result of treatment. Hence, one can infer that a prophylactic neck dissection would be equally noncontributory.

Second, in the majority of patients presenting with lymph nodes, the nodes are found to be fixed to the deep tissues in the neck and this generally means the carotid sheath; involvement of this sheath makes a neck dissection dangerous especially following radiotherapy.

Third, the retropharyngeal nodes, which are involved early in the disease, are not included in a routine neck dissection.

There are surgeons elsewhere who believe neck dissection is of value provided the nodes are limited in involvement and are not fixed and the procedure is done soon after radiotherapy. One oncologist[20] has advocated the "softening" of lymph nodes by the use of chemotherapy followed by surgical removal. However, the healing of a large wound following radiation therapy must necessarily be precarious. Nevertheless, a solitary node found after radiotherapy can be removed with advantage.

Chemotherapy

The use of chemotherapy for recurrent cancers of the nasopharynx has been disappointing. Simple drugs such as cyclophosphamide, methotrexate, or bleomycin have been utilized with poor response rates (less than 30 percent), and those cases that do respond do so only for brief periods.

The use of combination chemotherapy using cyclophosphamide, 5-fluorouracil, methotrexate, and vincristine does not seem to improve the response rate.[16] A combination termed BACON,[35, 44] consisting of bleo-

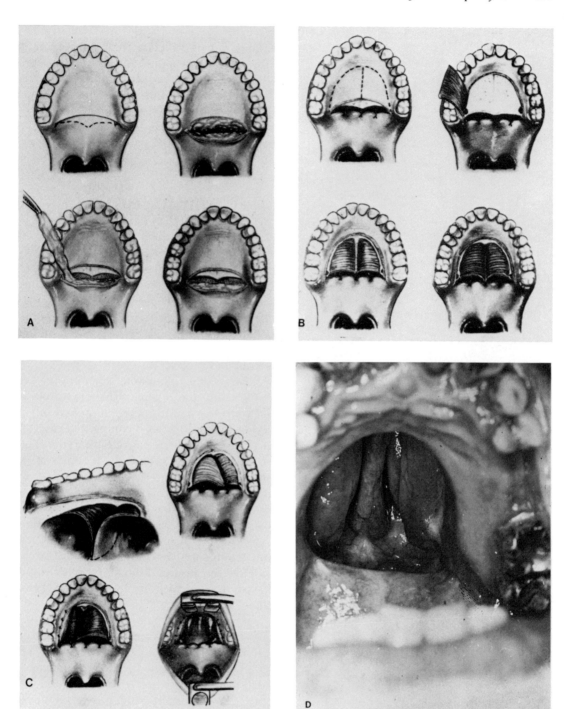

Fig. 16-35. (A) Technique of a temporary fenestration. (B) Fenestration technique, continued. (C) Fenestration technique, continued. (D) Completed permanent palatal fenestration. (Wilson, C. P. 1957. Observations on the surgery of the nasopharynx. Annals of Otology, Rhinology and Laryngology, 66:5.)

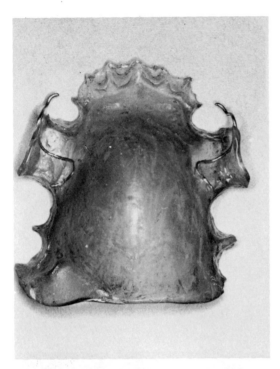

Fig. 16-36. Prosthesis for patient with teeth.

mycin, adriamycin, CCNU, Oncovin (vincristine), and nitrogen mustard, has been tried and not shown to improve the response rate either.

Cis-platinum, with and without bleo-

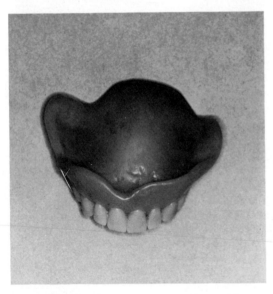

Fig. 16-37. Prosthesis for patient without teeth.

mycin, is presently being used, but the response rate is still less than 30 percent.[56] However, this response rate is with patients who have been treatment failures with radiation therapy and usually chemotherapy.

The poor response rate of chemotherapy may be related to the poor blood supply to the nasopharynx particularly following radiation.

COMPLICATIONS OF RADIOTHERAPY

Following radiotherapy, the usual complications such as dryness of the mouth exist. In years past, the skin of Chinese patients was badly blackened by the 250 kV machines, and this was one of the reasons some patients refused treatment. In addition, the following complications have been seen after radiation for NPC:

Ear. The tympanic membrane becomes white and opaque. Chronic suppurative otitis media with perforation and infection of the middle ear is common in cases of ulcerated lesions of the nasopharynx. The external auditory canal skin becomes atrophied, bone becomes exposed, and infection and sequestration may take place. Involvement of the internal ear with giddiness following radiation is not uncommon. High tone loss in hearing has been noted by me and confirmed by others.[28, 29, 32] Unfortunately, no histopathologic proof of damage to the cochlea in humans has been obtained.

Trismus. Trismus occurs as a consequence of postradiation fibrosis and cancer infiltration of the pterygoid muscles (Fig. 16-38). Surgeons can help in the management of these patients by stretching the jaw muscles periodically under general anesthesia or through the use of prosthetics (see Ch. 9). Regretfully, the majority of patients refuse to keep the muscles stretched following the procedure because it is a painful maneuver. The greatest problem with trismus is, of course, feeding. If the patient has a full set of teeth, adequate feeding is difficult and must be assisted by a nasal tube.

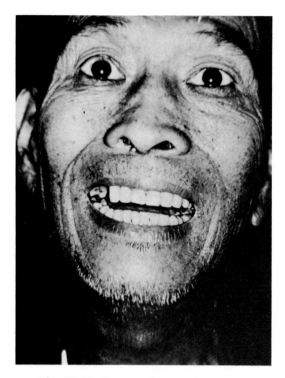

Fig. 16-38. Severe trismus after radiotherapy.

Bone. The atlas and the base of the skull may undergo necrosis. The roof of the postnasal space (body of sphenoid) may also undergo necrosis. Sequestration may take place. In the latter condition a foul discharge is present. These changes are the end result of tumor infiltration, sepsis, and radiation necrosis. Frequent cleansing with a modified Proetz technique is required. A palatal fenestration in these cases would greatly help in the hygiene of the nasopharynx. Trismus, of course, prevents success with such a procedure.

Nose. More than two-thirds of patients who have undergone radiotherapy, particularly those with an ulcerated lesion, develop a nasal infection. Maxillary sinusitis is very common. The causative factors must be the loss of nasal ciliary action in combination with sepsis in the nasopharynx.

Mild myelitis. Lhermitte sign, a sensation of pins and needles shooting down the body upon flexion of the neck, is reversible. Brown-Séquard syndrome, or a varying degree of transverse myelitis of the cervical cord, is irreversible and leads to quadraplegia.

Radiation caries. This condition is sometimes seen after radiotherapy. Dental care should always be given before, during, and after radiotherapy.

Ulceration of tongue. This is a rare complication following radiotherapy.

Permanent epilation of areas of the scalp can occur.

Rarely, *retinal atrophy* may occur.[30]

The above complications are becoming less common with the use of supervoltage machines in the treatment of NPC.

Management

Maxillary sinusitis is treated in the usual way with an appropriate antibiotic and antral lavages. No operative treatment is done within 18 months following radiotherapy for fear of causing osteomyelitis. Extensive bone necroses can occur in cases when surgery is done too soon. No tooth extraction should be done following radiotherapy for the same reason.

Epipharyngitis. Since most tumors are of the ulcerative type, a raw surface persists for some months following radiotherapy. The area may become septic, thus requiring frequent cleansing. This can be accomplished by using a modified Proetz procedure, i.e., normal saline is instilled into one nasal cavity and aspirated from the other with a Proetz apparatus.

Ear. When 250 kV machines were used in the past, the external auditory canal skin often became atrophic, revealing bone. Subsequent infection generally set in resulting in an osteomyelitis. Sequestration has been seen in the bony portion of the external canal. Over half of the patients developed otitis media that tends to be recurrent because of the sepsis in the nasopharynx and a malfunctioning eustachian tube. Cholesteatoma is unusual when chronic otitis media coexists with NPC. Nevertheless, there are cases in which extensive granulation takes place giving rise to an uncontrollable discharge from a mastoid involvement. These cases are treated surgically by means of radical mastoidectomy. No reconstruction is ever attempted, as even the healing of the postaural skin is often poor.

END RESULTS

The results by sex, age, and stage of all NPC patients treated in 1965 at Queen Mary Hospital with orthovoltage radiation therapy and at Queen Elizabeth Hospital with megavoltage therapy were reported in 1970.[22, 25] The 10-year cumulative actuarial survival and relapse-free curves of the 1965 series and the 5-year cumulative actuarial survival and relapse-free curves of the 1969 to 1971 series are shown in Figure 16-39. The 5-year treatment results of both groups are presented in Table 16-7.

The results when analyzed according to sex and age showed a significantly better crude or absolute survival in patients within age group 20 to 39 than those within 40 to 59, but no significant difference in survival was observed between the sexes[25] (Tables 16-8, and 16-9). Table 16-10 gives the 5-year relapse-free rate for the same group of patients. Stage IV patients were treated mostly at Queen Mary Hospital with orthovoltage radiation therapy, and the results, therefore, are not included.

Prognosis definitely seems to be related

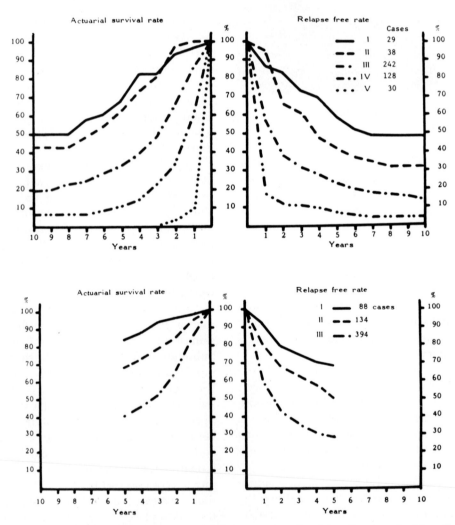

Fig. 16-39. Cumulative proportional actuarial survival and relapse-free survival by clinical stage. Top two graphs are for 1965; bottom two graphs for 1969 to 1971. (Reprinted with permission from International Journal of Radiation: Oncology, Biology, Physics, 4:181, Ho, H. C., An epidemiologic and clinical study of nasopharyngeal carcinoma. Copyright 1978, Pergamon Press, Ltd.)

TABLE 16-7. FIVE-YEAR TREATMENT RESULTS OF
NASOPHARYNGEAL CARCINOMA BY CLINICAL STAGE

Stage	Actuarial Survival Rate (%) 1965	1969–1971	Relapse-free* Rate (%) 1965	1969–1971
I	67.9	83.9	17/29(58.6)	60/88(68.2)
II	62.2	67.9	16/38(42.1)	67/134(50.0)
III	32.9	40.3	55/242(22.7)	114/394(28.9)
IV	11.0		9/128(7.0)	

*Relapse-free after a single course of radiation therapy.

TABLE 16-8. FIVE-YEAR CRUDE SURVIVAL RATES (%) FOR NASOPHARYNGEAL
CARCINOMA TREATED IN 1969–1971—ANALYSIS BY AGE, SEX, AND STAGE[25]

Stage	<40 years Male	Female	≥40 years Male	Female	Total Male	Female
I & II	34/43(79.1)	25/28(89.3)	66/105(62.9)	28/45(62.2)	100/148(67.6)	53/73(72.6)
III	40/87(46.0)	10/29(34.5)	58/189(30.7)	34/90(37.8)	98/276(35.5)	44/119(37.0)
Total	74/130(57.0)	35/57(61.4)	124/294(42.2)	62/135(46.0)	198/424(47.0)	97/192(50.6)

TABLE 16-9. FIVE-YEAR RESULTS OF NASOPHARYNGEAL CARCINOMA PATIENTS
TREATED IN 1969–1971—ANALYSIS BY AGE AND STAGE

Stage	RFR*(%) Age <40	≥40	Probability and Significance	Alive (%) Age <40	≥40	Probability and Significance
I	22/26 (84.6)	38/62 (61.3)	$\chi^2 = 4.59$ $P < 0.0321$ S.	25/26 (96.2)	47/62 (75.8)	$\chi^2 = 5.10$ $P < 0.0240$ S.
II	25/45 (56.6)	42.89 (47.2)	$\chi^2 = 0.84$ $P < 0.360$ N.S.	34/45 (75.6)	47/89 (52.8)	$\chi^2 = 6.47$ $P < 0.0110$ S.
III	39/116 (33.6)	75/278 (27.0)	$\chi^2 = 1.76$ $P < 0.185$ N.S.	49/116 (42.2)	92/278 (33.1)	$\chi^2 = 2.98$ $P < 0.0843$ N.S.
Total	86/187 (46.0)	155/429 (36.1)	$\chi^2 = 5.31$ $P < 0.0211$ S.	108/187 (57.8)	186/429 (43.4)	$\chi^2 = 10.8$ $P < 0.0010$ S.

*RFR, Relapse free rate after a single course of radiation therapy.

to the level of cervical node involvement as in Ho's classification and not so much to the laterality or mobility of the nodes. This is shown in Tables 16-11, 16-12, 16-13, and 16-14.

SUMMARY

Nasopharyngeal carcinoma is a unique disease in that it is definitely influenced by race and environment, its diagnosis is rarely made possible by the symptoms and signs arising from the primary lesion, and its treatment is almost entirely radiotherapeutic.

Its manner of spread is also unique in that the cancer may reach an advanced stage without affecting cervical lymph nodes. Yet in some cases, metastatic lymphadenopathy is the first presenting symptom. There is no relationship between the clinical behavior of the disease and the histopathology of the cancer.

NPC is a condition extremely difficult to treat because of the proximity of the cancer to vital structures, including the brain, the spinal cord, the eyes, and the ears, that are at the base of the skull.

It has been established beyond doubt that there is a definite relationship between the Epstein-Barr virus and nasopharyngeal carcinoma.

All otorhinolaryngologists should keep NPC in mind so as not to miss recognition of the disease. This is particularly true for clinicians practicing in a non-Chinese population. Like other cancers, only early detection will afford a reasonable prognosis.

Cervical node biopsy should not be the first procedure used to establish a diagnosis. A positive biopsy can be obtained from the primary lesion in 99 percent of cases.

ACKNOWLEDGEMENT

I am greatly indebted to Dr. H. C. Ho, M.D., Hon.D.Sc. (HK); F.R.C.P. (Lond.); F.F.R. (D. & T.); Hon. F.R.C.R.A; F.R.A.C.R; Chief in Radiology and Oncology, Medical

TABLE 16-10. FIVE-YEAR RELAPSE-FREE RATES (%) FOR NASOPHARYNGEAL CARCINOMA TREATED IN 1969–1971—ANALYSIS BY AGE, SEX, AND STAGE

Stage	<40 years Male	<40 years Female	≥40 years Male	≥40 years Female	Total Male	Total Female
I & II	27/43(62.8)	20/28(71.4)	55/105(52.4)	25/45(55.6)	82/148(55.4)	45/73(61.6)
III	32/87(36.8)	8/29(27.6)	48/189(25.4)	27/90(30.0)	80/276(29.0)	35/119(29.4)
Total	59/130(45.4)	28/57(49.1)	103/294(35.0)	52/135(38.5)	162/424(38.2)	80/192(41.7)

TABLE 16-11. FIVE-YEAR CRUDE SURVIVAL RATES FOR NASOPHARYNGEAL CARCINOMA WITH MOBILE CERVICAL NODE(S)—BY LEVEL AND LATERALITY OF INVOLVEMENT (1965–1967)

Level	Unilateral (%)	Bilateral (%)	Probability (Significance)
(T1 or T2) N1	40/62(64.5)	7/16(43.8)	$P < 0.14$ (N.S.)
(T1 or T2) N2	11/31(35.5)	12/33(36.4)	$P < 0.94$ (N.S.)
(T1 or T2) N3	1/8 (12.5)	5/19(26.3)	$P < 0.43$ (N.S.)

TABLE 16-12. FIVE-YEAR RELAPSE-FREE SURVIVAL
RATES FOR NASOPHARYNGEAL CARCINOMA WITH
MOBILE CERVICAL NODE(S)—ANALYSIS BY LEVEL AND
LATERALITY OR INVOLVEMENT (1965–1967)

Level	Unilateral (%)	Bilateral (%)	Probability (Significance)
(T1 or 2) N1	35/62(56.5)	6/16(37.5)	$P < 0.18$ (N.S.)
(T1 or 2) N2	11/31(35.5)	11/33(33.3)	$P < 0.86$ (N.S.)
(T1 or 2) N3	1/8 (12.5)	2/19(10.5)	$P < 0.88$ (N.S.)

TABLE 16-13. FIVE-YEAR CRUDE SURVIVAL RATES
FOR NASOPHARYNGEAL CARCINOMA WITH
UNILATERAL CERVICAL NODE(S)—ANALYSIS BY
LEVEL AND MOBILITY (1965–1967)

Level	Mobile (%)	Fixed (%)	Probability (Significance)
(T1 or 2) N1	40/62(64.5)	8/20(40.0)	$P < 0.055$ (N.S.)
(T1 or 2) N2	11/31(35.5)	19/63(30.2)	$P < 0.60$ (N.S.)
(T1 or 2) N3	1/8 (12.5)	5/46(10.9)	$P < 0.89$ (N.S.)

TABLE 16-14. FIVE-YEAR RELAPSE-FREE SURVIVAL
RATES FOR NASOPHARYNGEAL CARCINOMA WITH
UNILATERAL CERVICAL NODE(S)—ANALYSIS BY
LEVEL AND MOBILITY (1965–1967)

Level	Mobile (%)	Fixed (%)	Probability (Significance)
(T1 or 2) N1	35/62(56.5)	8/20(40.0)	$P < 0.20$ (N.S.)
(T1 or 2) N2	11/31(35.5)	16/63(25.4)	$P < 0.31$ (N.S.)
(T1 or 2) N3	1/8 (12.5)	2/46(4.3)	$P < 0.36$ (N.S.)

and Health Department, Institute of Radiology and Oncology, Queen Elizabeth Hospital, Kowloon, Hong Kong, for his cooperation and generosity in giving me a full text on radiotherapy; to Dr. T. B. Teoh, Ph.D., F.R.C.Path., Consultant Pathologist in charge at the Medical and Health Department, Institute of Pathology, Sai Ying Pun Jockey Club Clinic, Hong Kong, for his patience in helping me to prepare the pictures and his expert advice on the pathology; to Dr. Rudy Khoo, M.B: B.S.: D.M.R.T; F.R.C.R; Consultant in Radiotherapy and Oncology, Medical and Health Department, Institute of Radiology and Oncology, Queen Mary Hospital, Hong Kong for the information given in the section on chemotherapy; and to all the publishers and authors who have supplied excellent source material in their journals and textbooks; and to my personal secretary, Miss Helen Yuen, for typing the script.

REFERENCES

1. Ali M. Y. 1965. Histology of the human nasopharyngeal mucosa. Journal of Anatomy, 99: 657.

2. Ali M. Y. 1967. Distribution and character of the squamous epithelium in the human nasopharynx. In Muir, C. S., and Shanmugaratnam, K., Eds.: Cancer of the Nasopharynx. Munksgaard, Copenhagen, 138.

3. Bailar, J. C., III., 1967. Race, environment, and family in the epidemiology of cancer of the nasopharynx. In Muir, C. S., and Shanmugaratnam, K., Eds.: Cancer of the Nasopharynx. Munksgaard, Copenhagen, 101.

4. Batson, O. V. 1942. Veins of the pharynx. Archives of Otolaryngology, 36: 212.

5. Ch'en P'ei En. 1956. Clinical determination of urinary 17-ketosteroids: A preliminary report. Chinese Medical Journal, 74: 424.

6. Choa, G. 1974. Nasopharyngeal Carcinoma. Journal of Laryngology and Otology, 88: 145.

7. Clifford, P. 1967. Malignant disease of the nasopharynx and paranasal sinuses in Kenya. In Muir, C. S., and Shanmugaratnam, K., Eds.: Cancer of the Nasopharynx Munksgaard, Copenhagen, 82.

8. Clifford, P. 1970. A review on the epidemiology of nasopharyngeal carcinoma. International Journal of Cancer, 5: 287.

9. Daito, T., Sakamoto, H., and Hara, H. J. 1952. Neoplasm of the nasopharynx: Review of 86 cases which appeared in the Japanese literature. Archives of Otolaryngology, 56: 45.

10. Dawes, J. D., Harkness, D. G., Marshall, H. F., and Van Miert, P. J. 1969. Malignant disease of the nasopharynx. Journal of Laryngology and Otology, 83: 211.

11. De Schryver, A., Friberg, S., Jr., Klein, G. Henle, W., Henle, C., de-Thé, G., Clifford, P., and Ho, H. C. 1969. Epstein-Barr virus-associated antibody patterns in carcinoma of the postnasal space. Clinical and Experimental Immunology, 5: 443.

12. De Schryver, A., Lein, G., Henle, W., and Henle, G. 1974. EB virus-associated antibodies in Caucasian patients with carcinoma of the nasopharynx and in long-term survivors after treatment. International Journal of Cancer, 13: 319.

13. Desgranges, G., Wolf, H., de-Thé, G., Shanmugaratnam, K., Cammoun, N., Ellorey, R., Klein, G., Lennert, K., Minoz, N., and Zur Hausen, H. 1975. Nasopharyngeal carcinoma X: Presence of Epstein-Barr genomes in separated epithelial cells of tumours in patients from Singapore, Tunisia, and Kenya. International Journal of Cancer, 16: 7.

14. De-Thé, G., Ho, H. C., Ablashi, D. V., Day, N. E., Macario, A. J. L., Martin-Berthelon, M. C., Pearson, G., and Sohier, R. 1975. Nasopharyngeal carcinoma IX: Antibodies to EBVA and correlation with response to other EBV antigens in Chinese patients. International Journal of Cancer, 16: 713.

15. Godtfredsen, E. 1944. Ophthalmologic and Neurologic Symptoms of Malignant Nasopharyngeal Tumours: Clinical Study Comprising 454 Cases with Special Reference to Histopathology and Possibility of Earlier Recognition. Munksgaard, Copenhagen.

16. Hanham, I. W. F., Newton, K. A., and Westbury, G. 1971. Seventy-five cases of solid tumours treated by a modified quadruple chemotherapy regime. British Journal of Cancer, 25: 462.

17. Henderson, B. E., Louie, E., Bogdanoff, E., Henle, W., Alena, B., and Henle, G. 1974. Antibodies to herpes group viruses in patients with nasopharyngeal and other head and neck cancers. Cancer Research, 34: 1207.

18. Henle, W., Ho, H. C., Henle, G., and Kwan, H. C. 1973. Antibodies to Epstein-Barr virus-related antigen in nasopharyngeal carcinomas. Comparison of active cases and long-term survivors. Journal of the National Cancer Institute, 51: 361.

19. Henle, W., Henle, G., Ho, H. C., Burtin, P., Cachin, Y., Clifford, P., de Schryver, A., de-Thé, G., Diehl, V., and Klein, G., 1970. Antibodies to Epstein-Barr virus in nasopharyngeal carcinoma, other head and neck neoplasms, and control groups. Journal of the National Cancer Institute 33: 225.

20. Hiranandani, L. H. 1971. The management of cervical metastasis in head and neck cancers. Journal of Laryngology and Otology, 18: 1097.

21. Ho, H. C., 1967. Nasopharyngeal carcinoma in Hong Kong. In Muir, C. S., and Shanmugaratnam, K.; Eds.: Cancer of the Nasopharynx. Munksgaard, Copenhagen, 58.

22. Ho, H. C. 1970. The natural history and treatment of nasopharyngeal carcinoma. In Clark, L., Cumley, R. W., McCay, J. E., and Copeland, M. M., Eds.; Oncology, Vol. 4. Year Book Medical Publishers, Chicago, 1.

23. Ho, H. C. 1971. Genetic and environment factors in nasopharyngeal carcinoma. In Nakahara, W., Nishioka, K., Hirayma, T.,

and Ito, Y., Eds.: Recent Advances in Human Tumour Virology and Immunology, University of Tokyo Press, Tokyo, 275.

24. Ho, H. C. 1974. Diagnosis of nasopharyngeal carcinoma. Bulletin of the Hong Kong Medical Association, 26: 53.

25. Ho, H. C. 1975. Treatment of nasopharyngeal carcinoma. In Trujillo, M., Ed.: Progresos en Radiologia O.R.L. Editorial Marban, Madrid, 516.

26. Ho, H. C. 1976. Epstein-Barr virus and specific IgA and the IgG serus antibodies in nasopharyngeal carcinoma. British Journal of Cancer, 34: 655.

27. Ho, H. C. 1978. An epidemiologic and clinical study of nasopharyngeal carcinoma. International Journal of Radiation Oncology, Biology, Physics, 4: 181.

28. Kelemen, G. 1955. Experimental defects in the ear and upper airways induced by radiation. Archives of Otolaryngology, 61: 405.

29. Kelemen, G. 1964. Response of the Nervous System to Ionizing Radiation. Little, Brown, Boston.

30. Khoo, R. 1977. Personal communication.

31. Khoo, R. 1979. Personal communication.

32. Leach, W. 1965. Irradiation of the ear. Journal of Laryngology and Otology, 79: 870.

33. Lederman, M. 1961. Cancer of the Nasopharynx: Its Natural History and Treatment. Charles C. Thomas, Springfield, IL.

34. Lin, T. M., Yang, C. S., Ho, S. W., et al. 1971. Antibodies to herpes type virus. In Nakahara. W., et al., Eds.: Recent Advances in Human Tumour Virology and Immunology. University of Tokyo Press, Tokyo, 309.

35. Livingston, R. B., Einhorn, L. H., Burgess, M. A., Gottlieb, J. A., and Freireich, E. J. 1975. Advances in treatment of recurrent and disseminated squamous carcinoma of the lung, head and neck. In M. D. Anderson Hospital, Ed.: Cancer Chemotherapy. Year Book Medical Publishers, Chicago, 233.

36. McCabe, B. F., McGuirt, W. F. 1978. Significance of a neck node biopsy prior to definitive treatment for a metastatic cervical carcinoma. Laryngoscope, 88: 594.

37. Martin, H., and Quan, S. 1951. Racial incidence (Chinese) of nasopharyngeal cancer. Annals of Otology, Rhinology and Laryngology, 61: 168.

38. Martin, H., and Romieu, C. 1952. The diagnostic significance of a lump in the neck. Postgraduate Medicine, 11: 491.

39. Muir, C. S. 1972. Nasopharyngeal carcinoma in non-Chinese populations: Oncogenesis & herpes viruses. In Biggs, P. M., de-Thé, G., and Payne, L. N., Eds.: National Agency for Research on Cancer Publications, No. 2. Lyon, IARC, 367.

40. Old, L. J., Boyse, E. A., Oettgen, H. F., De-Harven, E., Geering, G., Williamson, B., and Clifford, P. 1966. Precipitation antibody in human serus to an antigen present in cultured Burkitt's lymphoma cells. Proceedings of the National Academy of Sciences, USA, 56: 1699.

41. Proetz, A. W. 1941. Essays of the Applied Physiology on the Nose. Annals Publishing Company, St. Louis.

42. Proetz, A. W. 1953. Respiratory air currents and their clinical aspects. Journal of Laryngology and Otology, 67: 1.

43. Reverchon, L., and Coutard, H. 1921. Bulletins et Memoirs de la Societé Française d'Otorhinolaryngologie 34: 209.

44. Richman, S. P., Livingston, R. B., Gutterman, J. U., Suen, J. Y., and Hersh, E. M. 1976. Chemotherapy versus chemoimmunotherapy of head and neck cancer: Report of a randomized study. Cancer Treatment Reports, 60: 535.

45. Rouviere, H. 1938. Anatomy of the Human Lymphatic System, Tobias, M. J. (translator) J. W. Edwards, Ann Arbor, MI.

46. Schmincke, A. 1921. Beitraege zur Pathologischen Anatomie and zur Allgemeinen Pathologie, 98: 161.

47. Shanmugaratnam, K., and Higginson, J. 1967. Aetiology of nasopharyngeal carcinoma. In Muir, C. S., and Shanmugaratnam, K., Eds.: Cancer of the Nasopharynx. Munksgaard, Copenhagen, 130.

48. Shanmugaratnam, K, Sobin, L. H., and pathologists in 10 countries. 1978. International Histological Classification of Tumours, No. 19 - Histological Typing of Upper Respiratory Tract Tumours, p. 19.

49. Sturton, S. D., Wen, H. L., and Sturton, O. G. 1966. Etiology of cancer of the nasopharynx. Cancer, 19: 1666.

50. Svoboda, D. J., Kirchner, F. R., and Shanmugaratnam, K. 1967. The fine structure of nasopharyngeal carcinomas. In Muir, C. S., and Shanmugaratnam, Eds.: Cancer of the Nasopharynx. Munksgaard, Copenhagen, 163.

51. Teoh, T. B. 1957. Epidermoid carcinoma of the nasopharynx among Chinese: A study of

31 necropsies. Journal of Pathology and Bacteriology, 73:   451.

52. Teoh, T. B. 1971. The pathologist and surgical pathology of head and neck tumours. Journal of the Royal College of Surgeons of Edinburgh, 16:   117.

53. U. I. C. C. 1973. Clinical Oncology—A Manual for Students and Doctors, edited by Committee on Professional Education of UICC. International Union Against Cancer, Geneva.

54. U. I. C. C. 1974. TNM Classification of Malignant tumours. 2nd ed. International Union Against Cancer, Geneva, 24.

55. Wilson, C. P. 1957. Observations on the surgery of the nasopharynx. Annals of Otology, Rhinology and Laryngology, 66:   5.

56. Wittes, R. E., Cvitkovic, E., Shah, J., Gerald, F. P., and Strong, E. W. 1977. Cis-dichlorodiammine platinum (II) in the treatment of epidermoid carcinoma of the head and neck. Cancer Treatment Reports, 61:   359.

57. Zippin, C., Tekawa, I. S., Bragg, K. U., Watson, D. A., and Linden, G. 1962 Studies on heredity and environment in cancer of the nasopharynx. Journal of the National Cancer Institute, 29:   483.

17 | Carcinoma of the Hypopharynx and Cervical Esophagus

Helmuth Goepfert, M.D.

The two goals in treatment of carcinoma of the hypopharynx and cervical esophagus are preservation of life and preservation or restoration of safe and useful laryngopharyngeal function. Selection of treatment is based upon a complete evaluation of the patient's condition, including regional and systemic disease, and knowledge of the natural history of the disease in the above-named locations.

Several features contribute to the poor prognosis associated with these carcinomas. Most of the patients who present for definitive treatment are chronic alcoholics who, are malnourished and have advanced malignant disease. The large size of the primary and the marked tendency toward submucosal spread requires extensive resection, which in most cases does not permit preservation of the larynx.[11, 30] The presence of large fixed ipsilateral or bilateral cervical lymph node deposits mitigates against regional control.

ANATOMY

The hypopharynx, or laryngopharynx, is generally regarded as extending from the free margin of the tip of the epiglottis to the lower border of the cricoid cartilage (Fig. 17-1A). A horizontal line drawn at the level of the hyoid bone is accepted as the border between the posterior oropharyngeal and hypopharyngeal walls. In the adult, the lower end of the hypopharynx corresponds approximately to the sixth cervical vertebra.

The cervical esophagus extends from the lower edge of the cricoid cartilage to the thoracic inlet.

The lumen of the hypopharynx is cone shaped, with the wider opening superior; it becomes more narrow in the postcricoid and cervical esophageal area. Within the hypopharynx, three distinct regions are recognized; the posterior pharyngeal wall, the pyriform sinuses, and the postcricoid area (Fig. 17-1B). The anterior wall of the hypopharynx opens directly into the larynx, and the posterior surfaces of the arytenoid cartilages form the upper boundary of the postcricoid area.

The wall of the hypopharynx is composed of four layers: an inner mucosal lining of stratified squamous epithelium over a loose stroma; a fibrous layer of pharyngeal aponeurisis; a muscular layer formed by the inferior constrictor muscle and, in the upper part, the distal portion of the middle constrictor, (the most distal fibers of the inferior constrictor condense into the cricopharyngeal muscle, and just proximal to this muscle is an area of relative weakness known as Killian's triangle); and an outer layer of fascia that derives from buccopharyngeal fascia.

Loose connective tissue separates the pharynx posteriorly from the deep cervical fascia which covers the underlying longus capitis and longus colli muscles and the fourth, fifth, and sixth cervical vertebrae.

The hypopharyngeal lumen is oval shaped. The two recesses lateral to the larynx are the pyriform sinuses. On horizontal

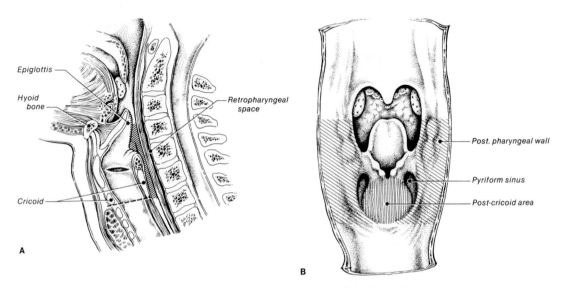

Fig. 17-1. (A and B) Anatomical regions of the hypopharynx.

cross section, the lumen is roughly triangular in shape, with the base posterior. The upper edges are at the pharyngoepiglottic folds and the lower edge is the upper border of the cricoid cartilage. Laterally, each pyriform sinus is bound by thyrohyoid membrane and by the thyroid ala. At the junction of the middle and lower thirds of the pyriform sinus, a mucosal fold is visible on the lateral wall that covers the internal branch of the superior laryngeal nerve. The proximity of this nerve accounts for the referred otalgia that is often found in lesions of this area and makes the nerve particularly vulnerable as a route of spread (Fig. 17-2). Medially, the pyriform sinuses are bound by the aryepiglottic fold and the arytenoid cartilages. The upper portion of the pyriform sinus is the vestibule.

On cross section, the postcricoid area is oval when noted on direct laryngoscopy. In the resting state, the lumen is closed by the cricopharyngeal muscle. The terminal portions of each recurrent laryngeal nerve are encountered between the fibers of this muscle and the posterior cricoarytenoid of the larynx. Motor and sensory nerve supply to the hypopharynx is provided through the pharyngeal plexus formed by branches of the glossopharyngeal and vagus nerves and the superior laryngeal nerves of the vagus. The arterial supply derives from branches

of the superior thyroid arteries to the larynx and collateral vessels from the lingual and ascending pharyngeal arteries.

There is a rich lymphatic network draining the pharynx and cervical esopha-

HYPOPHARYNX AND CERVICAL ESOPHAGUS

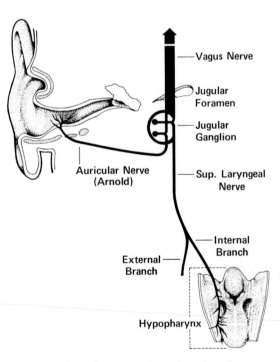

Fig. 17-2. Anatomical explanation for referred otalgia.

gus. The collecting channels of the pharyngeal wall drain primarily into the nodes along the internal jugular vein at the subdigastric, carotid triangle, and midjugular portions. There are lymphatic vessels draining the pyriform sinus; these vessels follow the superior laryngeal nerves through the cricothyroid membrane. The first echelon nodes draining the pyriform sinus are in the jugulocarotid triangle. The retropharyngeal nodes of Rouviere, close to the base of the skull, are the site of drainage for lymphatics of the posterior pharyngeal wall and, although seldom clinically obvious on initial examination because of their location, are microscopically positive in up to 40 percent of cancers that involve the posterior pharynx[4] (Fig. 17-3). The nodes along the recurrent nerves and the paratracheal nodes are preferred sites for metastasis of lesions originating in the lower portion of the hypopharynx and the cervical esophagus.[28]

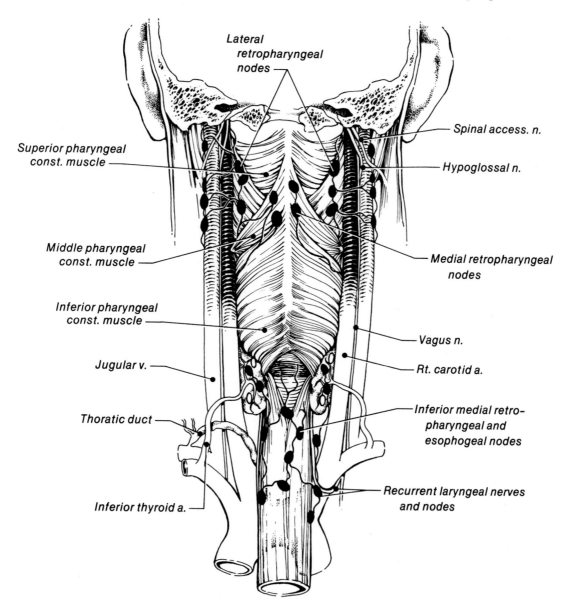

Fig. 17-3. Lymphatic drainage of hypopharynx and cervical esophagus as viewed from posterior.

The junction between the postcricoid area and the cervical esophagus is the narrowest portion of the upper alimentary tract and is called the cricopharyngeus. The esophagus is lined by nonkeratinizing squamous epithelium over a loose stroma and muscular layers consisting of an inner circular and an outer longitudinal layer covered by a fascial sheath. Between the cricopharyngeal and upper portion of the esophageal musculature is Lanier's triangle. The outermost layer of the cervical esophagus is continuous with the buccopharyngeal fascia. This layer separates the esophagus from the retroesophageal space posteriorly which is in continuity with the retropharyngeal space above and the posterior mediastinum below.

Anteriorly, the cervical esophagus is in direct relation to the trachea though it deviates slightly to the left of this organ. In the tracheoesophageal groove on both sides, the recurrent laryngeal nerves and the paratracheal nodes are found. The lateral lobes of the thyroid gland and, more lateral, the carotid sheaths and their contents are related to the cervical esophagus. The lobes of the thyroid gland may be involved by direct extension of tumors from the pyriform sinus. The nerve supply is provided by branches of the recurrent laryngeal nerves and the vascular supply by branches of the inferior thyroid arteries and ascending vessels from the thoracic esophagus. The lymphatic system drains primarily into the paratracheal and upper mediastinal lymph nodes and into the nodes on the lowest portion of the jugular chains.

ETIOLOGY

The etiology of cancer in this area is no more definitively established than it is for the other locations in the upper aerodigestive tract.[22] Excessive smoking and alcohol consumption along with associated nutritional deficiencies seem to be common denominators in most cases.[24] Alcohol by itself is probably not carcinogenic, but the associated vitamin deficiency may be cocarcinogenic.[43] In northern Europe, the high incidence of the Paterson-Brown-Kelly or Plummer-Vinson syndrome has been associated with a high incidence of postcricoid carcinoma, particularly in nonsmoking women. Correction of this disorder appears to have decreased the incidence of this cancer.[27]

At present, it is not known if any food additive or deficiency in early life is a causative factor. Further studies in this area and in the field of genetics are under way in different parts of the world, but information is difficult to accrue and no definitive explanations have been derived.[43] The possible influences of vitamin A and C deficiencies in the pathogenesis and progression of cancer in this area need further clarification.[10]

CLASSIFICATION

Practically all malignant neoplasms in this location are squamous cell carcinomas predominately of the poorly differentiated type. Most cancers of the hypopharynx originate in the pyriform sinus (66 to 75 percent), fewer in the posterior pharyngeal wall (20 to 25 percent), and fewer still in the postcricoid area. Occasionally a malignant tumor of salivary gland origin is encountered.[38] Benign or malignant mesenchymal tumors are rare.[36]

PATIENT EVALUATION

Symptoms

The triad of pain in the throat, referred otalgia (usually unilateral), and dysphagia is present in over one-half of patients with cancer of the hypopharynx. Hoarseness and other symptoms of laryngeal dysfunction occur in more advanced tumors of the pyriform sinus and pharyngeal wall as well as in cases of postcricoid or cervical esophageal cancer invading the recurrent laryngeal nerves or the arytenoid cartilages. Careful questioning will often reveal difficulty in swallowing, even for liquids, repeated "clearing of the throat," and a feeling of a foreign body lodged somewhere in the throat. In rare instances, the patient with a lesion of the postcricoid area or cervical esophagus manifests rapid progressive dysphagia from an early superficial, concentric, narrowing cancer without spread of the cancer outside of the organ. Progressive difficulty in deglutition is responsible for weight loss, which enhances the malnutrition that commonly accompanies cancer in these locations. Excessive salivation, often blood-tinged, is sometimes reported in more advanced lesions.

Up to 25 percent of patient with lesions of the pyriform sinus and/or the pharyngeal wall present to the physician with a palpable mass in the neck without symptoms referring to the primary tumor. The progressive enlargement of retropharyngeal nodes, although seldom an initial symptom, will produce occipital and nape-of-the-neck pain, often referred to the orbit; this pain is relieved by slight head flexion.

Signs

Indirect mirror examination will, in most cancers of the hypopharynx and pyriform sinuses, identify the primary lesion and its extent, although the distal extent of the tumor may be difficult to determine. Tumors of the postcricoid area and cervical esophagus may attain considerable size before any changes become visible by indirect laryngoscopy. The findings of edema and erythema of the postcricoid area and pooling of secretions in the hypopharynx are important indirect signs of the underlying pathology, as it may not be possible to visualize the pyriform sinus in late stages. The absence of laryngeal crepitus when mobilizing the laryngeal framework over the cervical spine indicates an abnormality between the structures. Vocal cord mobility and adequacy of laryngeal function should be established clinically to determine the extent of disease and to help decide upon a treatment modality.

Direct extension of the cancer into the tissues of the neck and into the prevertebral fascia should be searched for by manual examination, but may be difficult to differentiate from involvement from first-echelon lymph node metastasis. The pyriform sinus can be the site of a small primary tumor in a patient presenting with a mass in the neck, so this area should be one of the sites diligently examined under these circumstances. It may be necessary to use local anesthesia, systemic sedation, or both to perform an appropriate inspection on the initial visit.

The weight of the patient should be recorded and compared to the patient's usual weight to determine recent weight loss.

Patterns of Spread

Tumors of the pharyngeal wall and pyriform sinus can arise from any of the walls, rapidly become infiltrating and ulcerative, and show extensive submucosal spread (Fig. 17-4). It is not unusual to find up to 10 mm of submucosal extension beyond what can be clinically appreciated within the pyriform sinus, and up to 5 mm of submucosal spread in a postcricoid cancer is not unusual (Fig. 17-5). In the cervical esophagus, cancers are notorious for submucosal extension and apparent "skip areas." Furthermore, several areas of carcinoma in situ usually surround the main tumor. Synchronous primaries may be found in the hypopharynx and cervical esophagus.[11, 18, 26]

Cancers of the posterior pharyngeal wall usually become quite large before invading prevertebral fascia, muscles, or vertebral bodies. Tumors arising within the pyriform sinus often invade the medial wall and produce vocal cord fixation or they may extend laterally through the cricoid cartilage and may involve the thyroid gland or adjacent soft tissue. Cancers of the postcricoid area and cervical esophagus often impair laryngeal function by invading the recurrent laryngeal nerves. Cancers of the cervical esophagus may also grow into the tracheal wall and create tracheoesophageal fistulae.

The lymphatic vessels are frequently

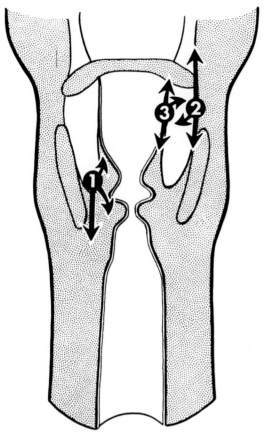

Fig. 17-4. Lesions in the pyriform sinus may extend into several adjacent structures, depending on their site of origin. Lesions located superiorly (2 or 3) are sometimes suitable for conservative surgery, and exophytic tumors in these locations are amenable to curative radiotherapy; tumors invading the apex (1) are not suitable for conservation surgery. (Fletcher, G. H., 1980. Textbook of Radiotherapy, 3rd edn., Lea and Febiger, Philadelphia, 358.)

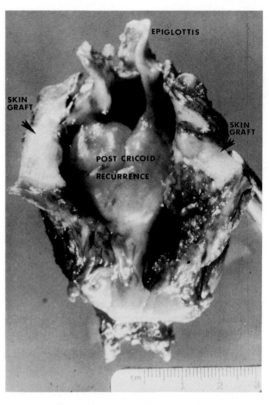

Fig. 17-5. A 61-year-old man underwent a transhyoid pharyngostomy and excision of a squamous cell carcinoma of the hypopharyngeal wall, extending from the tip of the epiglottis to the arytenoid and insinuating into the vestibule of the left pyriform sinus. Neck was negative for nodes. Split-thickness graft was used for repair. Postoperative radiotherapy was given in 6,000 rads over 6 weeks to primary and adjacent lymph node areas. Eight months later the patient returned with recurrent tumor in the pyriform sinus and retrocricoid area. A total laryngopharyngectomy was performed. Arrows point to previously skin-grafted areas in the specimen.

invaded, and extension along perineural spaces occurs erratically. Lymph nodes metastases, frequently bilateral, are found on initial examination in up to 60 percent of patients with cancer of the posterior pharyngeal wall.[28] Lymph node metastases from the pyriform sinus are present in 75 percent of the patients. Metastases from the postcricoid area and cervical esophagus may not be apparent because of early involvement of the paratracheal nodes, which are not easily palpable. Metastases to the nodes of Rouviere have been found in up to 44 percent of patients with disease involving the pharyngeal walls[5, 18] (Fig. 17-6).

Special Diagnostic Studies

RADIOLOGY

Soft-tissue radiographs of the neck, barium swallow esophograms, contrast laryngo-

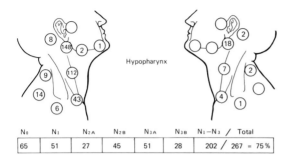

N₀	N₁	N₂ₐ	N₂ᵦ	N₃ₐ	N₃ᵦ	N₁–N₃ / Total
65	51	27	45	51	28	202 / 267 = 75%

Fig. 17-6. Distribution of clinically positive lymph nodes in patients with cancer of the hypopharynx. (Lindberg, R. D. 1972. Distribution of cervical lymph node metastases from squamous cell carcinoma of the upper respiratory and digestive tract. Cancer, 29:1446.)

grams, polytomograms, and computerized tomograms are important studies used in establishing the site of origin of the primary tumor, extension of disease, and impairment of function of the involved structures. It is important to employ only those studies that are necessary. Whenever possible, these should be done prior to endoscopic and biopsy maneuvers, as such maneuvers cause edema and may distort the structures, making radiologic assessments less than satisfactory. If endoscopic and biopsy examinations are performed first, a delay of 5 to 7 days is advisable before subjecting the patient to radiologic examination.

Lateral soft-tissue radiographs of the neck or lateral xerograms are useful in judging the thickness of the retropharyngeal and/or retroesophageal space in lesions of the pharyngeal wall or cervical esophagus as an indication of the direct extension of disease. These radiographs may also reveal direct extension and involvement of the cervical vertebrae.

Contrast laryngograms in the anteroposterior and lateral projections can establish the distal extent of the lesion and may detect tumor in the distal third of the pyriform sinus. They are particularly useful when conservation surgery is being considered. Contrast laryngograms may contribute important information such as failure of the pyriform sinuses to fill, distortion of the

radiographic architecture of the larynx, and absence of mobility of the vocal cords.

The barium swallow esophagram should also be recorded in at least two projections. Abnormalities include displacement of the contrast medium, obstruction of the barium column, aspiration of the barium into the larynx and trachea, and partial filling or nonfilling of any of the studied segments. With the exception of cases of total obstruction, this study permits establishment of the distal extent of lesions of the postcricoid area and cervical esophagus.

Coronal polytomograms may be helpful in determining the site of origin and extent of lesions of the pyriform sinus. Occasionally this study will show destruction of cartilage. It is a safe radiologic study that can be performed even in cases of impending upper airway obstruction.

Computerized tomograms may help delineate the extent of soft tissue involvement and can be an important adjunct in determining cartilage, or bone invasion or both.

ENDOSCOPY

Endoscopic examination helps to confirm the extent of the tumor, rule out the existence of synchronous primary cancers, and obtain a specimen for histologic diagnosis. Triple endoscopic examination may give important supplemental information and occasionally will uncover a synchronous primary tumor undetectable otherwise. I do not perform multiple biopsies around the tumor to establish its exact extent, as these may distort the regional anatomy and theoretically could implant tumor cells.

Other Evaluative Studies

The chest x-ray examination and a guided search for distant metastasis based upon history, symptoms, and signs completes the pretreatment evaluation. Because of chronic alcoholism, liver function studies are frequently abnormal in patients with head and neck cancers. Routine isotope scanning of the liver seldom identifies early metastasis.

If an operation is contemplated that will spare the larynx, evaluation of pulmonary function is mandatory.

In recent years, testing for delayed hypersensitivity to intradermally injected antigens and other immunologic studies has become more common. Most patients with advanced head and neck cancer are known to be anergic. It remains to be established if this anergy is due to the patient's tumor burden, is in part a response to malnutrition, or was present and was a contributing factor to the development of the cancer. The patient's nutritional status is established through determination of percentage of weight loss and level of serum albumin. Frequently, these patients need nutritional preparation and replenishment prior to or concomitantly with treatment.

Staging

According to the American Joint Committee for Cancer Staging and End Results Reporting,[2] primary lesions of the hypopharynx are classified as follows:

T1S   Carcinoma in situ;

T1   Tumor confined to the site of origin;

T2   Extension of tumor to adjacent regional site without fixation of the hemilarynx;

T3   Extension of tumor to adjacent regional site with fixation of the hemilarynx; and

T4   Massive tumor invading bone, and/or cartilage, and/or soft tissues of the neck.

For lesions of the cervical esophagus, the recommended staging system is the same as that used for the interthoracic portion of the esophagus:

T1S   Carcinoma in situ;

T1   Tumor that involves 5 cm or less esophageal length, produces no obstruction, and has no circumferential involvement or extraesophageal spread;

T2   Tumor that involves more than 5 cm of esophageal length, without extraesophageal spread, or any size tumor involving the entire circumference of the organ and that produces obstruction;

T3   Any tumor with evidence of extraesophageal spread as judged by clinical, roentgenologic, and endoscopic evidence, and/or fistula formation into the trachea, and/or venous obstruction in the thoracic inlet.

The nodal classification system for the hypopharynx is the same as for the other sites in the head and neck. However, for the esophageal primary lesions the following system is used: N0—no palpable nodes; N1—movable, unilateral, palpable nodes; N2—movable, bilateral, palpable nodes: and N3—fixed nodes.

SELECTION OF TREATMENT

The important factors in selecting treatment modalities or combinations thereof include patient factors, extent of disease, involvement of the laryngeal framework, and presence and extent of lymph node metastasis. Only a few patients with pharyngeal wall or pyriform sinus cancers are amenable to partial pharyngectomy or partial laryngopharyngectomy with satisfactory functional results (Figs. 17-7 A–C). The patient should not be endangered by ill-advised conservation procedures; therefore, most patients must undergo a laryngectomy as part of the ablative procedure.[8, 11, 20, 33]

Surgical resection and radiation therapy either alone or in combination provide the mainstays of curative treatment. Early lesions of the pharyngeal wall and pyriform sinus can be treated by either modality with good results and preservation of function. Radiation therapy has a definite place in the management of early primary (particularly exophytic) tumors of the pharyngeal wall and pyriform sinus.[32] This modality has infrequently cured patients with lesions of the postcricoid area and cervical esophagus.[23]

Surgical management of lesions of the pharyngeal wall allows preservation of a functioning larynx in fewer than one-half of

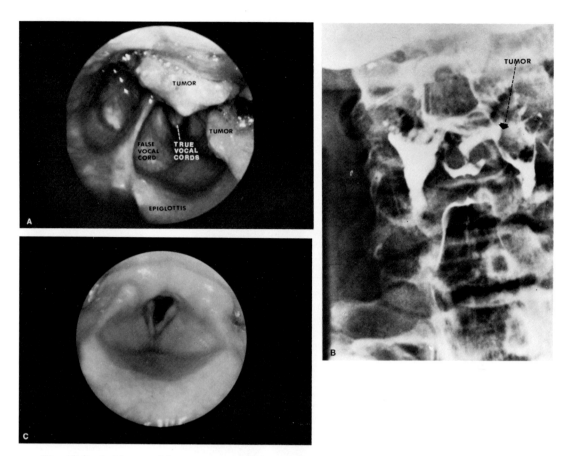

Fig. 17-7. A 64-year-old man presented in October 1975 with a 3-month history of a sore throat, during which time he had lost 14 pounds. (A and B) A lesion occupied the vestibule of the left pyriform sinus, with extension onto the posterior pharyngeal wall. One lymph node was palpable in the left side of the neck at the jugulocarotid area. At surgery, the patient was found to have a squamous cell carcinoma of the pyriform sinus vestibule extending onto the pharyngeal wall. He underwent a supraglottic laryngectomy, resection of the pharyngeal wall and part of the pyriform sinus, and a left modified neck dissection. He was given radiation treatment postoperatively: 6,000 rads in 6½ weeks to the upper neck and 5,000 rads to the lower. One year later the patient was free of disease. (C) A laryngoscopic picture shows the state of the larynx (Fletcher, G. H. and Goepfert, H. 1977. Irradiation in management of squamous cell carcinomas of the larynx. In English, G. M., Ed.: Otolaryngology. Vol. V. Harper & Row, Hagerstown, MD., Ch. 39.)

cases. In most instances, a total laryngo-pharyngectomy and reconstruction of the alimentary tract are necessary. Margins of excision should be checked by frozen-section evaluation to assure adequate removal of cancer. The selection of the reconstructive procedure depends upon the experience of the team caring for the patient and the availability of regional tissue or pedicled segments of the gastrointestinal tract that need to be brought into the surgically created defect (Figs. 17-8 A and B and 17-9).

Cancer of the pyriform sinus allows preservation of the larynx in less than 2 percent of cases, and this procedure is not feasible when disease extends into the lower third or apex of the pyriform sinus. The extent of regional lymph node involvement and the treatment modality chosen for the primary determine the mode of nodal ther-

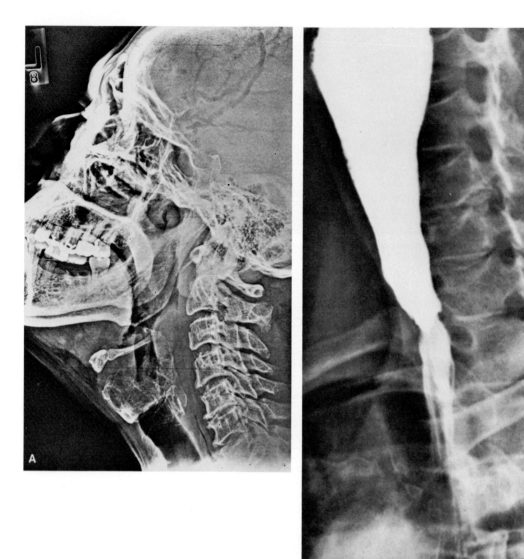

Fig. 17-8. (A) This is the lateral xerogram of a 57-year-old man with a squamous carcinoma extending from the right torus tubarius to the level of the arytenoids and involving 30 percent of the circumference of the pharyngeal wall. Direct extension into the neck was palpable, but no nodes were felt. A laryngopharyngectomy and neck dissection were performed for squamous carcinoma, grade III and metastatic disease was found in 1 of 35 cervical lymph nodes. Repair was accomplished by a deltopectoral flap. No other therapy was given. The patient has remained free of disease for 3 years. (B) Postoperative barium swallow.

apy. For further details on management of regional lymphatics, see Chapter 10.

Cancer of the cervical esophagus may seldom be treated by surgical resection and visceral bypass without removal of the lar-

ynx and upper portion of the trachea (Figs. 17-10 A and B). Cervical esophageal and postcricoid cancer usually require a pharyngoesophagolaryngectomy and reconstruction.[4, 12]

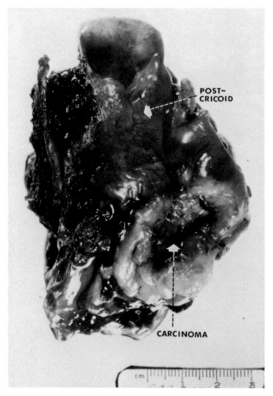

POST-
CRICOID

CARCINOMA

Fig. 17-9. Surgical specimen from a 60-year-old woman with a squamous cell carcinoma of the postcricoid area and a 25-year history of pernicious anemia. She had lost 4 pounds in one month. A total pharyngolaryngoesophagectomy was performed for a lesion that extended through the full thickness of the postcricoid pharyngeal wall. Colon interposition was performed, with the proximal anastomosis at the base of the tongue. The patient was able to swallow within 10 days and remained free of disease 2 years later.

A treatment program combining surgery and irradiation should be considered whenever the location and extent of the primary tumor and/or the number of lymph node metastases make microscopic subclinical disease likely (Figs. 17-11 A–C). Several studies on combined treatment indicate that whenever surgery and postoperative radiation are chosen, tolerance is superior to that of preoperative radiotherapy and sur-

gery.[25, 35, 36, 41] Most patients already have impaired deglutition, and the edema and local inflammation produced by preoperative radiotherapy further downgrades their nutritional status.

The use of total parenteral nutrition to carry these patients through part or all of their treatment has definitely enhanced therapeutic possibilities, but it remains to be seen if this will increase the overall scope and results of treatment. Consideration should be given to nutritional replenishment prior to any treatment whenever a patient presents with over 10 percent weight loss and/or serum albumin level below 3.5 percent. Experience with nutritional therapy thus far shows improvement in healing after surgery with fewer local and systemic complications; it still is not known if the change in the immunologic reactivity will affect the prognosis of these patients.

Systemic chemotherapy with single and multiple agents has been tried for over a decade for patients with advanced stage disease. Systemic chemotherapy has been recommended in recent years as an adjuvant before and/or after conventional treatment. Several schedules of single-drug and multiple-drug regimens are under evaluation, but there is no conclusive evidence yet that such adjuvant therapy has improved overall results. It should be noted that the addition of aggressive chemotherapy substantially increases the cost of patient care and very often results in considerable morbidity.

The field of immunology is rapidly developing, and several types of immunomodulation have been used to treat the impaired delayed hypersensitivity common to patients with head and neck cancer.[40] Trials with bacillus Calmette-Guérin in several forms have proved unsuccessful, and positive reports on any attempt at immunomodulation are lacking. The simplistic attitude originally adopted toward restoration of host-immunologic response has probably contributed to the failure thus far. Further work is necessary in this field.

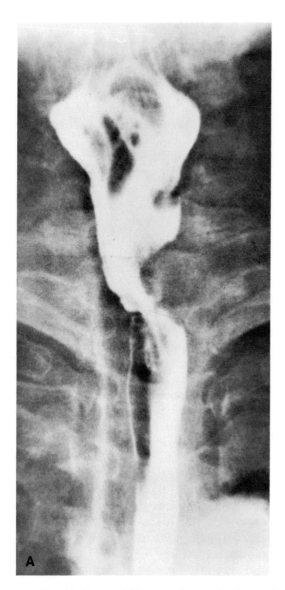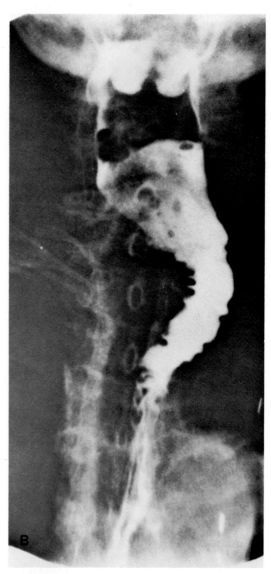

Fig. 17-10. (A) A 77-year-old man had a carcinoma of the cervical esophagus extending to the level of the thoracic inlet and causing partial obstruction. Cervical esophagectomy plus left thyroid lobectomy and regional node dissection were performed for an invasive carcinoma with metastasis to one regional node. (B) A colon interposition was performed, with anastomosis to the apex of the left pyriform sinus. The patient was able to swallow with 10 days and was given postoperative radiation therapy, 5,000 rads in 5 weeks, to a field that covered the primary mediastinum. A year and a half later, the patient was free of any recurrence or metastases.

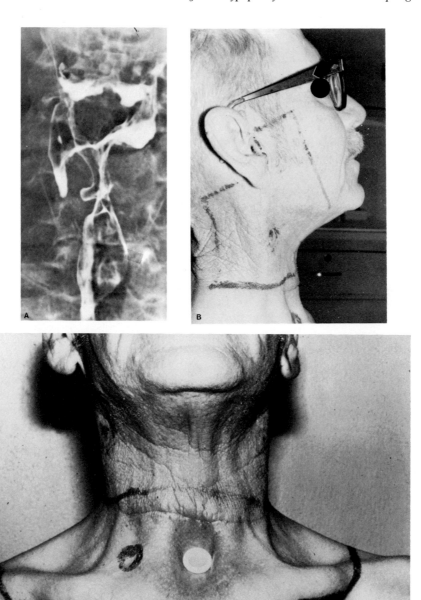

Fig. 17-11. A 62-year-old man presented in May 1974 with several clinically positive nodes in the left subdigastric and midjugular areas, another subdigastric node on the right side, and a lesion in the pyriform sinus. (A) Laryngogram shows obliteration of the pyriform sinus, ventricle, and subglottic angle on the left. Biopsy examination revealed squamous cell carcinoma. On May 20, 1974, the patient underwent a laryngectomy and partial pharyngectomy, left radical neck dissection, and right modified neck dissection. The specimen revealed in situ carcinoma at the lateral pharyngeal wall margin. (B and C) From June 11, 1974 to July 26, 1974, the patient received a tumor dose of 6,000 rads of radiation to the upper neck field and 5,000 rads to the lower neck fields. The parapharyngeal lymphatics received 5,000 rads. Because of extensive subglottic disease, the stoma was irradiated with a plastic stomal button in place. The patient had no evidence of disease as of November 17, 1976. (Fletcher, G. H., and Goepfert, H. 1977. Irradiation in management of squamous cell carcinomas of the larynx. In English, G. M., Ed.: Otolaryngology. Vol. V. Harper & Row, Hagerstown, MD, Ch. 39.)

SURGICAL RECONSTRUCTION

Split-thickness skin grafts and regional flaps have been used extensively in the reconstruction of defects in the hypopharynx and cervical esophagus.[4, 6, 7, 37] Small defects of the pharyngeal wall can be covered by skin grafts; but whenever a total circumferential replacement of the hypopharynx or cervical esophagus is required, the results are less favorable because of delayed healing and stricture formation at the site of the repair.

The use of regional flaps in the form of medially-based or laterally-based deltopectoral skin flaps usually requires a multistage procedure for completion; this adds to the recovery time and expense of hospitalization and delays effective postoperative radiation therapy for an undesirable period.[4] The use of myocutaneous flaps (pectoralis major, trapezius) has allowed reconstruction to be performed in a single stage procedure.[3]

For the reconstruction of defects following the resection of postcricoid and cervical esophageal carcinoma, either a regional skin flap, a pharyngogastric anastomosis with or without total esophagectomy, or a colon bypass should be considered.[1, 4, 12, 16, 17, 21, 31] One advantage of the two intestinal procedures is that the patient is subjected to only one surgical procedure in the neck, and although the operation initially is more extensive, the results are satisfactory—with acceptable morbidity and mortality rates—if the procedure is performed by an experienced, coordinated team.

The pharyngogastric anastomosis ("gastric pull-up"), which requires mobilization of the stomach and its advancement through the posterior mediastinum, can be done in conjunction with total esophagectomy. It seems to offer good therapeutic results for curative purposes and has also been recognized as a satisfactory means of palliation.[1, 21] Even with local recurrence, the large lumen at the anastomosis is rarely obstructed. Other advantages are that no anastomosis is required within the abdomen, and patients experience little or no regurgitation.

The colon bypass is preferred by some physicians because it entails less surgical intervention within the chest and can be performed even if the patient has previously had upper abdominal surgery. It has been found that selective mesenteric arteriography allows one to choose the most appropriate, well-vascularized colonic segment, and has greatly reduced the incidence of cervical anastomotic breakdowns.[42] For either the pharyngogastric anastomosis or colon bypass to be done expeditiously, two teams of surgeons are needed.

Free-vascularized intestinal transplants in the form of autografts have been studied experimentally using microvascular techniques, but in only a few cases has this procedure been successful in humans. Unfortunately, it is time consuming and often accompanied by unacceptable complications. It clearly needs further study and refinement.[16]

It is difficult to recommend a standard method of reconstruction, since this will vary according to the experience of the surgeon and the extent of the disease present. Some methods of reconstruction can be found in Chapter 27.

POSTOPERATIVE CARE AND REHABILITATION

An important part of nursing care, begun prior to surgery, consists of preparing the patient for future changes and giving him enough motivation for self-care. The more aggressive the nurses' teachings, the better the patient will be able to handle his own rehabilitation.

Adequate replacement of fluids lost during surgery and aggressive pulmonary cleansing are of paramount importance. The tracheostomy facilitates pulmonary care, and the nasogastric or gastrostomy tube is used for decompression until intestinal mobility has been resumed. Nasogastric or gastrostomy feeding can then be instituted gradually. Early ambulation is necessary to avoid complications secondary to stasis. Most patients should walk the morning after surgery.

Whenever a laryngeal-preservation procedure is performed, the teaching of deglutition is necessary and can often be performed by speech pathologists and/or physical therapists. It should be initiated after postoperative laryngopharyngeal edema has subsided and the nasogastric tube is removed. Patients who undergo a total laryngectomy need to be trained in some means of communication. Unfortunately, whenever the entire pharynx or cervical esophagus is replaced by skin pedicles or a viscus, the goal of oral communication is often incompletely achieved.

The presence of a segment of large bowel without the propulsory activity of the normal pharynx and esophagus occasionally presents deglutition problems especially when the segment has to be anastomosed at the level of the oropharynx. The consistency of foods should be adjusted to accommodate this shortcoming of the repaired segment.

Most of the early complications are due to leakage from the site of the pharyngo-esophageal wall repair. Previous radiation therapy—regardless of whether it was planned—is accompanied by the highest incidence of wound breakdown, especially if the patient is malnourished. If there is any doubt as to the patient's healing abilities, a controlled pharyngeal fistula should be established. Fistulization occurs frequently because of an over-zealous attempt to close the hypopharynx without having enough mucosa available. Complications secondary to partial laryngectomy, such as chronic aspiration and repeated pulmonary infection, may later require removal of the larynx.[15] (See Ch. 28 for more detailed discussion.)

END RESULTS

The literature regarding cancer of the hypopharynx and cervical esophagus contains abundant descriptions of surgical and reconstructive procedures for such lesions. Several authors have emphasized the reasons for treatment failures.[6, 9, 19, 34, 39] A tendency toward extensive microscopic regional infiltration and a high incidence of distant

TABLE 17-1. RESULTS OF TREATMENT OF CANCER OF THE HYPOPHARYNX

Study	Modality*	Survival Rate in Percent (Years)
Carpenter and	S	52 (3)
DeSanto[11]	S	47 (5)
Shah et al.[36]	S, S+X	25.9 (5)
	S, S+X	20 (10)
Rasack et al.[34]	S	28 (5)
	S+X	37.3 (5)
Vandenbrouck et al.[41]	X+S	56 (5)
Inoue and Shigematsu[23]	X	36 (3)
	X	25 (5)
MacComb and	S	15.9 (5)
Fletcher[29]	X	15.2 (5)
Stefani and Eells[39]	-----	9.1 (5)

*S, surgery, X, irradiation; S+X/X+S, combined.

metastases and second primaries are common with these lesions. In any series of patients, the method of treatment selection affects the results achieved. The analysis of reported results is further complicated by the fact that some series identify each location separately, whereas in other reports the hypopharynx is not subdivided (Table 17-1). Furthermore, cancer of the hypopharyngeal wall is often grouped with cancer of the oropharyngeal wall.

Unfortunately, the existing evidence regarding the value of planned combined treatment (surgery and irradiation) is conflicting, and although it seems that this combination helps reduce the incidence of recurrence above the clavicle, the overall survival rate has not shown improvement.[34, 36]

Hypopharyngeal Wall

Guillamondequi et al.[18] and Meoz-Mendez et al.[32] have recently reported on the results of radiation, surgery, and combined therapy for cancer of the hypopharyngeal wall. For early lesions, surgery and irradiation are equally effective. Control at the primary site can be expected, and laryngeal function can be preserved. About 75 percent of pa-

tients, however, present with large primary tumors and advanced nodal disease and, therefore, have a predictably worse prognosis. Aggressive combined therapy is required under such circumstances, but in spite of it, the survival rate is still quite low. Failure at the primary site is common. There is a 20 percent failure rate in the neck. Second primary cancers account for 15 percent of failures.

Postoperative irradiation frequently has to be postponed beyond the ideal time period because of delayed healing and prolonged repairs. This could decrease the local control rate, since gross disease may be present when the postoperative irradiation has begun.

Pyriform Sinus

Many discrepancies exist in the results reported for cancer of the pyriform sinus. Early lesions are handled equally well by a conservative laryngeal procedure and by irradiation.[13, 14, 29, 30, 33] The more common advanced lesions require total laryngectomy, and the best results reported for these lesions is a 41 percent 5-year survival rate for patients treated by surgery alone (Table 17-2). Very often this is the only modality

TABLE 17-2. RESULTS OF TREATMENT OF CANCER OF THE PYRIFORM SINUS

Study	Modality*	Survival Rate in Percent (Years)
McGavran et al.[30]	S	50 (3)
	S	41 (5)
MacComb and Fletcher[29]	S, S+X	26 (3)
	S, S+X	18.8 (3)
Kirchner[26]	S	29 (3)
	X+S	36 (3)
Jesse and Lindberg[25]	S	22 (5)
	S+X	33 (5)
Fletcher and Goepfert[14]	S+X	50(2)

*S, surgery, X, irradiation, S+X/X+S, combined.

of treatment a patient with an advanced lesion will tolerate. Surgery followed by radiotherapy has an acceptable morbidity rate and offers the best regional control of disease. The long-term survival rate is not substantially improved, in part because such patients develop distant metastases.[14] The overall 5-year survival rate by combination treatment is 40 to 50 percent in the best of circumstances (Table 17-2). Byers and Krueger[9a] in a recent review of patients with advanced carcinoma of the pyriform sinus (T3 and T4 with significant neck node metastases) treated by surgery and postoperative radiation therapy found only 23 percent free of disease after 2 years. Fifty-one percent of patients died of their cancer, including four patients with positive retropharyngeal node metastases and five of six patients with positive bilateral lymph node metastases. At present, an aggressive approach with preoperative chemotherapy is under evaluation by several cooperative groups, but no conclusive evidence is available yet that would indicate a substantial improvement in survival rates.

Postcricoid Area and Cervical Esophagus

Irradiation alone produces few satisfactory results with cancer of the postcricoid area and cervical esophagus. Whenever a surgical resection and bypass procedure is feasible, the results are better and the patient's comfort is markedly enhanced. Many of the failures are due to spread of disease beyond the scope of regional therapy. The review of existing literature shows a wide range in five-year survival figures reported, from 20 to 50 percent.[9] One has to wonder if these populations have different selection factors.

The information on combined treatment results is meager. Limited tolerance of irradiation of the interposed colonic segment is often a restricting factor. The use of indwelling esophageal stents for palliation seldom enhances the patient's comfort and often causes complications that defeat its purpose.

SUMMARY

The technical refinements and therapeutic innovations acquired by the head and neck cancer team during the last decade have enhanced the scope of therapy in the field of cancer of the hypopharynx and cervical esophagus. The improvement in survival, though, has been meager; and by and large the results continue to be disappointing.

To improve on the present results of therapy, means for earlier diagnosis and new modalities of treatment will have to be developed.

REFERENCES

1. Akiyama, H., Hiyama, M., Miyazono, H. 1975. Total esophageal reconstruction after extraction of the esophagus. Annals of Surgery 182: 547.

2. American Joint Committee for Cancer Staging and End Results Reporting. 1977. Manual for Staging of Cancer. American Joint Committee, Chicago.

3. Ariyan, S. 1979. The pectoralis major myocutaneous flap. A versatile flap for reconstruction in the head and neck. Plastic and Reconstructive Surgery, 63: 73.

4. Bakamjian, V. Y. 1965. A two-stage method for pharyngoesophageal reconstruction with a primary pectoral skin flap. Plastic and Reconstructive Surgery, 36: 173.

5. Ballantyne, A. J. 1964. Significance of retropharyngeal nodes in cancer of the head and neck. American Journal of Surgery, 108: 500.

6. Ballantyne, A. J. 1967. Principles of surgical management of cancer of the pharyngeal walls. Cancer, 20: 663.

7. Ballantyne, A. J. 1971. Methods of repair after surgery for cancer of the pharyngeal wall, postcricoid area, and cervical esophagus. American Journal of Surgery, 122: 482.

8. Briant, T. D. R., Bryce, D. P., and Smith, T. J. 1977. Carcinoma of the hypopharynx —a five-year follow-up. Journal of Otolaryngology, 6: 353.

9. Burdette, W. J., and Jesse, R. 1972. Carcinoma of the cervical esophagus. Journal of Thoracic and Cardiovascular Surgery, 63: 41.

9a. Byers, R. M., Krueger, W. W., and Saxton, J.

1979. Use of surgery and postoperative radiation in the treatment of advanced squamous cell carcinoma of the pyriform sinus. American Journal of Surgery, 138: 597.

10. Cameron, E., Pauling, L. Leibovitz, B. 1979. Ascorbic acid and cancer: A review. Cancer Research, 39: 663.

11. Carpenter, R. J., III and DeSanto, L. W. 1977. Cancer of the hypopharynx. Surgical Clinics of North America, 57: 723.

12. Fairman, H. D., Hadley, S. K. J., and John, H. T. 1964. Pharyngolaryngectomy and colonic reconstruction. A one-stage operation for cancer of the pharynx and cervical esophagus. British Journal of Surgery, 51: 663.

13. Fletcher, G. H. 1973. Textbook of Radiotherapy. 2nd edn. Lea & Febiger, Philadelphia.

14. Fletcher, G. H., and Goepfert, H. 1977. Irradiation in management of squamous cell carcinomas of the larynx. In English, G. M., Ed.: Otolaryngology. Vol. 5. Harper & Row, Hagerstown, MD, Ch. 39.)

15. Gall, A. M., Sessions, D. G., and Ogura, J. H. 1977. Complications following surgery for cancer of the larynx and hypopharynx. Cancer, 39: 624.

16. Grage, T. B., and Quick, C. A. 1978. The use of revascularized ileocolic autografts for primary repair after pharyngolaryngoesophagectomy. American Journal of Surgery, 136: 477.

17. Griffiths, J. D., and Shaw, H. J. 1973. Cancer of the laryngopharynx and cervical esophagus. Archives of Otolaryngology, 97: 340.

18. Guillamondegui, O. M., Meoz, R., and Jesse, R. H. 1978. Surgical treatment of squamous cell carcinoma of the pharyngeal walls. American Journal of Surgery, 136: 474.

19. Harrison, D. F. N. 1970. Pathology of hypopharyngeal cancer in relation to surgical management. Journal of Laryngology and Otology, 84: 349.

20. Harrison, D. F. N. 1972. Role of surgery in the management of postcricoid and cervical esophageal neoplasms. Annals of Otology, Rhinology and Laryngology, 81: 465.

21. Harrison, D. F. N. 1979. Surgical management of hypopharyngeal cancer. Particular reference to the gastric "pull-up" operation. Archives of Otolaryngology, 105: 149.

22. Higginson, J., Terracini, B., and Agthe, C. 1975. Nutrition and cancer: Ingestion of foodborne carcinogens. In Schottenfeld, D., Ed.: Cancer Epidermiology and Prevention: Current Concepts. Charles C Thomas, Springfield, IL, 177.

23. Inoue, T., and Shigematsu, Y. 1976. Hypopharyngeal carcinoma. Long-term survivors following radical radiation therapy. Acta Radiologica: Therapy (Stockholm), 15: 201.

24. Jayant, K., Balakrishnan, V., Sanghvi, L. D., and Jussawalla, D. J. 1977. Quantification of the role of smoking and chewing tobacco in oral, pharyngeal, and oesophageal cancers. British Journal of Cancer, 35: 232.

25. Jesse, R. H., and Lindberg, R. D. 1975. The efficacy of combining radiation therapy with a surgical procedure in patients with cervical metastases from squamous cancer of the oropharynx and hypopharynx. Cancer, 35: 1163.

26. Kirchner, J. A. 1975. Pyriform sinus cancer: A clinical and laboratory study. Annals of Otology, Rhinology and Laryngology, 84: 793.

27. Larsson, L. G., Sandstrom, A., and Westling, P. 1975. Relationship of Plummer-Vinson disease to cancer of the upper alimentary tract in Sweden. Cancer Research, 35: 3308.

28. Lindberg, R. 1972. Distribution of cervical lymph node metastases from squamous cell carcinoma of the upper respiratory and digestive tracts. Cancer, 29: 1446.

29. MacComb, W. S. and Fletcher, G. H. 1967. Cancer of the Head and Neck. Williams & Wilkins, Baltimore.

30. McGavran, M. H., Bauer, W. C., Spjut, H. J., and Ogura, J. H. 1963. Carcinoma of the pyriform sinus: The results of radical surgery. Archives of Otolaryngology, 78: 826.

31. McKeown, K. C. 1976. Total three stage oesophagectomy for cancer of the oesophagus. British Journal of Surgery, 63: 259.

32. Meoz-Mendez, R. T., Fletcher, G. H., Guillamondegui, O. M., and Peters, L. J. 1978. Analysis of the results of irradiation in the treatment of squamous cell carcinomas of the pharyngeal walls. International Journal of Radiation Oncology, Biology, and Physics, 4: 579.

33. Ogura, J. H., Jurema, A. A., and Watson, R. K. 1960. Partial laryngopharyngectomy and neck dissection for pyriform sinus cancer. Conservation surgery with immediate reconstruction. Laryngoscope, 70: 1399.

34. Razack, M. S., Sako, K., Marchetta, F. C., Calamel, P., Bakamjian, V., and Shedd, D. P.

1977. Carcinoma of the hypopharynx: Success and failure. American Journal of Surgery, 134: 489.

35. Schneider, J. J., Fletcher, G. H., and Barkley, H. T., Jr. 1975. Control by irradiation alone of nonfixed clinically positive lymph nodes from squamous cell carcinoma of the oral cavity, oropharynx, supraglottic larynx, and hypopharynx. American Journal of Roentgenology, Radium Therapy, and Nuclear Medicine, 123: 42.

36. Shah, J. P., Shaha, A. R., Spiro, R. H., and Strong, E. W. 1976. Carcinoma of the hypopharynx. American Journal of Surgery, 132: 439.

37. Shaw, H. J. 1972. Repair of the laryngopharynx and cervical oesophagus after irradiation. British Journal of Surgery, 59: 524.

38. Spiro, R. H., Hajdu, S. I., Lewis, J. S., and Strong, E. W. 1976. Mucus gland tumors of the larynx and laryngopharynx. Annals of Otology, Rhinology and Laryngology, 85: 498.

39. Stefani, S., and Eells, R. W. 1971. Carcinoma of the hypopharynx—a study of distant metastases, treatment failures, and multiple primary cancers in 215 male patients. Laryngoscope, 81: 1491.

40. Tarpley, J. L., Potvin, C., and Chretien, P. B. 1975. Prolonged depression of cellular immunity in cured laryngopharyngeal cancer patients treated with radiation therapy. Cancer, 35: 638.

41. Vandenbrouck, C., Sancho, H., LeFur, R., Richard, J. M., and Cachin, Y. 1977. Results of a randomized clinical trial of preoperative irradiation versus postoperative in treatment of tumors of the hypopharynx. Cancer, 39: 1445.

42. Ventemiglia, R., Khalil, K. G., Frazier, O. H., and Mountain, C. F. 1977. The role of preoperative mesenteric arteriography in colon interposition. Journal of Thoracic and Cardiovascular Surgery 74: 98.

43. Wynder, E. L. 1976. Nutrition and Cancer. Federation Proceedings, 35: 1309.

18 | Cancer of the Larynx

William Lawson, M.D.
Hugh F. Biller, M.D.

INTRODUCTION

While laryngeal malignancies are principally squamous cell carcinoma, a variety of other epithelial and nonepithelial tumors also occur. In order to determine the prognosis and to select therapy for a given lesion it is important to classify it with regard to histologic type, anatomic location, and extent of involvement. This requires a knowledge of the regional anatomy, patterns of spread, diagnostic techniques, systems of staging, tumor biology, and the results of the various therapeutic modalities available. Laryngeal cancer will be discussed with respect to each of these factors.

INCIDENCE, EPIDEMIOLOGY AND ETIOLOGY

Laryngeal carcinoma represents less than 1 percent of all malignant lesions. The incidence of carcinoma of the larynx has been estimated at 1 new case per 100,000 population.[17] However, analysis of reports from cancer registries reveals considerable variation in the incidence of laryngeal carcinoma in different countries. While significant geographic differences exist, they follow no definite geographic pattern.[16] Within Scandinavia it occurs with 3 times greater frequency in Finland (7.2 cases per 100,000) than in the other Scandinavian countries (1.8 to 2.3).[171] It is of interest to note that there has been no significant change in the mortality rates for carcinoma of the larynx over the past 25 years.[16] Also, the survival rate for either glottic or supraglottic cancer does not correlate with the primary treatment employed.[278]

There exists a sexual difference in the occurrence of carcinoma of the larynx, with it being more common in males. Furthermore, reports from most tumor registries indicate that the incidence of laryngeal carcinoma is increasing among males. Analysis of 46 geographic regions by Barclay and Rao[16] revealed a median incidence of 0.4 per 100,000 in females. The generally cited male to female ratio is about 10:1. However, the ratio varies with the country and in some regions it may be as high as 23:1 (Finland).

The peak age for the occurrence of laryngeal carcinoma is the sixth and seventh decades, with the vast majority of cases occurring between 40 and 69 years. Less than 1 percent of laryngeal cancers arise in patients under 30 years of age. Jones and Gabriel[124] collected 99 cases in persons under 20 years of age on review of the literature through 1969. Laryngeal carcinoma also tends to occur at a somewhat younger age in women.[16]

There also exist differences in the topographic incidence of laryngeal carcinomas (Table 18-1). The majority of tumors arise in the glottic region. In Finland, however, there is a preponderance of supraglottic lesions, which appear a decade earlier in affected individuals in this country.[171] Iwamoto[116] also found an increased incidence of supraglottic lesions among females in Japan.

The number of cases is generally proportional to the population, with an in-

TABLE 18-1. GEOGRAPHIC VARIATIONS IN THE ANATOMIC DISTRIBUTION OF
LARYNGEAL CARCINOMAS

Study	Country	Number of Cases	Supraglottic (%)	Glottic (%)	Subglottic (%)	Combined (%)
Krajina[142]	Croatia	704	19.7	19.3	0.9	60.1%
Iwamoto[116]	Japan	6,360	49	50	1	
Atkinson[13]	Australia	971	19–42	51–77	2–7	
Lauerma[148]	Finland	638	67	32	1	
Martensson[171]	Sweden	578	11	87	2	
Jankovic and Merkas[118]	Yugoslavia	722	62	35	3.5	
Smith et al.[252]	United States	1,645	34	65	1	

creased incidence reported in urban areas.[116, 171] However, some researchers have reported an increased occurrence in rural areas.[143] No correlation has been found between occupation and the occurrence of carcinoma of the larynx.[116, 143] However, some studies have noted a history of voice abuse and chronic laryngitis in affected patients.[116] Wynder[295] claimed an increased occupational risk for workers exposed to wood dust. An increased incidence of airway cancer including the larynx has been reported in employees in poison gas (nitrogen mustard) factories.[146] There also appears to be a relationship between laryngeal carcinoma and asbestosis. Stell and McGill[262] found a significantly increased incidence of cancer of the larynx in persons with exposure to asbestos. However, Morgan and Shettigara[188] noted that in their series the risk imposed by asbestos in the development of laryngeal carcinoma was confined to smokers. Dietary factors have also been cited as increasing susceptibility to laryngeal carcinoma. Stocks[267] correlated tea drinking with cancer of the larynx in females. Hiranandani[106] considered the slaked lime present in the Indian tea mixture to produce irritation leading to leukoplakia and postcricoid carcinoma.

Concerning social habits, epidemiologic studies have implicated cigarette smoking[115, 143] but not alcohol as a causal factor in the development of laryngeal cancer. Hiranandani[106] found on study of 1,000

Indian smokers that 30 percent failed to develop leukoplakia despite heavy smoking, 10 percent showed leukoplakia smoking 10 to 20 cigarettes per day for a few years, and 60 percent had intermediate changes. In the highly susceptible group, 20 percent developed cancer, whereas in the nonsusceptible group only 2 of 300 patients had cancer. Wynder et al.[296] concluded that cigarette smoking was the principle risk factor for the development of supraglottic and glottic carcinoma, with pipe and cigar smoking also increasing the risk. Heavy alcohol intake significantly enhanced the risk, especially to the supraglottis. However, in the absence of tobacco use, alcohol was not found to increase the risk of laryngeal carcinoma. Wynder[295] also believed that differences in incidence encountered in various religious, socioeconomic, and educational groups only reflected differences in the consumption of tobacco and alcohol. The observed increase in the sex ratio of the occurrence of laryngeal cancer in women from 14.9:1 in 1956 to 4.6:1 in 1973 was believed to reflect the increased smoking by women in the United States. However, Lowry[160] claimed a strong association between heavy alcohol intake and carcinoma of the supraglottic larynx, though not that of the vocal cords.

Histologic evidence exists supporting an irritative effect of smoking on the larynx that may be the forerunner of neoplastic transformation. Ryan et al.[230] documented excessive keratinization, epithelial hyperplasia, squamous metaplasia, edema, and chronic inflammation; and Auerbach et al.[14] documented the occurrence of atypia and carcinoma in situ in the larynx of smokers as compared to nonsmokers. Homberger[108] was even able to experimentally induce carcinoma of the larynx in laboratory animals by exposure to cigarette smoke.

Exposure to radiation has also been implicated as an etiologic factor in laryngeal cancer. Goolden[93] reported the occurrence of laryngeal malignancies in patients previously irradiated for benign diseases. Rabbett[224] noted instances of the conversion of laryngeal papillomatosis to carcinomatosis after irradiation. Lawson and Som[149] found the incidence of second primary cancer within the larynx to be more than double in individuals who had received radiotherapy as opposed to surgery for the management of the first lesion.

There also appears to be a genetic fac-tor operative in the development of laryngeal carcinoma. Iwamotto[116] found in 56 percent of his cases a positive family history for malignancy. However, in only 3 percent of other family members did the tumor also arise in the larynx. Daly and Strong[57] observed second primary malignancies in 19.5 percent of patients with glottic lesions, of which 4 percent also occurred in the head and neck. There also exist reports, principally in the Russian literature, of cases of familial laryngeal malignancies.[161]

ANATOMY

The larynx is that section of the respiratory tract composed of the epiglottis and the thyroid, cricoid, arytenoid, corniculate, and cuneiform cartilages, surrounded by the supporting and intrinsic muscles and soft tissues, and invested by the lining mucosa (Fig.

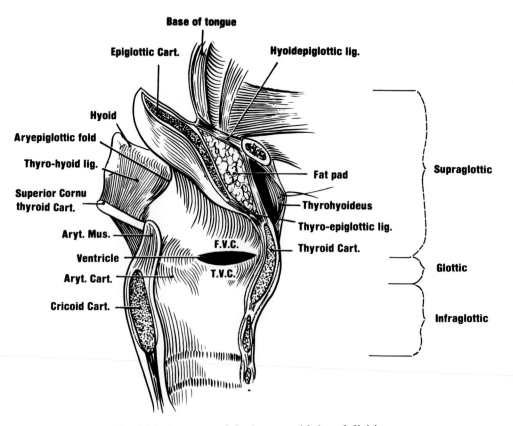

Fig. 18-1. Anatomy of the larynx, with its subdivisions.

18-1). Its superior borders are the free edge and lateral margins of the epiglottis, the aryepiglottic folds, the arytenoid regions, and the interarytenoid space. The inferior border is defined as a plane passing through the lower edge of the cricoid cartilage. Its anterolateral boundaries are the thyrohyoid membrane, thyroid lamina, cricothyroid membrane and muscles, and the anterior arch of the cricoid cartilage. Its posterior border is the arytenoid cartilages, interarytenoid space, and rostrum of the cricoid. The larynx may be further subdivided into three anatomic areas—the supraglottis, glottis, and subglottis—although there exists some controversy as to the exact borders of these three compartments.

The *supraglottic portion* of the larynx includes the laryngeal surface of the epiglottis, the aryepiglottic folds, the laryngeal surfaces of the arytenoids, the false (ventricular) folds, and the ventricles. The superior limit is generally accepted to be the hyoepiglottic ligament, while the anterior border is the thyrohyoid membrane. The hyoid bone itself is considered extralaryngeal. While the mucosa of the lingual surface of the tip of the epiglottis is considered laryngeal, the vallecular mucosa overlying the hyoepiglottic ligament is classified as oropharyngeal. Prior to 1972 the International Union Against Cancer (UICC)[285] classification recognized a marginal zone of the larynx, the epilarynx, comprising the suprahyoid portion of the epiglottis and aryepiglottic folds. While tumors arising there behave similarly to hypopharyngeal cancers, this region has been now included in the supraglottic larynx.

The exact location of the boundary through the ventricle to separate the supraglottic and glottic regions has had varying interpretations. While anatomically the superior arcuate line—where the squamous epithelium of the true cord joins the respiratory mucosa of the ventricle—is the actual boundary, the clinical junction is different. The lateral recess or angle of the ventricle is generally used as the clinical boundary, with the floor of the ventricle included in the glottic region and the roof of the ventricle and saccule considered supraglottic.

The *glottic portion* consists of both true cords and the anterior and posterior commissures, surrounding the glottic chink, or rima glottidis. The glottis has its greatest vertical dimension at the midportion of the vocal cord (about 5 mm). The anterior commissure where the true cords meet has a vertical height of 2 to 3 mm. The posterior commissure is a 5 mm high strip of mucosa extending posteriorly from the vocal process of one vocal cord across the interarytenoid area to the vocal process of the opposite cord.

The *subglottic portion* is the region of the larynx that is bounded by the vocal cords superiorly and the lower border of the cricoid cartilage inferiorly. The border between the glottic and subglottic areas is generally accepted as the lower edge of the strip of squamous epithelium that covers the vocal cords and is about 5 mm from the free margin of the vocal cord. However, the classification of the American Joint Committee[5] and International Union Against Cancer[285] places the undersurface of the vocal cords in the glottic region. This disparity has risen because the classification is based on clinical examination rather than anatomic features. While the upper limit of the subglottis is generally considered to be 5 mm below the free edge of the vocal cord, Kirchner[132] recommended that it should be placed 1 cm below the cord margin. Tucker[281] also described an anterior subglottic space whose apex was the anterior commissure ligament above. Lederman[151] divided the subglottis into an upper mobile portion and a lower fixed portion. The key structure in the subglottic space is the conus elasticus, or cricovocal ligament, which is a fibroelastic membrane extending superiorly from the upper border of the cricoid cartilage to form the vocal ligament.

This subdivision of the larynx into three anatomic areas has its basis in its embryologic derivation. In addition to serving as barriers to the vertical spread of tumors, the biologic behavior of neoplasms and their pattern of spread at each anatomic site is different. Consequently, these fundamental differences are important in the prognosis and management of tumors arising at each site. This compartmentalization of the larynx also provides an anatomic basis for partial laryngeal surgery.

While the supraglottic larynx arises from the buccopharyngeal anlage (arches III, IV), the glottic and subglottic portions are derived from the tracheobronchial anlage (arches V, VI).[100] As a consequence of these embryologic partitions, the various portions have an independent lymphatic circulation. Dye injection studies in man by Pressman et al.[220] have demonstrated that the submucosal lymphatics of the larynx are also compartmentalized and serve as an important influence in determining the spread of laryngeal neoplasms. Lymphatic spread from the epiglottis is to the false cord and ends abruptly along its inferior border. The ventricle appears to be a compartment isolated from the false cord. The true cord has a sparse lymphatic network and also serves as an additional barrier in the vertical lymphatic drainage of the larynx. Dye injected into the subglottic area ended sharply at the lower border of the cricoid cartilage. The left and right sides of the larynx also appear to be independent at all levels. The supraglottic lymphatics drain through the thyrohyoid space to cervical lymph nodes, whereas the infraglottic laryngeal lymphatics drain to the cervical nodes through the cricothyroid plexus. Anterior subglottic lesions spread readily to the cricothyroid lymph node. However, there is cross-flow in the superficial lymphatic drainage from the anterior commissure and anterior subglottic region.[122] There is no midline partition in the anterior neck and lesions that have spread to the prelaryngeal and pretracheal areas should be treated as a block.[281] With advanced supraglottic tumors, anatomic barriers based on embryologic development disappear and tumor dissemination may occur throughout the neck.[233] This is especially true with involvement of the preepiglottic space.[128] However, Johner[122] believed that the lack of direct lymphatic communication between the lower neck and mediastinum limited the metastatic extension of squamous cell carcinoma of the larynx for long periods of time.

Tucker[281] postulated that while both the supraglottic and subglottic areas are embryologically derived from wedge-shaped midline cell masses, the glottic structures arise from two lateral cell masses, which later fuse at the anterior commissure. Tucker[281] offered this X-concept to explain why glottic lesions remain unilateral for long periods of time, whereas supraglottic and subglottic lesions readily grow anteriorly to extend to the opposite side. However, Hast[100] cautioned that there is no embryologic basis for the vertical hemilaryngectomy.

There are other anatomic features that influence the spread of tumors within the larynx. The paraglottic and preepiglottic spaces and the anterior commissure ligament represent avenues for tumor dissemination. The paraglottic space is that portion of the larynx bounded by the thyroid ala anterolaterally, conus elasticus inferiorly, quadrangular membrane medially, and the pyriform mucosa posteriorly.[282] Primary paraglottic tumors can rise from the mucosa of the saccule and ventricle. However, the paraglottic space is usually involved secondarily by extension of tumor from the mucosa anywhere in the intrinsic larynx or from the anterior and medial walls of the pyriform sinus. The paraglottic space cannot be examined directly and involvement is inferred by the presence of edema or cord fixation or by radiographic evidence of fullness or bulging.[281] Lesions can extensively spread in this space laterally, extending even up into the preepiglottic space. Lateral supraglottic tumors can readily spread along the inner face of the thyroid cartilage for great distances. Tumor spread, however, is generally limited by the conus elasticus below.

In addition to vertical extension, Tucker[280] stressed the ability of tumors to grow posteriorly in the paraglottic space to reach the pyriform sinus. Subglottic tumors may also extend submucosally over the superior rim of the cricoid cartilage, medially to the cricoarytenoid joint, and just under the interarytenoid muscle. Consequently, in resecting extensive lesions with fixed cords and subglottic involvement, care must be taken not to leave residual tumor under the hypopharyngeal mucosa, inviting recurrence there.[280]

The terminology of the soft-tissue spaces within the larynx is also controversial. The preepiglottic space as classically described by Clerf[47] and Leroux-Robert[153] is a funnel-shaped area bounded by the upper thyroid cartilage and thyrohyoid membrane anteriorly, the hyoepiglottic ligament superiorly, and the epiglottis and quadrangular membrane posteriorly (Fig. 18-1). However, this fat-filled space anterior to the epiglottis can also extend in a horseshoe fashion about it posterolaterally. Since this space merges with the paraglottic space, it has been termed collectively the periepiglottic space by Maguire and Dayal.[168]

The region of the anterior commissure tendon is also a site for tumor spread. Where the two true cords meet to form the anterior commissure tendon, the internal perichondrium of the thyroid cartilage lies close to the glottic epithelium. There is also a gap in the tendon just superior to it where the ventricular commissural mucosa similarly lies close to the cartilage.[39, 283] Consequently, a tumor in this region may involve the supraglottic, glottic, and subglottic larynx in an anterior midsagittal plane. The epiglottic cartilage has numerous natural dehiscences, which facilitate tumor spread into the preepiglottic space. When cartilage invasion occurs, the ossified portion shows the least resistance to tumor spread.[196, 210] Micheau et al.[174] found that in 94 percent of 70 cases with cartilage invasion studied by whole organ section, the tumor involved the ossified areas. Similar observations were found with serial sections by Kirchner.[131] However, Norris et al.[196] found that while a poor survival accompanied cricoid and thyroid cartilage invasion (40 percent), this was not true of invasion of the epiglottis (90%).

The conus elasticus is an important barrier to tumor spread. The majority of glottic tumors remain superficial to it, with a mo-bile cord, thus permitting partial laryngectomy.[132] Tumors in the paraglottic space may grow extensively deep to the conus elasticus, producing cord fixation and extralaryngeal spread, with minimal mucosal changes. The conus elasticus also constrains the upward growth of subglottic lesions. However, with advanced glottic, transglottic, and subglottic carcinomas, penetration occurs.

It has also been suggested that the mucous glands of the larynx influence the spread of carcinoma.[37, 38] According to this theory, the absence of mucous glands within the vocal cord, at the anterior commissure, and in the ventricle, may explain the tendency of glottic carcinomas to remain localized and the apparent resistance to the spread of supraglottic tumors onto the vocal cords. However, the extensive system of tuboalveolar glands present in the anterior subglottis may facilitate tumor spread from the anterior commissure.[27, 77] Tumors of the false cord are also believed to extend into the preepiglottic space through such a glandular system.[37]

Some workers believe blood vessels also determine tumor spread. Microvascular studies reveal that the blood vessels of the vocal cords run linearly, whereas in the subglottis they become circumferential.[77] The anterior commissure appears to be an avascular area, with the parallel vocal cord vessels streaming inferiorly into the subglottis and there crossing the midline to communicate with the vessels of the opposite side. In the anterior subglottis these blood vessels also communicate with vessels from the cricothyroid artery, which penetrates the cricothyroid membrane. After a study of the human and primate larynx, Freeland[76] suggested that tumor spread was influenced by lines of least resistance created by these blood vessels. Olofsson[210] in a study of 130 specimens found 27 instances of vascular invasion by laryngeal tumors and 20 instances of perineural invasion by tumor. Glottic tumors were mainly responsible for blood vessel invasion.

The larynx has segmental sensory and motor innervation from the superior and recurrent laryngeal branches of the vagus nerves. While there are numerous free, tactile, and proprioceptive endings, intrinsic laryngeal lesions produce relatively few symptoms of sensory disturbances. Advanced lesions, particularly those with hypopharyngeal extension, cause discomfort on swallowing and pain referred into the ear. Infiltration along nerves is not a major route of tumor spread.

Patterns of Spread

The spread of laryngeal carcinoma is dependent on the site of origin of the tumor and anatomic barriers within the larynx. Consequently it is important to understand the compartmentalization of the larynx and the patterns of tumor growth, as they form the basis of conservation laryngeal surgery.

Tumors arising on the free margin of the membranous portion of the true vocal cord initially spread along the cord and involve Reinke's space. Infiltrative lesions may cause cord fixation by involvement of the intrinsic muscles. Exophytic lesions may bulge into the ventricle or spread into the subglottic space. They may extend anteriorly to involve the anterior commissure or posteriorly to the vocal process or anterior face of the arytenoid. From the anterior commissure, tumors may spread to the opposite vocal cord or into the anterior subglottic space. They can grow vertically, crossing the ventricle into the supraglottic larynx or the lateral subglottic region before spreading to the opposite hemilarynx. Growth outside the larynx occurs at anatomic points of weakness. Lesions involving the anterior commissure and subglottis can penetrate the cricothyroid membrane and extend extralaryngeally. Posterior growth permits penetration of the cricoid space with invasion of the thyroid or cricoid cartilages. The tumor may then extend medially or laterally to the arytenoid cartilage. Whole organ study by Oloffson[210, 212] of 73 advanced primary glottic lesions revealed that 13 remained limited to the glottis, whereas 60 underwent vertical spread (24 subglottic, 5

supraglottic, and 31 both supraglottic and subglottic). Contralateral spread occurred in 35 cases and generally accompanied extensive vertical spread. In 57 cases muscle invasion was found, and in 27 cases spread outside the larynx occurred. The latter was primarily by invasion of the thyroid cartilage in the midline and by anterior spread through the cricothyroid membrane. Another study of 36 laryngectomy specimens for advanced glottic carcinoma by Micheau et al.[174] revealed involvement of the false cords and invasion of the base of the epiglottis in 10 percent, invasion of the ventricle in 56 percent, involvement of the anterior commissure in 81 percent, destruction of the arytenoid cartilage in 72 percent, penetration of the conus elasticus in 78 percent, and subglottic extension in 58 percent.

Tumors arising in the supraglottic region vary in growth pattern with the site of origin. Lesions of the laryngeal surface of the epiglottis spread superficially and horizontally to the opposite side and also often invade the preepiglottic space through preformed channels in the epiglottis or by cartilaginous destruction or by disruption of the thyroepiglottic ligament (Figs. 18-2 A and B). Micheau et al.[174] found destruction of the thyroepiglottic ligament by tumor in 15 of 18 epiglottic lesions. They also found the hyoepiglottic ligament an effective barrier to tumor spread from the epiglottis unless the vallecula or the base of the tongue was involved. Epiglottic carcinomas are also capable of thyroid cartilage invasion. This should be suspected with lesions extending to the epiglottic petiole or anterior commissure, with poorly differentiated carcinoma, and with ulcerating tumors.[131] Kirchner[131, 132] found on serial section of 10 epiglottic tumors that 8 had invaded the epiglottic cartilage, 5 the thyroid cartilage, and 6 the preepiglottic space. Olofsson[210] and Olofsson and van Nostrand[212] reported that of 15 epiglottic carcinomas sectioned, 10 had invaded the epiglottic cartilage, 2 had destroyed the thyroid cartilage, and 10 had extended into the preepiglottic space. Tumors arising on the false cords tend to

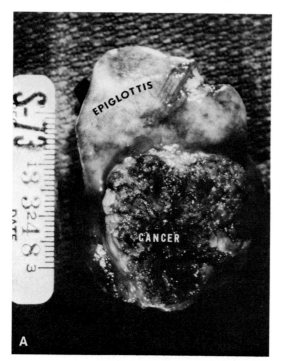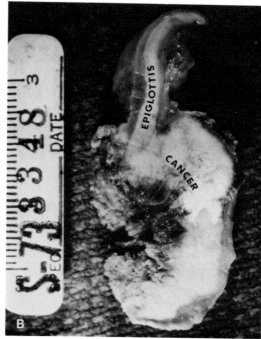

Fig. 18-2. Carcinoma of the epiglottis. (A) Lesion arising at the level of the petiole. (B) Sagittal section demonstrating invasion of preepiglottic space.

grow upward to the epiglottis, backward to the aryepiglottic folds and arytenoids, and forward to the anterior commissure. With involvement of the paraglottic space, tumors can spread extensively vertically and can involve the ventricles indirectly.

Carcinoma arising primarily in the ventricle is considered to be rare. However, lesions occurring at this site are capable of extensive supraglottic and transglottic spread. A study by Micheau et al.[174] of 23 laryngectomy specimens from patients with cancer of the ventricle revealed upward spread with destruction of the base of the epiglottis and involvement of the preepiglottic space (11 cases). Downward spread did involve the glottis superficially over the mucosa (9 cases) or deeply through the paraglottic space with penetration of the conus elasticus (16 cases). Contralateral spread across the anterior commissure ligament also occurs. While many supraglottic tumors show a pushing pattern of growth and tend to stop at the ventricle, some cross over it onto the

glottis.[210] Bocca et al.[33] found none of 160 supraglottic carcinomas to invade the floor of the ventricle or the vocal cord. However, Olofsson[210] and Olofsson and van Nostrand[212] found that of 25 primary supraglottic tumors, 11 remained localized in the supraglottis, 6 spread to the glottis, 6 spread to the vallecula, and 4 to the pyriform sinus. Nine tumors were bilateral, generally crossing the midline anteriorly, and the interarytenoid area was involved in 2 cases. Kirchner and Som[136] found 8 of 30 supraglottic carcinomas to extend below the anterior commissure, with 5 invading the thyroid cartilage.

Tumors arising primarily in the subglottic region are rare and tend to spread circumferentially, generally presenting when quite advanced (Fig. 18-3). Olofsson[210] and Olofsson and van Nostrand[212] found that of four primary subglottic tumors, three invaded the laryngeal cartilage and extended outside the larynx. All four tumors extended through the conus elasti-

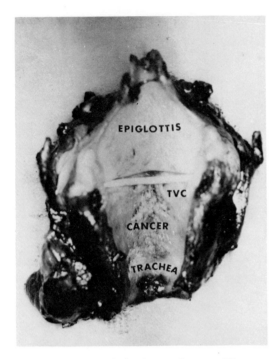

Fig. 18-3. Subglottic carcinoma. The wood splint is at the level of the true cords which were mobile. The tumor has spread downward to involve the upper two tracheal rings.

cus to invade the thyroarytenoid muscles without mucosal abnormality. Micheau et al.[174] reported that of four subglottic tumors three were bilateral and invaded the cricothyroid membrane and the thyroid gland. All involved the cricoid cartilage, but none spread above the glottis. Harrison[98] emphasized the ability of subglottic tumors to extend posteriorly above and below the cricoid cartilage and under the interarytenoid muscle, inviting recurrence in the hypopharynx and esophagus. Harrison[98] also stressed the ability of subglottic tumors to extend outside the larynx, producing invasion of the thyroid gland.

Olofsson[210] found direct invasion of the thyroid gland in only 7 of 110 specimens studied, all 7 being extensive lesions. He recommended removal of the isthmus and ipsilateral lobe of the thyroid for all subglottic, glottic-subglottic, and transglottic tumors, and for those with a fixed cord.

McGavran et al.[164] termed lesions that

crossed the ventricle, transglottic (Fig. 18-4). This type of lesion was originally described by Leroux-Robert[153] who believed it arose in the ventricle. However, vertical extension from the supraglottic and glottic regions may produce such lesions. These lesions often involve the paraglottic space and show an aggressive and infiltrative pattern of growth, cause cord fixation, and carry a poor prognosis. Kirchner et al.[138] found, on serial section of 19 transglottic lesions, that 15 had invaded cartilage (thyroid 8, cricoid 5, arytenoid 5) and 16 had reached or penetrated the cricothyroid membrane.

Tumors of the hypopharynx may also involve the larynx by continued growth. Carcinoma of the pyriform sinus may extend medially to invade the posterior cricoarytenoid and interarytenoid muscles and limit vocal cord mobility, may invade the thyroid cartilage laterally, or may extend forward into the paraglottic space and widely infiltrate transglottically. Carcinoma of

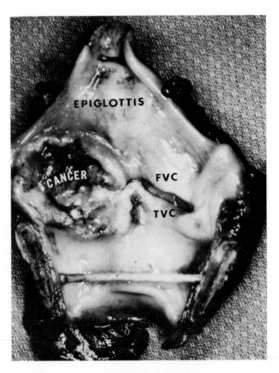

Fig. 18-4. Transglottic carcinoma crossing the ventricle to involve true and false cords.

the postcricoid region may directly invade the cricoid and arytenoid cartilages.

Vocal cord fixation is an indication of an advanced tumor and consequently carries a poor prognosis. In addition to deep invasion by a glottic carcinoma, vocal cord fixation can arise—with minimal mucosal findings—by extension from a primary lesion elsewhere in the larynx and hypopharynx through the paraglottic space. Kirchner[131, 135] reported that of 30 cases with a fixed cord, 11 were primarily of the glottis, 9 transglottis, and 4 pyriform sinus. Analysis of 26 cases of vocal cord fixation by Olofsson et al.[213] showed thyroarytenoid muscle invasion in all, with the tumor spreading along the muscle bundles. After radiotherapy, viable cells were still found scattered throughout the muscle. Other structures invaded included the lateral cricoarytenoid muscle (19), interarytenoid (11), posterior cricoarytenoid muscle (7), cricoarytenoid joint (17), thyroid cartilage (16), and extralaryngeal extension (18). Perineural invasion was present in 10 cases. While more than half of the cases had extension outside the larynx, this was apparent clinically in only 2 cases.

CLASSIFICATION AND STAGING

The system of laryngeal cancer staging and end results reporting published by the American Joint Committee in 1963 was revised in 1972[5] because of deficiencies that had appeared. A major objection was the poor survival of patients with fixed cord lesions as compared to bilateral cordal lesions, which were now classified as T3 lesions. Also, T4N0M0 tumors were changed from stage IV to stage III lesions. The system underwent a further minor modification in 1977 principally with regard to classification of lymph node metastasis. However, the 1972 version is used in this chapter as it is the one adopted by the Centennial Committee on Laryngeal Cancer in the reporting of results (Tables 18-2 and 18-3).

TABLE 18-2. CLASSIFICATION OF LARYNGEAL CANCER[5]

Supraglottis
T1S	Carcinoma in situ
T1a	Tumor confined to laryngeal surface of epiglottis, or an aryepiglottic fold or arytenoid, or ventricular cavity or bands.
T1b	Tumor arising on the epiglottis, aryepiglottic fold, arytenoids, or ventricular cavity or bands and extending to involve one or more adjacent supraglottic sites.
T2	Tumor of the epiglottis and/or arytenoids, aryepiglottic folds, ventricles, or ventricular bands and extending onto the vocal cords.
T3	Tumor limited to the larynx with vocal cord fixation.
T4	Tumor of supraglottis extending beyond larynx (i.e. to pyriform sinus, postcricoid area, vallecula, base of the tongue)

Glottis
T1S	Carcinoma in situ
T1a	Tumor confined to one vocal cord, with normal mobility
T1b	Tumor involving both cords, with normal mobility
T2	Tumor extending to supraglottic or subglottic region with normal or impaired cord mobility
T3	Tumor limited to the larynx with vocal cord fixation
T4	Tumor destroying cartilage or extending beyond the larynx

Subglottis
T1S	Carcinoma in situ
T1a	Tumor limited to one side of the subglottic region, exclusive of the undersurface of the vocal cord.
T1b	Tumor extending to two sides of the subglottis, exclusive of the undersurface of the cords.
T2	Tumor involving the subglottis and extending onto the vocal cords.
T3	Tumor limited to the larynx with vocal cord fixation.
T4	Tumor of subglottis extending beyond larynx (i.e. trachea, postcricoid area, skin)

Lymph Nodes
N0	Cervical nodes not palpable
N1	Homolateral nonfixed palpable lymph nodes

TABLE 18-2—CONTINUED

N2	Palpable bilateral, contralateral or midline lymph nodes, nonfixed
N3	Fixed cervical lymph nodes

Distant Metastasis
M0	No distant metastasis
M1	Distant metastasis present

TABLE 18-3. STAGING OF LARYNGEAL CANCER[5]

Stage	Tumor Classification
Stage I	T1N0
Stage II	T2N0
Stage III	T3N0
	T4N0
	T1 to T4 with N1
	T1 to T4 with N2
Stage IV	T1 to T4 with N3
	T1 to T4 with N0 to N3 with M1

PATHOLOGY

Squamous cell carcinoma represents 95 to 98 percent of reported laryngeal malignancies. Most of these carcinomas are of the keratinizing type. However, 60 percent of the series reported by Krajina[143] were of the nonkeratinizing type. The remainder of the tumors are verrucous carcinoma, anaplastic carcinoma, pseudosarcoma, adenocarcinoma, and sarcomas. These lesions will be considered individually because of their differences in biologic behavior and management. Sporadic cases of transitional cell, basal cells, and lymphoepithelial tumors have also been reported.[106, 116, 252]

Prognostic Features

Numerous attempts have been made to correlate the microscopic appearance of a tumor with its biologic behavior and prog-

nosis. McGavran et al.[164] in a study of 96 cases found the degree of differentiation of squamous cell carcinoma of the larynx to be inversely proportional to its metastatic spread. Cervical metastasis was found in 11 percent of well-differentiated tumors, 22 percent of moderately differentiated tumors, and 49 percent of poorly differentiated tumors. Kashima[128] also found 7 of 29 well-differentiated and 7 of 11 poorly differentiated laryngeal carcinomas to have regional metastasis. Similar observations were made with transglottic tumors by Kirchner et al.[138] While histologic grading of tumor differentiation, as traditionally judged by keratinization according to the system of Broder, has had limited prognostic value, multifactorial analysis of the cell population (structure, differentiation, nuclear polymorphism, mitosis) and tumor-host relationship (mode of invasion, stage of invasion, vascular invasion, cellular response) is more promising. Jakobsson[117] found on analysis of 230 glottic carcinomas that 5-year survival and recurrence was predicted better by histologic grading than by the TNM classification. Lauerma[148] on analysis of 638 laryngeal carcinomas found a cure rate of 59 percent for well-differentiated as compared with 44 percent for undifferentiated tumors. However, the single most important pathologic feature correlating with cervical metastasis appeared to be the nature of the tumor-host interface. Tumors with infiltrating margins had a poorer prognosis than those with pushing edges.[128, 164, 260] Staley and Herzon[260] also found that nerve sheath invasion increased the probability of lymph node metastasis.

Attempts have also been made to assess the immunologic response of the host to malignant disease. Kashima[128] found the incidence of metastasis from laryngeal cancers to be independent of the host cellular response as judged by lymphocytic infiltration. The occurrence of sinus histiocytosis and the presence or absence of reactive lymphocytic proliferation in regional lymph nodes have also been studied in patients with laryngeal malignancy. While Hiranandani[106] believed the presence of reticular hyperplasia in cervical lymph nodes was a good prognostic sign, McGavran and Bauer[162] found no correlation between the degree of lymph node sinus histiocytosis and the presence of cervical metastasis or survival in a carefully controlled study of transglottic tumors. Berlinger et al.[23] claimed that evidence of lymphocytic stimulation correlated well with 5-year survival, whereas patients with lymphocytic depletion virtually all succumbed to their disease. However, Gilmore et al.[82] found in a double blind retrospective study no correlation between lymph node morphology and survival or metastasis.

DIAGNOSTIC STUDIES

Endoscopy

Direct laryngoscopy and biopsy under general anesthesia is the principle diagnostic method employed for laryngeal lesions. The purpose of the examination is not only to obtain tissue for microscopic study but also to map out the extent of the lesion for proper staging and selection of therapy. This is of critical importance if partial laryngeal surgery is contemplated. In addition to evaluating the supraglottic, glottic, and subglottic regions, cord mobility should be noted and the pyriform sinuses, post-cricoid region, vallecula, and base of the tongue should be inspected. Biopsies should be taken from the body of the tumor, avoiding ulcerative and necrotic areas (which may reveal only chronic inflammation) or peripheral regions (which may show premalignant changes or carcinoma in situ).

Microlaryngoscopy may be a useful adjunct for small lesions of the membranous cord when vocal stripping may provide both diagnosis and treatment. Endoscopy is of limited value in determining cartilage invasion and in estimating the exact amount of subglottic extension. Consequently, radiographic studies are necessary to supplement the clinical examination.

Radiography

The radiographic diagnostic techniques generally employed in patients with laryngeal carcinoma are lateral soft-tissue roentgenography of the neck, frontal tomography of the larynx, and contrast laryngography. Radiologic studies supplement clinical examination and laryngoscopy in the assessment of laryngeal lesions, especially when conservation surgery is contemplated.

Lateral soft-tissue roentgenography mainly detects lesions in the sagittal plane that involve the base of the tongue, epiglottis, preepiglottic space, aryepiglottic folds, arytenoid, and posterior pharyngeal wall. It may also provide information about destruction of the thyroid cartilage. With bulky lesions involving the hypopharynx, additional information concerning tumor extent may be obtained by barium swallow. With frontal tomography, the tumor mass is seen in profile. However, this technique does not permit detection of small lesions and depends primarily on demonstrating asymmetry of the two sides.

Contrast laryngography is the most valuable radiographic technique. The laryngogram performed in the AP and lateral projections during phonation and with the Valsalva maneuver permits dynamic study of the larynx and yields the best visualization of tumor location and extent. It demonstrates soft-tissue thickening, mucosal irregularities, and vocal cord mobility and may reveal small glottic lesions in the AP view and involvement of the anterior commissure in the lateral inspiratory view. This technique is especially valuable in assessing both anterior and lateral subglottic extension (Fig. 18-5). Phonation demonstrates vocal cord mobility and reverse phonation fills the ventricle and may show involvement or distortion of the false cord.[121] While a carcinoma of the epiglottis may appear on the lateral soft-tissue radiograph, the laryngogram is indispensable in delimiting its inferior extent. Nevertheless, evidence of cartilage invasion outside the larynx may not be apparent by the latter technique.[214] How-

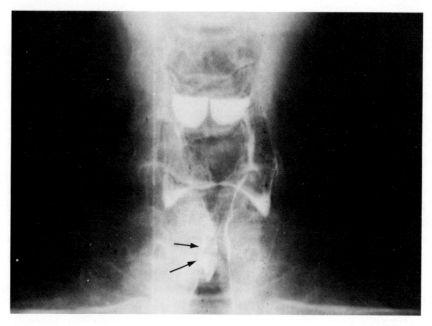

Fig. 18-5. Laryngogram revealing subglottic extension of a cordal carcinoma.

ever, cartilaginous destruction by tumor has been demonstrated with lateral xeroradiography.[226] Tantalum powder insufflation has been used as an alternative to conventional liquid media.[275] While it demonstrates the glottic and subglottic regions and bulky tumors better than do liquid media, it is not generally employed in contrast laryngography. The laryngogram may also show distortion or involvement of the vallecula and pyriform sinuses by lesions extending outside the larynx and with primary hypopharyngeal tumors.

Computerized tomography has been used to delineate laryngeal tumor extent. While it accurately demonstrates neoplastic involvement of laryngeal and paralaryngeal soft tissues, diagnosis of cartilage invasion is difficult because of nonuniform ossification and calcification.[7]

Transconioscopy

Martensson[170] popularized a method of retrograde examination of the subglottic space by introducing an optical system through the cricothyroid membrane. This technique, known as transconioscopy, was indicated for glottic carcinoma when subglottic extension was not visible by direct laryngoscopy but was contraindicated in cases with extensive spread or with primary subglottic tumors, which carry a risk of tumor penetration and seeding. Martensson[172] claimed only minimal subcutaneous emphysema and hematoma in over 400 cases in which transconioscopy was employed. Most workers, however, rely on contrast laryngography for the assessment of subglottic involvement.

Supravital Staining

Toluidine blue has been applied to the larynx at the time of microlaryngoscopy in an attempt to differentiate various lesions clinically.[270] While leukoplakia and keratosis do not fix the dye, carcinoma in situ and superficial carcinoma do. However, the staining of mucus, abrasions and ulcerations, and respiratory epithelium and the trapping of dye in papillary keratosis can produce false-positive and often confusing results.

Exfoliative Cytology

Cytologic smears have been made in the larynx similar to those made in the oral cavity in an attempt to establish the diagnosis of carcinoma by a noninvasive technique. Frable and Olsen[74] found exfoliative cytology to be diagnostic for malignancy in 8 of their 9 cases of laryngeal squamous cell carcinoma. However, in other, larger series a significant number of false-negative and false-positive readings occurred,[277] questioning the validity of this diagnostic method at the present time.

SQUAMOUS CARCINOMA—CLINICAL AND PATHOLOGIC FEATURES, MANAGEMENT, AND END RESULTS

The biologic behavior of squamous cell carcinoma of the larynx depends on the site of origin of the lesion, as the pattern of spread varies with the anatomic region. Tumor extent as well as tumor location influences lymph node metastases and ultimately prognosis. McGavran et al.[164] found no correlation between cartilage, vascular, and pre-epiglottic space invasion, cricothyroid membrane penetration, and soft-tissue extension with cervical lymph node metastasis. Norris et al.[196] correlated extralaryngeal involvement with decreased survival. Glottic carcinomas have a low incidence of cervical metastases, the majority of which are found with advanced lesions. In contradistinction, supraglottic tumors frequently produce ipsilateral and contralateral lymph node spread, even with early lesions.

Kirchner and Owen[134] found on study of 500 tumors of the larynx and laryngopharynx that the results of radiotherapy showed a steep gradient from T1 (82 percent) to T4 (5 percent) lesions, as compared to surgery (T1, 64 percent and T4, 40 percent). Moreover, this disparity in the effectiveness of radiotherapy was more pronounced at the glottic than at the supraglottic level. These observations were confirmed by Vermund.[288] Whereas surgery generally fails in the neck, radiotherapy fails at the primary site. However, Hendrickson et al.[102] contended after review of 498 T1 to T4 laryngeal lesions that when the results of salvage by radiotherapy or surgery are included, only small differences remain between the efficacy of the primary treatment.

The inability of radiotherapy to effectively control palpable lymph node metastasis as compared to surgery is of paramount importance, particularly with supraglottic tumors. Smith et al.[252] found on study of 1,645 laryngeal cancers, the survival with positive lymph nodes to be 51 percent, with negative lymph nodes 82 percent, with unilateral fixed nodes 26 percent, and bilateral fixed nodes 0 percent.

These fundamental differences in tumor spread and treatment responsiveness require carcinomas of the supraglottic, glottic, and subglottic larynx to be considered separately.

Supraglottic Carcinoma

The prominent presenting symptoms of supraglottic carcinoma are hoarseness, throat pain, dysphagia, and the occurrence of a neck mass. Other less common complaints are hemoptysis, ear pain, chronic cough, stridor, and the presence of an oral mass. Hoarseness may result from involvement of the false cord, extension onto the glottis, or by impaired vocal cord mobility due to involvement of the arytenoid cartilage, crico-arytenoid joint, or paraglottic space. Dysphagia generally represents extension into the hypopharynx or infiltration of the vallecula or base of the tongue. Occasionally, in a manner similar to lesions of the pyriform sinus, a small or asymptomatic supraglottic tumor may present with palpable cervical lymphadenopathy.

The majority of the lesions arise on the epiglottis, followed by the false cords and aryepiglottic folds. Cachin[42] found in his series of 72 early (T1, T2) supraglottic carcinomas that 56 developed on the infrahyoid epiglottis and false cords, 14 on the epilarynx, and 2 on the ventricle. Among the 221 tumors studied by Coates et al.,[48] 89 percent involved the epiglottis, 33 percent the false cords, 20 percent the aryepiglottic folds, and 7 percent the ventricles. The lesions were midline in 27 percent of the cases. Smith et al.[252] reported the distribution of 552 supraglottic carcinomas to involve the epiglottis (243), false cords (128), aryepiglottic folds (116), ventricle (38), and arytenoid (27).

Carcinoma of the supraglottic larynx has a significantly smaller 5-year survival rate when compared with carcinoma of the glottis. The prognosis depends on the extent and location of the primary lesion, the presence of cervical lymph node metastasis, and the nature of the primary therapy. Lymph node metastasis appears to be the most important determinant of survival. The development of nodal disease is influenced by the extent and location of the primary lesion. The occurrence of uncontrolled neck metastasis remains a constant source of therapeutic failure.

MARGINAL ZONE

Tumors of the marginal zone or epilarynx, which includes both the posterior surface of the suprahyoid portion of the epiglottis and the aryepiglottic folds, behave somewhat differently from tumors of the remainder of the supraglottic larynx. These tumors resemble hypopharyngeal cancers in that they spread early to involve the base of the tongue and the pharynx, have an increased incidence of metastatic spread, and less often involve the preepiglottic space. Carcinomas arising on the lingual surface of the epiglottis are considered extralaryngeal and behave like base of the tongue tumors. Sessions and Ogura[234] classified these lesions as superior hypopharyngeal tumors. This space was bounded by the epiglottis posteriorly, a line 1 cm posterior to the circumvallate papillae anteriorly, the glossoepiglottic folds laterally, and the vallecula inferiorly. Analyzing the overall survival rate (by partial and total laryngectomy) for

these tumors according to location, Sessions and Ogura[234] found the rate to be 53 percent (52 of 97 patients) for those with marginal lesions, 76 percent (134 of 177 patients) for supraglottic lesions, and 48 percent (12 of 25 patients) for lingual epiglottic lesions. Ogura et al.[207] described a 62 percent survival rate for those with the more limited lesions that were amenable to treatment by partial laryngopharyngectomy as compared to 28 percent for those requiring a total laryngectomy. The size of the lesions appeared to be a more important determinant of survival than the presence or absence of lymph node metastasis in this group. This reduced prognosis for tumors of the epilarynx has been confirmed by other workers. Taskinen[272] found on analysis of 932 supraglottic carcinomas, a 5-year survival rate of 40 percent for patients with epiglottic and false cord lesions and 25 percent for tumors of the arytenoid and aryepiglottic folds. Similar findings were reported by Cachin[42] (58 percent to 69 percent versus 43 percent).

LYMPH NODE METASTASIS

The extensive lymphatic network of the supraglottis expresses itself in the predilection of supraglottic carcinoma for regional lymph node spread. The incidence of regional metastasis generally reported varies from 25 to 50 percent. Ogura et al.[202] had described an incidence of regional spread of 29 percent, of which 12 percent were palpable and 17 percent were occult lymph nodes. Ogura et al.[206] later reported 23 percent of cases (41 of 177) to have clinically positive lymph nodes.

Fayos[67] reported a 25 percent incidence of lymph node metastasis among their 61 supraglottic tumors. Coates et al.[48] reported 72 of 221 cases (32 percent) to have palpable nodes. Bocca[32] cited the incidence of clinical and histologic cervical lymph node metastasis to be 35 percent of 240 cases. Hansen[95] reported clinically positive lymph nodes present in 41 percent of 511 lesions. Kirchner and Owen[134] reported an incidence of

48 percent palpable and 40 percent occult lymph node metastasis among 97 tumors. Smith et al.[252] observed 48 percent of 546 supraglottic tumors to have metastasized, with a high proportion of contralateral, bilateral, and fixed lymph nodes. Shah and Tollefsen[240] described 51 percent palpable and 34 percent (22 of 65 cases) occult metastasis in their series of 290 tumors. Som[254] reported lymph node metastasis in 32 percent of 75 patients, citing a 42 percent incidence of positive occult contralateral nodes in those patients with a positive palpable ipsilateral node greater than 2 cm. in diameter. Kirchner and Som[136] had 60 percent histologically proven cervical metastasis in 30 cases studied by serial sectioning.

The extent of the primary lesion influences the rate of metastasis. Cachin[42] found 27 percent of T1 lesions and 38 percent of T2 lesions to have palpable lymph nodes, of which 6 percent and 19 percent, respectively, were fixed. Taskinen[272] reported that 48 percent of all supraglottic tumors develop metastasis. However, this was only 13 percent for T1 lesions. Shah and Tollefsen[240] reported an incidence of cervical metastasis of 40 percent for T1, 42 percent for T2, 55 percent for T3, and 65 percent for T4 lesions.

The location of the primary is an additional determinant of metastasis, and tumors of the epilarynx behave similarly to those of the hypopharynx by having increased regional spread. Jankovic and Merkas[118] reported a 36.4 percent metastatic incidence for 88 lesions of the suprahyoid epiglottis, arytenoids, and aryepiglottic folds, as opposed to 15.3 percent for 391 infrahyoid epiglottic and false cord lesions. Shah and Tollefsen[240] found supraglottic tumors confined to the larynx had a 34 percent rate of metastasis (66 percent survival) whereas extension outside the larynx had a 69 percent spread (37 percent survival).

The high incidence of clinical and occult cervical lymph node metastasis associated with supraglottic tumors and the direct relationship of nodal disease to prognosis has prompted most authors to advocate routine ipsilateral and often contralateral radical neck dissection. Biller et al.[27] found a significant occurrence of contralateral spread with supraglottic carcinoma. In 143 cases studied, there were contralateral cervical metastases in 13 percent of T1, 23 percent of T2, 33 percent of T3, and 50 percent of T4 tumors. Consequently, contralateral standard or modified radical neck dissection is often employed when there is histologically proven tumor metastasis in the ipsilateral neck specimen.[136] Coates et al.[48] recommended elective radical neck dissection for all except T1 supraglottic lesions. Bocca[32] attributed the significant improvement in his 5-year cure rate for supraglottic carcinoma to the increased use of unilateral and bilateral modified neck dissection. Ogura et al.[202] observed an increase in survival from 74 percent to 78 percent with elective neck dissection and advocated its application regularly. However, Shah and Tollefsen[240] concluded that routine elective neck dissection was not warranted for supraglottic carcinoma after they observed a 5-year survival of 32 percent for patients with occult nodes as opposed to 27 percent for patients with palpable nodes. The subject of elective radical neck dissection for laryngeal carcinoma was reviewed by Staley and Herzon[260] with similar conclusions.

There is also some evidence that prophylactic radiotherapy to the neck can control occult nodal disease as seen by a decrease in the expected neck recurrence rate in patients so treated. Fletcher et al.[72] found only 1 of 69 N0 patients developed a metastatic node after elective neck irradiation. Goffinet et al.[86] reported that 81 percent of 31 irradiated patients with supraglottic tumors failed to develop cervical metastasis after 2 years. In 5 of the 6 failed cases the primary tumor was uncontrolled and presumably reseeded the nodes.

TREATMENT

The management of supraglottic carcinoma includes primary radiotherapy,[64] partial or total laryngectomy,[200, 254] and combined therapy.[291] Some surgeons irradiate early and selected advanced lesions for cure, reserving surgery to salvage failures. Others employ conservation surgery for early lesions amenable to partial laryngectomy and reserve total laryngectomy for advanced tumors. Some surgeons employ total laryngectomy for all operative candidates. Advocates of combined therapy utilize either preoperative or postoperative radiotherapy for patients who have advanced primary lesions or for those who have extensive neck metastases. These various therapeutic approaches will be considered individually because of the differences in reported end results.

Partial Laryngectomy. The supraglottic or subtotal horizontal laryngectomy represents a conservation laryngeal procedure in which the upper portion of the larynx is removed with preservation of its normal functions. The basis for this procedure rests in the embryologic derivation and subsequent anatomic compartmentalization of the larynx and its lymphatics, which limits tumor spread. The various studies supporting this basis have been cited in the section on anatomy. That this procedure is oncologically sound is confirmed clinically by a series of cases that show the 5-year tumor local control to be the same with supraglottic and total laryngectomy.[48, 200, 254] One of the important features of the procedure is resection of the preepiglottic space, which is an area of predilection of spread for tumors arising in this region. Supraglottic tumors may grow superiorly and laterally to invade the arytenoid, vallecula, base of the tongue, pyriform sinus, and lateral pharyngeal wall, and in selected cases these areas may be resected along with the supraglottic structures by the extended supraglottic laryngectomy. It should be noted that when a supraglottic tumor crosses the ventricle and spills onto the glottis it becomes transglottic, with a high probability of cartilage invasion and extension outside the larynx.[133] Patients with such lesions are no longer candidates for subtotal horizontal laryngectomy.

Selected cases of epiglottic carcinoma have been resected through a lateral pharyngotomy since the early part of this century. During the 1940's Alonso[3] in South America popularized the "partial horizontal laryngectomy." in which he excised lesions of the epiglottis and false cords along with the preepiglottic space, leaving a pharyngostomy. In 1958 Ogura[198] and in 1959 Som[253] reported in-continuity supraglottic resection and radical neck dissection for epiglottic tumors, with primary closure. Som[253] employed direct anastomosis and Ogura[198] used muscle flaps and a skin graft to resurface the pharyngeal defect. The procedure in its present form is decribed by Ogura and Biller.[200] Bocca[32] modified the standard procedure by preservation of the hyoid bone, with elevation of the periosteum off its inferior border to permit removal of the preepiglottic space; and closure of the pharyngostomy by approximation of the remaining thyroid alae to the hyoid bone with absorbable transfixing sutures. Bocca also considered the cricopharyngeal myotomy unnecessary.

Ogura and Biller[200] reported an 85 percent (17 of 20 cases) 3-year control rate for lesions confined to the epiglottis with supraglottic laryngectomy, but this rate dropped to 71 percent (23 of 32 cases) with extension onto the false cords. Som[254] described a 68 percent (51 of 75 cases) 5-year control rate with supraglottic laryngectomy. The same figure was reported by Coates et al.[48] with 30 treated cases.

Ogura et al.[206] reported an overall 3-year determinant survival rate of 76 percent for 177 supraglottic lesions treated by subtotal horizontal laryngectomy and radical neck dissection (some also received preoperative radiotherapy). With clinically positive lymph nodes, survival dropped to 57 to 66 percent, depending on the size of the primary lesion. In 30 patients recurrent tumor appeared, of which 47 percent could be salvaged by further radiotherapy or surgery. With supraglottic lesions extending onto an arytenoid and requiring its entire removal, Ogura et al.[203] reported a 75 percent 3-year survival rate among 59 patients undergoing extended supraglottic laryngectomy. However, all but 8 patients in this series had received preoperative radiotherapy (50 patients had 2,000 to 3,000 rads, 2 patients had 4,500 rads, 4 patients were radiotherapy failures after 5,000 to 7,000 rads). In 7 of the 20 patients with histologically positive lymph nodes, these nodes were occult. Analysis of recurrences revealed that most appeared within the first year of primary therapy, and all occurred within 3 years. Four of the twelve recurrences were salvaged by surgery, or radiotherapy, or a combination of both. Among the 4 patients with positive margins, 2 had recurrences. Increased recurrence and diminished survival also correlated well with the presence of positive lymph nodes. However, no correlation was found between the histopathologic cell type of the lesion and survival.

Bocca[32] claimed a 75 percent 5-year cure rate for 240 supraglottic tumors treated by supraglottic laryngectomy. He attributed this increased cure rate over his pervious series (60 percent) to both earlier diagnosis and the increased use of modified neck dissection. While Bocca's total series of cases numbers 240, among the 132 cases followed more than 5 years there was a 27 percent failure rate. The majority of recurrences appeared within the first postoperative year. Analysis of 27 recurrences showed 17 occurred in the larynx, 2 in the hypopharynx, and 8 in the base of the tongue. In 15 cases with intrinsic laryngeal recurrence, salvage was attempted by radiotherapy in 5 cases and total laryngectomy in 10. Three of the five irradiated patients and six of the ten laryngectomized patients were free of disease from 1 to 7 years posttherapy.

The complications of supraglottic laryngectomy include difficulties with swallowing rehabilitation and tracheal decannulation, which generally occur in proportion to the extent of the resection and the age and general medical condition of the patient. In elderly patients, those with chronic lung disease, or after procedures requiring the removal of an arytenoid or extensive portions of the base of the tongue or pharynx, prolonged aspiration and delayed tracheal decannulation are to be expected. Bocca[32] reported that in only 13 of 250 cases did dysphagia and dyspnea last for several weeks, with spontaneous recovery in all but one case, which required total laryngectomy. Bocca also reported only 6 instances of infection, 3 of fistula, and 3 of severe pneumonia among 223 cases. Prior high dose radiotherapy also increases postoperative complications, including infection, hemorrhage, fistula formation, and perichondritis.

Total Laryngectomy. Supraglottic carcinomas that have extended across the ventricle to become transglottic, have impaired vocal cord mobility, show invasion of the thyroid or cricoid cartilage or bilateral arytenoid involvement, or have spread outside the larynx with extensive invasion of the base of the tongue and hypopharynx should not be treated with partial subtotal horizontal laryngectomy and are best treated by total laryngectomy. Medical factors such as advanced age, debility, and chronic pulmonary disease, that compromise rehabilitation of deglutition, also contraindicate conservation surgery and such patients with supraglottic lesions are best treated by total laryngectomy to eliminate problems with postoperative aspiration.

While the earlier lesions are treated equally well by partial and total laryngectomy for control of disease at the primary site, the more advanced lesions requiring total laryngectomy have diminished survival because of extralaryngeal infiltrative growth and lymphatic spread. The increased occult and palpable lymph node disease that accompanies advanced supraglottic lesions requires radical neck dissection in addition to laryngectomy. Ogura et al.[206] reported a 3-year determinant survival rate of 66 percent for 35 supraglottic carcinomas with cord fixation (T3) treated by total laryngectomy and radical neck dissection. Coates et al.[48] found a 71 percent 5-year cure rate and a 3 percent local recurrence rate for 117 supraglottic tumors treated with total laryngectomy.

Radiotherapy. The overall survival rates reported with radiotherapy for the primary management of supraglottic carcinomas range from 30 to 70 percent. However, marked differences exist in treatment effectiveness depending on the size and location of the primary tumor and whether palpable cervical lymph node metastases are present. Larger primary lesions, tumors of the epilarynx, and the occurrence of regional metastases all significantly decrease survival. Ogura et al.[206] reported a 33 percent 3-year survival rate (22 cases) for those patients treated by radiotherapy alone. Taskinen[272] found an overall 5-year survival rate of 36.1 percent for 932 supraglottic lesions, the majority of which were treated by primary radiotherapy alone. The low survival rate, particularly with larger lesions, led them to later employ combined therapy. Jankovic and Merkas[118] reported a 39.2 percent 5-year survival rate for 439 supraglottic lesions treated primarily by radiotherapy. They claimed an additional 20 percent could be salvaged by a second course of radiation. Goffinet et al.[85] described a 46 percent control rate for radiotherapy alone (52 cases). However, with advanced primary lesions and positive neck nodes they noted that irradiation provided poor control. Olofsson et al.[215] reported a 47 percent 3-year survival rate for 30 cases (T1, T2) after primary radiotherapy. Coates et al.[48] reported a 47 percent control rate for 55 lesions, that were irradiated, with the remainder requiring salvage surgery. Hansen[95] also found primary radiotherapy to yield less than a 50 percent cure rate and treated more advanced lesions with combined therapy. Lederman[151, 152] reported a 53 percent control rate for T1 tumors and 64 percent for T2 tumors at 5 years among 70 cases lacking cervical metastasis. Lauerma[148] claimed cure rates of 69 percent (T1) and 48 percent (T2) for 101 similar cases. Henk[104] reported radical radiotherapy (5,000 rads in 3 weeks) to yield enhanced 5-year tumor control rates averaging 73 percent for T1 and T2 lesions and 51 percent for T3 and T4 tumors. Fletcher et al.[72] claimed 90 percent of T1 lesions were controlled by radiotherapy.

However, analysis by stage yields wide differences in the ability of radiotherapy to control supraglottic carcinomas. Kirchner and Owen[134] found control by radiotherapy to be 64 percent for T1, 67 percent for T2, and 5 percent for T4 tumors. On review of 544 supraglottic carcinomas, Vermund[288] reported radiotherapy to control 65 percent of T1, 61 percent of T2, 36 percent of T3, and 14 percent of T4 lesions. These figures for radiotherapy also include salvage surgery. Hansen[95] found the 5-year survival rate of 511 supraglottic carcinomas treated mainly by primary radiotherapy to be 68 percent for stage I, 57 percent for stage II, 35 percent for stage III, and 10 percent for stage IV tumors. However, Goepfert et al.[84] reported control of laryngeal disease with preservation of normal voice in 88.5 percent of T1, 77 percent of T2, 66 percent of T3, and 60 percent of T4 tumors by primary radiotherapy (147 cases).

While surgery and radiotherapy appear to yield comparable results for early lesions with negative necks,[134, 288] the effectiveness of radiotherapy in controlling advanced lesions diminishes markedly. Siirala et al.[245] reported an overall 5-year survival rate of 34 percent for 64 advanced (stage III and IV) supraglottic lesions. However, when analyzed by treatment modality the 5-year survival rate was 60 percent for surgery, 34 percent for combined therapy, and 20 percent for radiotherapy alone. Henry et al.[105] treated 183 T4 supraglottic tumors (1/3 with positive lymph nodes) primarily by radiotherapy with 42 percent free of disease at 3 years. Among 40 cases with recurrence, 22 were operated on and 10 of these were salvaged. They noted no improvement in the cure rate with supervoltage therapy compared to conventional radiation. Cachin[42] reported a 58 percent 5-year cure rate for radiotherapy (43 cases) for early supraglottic tumors, as opposed to 69 percent for high dose radiotherapy combined with partial laryngectomy (13 cases). However, the combined therapy group had greater lymph node disease. Wang et al.[291] reported 3-year cure rates of 74 percent for early (53 T1 and T2) and 23 percent for advanced (17 T3 and T4) supraglottic tumors with radiotherapy. The presence of palpable lymph nodes reduced survival from 63 to 22 percent. These observations led them to employ combined therapy for extensive primary and cervical metastatic disease. Vermund[288] reported a 32 percent 5-year survival rate after primary radiotherapy and a 64 percent survival rate with primary surgery for 544 T2 and T4 supraglottic carcinomas.

The location of the lesion also appeared to be an important survival factor. Cachin[42] reported that the cure rate for early lesions of the epilarynx (14 cases) treated by radiotherapy, surgery, or a combination fell from about 60 percent to 43 percent for the remainder of the supraglottic larynx. However, Fletcher et al.[71] reported a 64 percent control rate for early infrahyoid and false cord lesions and 69 percent for suprahyoid and aryepiglottic fold tumors. These authors stated that base of tongue and preepiglottic space involvement have been a continued source of failure with radiotherapy.

In view of the findings it appears that primary radiotherapy finds its greatest success in curing smaller and exophytic supraglottic tumors in patients with negative necks. In cases with smaller primary tumors and positive necks the larynx may be treated by irradiation for cure and a radical neck dissection performed. Prophylactic neck irradiation may be also given to the contralateral side for treatment of occult disease. The presence of an advanced tumor with cord fixation or cartilage destruction mandates surgery for cure. With lesions having infiltration into the pharyngeal wall or base of the tongue, which carry a high probability of local recurrence, or in patients with extensive neck metastasis, preoperative or postoperative radiotherapy may be employed to improve survival. It should also be noted that salvage surgery after radiation failure will probably require a total laryngectomy rather than a conservation procedure because of the increased incidence of chondritis and difficulty in assessing the extent of residual or recurrent disease.

Combined Therapy. Radiotherapy has been used preoperatively or postoperatively in conjunction with surgery to decrease the incidence of local and regional recurrences. Preoperative irradiation may also render patients with fixed neck lesions resectable.

Ogura and Biller[201] analyzed 69 operated supraglottic carcinomas (51 undergoing partial laryngectomy) of which one group had received 1,500 to 3,000 rads preoperative radiation and the other had received no radiation. There was no significant difference in survival at 3 years between the two groups. Cachin[43] reviewed 71 cases of horizontal partial laryngectomy receiving 4,000 rads preoperatively. The survival rate was 62 percent at 3 years and 53 percent at 5 years, which was comparable to the figures for nonirradiated cases. However, he noted a significant increase in complications and suggested that preoperative radiotherapy be eliminated with supraglottic laryngectomy.

Reddi and Mercado[225] reported 5-year survival rates of 75 and 50 percent respectively for early and late supraglottic lesions receiving combined therapy. They concluded that low dose (3,000 to 3,600 rads) preoperative radiation was of limited value in improving prognosis.

However, Cachin[42] reported increased survival for early lesions treated by combined therapy (69 percent survival rate) as opposed to primary radiotherapy (58 percent). The poor results with primary radiotherapy for advanced lesions and cases with metastatic disease led Wang et al.[290, 291] to employ 4,000 rads preoperatively followed by total laryngectomy and radical neck dissection. They reported the 3-year cure rate improved from 23 to 54 percent for T3 and T4 lesions and from 22 to 55 percent for cases with lymph node disease. Ogura et al.[206] observed fewer recurrences after treatment with preoperative radiotherapy in patients with supraglottic lesions having clinically positive lymph nodes. He also recommended the use of preoperative radiation for more extensive primary tumors, which carried a diminished 5-year survival rate. Hansen[95] and Goldman and Roffman[87] similarly reported increased cure and decreased recurrence with combined therapy for supraglottic tumors.

Fletcher et al.[71] advocated postoperative radiotherapy for patients with advanced primary lesions having extralaryngeal spread and for those with extensive neck disease. They reported increasing the 2-year cure rate from 38 to 71 percent for patients with advanced nodal disease. In a later publication[84] they reported the cervical recurrence rate fell to 15 percent with combined therapy from 45 percent with surgery alone in N2 and N3 patients. This group also substitutes removal of clinically involved nodes for standard radical neck dissection after high dose radiotherapy.

Glottic Carcinoma

The reported 5-year cure rate for glottic carcinoma averages 70 to 80 percent. However, it varies considerably with the stage of the disease (Table 18-4). Several factors contribute to the excellent cure rate of glottic carcinoma. The lesions are detected early because anatomic distortion of the vocal cord rapidly produces a change in vocal quality. The majority of the lesions arising on the true cord are well-differentiated squamous carcinomas that generally tend to be exophytic. The sparse lymphatic drainage of the true cord limits metastatic spread. Also, immunologic factors may be operative as an inflammatory infiltrate often surrounds the developing tumor. With advanced lesions, penetration into adjacent tissue opens anatomic pathways for local and metastatic spread and compromises survival.

The glottis is generally the most common site reported for the development of a laryngeal carcinoma. Hoarseness appears early because of interference with vibratory motion of the vocal cords. It is only with advanced lesions that dyspnea appears because of vocal cord fixation and obstruction of the glottic chink by tumor bulk. The tumor generally arises on the anterior two-thirds of the membranous portion of the cord and spreads slowly anteriorly, posteriorly, vertically, and laterally as already outlined. Tumors arising primarily at the anterior commissure and posterior third of the vocal cord are uncommon and have a somewhat different biologic behavior at these sites. Also, the behavior, prognosis, and management of glottic carcinoma varies with its extent. Consequently, each type of glottic carcinoma will be considered individually. While the results of radiotherapy and surgery are seemingly comparable for early lesions, marked differences appear when there is a transglottic tumor compared to those with impaired cord mobility. Kirchner and Owen[134] found that control by surgery versus radiotherapy was 80 vs. 83 percent for T1 tumors, but it dropped to 88 vs 35

TABLE 18-4. SURVIVAL OF PATIENTS WITH GLOTTIC CARCINOMA ACCORDING TO STAGE

Study	Number of Cases	Overall Survival Rate (%)	5-Year Survival Rate (%)			
			T1	T2	T3	T4
Leroux-Robert[153]	620	72	93	85	56	26
Skolnik et al.[249]	264	70	82	70	48 (T3 and T4 as one category)	
Ennuyer and Bataini[65]	214	77	82	51	48	
Stewart et al.[266]	291	70	90	73	57	30
Hawkins[101]	800	80	96	72	50	25
Daly et al.[57]	464	81.5	89	85	59	0

percent for T2 tumors, and 72 vs 25 percent for T3 tumors.

MEMBRANOUS CORD LESIONS

Carcinoma of the midportion of the true cord with good mobility is treated with about equal success by radiotherapy and conservation laryngeal surgery. Radiotherapy is generally employed because it provides better preservation of voice quality without compromising survival. The 5-year cure rates reported with primary radiotherapy for early glottic tumors range from 82 to 98 percent. However, it should be noted that these figures represent net tumor control after salvage surgery, and that recurrence rates of 9 to 21 percent have been reported after irradiation (see Table 18-5). There are other factors that also make the apparent curability of glottic carcinoma by radiotherapy falsely high. The finding of Stutsman and McGavran[271] that in about 20 percent of the patients undergoing hemilaryngectomy there was no tumor in the specimen suggests that the lesion was totally removed by the biopsy. Also, when radiotherapy end results are reported, distinction is often not made between carcinoma in situ, superficially invasive carcinoma, and invasive carcinoma.

The results of primary surgery for T1 glottic tumors are comparable or greater than those achieved by irradiation. Laryngo-fissure and cordectomy has yielded cure rates of 84 to 98 percent.[57, 155, 235, 259] Lillie and DeSanto[158] initially reported 98 cases of in situ or early carcinoma treated by transoral excision with control of the disease in all cases. DeSanto[60] later described 4 patients among 50 cases of carcinoma in situ and 53 early invasive carcinomas of the glottis who required laryngectomy 5 or more years after initial therapy. Laryngofissure and cordectomy was also employed for 197 similar glottic tumors with approximately 90 percent actuarial survival at 5 years. However, hemilaryngectomy has supplanted cordectomy in the operative management of glottic carcinoma, as it gives a wider margin of resection and can be used for more extensive lesions with greater local control. This procedure also provides a stronger voice than laryngofissure. Peroral cryosurgery[180] and laser excision[268] have also been used successfully with some early lesions.

With extension of the tumor to the anterior commissure or posteriorly behind the vocal process, greater controversy exists as to the superior modality of primary treatment. Radiotherapy for these lesions yields an even lessened tumor control. Wang[290] reported 5-year recurrence-free rates of 92 percent for lesions of the anterior two-thirds of the vocal cord, 81 percent for those with anterior commissure involvement, and 76 percent for those with posterior third extension. However, advocates of radiation ther-

TABLE 18-5. RADIOTHERAPY RESULTS WITH T1 GLOTTIC CARCINOMA

Study	Number of Cases	Radiation Failures	Surgical Salvage	Net 5-Year Survival Rate
Constable et al.[55]	107	9% (10)	100% (6)	83% (89)
Wang[289]	325	13% (43)	82% (40)	87% (282)
Jorgensen[125]	44	14% (6)	100% (6)	93% (41)
Ennuyer and Bataini[65]	71	14% (10)	70% (10)	82% (58)
Fletcher et al.[72]	210	14% (30)	90% (29)	98% (206)
Hawkins[101]	260	21% (54)	68% (54)	80% (207)

apy claim that salvage is still possible in 55 to 75 percent of the radiation failures[15, 181, 219, 250] resulting in a greater proportion of retained larynges. However, it should be noted that salvage surgery is generally by total laryngectomy because many of the patients are no longer candidates for conservation surgery. Ballantyne and Fletcher[15] were able to perform partial surgery in only 15 percent of radiation failures. After radiotherapy the actual extent of the disease is more extensive than it appears clinically, since scattered nests of submucosal tumor are present.[30] Also the majority of recurrences after radiotherapy are larger than the original lesion, making fewer patients candidates for conservation procedures. Moreover, after radiotherapy the rate of operative complications (wound infection, flap necrosis, carotid rupture, hemorrhage, salivary fistula) increases markedly (from 10 to as high as 54 percent[249]), although this is denied by some workers.[55] The occurrence of perichondritis after partial surgery for radiation failure may result in delayed decannulation or even total laryngectomy. However, Biller, et al.[30] reported hemilaryngectomy to control 14 of 18 (78 percent) postradiation carcinomas of the true cords. Case selection was important with local failure occurring principally in patients with greater than 5 mm of subglottic extension.

Radiotherapy should be used in selected cases of early glottic carcinoma. However, with lesions extending beyond the confines of the membranous cord, hemilaryngectomy becomes the treatment method of choice. While Vermund[288] reported a control rate for surgery of 83 percent and for radiotherapy of 78 percent on review of 1,425 T1 glottic lesions, DeSanto[60] reported only 37 percent of 57 cases of T1b invasive cord carcinomas to be cured by radiation alone. Biller et al.[29] found hemilaryngectomy to provide a 77 percent 5-year cure rate for 58 similar lesions. Kirchner and Owen[134] claimed a 78 percent control rate (14 of 18 cases) by partial laryngectomy. Ogura et al.[205] reported 87 percent of T1

lesions (205 cases) to be free of disease at 3 years after hemilaryngectomy. Moreover, 74 percent of the failures could be salvaged by total laryngectomy. Brandenburg and Rutter[36] found that T1 and T2 patients treated by partial surgery had a lower incidence of local residual disease than those who were initially radiated. However, Hendrickson et al.[102] concluded after a study of 210 patients with radiated and 84 with operated cordal carcinomas that comparable results are achieved (95 percent 5-year cure rate) after salvage procedures, and that selection of therapy should be based on the expected morbidity. While radiotherapy is preferable to total laryngectomy in the management of these more extensive unilateral mobile cordal lesions, the better local control provided by hemilaryngectomy ultimately results in more retained larynges and makes it the preferred mode of treatment.

ANTERIOR COMMISSURE LESIONS

Involvement of the anterior commissure promotes early invasion and spread of glottic tumors. This is due to the close relationship between the mucosa and cartilage at this point, the extension of the anterior commissure ligament into the cartilage without an intervening perichondrium, and the access to the cricothyroid membrane which lies just below subglottically. Study of serially sectioned larynges has demonstrated that extralaryngeal spread and invasion of the laryngeal framework occurs primarily anteriorly through the cricothyroid membrane and adjacent thyroid cartilage. Olofsson and Von Nostrand[212] found on sectioning 73 glottic carcinomas that 21 of the 26 invading the thyroid cartilage did so at the anterior commissure and 22 of the 27 extending outside the larynx did so through the cricothyroid membrane. However, Kirchner and Fischer[133] found that tumor spread forward and laterally was resisted by the anterior commissure tendon and the conus elasticus, respectively. In only 2 of their 13 cases was cartilage invasion found. Also, submucosal spread was not observed beyond the surface appearance of the tumor.

The majority of tumors involving the anterior commissure occurred as a result of spread from the vocal cord whereas lesions arising in the anterior commissure primarily are exceedingly rare. Olofsson[211] reported 9 percent (96) of 746 glottic tumors to involve the anterior commissure, with only 2 cases arising there primarily. Sessions et al.[238] found on their review of 591 glottic and subglottic tumors that 25 percent (175) secondarily involved the anterior commissure whereas 1 percent (5 cases) arose there primarily. Smith et al.[252] reported 2.2 percent (24) of 1,060 glottic carcinomas to be limited to the anterior commissure with another 6.7 percent combined with a cordal lesion. The incidence of lymph node metastasis with anterior commissure involvement is low. Olofsson[211] reported 4 percent and Sessions et al.[238] 8 percent cervical metastasis in their series.

Lesions involving the anterior commissure have been treated both by surgery and radiotherapy. Som and Silver[257] reported a 68 percent cure rate (over 3 years) for 38 patients with partial laryngectomy, which was increased to 81 percent with salvage surgery. Kirchner and Som[137] later reported a success rate of 69 percent for 58 lesions followed from 4 to 19 years. However, in 3 cases total laryngectomy was required for salvage. In their series, 7 of the 8 local recurrences appeared subglottically. Metastasis appeared in 9 patients (cervical nodes 5, Delphian node 3, systemic 1), of which 6 resulted in death. Three of the eleven patients in the series who were operated on after radiotherapy failure developed perichondritis. Five of their specimens studied by serial section failed to show invasion of the thyroid cartilage even though the vocal cords had limited mobility in 3 cases. Sessions et al.[238] found the survival and recurrence rates of anterior commissure lesions to correlate with the size and stage of the tumor. In their experience subglottic extension did not influence survival. They reported absolute 3-year survival rates of 76 percent (57 of 75 cases) for those with unilateral vocal cord lesions involving the anterior commissure and 61 percent (59 of 96 cases) for horseshoe lesions, those involving both vocal cords. Sessions et al.[237] found hemilaryngectomy to provide a 5-year survival rate of 74 percent (45 of 61 cases) for those with stage I and II lesions. Patients with stage III and IV glottic lesions (82 cases) treated by total laryngectomy had a 62 percent 5-year survival rate.

Several authors have also reported good control of anterior commissure tumors by radiotherapy, with minimal complications. Olofsson et al.[216] claimed an 80 percent 5-year crude survival rate for 57 patients with anterior commissure lesions treated primarily with radiation. However, 15 of the 57 patients had residual or recurrent tumor, of which 10 underwent total laryngeotomy. Salvage was accomplished in 8 of these 10 patients. Kirchner and Fischer[133] reported equal control (85 percent) of anterior commissure cancer by radiotherapy (19 cases) and surgery (20 cases). However, the lesions in the surgically treated group were far more advanced, many with cord fixation. Jesse et al.[120] claimed an 8.8 percent failure rate for radiation treatment of 91 T1 and T2 glottic tumors with anterior commissure extension. However, recurrent cancer developed in 22 patients, the majority having lesions with subglottic extension and anterior commissure involvement. They considered this latter group to require surgery (8 of 11).

POSTERIOR CORD LESIONS

Extension of a membranous cord lesion posteriorly to involve the vocal process and anterior face of the arytenoid changes the biologic behavior of the tumor and decreases survival. Further infiltrative growth posteriorly may involve the thyroarytenoid muscle or cricoarytenoid joint with impaired cord mobility, or growth may invade the cricoid cartilage and extend to the pharynx giving an even decreased curability.

As with extension to the anterior commissure, posterior growth of a glottic tumor diminishes control by radiotherapy. This decreased radiocurability has reinforced the contention of advocates of partial laryngectomy that surgery should be the primary treatment modality in these cases, as it will ultimately yield more functional larynges. Analysis of 104 cases of glottic carcinoma extending onto the vocal process and face of the arytenoid by Som[255] showed a curability of 74 percent with extended hemilaryngectomy. Ogura et al.[204] reported a 3-year control rate of 90 percent for hemilaryngectomy of 79 tumors with arytenoid extension. One patient had clinically positive lymph nodes. There were 6 recurrences, 3 occurring locally and 3 in the neck. Three of these patients were salvaged by radiation or surgery. Two of the three patients who died of disease were radiation failures secondarily treated by hemilaryngectomy.

T2 LESIONS

Vertical extension of a glottic cancer to the supraglottic and subglottic regions alters its behavior and decreases survival (Table 18-4). Treatment by radiotherapy now yields a failure rate of about 30 to 45 percent[35] (Table 18-6). Estimates of 5-year survival rates after primary radiotherapy followed by salvage surgery range from as low as 52 to 57 percent[65, 118] to as high as 85 to 90 percent[72, 117]. Vermund[288] found a 50 percent absolute 5-year survival rate after initial

radiation as compared to 61 percent for initial surgery and concluded that the difference did not justify total laryngectomy as primary management of such tumors. However, Ogura et al.[205] reported an 82 percent control of 55 T2 lesions by hemilaryngectomy.

Since the surgical management differs for subglottic and transglottic lesions they will be considered separately.

SUBGLOTTIC LESIONS

Growth of a glottic tumor into the subglottis more than 10 mm anteriorly and 5 mm posterolaterally places it in contact with the cricothyroid membrane and cricoid cartilage respectively, making available to it new avenues of spread. The extensive system of subglottic lymphatics also provides pathways for extralaryngeal extension. Olofsson[210] found metastasis to the prelaryngeal (Delphian) lymph node in 8 of 110 laryngectomy specimens studied. In all cases the tumor had invaded the subglottic space and in 6 there was extension through the cricothyroid membrane.

As do cordal carcinomas with anterior and posterior extension, subglottic involvement also lessens radiocurability. Sessions et al.[236] found 22 percent (132 of 585) of glottic tumors to extend subglotically. In 5 percent there was lymph node metastasis. When analyzed by treatment modality, the 3-year survival rate was 83 percent for hemi-

TABLE 18-6. RADIOTHERAPY RESULTS WITH T2 GLOTTIC CARCINOMA

Study	Number of Cases	Radiation Failures	Surgical Salvage	Net 5-Year Survival Rate
Wang[289]	90	28% (25)	78% (23)	72% (65)
Fletcher et al.[72]	120	29% (35)	74% (31)	90% (108)
Ennuyer and Bataini[65]	27	33% (9)	57% (7)	52% (14)
Hawkins[101]	73	37% (27)	41% (27)	60% (44)
Jorgensen[125]	25	44% (11)	72% (25)	72% (18)

laryngectomy (63 cases), 63 percent for total laryngectomy (46 cases), and 63 percent for radiotherapy (16 cases). However, the end results were related to the extent of the tumor. While unilateral lesions with anterior commissure involvement and less than 10 mm of subglottic extension had a survival of 90 percent, it dropped to 50 percent with more than 10mm. of subglottic extent. Recurrences occurred in 19 percent of the series and were most frequent with subglottic lesions extending more than 20 mm.

TRANSGLOTTIC LESIONS

When a glottic carcinoma extends upward across the ventricle to the supraglottic larynx there is an appreciable diminution in survival. Such transglottic lesions have access to the paraglottic space, which permits extensive spread and cartilage invasion.[138] Cartilage invasion and regional lymph node metastasis increase in frequency with lesions greater than 3 to 4 cm in diameter.

Radiotherapy is the primary treatment modality for patients with these lesions, as these patients are not candidates for partial laryngeal surgery. Total laryngectomy is generally reserved for radiotherapy failures. Care must be taken in assessing transglottic lesions, as impaired cord mobility or cartilage invasion would reclassify them as T3 and T4 tumors respectively and require total laryngectomy for effective local control.

FIXED CORD LESIONS

Fixation of the vocal cord is a grave prognostic sign generally signifying extensive laryngeal infiltration by advanced glottic, transglottic, subglottic, or hypopharyngeal tumors with paraglottic space extension. Many of these lesions are associated with cartilage destruction and increased lymphatic spread, lessening control locally or regionally by both radiation and surgery. Olofsson et al.[213] found on serially sectioning 28 larynges with fixed cords that 50 percent were clinically underassessed, particularly with regard to extralaryngeal extension. While the main cause of fixation is by invasion of the thyroarytenoid muscle,[135, 213] fixation may also result from involvement of the cricoarytenoid joint and the other intrinsic laryngeal muscles.

With the presence of cord fixation, surgery is clearly superior to radiotherapy in the management of laryngeal carcinoma (see Table 18-7). Primary treatment by radiation generally yields tumor control in about 25 to 30 percent of the cases.[65, 134, 181, 290] This may be improved by salvage surgery to yield 5-year survival rates averaging about 50 percent[65, 101, 241, 266] The generally accepted treatment is total laryngectomy, with radical neck dissection if palpable cervical lymph nodes are present. However, Kirchner and Som[135] found that in 18 of 23 total laryngectomy specimens of fixed cord lesions, the tumor was limited to the vocal cord, with no specimens showing in-

TABLE 18-7. CONTROL OF FIXED CORD LESIONS BY RADIOTHERAPY AND SURGERY

Study	Number of Cases	5-Year Survival Rate (%)	
		Radiotherapy	Surgery
Marchetta et al.[169]	81	20	62
Martensson et al.[173]	72	24	55
Kirchner et al.[134]	31	25	72
Vermund[288]	76	29	55

vasion of the thyroid and cricoid cartilages. This prompted them to perform hemi-laryngectomy in selected cases with cord fixation, with a 60 percent (13 of 22) cure rate. Three of the 9 recurrences were salvaged by total laryngectomy. Recurrences appeared in 4 of the 5 patients with subglottic extension. In a later study Som[255] reported a 58 percent curability in 26 patients with selected T3 glottic tumors treated by partial laryngectomy.

ADVANCED LESIONS

Glottic carcinomas that destroy the thyroid cartilage and extend outside the larynx are classified as T4 lesions. Jesse[119] analyzed the results of treatment of 48 of 51 patients with such advanced tumors (3 had distant metastasis and were untreated). There were clinically positive lymph nodes in 19 percent and occult metastases in another 20 percent. About 30 percent of the patients required an emergency tracheostomy. The minimal therapeutic procedure was total laryngectomy, with 16 patients also receiving radiotherapy. The 4-year cure rate was 54 percent. However, in those cases with positive lymph nodes, pharyngeal extension, and a prior tracheostomy it dropped to 38 percent. In 5 patients there was local recurrence and in 2 lymph node metastasis. Two others who had both local and regional control developed distant metastasis. While 63 percent of the patients receiving combined therapy survived, the benefits of postoperative radiotherapy in eliminating recurrence remained to be established. Table 18-4 reveals the poor 5-year survival of patients with such lesions, as encountered in various studies employing both radiotherapy and surgery in their management.

LYMPH NODE METASTASIS

Tumors confined to the membranous portion of the vocal cord rarely produce regional metastases because of the scarcity of lymphatics. However, with extension of the primary tumor beyond these confines the incidence of lymph node metastasis increases proportionately. Jakobsson[117] reported less then 1 percent incidence (2 out of 230 cases), of which there was one T1 and one T3 tumor. Leroux-Robert[155] reported 15 metastasis in 620 cases (2.5 percent incidence), of which one was with a T2 lesion, 7 with T3 lesions, and 7 with T4 lesions. Till et al.[278] noted 396 metastases among 10,989 cases collected from various tumor registries for an incidence of 3.5 percent. Kirchner and Owen[134] reported 8 metastases among 209 glottic lesions (all among the 73 T2 and T3 tumors). Jankovic and Merkas[118] found secondary spread in 5.5 percent of 271 glottic carcinomas (1 T1, 10 T2, 4 T3 lesions). Hawkins[101] reported 7 percent lymph node metastasis among 800 glottic carcinomas, the majority being T3 and T4 lesions. Daly and Strong[57] also reported the incidence of lymph node metastasis to be related to the extent of the primary. Metastases occurred in 5 percent of T1, 8 percent of T2 and 15 percent of T3 lesions. An additional 11 percent of the T3 patients required a second neck dissection for proven metastases.

While the incidence of lymph node metastasis is too low to justify elective neck dissection, the presence of a palpable lymph node mandates radical surgery because radiotherapy is ineffective for control.[288] Some surgeons advocate resection of the paratracheal tissues or thyroid gland[99] for tumors having extensive subglottic extension.

Subglottic Tumors

Carcinoma involving the subglottic region may arise there primarily or by extension from the glottis. While involvement of the subglottic space permits the tumor access to new anatomic pathways of spread, both types of lesions have their own patterns of biologic behavior. Tumor has also been reported there as a result of distant metastasis.[263] The reported incidence of primary subglottic carcinoma generally ranges from 1 to 8 percent in the larger series,[98, 152, 212, 236, 263] averaging about 1 to 2 percent. Stell[261] reported 40 primary subglottic tumors among 1,011 laryngeal cancers for an incidence of 4.1 percent. Estimates of the occurrence of secondary subglottic spread from the true cord varies between 11 and 33 percent. Rates reported were 11.4 percent (19 of 166 cases) by Stell and Tobin,[263] 13.2 percent (52 of 468 cases) by Stell,[261] 20.5 percent (62 of 306 cases) by Shaw,[241] 22 percent (132 of 591 cases) by Sessions et al.,[236] and 33 percent (24 of 73 cases) studied by serial section by Olofsson.[211] This disparity is believed to be due to difficulties in assessing the extent of laryngeal lesions relying on direct laryngoscopy and tomography alone. This is underscored by the report of Martensson[172] in which 10 of 22 cases studied by transconioscopy showed subglottic extension that had been missed by laryngoscopy and laryngography. Sorenson[258] similarly detected subglottic spread by this method in 11 cases of laryngeal carcinoma, of which 4 had been missed by endoscopic and radiographic examination.

The reported incidence of regional lymph node metastasis with subglottic carcinoma is generally under 10 percent. Lederman[151, 152] reported an occurrence of 4.3 percent (6 of 140 cases); Pietrantoni et al.,[218] 9.25 percent (5 of 54 cases); and Martensson et al.,[173] 10 percent (1 of 10 cases). However, Stell and Tobin[263] reported 16 percent of primary subglottic tumors and 5.5 percent of secondary tumors to have palpable cervical lymph nodes on study of 45 patients. Stell[261] found on review of 104 subglottic tumors an incidence of 21.9 percent among 42 true subglottic lesions and 19.3 percent among 62 tumors with subglottic spread. Subglottic carcinoma apparently spreads initially to the paratracheal region before producing palpable lateral cervical metastasis. Consequently, the actual metastatic activity of these tumors is probably clinically underestimated. Harrison[98] cited an incidence of paratracheal node involvement as high as 50 percent. Radioisotope study of the lymphatics of the subglottic region in man by Welsh[292] revealed 96 percent drained to ipsilateral paratracheal nodes, 2.6 percent to contralateral nodes, and 0.2 percent to the superior mediastinum. Three lymphatic pedicles were identified: an anterior one, which penetrated the cricothyroid membrane and drained into the prelaryngeal (Delphian) node and in turn into the pretracheal and supraclavicular nodes; and 2 posterolateral ones, which penetrated the cricotracheal membrane with drainage to the paratracheal nodes and to the superior mediastinum.

On review of larger series there appears to be a preponderance of women developing subglottic cancer. Stell and Tobin[263] found that 44 percent of their 25 primary subglottic tumors occurred in women. Lederman[151] reported 16.4 percent of his series to be women. Subglottic carcinoma also appears to arise at a somewhat earlier age in women.

Concerning presenting symptoms, patients with primary subglottic tumors generally demonstrate airway obstruction, with stridor and dyspnea; whereas in those with tumors with secondary spread, hoarseness is more prominent. Stell and Tobin[263] found one-third of their primary tumor cases to require emergency tracheotomy, whereas only 1 of 19 secondary tumors required tracheotomy. The incidence of vocal cord fixation at the time of diagnosis is also high with subglottic tumors. Stell[261] reported 35 of 42 true subglottic tumors and 34 of 62 tumors with subglottic spread to show vocal cord fixation.

There is also a high incidence of local recurrence and distant metastasis with primary subglottic tumors. Stell and Tobin[263] reported 21 of 45 subglottic tumors developed recurrence, the majority within one year. There were 9 incidences of distant metastasis, of which 8 occurred among 25 primary tumors and one among 19 secondary tumors. The sites of metastasis were bone (4), lung (4), and mediastinum (1).

Olofsson[210] stressed the ability of primary subglottic tumors to produce extensive circumferential growth, invade cartilage, and spread outside the larynx. In a study of 110 serially sectioned larynges, he identified 4 primary subglottic and 24 glottic-subglottic lesions. Of the 4 primary tumors, all extended through the conus elasticus to involve the true cord submucosally, 3 spread to the opposite side, all invaded the vocalis muscle (2 the lateral cricoarytenoid muscle, 1 the posterior cricoarytenoid muscle, and 1 the interarytenoid muscle), 2 invaded the thyroid cartilage, and 3 extended outside the larynx. Spread may occur posteriorly along the cricotracheal space and, if undetected, results in residual tumor in the hypopharynx and the development of a stomal recurrence. Anterior spread occurs directly through the cricothyroid membrane or along blood vessels and lymphatics. Among the 24 glottic-subglottic tumors in the series, 6 invaded the vocalis muscle and produced cord fixation; 3 invaded the thyroid cartilage, 4 the cricoid cartilage, and 8 the arytenoid cartilages; and 7 spread outside the larynx anteriorly through the cricothyroid membrane.

Histologically the majority of tumors arising in the subglottis are squamous cell carcinomas. However, the occurrence of primary and metastatic adenocarcinoma has been reported in this region.[263]

Attempts have been made to control these tumors with both radiotherapy and surgery. However, the prognosis of primary subglottic tumors remains poor. In addition to wide field laryngectomy, Harrison[99] has advocated removal of the manubrium and resection of the paratracheal nodes with low tracheal resection in an attempt to eliminate tracheal and stomal recurrences. However, Stell and Tobin[263] did not endorse mediastinal dissection because of the low incidence of mediastinal metastasis in their series. An elective radical neck dissection is not generally performed for subglottic carcinomas. Harrison[98, 99] also favored excision of the thyroid isthmus and one or both lobes for tumors involving the subglottic region. While serial section studies[210] show a relatively low incidence of thyroid gland spread and metastasis, partial resection of the thyroid gland is generally performed, as neoplastic involvement cannot be assessed clinically.

Stell and Tobin[263] reported 44 percent of patients with primary subglottic and 31 percent of patients with secondary subglottic tumors to succumb despite the modality of therapy. Vermund[288] and Harrison[98] both reported mortality figures of approximately 60 percent.

OTHER EPITHELIAL MALIGNANT TUMORS

The normal nonkeratinizing squamous epithelium of the vocal cord may undergo a spectrum of changes ranging from transformation to a keratinizing epithelium through frank carcinoma. While they may not be clinically distinguishable, the various lesions have different biologic behaviors and their microscopic recognition is important because it influences the selection of therapy.

Premalignant Lesions

The laryngeal mucosa may become hyperplastic and convert to a keratinizing squamous epithelium, which has been also described as keratosis, hyperkeratosis, pachyderma laryngis, and leukoplakia. Microscopically, the epithelium shows an orderly maturation. However, when there are cells with nuclear aberations present these changes have been classified as atypia.

Both laryngeal keratosis and atypia have been cited as examples of premalignant change. However, only a small number of patients with these changes develop carcinoma. The presence of atypia actually places the individual at greater risk. Gabriel and Jones[80] found that of 30 patients with laryngeal keratosis, none of the 13 without atypia developed carcinoma, whereas one of 17 with atypia did. Norris and Peale[195] reported 1 of 30 patients with keratosis alone who developed carcinoma. However, 11 of 86 also having atypia did. McGavran et al.[163] noted that 3 of 84 cases of keratosis developed laryngeal carcinoma, of which 2 also had atypia. Keratosis and atypia represent reactive epithelial changes and may accompany chronic inflammation as well as tumor. There is statistical evidence that smoking promotes the development of atypia in the laryngeal epithelium.[14] Auerbach et al.[14] reported that 16 percent of 644 cigarette smokers had evidence of carcinoma in situ of the larynx at autopsy, and 99 percent also had atypia. None of the ex-cigarette smokers studied showed carcinoma in situ and 25 percent had only mild atypia, similar to nonsmokers.

Carcinoma in Situ

In carcinoma in situ the squamous epithelium shows disordered maturation with replacement by malignant-appearing cells that do not invade the basement membrane. The occurrence of carcinoma in situ in the larynx at an earlier age than invasive carcinoma was interpreted by Miller[178] as support for the concept that it is only the predecessor of invasive carcinoma. Bauer[21] showed that 49 percent of 354 laryngeal cancers studied by step sections also contained carcinoma in situ. It more commonly accompanied nonkeratinizing carcinoma (76 percent) than keratinizing carcinoma (29 percent). Because of the presence of carcinoma in situ at the edge of the lesions, Bauer[21] suggested that it may represent a method of intramucosal spread. The report of carcinoma in situ should alert the clinician that invasive carcinoma may be present in an adjacent area.

The definite malignant potential of this lesion is underscored by the report of Miller and Fischer[179] who found that vocal cord stripping failed to control 25 cases of carcinoma in situ in the larynx, 13 of which recurred as invasive carcinoma and 12 as carcinoma in situ. However, Som[256] reported that vocal cord stripping controlled 20 of 24 cases. Four recurred as invasive carcinoma. While Holinger and Schild[107] reported good results with radiotherapy for laryngeal carcinoma in situ, other groups described relatively poor contol. Miller and Fisher[179] reported a failure rate of 51 percent of 43

cases, and De Santo[60] of 28 percent of 29 cases, for which salvage surgery was required for residual or reucrrent disease. Miller[178] found 18 of 22 radiation failures to recur as invasive carcinoma and 4 as carcinoma in situ. The interval for invasive carcinoma to develop ranged from several months to as long as 9 years. Analysis of 203 treated cases of laryngeal carcinoma in situ by Miller and Fisher[179] yielded the following results: 75 percent cure of 100 lesions managed by vocal cord stripping; 93 percent cure of 60 lesions having laryngofissure and cordectomy; and 49 percent cure of 43 lesions receiving radiotherapy. Cryosurgery[182] and the laser beam[269] have been also employed with some success as initial therapy or after radiation failure for carcinoma in situ as well as for premalignant lesions.

Superficially Invasive Carcinoma

In superficially invasive carcinoma (also called microinvasive carcinoma) there are, in addition to malignant-appearing cells within the epithelium, scattered foci of invasion through the basement membrane. While representing true neoplastic transformation, this lesion has a level of malignancy less than that of true invasive carcinoma. McGavran et al.[163] reported that only 1 of 15 patients with superficially invasive carcinoma of the true cord failed to be cured by biopsy alone. This is in keeping with the report of Stutsman and McGavran[271] that 20 percent of hemilaryngectomy specimens were free of residual tumor after endoscopic biopsy. These results were interpreted as supporting ultraconservative management (vocal cord stripping) of this type of laryngeal lesion. However, many surgeons endorse irradiation or excision by laryngofissure or hemilaryngectomy as the treatment of choice.

Verrucous Carcinoma

Verrucous carcinoma was originally recognized as an entity in the oral cavity[2] and later in the larynx.[28, 145] Clinically, it presents as a grey-white, exophytic, warty growth with fine papillary projections (Fig. 18-6). Microscopically, it consists of a well-differentiated keratinizing squamous epithelium penetrating the adjacent tissues with finger-like processes. The tumor has pushing margins and often provokes an intensive inflammatory reaction. The epithelium maintains a normal stratification and the cells show none of the cytoplasmic or nuclear features of squamous cell carcinoma, despite extensive penetration into surrounding tissues. Because of this, biopsies are often interpreted as representing only benign keratosis and close collaboration between the clinician and pathologist is necessary to establish the correct diagnosis in these cases.

The reported incidence of verrucous carcinoma of the larynx is 1 to 2 percent. Van Nostrand and Olofsson[286] calculated it at 1.3 percent of 800 cases; Rider[227] at 1.6 percent of 1,000 cases; Kraus and Perez-Mesa[145] at 2 percent of 600 cases. However, Fisher[69] found an incidence of 11 percent in 276 cases. There appears to be a preponderance of males in the ratio of 3:1, and a peak incidence at ages 40 to 69 years. The majority of the cases arise on the true cords and supraglottic larynx. Fisher[69] believed the sharp margin and deep clefts seen on the cut surface of the tumor are almost diagnostic of this lesion.

The biologic behavior of verrucous carcinoma of the larynx is similar to that encountered in the oral cavity. The clinical course is characterized by slow growth and local invasion, without the formation of regional or distant metastasis.[28] Verrucous carcinoma of the oral cavity appears to have limited responsiveness to radiotherapy. Ackerman[2] reported 7 failures among 7 irradiated cases and Kraus et al.[145] 17 failures among 17 cases so treated. Moreover, there appears to be evidence that irradiation promotes the transformation of verrucous carcinoma into anaplastic cancer. This was observed in 10 of 35 radiated oral cavity lesions.[73, 145, 217] In the larynx[63, 286] 2 of the 4 radiated cases also failed, with one patient subsequently developing anaplastic carcinoma. However, Rider[227] reported 6 of 7 patients with laryngeal lesions treated by radiation to be free of disease 1 to 7 years later. He states that one patient treated palliatively succumbed to distant metastasis by an anaplastic carcinoma 10 months later. Analysis of 25 surgically treated cases reported in the literature[59, 63, 286] revealed 23 to be disease-free for 1 to 10 years and 2 to be failures. There were no instances of anaplastic transformation. Consequently, it was concluded that surgery either by partial or total laryngectomy was the treatment modality of choice.[25] Radical neck dissection was not necessary, since in the absence of prior radiation it is questionable whether lymph node metastasis occurs with verrucous carcinoma. Hyams[112] states that there were no cervical metastases in his series of 29 cases from the Armed Forces Institute of Pathology. However, Fisher[69] reported 5 instances of cervical lymph node metastasis in his series of 31 cases. In 3 cases the tumor in the lymph node appeared verrucous, while in 2 it was squamous cell carcinoma. Two of his patients died of disease. However, they had both received radiotherapy.

Pseudosarcoma

This lesion is also known as the carcinosarcoma, spindle cell carcinoma, pleomorphic carcinoma, squamous cell carcinoma with pseudosarcomatous stroma, and collision tumor, and arises as uncommonly in the lar-

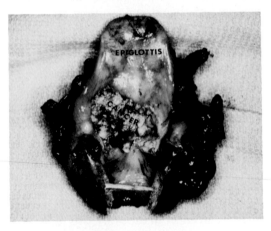

Fig. 18-6. Verrucous carcinoma invading the thyroid cartilage.

ynx as it does in the remainder of the aero-digestive tract. The nomenclature reflects the confusion in understanding the pathogenesis of this lesion. As the name implies, the lesion has both epithelial and mesenchymal components. The epithelial portion may resemble a well-differentiated squamous cell carcinoma or it may be so inconspicuous as to be overlooked in the sarcoma-like stroma. Despite its histologic appearance, most pathologists view this neoplasm as basically a squamous cell carcinoma with a histologically dominant stroma. The latter may be composed of spindle cells that may appear markedly anaplastic and sarcomatous or may resemble an inflammatory fibroblastic proliferation. The mesenchymal elements have been variously interpreted as representing a reactive stromal hyperplasia (pseudosarcoma) or as representing elements of true neoplasm. The concept of this tumor as a pseudosarcoma[147] is underscored by the presence of these spindle cells in both regional and distant metastasis.[111] Electron microscopic studies appear to confirm the squamous cell origin of these spindle elements.[157] Several researchers have also demonstrated a morphologic transition from the squamous cell to the spindle cell elements, supporting the concept of this lesion as a pleomorphic or spindle cell carcinoma.[6, 17, 111, 244] However, Goellner et al.[83] concluded after ultrastructural and histochemical study that the spindle elements represented reactive hyperplasia.

Some researchers believed these lesions were of a low order of malignancy, with the aggressive cases representing carcinosarcomas.[83] In addition, Batsakis[17] believed these sarcoma-like cells are derived from the laryngeal epithelium, thus making the lesion a true pleomorphic carcinoma. However, he acknowledged that proliferating fibroblasts could contribute to the stromal mass. Batsakis[17] recognized, in addition to the pleomorphic anaplastic carcinoma or carcinoma with a pseudosarcomatous reaction, a true carcinosarcoma in which two independent neoplasms have collided and intermingled.

Clinically, pseudosarcoma may appear as either a polypoid or infiltrative lesion. According to Batsakis[17] the different gross appearances are significant, as the biologic behavior of each type of neoplasm is different. The polypoid type is characterized as a slow-growing lesion that uncommonly metastasizes, whereas the infiltrative type behaves similarly to an invasive squamous cell carcinoma. A review of 39 cases by Hyams[111] revealed 23 tumors to arise on the vocal cords, 4 in the pyriform sinuses, and the remainder scattered throughout the supraglottic and subglottic larynx. There was a male predominance in the ratio of 12:1 in the series of Hyams,[111] and the mean age of their patients was 68 years. These tumors generally appear polypoid, with a smooth glistening surface, and have a pedunculated or sessile base. Study of the gross specimen generally does not reveal invasion beyond the submucosa.

Careful microscopic search of the specimen usually reveals an often inconspicuous focus of squamous cell carcinoma of variable grade, generally present in the stalk of the lesion.[111] The spindle cell component, which comprises the greatest portion of the lesion, also varies widely in its histologic differentiation. In some areas it may resemble a fibrosarcoma, in others merely reactive hyperplasia. Hyams[111] found tumor giant cells in about half of his cases. Biopsy made of a polypoid laryngeal lesion may reveal only the spindle cells and thus invite diagnostic confusion with a true sarcoma.

However, Hyams[111] considered the virulence of these tumors to be underrated. He cited 10 instances of regional lymph node metastasis in a series of 39 cases and a 40 percent 2-year mortality rate. Tumor control has been achieved by both simple excision and laryngectomy. However, radiotherapy appears to be of a limited effectiveness in curing these tumors.[111]

Small Cell Carcinoma

Several cases of small cell or oat cell carcinoma histologically identical with those arising in the bronchial tree have been reported in the larynx. Definitive diagnosis is made in these cases by the demonstration by electronmicroscopy of neurosecretory granules in the cytoplasm of the cells. The lesions can arise anywhere in the larynx and can produce extensive regional and distant metastases. In the majority of cases the tumor causes death within a year despite radical surgery. To prolong survival the use of chemotherapy and radiotherapy has been suggested based on its effectiveness with lung tumors.[190]

Adenocarcinoma

Adenocarcinomas represent less than 1 percent of laryngeal neoplasms. Cady et al.[44] found 17 adenocarcinomas among 2,500 laryngeal malignancies for an incidence of 0.6 percent. Sessions et al.[239] reported 9 cases among 888 laryngeal neoplasms (incidence of about 1 percent). Eschwege et al.[66] reported 5 adenocarcinomas (all cylindromas) among 1,342 laryngeal carcinomas (0.4 percent incidence). These tumors are derived from mucous glands present in the lining mucosa of the larynx; these glands are especially numerous in the ventricular folds and below the anterior commissure, sparse on the free portion of the epiglottis and aryepiglottic folds, and absent on the true cords.[191] The distribution of tumors reflects the relative incidence of mucous glands.

The histologic patterns formed by these laryngeal tumors are identical to those arising in the major and minor salivary glands. The majority are nonspecific adenocarcinomas, followed in frequency by cylindromas and mucoepidermoid carcinomas. Whicker et al.[294] reported their series of 27 glandular laryngeal malignancies to consist of 12 adenocarcinomas, 9 cylindromas, and 6 mucoepidermoid carcinomas.

NONSPECIFIC ADENOCARCINOMA

These tumors may vary widely in the degree of differentiation of acinar and ductal ele-

ments and the extent of pleomorphism present, but they form no distinctive histologic pattern. They show a predilection for elderly males and arise primarily in the supraglottic and transglottic regions.[279] Presenting symptoms include hoarseness, pain, cough, and a palpable cervical mass. Direct laryngoscopy usually reveals a bulky, smooth mass bulging into the laryngeal lumen. About 50 percent of the patients with these tumors will develop cervical metastases.[44] The majority of patients have been treated by total laryngectomy and radical neck dissection. Despite aggressive treatment most patients die from distant metastasis, primarily to the lungs and liver, within 2 years.[68]

ADENOID CYSTIC CARCINOMA (CYLINDROMA)

This lesion is histologically characterized by nests and cords of cells, which often form tubular structures enclosing acellular hyalinized material. Fechner[68] cautioned that myxoid degeneration of the stroma of these lesions may invite misdiagnosis of malignant mixed tumor, a lesion whose existence has not been definitely established within the larynx. About two thirds of the cases arise in the subglottis, with the remainder occurring mainly in the supraglottic region. There appears to be a slightly increased incidence in elderly females. Presenting symptoms include dyspnea, pain, cough, and hemoptysis. Direct laryngoscopy will generally reveal a smooth, firm mass. Treatment has consisted of simple excision, partial or total laryngectomy, and radiation. Local excision generally results in recurrence within a few years. Laryngectomy often prevents recurrence but does not appear to influence survival.[239] However, prolonged survival has been reported after treatment only by laryngofissure.[154, 156] Many workers employ radiotherapy routinely following surgery.[66, 154, 156]

Regional lymph node metastases are generally not prominent with laryngeal cylindromas. The majority of patients succumb to distant metastasis within a few years. However, like cylindromas arising at other sites, survival may be prolonged for many years despite extensive distant metastasis.[66]

MUCOEPIDERMOID CARCINOMA

Tumors composed of malignant-appearing glandular and squamous elements that assume a variety of histologic patterns have been reported to arise in the larynx.[44, 81, 276] Some of these tumors produce mucin and can be strictly classified as mucoepidermoid carcinomas, whereas others have been designated as adenosquamous carcinomas, stressing their aggressive nature.[81] There appears to be a male preponderance; however, too few cases have been reported to establish this with certainty. Tumor control has been reported both with laryngectomy[81] and radiotherapy,[276] but long-term followup is lacking in the reported cases.

UNUSUAL TUMORS

Other uncommon glandular- or alveolar-appearing tumors that have been reported in the larynx and may show malignant behavior include the oncocytoid carcinoma[123] and the paraganglioma.[150] The latter tumor, despite its organoid appearance, is probably of neural crest origin, with approximately 40 percent of the 30 reported cases in the larynx showing malignant behavior.

METASTATIC TUMORS

There are reports of glandular tumors metastasizing to the larynx. These are primarily renal cell carcinomas, but metastasis from breast, lung, prostate, and gastrointestinal adenocarcinomas has been described.[293] These lesions may occur in the soft tissues of the supraglottic, glottic, or subglottic regions and may mimic a primary neoplasm. Metastasis may also involve the laryngeal framework both clinically[223] and occultly,[62] generally spreading to the ossi-

fied portions of the thyroid and cricoid cartilages.

NONEPITHELIAL MALIGNANT TUMORS

Sarcomas

Mesenchymal malignant tumors comprise about 1 to 2 percent of laryngeal cancers.[19] Krajina[142] reported 20 sarcomas among 6,067 laryngeal malignancies, for an incidence of 0.3 percent. More than half of the sarcomas are fibrosarcomas, with the remainder being chondrosarcomas, rhabdomyosarcomas, and more unusual tumors. These lesions generally have a predilection for occurring in men. In the series of Krajina,[142] 18 of the 20 patients were men. They also tend to be highly lethal tumors, with only 4 of the 20 cases of Krajina[142] surviving more than 5 years. Partial and total laryngectomy has resulted in patients surviving for several years, whereas almost all patients treated by radiotherapy have died within 1 year.

FIBROSARCOMAS

Fibrosarcomas of the larynx show a predilection for occurring in elderly men. However, a case has even been reported in infancy.[228] The majority arise from the anterior portion of the vocal cords and anterior commissure, presenting as a nodular or pedunculated mass.[17] These tumors have also been described as arising in the ventricle and subglottis. A review of 29 laryngeal fibrosarcomas by Flanagan et al.[70] indicated a correlation between the histologic grade of the tumor and prognosis. These tumors spread by infiltration locally and do not commonly metastasize to regional lymph nodes. Consequently, small and well-differentiated tumors can be locally resected by laryngofissure or partial laryngectomy, whereas bulky, infiltrative, and anaplastic lesions should be excised by widefield laryngectomy.

CHONDROSARCOMAS

About one fifth of the approximately 150 cartilaginous neoplasms reported in the larynx are malignant. Cartilaginous laryngeal tumors have a marked male predominance, generally arising in those between 40 to 60 years of age. The majority (70 percent) arise from the posterolateral aspect of the cricoid cartilage, followed by the thyroid (20 percent) and arytenoid cartilages. Consequently, the clinical picture may be dominated by airway obstruction rather than hoarseness. Direct laryngoscopy reveals a smooth submucosal bulge, generally in the subglottis. Biopsy is usually unrewarding because of the firmness of the mass. Radiographs will demonstrate a homogenous density, often flecked with calcification. The criteria for histologic diagnosis of chondrosarcoma of the larynx is similar to those used with bone lesions.[110, 113] These are the presence of nuclear pleomorphism, and large binucleate and giant cells in the specimens. Huizenga and Balogh[110] subclassified laryngeal chondrosarcomas microscopically into low grade and high grade tumors and added the diagnostic feature of irregular clumping of cells (cluster disarray). Treatment consists of resection of the tumor, its perichondrial capsule, and a margin of normal tissue. Both the benign and malignant forms show slow growth with a definite tendency for recurrence. However, rare incidences of local and distant metastasis from laryngeal chondrosarcomas have been reported.[113] A partial laryngectomy may be employed. However, total laryngectomy may be necessary if more than half of the cricoid cartilage is removed because of the complication of laryngeal collapse and stenosis.

RHABDOMYOSARCOMA

Malignant skeletal muscle tumors of the larynx are extremely rare. Batsakis and Fox[18] found only 5 acceptable cases on review of the literature, to which they added another. All were histologically of the embryonal type and their biologic behavior appeared to be less aggressive than those arising at other anatomic sites in the head and neck. As with other rhabdomyosarcomas, the majority of the laryngeal lesions arose in the pediatric age group. Total laryngectomy is the treatment of choice.

OTHER SARCOMAS

Other histologic types of mesenchymal tumors are extremely rare in the larynx. These include the leiomyosarcoma,[129] hemangiosarcoma,[79] giant cell sarcoma,[79] and lymphosarcoma.[142]

TREATMENT

Surgery

LARYNGOFISSURE

Laryngofissure and cordectomy was the earliest conservation surgical procedure for the larynx. However, it has been supplanted in the management of glottic carcinoma by hemilaryngectomy and radiotherapy. It is indicated for an early carcinoma of the membranous portion of a completely mobile true vocal cord. Reported cure rates for such early T1 glottic lesions range from 84 to 98 percent[57, 155, 235, 259]. Despite the high percentage of cure the procedure has been replaced by hemilaryngectomy, which provides wider margins in the resection of the lesion and usually gives a stronger voice than that obtained by laryngofissure. Comparable cure rates by radiotherapy for very early lesions of the membranous cord, with preservation of normal voice quality, probably have made radiotherapy the treatment of choice for these lesions.

Technique. The procedure is performed under general anesthesia usually after a preliminary tracheostomy through the second or third tracheal ring has been performed with local anesthesia; an endotracheal tube is inserted through the tracheostomy. In some cases the patient may be anesthetized initially through endotracheal intubation, with the tube, later transferred into a tracheostomy. A horizontal midline incision is utilized, the subplatysmal flaps elevated, and the strap muscles retracted. The perichondrium over the thyroid cartilage is incised in the midline and elevated a few millimeters in either direction. The thyroid cartilage is then cut sagittally with an oscillating saw. The larynx is entered through an incision in the cricothyroid membrane at the upper border of the cricoid cartilage. The cricothyroid membrane is retracted with hooks and a vertical incision is made upward into the cartilaginous cut, visualizing the glottis from below. With the patient paralyzed, the glottis is divided in the midline through the anterior commissure ligament and both thyroid laminae are retracted with double-pronged hooks. With cordectomy, horizontal incisions are made above and below the true cord and joined posteriorly by an incision made at the tip of the vocal process. The entire true cord including the vocalis muscle is excised just external to the perichondrium. A mucosal flap is advanced from the area of the false cord to cover the resection site and promote the formation of a pseudocord. This flap is sutured to the perichondrium with fine absorbable sutures. The cut edges of the thyroid cartilage are approximated and held in position by suturing the overlying soft tissues. The neck wound is closed in layers over a Penrose drain placed subcutaneously. The endotracheal tube is removed and replaced with a cuffed tracheostomy tube, which is maintained for several days until the patient can be safely decannulated. In the initial postoperative period the cuff is kept inflated to prevent aspiration of blood and to minimize subcutaneous emphysema.

PARTIAL LARYNGECTOMY

The most significant advance in the treatment of laryngeal cancer in the past 50 years has been the introduction of techniques that allow preservation of the functions of the larynx without decreasing the curability.[200]

However, accurate preoperative assessment of the extent of tumor involvement is essential. Additionally, reconstructive procedures must be performed that insure an adequate airway and glottic competence to prevent aspiration.

Hemilaryngectomy. Hemilaryngectomy has found its widest application in the management of glottic carcinoma with extension anteriorly to involve the anterior commissure and extension posteriorly to involve the vocal process and anterior surface of the arytenoid, because it offers a higher degree of curability than radiotherapy.

The vertical hemilaryngectomy as originally performed consisted of division of the larynx sagittally in the midplane, with resection of half of the anatomic larynx. However, division of the cricoid cartilage has a devastating effect on laryngeal function. The term as presently used (vertical frontolateral hemilaryngectomy) denotes a thyrotomy sagittally at the midline or slightly to the contralateral side when the anterior commissure is involved, as well as a posterior thyrotomy, with resection, in-continuity of the thyroid lamina, involved true cord, ventricle, and false cord. The extended frontolateral hemilaryngectomy is employed with cordal lesions that have extended posteriorly behind the vocal process onto the anterior face of the arytenoid. In this procedure all or nearly all of the thyroid lamina is removed along with the arytenoid cartilage and the overlying soft tissues. A modification of this procedure has been devised by Biller et al.[26] for lesions with posterior subglottic extension; in this modification a portion of the cricoid cartilage is removed. Since resection of the posterior aspect of the cricoid cartilage is associated with severe aspiration, this technique employs rotation of the posterior portion of the thyroid cartilage to fill the defect posteriorly.

The anterior commissure technique is employed for lesions involving the anterior commissure with bilateral cordal involvement. It involves a bilateral anterior sagittal thyrotomy and resection of both vocal cords a variable distance backwards toward the vocal process, with the placement of a keel to prevent webbing of the larynx anteriorly.

A variety of subtotal laryngectomy procedures have been proposed for the resection of the transglottic tumors. The method of Iwai[114, 115] for cases with a fixed vocal cord employs supraglottic laryngectomy as well as resection of the vertical half of the larynx including the cricoid arch and uses the lateral portion of the thyroid lamina and superior horn to reconstruct the posterior laryngeal defect. He reported tumor cure in 5 of 9 cases using this method.

Contraindications of Vertical Frontolateral Hemilaryngectomy[194, 209]

1. Tumor extension from the ipsilateral vocal cord across the anterior commissure to involve more than one third of the contralateral vocal cord.

2. Extension subglottically greater than 10 mm anteriorly and more than 5 mm posterolaterally.

3. This technique can still be used if the vocal process and anterior surface of the arytenoid are involved, but involvement of the cricoarytenoid joint, interarytenoid area, opposite arytenoid, or rostrum of the cricoid is a contraindication.

4. Extension across the ventricle to the false cord.

5. Thyroid cartilage invasion.

6. Impaired vocal cord mobility is a relative contraindication.

Lesions to be considered appropriate for partial laryngectomy should fit the requirements before radiotherapy. One must be extremely cautious with postradiotherapy recurrences, particularly in the subglottic area, when contemplating conservation surgery.[30]

Technique. A preliminary tracheostomy is performed through a transverse incision with the patient under local anesthesia. Following induction of general anesthesia through the tracheotomy site, the transverse tracheostomy incision is extended bilaterally beyond the external jugular veins and the flap is elevated deep to the platysma to the level of the hyoid bone. The strap muscles are separated in the midline, exposing the cricoid and thyroid cartilages (Fig. 18-7A). The perichondrium of the thyroid cartilage is incised in the midline and elevated from the thyroid ala on the involved side (Fig. 18-7B). The perichondrium on the contralateral side is elevated 1 or 2 mm. If the tumor does not involve the anterior commissure, the thyroid cartilage is cut in the midline. If the tumor involves the anterior commissure, the thyroid cartilage cut is 1 cm lateral to the midline on the contralateral side. The cartilage cut is made with a Stryker saw and does not section the internal perichondrium. The second cartilage cut on the side of the lesion is performed 1 cm anterior to the posterior border of the thyroid cartilage. The cricothyroid membrane is then incised at the upper border of the cricoid cartilage. The patient is paralyzed and the subglottis and the extent of the tumor are visualized through the cricothyroid space. The thyrotomy is completed from below under direct vision (Fig. 18-7C). The hemilarynx to be excised is mobilized by incising the lateral subglottis just above the cricoid cartilage to the area of the vocal process (Fig. 18-7D). Superiorly, an incision that divides the thyrohyoid membrane and detaches the epiglottis is made along the upper border of the thyroid lamina above the false cord. The superior laryngeal vessels are clamped, divided, and ligated. The posterior cut is made with an angled scissors, and depending on tumor extent, the cut either sections the vocal process or removes the entire arytenoid. With the extended hemilaryngectomy, the cricoarytenoid joint is severed with a scissors. An incision is next made through the interarytenoid mucosa and muscle down to the cricoid cartilage, taking care not to injure the mucosa over the posterior aspect of the arytenoid. With dissection of the arytenoid from the pharyngeal mucosa the specimen is now free.

After removal of the specimen, various reconstructive procedures are required. If the arytenoid cartilage has been removed, replacement with a free or pedicled muscle,[200] tendon, or cartilage graft[31, 255] is re-

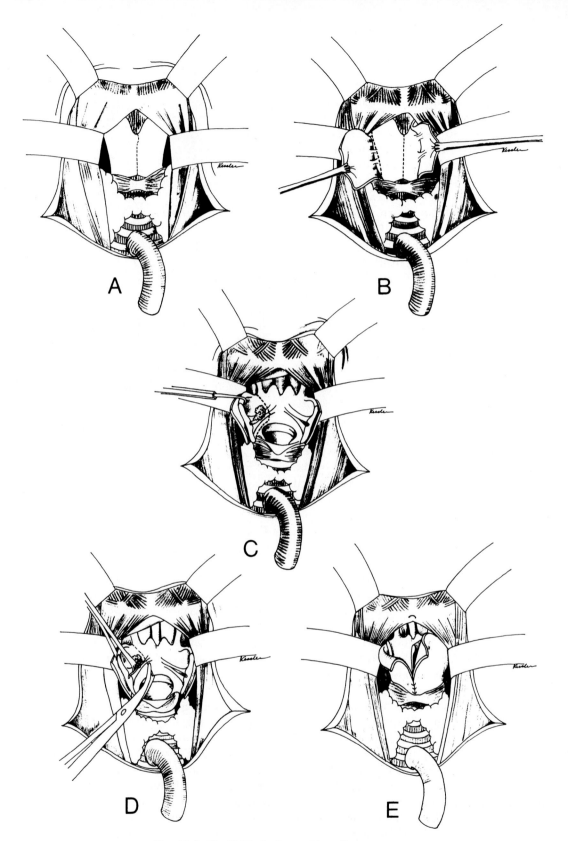

Fig. 18-7. (A–E) Technique of hemilaryngectomy.

quired to obtain glottic closure posteriorly to prevent postoperative aspiration. After its placement, the area is resurfaced by advancing the pyriform sinus mucosa and suturing the flap to the cricoid cartilage with fine absorbable sutures. If a portion of the contralateral cord has been removed, the remainder must be reattached anteriorly to the inner thyroid perichondrium. In order to reset the petiole anteriorly it must be sutured to the hyoid bone. Closure of the larynx is accomplished by reapproximating the perichondrium and strap muscles (Fig. 18-7E). While Norris[192] originally employed a skin graft and stent with the extended partial procedures to prevent laryngeal stenosis, this is not necessary as adequate thyroid cartilage remains. A Penrose drain is placed and the skin flaps are sutured together in layers.

The patient is fed by a nasogastric tube for 1 week, after which time the tracheostomy tube is occluded and the patient is started on oral feedings. The tracheostomy tube is usually removed in the next few days. Occasionally, persistent edema of the glottis occurs and decannulation is delayed for 4 to 6 weeks. Aspiration is usually not a complication, if arytenoid replacement has been performed. The voice is usually husky, but with subsequent scarring, the voice may become breathy. In such cases, voice improvement can be obtained with Teflon injection of the pseudocord. Lesions that are amenable to hemilaryngectomy have a low incidence of cervical metastasis and elective neck dissection is not indicated.

Anterior Commissure Modification. Glottic carcinoma that extends in horseshoe fashion across the anterior commissure requires modification of the standard vertical partial laryngectomy technique. The application of this technique is generally limited by either extension of the tumor on one side beyond the vocal process of an arytenoid, subglottic extension greater than 10 mm, supraglottic extension anteriorly or laterally, limited vocal cord mobility, or evidence of thyroid cartilage invasion (Fig. 18-8). It may be employed after radiation failure

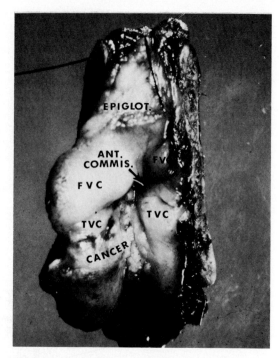

Fig. 18-8. Partial Laryngectomy—anterior commissure technique specimen. Note involvement of left true cord, anterior commissure, and anterior subglottic space.

only for those patients who were originally candidates for this procedure.

Technique.[137, 257]   After the induction of general anesthesia through a tracheostomy, the transverse incision is extended laterally and flaps are raised deep to the platysma. The strap muscles are separated in the midline. The perichondrium of the thyroid cartilage is also incised in the midline and is elevated bilaterally. Bilateral vertical thyrotomy incisions are made with an oscillating saw approximately 1 cm to either side of the midline. An incision is made through the cricothyroid membrane horizontally just above the cricoid cartilage and is carried vertically upward to the thyrotomy incision on the side of lesser involvement. With lesions with subglottic extension of 1 cm or greater, an additional margin may be obtained inferiorly by partial resection of the anterior portion of the cricoid cartilage. The severed thyroid cartilage is retracted by hooks and the lesion is visualized from below. The true and false cords are divided up to the thyrohyoid membrane. Both halves of the larynx are now retracted with double hooks; and under direct visualization, the interior of the larynx is incised on the side of greater involvement. A subperichondrial dissection is performed to the thyrotomy and the surgical specimen is removed. Because there remains insufficient mucosa for primary repair, skin grafts,[192] skin flaps,[52] and the placement of a keel have been utilized to prevent anterior webbing and stenosis of the larynx.

A tantalum or Silastic keel flanged anteriorly is positioned to extend between both vocal processes but not to impinge on the cricoid cartilage posteriorly. The keel is maintained in position by wire sutures to the thyroid alae. The strap muscles are approximated anteriorly over the operative defect, and the tracheostomy tube replaces the endotracheal tube. After 4 to 6 weeks the keel is removed and the patient can be decannulated.

Supraglottic Laryngectomy. The horizontal partial laryngectomy (supraglottic resection) is performed for carcinoma involving the epiglottis and false cords. This procedure can be extended to include carcinomas of the aryepiglottic fold and anterior and lateral walls of the pyriform sinus and selected lesions involving the vallecula and base of the tongue. An elective neck dissection is usually performed, in view of the high incidence of occult nodes.

Contraindications of the Supraglottic Laryngectomy

1. Tumor extension onto the cricoid cartilage.

2. Bilateral arytenoid involvement.

3. Arytenoid fixation.

4. Extension onto the glottis or the presence of impaired vocal cord mobility.

5. Thyroid cartilage invasion.

6. Involvement of the apex of the pyriform sinus or postcricoid region.

7. Involvement of the base of the tongue more than 1 cm posteriorly to the circumvallate papillae.

Involvement of the perichondrium or anterior commissure indicates a transglottic lesion and if this is found at the time of surgery total laryngectomy should be performed. Subtotal horizontal laryngectomy may be also contraindicated in patients with chronic lung disease or in the elderly or debilitated patient in whom postoperative aspiration may be a problem. Failure to achieve rehabilitation of swallowing may eventually require a total laryngectomy in such patients.

Technique. After a Y type incision (Fig. 18-9A), the suprahyoid muscles are severed from the hyoid bone, from the lesser cornu on the contralateral side to the tip of the greater cornu on the involved side (Fig. 18-9B). The hyoid bone is then cut at the contralateral lesser cornu. The strap muscles on the ipsilateral side are severed at the superior border of the thyroid cartilage, exposing the thyroid perichondrium. On the opposite side, the strap muscles are severed only medially, exposing the perichondrium midway from the notch to the posterior aspect. The perichondrium is incised and reflected inferiorly to the lower border of the thyroid ala (Fig. 18-9C).

The proposed cartilage cuts are outlined with methylene blue dye. The anterior cut is made at the junction of the upper one-third and the lower two-thirds as measured from the base of the thyroid notch to the inferior margin of the thyroid cartilage. From this point, on the side of the lesion, the cut is extended straight posteriorly, bisecting the posterior border of the thyroid cartilage approximately midway between the origin of the superior cornu and the inferior cornu. On the contralateral side the thyroid cartilage cut extends superiorly, bisecting the upper edge of the thyroid ala midway between the notch and the superior cornu (Fig. 18-9D).

Entrance into the pharynx is through the vallecula, provided the tumor does not involve the lingual surface of the epiglottis; if the vallecula, base of the tongue, or lingual surface of the epiglottis is involved by tumor then entrance is through the pyriform sinus. After the pharynx is entered,

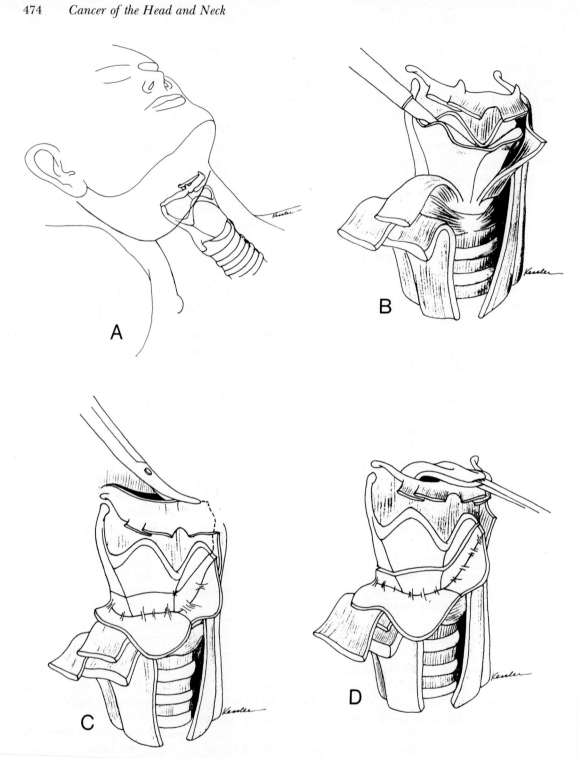

Fig. 18-9. (A–D) Technique of supraglottic resection.

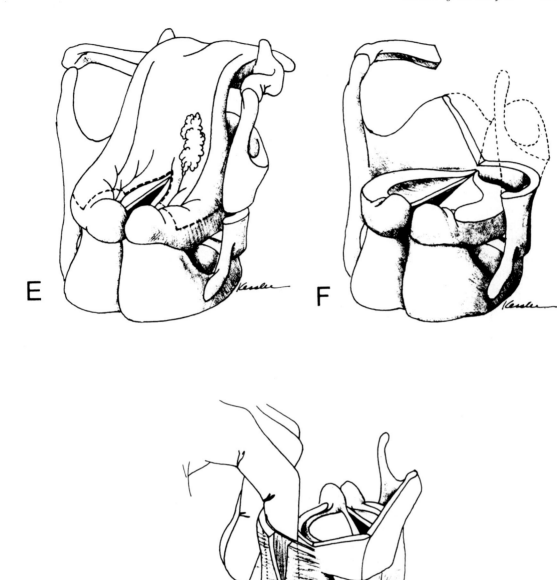

Fig. 18-9 continued. (E–G) Technique of supraglottic resection.

the epiglottis is grasped with a tenaculum, the patient is paralyzed, and the resection is initiated on the uninvolved side. The ary-epiglottic fold is severed above the aryte-noid, followed by sectioning of the false cord from the true cord at the level of the ventricle. After the anterior commissure is reached, the resected portion of the supra-glottis can be rotated to expose the side of major tumor involvement. Assessment at this time determines whether the arytenoid should be resected partially, totally, or not at all. The aryepiglottic fold on the involved side is sectioned, and the resection is completed by traversing the arytenoid to the ventricle and then to the anterior commissure (Fig. 18-9E). The resected supraglottis is then removed (Fig. 18-9F). A cricopharyngeal myotomy is then performed, with the surgeon being careful not to injure the recurrent laryngeal nerve (Fig. 18-9G). If the recurrent laryngeal nerve is not identified, the myotomy should be performed posteriorly to avoid inadvertent injury.

If the arytenoid cartilage has been partially or totally removed, it is necessary to fix the residual cord to the midline in order to obtain adequate glottic closure postoperatively. Fixation of the cord in the midline is performed by suturing the vocal process to the cricoid. If there is insufficient length, a piece of cartilage is used to replace the extirpated arytenoid. The vocal cord is then fixed to this cartilage. A small mucosal flap from the pyriform sinus is sutured over the cartilage transplant. The supraglottic resection may be extended to include the lateral wall of the pyriform sinus and lateral and posterior pharyngeal walls. These hypopharyngeal mucosal defects may be resurfaced by the use of a split-thickness skin or dermal graft supported by a Negus stent. In patients who have received high dose preoperative radiation, the transfer of a regional pedicled flap is necessary, with the creation of a pharyngostome.

Closure is obtained by approximating the perichondrium and strap muscles to the base of the tongue. This closure is performed with nonabsorbable interrupted sutures. Hemovacs are inserted, a dermal graft may be utilized to cover the carotid artery, and the skin flaps are reapproximated and sutured. The patient's head is flexed during the postoperative period and he is fed by nasogastric tube. At 14 days the tracheostomy tube is corked, and it is removed the following day if the airway is adequate. The tracheostomy site is allowed to heal and oral feedings are started by the third postoperative week. Initially, a pureed diet is started and after a few days liquids are introduced. Minimal aspiration occurs during the first few days of oral feedings.

The complications associated with this procedure are those associated with wound healing and rehabilitation of deglutition. If a fistula forms, rotation of pedicled flaps is usually required for closure. Persistent aspiration occurs more frequently when the supraglottic resection is extended to include the base of the tongue or to the pyriform sinus. In these cases, deglutition may be delayed for an additional 4 to 8 weeks. Adequate glottic closure is essential for deglutition without aspiration. Since initiation of normal deglutition requires strenuous activity and since certain patients require additional time to gain weight, nasogastric feedings may be necessary for an additional 3 to 6 weeks before successful deglutition is accomplished.

TOTAL LARYNGECTOMY

Total laryngectomy, without neck dissection, is performed for carcinomas that have a low incidence of occult cervical metastasis. This would include bilateral vocal cord lesions following failure of radiation therapy, vocal cord carcinomas with fixation, interarytenoid lesions, and small lesions involving the true and false vocal cords. Total laryngectomy should be performed with elective neck dissection for tumors that involve the epiglottis, pyriform sinus, postcricoid area, the base of the tongue, or for large transglottic tumors.

Technique. A low collar incision is utilized for laryngectomy without neck dissection, and a hockey stick incision is utilized for laryngectomy with neck dissection. A preliminary tracheostomy is performed with the patient under local anesthesia, following which general anesthesia is maintained through the tracheostomy site. The flaps are elevated deep to the platysma muscle. If a neck dissection is performed, the specimen is left attached along the lateral aspect of the thyroid and cricoid cartilages.

The strap muscles are severed 1 finger-breadth above the suprasternal notch, and the thyroid gland is exposed (Fig. 18-10A). The thyroid lobe on the side of the lesion is mobilized and the inferior thyroid vessels are identified, clamped, and ligated. The thyroid lobe is left attached to the cricoid superiorly. The isthmus is divided on the contralateral side of the tumor. The thyroid lobe on the contralateral side of the tumor is separated from the trachea and the underlying cricoid cartilage (Fig. 18-10B). The sternomastoid muscle is retracted laterally and the posterior border of the thyroid cartilage is rotated anteriorly. The omohyoid muscle is divided and the inferior constrictor muscle is sectioned along the posterior border of the thyroid ala (Fig. 18-10D). The superior thyroid artery is identified, clamped, and ligated. The superior cornu of the thyroid cartilage is separated from the underlying pharyngeal mucosa. The thyroid cartilage and the superior thyroid artery are similarly dissected on the opposite side. The hyoid bone is then skeletonized by cutting the suprahyoid musculature (Fig. 18-10C).

The pharynx is entered through the vallecula, provided the tumor does not involve the lingual surface of the epiglottis. If the lingual surface of the epiglottis, or vallecula, is involved with tumor, entrance into the pharynx is through the pyriform sinus. Once the pharynx is entered, the epiglottis is grasped and the dissection proceeds on the side contralateral to the tumor (Fig. 18-10D). The incision continues down the lateral wall of the epiglottis and then to the anterior lateral pharyngeal wall, preserving the pyriform sinus mucosa. The mucosa is incised in the postcricoid area at the inferior border of the cricoid cartilage. The larynx can then be rotated anteriorly, giving excellent exposure to the contralateral, and sometimes involved, pyriform sinus. The opposite side is then resected with an adequate margin of normal tissue. The inferior aspect of the mucosal excision should be at the level of the inferior border of the cricoid cartilage. The proximal trachea is separated

from the esophagus, and the trachea is transected at the third tracheal ring (Fig. 18-10E).

The pharynx is closed in a T fashion, either with a continuous inverting chromic suture reinforced with a second layer of interrupted nonabsorbable sutures or with all interrupted nonabsorbable sutures (Figs. 18-10F and 18-10G). A generous portion of the skin is resected from the lower and upper flaps at the site of the tracheostoma. The skin flap is resutured in layers, and the skin margin is carefully approximated to the tracheostoma with interrupted sutures. The patient is fed by nasogastric tube for approximately 7 days, and then oral feeding is instituted.

Complications.   The complications of total laryngectomy include wound breakdown and fistula formation. Small fistulas close spontaneously; the larger ones require pedicle flap closure. Stenosis of the pharynx occasionally occurs and is adequately treated by dilation. Esophageal speech training is instituted at the third postoperative week. Patients who fail to develop esophageal speech can utilize one of the electronic vibrators. In selected patients who cannot develop esophageal speech, surgical rehabilitation procedures may be performed.

Radiotherapy

Radiotherapy for laryngeal carcinoma presently employs megavoltage radiation with a cobalt 60 teletherapy unit or a linear accelerator. This permits delivery of a high dosage accurately to a limited area with sparing of the surrounding soft tissues and overlying skin. Tumor doses in the range of 6,000 to 7,000 rads are required for tumor control, with the portal size determined by the location of the tumor.[290] With glottic lesions, which have a low incidence of regional lymph node metastasis, the portals are small. However, with supraglottic lesions, which have a high incidence of regional metastases, the portals may be enlarged to in-

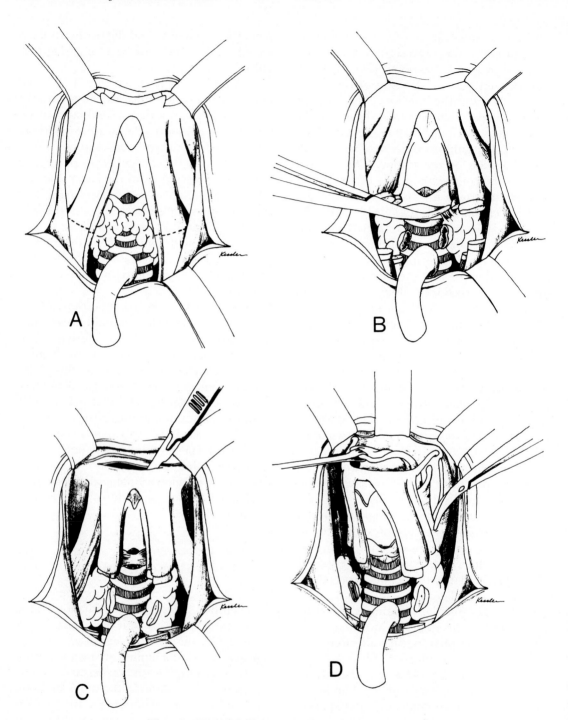

Fig. 18-10 (A–D) Technique of total laryngectomy.

clude the neck as well as the supraglottis, as there is some evidence that elective neck irradiation decreases the observed lymph node metastasis in patients with laryngeal carcinomas and negative necks.[72, 86] Bran-denburg and Rutter[36] found advanced laryngeal (T3 and T4) tumors treated by radiotherapy to have a local recurrence rate of 80 percent and a lymph node metastatic rate of 9 percent. Similar lesions treated primar-

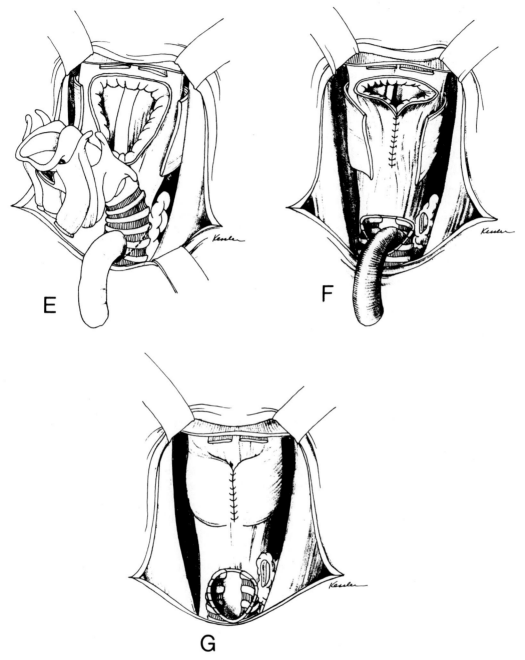

Fig. 18-10 continued. (E–G) Technique of total laryngectomy.

ily by surgery had a local failure rate of 16 percent and a regional recurrence rate of 23 percent, findings that also suggest that radiation may prevent lymph node metastasis. In the management of patients with clinically positive lymph node metastases, radiation has little to offer.

The end results of radiotherapy with squamous cell carcinoma of the supraglottic, glottic, and subglottic larynx, as well as with other epithelial and nonepithelial malignancies, have been already discussed in their respective sections. Attempts have been made to increase the effectiveness of radiation by combining it with hyperbaric oxygen in hopes of eliminating the more radioresistant hypoxic cells. Freeland[76] demonstrated angiographically the presence in laryngeal carcinomas of avascular areas that were not present in the normal organ. However, Henk[104] found that while combining irradiation with hyperbaric oxygen enhanced local tumor control significantly, survival was not changed when compared to the control group (patients irradiated in air). This enhanced control was attributed to the great application of salvage surgery to conventionally irradiated patients, whereas in the hyperbaric group radiation effects masked persistent neoplasm until surgery could not be performed. The vulnerability of laryngeal cartilage to radiation was also evidenced by a marked increase in the incidence of perichondritis and edema requiring tracheostomy in the hyperbaric group. Radical radiotherapy (5,000 rads in 3 weeks) yielded control of glottic and supraglottic carcinomas comparable to conventional methods.[104]

The changes produced in the larynx by therapeutic radiation range from mild soft tissue enlargement[226] to total organ necrosis. Edema of the larynx, particularly of the arytenoids, is a frequent sequela of radiotherapy. However, swelling persisting more than 6 months should suggest residual or recurrent disease,[41] which may require multiple deep biopsies for diagnosis.[126] Persistent or recurrent hoarseness, ulceration, and alteration of cord mobility all indicate recurrence.[15] While Fayos[67] reported no complications after megovoltage treatment of 192 laryngeal carcinomas, Goffinet et al.[85] described a 9 percent incidence (19 of 213 cases) of complications such as prolonged and permanent tracheostomy, chondritis, myositis, and extensive cervical and pharyngeal fibrosis. Vermund[288] calculated a 5 percent incidence of chondronecrosis among 474 cases.

Combined Therapy

Planned preoperative radiotherapy in varying doses has been combined with surgery in an attempt to improve survival of those patients with advanced laryngeal tumors. The rationale for low dose preoperative radiotherapy is that even small amounts of radiation inactivate most tumor cells without significantly interfering with wound healing. High dose preoperative radiotherapy combines the full tumoricidal effect of radiation with surgical excision.

Proponents of high dose combined therapy (Goldman et al.)[87-90] cite radiobiologic, histopathologic, and clinical evidence in support of this vigorous therapeutic approach. Friedman and Goldman[78] showed that even after 5,500 rads, laryngeal tumor cells are capable of synthesizing DNA. Microscopically, 8 of 13 larynges that appeared to be clinically free of disease showed residual tumor on serial sectioning. Nine of the 26 larynges were sterilized by radiation, demonstrating the efficacy of higher doses in protecting against local spread. However, rather than supporting the concept of primary treatment by radiotherapy and reserving surgery for recurrence as advocated by some workers,[40] Goldman et al.[87-90] argued that the demonstration of widely scattered foci of viable tumor cells beneath intact mucous membranes and the difficulty in clinically determining the presence of residual cancer made it impossible to predict who would develop recurrent or metastatic disease. Consequently, all patients were operated upon, rather than waiting for recurrent disease to appear with the diminished survival rate accompanying salvage surgery.

However, different studies evaluating the effectiveness of low and high dose combined therapy in controlling carcinoma of the larynx and laryngopharynx have yielded varying and even conflicting results. Hendrickson and Liebner[103] found low dose preoperative radiation as effective as high dose radiation in improving survival of those with operable supraglottic tumors. Skolnick et al.[251] reported no difference in the survival of patients with laryngeal and hypopharyngeal cancers in a randomized study using 2,000 rads and 5,000 rads preoperatively. In a later expanded study of 92 advanced supraglottic and glottic tumors by

Skolnick et al.[250], low dose planned preoperative radiation improved survival (42 and 54 percent, respectively) when compared to the high dose group (21 and 27 percent, respectively). The presence of histologically positive lymph nodes strongly influenced survival. Skolnick et al.[250] found 52 and 23 percent 5-year survival rates for patients with negative and positive nodes, respectively.

Ogura and Biller[201] reported decreased local recurrence for advanced laryngeal and hypopharyngeal lesions using low dose (1,500 to 3,000 rads) preoperative radiation. However, Constable et al.,[56] using doses between 4,500 and 6,000 rads for 72 advanced lesions, reported the recurrence rate to be directly related to the radiation dosage, with larger numbers of failures occurring with lower doses. This latter group found that combined therapy resulted in an 82 percent local control rate, as compared to 71 percent in cases treated by surgery alone.[54] However, the surgical group had smaller lesions and in some instances received postoperative radiation. In contradistinction, Brandenburg and Rutter[36] reported no significant difference in the recurrence rate or overall survival rate between patients receiving surgery and those receiving combined therapy with 5,000 rads preoperative radiation.

The appearance of postoperative complications, principally fistula formation, appears to be dose-related.[56] While some surgeons report low morbidity operating on heavily irradiated tissues,[229] generally a significant increase in morbidity is observed in patients receiving high dose preoperative radiation.[56, 250] It has been suggested that the poorer survival observed in some series employing high dose preoperative radiation may be due to obscured nodal metastasis by partial tumor suppression or interference with the host's immunologic response.[250]

Constable et al.[56] reported an absolute 5-year survival rate of 64 percent and a determinate survival rate of 78 percent with intermediate dose combined therapy. Goldman et al.[87] reported an actuarial 5-year survival rate of 59 percent and a determinate survival rate of 86 percent with high dose combined therapy. However, Bryce and Rider[40] claimed a 52 percent cure rate with high dose combined therapy as opposed to 56 percent for the control group. This latter group received radiotherapy and salvage surgery, with 61 percent retaining their larynges. These authors did not feel the difference in survival justified routine laryngectomy after radiation.

Chemotherapy

Chemotherapy has generally been employed for patients with extensive and inoperable laryngeal lesions, either for palliation or to induce tumor regression in an attempt to make the lesion resectable. While a tumor response has been observed, the 5-year survival rate has not been significantly altered and most studies suffer from the criticism of not being properly randomized. Rygard and Hansen[232] reported 12 of 44 patients with laryngeal carcinoma treated with bleomycin to have complete tumor regression for 4 to 42 months. Berdal et al.[22] also reported total regression in 2 of 16 cases. In most cases, however, less than 50 percent regression occurred and recurrence rapidly appeared. The combined use of chemotherapy and radiotherapy has also been applied to laryngeal cancer. Rygard and Hansen[231] reported a total regression in 44 percent (13 of 29) and Berdal et al.[22] in 62 percent (51 of 82) of laryngeal carcinomas treated simultaneously with bleomycin and radiation. While recurrences rapidly developed, in some cases the tumor became resectable with total laryngectomy. However, Kramer[144] found no significant differences in the survival of 76 cases of supraglottic carcinoma treated with methotrexate and radiation as compared with radiation alone.

Palliative Treatment

The patient with an advanced laryngeal carcinoma who (1) has infiltrative growth at the primary site or in regional lymph nodes that is so extensive that control of the lesion by surgery alone or in combination with radiotherapy is impossible, or (2) refuses definite treatment, or (3) is in such poor general medical condition so as not to tolerate definitive treatment, may be offered therapeutic measures to improve the duration and quality of life. Such measures, which are commonly termed palliative care, are directed toward pain, tumor bulk, maintenance of vital function (respiration, deglutition), and the social needs of the patient.

Pain is generally controlled by the use of analgesics, with regional nerve blocks and neurosurgical procedures—such as cordotomy or stereotactic surgery—not commonly employed.

Maintaining the airway for patients with obstructive lesions or providing pulmonary toilet for patients with aspiration through an incompetent larynx is generally achieved by tracheostomy. Total laryngectomy is not commonly indicated but may be indicated in cases with persistent aspiration and secondary pneumonia. Alimentation is achieved by nasogastric tube feeding when the esophagus is patent or by feeding gastrostomy when it is not.

For patients with unresectable lesions or those with postoperative recurrence, radiotherapy is most often employed in an attempt to control tumor growth, to induce regression in tumor mass, or to alleviate pain. Further irradiation has been employed in radiotherapy failures by delivering booster doses by external beam to small areas or by an interstitial implant into primary or metastatic lesions.[49]

Cryosurgery has been used for palliation of head and neck malignancies because of its ability to decrease pain, bleeding, and tumor bulk. However, it has limited application for patients with advanced laryngeal malignancies.

Chemotherapy has not been widely used for laryngeal carcinomas because although remissions have been obtained in a significant number of cases, they generally are incomplete and short-lived. The agents most commonly employed in treating advanced head and neck malignancies are methotrexate, bleomycin, and hydroxyurea. Methotrexate has been employed in intermediate dosage schedules and in high dose with leucovorin rescue.

Bertino[24] found that 6 of 18 cases of laryngeal carcinoma responded to methotrexate therapy, with an average response time of 3.8 months. His impression was that epidermoid carcinoma of the larynx was less responsive to this agent than were oral cavity lesions. Combination chemotherapy with methotrexate and bleomycin was attempted but discontinued because of severe toxicity.

STOMAL RECURRENCE

Suggested causes of the development of stomal recurrence following laryngectomy include submucosal extension of tumor or lymphatic spread, paratracheal lymph node metastasis, tumor implants at the site of surgery, or origin from a new primary tumor. The last cited cause is uncommon and was found in only 1 of 20 stomal recurrences studied by Batsakis et al.[20] Batsakis[17] noted that patients having specimens with surgical margins of clearance of 2 mm or less have a 5-year survival rate equal to those with a positive margin, whereas those with margins greater than 2 mm have a prognosis almost equal to widely resected lesions. Stomal recurrences are often found with tumors arising or extending subglottically[97, 193] but are uncommon with supraglottic lesions. Harris and Butler[97] stressed the importance of pretracheal, prelaryngeal, and recurrent laryngeal lymphatic spread with subglottic and pyriform apex tumors and advocated resection of the pretracheal fascia and fat as far inferior as the sternal notch with such lesions. It is controversial whether tracheostomy prior to laryngectomy influences stomal recurrence. Most surgeons have observed an increased incidence of such recurrence following preliminary tracheostomy[130, 159, 264, 265] whereas others[184, 196] relate it only to the increased size of such obstructive lesions. Consequently, emergency laryngectomy has been recommended for bulky tumors in an attempt to decrease peristomal recurrence.[109] Endotracheal intubation does not appear to have a significant role in the development of stomal recurrence.[261]

The incidence varies between 1.7 and 14.7 percent in large reported series, averaging about 5 percent. The majority of stomal recurrences appear within 6 months of surgery. Radiotherapy generally provides only temporary benefit in the management of this complication. Salvage surgery is employed for those cases that have limited extension into the mediastinum and are still resectable. The operative procedure advocated by Sisson[247] employs wide local resection of the tumor along with the manubrium and clavicular heads, creation of a new tracheostomy at a lower level, and closure of the operative defect with regional flaps. However, the procedure itself is accompanied by significant mortality and morbidity rates from infection and secondary great vessel rupture.

DISTANT METASTASES

The reported incidence of distant metastasis varies with the site of the primary lesion and whether calculations are made from clinical or autopsy material. In the study of Harrer and Lewis[96] 16 of 18 patients with carcinoma of the larynx had diffuse metastasis at autopsy. O'Brien et al.[197] reported 18 of 29 patients (62 percent) with laryngeal carcinoma to show distant spread. Abramson et al.[1] found 34 percent of 650 patients (75 autopsied) with laryngeal malignancy to have distant metastasis. The latter two studies showed that supraglottic lesions had the greatest potential for distant spread. This was confirmed by Alonso[4] who found that supraglottic tumors comprised 59 percent and glottic tumors 24 percent of a series of 107 laryngeal and hypopharyngeal cancers with distant metastasis. Goffinet et al.[85] reported 18 percent of 67 supraglottic and 6 percent of 146 glottic tumors to produce

distant metastasis. Fletcher et al.[72] observed an incidence of 19 percent for 267 supraglottic lesions. Subglottic tumors probably have a rate of distant metastasis intermediate between supraglottic and glottic carcinomas.[20]

Failure to control the primary tumor or cervical lymph node disease contributes most to the formation of distant metastasis and to death.[1, 221] Abramson et al.[1] found that 80 percent of the patients with distant spread had tumor locally in the neck at autopsy. If the primary tumor is controlled, the initial method of treatment has no influence on distant spread. Alonso[4] found that radiotherapy did not influence the spread rate. Biopsy does not contribute to dissemination. However, tracheostomy with endoscopy carries the theoretical risk of seeding into the lower respiratory tract. The size of the primary lesion also does not appear to correlate with the rate of metastasis.[221] Similarly, age, sex, and the physical condition of the patient do not seem to influence distant spread. Histologic differentiation also does not affect the ability to disseminate.[20] The most common site of spread is to the lungs, where the lesions appear as small and multiple nodules. Abramson et al.[1] found only 1 of 26 patients with distant spread to lack pulmonary metastases. Other sites of spread in decreasing order of frequency are the mediastinal lymph nodes, skeleton, and liver. Spread may occur to other viscera including the heart.[96] While Fletcher et al.[71] reported that the great majority of distant metastases appeared within 2 years, Batsakis et al.[20] estimated that 40 percent appeared within 5 years after treatment of the primary tumor. However, once metastases are manifest, the vast majority of patients succumb rapidly.

REHABILITATION

Vocal rehabilitation following total laryngectomy consists of learning esophageal speech, using an artificial larynx, or undergoing a reconstructive operative procedure.

The latter includes the creation of a fistula, the use of a laryngeal prosthesis, and a laryngoplasty with neoglottic reconstruction. Surgical rehabilitative measures may be performed immediately at the time of the ablative procedure or delayed until there is failure to develop esophageal speech, or a dissatisfaction with the results of esophageal speech or of an external mechanical vibrator. Estimates of the number of patients failing to develop adequate esophageal speech range from 17 to 50 percent.[91] Many patients also fail to use the electronic transcervical artificial larynx.[222] It is in these aphonic patients that surgical vocal rehabilitation has its greatest application.

Artificial Larynx

Artificial larynges are of two basic types. The transcervical type is a handheld, battery operated device that causes the neck tissues to vibrate creating a low pitched sound in the hypopharynx that is modulated into speech by the tongue, lips, teeth, and palate as articulators. While it can produce a loud and intelligible voice, it is mechanical in quality. Some patients cannot use this type of vibrator because of changes in the soft tissues of the neck resulting from surgery or radiotherapy that render them too rigid to vibrate.

The transoral type may be either an electric or pneumatic device. The electric type is a battery powered oscillator that passes sound through a tube into the mouth where it is articulated into speech. While it produces a loud sound, the sound is not as intelligible as that of the transcervical type. The mouth tube also becomes blocked by saliva. The pneumatic type (Tokyo larynx) uses expired air from the trachea to vibrate a reed or diaphragm that passes into the mouth by a tube. This device produces loud natural speech, but is conspicuous and becomes clogged. Goode[92] described an artificial larynx that could be concealed by incorporation into a denture.

Fistulas and Shunts

Fistula speech employs the surgical creation of a tracheopharyngeal or tracheoesophageal fistula in which the expired air moves a soft tissue pseudoglottis or a mechanical reed vibrator. Fistula speech has a more natural vocal quality and is of higher pitch than that of the artificial larynges. However, the formation of a fistula is often a multistage procedure, is generally contraindicated by prior radiotherapy, and is complicated by stenosis, salivary leakage and aspiration, and disturbance of pharyngeal function.[61] There are basically two types of shunts that can be formed. The external or indirect fistula requires a connecting prosthesis, which may incorporate a mechanical vibrator.[242, 274] With the internal or direct fistula the air is shunted by a finger over the tracheostoma[11, 12, 177] into a soft tissue tube entering the pharynx.

Asai[11] described the creation of a skin-lined tube between the tracheostoma and hypopharynx; the procedure involved several stages and used local tissues. Asai[12] later reported the results with three methods of fistula formation in 72 patients. While good speech was usually obtained, there was rupture of the dermal tube in 10 cases, stenosis of the fistula in 10 cases, and aspiration pneumonia in 2 cases. Miller[175–177] utilized this method of reconstruction but reported excellent speech in only 20 percent of 40 cases.[177] Karlan[127] modified the Asai technique into a two-stage operation and used a valved tracheostomy tube to eliminate the need for digital occlusion of the trachea opening.

In addition to shunt stenosis and aspiration, prior radiotherapy also increases the risk of flap necrosis and carotid rupture and is a contraindication to this method of repair. McGrail and Oldfield[167] attempted to overcome these problems by using a medially based deltopectoral flap to form the tracheopharyngeal skin tube. McGrail[166], however, reported achieving an excellent voice in only 3 of 34 patients treated by this one-stage procedure; in addition, aspiration continued to be a major problem. Fredrickson et al.[75] described a modification in which the hyoid bone was retained and the tubed flap brought over it, eliminating aspiration. Montgomery and Lavelle[186] also transposed the sternomastoid muscle across and above the hypopharyngeal tube to provide sphincteric function for phonation and to eliminate aspiration. Other modifications of the internal type shunt employ a mucosal lined tube[185, 187] and skin[53] and vein[50] grafts. Conley[51] comments that while 43 patients in which he created fistulas developed speech, many complications (including mediastinitis) limited the usefulness of this technique.

Tracheoesophageal shunts have also been created by simple[140] and tubed[46] esophageal mucosal flaps that communicate with the posterior wall of the trachea. Komorn[141] was able to obtain useful speech with the creation of such a fistula in 19 of 30 patients and Calcaterra[45] in 2 of 7 patients. Aspiration and stenosis complicated this type of shunt also.

Laryngeal Prosthesis

External mechanical laryngeal prosthesis have also been placed between the tracheostome and a surgically created esophageal or hypopharyngeal fistula in an attempt to produce intelligible speech with the elimination of digital occlusion. Air from the trachea may simply pass through the prosthesis and enter the fistula causing vibration of a pseudoglottis, or a vibrating mechanism may be present in the prosthesis that creates a pseudovoice that enters the vocal tract through the fistula.

Neoglottic Reconstruction

European workers have popularized laryngoplastic procedures that create a neoglottis by subtotal excision of the larynx with transposition of the hypopharyngeal mucosa to the remaining laryngeal or tracheal cartilage. The type of lesion present must permit subtotal laryngectomy without compromising survival but must be more extensive than those resectable by conventional conservation laryngeal procedures. Extension outside the larynx, metastatic spread, and prior radiotherapy are generally considered contraindications.

In the method of Serafini and Arslan[8-10] a tracheopharyngeal anastomosis is performed with the anterior tracheal wall attached to the epiglottis. The neoglottis is formed by the external laryngeal perichondrium and cricopharyngeal muscles, which have been preserved and brought together in the midline within the tracheal lumen. Arslan reported excellent speech and minimal aspiration in 35 patients. However, local recurrence developed in 4 patients.

Vega[287] adopted the technique of Serafini,[10] modifying it in individual cases by leaving the hyoid bone or portions of the cricoid cartilage.

Staffieri[259a] performed a tracheopharyngeal anastomosis and created a neoglottis from the hypopharyngeal mucosa. While phonation was excellent, aspiration was a major problem.

Mozolewski et al.[189] performed an "arytenoid vocal shunt" (supracricoid laryngectomy also leaving one or both arytenoids) and were able to achieve phonation in 22 of 25 patients.

Iwai and Koike[115] reported a method of "primary laryngoplasty" in which the lateral halves of the thyroid cartilage were preserved, brought together in the midline, and relined with hypopharyngeal mucosa to form a neoglottis. Good voice and minimal aspiration were reported in all 19 cases so treated.

Historically, it is of interest to note that the earliest attempt at vocal rehabilitation was performed by attempting to create a tracheoesophageal shunt by Gussenbauer on the first laryngectomy patient of Bilroth. He devised a modified valved tracheostomy tube that delivered air from the trachea to the hypopharynx through a pharyngostomy.

Taub[273, 274] employed an air bypass prosthesis that allowed the patient to breathe and speak without any manual adjustments. The expired air passed through the esophago-cutaneous fistula and produced a vibratory column of air at the cricopharyngeus that was articulated into speech. He reported the successful use of this device in 13 of 26 patients. However, fistula leakage, skin slough, and carotid hemorrhage in two radiated cases were complications encountered with this technique. Shedd et al.[243] employed the Tokyo artificial larynx in their reed-fistula prosthetic appliance, which entered a pharyngocutaneous fistula. They claimed satisfactory results in 6 of 10 patients. Again salivary leakage and poor vocal quality have been problems with this method. Sisson et al.[248] created a hypopharyngeal fistula, the location of which depended on the position of the patient's pseudoglottis. This was determined by fluoroscopy, which indicated the site of maximum vibration of the mucous membranes. The connecting prosthesis (Northwestern laryngeal vocal prosthesis) extended between the laryngectomy tube and fistula and lacked a vibrator. A good voice was produced in 7 of their 8 patients. Edwards[61] similarly employed a simple valved connecting prosthesis and a hypopharyngeal fistula. Singer and Blom[246a] have devised a tracheo-esophageal fistula prosthesis (sometimes referred to as the "duckbill" prosthesis) which has been used in over 60 cases with greater than 90 percent success. The complication rate has been low and at present this procedure is the safest and simplest method of surgical voice rehabilitation.

Laryngeal Transplantation

The application of laryngeal transplantation to achieve vocal rehabilitation has been limited by problems in revascularization, reinnervation, and host rejection. Laryngeal transplantation has been performed in dogs[208, 246] with microvascular techniques achieving revascularization and a viable organ. However, failure to achieve reinnervation results in a functionless organ with serious aspiration problems. Kluyskens et al.[139] performed the transplantation of a cadaver larynx to a patient undergoing subtotal laryngectomy. While the larynx remained viable despite lack of direct vascular anastomosis, the patient developed widespread tumor dissemination while on immunosuppressive therapy. The subject of laryngeal transplantation has been reviewed by Tucker.[284]

SUMMARY

While cancers of the larynx are relatively uncommon, their effects may be devastating because of disturbance of the phonatory, respiratory, and protective functions of the larynx.

The majority of laryngeal cancers are squamous cell carcinomas; however, their topographic occurrence within the larynx is of paramount importance because the location of the neoplasm influences prognosis and selection of therapy. The subclassification of laryngeal malignancies into supraglottic, glottic, and subglottic carcinomas is based on the embryologic compartmentalization of the larynx, which produces barriers to their growth and lymphatic dissemination from each site. Such anatomic features as the anterior commissure ligament, preepiglottic and paraglottic spaces, conus elasticus, mucous glands, blood vessels, lymphatics, and the cartilages themselves influence tumor spread.

The resulting fundamental differences in the clinical behavior of tumors at the different regions in the larynx, combined with their extent (stage), determine whether surgery, radiotherapy, or both, are to be employed in their management. The techniques of vertical and horizontal partial laryngectomy permit tumor resection with preservation of laryngeal function in properly selected cases. While radiotherapy provides tumor control comparable to surgery for early cases of laryngeal cancer, for more advanced lesions surgery becomes clearly superior. Cervical metastases are a prominent feature of supraglottic lesions and palpable nodal disease mandates radical neck dissection. Tumors having extensive subglottic spread and paratracheal metastases favor the development of stomal recurrences. Distant metastases are also found more often with supraglottic tumors. At the present time, chemotherapy is of limited palliative value for those with laryngeal malignancies.

In the totally laryngectomized patient, vocal rehabilitation may be attempted by the development of esophageal speech, use of an artificial device, the surgical creation of a shunt, or a laryngoplastic procedure with neoglottic reconstruction.

REFERENCES

1. Abramson, A. L., Parisier, S. C., Zamansky, M. J., and Sulka, M. 1971. Distant metastases from carcinoma of the larynx. Laryngoscope, 81: 1503.

2. Ackerman, L. V. 1948. Verrucous carcinoma of the oral cavity. Surgery, 23: 670.

3. Alonso, J. M. 1947. Conservative surgery of cancer of the larynx. Transactions of the American Academy of Ophthalmology and Otolaryngology, 51: 633.

4. Alonso, J. M. 1967. Metastasis of laryngeal and hypo-pharyngeal carcinoma. Acta Otolaryngologica, 64: 353.

5. American Joint Committee (AJC) for Cancer Staging and End Results Reporting. 1972. Clinical Staging System for Carcinoma of the Larynx. American Joint Committee; Chicago.

6. Appelman, H. D., and Oberman, H. A. 1965. Squamous cell carcinoma of the larynx with sarcoma-like stroma. A clinicopathologic assessment of spindle cell carcinoma and "pseudosarcoma." American Journal of Clinical Pathology, 44: 135.

7. Archer, C. R., Friedman, W. H., Yeager, V. L., and Katsantonis, G. P. 1978. Evaluation of laryngeal cancer by computed tomography. Journal of Computer Assisted Tomography, 2: 618.

8. Arslan, M. 1972. Reconstructive laryngectomy. Report on the first 35 cases. Annals of Otology, Rhinology and Laryngology, 81: 479.

9. Arslan, M. 1975. Techniques of laryngeal reconstruction. Laryngoscope, 85: 862.

10. Arslan, M., and Serafini, I. 1972. Restoration of laryngeal functions after total laryngectomy. Report on the first 25 cases. Laryngoscope, 82: 1349.

11. Asai, R. 1960. Laryngoplasty. Journal of the Japanese Broncho-Esophagological Society, 12: 1.

12. Asai, R. 1972. Laryngoplasty after total laryngectomy. Archives of Otolaryngology, 95: 114.

13. Atkinson, L. 1975. Some features of the epidemiology of cancer of the larynx in Australia and Papua, New Guinea. Laryngoscope, 85: 1173.

14. Auerbach, O., Hammond, E. C., and Garfinkel, L. 1970. Histologic changes in the larynx in relation to smoking habits. Cancer, 25: 92.

15. Ballantyne, A. J., and Fletcher, G. H. 1974. Surgical management of irradiation failures of nonfixed cancers of the glottic region. American Journal of Roentgenology, Radium Therapy and Nuclear Medicine, 120: 164.

16. Barclay, T. H. C., and Rao, N. N. 1975. The incidence and mortality rates for laryngeal cancer from total cancer registries. Laryngoscope, 85: 254.

17. Batsakis, J. G. 1974. Tumors of the Head and Neck: Clinical and Pathological Considerations. Williams and Wilkins, Baltimore.

18. Batsakis, J. G., and Fox, J. E. 1970. Rhabdomyosarcoma of the larynx. Report of a case. Archives of Otolaryngology, 91: 136.

19. Batsakis, J. G., and Fox, J. E. 1970. Supporting tissue neoplasms of the larynx. Surgery, Gynecology and Obstetrics, 131: 989.

20. Batsakis, J. H., Hybels, R., and Rice, D. H. 1976. Laryngeal carcinoma: Stomal recurrences and distant metastases. In Alberti, P. W., and Bryce, D. P., Eds.: Workshops from the Centennial Conference on Laryngeal Cancer. Appleton-Century-Crofts, New York, 868.

21. Bauer, W. C. 1976. Concomitant carcinoma in situ and invasive carcinoma of the larynx. In Alberti, P. W., and Bryce, D. P., Eds.: Workshops from the Centennial Conference on Laryngeal Cancer. Appleton-Century-Crofts, New York, 127.

22. Berdal, P, Iversen, O. H., and Weyde, R. 1976. Simultaneous intermittent bleomycin and radiological treatment of laryngeal cancer. In Alberti, P. W., and Bryce, D. P., Eds.: Workshops from the Centennial

Conference on Laryngeal Cancer. Appleton-Century-Crofts, New York, 333.

23. Berlinger, N. T., Tsakraklides, V., Pollak, K., Adams, G. L., Yang, M., and Good, R. A.: 1976. Prognostic significance of lymph node histology in patients with squamous cell carcinoma of the larynx, pharynx, or oral cavity. Laryngoscope, 86: 792.

24. Bertino, J. R. 1976. Chemotherapeutic approaches to advanced carcinoma of the larynx. In Alberti, P. W., and Bryce, D. P., Eds.: Workshops from the Centennial Conference on Laryngeal Cancer, Appleton-Century-Crofts, New York, 548.

25. Biller, H. F., and Bergman, J. A. 1976. Verrucous carcinoma of the larynx. In Alberti, P. W., and Bryce, D. P., Eds.: Workshops from the Centennial Conference on Laryngeal Cancer. Appleton-Century-Crofts, New York, 462.

26. Biller, H. F., Blaugrund, S. M., and Som, M. L. 1976. Decreasing limitations of partial laryngectomy for vocal cord cancer. In Alberti, P. W., and Bryce, D. P., Eds.: Workshops from the Centennial Conference on Laryngeal Cancer, Appleton-Century-Crofts, New York, 424.

27. Biller, H. F., Davis, W. H., and Ogura, H. H. 1971. Delayed contralateral cervical metastases with laryngeal and laryngopharyngeal cancers. Laryngoscope, 81: 1499.

28. Biller, H. F., Ogura, J. H., and Bauer, W. C. 1971. Verrucous cancer of the larynx. Laryngoscope, 81: 1323.

29. Biller, H. F., Ogura, J. H., and Pratt, L. 1971. Hemilaryngectomy for T_2 glottic cancers. Archives of Otolaryngology, 93: 238.

30. Biller, H. F., Barnhill, F. R., Ogura, J. H., and Perez, C. A. 1970. Hemilaryngectomy following radiation failure for carcinoma of the vocal cords. Laryngoscope, 80: 249.

31. Blaugrund, S. M., and Kurland, S. R. 1975. Replacement of the arytenoid following vertical hemilaryngectomy. Laryngoscope, 85: 935.

32. Bocca, E. 1975. Supraglottic cancer. Laryngoscope, 85: 1318.

33. Bocca, E., Pignataro, O., and Mosciaro, O. 1968. Supraglottic surgery of the larynx. Annals of Otology, Rhinology and Laryngology, 77: 1005.

34. Bonneau, R. A., and Lehman, R. H. 1975. Stomal recurrence following laryngectomy. Archives of Otolaryngology, 101: 408.

35. Bosch, A., Kademian, M. T., Frias, Z. C., and Caldwell, W. L. 1978. Failures after irradiation in early vocal cord cancer. Laryngoscope, 88: 2017.

36. Brandenburg, J. H., and Rutter, S. W. 1977. Residual carcinoma of the larynx. Laryngoscope, 87: 224.

37. Bridger, G. P. 1976. Mucous gland involvement in cancer at the anterior commissure. In Alberti, P. W., and Bryce, D. P., Eds.: Workshops from the Centennial Conference on Laryngeal Cancer. Appleton-Century-Crofts, New York, 101.

38. Bridger, G. P., Nassar, V. H. 1972. Cancer spread in the larynx. Archives of Otolaryngology, 95: 497.

39. Broyles, E. N. 1943. The anterior commissure tendon. Annals of Otology, Rhinology and Laryngology, 52: 342.

40. Bryce, D. P., and Rider, W. D. 1971. Preoperative irradiation in the treatment of advanced laryngeal carcinoma. Laryngoscope, 81: 1481.

41. Bryce, D. P., Ireland, P. E., and Rider, W. D. 1963. Experience in the surgical and radiological treatment in 500 cases of carcinoma of the larynx. Annals of Otology, Rhinology and Laryngology, 72: 416.

42. Cachin, Y. 1975. Supraglottic carcinomas: The early cases. Laryngoscope, 85: 1617.

43. Cachin, Y. 1976. Limitations of horizontal partial laryngectomy. In Alberti, P. W., and Bryce, D. P., Eds.: Workshops from the Centennial Conference on Laryngeal Cancer. Appleton-Century-Crofts, New York. 385.

44. Cady, B., Rippey, J. H., and Frazell, E. L. 1968. Non-epidermoid cancer of the larynx. Annals of Surgery, 167: 116.

45. Calcaterra, T. C. 1976. Tracheo-esophageal shunt for speech rehabilitation after total laryngectomy. In Alberti, P. W., and Bryce, D. P., Eds.: Workshops from the Centennial Conference on Laryngeal Cancer, Appleton-Century-Crofts, New York, 576.

46. Calcaterra, T. C., and Jafek, B. W. 1971. Tracheo-esophageal shunt for speech rehabilitation after total laryngectomy. Archives of Otolaryngology, 94: 124.

47. Clerf, L. H. 1944. The pre-epiglottic space and its relation to carcinoma of the epiglottis. Archives of Otolaryngology, 40: 177.

48. Coates, H. L., DeSanto, L. W., Devine, K. D., and Elveback, L. A.: 1976. Carcinoma of the supraglottic larynx. A review of

221 cases. Archives of Otolaryngology, 102: 686.

49. Collins, V. P. 1976. Comments on the radiotherapeutic approach to advanced disease. In Alberti, P. W., and Bryce, D. P., Eds.: Workshops from the Centennial Conference on Laryngeal Cancer. Appleton-Century-Crofts, New York, 523.

50. Conley, J. J. 1959. Vocal rehabilitation by autogenous vein graft. Annals of Otology, Rhinology and Laryngology, 68: 990.

51. Conley, J. 1969. Surgical techniques for the vocal rehabilitation of the postlaryngectomized patient. Transactions of the American Academy of Ophthalmology and Otolaryngology, 73: 288.

52. Conley, J. 1975. Regional skin flaps in partial laryngectomy. Laryngoscope, 85: 942.

53. Conley, J. J., De Amesti, F., and Pierce, M. K. 1958. A new surgical technique for the vocal rehabilitation of the laryngectomized patient. Annals of Otology, Rhinology and Laryngology, 67: 655.

54. Constable, W. C., Marks, R. D., Jr., Robbins, J. P., and Fitz-Hugh, G. S.: 1972. High dose preoperative radiotherapy and surgery for cancer of the larynx. Laryngoscope, 82: 1861.

55. Constable, W. C., White, R. L., El-Mahdi, A. M., Fitz-Hugh, G. S. 1975. Radiotherapeutic management of the cancer of the glottis, University of Virginia, 1956-1971. Laryngoscope, 85: 1494.

56. Constable, W. C., White, R. L., El-Mahdi, A. M., and Fitz-Hugh, G. S. 1976. Intermediate dose preoperative radiotherapy for cancer of the larynx—end results. In Alberti, P. W., and Bryce, D. P., Eds.: Workshops from the Centennial Conference on Laryngeal Cancer. Appleton-Century-Crofts, New York. 360.

57. Daly, C. J., and Strong, E. W. 1975. Carcinoma of the glottic larynx. American Journal of Surgery, 130: 489.

58. Daly, J. F., and Kwok, F. N. 1975. Laryngofissure and cordectomy. Laryngoscope, 85: 1290.

59. Demian, S. D. E., Bushkin, F. L., and Echevarria, R. A. 1973. Perineural invasion and anaplastic transformation of verrucous carcinoma. Cancer, 32: 395.

60. De Santo, L. W. 1976. Selection of treatment for in situ and early invasive carcinoma of the glottis. In Alberti, P. W., and Bryce, D. P., Eds.: Workshops from the Centennial Conference on Laryngeal Cancer. Appleton-Century-Crofts, New York, 146.

61. Edwards, N. 1975. Post-laryngectomy vocal rehabilitation using expired air and an external fistula method. Laryngoscope, 85: 690.

62. Ehrlich, A. 1954. Tumor involving the laryngeal cartilages. Archives of Otolaryngology, 59: 178.

63. Elliott, G. B., MacDougall, J. A., and Elliott, J. D. A. 1973. Problems of verrucous squamous carcinoma. Annals of Surgery, 177: 21.

64. Ennuyer, A., and Bataini, P. 1965. Treatment of supra-glottic carcinomas by telecobalt therapy. British Journal of Radiology, 38: 661.

65. Ennuyer, A., and Bataini, P. 1975. VI. Laryngeal Carcinomas. Laryngoscope, 85: 1467.

66. Eschwege, F., Cachin, Y., and Micheau, C. H. 1976. Treatment of adenocarcinomas of the larynx. In Alberti, P. W., and Bryce, D. P., Eds.: Workshops from the Centennial Conference on Laryngeal Cancer. Appleton-Century-Crofts, New York, 472.

67. Fayos, J. V. 1975. Carcinoma of the endolarynx: Results of irradiation. Cancer, 35: 1525.

68. Fechner, R. E. 1976. Adenocarcinoma of the larynx. In Alberti, P. W., and Bryce, D. P., Eds.: Workshops from the Centennial Conference on Laryngeal Cancer. Appleton-Century-Crofts, New York, 466.

69. Fisher, H. R. 1976. Verrucous carcinoma of the larynx—A study of its pathologic anatomy. In Alberti, P. W., and Bryce, D. P., Eds.: Workshops from the Centennial Conference on Laryngeal Cancer. Appleton-Century-Crofts, New York, 452.

70. Flanagan, P., Cross, R. M., and Libcke, J. H. 1965. Fibrosarcoma of the larynx. Journal of Laryngology and Otology, 79: 1049.

71. Fletcher, G. H., Jesse, R. H., Lindberg, R. D., and Koons, C. A. 1970. The place of radiotherapy in the management of the squamous cell carcinoma of the supraglottic larynx. American Journal of Roentgenology, 108: 19.

72. Fletcher, G. H., Lindberg, R. D., Hamberger, A., and Horiot, J. C. 1975. Reasons for irradiation failure in squamous cell carcinoma of the larynx. Laryngoscope, 85: 987.

73. Fonts, E. A., Greenlaw, R. H., Rush, B. F., and Rovin, S. 1969. Verrucous squamous

cell carcinoma of the oral cavity. Cancer, 23: 152.

74. Frable, W. J., and Olson, N. R. 1967. Cytology: An adjunct in the diagnosis of carcinoma of the larynx. Archives of Otolaryngology, 85: 50.

75. Fredrickson, J. M., Bryce, D. P., and Williams, G. T. 1973. Laryngeal reconstruction to prevent aspiration. Archives of Otolaryngology, 97: 457.

76. Freeland, A. P. 1976. Microfil angiography: A demonstration of the microvasculature of the larynx with reference to tumor spread. In Alberti, P. W., and Bryce, D. P., Eds.: Workshops from the Centennial Conference on Laryngeal Cancer. Appleton-Century-Crofts, New York, 279.

77. Freeland, A. P., and Van Nostrand, A. W. 1976. The applied anatomy of the anterior commissure and subglottis. In Alberti, P. W., and Bryce, D. P., Eds.: Workshops from the Centennial Conference on Laryngeal Cancer. Appleton-Century-Crofts, New York, 652.

78. Friedman, W. H., and Goldman, J. L. 1969. Tritiated thymidine studies of radiated laryngeal cancer. Archives of Otolaryngology, 89: 766.

79. Friedmann, I. 1976. Sarcomas of the larynx. In Alberti, P. W., and Bryce, D. P., Eds.: Workshops from the Centennial Conference on Laryngeal Cancer. Appleton-Century-Crofts, New York, 479.

80. Gabriel, C. E., and Jones, D. G. 1962. Hyperkeratosis of the larynx. Journal of Laryngology and Otology, 76: 947.

81. Gerughty, R. M., Hennigar, G. R., and Brown, F. M. 1968. Adenosquamous carcinoma of the nasal, oral and laryngeal cavities. A clinicopathologic survey of ten cases. Cancer, 22: 1140.

82. Gilmore, B. B., Repola, D. A., and Batsakis, J. G. 1978. Carcinoma of the larynx: Lymph node reaction patterns. Laryngoscope, 88: 1333.

83. Goellner, J. R., Devine, K. D., and Weiland L. H. 1973. Pseudosarcoma of the larynx. American Journal of Clinical Pathology, 59: 312.

84. Goepfert, H., Jesse, R. H., Fletcher, G. H., and Hamberger, A. 1975. Optimal treatment for the technically resectable squamous cell carcinoma of the supraglottic larynx. Laryngoscope, 85: 14.

85. Goffinet, D. R., Eltringham, J. R., Glatstein, E., and Bagshaw, M. A. 1973. Carcinoma of the larynx: Results of radiation therapy in 213 patients. American Journal of Roentgenology, Radium Therapy and Nuclear Medicine, 117: 553.

86. Goffinet, D. R., Gilbert, E. H., Weller, S. A., and Bagshaw, M. A. 1976. Irradiation of clinically uninvolved cervical lymph nodes. In Alberti, P. W., and Bryce, D. P., Eds.: Workshops from the Centennial Conference on Laryngeal Cancer. Appleton-Century-Crofts, New York, 889.

87. Goldman, J. L., and Roffman, J. D. 1976. Combined pre-operative irradiation and surgery for advanced cancer of the larynx and laryngopharynx. (A 14-year correlative statistical and histopathological study). In Alberti, P. W., and Bryce, D. P., Eds.: Workshops from the Centennial Conference on Laryngeal Cancer. Appleton-Century-Crofts, New York, 365.

88. Goldman, J. L., and Silverstone, S. M. 1961. Combined radiation and surgical therapy for cancer of the larynx and laryngopharynx. Transactions of the American Academy of Ophthalmology and Otolaryngology, 65: 496.

89. Goldman, J. L., Cheren, R. V., Zak, F. G., and Gunsberg, M. 1966. Histopathology of larynges and radical neck specimens in a combined radiation and surgery program for advanced carcinoma of the larynx and laryngopharynx. Annals of Otology, Rhinology and Laryngology, 75: 313.

90. Goldman, J. L., Zak, F. G., Roffman, J. D., and Birken, E. A.: 1972. High dosage preoperative radiation and surgery for carcinoma of the larynx and laryngopharynx. Annals of Otology, Rhinology and Laryngology, 81: 488.

91. Goode, R. L. 1969. The development of an improved artificial larynx. Transactions of the American Academy of Ophthalmology and Otolaryngology, 73: 279.

92. Goode, R. L. 1975. Artificial laryngeal devices in post-laryngectomy rehabilitation. Laryngoscope, 85: 677.

93. Goolden, A. W. G. 1951. Radiation cancer of the pharynx. British Medical Journal, 2: 1110.

94. Gussenbauer, C. 1874. Uber die erste durch Th. Billroth am menschen ausgefuhrte Kehlkopf-Exstirpation und die Anwendung eines Kunstlichen Kehlkopfes. Archiv für Klinische Chirurgic (Berlin), 17: 343.

95. Hansen, H. S. 1975. Supraglottic carcinoma of the aryepiglottic fold. Laryngoscope, 85: 1667.

96. Harrer, W. V., and Lewis, P. L. 1970. Carci-

noma of the larynx with cardiac metastases. Archives of Otolaryngology, 91: 382.

97. Harris, H. H., and Butler, E. 1968. Surgical limits in cancer of the subglottic larynx. Archives of Otolaryngology, 87: 490.

98. Harrison, D. F. N. 1971. The pathology and management of subglottic cancer. Annals of Otology, Rhinology and Laryngology, 80: 6.

99. Harrison, D. F. N. 1975. Laryngectomy for subglottic lesions. Laryngoscope, 85: 1208.

100. Hast, M. H. 1976. Applied embryology of the larynx. In Alberti, P. W., and Bryce, D. P., Eds.: Workshops from the Centennial Conference on Laryngeal Cancer. Appleton-Century-Crofts, New York, 6.

101. Hawkins, N. V. 1975. VIII. The treatment of glottic carcinoma: An analysis of 800 cases. Laryngoscope, 85: 1485.

102. Hendrickson, F. R., Kline, T. C., Jr., and Hibbs, G. G. 1975. Primary squamous cell carcinoma of the larynx. Laryngoscope, 85: 1650.

103. Hendrickson, F. R., and Liebner, E. 1968. Results of pre-operative radiotherapy for supraglottic larynx cancer. Annals of Otology, Rhinology and Laryngology, 77: 222.

104. Henk, J. M. 1975. The influence of oxygen and hypoxia on laryngeal cancer management. Laryngoscope, 85: 1134.

105. Henry, J., Balikdjian, D., Storme, G., Lustman-Marechal, J., and Degandt, J. B. 1975. Radiotherapy in the treatment of T3-T4 supraglottic tumors. Laryngoscope, 85: 1682.

106. Hiranandani, L. H. 1975. Panel on epidemiology and etiology of laryngeal carcinoma. Laryngoscope, 85: 1197.

107. Holinger, P. H., and Schild, J. A. 1976. Carcinoma in situ of the larynx. In Alberti, P. W., and Bryce, D. P., Eds.: Workshops from the Centennial Conference on Laryngeal Cancer. Appleton-Century-Crofts, New York, 143.

108. Homburger, F. 1975. "Smokers' Larynx" and carcinoma of the larynx in Syrian hamsters exposed to cigarette smoke. Laryngoscope, 85: 1874.

109. Hoover, W. B., and King, G. D. 1954. Emergency laryngectomy. Archives of Otolaryngology, 59: 431.

110. Huizenga, C., and Balogh, K. 1970. Cartilaginous tumors of the larynx: A clinicopathologic study of 10 new cases and a review of the literature. Cancer, 26: 201.

111. Hyams, V. J. 1976. Spindle cell carcinoma of the larynx. In Alberti, P. W., and Bryce, D. P., Eds.: Workshops from the Centennial Conference on Laryngeal Cancer. Appleton-Century-Crofts, New York, 489.

112. Hyams, V. J. 1976. In discussion, Biller, H. F., and Bergman, J. A. Verrucous carcinoma of the larynx. In Alberti, P. W., and Bryce, D. P., Eds.: Workshops from the Centennial Conference on Laryngeal Cancer. Appleton-Century-Crofts, New York, 462.

113. Hyams, V. J., and Rabuzzi, D. D. 1970. Cartilaginous tumors of the larynx. Laryngoscope, 80: 755.

114. Iwai, H. 1976. Limitations of conservation surgery in carcinoma involving the arytenoid. In Alberti, P. W., and Bryce, D. P., Eds.: Workshops from the Centennial Conference on Laryngeal Cancer. Appleton-Century-Crofts, New York, 426.

115. Iwai, H., and Koike, Y. 1975. Primary laryngoplasty. Laryngoscope, 85: 929.

116. Iwamoto, H. 1975. An epidemiological study of laryngeal cancer in Japan (1960–1969). Laryngoscope, 85: 1162.

117. Jakobsson, P. A. 1976. Histologic grading of malignancy and prognosis in glottic carcinoma of the larynx. In Alberti, P. W., and Bryce, D. P., Eds.: Workshops from the Centennial Conference on Laryngeal Cancer. Appleton-Century-Crofts, New York, 847.

118. Jankovic, I., and Merkas, Z. 1976. Radiotherapy as the primary approach in the treatment of laryngeal cancer. In Alberti, P. W., and Bryce, D. P., Eds.: Workshops from the Centennial Conference on Laryngeal Cancer. Appleton-Century-Crofts, New York, 881.

119. Jesse, R. H. 1975. I. The evaluation of treatment of patients with extensive squamous cancer of the vocal cords. Laryngoscope, 85: 1424.

120. Jesse, R. H., Lindberg, R. D., and Horiot, J. C. 1971. Vocal cord cancer with anterior commissure extension, choice of treatment. American Journal of Surgery, 122: 437.

121. Jing, B. S. 1976. Roentgen examination of laryngeal cancer: A critical evaluation. In Alberti, P. W., and Bryce, D. P., Eds.: Workshops from the Centennial Conference on Laryngeal Cancer. Appleton-Century-Crofts, New York, 232.

122. Johner, C. H. 1970. The lymphatics of the larynx. Otolaryngologic Clinics of North America, 3: 439.

123. Johns, M. E., Batsakis, J. G., and Short,

C. D. 1973. Oncocytic and oncocytoid tumors of the salivary glands. Laryngoscope, 83: 1940.

124. Jones, G. D., and Gabriel, C. E. 1969. The incidence of carcinoma of the larynx in persons under twenty years of age. Laryngoscope, 79: 251.

125. Jorgensen, K. 1974. Carcinoma of the larynx. III. Therapeutic Results. Acta Radiologica: Therapy, Physics, Biology (Stockholm) 13: 446.

126. Kagan, A. R., Calcaterra, T., Ward, P., and Chan, P. 1974. Significance of edema of the endolarynx following curative irradiation for carcinoma. American Journal of Roentgenology, Radium Therapy and Nuclear Medicine, 120: 169.

127. Karlan, M. S. 1968. Two stage Asai laryngectomy utilizing a modified Tucker valve. American Journal of Surgery, 116: 597.

128. Kashima, H. K. 1976. The characteristics of laryngeal cancer correlating with cervical lymph node metastasis. In Alberti, P. W., and Bryce, D. P., Eds., Workshops from the Centennial Conference on Laryngeal Cancer. Appleton-Century-Crofts, New York, 855.

129. Kawabe, Y., and Kondo, T. 1967. Laryngeal leiomyosarcoma. Evaluation of the authors' case and observation of the literature. Journal of Otolaryngology of Japan (Tokyo), 39: 427.

130. Keim, W. F., Shapiro, M. J., and Rosin, H. D. 1965. Study of postlaryngectomy stomal recurrence. Archives of Otolaryngology, 81: 183.

131. Kirchner, J. A. 1969. One hundred laryngeal cancers studied by serial section. Annals of Otology, Rhinology and Laryngology, 78: 689.

132. Kirchner, J. A. 1976. Growth and spread of laryngeal cancer as related to partial laryngectomy. In Alberti, P. W., and Bryce, D. P., Eds.: Workshops from the Centennial Conference on Laryngeal Cancer. Appleton-Century-Crofts, New York, 54.

133. Kirchner, J. A., and Fischer, J. J. 1976. Anterior commissure cancer—a clinical and laboratory study of 39 cases. In Alberti, P. W., and Bryce, D. P., Eds.: Workshops from the Centennial Conference on Laryngeal Cancer. Appleton-Century-Crofts, New York, 645.

134. Kirchner, J. A., and Owen, J. R. 1977. Five hundred cancers of the larynx and pyriform sinus. Results of treatment of radiation and surgery. Laryngoscope, 87: 1288.

135. Kirchner, J. A., and Som, M. L. 1971. Clinical significance of fixed vocal cord. Laryngoscope, 81: 1029.

136. Kirchner, J. A., and Som, M. L. 1971. Clinical and histological observations on supraglottic cancer. Annals of Otology, Rhinology and Laryngology, 80: 638.

137. Kirchner, J. A., and Som, M. L. 1975. The anterior commissure technique of partial laryngectomy: Clinical and laboratory observations. Laryngoscope, 85: 1308.

138. Kirchner, J. A., Cornog, J. L., and Holmes, R. E. 1974. Transglottic cancer: Its growth and spread within the larynx. Archives of Otolaryngology, 99: 247.

139. Kluyskens, P., and Ringoir, S. 1970. Follow-up of a human larynx transplantation. Laryngoscope, 80: 1244.

140. Komorn, R. M. 1976. Tracheo-esophageal shunt vocal rehabilitation. In Alberti, P. W., and Bryce, D. P., Eds.: Workshops from the Centennial Conference on Laryngeal Cancer. Appleton-Century-Crofts, New York, 571.

141. Komorn, R. M., Weycer, J. S., Sessions, R. B., and Malone, P. 1973. Vocal rehabilitation with a tracheo-esophageal shunt. Archives of Otolaryngology, 97: 303.

142. Krajina, Z. 1976. Laryngeal sarcoma. In Alberti, P. W., and Bryce, D. P., Eds.: Workshops from the Centennial Conference on Laryngeal Cancer. Appleton-Century-Crofts, New York, 485.

143. Krajina, Z., Kulcar, Z., and Konić-Carnelutti, V. 1975. Epidemiology of laryngeal cancer. Laryngoscope, 85: 1155.

144. Kramer, S. 1976. Methotrexate and radiation therapy in the treatment of advanced squamous cell carcinoma of the oral cavity, oropharynx, supraglottic larynx, and hypopharynx. (Preliminary report of a controlled clinical trial of the Radiation Therapy Oncology Group). In Alberti, P. W., and Bryce, D. P., Eds.: Workshops from the Centennial Conference on Laryngeal Cancer. Appleton-Century-Crofts, New York, 327.

145. Kraus, F., and Perez-Mesa, C. 1966. Verrucous carcinoma: Clinical and pathological study of 105 cases involving oral cavity, larynx and genitalia. Cancer, 19: 26.

146. Kurozumi, S., Harada, Y., Sugimoto, Y., and Sasaki, H. 1977. Airway malignancy in poisonous gas workers. Journal of Laryngology and Otology, 91: 217.

147. Lane, N. 1957. Pseudosarcoma (Polypoid

sarcoma-like masses) associated with squamous-cell carcinoma of the mouth, fauces, and larynx; report of ten cases. Cancer, 10: 19.

148. Lauerma, S. 1967. Treatment of laryngeal cancer. A study of 638 cases. Acta Oto-Laryngologica, suppl., 225: 1.

149. Lawson, W., and Som, M. 1975. Second primary cancer after irradiation of laryngeal cancer. Annals of Otology, Rhinology and Laryngology, 84: 771.

150. Lawson, W., and Zak, F. G. 1974. The glomus bodies ("Paraganglia") of the human larynx. Laryngoscope, 84: 98.

151. Lederman, M. 1970. Radiotherapy of cancer of the larynx. Journal of Laryngology and Otology, 84: 867.

152. Lederman, M. 1971. Cancer of the larynx. Part I: Natural history in relation to treatment. (Part II (with Whall, M. A.): The techniques of radiation treatment.) British Journal of Radiology, 44: 569.

153. Leroux-Robert, J. 1936. Les epitheliomas intralarynges. Formes anatomo-cliniques. Voies d'extension. These pour le doctorat en medicine. Gaston Dion Cie, Paris.

154. Leroux-Robert, J. 1970. Cylindromes et pseudo-cylindromes O.R.L. Évolution et pronostic des cylindromes vrais. Á propos de 32 cas observés il y a plus des ans. Annales d'Oto-Laryngologie et de Chirurgie Cervico-Faciale, 87: 713.

155. Leroux-Robert, J. 1975. IV. A statistical study of 620 laryngeal carcinomas of the glottic region personally operated upon more than five years ago. Laryngoscope, 85: 1440.

156. Leroux-Robert, J., and Courtial, C. L. 1965. Tumeurs mixtes et cylindromes du larynx. Annales d'Oto-Laryngologie et de Chirurgie Cervico-Faciale (Paris), 82: 1.

157. Lichtiger, B., Mackay, B., and Tessmer, C. F. 1970. Spindle-cell variant of squamous carcinoma. A light and electrical Microscopic Study of 13 cases. Cancer, 26: 1311.

158. Lillie, J. C., and DeSanto, L. W. 1973. Transoral surgery of early cordal carcinoma. Transactions of the American Academy of Ophthalmology and Otolaryngology, 77: ORL 92.

159. Loewy, A., and Laker, H.I. 1968. Tracheal stoma problems. Archives of Otolaryngology, 87: 477.

160. Lowry, W. S. 1975. Alcoholism in cancer of the head and neck. Laryngoscope, 85: 1275.

161. Luk'ianchenko, A. G. 1975. 3 Cases of familial laryngeal cancer. (Russian) Zhurnal Ushnykh, Nosovykh I Gorlovykh Boleznei, 4: 98.

162. McGavran, M. H., and Bauer, W. C. 1976. Sinus histiocytosis and cervical lymph node metastases from transglottic epidermoid carcinoma of the larynx. In Alberti, P. W., and Bryce, D. P., Eds.: Workshops from the Centennial Conference on Laryngeal Cancer. Appleton-Century-Crofts, New York, 865.

163. McGavran, M. H., Bauer, W. C., and Ogura, J. H. 1960. Isolated laryngeal keratosis. Its relation to carcinoma of the larynx based on a clinicopathologic study of 87 consecutive cases with long-term follow-up. Laryngoscope, 70: 932.

164. McGavran, M. H., Bauer, W. C., and Ogura, J. H. 1961. The incidence of cervical lymph node metastases from epidermoid carcinoma of the larynx and their relationship to certain characteristics of the primary tumor. A study based on the clinical and pathological findings for 96 patients treated by primary en bloc laryngectomy and radical neck dissection. Cancer, 14: 55.

165. McGavran, M. H., Stutsman, A. C., and Ogura, J. H. 1976. Superficially invasive epidermoid carcinoma of the true vocal cord. In Alberti, P. W., and Bryce, D. P., Eds.: Workshops from the Centennial Conference on Laryngeal Cancer. Appleton-Century-Crofts, New York, 120.

166. McGrail, J. S. 1976. Vocal rehabilitation at or following laryngectomy. In Alberti, P. W., and Bryce, D. P., Eds.: Workshops from the Centennial Conference on Laryngeal Cancer. Appleton-Century-Crofts, New York, 560.

167. McGrail, J. S., and Oldfield, D. L. 1971. One-stage operation for vocal rehabilitation at laryngectomy. Transactions of the American Academy of Ophthalmology and Otolaryngology, 75: 510.

168. Maguire, A., and Dayal, V. S. 1976. Supraglottic anatomy: The pre- or the periepiglottic space? In Alberti, P. W., and Bryce, D. P., Eds.: Workshops from the Centennial Conference on Laryngeal Cancer. Appleton-Century-Crofts, New York, 26.

169. Marchetta, F. C., Sako, K., and Mattick, W. L. 1968. Squamous cell carcinoma of the larynx. American Journal of Surgery, 116: 491.

170. Martensson, B. 1967. Transconioscopy in cancer of the larynx. With special reference to the detection of subglottic extension. Acta Oto-Laryngologica, suppl., 224: 476.

171. Martensson, B. 1975. Epidemiological aspects on laryngeal carcinoma in Scandinavia. Laryngoscope, 85: 1185.

172. Martensson, B. 1976. Indications for transconiscopy. In Alberti, P. W., and Bryce, D. P., Eds.: Workshops from the Centennial Conference on Laryngeal Cancer. Appleton-Century-Crofts, New York, 668.

173. Martensson, B., Fluur, E., and Jacobsson, F. 1967. Aspects on treatment of cancer of the larynx. Annals of Otology, Rhinology and Laryngology, 76: 313.

174. Micheau, C., Luboinski, B., Sancho, H., and Cachin, Y. 1976. Modes of invasion of cancer of the larynx. A statistical, histological, and radioclinical analysis of 120 cases. Cancer, 38: 346.

175. Miller, A. H. 1967. First experiences with the Asai technique for vocal rehabilitation after total laryngectomy. Annals of Otology, Rhinology and Laryngology, 76: 829.

176. Miller, A. H. 1968. Further experiences with the Asai technique of vocal rehabilitation after laryngectomy. Transactions of the American Academy of Ophthalmology and Otolaryngology, 72: 779.

177. Miller, A. H. 1976. Experiences with the Asai technique. In Alberti, P. W., and Bryce, D. P., Eds.: Workshops from the Centennial Conference on Laryngeal Cancer. Appleton-Century-Crofts, New York, 557.

178. Miller, A. H. 1976. Carcinoma in situ of the larynx—clinical appearance and treatment. In Alberti, P. W., and Bryce, D. P., Eds.: Workshops from the Centennial Conference on Laryngeal Cancer. Appleton-Century-Crofts, New York, 161.

179. Miller, A. H., and Fisher, H. R. 1971. Clues to the life history of carcinoma in situ of the larynx. Laryngoscope, 81: 1475.

180. Miller, D. 1975. Cryosurgery as a modality in the treatment of carcinoma of the larynx. Laryngoscope, 85: 1281.

181. Miller, D. 1975. III. Management of glottic carcinoma. Laryngoscope, 85: 1435.

182. Miller, D. 1976. Management of keratosis and carcinoma in situ with cryosurgery. In Alberti, P. W., and Bryce, D. P., Eds.: Workshops from the Centennial Conference on Laryngeal Cancer. Appleton-Century-Crofts, New York, 151.

183. Minckler, D. S., Meligro, C. H., Norris, H. T. 1970. Carcinosarcoma of the larynx. Case report with metastases of epidermoid and sarcomatous elements. Cancer, 26: 195.

184. Modlin, B., and Ogura, J. H. 1969. Postlaryngectomy tracheal stomal recurrences. Laryngoscope, 79: 239.

185. Montgomery, W. W. 1972. Postlaryngectomy vocal rehabilitation. Archives of Otolaryngology, 95: 76.

186. Montgomery, W. W., and Lavelle, W. G. 1974. A technique for improving esophageal and tracheopharyngeal speech. Annals of Otology, Rhinology and Laryngology, 83: 452.

187. Montgomery, W. W., and Toohill, R. J. 1968. Voice rehabilitation after laryngectomy. Archives of Otolaryngology, 88: 499.

188. Morgan, R. W., and Shettigara, P. T. 1976. Occupational asbestos exposure, smoking, and laryngeal carcinoma. Annals of the New York Academy of Sciences, 271: 308.

189. Mozolewski, E. S., Zietek, E., Wysocki, R., Jach, K., and Jassem, W. 1975. Arytenoid vocal shunt in laryngectomized patients. Laryngoscope, 85: 853.

190. Myerowitz, R L., Barnes, E. L., and Myers, E. 1978. Small cell anaplastic (oat cell) carcinoma of the larynx: Report of a case and review of the literature. Laryngoscope, 88: 1697.

191. Nassar, V. H., Bridger, G. P. 1971. Topography of the laryngeal mucous glands. Archives of Otolaryngology, 94: 490.

192. Norris, C. M. 1958. Technique of extended fronto-lateral partial laryngectomy. Laryngoscope, 68: 1240.

193. Norris, C. M. 1959. Causes of failure in surgical treatment of malignant tumors of the larynx. Annals of Otology, Rhinology and Laryngology, 68: 487.

194. Norris, C. M. 1976. Role and limitations of vertical hemilaryngectomy. In Alberti, P. W., and Bryce, D. P., Eds.: Workshops from the Centennial Conference on Laryngeal Cancer. Appleton-Century-Crofts, New York, 418.

195. Norris, C. M., and Peale, A. R. 1963. Keratosis of the larynx. Journal of Laryngology and Otology, 77: 635.

196. Norris, C. M., Tucker, G. F., Jr., Kuo, B. F., and Pitser, W. F. 1970. A correlation of clinical staging, pathological findings and

five year end results in surgically treated cancer of the larynx. Annals of Otology, Rhinology and Laryngology, 79: 1033.

197. O'Brien, P. H., Carlson, R., Steubner, E. A., Jr., and Staley, C. T.: 1971. Distant metastases in epidermoid cell carcinoma of the head and neck. Cancer, 27: 304.

198. Ogura, J. H. 1958. Supraglottic subtotal laryngectomy and radical neck dissection for carcinoma of the epiglottis. Laryngoscope, 68: 983.

199. Ogura, J. H., and Biller, H. F. 1969. Glottic reconstruction following extended frontolateral hemilaryngectomy. Laryngoscope, 79: 2181.

200. Ogura, J. H., and Biller, H. F. 1969. Conservative surgery in cancer of the head and neck. Otolaryngologic Clinics of North America, 2: 641.

201. Ogura, J. H., and Biller, H. F. 1970. Preoperative irradiation for laryngeal and laryngopharyngeal cancers. Laryngoscope, 80: 802.

202. Ogura, J. H., Biller, H. F., and Wette, R. 1971. Elective neck dissection for pharyngeal and laryngeal cancers: An evaluation. Annals of Otology, Rhinology and Laryngology, 80: 646.

203. Ogura, J. H., Sessions, D. G., and Ciralsky, R. H. 1975. Supraglottic carcinoma with extension to the arytenoid. Laryngoscope, 85: 1327.

204. Ogura, J. H., Sessions, D. G., and Ciralsky, R. H. 1975. Glottic cancer with extension to the arytenoid. Laryngoscope, 85: 1822.

205. Ogura, J. H., Sessions, D. G., and Spector, G. J. 1975. Analysis of surgical therapy for epidermoid carcinoma of the laryngeal glottis. Laryngoscope, 85: 1522.

206. Ogura, J. H., Sessions, D. G., and Spector, G. J. 1975. Conservation surgery for epidermoid carcinoma of the supraglottic larynx. Laryngoscope, 85: 1808.

207. Ogura, J. H., Spector, G. J., and Sessions, D. G. 1975. Conservation surgery for epidermoid carcinoma of the marginal area (aryepiglottic fold extension). Laryngoscope, 85: 1801.

208. Ogura, J. H., Kawasaki, M., Takenouchi, S., and Yagi, M. 1966. Replantation and transplantation of the canine larynx. Annals of Otology, Rhinology and Laryngology, 75: 295.

209. Ogura, J. H., Sessions, D. G., Spector, G. J., and Alonso, W. A. 1976. Roles and limitations of conservation surgical therapy for laryngeal cancer. In Alberti, P. W., and Bryce, D. P., Eds.: Workshops from the Centennial Conference on Laryngeal Cancer. Appleton-Century-Crofts, New York, 392.

210. Olofsson, J. 1976. Growth and spread of laryngeal carcinoma. In Alberti, P. W., and Bryce, D. P., Eds.: Workshops from the Centennial Conference on Laryngeal Cancer. Appleton-Century-Crofts, New York, 40.

211. Olofsson, J. 1976. Specific features of laryngeal carcinoma involving the anterior commissure and the subglottic region. In Alberti, P. W., and Bryce, D. P., Eds.: Workshops from the Centennial Conference on Laryngeal Cancer. Appleton-Century-Crofts, New York, 626.

212. Olofsson, J., and van Nostrand, A. W. P. 1973. Growth and spread of laryngeal and hypopharyngeal carcinoma with reflections on the effect of preoperative irradiation. 139 cases studied by whole organ serial sectioning. Acta Oto-laryngologica (Stockholm), suppl., 308: 1.

213. Olofsson, J., Lord, I. J., and van Nostrand, A. W. P. 1973. Vocal cord fixation in laryngeal carcinoma. Acta Oto-Laryngologica (Stockholm), 75: 496.

214. Olofsson, J., Freeland, A. P., Sokjer, Renouf, J. H., et al. 1976. Radiologic-pathologic correlations in laryngeal carcinoma. In Alberti, P. W., and Bryce, D. P., Eds.: Workshops from the Centennial Conference on Laryngeal Cancer. Appleton-Century-Crofts, New York, 254.

215. Olofsson, J., Williams, G. T., Bryce, D. P., and Rider, W. D. 1972. Radiotherapy vs. conservation surgery in the treatment of selected supraglottic carcinomas. Archives of Otolaryngology, 95: 240.

216. Olofsson, J., Williams, G. T., Rider, W. D., and Bryce, D. P. 1972. Anterior commissure carcinoma. Primary treatment with radiotherapy in 57 patients. Archives of Otolaryngology, 95: 230.

217. Perez, C. A. Kraus, F. T., Evans, J. C., et al. 1966. Anaplastic transformation in verrucous carcinoma of the oral cavity after radiation therapy. Radiology, 86: 108.

218. Pietrantoni, L., Agazzi, C., and Fior, R. 1962. Indications for surgical treatment of cervical lymph nodes in cancer of the larynx and hypopharynx. Laryngoscope, 72: 1511.

219. Poncet, P. 1975. II. Total laryngectomy for salvage in cancers of the glottic region. Laryngoscope, 85: 1430.

220. Pressman, J. J., Simon, M. B., and Monell C. 1970. Anatomical studies related to the dissemination of cancer of the larynx. Transactions of the American Academy of Ophthalmology and Otolaryngology, 64: 628.

221. Probert, J.C., Thompson, R. W., and Bagshaw, M. A. 1974. Patterns of spread of distant metastases in head and neck cancer. Cancer, 33: 127.

222. Putney, F. J. 1958. Rehabilitation of the post laryngectomized patient; specific discussion of failures: Advanced and difficult technical problems. Annals of Otology, Rhinology and Laryngology, 67: 544.

223. Quinn, F.B., Jr, and McCabe, B.F. 1957. Laryngeal metastases from malignant tumors in distant organs. Annals of Otology, Rhinology and Laryngology, 66: 139.

224. Rabbett, W.F. 1965. Juvenile laryngeal papillomatosis: The relation of irradiation to malignant degeneration in this disease. Annals of Otology, Rhinology and Laryngology, 74: 1149.

225. Reddi, R. P., and Mercado, R., Jr. 1979. Low-dose preoperative radiation therapy in carcinoma of the supraglottic larynx. Radiology, 130: 469.

226. Rideout, D.F. 1976. Appearances of the larynx after radiation therapy. In Alberti, P.W., and Bryce, D. P., Eds.: Workshops from the Centennial Conference on Laryngeal Cancer. Appleton-Century-Crofts, New York, 266.

227. Rider, W. D. 1976. Toronto experience of verrucous carcinoma of the larynx. In Alberti, P. W., and Bryce, D. P., Eds.: Workshops from the Centennial Conference on Laryngeal Cancer. Appleton-Century-Crofts, New York, 460.

228. Rigby, R. G., and Holinger, P. H. 1943. Fibrosarcoma of the larynx in an infant. Archives of Otolaryngology, 37: 425.

229. Robbins, J. P., Marks, R. M., Fitz-Hugh, G. S., and Constable, W. C. 1972. Immediate complications of laryngectomy following high-dose preoperative radiotherapy. Cancer, 30: 91.

230. Ryan, R. F., McDonald, J. R., and Devin, K. D. 1955. The pathologic effects of smoking on the larynx. Archives of Pathology, 60: 472.

231. Rygard, J., and Hansen, H. S. 1976. Combined bleomycin and irradiation. In Alberti, P. W., and Bryce, D. P., Eds.: Workshops from the Centennial Conference on Laryngeal Cancer. Appleton-Century-Crofts, New York, 323.

232. Rygard, J., and Hansen, H. S. 1976. Use of chemotherapy—Bleomycin. In Alberti, P. W., and Bryce, D. P., Eds.: Workshops from the Centennial Conference on Laryngeal Cancer. Appleton-Century-Crofts, New York, 189.

233. Sekula, J., and Horzela, T. 1971. Studies on the cervical lymph nodes. Utilizing iodinated I 131 serum albumin in patients with carcinoma of the larynx. Archives of Otolaryngology, 94: 118.

234. Sessions, D. G., and Ogura, J. H. 1976. Classification of laryngeal cancer. In Alberti, P. W., and Bryce, D. P., Eds.: Workshops from the Centennial Conference on Laryngeal Cancer. Appleton-Century-Crofts, New York, 83.

235. Sessions, D. G., Maness, G. M., and McSwain, B. 1965. Laryngofissure in the treatment of carcinoma of the vocal cord: A report of forty cases and a review of the literature. Laryngoscope, 75: 490.

236. Sessions, D. G., Ogura, J. H., and Fried, M. P. 1975. Carcinoma of the subglottic area. Laryngoscope, 85: 1417.

237. Sessions, D. G., Ogura, J. H., and Fried, M. P. 1974. The anterior commissure in glottic carcinoma. Laryngoscope, 85: 1624.

238. Session, D. G., Ogura, J. H., and Fried, M. P. 1976. Laryngeal carcinoma involving anterior commissure and subglottis. In Alberti, P. W., and Bryce, D. P., Eds.: Workshops from the Centennial Conference on Laryngeal Cancer. Appleton-Century-Crofts, New York, 674.

239. Sessions, D. G., Murray, J. P., Bauer, W. C., and Ogura, J. H. 1976. Adenocarcinoma of the larynx. In Alberti, P. W., and Bryce, D. P., Eds.: Workshops from the Centennial Conference on Laryngeal Cancer, Appleton-Century-Crofts, New York, 475.

240. Shah, J. P., and Tollefsen, H. R. 1974. Epidermoid carcinoma of the supraglottic larynx. Role of neck dissection in initial surgical treatment. American Journal of Surgery, 128: 494.

241. Shaw, H. J. 1965. Glottic cancer of the larynx. 1947–1956. Journal of Laryngology and Otology, 79: 1.

242. Shedd, D., Bakamjian, V., Sako, K., Mann, M., Barba, S., and Schaaf, N. 1972.

Reed-fistula method of speech rehabilitation after laryngectomy. American Journal of Surgery, 124: 510.

243. Shedd, D., Bakamjian, V., Sako, K., Mann, M., Weinberg, B., and Schaaf, N. 1976. Further appraisal of Reed-fistula specific following pharyngolaryngectomy. In Alberti, P. W., and Bryce, D. P., Eds.: Workshops from the Centennial Conference on Laryngeal Cancer. Appleton-Century-Crofts, New York, 591.

244. Sherwin, R. P., Strong, M. S., and Vaughn, C. W., Jr. 1963. Polypoid and junctional squamous cell carcinoma of the tongue and larynx with spindle cell carcinoma ("pseudosarcoma"). Cancer, 16: 51.

245. Siirala, U., and Paavolainen, M. 1975. The problem of advanced supraglottic carcinoma. Laryngoscope, 85: 1633.

246. Silver, C., Liebert, P. S., and Som, M. L. 1967. Autologous transplantation of the canine larynx. Archives of Otolaryngology, 86: 95.

246a. Singer, M. I., and Blom, E. D. An endoscopic technique for restoration of voice after laryngectomy. Presented at annual meeting of the American Laryngological Association, West Palm Beach, Florida, April 15, 1980. Annals of Otology, Rhinology and Laryngology (in press).

247. Sisson, G. A. 1970. Mediastinal dissection for recurrent cancer after laryngectomy. Transactions of the American Academy of Ophthalmology and Otolaryngology, 74: 767.

248. Sisson, G. A., McConnel, F. M., and Logemann, J. A. 1976. Rehabilitation after laryngectomy with hypopharyngeal voice prosthesis. In Alberti, P. W., and Bryce, D. P., Eds.: Workshops from the Centennial Conference on Laryngeal Cancer. Appleton-Century-Crofts, New York, 596.

249. Skolnik, E. M., Yee, K. F., Wheatley, M. A., and Martin, L. O. 1975. V. Carcinoma of the laryngeal glottis: Therapy and end results. Laryngoscope, 85: 1453.

250. Skolnick, E. M., Martin, L. O., Wheatley, M. A., Yee, K. F., and Kotler, R. 1976. Combined therapy in the management of laryngeal carcinoma. In Alberti, P. W., and Bryce, D. P., Eds.: Workshops from the Centennial Conference on Laryngeal Cancer. Appleton-Century-Crofts, New York, 350.

251. Skolnick, E. M., Soboroff, B. J., Tenta, L. T., Saberman, M. N., and Jones, H. C. 1968. Preoperative radiation of head and neck cancer. Transactions of the American Academy of Ophthalmology and Otolaryngology, 72: 937.

252. Smith, R. R., Caulk, R., Frazell, E., Holinger, P. H., MacComb, W. S., Russell, W. O., Schulz, M. D., and Tucker, G. F. 1973. Revision of the clinical staging system for cancer of the larynx. Cancer, 31: 72.

253. Som, M. L. 1959. Surgical treatment of carcinoma of the epiglottis by lateral pharyngotomy. Transactions of the American Academy of Ophthalmology and Otolaryngology, 63: 28.

254. Som, M. L. 1970. Conservation surgery for carcinoma of the supraglottis, Journal of Laryngology and Otology, 84: 655.

255. Som, M. L. 1975. Cordal cancer with extension to vocal process. Laryngoscope, 85: 1298.

256. Som, M. L. 1976. Surgery in premalignant lesions. In Alberti, P. W., and Bryce, D. P., Eds.: Workshops from the Centennial Conference of Laryngeal Cancer. Appleton-Century-Crofts, New York, 145.

257. Som, M. L., and Silver, C. E. 1968. The anterior commissure technique of partial laryngectomy. Archives of Otolaryngology, 87: 138.

258. Sorenson, H. 1970. Transconioscopy in laryngeal carcinoma. Archives of Otolaryngology, 92: 28.

259. Southwick, H. W. 1973. Cancer of the larynx: Surgical management. Seventh National Cancer Conference Proceedings. J. B. Lippincott, Philadelphia, 155.

259a. Staffieri, M., and Serafini, I. 1976. La riabilitazione chirurgica della voce e della respirazione dopo laringectomia totale. Atti Del xxix Congresso Nazionale, Bologna, Italia, Sept. 1976.

260. Staley, C., and Herzon, F. S. 1970. Elective neck dissection in carcinoma of the larynx. Otolaryngologic Clinics of North America, 3: 543.

261. Stell, P. M. 1976. The subglottic space. In Alberti, P. W., and Bryce, D. P., Eds.: Workshops from the Centennial Conference on Laryngeal Cancer. Appleton-Century-Crofts, New York, 682.

262. Stell, P. M., and McGill, T. 1973. Asbestos and laryngeal carcinoma. Lancet, 2: · 416.

263. Stell, P. M., and Tobin, K. E. 1976. The behavior of cancer affecting the subglottic space. In Alberti, P. W., and Bryce, D. P., Eds.: Workshops from the Centennial Conference on Laryngeal Cancer. Appleton-

Century-Crofts, New York, 620.

264. Stell, P. M., and Van Den Broek, P. 1971. Stomal recurrence after laryngectomy: Aetiology and management. Journal of Laryngology and Otology, 85: 131.

265. Stell, P. M., Bickford, B. J., and Brown, G. A. 1970. Thoracotracheostomy after resection of the larynx and cervical trachea for cancer. Journal of Laryngology and Otology, 84: 1097.

266. Stewart, J. G., Brown, J. R., Palmer, M. K., and Cooper, A. 1975. VII. The management of glottic carcinoma by primary irradiation with surgery in reserve. Laryngoscope, 85: 1477.

267. Stocks, P. 1970. Cancer mortality in relation to national consumption of cigarettes, solid fuel, tea and coffee. British Journal of Cancer, 24: 215.

268. Strong, M. S. 1975. Laser excision of carcinoma of the larynx. Laryngoscope, 85: 1286.

269. Strong, M. S. 1976. Laser management of premalignant lesions of the larynx. In Alberti, P. W., and Bryce, D. P., Eds.: Workshops from the Centennial Conference on Laryngeal Cancer. Appleton-Century-Crofts, New York, 154.

270. Strong, M. S., Vaughan, C. W., and Incze, J. 1970. Toluidine blue in diagnosis of cancer of the larynx. Archives of Otolaryngology, 91: 515.

271. Stutsman, A. C., and McGavran, M. H. 1971. Ultraconservative management of superficially invasive epidermoid carcinoma of the true vocal cord. Annals of Otology, Rhinology and Laryngology, 80: 507.

272. Taskinen, P. J. 1975. The early case of supraglottic carcinoma. Laryngoscope, 85: 1643.

273. Taub, S. 1976. Air bypass voice prosthesis for vocal rehabilitation of laryngectomees. In Alberti, P. W., and Bryce, D. P., Eds.: Workshops from the Centennial Conference on Laryngeal Cancer. Appleton-Century-Crofts, New York, 587.

274. Taub, S., and Bergner, L. H. 1973. Air bypass voice prosthesis for vocal rehabilitation of laryngectomees. American Journal of Surgery, 125: 748.

275. Tegtmeyer, C. J., Smith, N. J., El-Mahdi, A. M., Fitz-Hugh, G. S., and Constable, W. C. 1976. The value of tantalum powder as a contrast medium in laryngography. In Alberti, P. W., and Bryce, D. P., Eds.: Work-

shops from the Centennial Conference on Laryngeal Cancer. Appleton-Century-Crofts, New York, 249.

276. Thomas, K. 1971. Mucoepidermoid carcinoma of the larynx. Journal of Laryngology and Otology, 85: 261.

277. Thomsen, J., Olsen, J., and Sorensen, H. 1976. Replica cytology in cancer of the larynx: An evaluation of a replica method in the diagnosis of laryngeal malignancy. Journal of Otolaryngology, (Toronto) 5: 403.

278. Till, J. E., Bruce, W. R., Elwan, A., Till, M. J., Niederer, J., Reid, J., Hawkins, N. V., and Rider, W. D. 1975. A preliminary analysis of end results for cancer of the larynx. Laryngoscope, 85: 259.

279. Toomey, J. M. 1967. Adenocarcinoma of the larynx. Laryngoscope, 77: 931.

280. Tucker, G. F., Jr. 1963. Some clinical inferences from the study of serial laryngeal sections. Laryngoscope, 73: 728.

281. Tucker, G. F., Jr. 1976. The anatomy of laryngeal cancer. In Alberti, P. W., and Bryce, D. P., Eds.: Workshops from the Centennial Conference on Laryngeal Cancer. Appleton-Century-Crofts, New York, 11.

282. Tucker, G. F., and Smith, H. R. 1962. A histological demonstration of the development of laryngeal connective tissue compartments. Transactions of the American Academy of Ophthalmology and Otolaryngology, 66: 308.

283. Tucker, G. F. Alonso, W. A., Tucker, J. A., Cowan, M., and Druck, N. 1973. The anterior commissure revisited. Annals of Otology, Rhinology and Laryngology, 82: 625.

284. Tucker, H. M. 1975. Laryngeal transplantation: Current status 1974. Laryngoscope, 85: 787.

285. Union Internationale Contre le Cancer, American Joint Committee on Cancer Staging and End Results Reporting. Supplement to TNM Classification of Malignant Tumors. Geneva, 1973.

286. Van Nostrand, A. W. P., and Olofsson, J. 1972. Verrucous carcinoma of the larynx. A clinical and pathologic study of 10 cases. Cancer, 30: 691.

287. Vega, M. F. 1975. Larynx reconstructive surgery—A study of three-year findings—A modified surgical technique. Laryngoscope, 85: 866.

288. Vermund, H. 1970. Role of radiotherapy in

cancer of the larynx as related to the TNM system of staging. A review. Cancer, 25: 485.

289. Wang, C. C. 1974. Treatment of glottic carcinoma by megavoltage radiation therapy and results. American Journal of Roentgenology, Radium Therapy and Nuclear Medicine, 120: 157.

290. Wang, C. C. 1978. Treatment of squamous cell carcinoma of the larynx by radiation. Radiologic Clinics of North America, 16: 209.

291. Wang, C. C., Schulz, M. D., and Miller, D. 1972. Combined radiation therapy and surgery for carcinoma of the supraglottic and pyriform sinus. American Journal of Surgery, 124: 551.

292. Welsh, L. W. 1964. The normal human laryngeal lymphatics. Annals of Otology, Rhinology and Laryngology, 73: 569.

293. Whicker, J. H., Carder, G. A., and Devine K. D. 1972. Metastasis to the larynx. Report of a case and review of literature. Archives of Otolaryngology, 96: 182.

294. Whicker, J. H., Neel, H. B., III, Weiland, L. H., and Devine, K. D. 1974. Adenocarcinoma of the larynx. Annals of Otology, Rhinology and Laryngology, 83: 487.

295. Wynder, E. L. 1975. Toward the prevention of laryngeal cancer. Laryngoscope, 85: 1190.

296. Wynder, E. L., Bross, I. J., and Day, E. 1956. Epidemiological approach to the etiology of cancer of the larynx. JAMA, 160: 1384.

19 | Tumors of the Cervical Trachea

Hermes C. Grillo, M.D.

INTRODUCTION

The rarity of primary tumors of the trachea, recently estimated in a circumscribed population to be 2.7 new cases per million per year,[28] explains the relatively small experience that has been accumulated even in major institutions. Fifty-three primary cancers of the trachea were reported over a 30-year period from the Mayo Clinic,[17] 41 over a 33-year period from the Memorial Hospital for Cancer and Allied Diseases in New York,[15] 37 primary tumors of the trachea from the Toronto General Hospital in a 20-year period,[25] and 28 resections for tracheal tumors from 12 French and 2 Soviet groups.[4] At the Massachusetts General Hospital, between the years 1940 and 1977, 90 patients have been seen with either benign or malignant primary tumors of the trachea.[12] Sixty-three of these have been seen in the last 15 years of that 37-year period—a reflection of my special interest in this subject.

There is a paucity of experience, both in the behavior of primary tracheal tumors and in their response to modern surgical treatment and radiotherapy. Only recently have techniques permitting resection with primary reconstruction of the trachea been developed. Only a small number of series involving cases[4, 12, 25, 27] surgically managed by these more radical techniques are available for study and these did not include long-term follow-up. A similar lack of prolonged follow-up is a problem in analyzing results of treatment with radical radiotherapy.[28]

The surgical approach to tumors involving the cervical trachea obviously differs from those of the more distal trachea and carina. There are also differences in the distribution of tumors between the upper and lower trachea, although differences in behavior of given pathologic types does not appear to depend upon location. Although this chapter is directed toward the special problems of the cervical trachea, generalizations must be made from the total experience with tracheal tumors. It is a fallacy in most cases to consider the treatment of the tumors of the cervical trachea apart from the general problem of tracheal management as a whole. This statement is supported by the surgical anatomy of the trachea, the pathologic occurrence and behavior of the tumors, and the surgical techniques which have been developed for their management.

SURGICAL ANATOMY OF THE TRACHEA

The trachea commences at the lower border of the cricoid cartilage where the uppermost tracheal cartilage is partly inset beneath the cricoid cartilage. It terminates where the lateral walls of the right and left main bronchi flair out from the lower trachea. The carinal spur is useful as a more definite landmark for the termination of the trachea, since it is clearly definable bronchoscopically and radiologically. The average adult human trachea measures 11 cm in length, varying roughly in proportion to the height of the patient.[14] There are approximately two tracheal cartilaginous rings per centimeter of the trachea, and thus, the total number of rings ranges from 18 to 22. It must be remembered that the subglottic laryngeal airway measures 1.5 to 2.0 cm in length before the trachea is reached. Except for some cases of congenital stenosis with circumferential rings of the trachea,[8] the only completely circular cartilage in the upper airway is the cricoid with its broad posterior plate.

The potential for presentation of the trachea in the neck is of critical importance not only from the standpoint of surgical access to the trachea, but also from the standpoint of the ease of reconstruction following the resection of any length of the trachea. In the young individual, particularly in the absence of obesity, hyperextension of the neck will deliver more than 50 percent of the trachea into the neck.[9, 16] In a kyphotic, aged person, particularly an obese one, the cricoid cartilage may be located at the level of the sternal notch and even the most vigorous hyperextension may fail to deliver any of the trachea into the neck. In both the young and aged, the anatomic position of the trachea changes from an essentially subcutaneous position at the cricoid level to a prevertebral position at the carinal level. The course is thus obliquely caudad and dorsal when the patient stands in the erect position. In the kyphotic, aged patient, lateral projection becomes increasingly hori-

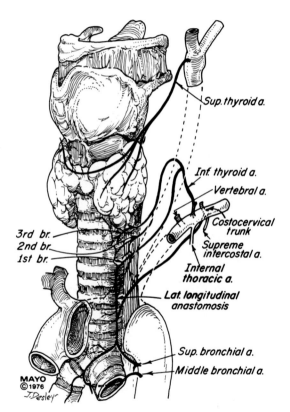

Fig. 19-1. Left anterior view of vessels supplying the trachea. In this specimen the lateral longitudinal anastomosis links branches of the inferior thyroid, costocervical trunk, and bronchial arteries. (Salassa, J. R., Pearson, B. W., and Payne, W. S. 1977. Growth and microscopical blood supply of the trachea. Annals of Thoracic Surgery, 24: 100–107.)

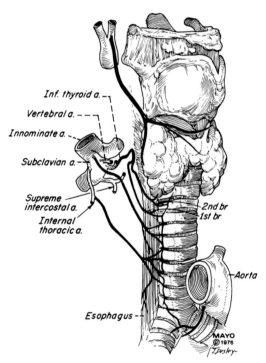

Fig. 19-2. Right anterior view of vessels supplying the trachea. In this specimen the lateral longitudinal anastomosis links branches from the inferior thyroid, the subclavian, the internal thoracic, and the superior bronchial arteries. (Salassa, J. R., Pearson, B. W., and Payne, W. S. 1977. Growth and microscopical blood supply of the trachea. Annals of Thoracic Surgery, 24: 100–107.)

zontal. The slight extensibility and flexibility of the trachea in youth diminishes with increasing age. Calcification of the cartilages also occurs with age and with injury.

The blood supply of the trachea is of special importance in resection and reconstruction of the trachea. The upper trachea is principally supplied by branches of the inferior thyroid artery.[21] The lower trachea is supplied by branches of the bronchial artery with contributions from the subclavian, supreme intercostal, internal thoracic, and innominate arteries[29] (Figs. 19-1 and 19-2). The vessels supply branches anteriorly to the trachea and posteriorly to the esophagus, arriving at the trachea through lateral pedicles of tissue. The longitudinal anastomoses between these vessels are very fine. Transverse intercartilaginous arteries branch ultimately into a submucosal capillary network (Fig. 19-3). Excessive division of the lateral tissues by circumferential dissection of the trachea can easily destroy this blood supply and thus lead to serious and sometimes disastrous complications.[10]

The relationship of the recurrent nerves to the trachea and the esophagus and the point of entry of these nerves into the larynx have been well described[14] and need not be repeated here. The close relationship of the trachea to the thyroid gland is similarly well known. The isthmus crosses the trachea at the second and third cartilaginous rings. Intimate adherence of the medial portions of both lobes of the thyroid to the trachea is observed at this same level laterally. Because of this intimate adherence, it may become necessary to remove a lobe or sometimes the entire thyroid gland when surgically managing a tumor in the upper

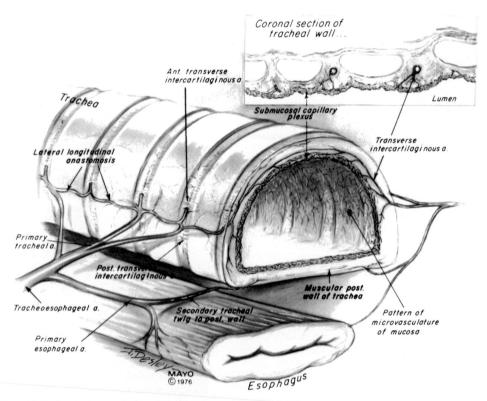

Fig. 19-3. Semischematic view of the tracheal microscopic blood supply. Transverse intercartilaginous arteries derived from the lateral longitudinal anastomosis penetrate the soft tissues between each cartilage to supply a rich vascular network beneath the endotracheal mucosa. (Salassa, J. R., Pearson, B. W., and Payne, W. S. 1977. Growth and microscopical blood supply of the trachea. Annals of Thoracic Surgery, 24:   100–107.)

trachea. Posteriorly, the esophagus has a common interface through areolar tissue with the membranous wall of the trachea. The blood supply of the esophagus and membranous tracheal wall are intimately linked. Anteriorly, the innominate artery courses obliquely across the anterior surface of the trachea; below this level the aorta arches backward across the left tracheo-bronchial angle where the left recurrent laryngeal nerve arrives at its place in the tracheoesophageal groove.

The lymph nodes adjacent to the trachea are stations in the pathways from the lungs and mediastinum and are well known to the surgeon who treats thoracic neoplasms. The lymphatics of the trachea have been less well studied. Gross observations of the clinical behavior of tumor metastatic from the trachea have been made. Metastases appear to involve the most closely adjacent groups of tracheal lymph nodes. Metastases to the nodes on the opposite side from where the primary tumor lies or to the carina from lower tracheal tumors are common. More remote metastases to scalene nodes or to other cervical nodes have not often been seen.

CLASSIFICATION OF TUMORS

Squamous cell carcinoma is the most common primary tumor of the trachea. Forty-two of the 90 patients in my series had this diagnosis[12] (see Table 19-1). Squamous carcinoma of the larynx, esophagus, and lung were not included in this series. Twenty-nine patients in this series had adenoid cystic carcinoma, which was formerly called by the mistakenly benign-sounding term of "cylindroma." Ten additional patients presented with various other malignant tumors including chondrosarcoma, carcinosarcoma, carcinoid tumor, spindle cell sarcoma, adenosquamous carcinoma, adenocarcinoma, and monocytic leukemia. Nine patients in this series had primary benign tumors including chondroma, chondroblastoma, squamous papilloma, granular cell tumor, hemangioma, and fibroma. Since the time of this report, I have also encountered mucoepidermoid carcinomas, plexiform neurofibroma, and a unique myxoid spindle cell sarcoma.

Other malignant tumors in the trachea have been reported, including small cell undifferentiated carcinoma, lymphoma, Hodgkin disease, plasma cell myeloma, and leiomyosarcoma.[2] As categories are subdivided, the numbers of cases become even smaller. Adenoid cystic carcinoma is relatively common in the trachea, but extremely rare in the main bronchi; while carcinoid tumors, which are found in the main bronchi and peripherally in lung, are extraordinarily rare in the trachea. I have seen three carcinoid tumors primary in the trachea and a fourth that was recurrent from a proximal main bronchial lesion.[1] Cartilaginous tumors, rare in the larynx, are even rarer in the trachea.[34]

TABLE 19-1. PRIMARY TRACHEAL TUMORS IN 90 PATIENTS[12]

Type	Number of Cases*
Malignant	
Squamous cell carcinoma	42
Adenoid cystic carcinoma	29
Carcinoid tumor	3
Carcinosarcoma	
Spindle cell sarcoma	
Myxoid spindle cell sarcoma	
Adenosquamous carcinoma	
Adenocarcinoma	
Mucoepidermoid carcinoma	
Chondrosarcoma	
Monocytic leukemia	
Benign	9
Chondroma	
Chondroblastoma	
Granular cell tumor	
Squamous papilloma	
Hemangioma	
Fibroma	

*Numbers provided only for those diagnoses with 3 or more cases in this series.

The peak incidence of squamous carcinoma of the trachea is between 50 and 60 years of age, while the incidence of adenoid cystic carcinoma is approximately a decade earlier. In the pediatric age group, the most common tumors of the trachea are squamous cell papilloma, hemangioma, and fibroma.[6] Preceding or subsequent primary neoplasms in respiratory and digestive tracts appear to be quite common with tracheal carcinoma.[15]

No definitive statement about the patterns of distribution of each of these types of tumors in the trachea can be made from available data. In my series, 10 patients with squamous cell carcinoma were treated by resection: two had tumors in the upper half of the trachea, one exactly in the midtrachea, five in the lower trachea, and two involving the carina. Of the nine patients with adenoid cystic carcinoma treated by resection and primary reconstruction, two had tumors in the cervical trachea, one in the lower trachea, and six at the carina with varying extensions to right or left main bronchi. In two of these cases, additional adenoid cystic carcinomas invaded the lower portion of the larynx as well. Of the group of 12 patients with miscellaneous tumors, 5 presented with lesions in the upper trachea; this group of lesions consisted of chondroma, low-grade chondrosarcoma, spindle cell tumor, granular cell tumor, and an unusual malignant lesion that contained both adenoid, squamous, and papillary components and further involved the larynx extensively. Tumors found in the lower trachea of 5 other patients in the group of 12 were two carcinoids, one squamous papilloma, one carcinosarcoma, and one chondroblastoma (essentially in midtrachea). In two cases, tumors were found at the carina: one was a highly malignant and invasive carcinoid; the other a myxoid spindle cell sarcoma. One patient with granular cell tumor in the upper trachea had a second tumor of the same type in the bronchus intermedius.

Neoplasms may also involve the trachea secondarily. Carcinomas of the esophagus, thyroid, lung, and larynx have a propensity for invasion of the trachea; carcinoma from the lung usually represents direct extension upward from a proximal main bronchial lesion. It is also not uncommon, particularly in undifferentiated lesions such as "oat-cell" carcinoma, to have invasion of the trachea from metastatic lymph nodes in the paratracheal region. Carcinoma of the esophagus may invade at any point from the postcricoid level to the carina. Fistulization from either spontaneous necrosis of esophageal tumor or following irradiation is a well known and often disastrous complication. A variety of types of thyroid cancer may invade the trachea, sometimes presenting with hemoptysis. In my experience, when the trachea was involved by primary carcinoma of the thyroid a secondary tumor more often represents a recurrence following incomplete surgical removal of the primary tumor. Tracheal invasion by thyroid carcinoma has been seen with papillary adenocarcinoma, follicular adenocarcinoma, mixed patterns, giant cell carcinoma, and carcinosarcoma.[11, 18] Direct extension of subglottic laryngeal carcinoma into the trachea has been often noted. The apparent recurrence of carcinoma at the tracheal stoma following laryngectomy may well derive from involvement of paratracheal lymphatics rather than from implantation at the time of tracheotomy as has been suggested. Attempts at extirpation by further surgical resection of the trachea in such cases often fail.

Primary *squamous cell cancer* of the trachea may present as an exophytic lesion that is quite circumscribed or as a spreading lesion involving a considerable length of trachea. It may also present as an apparently discontinuous lesion at several points in the trachea. Ulcerative presentation also occurs. The tumor may grow into the mediastinum and may be noted radiographically as a bulky extratracheal mass. Metastases to paratracheal and subcarinal lymph nodes and direct invasion of mediastinal structures may also occur. Over the last 15 years, one-half of my patients who had a squamous cell carcinoma primary in the trachea were deemed to be beyond the bounds of segmental or radical extirpation.

Adenoid cystic carcinoma may present as an exophytic lesion, often with poorly defined margins. A bulky extratracheal mass may often be demonstrated. At exploration, the tumor mass is often found to have compressed and displaced adjacent structures within the mediastinum rather than to have invaded them directly. In the cervical trachea, however, direct invasion of the thyroid gland does occur. The esophagus may be invaded. Although lymph nodes immediately adjacent to the trachea may be involved by metastatic tumor in adenoid cystic carcinoma, this is much less common than it is for squamous cell carcinoma. There is apparently a wide variation in the metastatic potential of adenoid cystic carcinoma. Marked characteristics of this neoplasm are submucosal extension and perineural invasion over long distances. The submucosal extent is often not visible to the naked eye even after transection of the trachea. Frozen-section control during surgery therefore becomes vital, and the extent of the tumor may present the surgeon with an enormous problem that was not predictable preoperatively. If the lesion is located in the upper trachea, the larynx may have been invaded. Multiple pulmonary metastases are not uncommon. Such metastases may not become apparent for years and may not even be symptomatic when discovered. Metastases to bone, brain, and other organs also occur in cases of the more aggressive tumors.

The paucity of experience with other tumors makes it difficult to predict their biologic behavior. This very lack of information may, however, justify the aggressive surgical approach. My study of the information available in the literature demonstrated that a few patients who reported with carcinosarcoma of the trachea had died of strangulation obstruction without evidence of distant metastases or invasion of the mediastinum. My only patient with this tumor was therefore treated by radical surgery and has had no recurrence after many years.

EVALUATION OF PATIENTS

The symptoms of tracheal tumor, even when there is already a high degree of airway obstruction, may be insidious. The order of frequency of symptoms in the series of Weber and myself was dyspnea, hemoptysis, cough, wheezing, dysphagia, change in voice or hoarseness, stridor, and pneumonia[33] (Table 19-2). Most often there is a history of slowly progressive dyspnea on exertion. All too often the patient who has simply developed shortness of breath and wheezing has an apparently normal chest roentgenogram and is diagnosed as suffering from adult-onset asthma. Some patients have been treated with steroids for long periods of time prior to the recognition of a slowly growing tumor. One patient could only breathe while sitting upright in bed and could barely gasp a few words at a time; her symptoms had been present for $2^1/_2$ years and were due to a slowly growing adenoid cystic carcinoma. Many patients will produce hemoptysis from malignant neoplasms. This often leads to appropriate bronchoscopic diagnosis. An irritative cough that

TABLE 19-2. SYMPTOMS OF TRACHEAL TUMORS IN 84 PATIENTS

Symptom	Number of Cases
Dyspnea	44
Hemoptysis	28
Cough	22
Wheeze	16
Dysphagia	13
Change in voice, hoarseness	13*
Stridor	12
Pneumonia	10

*8 of 13 had vocal cord paralysis.
(Based on data from Weber, A. L., and Grillo, H. C. 1978. Tracheal tumors: A radiological, clinical, and pathological evaluation of 84 cases. Radiologic Clinics of North America, 16: 227.)

may or may not be productive and that in time may be associated with hemoptysis is frequently seen. Involvement of one of the recurrent nerves leads to hoarseness, which may also be insidious in its onset. Stridor may be detected later in the course of the disease. Forced inspiration or expiration with mouth open will heighten the stridor. A few patients, particularly those with more distal tumors and carinal tumors, have presented with either unilateral or, occasionally, bilateral pneumonitis. This may resolve in response to antibiotics, only to recur later.

Diagnostic Studies

The presence of any of the above symptoms or signs without adequate explanation is justification for simple but careful radiologic studies.[19, 22] These studies will define the presence and extent of tumor in almost every case. The use of an intratracheal contrast medium is generally unnecessary. I obtain the following studies: (1) preliminary chest x-rays (posteroanterior, lateral, and oblique) centered high enough to obtain good views of the trachea; (2) anteroposterior, overpenetrated, high kV view including the larynx and trachea to the carina; (3) lateral view of the neck in extension with swallowing to elevate the upper trachea; (4) fluoroscopy of the larynx and trachea with necessary spot films and opacification of the esophagus with barium; and (5) anteroposterior, lateral, and oblique linear laminography of the trachea, if necessary, following the prior views.

The overpenetrated view is often the most useful view for obtaining a general picture of the extent of the tumor and its involvement of the trachea, its extension into the mediastinum, and its relationship to the normal portions of the airway. The fluoroscopic views provide information on the involvement of the recurrent laryngeal nerves, any variability in the airway, and, also, involvement of the esophagus. Laminography may give additional precise information about invasion of tracheal and laryngeal walls and the extent of mediastinal and

carinal involvement. Some patients may be nearly obstructed and thus, the use of even a topical anesthesia and liquid contrast media may be contraindicated. While insufflated tantalum studies may have usefulness, in general the quality of the information obtained from the simple x-ray studies described is such that no further data are required in order to plan the next diagnostic and therapeutic steps. Xerography studies provide very much the same information that x-ray studies do, but the former are often dramatic in quality. If there is a question of involvement of the superior vena cava, innominate artery, or pulmonary arteries, angiography occasionally becomes helpful. Computed tomography has thus far added little additional information to the examination of the trachea.[22]

Functional studies have been of limited usefulness, although of considerable theoretic importance.[20] Changes in peak flow rates and flow volume loops and the description of the physiology by flow volume loop has in a few cases called attention to the presence of an obstructing lesion when clinical signs had been overlooked.[31] Pulmonary function studies may also give some information about the status of the parenchyma distal to the upper airway obstruction. This is rarely of crucial importance, since an obstructing airway lesion requires treatment almost regardless of the state of the lungs. It may, however, have importance in deciding upon what magnitude of surgical procedure can be tolerated, particularly if the operation is to be an intrathoracic procedure for a tumor of the lower trachea or carina.

Endoscopy is required at some point during evaluation of the patient. The use of a flexible bronchoscope to make the initial diagnosis in patients who present with obscure symptoms is certainly to be praised. The usual precautions against hypoxia are, of course, essential, and no effort should be made to instrument or pass beyond a tumor if there is a high degree of obstruction and if preparations have not been made to proceed directly with surgery. I prefer, usually, to obtain radiologic definition of a mass and to reserve endoscopy for the time of definitive therapy when a tumor appears to be surgically treatable. Separate endoscopy is more often utilized in cases in which it is probable that the tumor is not resectable. If endoscopy is to be performed at the time of a proposed surgical intervention, adequate facilities for dependable frozen sections must be available because resection of tracheal tumors should not be performed without accurate diagnosis and meticulous control of the margins of resection.

If a tumor appears to be excessively vascular, it is wiser not to biopsy but to proceed with the necessary surgical exposure and obtain a histologic diagnosis later, when the field is under direct control. In a few cases it is better not to biopsy at all. For instance, one of my patients presented with a lesion that appeared to be a hemangioma. Following the direct examination, angiographic studies demonstrated a huge, presumably congenital, vascular malformation extending from the lower border of the larynx to the carina bilaterally with enormous feeding vessels. Only a small portion presented intratracheally as an apparently isolated tumor.

In general, the necessity to establish an airway by removal of bits of tumor or to obtain more adequate biopsy for diagnosis by frozen section justifies the use of rigid bronchoscopes (with appropriate magnifying telescopes) in preference to the flexible instrument. The flexible bronchoscope has particular use for passing beyond the margin of an obstructing tumor at the carinal level to obtain biopsies distal to the gross lower limits of an adenoid cystic carcinoma. In such cases I have obtained positive biopsies as far as the upper lobes bilaterally, indicating surgical unresectability. Esophagoscopy is also done if the prior barium esophagogram suggests involvement.

If the radiologic identification of a tumor has been made, it is far better not to proceed too far with endoscopic diagnostic studies if the institution where the diagnosis has been made is not prepared to do adequate surgery. Certainly, emergency tracheostomies and other interferences with the surgical field should be avoided if possible.

I prefer to use the rigid bronchoscope to study these tumors. The patient is usually examined under general anesthesia after a slow and careful induction with halothane.[5] The surgeon is at hand when anesthesia is induced, since patients with high degrees of obstruction may become more severely obstructed even with a careful induction. Pediatric bronchoscopes are available as well as the larger adult sizes. A smaller bronchoscope can usually be insinuated past a tumor if an emergency arises. In most cases there is an uninvolved portion of the tracheal wall that permits this to be done. Only rarely is there complete circumferential involvement. In such a case one must be prepared to use the small bronchoscopes serially as dilators until a more adequate airway can be established; if necessary, bits of tumor can be removed with the biopsy forceps through the larger bronchoscope in order to establish the airway.

Staging

No formal TNM system has evolved for tracheal carcinoma yet, so none will be presented here.

SELECTION OF TREATMENT

Localized Tumors

At present there is no question but that the best treatment for a benign tumor of the trachea is its complete surgical extirpation with primary end-to-end reconstruction.[4, 12, 27] This is almost always feasible in benign lesions even if they are relatively extensive. Complete removal, usually by circumferential segmental resection, must be emphasized. Lateral resection is rarely acceptable. Repair following lateral resection, which cannot be closed primarily without distortion, demands patches and is often complex. This leads to cicatricial healing, and there is a greater danger of postoperative leakage and sepsis. Removal is less often complete, and recurrence follows.

The same rationale applies to the management of low-grade malignant tumors of the trachea. Segmental resection and reconstruction done in a single stage appears to offer the best chance for cure or extended palliation for both squamous cell carcinoma and adenoid cystic carcinoma of the trachea. Presently, available data suggest that cure is indeed possible when complete surgical extirpation has been accomplished. Few true cures have been demonstrated by radiation therapy alone. Although the advisability of adding either preoperative or postoperative irradiation is not yet statistically proven, early evidence indicates its usefulness.[12, 26]

Tracheal resection and reconstruction in a single stage has limited application for tumors involving the trachea secondarily. However, when the tumor is localized and when the primary lesion was of low-grade malignancy as in papillary and certain follicular carcinomas of the thyroid, tracheal resection may lead either to cure or long-term palliation. Many of these tumors respond poorly to irradiation, and surgical resection therefore certainly offers the best hope for cure to the patient.[12, 18] Occasionally in other tumors (neoplasm of the esophagus or lung) with apparent localization but with involvement of the trachea, carefully planned palliative resection also appears to be indicated.

Primary resection of adenoid cystic carcinoma of the trachea that seems locally curable by resection may sometimes be justified in a patient who has pulmonary metastases. Many of these pulmonary metastases will grow very slowly over many years before becoming symptomatic. For this reason Eschapasse[4] proposed surgical treatment of these lesions.

Extensive Contained Disease

Involvement of the majority of the trachea by longitudinal extension of adenoid cystic carcinoma creates a special problem. At the present time we assume that surgical extir-

pation of the primary tumor, it if can be done completely, is the best method of treatment—with or without preoperative or postoperative irradiation. The limited statistics available[12, 26] support the validity of this approach, although there have been voices raised in favor of irradiation alone.[28] Modern techniques of resection with primary reconstruction using the patient's own tissues do not usually allow for removal of more than approximately one-half of the trachea, although greater lengths have indeed been resected in individual cases. For cases involving more than one-half of the trachea, either a complex staged reconstruction or the insertion of a prosthesis must be used. Such methods carry a high incidence of major complications. Each case must be carefully evaluated with consideration of the extent of the disease, the potential for cure, the magnitude and complexity of the reconstruction, the actual experience that is available with each of these techniques, and the experience of the team providing the treatment. When primary reconstruction is not feasible, it may well be better judgment—for the present time—to apply "curative" doses of radiotherapy to achieve prolonged palliation. If the larynx is also involved, resection with mediastinal tracheostomy becomes acceptable.[8]

Advanced, Invasive Disease

In a 15-year period a group of 27 patients with primary squamous cell carcinoma of the trachea were seen. Thirteen were treated by attempts at surgical extirpation, and 14 were considered to be beyond the bounds of surgery, except for tracheostomy in some cases.[12] The decision against surgery was based in most cases upon identification of tumor involving very long segments of trachea or carina (50 to 60 percent and over), extension into the mediastinum (determined radiologically), or extension involving the main bronchi. The patients with unresectable tumor were treated with irradiation. In a few cases, tumor was cored out through the rigid bronchoscope to provide an adequate airway. Bleeding is usually not excessive. Other physical modalities of tissue destruction such as cryoprobes, electrocoagulation, and laser beams can be similarly utilized with the same net effect.

These considerations apply particularly in tumors of the lower trachea where simple tracheostomy will not solve the problem even if a long tube is placed. If massive tumor is present in the upper trachea, an alternative is to insert a tracheostomy tube and if necessary to core out tumor so that the tube passes into normal trachea. Radiation can then be administered with the tube in place. Earlier in my experience, several patients were subjected to mediastinal tracheostomy distal to an obstructing tumor of the upper trachea. Such an extensive procedure is unjustified in view of the final expectations. Distant metastases may occur to any of the usual sites where carcinoma of the lung metastasizes. For the most part, in these cases death resulted from extension of local disease.

During this same 15-year period, 22 patients were seen with adenoid cystic carcinoma. Sixteen were subjected to attempts at surgical extirpation, but only 6 were treated primarily with radiotherapy. In two cases, the exploration showed such extensive disease that removal was impossible. Two other patients had undergone extensive radiotherapy previously (5 and 7 years) and developed local recurrence at the site of the original tumor. Further radiotherapy was deemed to be impossible in these patients and surgery could not be done for fear of inadequate healing.

Both of the most common types of carcinoma of the trachea, namely squamous and adenoid cystic, are generally responsive to irradiation. Recurrence occurs earlier in squamous lesions, whereas very prolonged palliation may be obtained from full dose irradiation of adenoid cystic carcinoma. When squamous cell carcinoma massively involves the mediastinum, little palliation can be expected. Most of the other types of primary tumors of the trachea, whether of low-grade malignancy or benign, produce symptoms of airway obstruction before there is a massive bulk of tumor or mediastinal invasion. When carcinoma of lung or esophagus involves the trachea extensively, little can be done therapeutically.

SURGICAL RECONSTRUCTION

There is usually only one good opportunity to extirpate a tracheal tumor and that is at the initial operation. The responsibility lies with the principal surgeon to make provision at that sitting for adequate resection and reconstruction. If he has any question about his abilities to handle one or another aspect of the surgery, he should obtain adequate help in advance of the operating date or, more appropriately, should refer the patient to a center where such surgery is done more frequently. For the surgeon to use staged reconstruction to restore a large gap in the upper trachea simply because he is not prepared to extend his field into the mediastinum is unacceptable.

The surgeon embarking upon the treatment of a tracheal tumor should have at his command a full understanding of the techniques of management of the entire upper airway. His knowledge should include familiarity with the larynx, the techniques of laryngeal release, the methods of obtaining a tensionless anastomosis following resection of the cervical trachea, and the techniques of extension of the exposure (even when this has not been anticipated preoperatively) to include the mediastinal trachea. He should also have the foresight to be prepared for intrathoracic extension if necessary for carinal mobilization. The special knowledge of the tracheal blood supply, the intimate course of the recurrent laryngeal nerves, and the acceptable types of repair must clearly be available to the surgeon and be the product of careful study prior to undertaking such a reconstruction. Over the years I have seen far too many patients condemned to multiple attempts at surgical correction of unnecessary complications of inadequate surgery for tumors that could have been removed effectively at an initial procedure.

Circumferential Resection and Reconstruction

In this section I shall deal with resection and reconstruction of the upper trachea, but the reader should keep in mind constantly that this is a thoroughly artificial division of a single field of expertise—tracheal surgery. The operations are carried out under spontaneous or assisted ventilation, without respiratory paralysis.[5] A cardiopulmonary bypass procedure is unnecessary even for relatively complex reconstructions of the cervical or intrathoracic trachea or carina. If a carinal reconstruction is so complicated by other attendant problems that a bypass procedure appears indicated, the very manipulation that has to be done under heparinization will lead to potentially lethal parenchymal hemorrhage. Occasionally, a bypass procedure is required for a *portion* of an operation when, for example, partial resection or reconstruction of the pulmonary artery is required; but the bypass would not be required for the *entire* operation.

The use of the initial diagnostic endoscopy has already been discussed. Intubation can usually be accomplished around the tumor even if there is a high degree of obstruction. It is rare to have a circumferential tumor that does not leave some portion of tracheal wall uninvolved against which a tube may be insinuated. The anesthetist should also examine the airway through the bronchoscope after the surgeon has inserted it so that he will know what size tube to select and how to direct it. In the initial phases, if necessary, a bronchoscope may be passed beyond the tumor until anesthesia is deepened.

The usual initial approach for tumors in the upper half of the trachea is through an anterior collar incision placed low on the neck for cosmetic reasons. The patient is usually positioned supine on the table with an inflatable bag beneath the shoulders so that the neck may be easily and reversibly hyperextended during the operation. The field must include the entire area from the chin to the xyphoid, to permit partial median sternotomy if required. If further intrathoracic extension is necessary beyond a mediastinal extension, the patient is tilted on the table so that the right hemithorax is available. The right arm is abducted at the shoulder with elbow flexed so that the field may extend to the posterior axillary line. Lateral tilting of the table restores the patient to the horizontal position while maintaining a potential for intrathoracic extension. A totally different position is used when the entire trachea must be approached but with emphasis on the lower or carinal portion.[9]

A bronchoscopic biopsy is submitted for frozen section if histologic definition of the lesion has not been obtained previously. The biopsy is omitted only if there appears to be significant danger of unusual hemorrhage. Flaps of skin and platysma are elevated to a point above the cricoid cartilage and below the sternal notch. Unless the tumor is primarily of the thyroid or is of unusual magnitude, the strap muscles are not excised with the specimen but are elevated after opening the midline fascia. If there is any question of invasion, the strap muscles are appropriately detached and removed with the tumor mass. If the tumor is largely intraluminal, a pretracheal plane is established, with the surgeon taking care not to approach a presenting surface of tumor too closely. If the tumor is malignant or of questionable malignancy and has invaded the tracheal wall, an entire lobe or a portion of a lobe of the thyroid gland is also excised to provide a margin beyond the tumor. It has usually been unnecessary to remove the entire thyroid gland, except in primary thyroid malignancy and in massively invasive adenoid cystic carcinoma of the upper trachea. In most cases a pretracheal plane is established all the way to the carina even in the case of upper tracheal tumors. This adds a certain mobility to the lower trachea for the reconstruction after resection. Exposure of the innominate artery is avoided by keeping the dissection close to the trachea. However, if there is tumor at this level it is necessary to dissect closer to the innominate artery. This dissection is not as hazardous for a tumor as it is for postinflammatory strictures since the artery is not itself pathologically damaged.

If dissection becomes difficult because of inadequate transcervical exposure, the incision is extended vertically from the midpoint of the collar incision downward over the sternum to a point 1 or 2 cm below the sternal angle. If wider access to the upper mediastinum is necessary, the sternum may be divided either with the Lebsche knife or power saw. Division of the entire sternum is not necessary, since the trachea terminates at the level of the sternal angle; and moreover, such division may be hazardous, since the great vessels and the heart are immediately beneath the sternum anteriorly at this level. The pleural space is not opened unless there is a special indication.

The amount of paratracheal tissue, including paratracheal lymph nodes, that needs to be excised varies with the pathology. A compromise must be made between leaving behind paratracheal tissue that may contain positive lymph nodes and avoiding devascularization of the trachea. Isolation of the portion of the trachea containing the tumor is begun on the side of the trachea away from the tumor. An effort is made to include appropriate lymph node masses. For example, with a thyroid neoplasm, the inferior thyroid lymph nodes in the "V" between the innominate and the left common carotid arteries are included with the specimen. The recurrent nerves are usually isolated and carefully dissected at a point inferior to the tumor. The nerves are spared if possible, but they may need to be sacrificed deliberately if the tumor clearly involves a nerve at a higher level; this method of nerve dissection is very much in contrast to the techniques used in dissection of a benign stricture.

The esophagus is most often left intact, but sometimes a full-thickness segment of the anterolateral wall of the esophagus must be excised; in other cases, however, just the muscularis is removed. If only a portion of the wall is removed either in depth or circumferentially, the esophagus is reconstructed with double layers of fine interrupted sutures as a narrowed tube. The tube serves as a duct for salivary secretions and for alimentation, and it often dilates in time without requiring additional reconstruction. If a segment must be excised, it is usually predictable in advance; and appropriate preparation is made for advancement of a substernal colon bypass at this initial procedure. This situation is quite uncommon with esophageal cancer but does occur at times with thyroid carcinoma.

In tumors of the upper half of the trachea, the trachea is dissected circumferentially inferior to the lowermost extent of the tumor. It is often possible to palpate the tumor extrinsically even if it has not invaded through the cartilage. Rarely is it difficult to define the limits of the tumor, but if so the patient can be rebronchoscoped during the operation and the level of gross tumor marked by the assistant with a fine suture in response to the indications of the bronchoscopist. Care is taken not to dissect the trachea circumferentially for any distance inferior to the point where the division will be made. While 1 or even 2 cm may be dissected circumferentially, further dissection may endanger the blood supply.

Midlateral traction sutures of 2-0 silk are placed through the full thickness of the tracheal wall approximately 2 cm distal to the expected point of transection. Preparations are made with sterile tubing for connecting to an endotracheal tube in the operative field. The trachea is opened on the side opposite the tumor to avoid cutting across tumor; and if it appears that the division will be at an appropriate level, the transection is completed. If the cut is too close to tumor, a second level is selected under direct vision. Following division of the trachea, the patient is intubated across the operative field with a flexible armored tube (Tovell) and then the operation is continued. An assistant usually exerts traction on the two tracheal-holding sutures and keeps the tube positioned with its cuff inflated so that blood and secretions will not run into the lungs and so that the tube will remain at an appropriate position in the trachea. The divided end of the trachea is carefully examined. It is grasped with forceps and held away from the esophagus. The distal tracheal wall is biopsied to be certain that it is free of microscopic tumor.

The proximal endotracheal tube is withdrawn above the level of transection. A catheter is sutured to the tip of the proximal endotracheal tube so that if the tube has to be withdrawn through the vocal cords, it can be easily brought back down again with the catheter acting as a guide. The proximal specimen is dissected upward, thus separating it from the esophagus. Transection proximal to the tumor specimen is done in the same manner as was the distal transection. Careful examination is made to see whether the tumor has been totally encompassed. Proximal lateral traction sutures are also placed, very often in the lateral margins of the larynx in cervical resections.

It is very difficult on initial bronchoscopy always to be certain that the proximal end of a superiorly situated tracheal tumor is not within the inferior portion of the larynx. It is also very difficult to be certain, particularly in adenoid cystic carcinoma, whether there is microscopic disease in the submucosa of the larynx. If preoperative examination and biopsies have not established such involvement, the full extent of disease must be established during operation. Patients with adenoid cystic carcinoma in the most superior aspect of the trachea must be warned in advance about the possibility of partial or complete laryngectomy.

It may be necessary to bevel the resection margin into the inferior aspect of the larynx, taking portions of the anterior and lateral and sometimes even posterior cricoid cartilage along with the overlying mucosa. The recurrent nerve may have to be sacrificed because of direct extension posterolaterally by tumor, even though preoperatively vocal cord function was not impaired. It is possible in some cases to salvage the nerve posteriorly, since only the mucosa and not the cartilage is involved with tumor. A nerve stimulator may help to determine whether the function of the vocal cord has been preserved in such exceedingly high resections. Improvisation may be necessary. For example, in one recent case of granular cell tumor it was necessary to resect mucosal and submucosal tissue posteriorly over the cricoid plate almost to the posterior commissure. The membranous wall of trachea was correspondingly tailored to provide a covering flap to restore this area in the reconstruction. If the anterior portion, or a lateral segment, of cricoid cartilage has been removed, the distal end of the trachea can be beveled so that it will fit into this otherwise atypical suture line. The anastomotic line, however, is kept as simple as possible to insure noncicatricial healing.

No matter how well planned and thorough the resection has been either the proximal or distal biopsies may show tumor still present in the resection margins. This occurs more frequently with adenoid cystic carcinoma than with squamous cell carcinoma. Additional segments of the trachea must be resected in such cases. This type of occurrence leads to difficulties for the occasional tracheal surgeon and for the tracheal surgeon who is restricted in his approach to cervical procedures only.

Following completion of resection, with proof of uninvolved margins, attention is turned to the reconstruction (Fig. 19-4). Simple traction by the surgeon and his assistant on the proximal and distal lateral-holding sutures, with the neck provisionally flexed, may demonstrate that the trachea will come together easily without excessive tension. Experimentally, a pull of 1,200 grams or more creates major risk of dehiscence in the adult. I have tried to use lesser tensions. Although measurements have been made, in practice I have made a qualitative judgment that leans to the side of less tension. The simplest way of relaxing tension is to flex the patient's neck so that the chin approaches the sternum. As the patient becomes older, more kyphotic, or far more obese, the length of resection increases and simple flexion will be insufficient. Only a limited amount of length can be gained distally. The arch of the aorta holds the lower trachea quite fixed by arching over the left main bronchus. Extension of blunt pretracheal dissection over the anterior surface of the right and left main bronchi will help a little. This dissection usually is carried only a short distance in order to avoid injury to the blood supply.

Laryngeal release may be necessary if tension is excessive during the tracheal reconstruction. A second short horizontal incision over the hyoid bone is preferred, since U-shaped flaps or lateral extensions of the collar incision provide less satisfactory cosmetic results. The field must be made continuous beneath the platysma from the lower to the upper incision. The thyrohyoid release described by Dedo and Fishman[3] was used earlier in this series, but this has been replaced with Montgomery's[23] suprahyoid release. Postoperative problems with swallowing have been minimal, aspiration rare, and recovery from minimal dysphagia very prompt with the latter procedure. Laryngeal release may provide 1 to 3 cm anteriorly where the maximum amount of relaxation is needed. In rare cases further maneuvers will be required, including entry into the thorax. For the latter situation the sternal incision is carried more distally and angled into the right fourth intercostal space. Mobilization of the inferior pulmonary ligament and the right hilum intrapericardially if need be, as described previously,[8] provides further upward mobility. Bronchial transplantation is only very rarely required to facilitate proximal tracheal resection.

Once it has been demonstrated that approximation may be obtained without excessive tension, the patient's neck is again extended and the anastomosis completed. The sutures are placed individually so that the knots will lie outside the lumen. Sutures are spaced approximately 4 mm from the cut margins of larynx or trachea and at 4 mm intervals. The posterior midline suture is placed first, clamping it and fixing it to the drapes. Successive sutures are serially positioned from the midline of the posterior trachea to a point just in front of the midlateral line on one side and then on the opposite side. Anterior sutures are placed thereafter. It is theoretically attractive to complete the posterior part of the anastomosis first. In cases of extensive resection, however, where acute flexion of the neck is necessary to obtain a tensionless anastomosis, the field will nearly "disappear" at this point. In general, it is best to place all sutures prior to tying any of them. Fine, strong suture material is selected. One must slide the posterior sutures by touch, since this portion of the anastomosis will not be visible. The sutures must not break while being tied, since the cervical flexion makes them irreplaceable. Currently I use 4-0 Vicryl, an absorbable polymer, in order to avoid postoperative suture line granulomas. It is satisfactory, although more difficult to use than nonabsorbable sutures such as Tevdek.

Once all the anastomotic sutures have been placed and carefully clipped to the drapes, the patient's neck is securely supported in flexion by the anesthetist. The tube across the operative field is removed and the one from above advanced, after the distal airway is carefully cleaned with suction. The lateral traction sutures are pulled together and tied by the surgeon and his assistant, approximating but not intussuscepting the tracheal ends. The anastomotic sutures are tied from front to back. The anastomosis is then tested under saline for air-tightness by deflating the cuff and applying high pressures through the endotracheal tube. If the thyroid isthmus is intact, it may be sutured back over a high anastomosis. Although it is not necessary to interpose a pedicled strap muscle between the innominate artery and the anastomosis, some surgeons may desire the added measure of security that this theoretically affords.

Suction drains are placed in the sub-

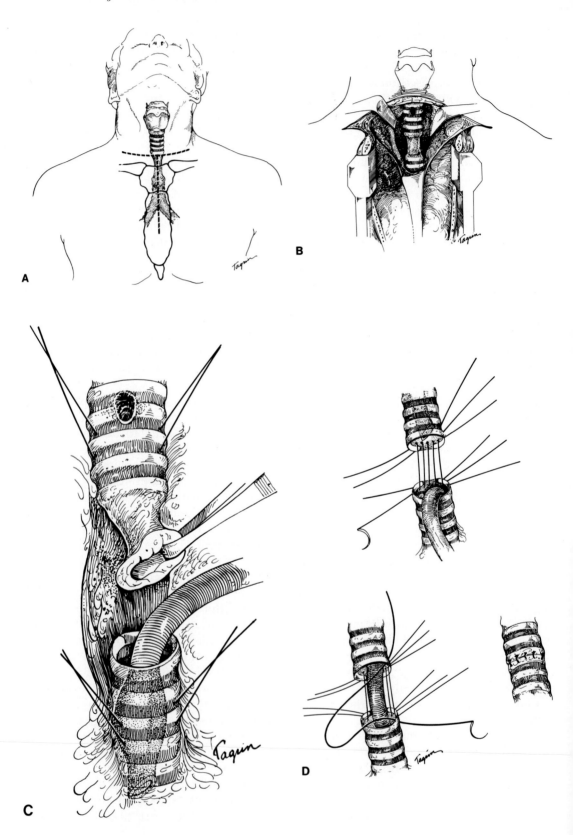

A

B

C

D

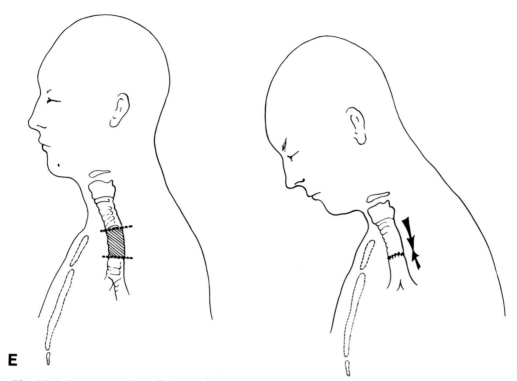

E

Fig. 19-4. Reconstruction of the upper trachea. (A) Collar incision and extension for upper sternotomy. Essentially all benign strictures as well as upper tracheal neoplasms may be most easily reconstructed through this approach. (B) Dissection is carried anteriorly to the level of the carina. Nothing is gained by dividing the innominate vein. The innominate artery may be gently retracted downward. The pleura is intact. (C) Circumferential dissection has been carried out only immediately beneath the lowermost level of the pathology. Traction sutures are in place and the patient has been intubated distal to the lesion. The lesion is now being retracted upward to facilitate dissection from the underlying esophagus. (D) Details of the anastomotic technique. The sutures are placed beginning posteriorly and working anteriorly. In recent years I have tended to place all the sutures prior to advancing the tube from above into the distal trachea. All the knots are on the outside. This diagrammatic representation must be recognized not to indicate complete circumferential dissection of the lengths of trachea shown. (E) This diagram indicates that the maximum amount of approximation is obtained by cervical flexion rather than by upward traction on the carina in the anterior approach. (Fig. 19-4 A–D reproduced with permission from Grillo, H. C. Surgery of the trachea. In Ravitch M. M., et al., Eds.: Current Problems in Surgery. Copyright © 1970 by Year Book Medical Publishers, Inc., Chicago. Fig. 19-4 E from Grillo, H. C. 1976. Congenital lesions, neoplasms and injuries of the trachea. In Sabiston, D. C., Jr, and Spencer, F. C., Eds.: Gibbon's Surgery of the Chest. 3rd edn. Saunders, Philadelphia, 256).

sternal and paratracheal areas. Closure is made by approximating sternum, strap muscles, and platysma serially. One or two heavy sutures are then placed from the crease just below the chin to the presternal skin to serve as guardian sutures in the postoperative phase, reminding the patient not to hyperextend his neck suddenly, either awake or asleep. This may seem brutal but, when explained in advance, is truly much kinder than splints, collars, braces, or straps.

The patients are allowed to wake up in the operating room, and they are extubated while still on the operating table. This allows the anesthetist and surgeon to be certain that the anastomosis is satisfactory. If it is not functional at this time, it is not likely to be so later on. Tracheostomy is rarely needed after tracheal reconstruction unless complex laryngeal repair has been concomitantly required. If a tracheostomy is necessary, the tube must not impinge upon either the suture line above or the innominate artery below. A centimeter and preferably more should remain between the suture line and the placement, through a tiny vertical incision, of a number 4 or 5 Jackson tube.

If there is a problem about the placement of such a tube because of the length of trachea resected, it is preferable to wall off both the tracheal incision and the innominate artery by thyroid and pedicled strap muscles. A tiny area of trachea is thus defined for later tracheostomy. A *small* endotracheal tube is passed through the vocal cords from above with a low-pressure cuff placed well away from the anastomosis and preferably not inflated. After several days this tube may be removed in the operating room under optimal conditions. If the patient still requires a temporary airway, a small tracheostomy tube may be inserted in the premarked and isolated area. Since by this time the anastomosis and the artery are sealed off, introduction of the tube may be made more safely. Under no circumstances is the tube ever placed through the anastomosis itself. In most cases, however, even if there is some airway compromise because of deliberate paralysis of a recurrent nerve or because of laryngeal repair, a careful regimen of fluid restriction and the use of racemic epinephrine, topical steroids, elevation of the head, and humidified oxygen will allow one to tide the patient over the first 4 to 6 difficult days until the edema subsides.

In 38 tracheal resections with end-to-end reconstruction done for both primary and secondary tumors, 15 tumors were of the upper trachea, 3 of the midtrachea, 9 of the lower trachea, and 11 of the carina. Five patients with upper tracheal tumors not of thyroid origin required hemithyroidectomy. In one of these cases, the recurrent nerve was deliberately sacrificed because it was invaded by tumor. Thyroidectomy was, of course, also done in patients with primary thyroid lesions, including sacrifice of a paralyzed nerve in one case and block removal of strap muscles in most cases.

Of the 15 patients with lesions in the upper trachea, all except two patients were operated on through the cervical approach alone. These two patients required a cervicomediastinal approach with partial division of the sternum and one required a transthoracic exposure for additional mobilization for reconstruction. Two of the three lesions in the middle trachea required cervicomediastinal exposure and one was done through a posterolateral thoracotomy.

Tumors of the lower trachea and carina were all approached transthoracically, sometimes with the use of a "trapdoor" incision or an adjunctive cervical incision for laryngeal release. The length of resection in the upper tracheal group varied from 3 to 4 cm, in the cervicomediastinal group from 2 to 6 cm, and in the transthoracic group from 2 to 7 cm. Carinal resections varied from 2 to 6 cm. Overall, primary resection required 0 to 2 cm in 5 patients, 2 to 4 cm in 20 patients and 4 to 7 cm in 7 patients.[12]

Of the 38 patients who have undergone reconstruction as described above, laryngeal release was required in only 4. It was not required in any of the cervical or cervicomediastinal groups. In only one patient in the entire upper tracheal tumor series was a lateral "window" resection possible. This patient had a tiny recurrence of papillary carcinoma of the thyroid. All of the others required circumferential resection with direct anastomosis.

Destructive Resection (Laryngotrachectomy)

In a small number of patients, an upper airway tumor will sufficiently invade and involve the larynx so that partial laryngectomy may not be effective and laryngotracheotomy is required. Even though it may not be possible to determine this until operation, the patient must be adequately prepared.

A permanent tracheostoma is created in the base of the neck. The problem is compounded if the tumor requires removal of a significant portion of trachea. In such a case, the distal trachea will not reach the base of the neck and excessive tension will develop. Mediastinal tracheostomy is indicated for such patients.

Techniques for mediastinal tracheostomy have failed often due to separation of the suture line with subsequent massive hemorrhage from erosion of the innominate artery or aortic arch.[30, 32] In an effort to avoid these problems, some years ago a technique was described[8] that consisted of removal of portions of the anterior bony chest wall to allow a full-thickness, well-vascularized bipedicled skin flap to be brought down to the stump of the trachea after fashioning a simple circular suture line. This technique was accomplished by extrapleural resection of the medial ends of the clavicles (resection of the upper sternum to a point below the sternal angle through the second interspace) and removal of the first and second costal cartilages on both sides. The procedure was done through a long horizontal incision at the base of the neck extending laterally over the upper borders of the clavicles and a second horizontal incision placed below this on the chest wall. The flap was elevated over the pectoral fascia, saving the lateral blood supply, and brought down into the mediastinum where it was sutured to the trachea at a midpoint opening of the latter. Full-thickness skin was advanced over the entire sternal defect by a third horizontal relaxing incision over the lower sternum. The resulting defect was closed by skin grafting. Initial success with this procedure was followed nonetheless by a number of cases in which separation occurred at the tracheocutaneous suture lines with subsequent hemorrhage. This occurred particularly in cases in which resection of the trachea had to be done a few centimeters from the carina. This technique is still in an evolutionary phase and attempts are being made to correct the separation-hemorrhage problem by angiographically and electroencephalographically monitored division of the in-nominate artery and by substernal advancement of pedicled omental grafts to protect the great arteries.

Even more difficult circumstances arise in some cases even when it is possible to extirpate a tumor by subtotal removal of the trachea, such as in the case of a submucosally infiltrating adenoid cystic carcinoma of the trachea that has not invaded mediastinal structures. The larynx may not be invaded, and there may or may not be involvement of recurrent laryngeal nerves. Following the resection, so little trachea remains and the gap is so great that no mobilization or laryngeal release can possibly bridge the defect. The alternatives in this situation are to avoid surgery altogether and use irradiation, to settle for a mediastinal tracheostomy with its attendant hazards, or to use a prosthesis.[24] The use of a prosthesis has known hazards of erosion of great vessels and granulation tissue obstruction. Staged reconstruction presents similar hazards. In a small number of cases, the technique of mediastinal tracheostomy by removal of portions of the sternum and the interposition of skin flaps has been carried out. At a later date the skin is inverted using specially devised subcutaneous plastic rings[7] to provide stability to the thus formed skin tube. Success has been obtained in several cases, but in an equal number of cases the procedure has been impossible to complete because of stenosis at the tracheocutaneous anastomosis or because of separation, sepsis, and fatal hemorrhage. At present there is no totally satisfactory solution for this rare type of tumor involvement. Over a period of 15 years during which the 38 reconstructions described were performed as well as number of laryngotracheotomies, approximately 10 patients were seen who appeared to be appropriate candidates for subtotal resection of the trachea with reconstruction. The problem merits continuing attention.

POSTOPERATIVE CARE

Throughout the performance of tracheal reconstruction careful attention is given to preventing blood and secretions from running into the tracheobronchial tree. This prevention is essential in order to avoid postoperative shunting and pneumonitis, which might require ventilation—a procedure extraordinarily hazardous to any recently complete tracheal reconstruction. One must not depend entirely upon an inflated cuff in the distal trachea to prevent intraoperative aspiration. Blood will pass between the interface of the cuff and the tracheal wall. An assistant must suction the area above the cuff continuously. Postoperatively, the patient maintains airway clearance by gentle coughing. He has been instructed preoperatively in the techniques of chest physiotherapy. If these techniques are inadequate, tracheal suctioning is done. The flexible bronchoscope is employed if tracheal suctioning fails to keep the airway clear. This scope can easily be passed with safety through the nose without disturbing the flexed position. Little difficulty in airway clearance has been encountered postoperatively in cases of reconstructions of the upper trachea. Most of the problems follow complex carinal reimplantations.

Cervical fixation with sutures is maintained empirically for one week postoperation. Following this period, the sutures are removed and the patient instructed not to extend the neck actively for one week further. After this second week, there is no need for further restriction. The larynx will remain in its devolved position with the trachea fixed by the carina at the aortic arch. Full extension of the neck is ultimately obtained, but the larynx always remains in the more caudad position. Occasionally, when the trachea has been markedly shortened the patient will have to swallow with his neck in the slightly flexed position.

COMPLICATIONS

Following the tracheal reconstructions in my series, particularly those of the upper trachea, there have been few early complications. Major problems have more often followed carinal reconstructions or laryngotracheal resections without restoration of continuity. Laryngeal edema has been mentioned and its management noted. This usually regresses within a week. Pneumonia has been extremely rare following the upper tracheal reconstructions because proper attention has been given to intraoperative management and to postoperative physiotherapy. All patients spend one or more days in a respiratory intensive care unit familiar with the management of such problems.

Suture line leakage has been extremely rare also. If an airtight anastomosis without tension has been achieved at the operating table, separation almost never occurs. Minimal air leakage at a suture line may occur, although this is also exceedingly rare. Minimal leakage can be managed through suction drains and will seal without further event. One patient with end-to-end anastomosis did develop leakage after an extended transthoracic resection in the lowermost trachea. This leakage ultimately healed with subsequent stenosis, which required reoperation. Problems following carinal reconstruction are not pertinent to this discussion.

Were tracheal separation to occur in the immediate postoperative phase, there would be reason to conclude that there had been a serious technical error. Reoperation might be considered even in the acute phase. If this happened following resection in the upper trachea, the simplest management might well be tracheostomy or insertion of a T-tube with corrective surgery after months of healing. Such separation has occurred in only one patient in my series (early in my experience) for whom the unfortunate decision was made to attempt resection for recurrent thyroid cancer 6 years after massive irradiation. Resection should not be tried under these circumstances.

Innominate artery hemorrhage has not occurred following tracheal resection for tumor and end-to-end anastomosis particularly above the carinal level. In fact this occurred in only one patient in over 200 cases for benign stenosis. Careful management of the artery as described should avoid this problem.

The most common later complication has been the formation of granulations at the suture line. This has been less of a problem in patients having resections for tumor than in patients who have had tracheal reconstructions for inflammatory disease, as residual inflammation may be present in such cases. Granulations may usually be managed by bronchoscopic removal under light anesthesia. Often a suture is found to have worked its way into the lumen at the base of the granulations. Removal of the suture leads to ultimate healing. In some cases multiple bronchoscopies are necessary over a period of time. Formation of granulations may be seen radiologically but is most often manifested by wheezing or minor hemoptysis. The patient must be warned in advance that this is not a cause for alarm or he will assume that he has recurrent tumor. Triamcinolone may be injected into the base of such granulations, but there is no clear evidence supporting its efficacy. Use of absorbable Vicryl sutures appears to prevent the problem.

Stenosis at the suture line has been seen following resection of benign strictures, particularly when a massive amount of inflammation has been present. Sometimes the formation of a ring of granulations will precede such re-stenosis. Stenosis has been rare following resection for tumors. Partial anastomotic stenosis occurred in one patient who was operated on for a tumor of the midtrachea while still on 50 mg per day of prednisone. He has a 30 percent cross sectional airway that may have to be corrected at a later date. It is my feeling that a partial separation occurred in this case because of the steroids. Operation was done at that time because of the patient's very marginal airway. Reoperation because of recurrent tracheal stenosis must always be done after a considerable interval to allow tracheal and paratracheal inflammation to subside.

The massive problems that can occur following low mediastinal tracheostomy or extended resections with either staged or prosthetic reconstruction have already been presented. The key problems are nonhealing, mediastinal sepsis and erosion of the major vessels deep in the mediastinum. With the use of prosthetics, the formation of granulations with obstruction and pulmonary sepsis are too common. Late hemorrhage from vascular erosion has complicated many attempts at prosthetic replacement of the trachea. This may occur even a year or more after placement of the prosthesis.

END RESULTS

From the foregoing it may be seen that we remain in a period of data gathering. There is not sufficient information available on which to base categorical statements about the ideal method of treatment of both primary and secondary tumors involving the trachea. The surgeon's goal is relief of airway obstruction and, if possible, the achievement of cure. With the relatively recent development, essentially in the last 17 years, of more dependable techniques for extended tracheal resection and reconstruction, it is now possible to approach many of these tumors more aggressively. In 1974 Eschapasse[4] published a collected series of 152 primary tracheal tumors treated by 14 groups of French and Russian surgeons. Thirty-two of the patients were treated by cylindrical resection and primary anastomosis and 18 of the patients received carinal reconstructions. Half of this group of resections (15 cylindrical and 10 carinal) were the work of Perelman.[27] The series of 152 cases also included 22 window resections. There were 18 early postoperative deaths in 162 operations. The greatest mortality was with squamous cell carcinoma. In the long term, the best results were with benign tumors, as might be expected, and with carcinoid tumors. Surgery for squamous cell carcinoma produced the worst results. Prolonged survival was achieved in treatment of adenoid cystic carcinoma but a considerable number of the late recurrences occurred.

Pearson et al.[26] reported a series of 16 patients with adenoid cystic carcinoma; 14 patients were treated by circumferential resection and 2 by lateral resection. While 6 patients were given prostheses and 3 were given laryngotrachectomies, only 5 were treated with primary anastomoses. Eight of the 16 were alive and well and apparently free of tumor 2 to 18 years postoperation. A limited series of resections were also reported by Houston et al.[17]

Up to 1977 our series[12] consisted of 36 patients with both primary and secondary tumors and listed 5 perioperative deaths. Only one death was in a patient who had a tumor of the upper trachea. This was the result of necrosis in a patient who underwent operative resection many years after high-dose irradiation of the trachea. Healing failed to occur. The other deaths were of patients with tumors of the distal trachea and more frequently of those with complex carinal reconstructions. Eight of the 31 surviving patients required one or more bronchoscopies for removal of granulations and sutures. Almost all of these patients had nonabsorbable suture material used for anastomosis. The development of stenosis following resection in a patient who was on high-dose steroids has already been mentioned. This was a midtracheal lesion. The only inadvertent nerve injury occurred in a patient who had an extensive lower mediastinal dissection in which the left recurrent nerve was injured.

Recurrence and survival rates of the entire group should be reviewed first, because of the small numbers of patients available (Table 19-3). Of the patients who had resection with primary reconstruction in the 15-year period between 1962 and 1977, there were 5 squamous cell carcinoma patients alive and without disease for periods ranging from 10 months to almost 14 years postoperation. Another patient was alive with disease at 1 year and 6 months. One had died without disease at 2 years, and another had died at 2 years and 8 months free from disease.

Of the group with adenoid cystic carcinoma, there were 6 patients surviving from 1 year and 3 months to over 15 years. There were 2 alive with disease, one at 1½ years and one at over 5½ years. No deaths have occurred in this group. The third group —7 patients with primary tumors, consisting of benign tumors and a small number of low-grade malignancies—were all alive at periods varying from over 1 year to over 15 years.

When we consider these limited results, supported by the findings of Eschapasse,[4] Perelman,[27] and Pearson,[26] we may conclude that tracheal resection with primary reconstruction is the method of choice for benign tumors of the trachea and for tumors of low-grade malignancy. We may also conclude that there is a great palliative value and very likely curative value in resection of adenoid cystic carcinoma. This is based on the fact that only one patient in our experience had ever achieved a cure or long survival in the period prior to radical resection. The group with squamous cell carcinoma, while carefully selected, is also doing quite well when compared with those who have squamous cell carcinoma of the lung or esophagus.

Only two of the small group of patients with secondary tumors operated upon in this series were alive without disease; one at 10 months and one at 4 years and 4 months. Five had died with disease after previous resections. However, the period of palliation ranged as follows: 6 months, 2 years, 3½ years, 6½ years, 8 years. This is a selected series, but it shows the value of palliative resection in secondary lesions.

Rostum and Morgan[28] reported a series of 44 patients with primary tumors of the trachea treated over a 25-year period primarily with irradiation. Thirty percent were alive and well (4.4 to 11 years) or had died of intercurrent disease (average of 4 years). This was a mixed group: 28 patients with squamous cell carcinoma; 3, adenoid cystic carcinoma; 4, adenocarcinoma; 3, oat cell carcinoma; 4, undifferentiated carcinoma; 1, Hodgkin disease; and 1, chondrosarcoma. A similar calculation in my series of patients

TABLE 19-3. RESULTS FROM PRIMARY RESECTION AND
ANASTOMOSIS OF TUMORS INVOLVING THE TRACHEA
(1962–1977)

Outcome	Squamous Cell Carcinoma	Adenoid Cystic Carcinoma	Other Tumors	Secondary Tumors
Postoperative deaths	2	1	1	1
Alive without disease	13 yr 7 mo 7 yr 7 mo 2 yr 5 mo 1 yr 11 mo 10 mo	15 yr 1 mo 7 yr 3 mo 5 yr 8 mo 4 yr 3 mo 1 yr 5 mo 1 yr 3 mo	15 yr 1 mo 8 yr 7 yr 3 mo 3 yr 6 mo 2 yr 9 mo 2 yr 5 mo 1 yr 10 mo 1 yr 1 mo	4 yr 4 mo 10 mo
Alive with disease	1 yr 6 mo	5 yr 8 mo 1 yr 6 mo	————	————
Dead without disease	2 yr	————	————	————
Dead with disease	2 yr 8 mo	————	————	8 yr 6 yr 6 mo 3 yr 6 mo 2 yr 6 mo

(Grillo, H. C. 1978. Tracheal tumors: Surgical management. Annals of Thoracic Surgery, 26: 112–125.)

with primary tumors (27 cases) revealed 19 alive and well or dead of other diseases at the end of a 15-year period, for a survival at that time of 70 percent. These are obviously noncomparable series both in composition and selection. However, in view of the number of patients whom I and others have seen with recurrent adenoid cystic carcinoma many years after full-course irradiation, it seems reasonable to propose resection, probably with adjuvant radiotherapy, as a more effective means of cure.

The 15 patients with upper tracheal and 3 with midtracheal tumors who underwent resection and end-to-end anastomosis are separately analyzed here. Of 3 with squamous cell carcinoma, one suffered recurrence extratracheally—presumably in a lymph node—over 2½ years after his resection and obtained a further period of pallia-

tion with radiotherapy prior to dying of his disease. The other two are alive and without disease at this time. Two with adenoid cystic carcinoma are alive without disease even though one patient required partial laryngeal resection and postoperative irradiation because of narrow margins. The six patients with other tumors—chondrosarcoma, chondroma, chondroblastoma, spindle cell tumor, carcinosarcoma, and granular cell tumor—are all alive and well although the patient with low-grade chondrosarcoma probably has subcutaneous metastases, for which he has refused excision or biopsy thus far. In addition, there was a group of 5 patients with thyroid lesions, one with a lung lesion apparently recurrent in high paratracheal lymph nodes and one with a localized lesion in the esophagus involving the trachea. Of those with thyroid lesions, one who had high-dose radiation years before a resection had been described as a failure of healing. A second patient achieved many years of palliation prior to dying of bony metastases. One died many years later without recurrent disease, and the other two are being followed presently without evidence of disease.

SUMMARY

The volume of data available on treatment of tumors involving the cervical trachea is such that categorical statements cannot be made. Available data do indicate clearly that benign primary tumors of the trachea and low-grade malignant tumors should be treated by resection and end-to-end single-stage reconstruction. The chances of excellent palliation and cure are high. Resection and reconstruction (when possible in a single stage) with the addition of postoperative irradiation appear to offer the best palliation and chance of cure for squamous cell carcinoma and adenoid cystic carcinoma of the trachea. Resection for secondary tumor with primary reconstruction may provide good palliation in carefully selected cases, chiefly in low-grade thyroid carcinoma. The necessity for considering the trachea as a single organ subject to a spectrum of surgical techniques rather than arbitrarily dividing it into the cervical and thoracic trachea is clearly evident.

REFERENCES

1. Briselli, M., Mark, G. J., and Grillo, H. C. 1978. Tracheal carcinoids. Cancer, 42: 2870.

2. Caldarola, V. T., Harrison, E. G., Jr., Clagett, O. T., and Schmidt, H. W. 1964. Benign tumors and tumorlike conditions of the trachea and bronchi. Annals of Otology, Rhinology, and Laryngology, 73: 1042.

3. Dedo, H. H., and Fishman, N. H. 1969. Laryngeal release and sleeve resection for tracheal stenosis. Annals of Otology, Rhinology, and Laryngology, 78: 285.

4. Eschapasse, H. 1974. Les tumeurs trachéales

primitives. Traitement chirurgical. Revue Française Maladies Resp., 2: 425.

5. Geffin, B., Bland, J., and Grillo, H. C. 1969. Anesthetic management of tracheal resection and reconstruction. Anesthesia and Analgesia (Cleveland), 48: 884.

6. Gilbert, J. G., Mazzarella, L. A., and Feit, L. J. 1953. Primary tracheal tumors in the infant and adult. Archives of Otolaryngology, 58: 1.

7. Grillo, H. C. 1965. Circumferential resection and reconstruction of mediastinal and cervical trachea. Annals of Surgery, 162: 374.

8. Grillo, H. C. 1966. Terminal or mural tracheostomy in the anterior mediastinum. Journal of Thoracic and Cardiovascular Surgery, 51: 422.

9. Grillo, H. C. 1976. Congenital lesions, neoplasms and injuries of the trachea, In Sabiston, D.C., Jr., and Spencer, F.C., Eds.: Gibbon's Surgery of the Chest, 3rd edn. W. B. Saunders, Philadelphia, 256.

10. Grillo, H. C. 1977. Tracheal blood supply. (editorial) Annals of Thoracic Surgery, 24: 99.

11. Grillo, H. C. 1977. Tracheal tumors. In Hardy, J. D., Ed.: Rhoads Textbook of Surgery: Principles and Practice. 5th edn. J. B. Lippincott, Philadelphia, 1364.

12. Grillo, H. C. 1978. Tracheal tumors: Surgical management. Annals of Thoracic Surgery, 26: 112.

13. Grillo, H. C.: Surgery of the Trachea. In Keen, G., Ed.: Operative Surgery and Management. John Wright, Bristol. (in press).

14. Grillo, H. C., Dignan, E. F., and Miura, T. 1964. Extensive resection and reconstruction of mediastinal trachea without prosthesis or graft: An anatomical study in man. Journal of Thoracic and Cardiovascular Surgery, 48: 741.

15. Hajdu, S. I., Huvos, A. G., Goodner, J. T., Foote, F. W., Jr., and Beattie, E. J., Jr. 1970. Carcinoma of the trachea. Clinicopathologic study of 41 cases. Cancer, 25: 1448.

16. Harris, R. S. 1959. The effect of extension of the head and neck upon the infrahyoid respiratory passage and the supraclavicular portion of the human trachea. Thorax, 14: 176.

17. Houston, H. E., Paynes, W. S., Harrison, E. G., Jr., and Olsen, A. M. 1969. Primary cancers of the trachea. Archives of Surgery, 99: 132.

18. Ishihara, T., Kikuchi, K., Ikeda, T., Inoue, H., Fukai, S., Ito, K., and Mimura, T. 1978.

Resection of thyroid carcinoma infiltrating the trachea. Thorax, 33: 378.

19. Janower, M. L., Grillo, H. C., MacMillan, A. S., Jr., and James, A. E., Jr. 1970. The radiological appearance of carcinoma of the trachea. Radiology, 96: 39.

20. Miller, R. D., and Hyatt, R. E. 1973. Evaluation of obstructing lesions of the trachea and larynx by flow-volume loops. American Review of Respiratory Disease, 108: 475.

21. Miura, T., and Grillo, H. C. 1966. The contribution of the inferior thyroid artery to the blood supply of the human trachea. Surgery, Gynecology, and Obstetrics, 123: 99.

22. Momose, K. J., and MacMillan, A. S., Jr. 1978. Roentgenologic investigations of the larynx and trachea. Radiologic Clinics of North America, 16: 321.

23. Montgomery, W. W. 1974. Suprahyoid release for tracheal anastomosis. Archives of Otolaryngology, 99: 255.

24. Neville, W. E., Bolanowski, P. J., and Soltanzadeh, H. 1976. Prosthetic reconstruction of the trachea and carina. Journal of Thoracic and Cardiovascular Surgery, 72: 525.

25. Pearson, F. G. 1974. Techniques in the surgery of the trachea. In Smith, R. E., and Williams, W. G., Eds.: Surgery of the Lung: The Coventry Conference. Proceedings of a conference held at the Postgraduate Medical Centre, Coventry, on 10th and 11th July, 1973. Butterworths; London, 91.

26. Pearson, F. G., Thompson, D. W., Weissberg, D., Simpson, W. J. K., and Kergin, F. G.

1974. Adenoid cystic carcinoma of the trachea. Experience with 16 patients managed by tracheal resection. Annals of Thoracic Surgery, 18: 16.

27. Perelman, M. I. 1976. Surgery of the Trachea. Mir, Moscow.

28. Rostom, A. Y., and Morgan, R. L. 1978. Results of treating primary tumours of the trachea by irradiation. Thorax, 33: 387.

29. Salassa, J. R., Pearson, B. W., and Payne, W. S. 1977. Gross and microscopical blood supply of the trachea. Annals of Thoracic Surgery, 24: 100.

30. Sisson, G. A., Straehley, C. J., Jr., and Johnson, N. E. 1962. Mediastinal dissection for recurrent cancer after laryngectomy. Laryngoscope, 72: 1064.

31. Strieder, D. J. 1975. Case records of the Massachusetts General Hospital, Case 42—1975. New England Journal of Medicine, 293: 866.

32. Waddell, W. R., and Cannon, B. 1959. A technic for subtotal excision of the trachea and establishment of a sternal tracheostomy. Annals of Surgery, 149: 1.

33. Weber, A. L., and Grillo, H. C. 1978. Tracheal tumor: Radiological, clinical and pathological evaluation. Advances in Otorhinolaryngology, 24: 170.

34. Weber, A. L., Shortsleeve, M., Goodman, M., Montgomery, W., and Grillo, H. C. 1978. Cartilaginous tumors of the larynx and trachea. Radiologic Clinics of North America, 16: 261.

20 | Cancer of the Salivary Glands

John Conley, M.D.
Daniel C. Baker, M.D.

INTRODUCTION

Although tumors of the salivary glands comprise less than 3 percent of all neoplasms in the head and neck region, they are of unusual interest and challenge to the surgeon because of their complex and varying array of histologic types and their regional anatomic relationships. The incidence is approximatley 1.5 to 2 per 100,000 population in the United States. The American Cancer Society reported nearly 650 deaths from salivary gland malignancies for the year 1977.[19]

The salivary glands are usually divided into two groups: the major salivary glands, which are the paired parotid, submandibular, and sublingual glands; and the minor salivary glands, which are located in the mucous membrane of the respiratory tract and upper digestive tract. The frequency of tumors occurring in the various glands is similar in most of the large series. Approxi-

TABLE 20-1. PERCENTAGE OF MALIGNANCY FOR 1,280 SALIVARY GLAND TUMORS TREATED AT THE COLUMBIA-PRESBYTERIAN MEDICAL CENTER, NEW YORK CITY

Location of Tumor	Percent Malignant
Parotid gland	20 to 30
Submandibular gland	30 to 50
Sublingual gland	80 to 90
Minor salivary gland	40 to 65

mately 80 to 85 percent of all salivary gland neoplasms occur in the parotid gland, 10 to 15 percent in the submandibular gland, and approximately 5 percent occur in the sublingual and minor salivary glands.[2, 6, 12] In terms of malignancy, a recent review of 1,280 salivary gland tumors treated at the Columbia-Presbyterian Medical Center in New York City yielded findings similar to other series reported in the literature[12, 18] (see Table 20-1). In general, as the size of the salivary gland decreases, the incidence of malignancy increases.

ANATOMY

Parotid Gland

A fundamental knowledge of the surgical anatomy of the parotid gland and facial nerve is the sine qua non for adequate management.

The parotid gland is paired and situated immediately inferior and anterior to the lower part of the ear ("parotid" is derived from two Greek words meaning "near the ear") (Fig. 20-1). Its superior limit is at the zygoma; its inferior limit is below the angle of the mandible. It extends anteriorly to a variable extent over the masseter muscle; posteriorly, it is bordered by the external auditory meatus, the mastoid and styloid processes, and the sternocleidomastoid and posterior digastric muscles. The deep portion of the gland extends in along the bony external auditory meatus behind the ascending ramus toward the base of the skull.

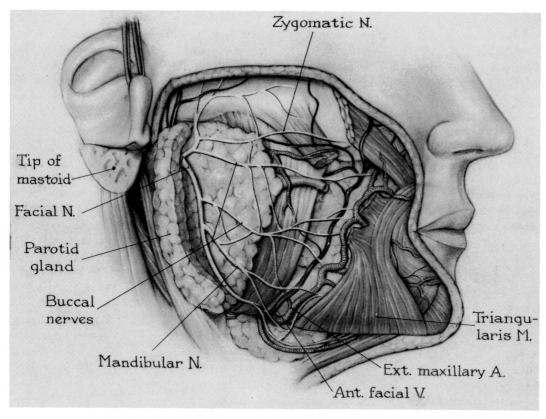

Fig. 20-1. Parotid gland and its anatomic relationship to the facial nerve, muscles, vessels, and ear. (Conley, J. 1975. Salivary Glands and the Facial Nerve. Georg Thieme, Stuttgart.)

The parotid (Stensen's) duct is approximately 6 cm long and opens into the mouth by a small orifice opposite the upper second molar. The direction of the duct corresponds to a line drawn across the face from the lower part of the concha to midway between the free margins of the upper lip and nasal ala, about one finger's breadth below the zygoma. The fascia of the gland is attached to the zygomatic arch above and to the fascia of the masseter and sternocleidomastoid muscle below.[17] In different regions about the parotid this fascia varies in thickness and fixation as it comes in contact with various muscles, bone, cartilage, blood vessels, and nerves.

The larger superficial segment of gland, which comprises 70 to 80 percent of the entire gland, lies lateral to the facial nerve branches, and the smaller deep portion lies medial to these branches. The portion of the gland embraced near the origin of the the two major nerve divisions is called the isthmus.[32] Although disputed by McKenzie,[21] there is good evidence, from a developmental point of view, that the parotid is anatomically collar-button shaped, with two lobes and a connecting short, slender isthmus;[20, 22] but, from a surgical point of view, the lobes seem more or less fused, yet are separable with careful surgical technique. In addition, the deep lobe has a retromandibular portion of variable size that hooks around the posterior portion of the mandible and extends medially into the loose areolar tissues of the upper lateral pharyngeal area in close relation to the internal carotid artery and internal jugular vein. Tumors arising in the retromandibular portion of the parotid have the potential to expand into the parapharyngeal space and base of the skull and to reach massive size prior to clinical presentation.

The facial nerve emerges from the skull through the stylomastoid foramen and passes 0.5 to 1.5 cm inferiorly with a slight anterolateral inclination to enter the parotid gland (Fig. 20-2). The facial nerve branches are given off after it has entered the parotid, with the exception of muscular rami to the occipital, auricular, posterior digastric, and stylohyoid muscles. In this short passage from foramen to gland, the nerve passes anterior to the posterior belly of the digastric muscle and lateral to the styloid process, external carotid artery, and posterior facial vein.[20] Shortly after entering the gland and at a point posterior and slightly medial to the ramus of the mandible, the nerve splits into two main divisions, the temporofacial and the cervicofacial portions (Fig. 20-3). These two divisions then sub-branch to form five main branches. The facial nerve emerges from beneath the superficial parotid lobe in five branches: the temporal, zygomatic, buccal, mandibular, and cervical. The terminal nerve branching (the so-called "pes anserinus," meaning "goose's foot") and possible anastomotic connections are complex, but several important facts emerge:[10]

1. In 13 percent of cases there are no anastomotic connections between terminal nerve branches.

2. In 70 percent of cases, anastomotic connections between the two major divisions exist.

3. Anastomoses between terminal branches of the three temporofacial divisions are frequent; anastomoses between the two branches of the cervicofacial division are infrequent. Hence, injury to the temporofacial division is less likely to result in permanent paralysis than is injury to the cervicofacial division.

4. Where nerve anastomoses between the temporofacial division do exist, they are often closely related to the parotid duct and can be readily injured when the duct is divided during surgery.

Our clinical experience, in several thousand parotidectomies and radical neck dissections, is that the lowest mandibular branch of the facial nerve usually lies from 1 to 3 cm below the lower border of the mandible, especially in the older patient with excessive cervical skin and tissue laxity. An important anatomic point made by Dingman and Grabb[11] is that the lowest mandibular branch, as it skirts the posterior portion of the angle of the mandible, lies above the lower border of the mandible 80 percent of the time; in the remaining 20 percent at least one branch of the ramus lies below, but within 1 cm, of the mandible. It is important to realize, however, that this excellent study was performed in fixed cadaver specimens where the tissues have been altered and are generally less mobile.

VASCULAR SUPPLY

The arterial supply in the region of the parotid gland is exceptionally rich. The gland receives tributaries from the external facial, occipital, posterior auricular, internal maxillary, transverse facial, and superficial tem-

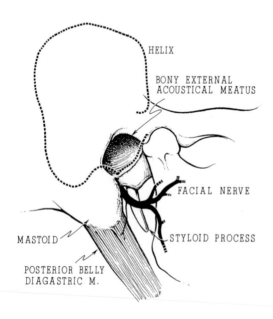

Fig. 20-2. The facial nerve as it emerges from the stylomastoid foramen. (Conley, J. 1975. Salivary Glands and the Facial Nerve. Georg Thieme, Stuttgart.)

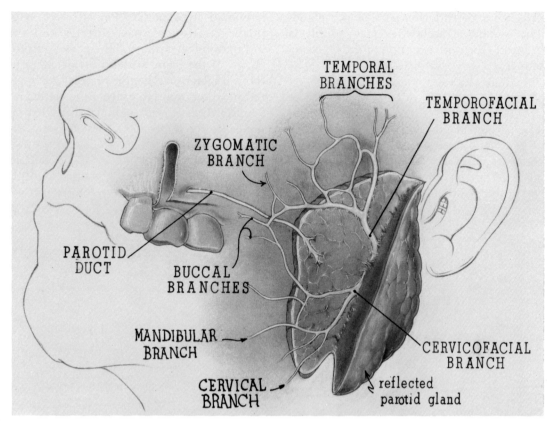

Fig. 20-3. The facial nerve divisions and their branches. (Conley, J. 1975. Salivary Glands and the Facial Nerve. Georg Thieme, Stuttgart.)

poral arteries. These vessels supply the muscles of the upper neck, mandible, ear, skin of the lateral face, scalp, and parotid gland in a vast and efficient interlacing network of arterial anastomoses. The control of arterial and venous bleeding during an operation on the gland is a painstaking and tedious procedure. Hypotensive anesthesia is preferred whenever feasible as this minimizes blood loss, facilitates dissection, and reduces risk of injury to the facial nerve.

Venous drainage about the parotid gland generally parallels the arterial system. The principal vein in the gland is the posterior facial, which is formed from a union of the superficial temporal and internal maxillary veins. The gland also receives a tributary from the posterior auricular area. As the posterior facial vein approaches the inferior aspect of the gland it divides into an an-

terior and posterior division. The posterior branch becomes continuous with the external jugular vein; the anterior branch unites with the anterior facial vein to form the common facial vein, which drains into the internal jugular vein. The position of the posterior facial vein is important clinically in that it is lateral to the superficial temporal artery and medial to the facial nerve, and that inferiorly it is a reliable landmark for branches of the facial nerve. The cervicofacial division of the facial nerve crosses the posterior facial vein and places at least one neural branch on the lateral wall of the vein. The cervical branch descends into the neck to innervate the midportion and lower portion of the platysma muscle. The ramus mandibularis is in occasional association with this branch but is usually separate and anterior to it where the posterior facial vein exits from the inferior part of the gland. The ramus mandibularis may supply a branch to the upper portion of the platysma muscle.

LYMPH SUPPLY

The parotid gland contains a rich network of lymphatic vessels in its parenchyma and about its periphery (Fig. 20-4). There are 20 to 30 lymph follicles and lymph nodes within the gland, all of which may undergo lymphoid hyperplasia. The afferent lymphatic vessels may pass directly into the intraparotid lymph nodes in the parenchyma of the gland without involvement of the paraglandular lymph nodes. Other afferent vessels may circumvent the gland and connect directly with paraglandular lymph nodes. In some instances, these two systems are interconnected. The dominant group of paraglandular lymph nodes is situated in the pretragal and supratragal area, and this is a frequent repository for cancerous

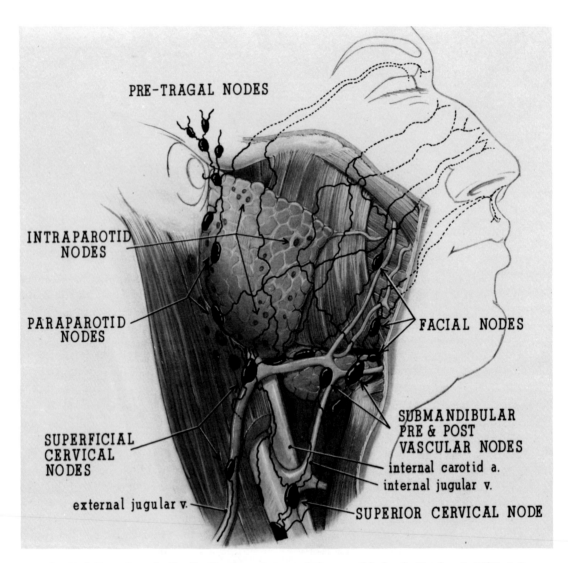

Fig. 20-4. Lymph node distribution in and around the parotid gland. (Conley, J. 1975. Salivary Glands and the Facial Nerve. Georg Thieme, Stuttgart.)

spread from the temple, scalp, and ear. There is a smaller number of nodes in association with the lateral, posterior, and inferior portions of the gland. There are no lymph nodes in the paraglandular region of the deep lobe. The efferent lymph channels from the parenchyma of the gland drain primarily into the superior deep jugular chain and also have connections with the spinal accessory, submandibular, and superficial lymph node systems.

THE NERVES

Great Auricular Nerve. This nerve arises from the cervical plexus, more specifically from the anterior divisions of the upper branches of C2 and C3. It perforates the deep cervical fascia, winds around the midposterior border of the sternocleidomastoid muscle, and then moves superiorly on this muscle in the superficial fascia deep to the platysma muscle toward the tail of the parotid gland. Close to the tail of the gland, the great auricular nerve divides into anterior and posterior branches. These branches are responsible for all major sensory perceptions in the region of the parotid gland and mediate the exquisite sensation of pain felt in the gland in suppurative processes. The anterior branch supplies the skin of the face over the parotid gland and frequently communicates with a minor division of the facial nerve in the gland. The posterior branch supplies the lower portion of the ear and the posterior aspect of the ear and lobule and communicates with the posterior auricular branch of the facial nerve, the auricular branch of the vagus nerve, and the lesser occipital nerve which arises from the cervical plexus. The great auricular nerve is routinely ablated in a resection of the parotid gland with resultant diminution in sensation in all of the associated regions.

Auriculotemporal Nerve. This nerve arises from the mandibular division of the 5th cranial nerve as it exits from the foramen ovale. These delicate branches pass forward encircling the middle meningeal artery at the base of the skull to form a single nerve at a point somewhat superior and parallel to the internal maxillary artery. The auriculotemporal nerve communicates with the facial nerve and the otic ganglion. It passes posteriorly beneath the neck of the mandible and the external pterygoid muscles in close proximity to the adjacent deep portion of the parotid gland where it communicates with the facial nerve. It then swings superiorly and egresses from the upper deep portion of the parotid gland near the root of the zygoma along with the superficial temporal artery and vein. It carries the parasympathetic secretory fibers to the parotid gland from the otic ganglion; interference with these fibers may precipitate the Frey syndrome. The auriculotemporal nerve is also responsible for sensory perception to the skin of the anterior upper ear, the external acoustic meatus, and the temporomandibular joint. The superficial temporal branches supply sensory perception to the region of the temple all the way to the top of the scalp. These latter branches also communicate with the facial and the zygomaticotemporal nerves.

External Carotid Nerves. The sympathetic plexus of the external carotid artery sends branches directly into the parotid gland; these branches communicate with the other nerves in a rich arborization of neural pathways within the gland.

Submandibular Gland

The submandibular gland resembles the parotid gland in color, but the former has slightly larger lobulations. The surgical anatomy of the submandibular gland makes it readily available for clinical examination and operative techniques. Bimanual palpation gives an accurate evaluation of the size, consistency, presence of calculi or neoplasm, and regional involvement. This gland occupies a strategic position in the posterior floor of the mouth between the tongue, mandible, and hyoid bone. Wharton's duct passes on the oral side of the mylohyoid muscle, along with an anterior extension of the gland, toward the puncta at the midline of the floor of the mouth. Posteriorly, the main body of the gland is compact, spheroid, and covered with a capsule and fascial attachments. It has an intimate relationship to the mandible, hypoglossal nerve, mylohyoid, posterior belly of the digastric and stylohyoid muscles, hyoid bone, and facial artery and vein. Its proximity to the lingual and mylohyoid nerves and, to a lesser degree, to the hypoglossal and alveolar nerves creates a facility for perineural extension of adjacent cancers. The submandibular gland also approximates the tail of the parotid gland, the sublingual gland, and the minor salivary glands in the floor of the mouth.

In surgery of the submandibular triangle, the marginal mandibular nerve is the only branch of the facial nerve liable to injury, since it dips below the lower border of the mandible and crosses the submandibular triangle deep to the platysma muscle; this branch can be located and preserved at the point where it passes superficially to the facial artery.

The lymph systems associated with the submandibular gland differ from those in the parotid gland. The submandibular gland does not contain lymph nodes or lymphoid follicles, whereas the parotid gland is richly supplied. Efferent lymph vessels from the capsule of the submandibular gland are connected primarily with the deep jugular system and the prevascular and postvascular nodes. Since these nodes also receive drainage from the lips, skin of the face, nose, scalp, floor of the mouth, and a portion of the tongue, enlargement of these nodes may cause confusion in the differential diagnosis between primary submandibular tumors, metastases from facial or intraoral cancers, and inflammatory processes. Indeed, 80 to 90 percent of all swellings in the submandibular space are inflammatory in origin.[6]

Sublingual Gland

The sublingual gland is less than one-half the size of the submandibular gland and is paired, with each gland weighing 3 to 4 grams. It rests against the sublingual fossa of the mandible, close to the symphysis, on the mylohyoid muscle. Here it is in close relationship to the submandibular duct, the lingual vessels and nerve, the hypoglossal nerve, and the mucosa of the floor of the mouth. There are some 20 excretory ducts (ducts of Rivinus) from the gland that separately empty into the floor of the mouth. An occasional duct (duct of Bartholin) may empty into the submandibular duct. The facial artery supplies the gland, with draining veins accompanying the arteries. Although the lymphatic drainage from the anterior portion of the gland is to the submandibular nodes, the predominant lymphatic drainage is to the jugulodigastric and deep jugular nodes.[17]

ETIOLOGY

Exposure to irradiation is associated with an increase in cancer of the salivary glands. No other significant factor associated with eating habits or the physiological function of these glands has been connected with the development of neoplasia.

CLASSIFICATION

Salivary gland tumors present difficulties in histologic diagnosis, nomenclature, and classification. The first reliable classification was presented by Foote and Frazell in 1953[15] and was based on a study of 877 patients with salivary gland tumors seen at Memorial Hospital in New York City from 1930 through 1949. Their work remains the foundation on which many others have built and has largely stood the test of time and practical usage throughout the world.

Various attempts have been made to classify salivary gland tumors on a scientific and histogenic basis, but most classifications in general use are based on combined histologic and behavioral features.[35] In recent

TABLE 20-2. CLASSIFICATION OF
SALIVARY GLAND TUMORS

Epithelial tumors
  Adenomas
    Pleomorphic adenoma (mixed tumor)
    Monomorphic adenomas
      Adenolymphoma
      Oxyphilic adenoma
      Other types
  Mucoepidermoid tumor
  Acinic cell tumor
  Carcinomas
    Adenoid cystic
    Adenocarcinoma
    Epidermoid carcinoma
    Undifferentiated
    Carcinoma in pleomorphic adenoma
      (Malignant mixed tumor)

Nonepithelial tumors

Unclassified tumors

Allied conditions
  Benign lymphoepithelial lesion
  Sialosis
  Oncocytosis

(Thackray, A. C., and Sobin, L. H. 1972. Histologic Typing of Salivary Gland Tumors. World Health Organization, Geneva, 16.)

years, the classification that has gained the most general acceptance is the one put forth by the World Health Organization[36] (see Table 20-2), which differs only slightly from that of Foote and Frazell. This classification is relatively simple, yet sufficiently flexible and applicable to be useful to clinicians and pathologists.

TNM Staging

Until recently, the TNM concept of tumor classification had not been applied to salivary gland neoplasms. In 1975, Spiro, Huvos, and Strong[30] proposed a clinical staging system that may offer a more predictable survival estimate than does histologic classification alone. Their system, which is divided into three clinical stages, is based on the size of the primary lesion, the presence of tumor fixation or ulceration, and the status of the facial nerve and the cervical lymph nodes. Of the 238 cases of previously untreated parotid cancer seen at the Memorial Hospital over a 30-year period that they reviewed, the 5-year survival rate was 85 percent in stage I disease, 67 percent in stage II, and only 10 percent in stage III. Moreover, when analyzing separately 81 cases of intermediate and high grade mucoepidermoid cancer according to stage of disease, the 5-year survival rate in stage I was 100 percent, in stage II 65 percent, and in stage III 10 percent. Thus the data suggest that clinical staging may influence survival more significantly than does histologic tumor appearance. However, whether their proposed classification will eventually be accepted is uncertain. At the present time a retrospective study of malignant salivary gland tumors is under way at various in-

TABLE 20-3. TNM STAGING SYSTEM FOR SALIVARY GLAND CANCER AS PROPOSED BY THE AMERICAN JOINT COMMITTEE FOR CANCER STAGING AND END RESULTS REPORTING 1976

T1	T2	T3
0–3 cm and solitary and freely mobile, and facial nerve intact*	3.1–6 cm and solitary and freely mobile or skin fixation and facial nerve intact*	>6 cm or multiple nodules or ulceration or deep fixation or facial nerve dysfunction*

*Applicable with parotid tumors only.
(Modified from American Joint Committee for Cancer Staging and End Results Reporting. 1976. Manual for Staging of Cancer. American Joint Committee, Chicago.)

stitutions to further analyze and develop this classification and staging system (see Table 20-3).

PATIENT EVALUATION— GENERAL CONSIDERATIONS

Tumors of the salivary glands are treated by a variety of surgeons and radiotherapists employing a wide scope of philosophic and therapeutic measures. The otolaryngologist, general surgeon, plastic surgeon, and maxillofacial surgeon each come from a different surgical background, which is evident in their technique. A similar situation exists in the schools of radiotherapy. For each patient this training background is modified by the surgeon's emotional attitude regarding the possible creation of a facial paralysis.

The vast majority of tumors of the parotid gland present as a painless mass. In such cases the patient should be advised regarding the physiology of the gland, the relationship of the facial nerve to the gland and the tumor, and the diagnostic possibilities, including the malignant potentialities of the biologic process. The final diagnosis is attained by exploration of the parotid gland and by the application of the technique of lateral lobectomy in the vast majority of cases. The surgeon should be prepared to finalize the surgical management on the basis of frozen-section examination. Every precaution must be taken to protect the patient's security. The patient must be informed preoperatively of the various possibilities and have given his knowledgeable consent for definitive treatment. When these criteria are not fulfilled, the operative procedure must be staged when the biologic facts have been established.

The initial concept in the management of a mass in the submandibular triangle fails to emphasize the fact that almost half are malignant. This failure leads the surgeon into the trap of presuming that he is dealing with inflammatory disease or a benign tumor. The unexpected finding of a malignancy upon frozen section, or the disconcerting report several days after operation that the excised tumor was malignant then comes as a shock to the surgeon. The surgeon may then elect, for a variety of reasons, to hope that he "got it all." Such an approach often proves disastrous in the aggressive tumor, and excision of the gland should be considered a formal biopsy technique only. It is more rational to discuss the possibility of malignant neoplasia in preparation for the primary operation and be prepared, within the criteria of frozen section, to execute an adequate primary resection. The rare sublingual neoplasm carries a higher incidence of malignancy and is managed in a similar manner.

The ubiquitous minor salivary gland tumor presenting as a submucosal mass is a tempting surgical exercise for all surgeons and dentists. A total or partial excision is usually carried out under local anesthesia on an outpatient basis. In view of the fact that approximately 40 to 65 percent of these tumors are malignant, the surgeon must insist that all of the tissues be examined microscopically and that any primary procedures be considered as biopsies only, especially when the lesion subsequently proves to be malignant. A definitive procedure is then planned. The alternative is a formal, planned excisional biopsy, with frozen section and compliance with all criteria for this technique.

Biopsy

Needle aspiration biopsy is accurate in a high percentage of cases, but should never be used as the only method of diagnosis in planning a mutilating operation on a patient with a salivary gland tumor. The success is fully dependent upon the needle being inserted into the germane part of the neoplasm, obtaining a representative portion of it, and finally having these small and irregular sections of tissue interpreted by a competent pathologist who is not only willing to subject himself to this exercise but who has the inherent instinct and talent for it. It is realistic to appreciate that, in a group of salivary gland tumors where microscopic pleomorphism is a common occurrence, the needle-aspirated material may be nonrepresentative and therefore misleading.

In order to lend greater accuracy to the diagnostic program in parotid tumors, the technique of lateral lobectomy—when feasible—will provide the tumor and the lateral lobe for examination by the pathologist. It is fortunate that the vast majority of tumors occur in the lateral lobe or the isthmus. Immediate frozen section on this generous specimen is, of course, not immune to error. The diagnosis may be modified as the permanent microscopic sections are reviewed.

There are exceptions to the above criteria. If the tumor has ulcerated through the skin or is extremely superficial in its relationship to the skin and malignancy is suspected, then a preoperative biopsy may be easily obtained by incisional technique. Otherwise, the formal incisional biopsy has been essentially abandoned, and although aspiration biopsy has some strong advocates, it has been largely replaced by the technique of lateral lobectomy with immediate frozen section. Whenever there is doubt or confusion concerning the diagnosis on the part of the pathologist, as there will be on occasion, the surgeon is obligated to wait for clarification. Conceivably, this could have harmful effects on the patient, but it is no more dangerous than either unnecessary or erroneous surgical intervention.

Changes in Diagnosis

In the management of tumors of the salivary glands it is not unusual for the pathologist to change the microscopic diagnosis after reviewing the permanent sections, particularly in dealing with malignant tumors. This occurred in 18 percent of the cases when a large group of slides from various hospitals were reviewed by other pathologists. This unsettling information is not always to the patient's disadvantage, and is resolved by a realistic reappraisal of the new data. A change may occur following a frozen section when the original areas examined were not representative of the tumor as a whole. The change may also follow the fact that a relatively inexperienced pathologist may carry out the frozen section and not be well acquainted with the vagaries of malignant neoplasia in these glands, and therefore the discrepancy is due, essentially, to his lack of experience. It is also possible, at frozen section, that more than one pathologist may examine the tissue and there may be a difference of opinion. Under these circumstances, the surgeon must wait for clarification.

It is mandatory that the surgeon assume the responsibility for gaining the greatest security for the patient. He must examine the specimen grossly, consult with the pathologist, advise the pathologist about the dangers and risks of proceeding with a mutilating procedure, seek the advice and counsel of the pathologist about proceeding, and then receive a report in writing with the pathologist's signature.

The changes in microscopic diagnosis that may be presented to the surgeon anywhere from 3 days to 3 weeks after the operation has been completed are disconcerting, awkward, and sometimes difficult to fit into the strategy of management. The patient should always be forewarned that a frozen-section diagnosis is not the final one and that there may be a change, either increasing or lessening the gravity of the situation.

In a series[6] of 278 malignant tumors the original pathologic diagnosis was changed in 18 percent of all of the cases (Table 20-4). This percentage varied from a high of 30 percent for undifferentiated carcinoma to 10 percent for squamous carcinoma and zero for lymphoma, melanoma, and miscellaneous tumors.

TABLE 20-4. FINAL PATHOLOGIC DIAGNOSIS
OF 278 PATIENTS WITH MALIGNANT
TUMOR OF THE PAROTID GLAND
PRESENTING AT PACK MEDICAL
FOUNDATION BETWEEN 1934–1972

Final Pathologic Diagnosis	No. of Cases	Percent
Mucoepidermoid carcinoma	81	29
High grade	21 (26%)	
Low grade	60 (74%)	
Adenocarcinoma	40	14
Adenoid cystic carcinoma	37	13
Malignant mixed tumor	37	13
Undifferentiated carcinoma	30	11
Squamous cell carcinoma	21	8
Acinic cell carcinoma	17	6
Lymphosarcoma	6	
Melanoma	1	6
Other	8	
Total	278	100

(Conley, J. 1975. Salivary Glands and the Facial Nerve. Georg Thieme, Stuttgart.)

MALIGNANT TUMORS OF THE PAROTID GLAND

All tumors in the parotid gland are important because of their biologic significance and their relationship to the facial nerve. The overriding consideration lies in the fact that approximately 20 to 25 percent of these tumors are malignant. Both the cell type and the stage of disease when the patient is first seen markedly affect the prognosis.[27, 30] Fortunately, the majority of these cancers are not highly aggressive. Unfortunately, the anaplastic cancers, and occasionally even the longstanding low grade cancers, show invasion of adjacent structures, including the facial nerve, spread to regional nodes, and blood-borne metastases.

Signs and Symptoms

Fifty-eight percent of the patients in our series (Table 20-5) presented with a mass and no other complaint. This group was dominated by the mucoepidermoid carcinomas (79 percent) and the acinic cell cancers (76 percent). Eighteen percent complained of some degree of nerve palsy. Thirty-two percent complained of a mass with pain. These latter two groups were dominated by the squamous cell carcinomas (52 percent) and the adenoid cystic cancers (54 percent). These statistics underscore the gravity and advanced state of neoplastic development seen in over one-third of the patients.

Although more than half of the patients presented with tumors that varied between

TABLE 20-5. PRESENTING SIGNS AND SYMPTOMS FOR 278
PATIENTS WITH TUMORS OF THE PAROTID GLAND

Presenting Signs and Symptoms	Number of Cases	Percent of Total
Mass only	163	58
Mass with pain	55	20
Mass with facial palsy or weakness	16	6
Mass with pain and palsy	34	12
Mass with trismus	5	2
Mass with sensory nerve change	2	1
Mass with fixation	3	1
Total	278	100

(Conley, J. 1975. Salivary Glands and the Facial Nerve. Georg Thieme, Stuttgart.)

2 to 4 cm in size, the remainder had tumors ranging from 6 to 15 cm. Bulkiness did not affect curability in the low grade cancers to a significant degree, but this characteristic was absolutely relevant in the high grade neoplasms.

Location of the Tumor

Forty-three percent of the tumors occupied the lateral lobe, only 10 percent were limited to the deep lobe, 27 percent involved both lobes and the isthmus, and 20 percent extended beyond the confines of the gland. This distribution of neoplasia throughout the gland challenges the possibility of a single operation being adequate to accommodate all varieties of parotid tumors. It is reasonable to state that only the tumors occurring in the lateral lobe would offer any chance for conservation of the facial nerve, and even they should be analyzed from the point of view of size, proximity to the nerve, and aggressiveness of the biologic process.

Metastasis

Metastasis proved to be the most significant factor in prognosis. Thirty-three percent of the patients presented with metastasis.

Approximately half of the metastases presented in the deep jugular chain, and the remainder occurred in the parotid, paraparotid, and posterior cervical nodes. The primary lymphatic drainage pattern favors the superior deep jugular chain and, to a lesser degree, the intraglandular and paraglandular lymph nodes.

In a series of 289 parotid malignancies treated at Memorial Hospital,[30] 20 percent of cervical nodes contained histologic evidence of metastatic carcinoma at the time of initial treatment and another 6 percent became involved later (Table 20-6). The incidence of regional nodal spread varied according to the histology of the primary lesion.

Mucoepidermoid Carcinoma

This cancer comprises about 5 percent of parotid tumors and 25 percent of malignant parotid tumors.[3] In most series this is the most common parotid cancer. Based upon the degree of tumor differentiation, these tumors are usually divided into a low grade or moderately malignant group and a highly malignant group. The low grade group occurs 10 times more frequently than the highly malignant group, and the 5-year

TABLE 20-6. CERVICAL LYMPH NODE METASTASIS ACCORDING TO HISTOLOGIC
FINDINGS IN PAROTID TUMORS

Lesion	Total Patients	Palpable on Admission	Occult	Appeared Later	Percent Positive
Mucoepidermoid carcinoma Low Grade	56	—	—	—	0
Mucoepidermoid carcinoma Intermediate and High Grade	89	25	10	4	44
Malignant mixed tumor	53	5	—	6	21
Acinic cell carcinoma	33	2	2	2	18
Adenocarcinoma	28	5	2	3	36
Adenoid cystic carcinoma	20	1	—	1	10
Squamous cell carcinoma	10	1	4	2	70
Total	289	39	18	18	26

(Spiro, R. H., Huvos, A. G., and Strong, E. W. 1975. Cancer of the parotid gland. A clincopathologic study of 289 primary cases. American Journal of Surgery, 130: 452.)

survival rate after surgery in the former group is about 90 percent, but only about 20 to 33 percent in the latter group.[23, 26, 31] However, it is misleading to rigidly imply that there is a clear distinction between these two groups, because even the best differentiated of these tumors can metastasize and behave in an unpredictable fashion. It may present such a variety of cellular patterns in various evolutionary stages that it can be difficult for the pathologist to correlate all of these histologic pictures consistently with the clinical course of the disease.

TREATMENT

Small, low grade tumors confined to the lateral lobe can be treated by total parotidectomy with preservation of the facial nerve (Figs. 20-5 A–C).

All low grade tumors that approximate the facial nerve and all recurrent tumors are treated by radical parotidectomy with an associated muscle cuff and immediate nerve-grafting.

The treatment of the undifferentiated mucoepidermoid carcinoma (21 cases)[6]

should include classic radical composite resection of the total parotid, associated muscles, and lateral neck contents. In the more extensive cases, an augmented radical operation may be applied, including a portion of the temporal bone, mandible, skin, auricle, and lateral neck. A full course of postoperative irradiation is advised to the region of the primary site and neck. Nerve grafting is not indicated in the advanced cases.

Adenoid Cystic Carcinoma (Cylindroma)

This is the second most common parotid malignancy in our series (37 cases).[6] The adenoid cystic carcinoma is one of the most biologically destructive and unpredictable tumors in the region of the head and neck. The subtlety of its presence, its mimicry of benign tumors, the unexpected extensions, the high incidence of unrecognized and local recurrence, and the systematic spread camouflage its pernicious nature. It is slow-growing but has a special proclivity to invade perineural spaces and lymphatics and causes pain and facial nerve paralysis.

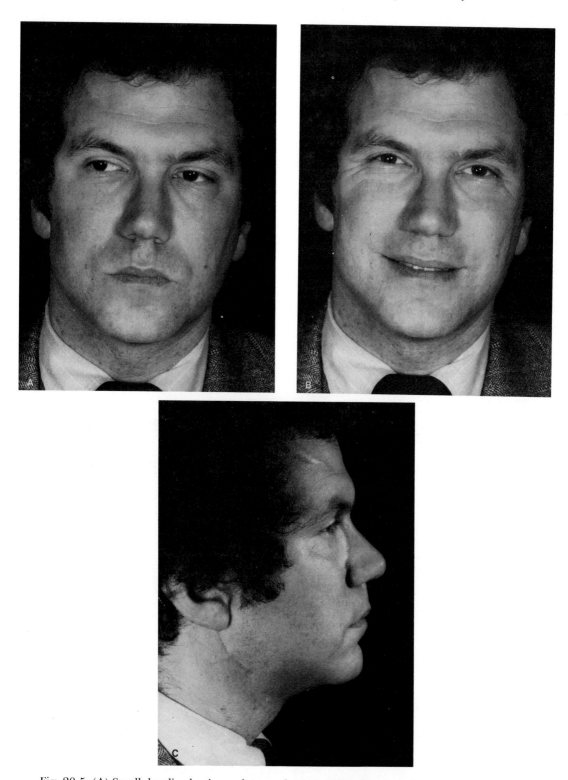

Fig. 20-5. (A) Small, localized primary low grade mucoepidermoid carcinoma treated by total parotidectomy and preservation of the facial nerve. (B) Normal facial movement. No post-operative irradiation was given. (C) Lateral view.

This tumor has a remarkable capacity for both local recurrence and ultimately wide dissemination. Regional metastasis was present at the time of the first examination in 7 percent of the cases.

In a review of 134 adenoid cystic carcinomas[7] of major and minor salivary gland origin, 50 percent of the patients had metastasis at the time of the review. Forty-two percent of the patients had at least one local recurrence. The majority had more than one recurrence, however, and some had as many as twelve. Sixty-seven percent of the patients with major salivary gland tumors manifested metastasis and recurrences, whereas 92 percent of the patients with minor salivary gland tumors manifested these extensions. The primary sites for extension and metastasis were the lungs, brain, lateral neck, and bones. It is stressed that recurrences of this particular cancer have been reported as late as 10 or even 20 years after surgery.

TREATMENT

The treatment of adenoid cystic carcinoma is usually multiphasic, extending over an interval of from 2 to 35 years. Local resection, regional and distant metastasis, chronic morbidity, and a broad range of age groups establishes the fact that no single type of management will prove adequate for this variety of circumstances. Primary adequate surgery, control of local recurrences and regional metastasis, philosophy regarding distant metastasis, the value of radiotherapy, and the principle of the "strategic retreat" are usually all utilized during the course of this disease. There is little wonder that there are mixed feelings regarding management, but certain basic factors are germane:

An adequate operation usually comprehends an ablative procedure larger than one would employ for epithelial cancer or sarcoma (Figs. 20-6 A and B). It includes the largest cuff of grossly normal tissue that can

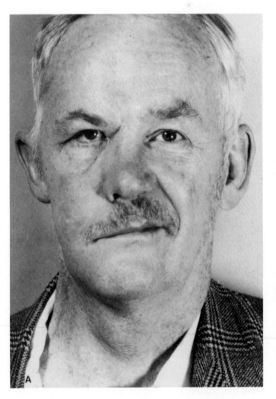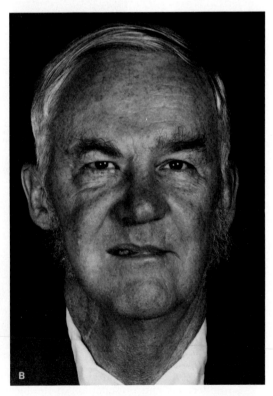

Fig 20-6. (A) Postoperative view of radical parotidectomy for adenoid cystic carcinoma. Immediate nerve graft was done. (B) Good movement of face one year later.

be rationally developed about the perimeters of the primary cancer. This concept represents the best opportunity for cure and for prevention or delay of local recurrence.

Advanced, grossly incurable disease is treated by a palliative program of irradiation. Conservative surgical intervention combined with irradiation may also have a place. The therapeutic decisions relative to these responsibilities are often frustrating and disappointing.

In the older patient, the rationale of preserving physiology and aesthetics has increased weight in the therapeutic decision.

Radical neck dissection is not included in the primary operation unless there is gross metastasis or the necessity of including a large soft tissue cuff about the primary neoplasm.

Irradiation is an effective form of treatment and in our series proved to be indispensable in the management of these problems. It was used in the treatment of nonresectable recurrences, to augment surgical management when the margins were not free of tumors, as palliation in the inoperable patient, to gain temporary local control in the surgically inaccessible tumors, and in the physiologically infirm patient. There was some degree of favorable response in every case in which irradiation was used as the sole method of treatment. Favorable responses extended over a period of 2 to 14 years. It is obvious that this is an effective instrument with which to buy time for the patient.

PROGNOSIS

For the full biologic effects of the adenoid cystic carcinoma to be appreciated, it must be evaluated over an interval of 20 to 30 years. Its behavior is both capricious and pernicious, with some individuals dying within an interval of 5 years and others surviving over 30 years.

A recent study by Perzin, Gullane, and Clairmont[24] of 62 cases indicates the importance of histologic pattern as a prognostic factor. They found no recurrences in 41 percent of patients with a predominantly "tubular" histologic pattern, as compared to no recurrences in only 11 percent of "cribriform" lesions, and all of the patients with the "solid" neoplasms having recurrence. The probability of dying from this tumor within the first 5 years after initial treatment, as calculated by standard life table methods, is 31 percent, and, by the end of 15 years, is 62 percent. The same analysis applied only to major salivary gland tumors shows a definite improvement in outlook to 24 percent and 43 percent, respectively. An analysis for only the minor salivary gland tumors is less favorable with probabilities of 36 percent and 76 percent respectively.

Malignant Pleomorphic Adenoma (Mixed Tumor)

There are two varieties of malignant mixed tumors which can be identified microscopically at different stages in their evolution. The first is the carcinoma arising in an old, long-standing benign mixed tumor and presenting with multiple foci of undifferentiated growth. This rare phenomenon suggests the development of new malignant foci within the old benign mixed tumor. The second type of malignant mixed tumor is quite different, and almost all of the cells appear malignant in a solid, massive conglomeration associated with only small remnants of benign mixed tumor. This would appear to be more on a "de novo" basis, and could be classified as being closer histopathologically to the pure variety of malignant mixed tumor. The time interval in the development of this latter variety of neoplasm is much shorter than that associated with the focal malignant changes. It is conceivable to have an overlapping of the growth patterns of the first type with the second.

TREATMENT

There is no place for conservative treatment in the management of this tumor. Suspicions are immediately aroused when the patient proffers a history of rapid growth and pain in a tumor that has been present for years. If malignancy is confirmed, a radical parotidectomy and paraglandular dissection is the minimal technique. An autogenous nerve graft is used to rehabilitate the face.

PROGNOSIS

There were 37 cases in this series.[6] When all cases are considered, the probability of dying within 5 years was 23 percent; when only the cases that had no previous treatment are considered, the probablity of dying within 5 years was 14 percent. These rather optimistic figures are balanced in the standard life tables by 21 percent living without recurrence, 29 percent living with at least one recurrence, 7 percent dead with at least one recurrence, and 43 percent dead without local recurrence.

Undifferentiated Carcinomas

In this group of 30 cases[6] the pathologists elected to classify them as high grade undifferentiated carcinomas rather than a specific histologic type. All agreed, however, that these tumors were anaplastic and undifferentiated, and microscopically represented a dangerous situation for the patient. It is recognized that many of these neoplasms, if viewed by only one pathologist in one institution, would fall into the classification of high grade mucoepidermoid cancer, adenocarcinoma, and anaplastic mixed tumor. Many of them had certain histologic features suggestive of such grouping.

TREATMENT

The basic treatment consists of augmented composite resections combined with irradiation. It is difficult to control these tumors by any combination of treatments. All of these tumors are aggressive clinically, may cause pain, become fixed and ulcerate the skin, and develop facial nerve palsy and regional metastases.

PROGNOSIS

The probability of dying within 5 years for all cases was 70 percent.[6] The probability of dying within 5 years for cases that had no previous treatment was 67 percent. Standard life tables show 10 percent living without recurrence, 20 percent dead with at least one recurrence, and 70 percent dead without recurrence. These were by far the most lethal tumors in the parotid gland.

Squamous Cell Carcinoma

There is little difficulty in the microscopic documentation of this high grade malignant neoplasm. It is usually aggressive from its inception, grows rapidly, infiltrates, causes pain, and ulcerates the skin. Approximately one-third of the patients had a facial paresis when first seen. Only eight percent (21 cases) of the carcinomas of the parotid gland proved to be squamous cell carcinomas.[6] One of the most striking features of this neoplasm is early aggressiveness and local and regional infiltration.

TREATMENT

All of these patients should be treated with an aggressive composite resection of the lateral neck contents and a total radical parotidectomy with a muscle cuff. In many instances, resection of the ear, a portion of the temporal bone and mandible, along with the local skin, must be included in the gross specimen. Many of the areas must be rehabilitated with regional flaps. Postoperative irradiation is recommended routinely at the primary site and neck.

PROGNOSIS

The probability of dying within 5 years for all cases was 58 percent. The probability of dying within 5 years for cases receiving no previous treatment dropped to 18 percent. Standard life tables showed 57 percent living with no recurrence, 14 percent dead with at least one recurrence, and 29 percent dead with no recurrence.

Acinic Cell Tumors

It is assumed that the acinic cell tumors originate from the serous cells of the acini of the parotid gland. Upon rare occasions they may be associated with the benign pleomorphic adenoma and the benign lymphoepithelial tumor. Although the acinic cell is quite characteristic, the specific cellular characteristics are varied. Some of the clear cell varieties may be mistaken for mucoepidermoid tumors, well-differentiated adenocarcinoma, hypernephroma, or parathyroid adenoma. It is unfortunate that the pathologists cannot state in all instances which of the acinic cell tumors will behave in either a benign or a malignant style. The clinician may be put in the position of treating them all as carcinomas or of forming his own judgment on their clinical behavior. Neither of these methods is completely satisfactory in tumor management. Acinic cell tumors comprised 6 percent (17 cases) of the tumors of the parotid gland in our study.[6]

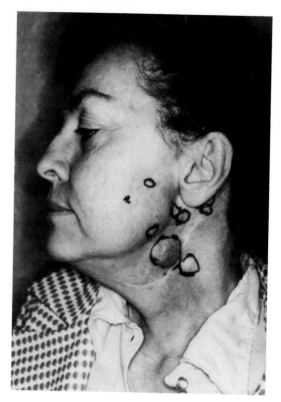

Fig. 20-7. Gross, multiple recurrent acinic cell carcinoma. Patient refused radical ablation.

TREATMENT

The majority of these neoplasms are managed by radical parotidectomy and paraglandular resection. A conservative approach can be considered for small tumors in the lateral lobe. If there is a recurrence, an augmented radical operation is advised. This strong therapeutic position is advocated primarily because of the uncertainty with the smaller pernicious group in this series (Fig. 20-7).

PROGNOSIS

Standard life tables indicated that the probability of dying within 5 years was 14 percent. The small group that we studied does not exhibit all of the dangers in dealing with this tumor.

Adenocarcinoma

Those tumors that did not fit into other specific categories are represented as a group of adenocarcinomas, which show considerable variation in their histologic pattern but have a rather consistent aggressive biologic predisposition. They comprise 14 percent (40 cases) of our group.[6]

TREATMENT

There is no conservative operation that will control these neoplasms, and the clinician should be prepared to expect a predictably relentless advancement of the tumor. A wide composite resection, including the lateral neck and a radical parotidectomy with a muscle cuff, is the minimum technique advised (Figs. 20-8 A and B). In the advanced cases, this technique is augmented at the primary site to include the mandible, the

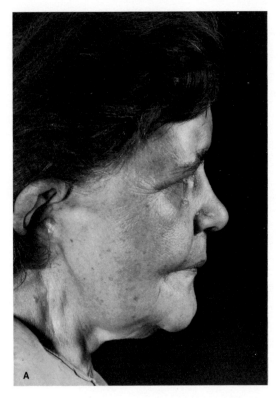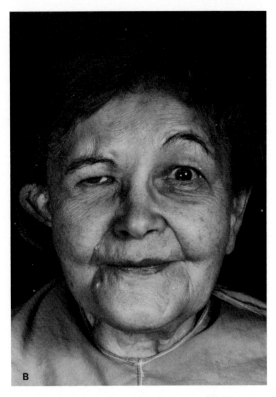

Fig. 20-8. (A) Extended radical resection for recurrent adenocarcinoma. The patient had an immediate nerve graft. (B) Good movement of face after one year.

ear, and a portion of the temporal bone. Postoperative irradiation is indicated.

PROGNOSIS

The probability of dying within 5 years for all cases was 51 percent, and within ten years was 59 percent. The probability of dying within 5 years for those with no previous treatment was reduced to 41 percent. Fifty percent of those dying had at least one recurrence, and seven percent with at least one recurrence were living with tumor. Twenty percent were dead without local recurrence.

SURGICAL TECHNIQUES: PAROTID GLAND TUMORS

The surgical treatment of tumors of the parotid gland is divided into techniques that

are planned to accommodate the biologic process and the facial nerve system. Five basic techniques are available for the management of these problems.

Enucleation

The original technique of enucleation, which attempted to ignore identification of the facial nerve by limiting the dissection to the "capsule" of the tumor, fell into ill repute because of the high local recurrence rate in the benign tumors and an insignificant cure rate in the malignant tumors. The concept of modified enucleation has been partially revived, however, in certain instances. The key to success is an understanding of the anatomy and gross pathology of these neoplasms in situ and a meticulous dissection, using the operating microscope to identify the characteristics of the margins of the tumor, its encapsulation phenomenon, any aberrant lobulations and, most important, any gross violation by local or diffuse infiltration into the adjacent glandular tissue. If the latter should appear under the microscope during the execution of this particular technique, then that operation should be immediately changed to a more adequate resection.

Lateral Lobectomy

The lateral lobectomy has gradually evolved into the basic operation for tumors of the parotid gland. Its practicality stems from the fact that the majority of tumors of the parotid gland are benign and occur in the lateral lobe. In addition, the technique may be adjusted to accommodate benign tumors of the isthmus and deep lobe. It may also be applied to small, well-differentiated, low grade malignant neoplasms of the lateral lobe that have not compromised the facial nerve. The technique of lateral lobectomy and its modifications satisfies the biologic requirements and facial nerve obligations in 80 to 85 percent of all of the tumors that occur in this gland. Any procedure that accomplishes this magnitude of success as an immediate diagnostic technique in every instance, and has a therapeutic effect in such a gratifyingly high incidence, is established as the initial operation of choice in the overwhelming majority of these problems.

Total Parotidectomy with Preservation of the Facial Nerve

Total parotidectomy with preservation of the facial nerve is more of a concept than a precise technical exercise. The very fact that the facial nerve remains intact makes a euphemism of the statement, as there are usually small islands of parenchyma remaining at the periphery of the gland. These isolated segments may be expected to atrophy if their drainage facility is destroyed, and in some instances this will create the effect of a total parotidectomy.

The indications for this technique are in the recurrent, multiple, benign tumors, the large benign tumors of the isthmus and deep lobe, and in some low grade malignant tumors of the lateral lobe.

Total Parotidectomy, Including the Facial Nerve

The operation of total parotidectomy including the facial nerve is frequently classified as a radical parotidectomy, not because of its surgical scope, primarily, but more because of the resultant facial paralysis. There is an understandable anxiety and resistance on the part of the patient to accept facial paralysis and, in some instances, for the doctor to recommend it. This could be reflected in the treatment and prognosis.

Certain varieties of mucoepidermoid tumors have been classified as low grade cancers with a very low incidence of local recurrence and regional metastasis. If they are large, situated in the isthmus or deep lobe, are recurrent, have just undergone gross subtotal resection, or have compromised any portion of the facial nerve system, they qualify for radical parotidectomy. Acinic cell adenocarcinoma has been reported as a low grade tumor, but qualifies for radical parotidectomy in some instances. It should be recognized, however, that repeated local recurrences with this tumor make it difficult to cure. Early malignant mixed tumors, early ductal carcinomas, and sebaceous carcinomas also qualify for radical parotidectomy. It is, of course, conceivable that some of these cancers could be cured without sacrifice of the facial nerve. However, until more hard data are presented to substantiate this, one may be taking an unnecessary risk in doing a smaller operation and preserving the facial nerve, particularly in view of the advancements made in the immediate rehabilitation of the facial nerve, which has now become an integral part of this operative technique. There also is no doubt that if the nerve is saved and the cancer has approximated it, postoperative irradiation enhances the cure rate.

The concept of this operation is to establish a specimen containing the entire parotid gland with its intraglandular lymphatics, the paraglandular lymphatics, and a cuff of normal tissue about the specimen. Externally, the specimen is covered by superficial fascia and platysma muscle. The masseter muscle gives a partial deep cuff, along with the posterior belly of the digastric and stylohyoid muscles. The tip of the mastoid and a portion of the sternocleidomastoid muscle supply a posterior cuff. The deep portion of the tail of the parotid is covered with the lymphatics and associated fat and areolar tissues of the superior internal jugular chain of lymph nodes. The spinal accessory, hypoglossal, and vagus nerves remain intact. The facial nerve deficiency is immediately rehabilitated by a free autogenous nerve graft procured from C3 or C4 of the ipsilateral cervical plexus. The ipsilateral side is used as a matter of convenience and is considered biologically safe under the conditions enumerated. If the tumors are high grade or if regional metastasis is present, the contralateral cervical plexus or a sural nerve should be used. The technique of nerve grafting should be considered in every instance following these resections and has greatly ameliorated the disadvantages of facial paralysis (Fig. 20-5).

Radical Parotidectomy and Radical Neck Dissection

The operation of radical parotidectomy with radical neck dissection has been developed with the hope of reducing the high incidence of local recurrence in the undifferentiated tumors of the parotid gland and in those tumors with a significant capacity for metastasis to the regional lymph nodes. It obviously has its best opportunity for success when applied as a primary procedure. It is also indicated for aggressive recurrent neoplasms. Its use is considered for the malignant tumors of the deep lobe, which are often advanced when first diagnosed and difficult to engage technically.

It is unfortunate that many cases of recurrent malignant tumors of the parotid gland are much more advanced than is clinically discernible. This is particularly true if irradiation has been used and the tumor has "gone underground." Under these adverse conditions it may be necessary to include the ear, mastoid, mandible, and associated skin in the specimen. Nerve grafting is hardly realistic in these latter cases, as the quality of the tissue bed, size of the wound, and general physiological circumstances often militate against it. It is desirable, however, in all primary ablative cases. The large skin deficiency created is corrected by free skin grafting or pedicle transfer. Although free skin grafting is the easiest and shortest method of dressing one of these extensive wounds, flap transfer is more desirable. Indeed, it is essential if postoperative irradiation is planned.

High grade mucoepidermoid carcinomas, squamous cell cancers, undifferentiated adenocarcinomas, advanced malignant mixed tumors, advanced acinic cell carcinomas, all large or aggressively recurrent malignant tumors, recurrent adenoid cystic carcinomas, all cancers with facial nerve paralysis, and all cancers with gross metastases qualify for the radical parotidectomy with radical neck dissection. It is obvious that this potpourri of carcinomas and biologic situations covers the advanced and serious aspects of malignant neoplasia in the parotid gland. It is therefore appropriate to consider postoperative irradiation as an additional palliative measure in these instances.

IRRADIATION

Irradiation occupies a specific and significant place in the treatment of tumors of the salivary glands. Its role in the management of these problems has changed dramatically from a position of dominance four decades ago to a more realistic position now. This evolution has been established on the basis of a more meaningful classification of these tumors with respect to response to radiotherapy, in addition to the development of surgical techniques that comply with the surgical anatomy of these structures and the biologic behavior of these neoplasms. Fletcher's contributions have been stimulating and significant.[13, 14]

The specific use of irradiation in the management of malignant tumors in the salivary glands is as follows:

1. In all of the lymphomas it is the primary method of treatment. The lymphoma presents as a mass either within the gland or adjacent to it, thereby necessitating removal for diagnostic purposes. The microscopic diagnosis is hopefully attained by frozen-section technique, thus terminating the operative procedure at that stage. The patient undergoes a general physiological survey for staging of this type of neoplasm and is then treated definitively with radiotherapy and/or chemotherapy. In approximately 90 percent of the cases the primary site is controlled by this method of management. The accurate classification and staging of lymphomas, combined with an aggressive radiotherapeutic program complemented by chemotherapy, has resulted in a significant improvement in the control of and in the curability factors of the lymphomas in the head and neck.

2. Irradiation is also of value as a complement to the surgical anatomy, surgical technique, and biologic characteristics of the malignant tumors in the following ways:

a. It is rational to augment the treatment of all malignant tumors of the deep lobe of the parotid gland with irradiation because of the difficulty in attaining a significant cuff of normal tissue about the tumor in this region. The same philosophy would apply with respect to the limitations of surgical anatomy in salivary gland tumors in other regions of the head and neck.

b. Postoperative irradiation may be helpful when the surgeon has preserved the facial nerve system in the parotid gland at the insistence of the patient who has a malignant tumor that is perilously close to the nerve.

c. When an operation is recognized as being inadequate, there must be consideration for the application of irradiation.

d. The local recurrence rate of 20 to 40 percent in cases of high grade cancers and in previously operated cancers of the salivary gland lends support to the consideration for the application of elective postoperative irradiation. There is evidence that this combination of therapeutic actions enhances cure rate and local control. The use of irradiation postoperatively has the advantage of application on the basis of information produced as a result of surgical intervention, and is preferred over elective preoperative irradiation in these regions (Figs. 20-9A and B).

e. The use of irradiation as a palliative tool with inoperable, recurrent, and uncontrolled cancers of the salivary glands is well recognized.

f. Irradiation should not be used as a substitute or excuse for adequate surgery.

In our series of 278 malignant tumors of the parotid gland, 55 percent received irradiation. Forty-two percent received it therapeutically. In 40 percent it was given postoperatively. In seven percent it was given as the only method of treatment, and in six percent it was given for palliation only. The outline of the field, the dosage, the targeting, and the general radiotherapeutic program requires the astute planning and direction of an experienced radiotherapist.

THE FACIAL NERVE IN PAROTID NEOPLASIA

Facial nerve paresis in the presence of a parotid tumor is almost always pathognomonic of cancer. This one sign portends a serious prognosis. Of 34 cases presenting this sign, 30 have been followed for at least five years.[8] Of these 30 patients, 21 are dead of tumor, one is dead of other causes at 7 years, one is living with tumor, and eight are free of tumor. Five of these eight have been followed over 10 years. Sixty percent of these patients had cervical metastasis. Eighty-four percent of those dying in less than 5 years had cervical metastasis, and 36 percent of those surviving over 5 years had cervical

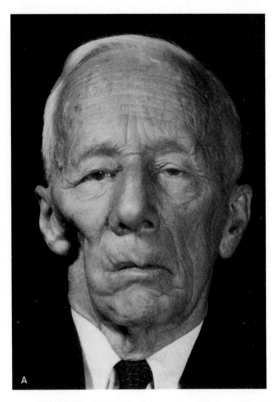
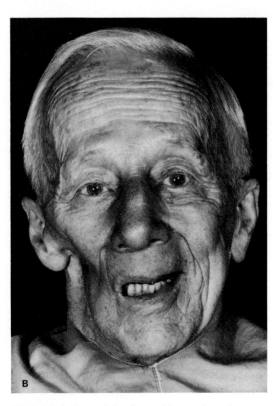

Fig. 20-9. (A) Radical resection of the parotid and lower portion of the face with preservation of the upper division of the facial nerve. Treated postoperatively with irradiation. (B) Five years postoperation.

metastasis. It is recognized that although the prognosis is very serious, it is not hopeless. Twenty-nine percent survived over 5 years, and 14 percent survived over 10 years.

The following classification shows the indications for resection and preservation of the facial nerve:

1. Indications for *resection* of the facial nerve in the treatment of tumors of the parotid gland:

   a. High grade malignant tumors;

   b. Large malignant tumors occupying a major portion of the parotid gland;

   c. Malignant tumors of the deep lobe;

   d. Malignant tumors presenting with facial nerve paresis;

   e. Recurrent malignant tumors;

   f. Certain recurrent benign mixed tumors that occupy the entire residuum of parotid gland and compromise the facial nerve.

2. Indications for *preservation* of the fa-

cial nerve in the treatment of tumors of the parotid gland:

   a. All benign tumors and cysts;

   b. Early low grade malignant tumors of the lateral lobe. These may require segmental resection of the facial nerve, total parotidectomy and, in some instances, postoperative irradiation.

   c. Recurrent benign mixed tumors. These may require a segmental resection of the facial nerve and total parotidectomy.

Nerve Grafting

Nerve grafting is one of the most significant advances in the rehabilitation of the paralyzed face and in the treatment of malignant tumors of the parotid gland. It is applicable when there is a loss of the main trunk of the facial nerve or of the peripheral facial nerve system. It is obvious that if the ablation extends into the internal auditory meatus medially it is technically unrealistic to attempt to anastomose a nerve graft to the proximal stump as part of an extracranial technique without appropriate neurosurgical preparation. If the distal part of the facial nerve system and its muscle bed is ablated in a radical technique involving the mimetic muscles, then peripheral nerve anastomosis would be unrealistic and another concept of rehabilitation would have to be used. The majority of ablative procedures dealing with cancer of the parotid gland, and some traumatic and iatrogenic circumstances, lend themselves ideally to free autogenous nerve grafting. Again, the best time to carry out nerve anastomosis under these circumstances is at the time of the primary operation.

The usual donor areas are the sensory branches of the cervical plexus, with a segment of nerve containing four or five branches. This graft is approximated to the proximal facial nerve stump with 8-0 to 10-0 atraumatic monofilament suture material. The peripheral branches are usually approximated with one suture. There is no question but that magnification with loupes or the dissecting microscope increases the precision of nerve approximation. Many of these grafts, however, have been placed without the aid of magnification with excellent return of function. The nerve graft is generous in length, thus eliminating any possibility of tension on the suture line. The suture line is encased in a soft nonconstrictive silicone tube, 1 cm long. All of these wounds must be drained.

When the above criteria are applied, one can expect some degree of movement in the face in 95 percent of the cases. The first signs of return of movement appear in the cheek and about the commissure of the mouth. The interval of time is from 6 to 12 months, depending upon the length of the graft, the accuracy of the anastomosis, and the volume of regenerating axons (Figs. 20-10A–C). The tone of the face during this interval is better than one would expect in a paralyzed face, and many individuals do not require an elective tarsorrhaphy. The move-

ment spreads from the middle third of the face into the cheek and about the orbit. The forehead and platysma movement usually do not return. Improvement in tone, movement, and coordination continues for another 2 years. The movement is always weaker than that on the normal side. It is basically mass movement in character and it exhibits varying degrees of dyskinesia. The natural response to emotional expression on the paralyzed side of the face is markedly limited but can be improved by persistent training and awareness.

TUMORS OF THE SUBMANDIBULAR AND SUBLINGUAL GLANDS

Submandibular Gland

CLASSIFICATION

Submandibular tumors, benign and malignant, are about one-ninth as common as parotid tumors, and one-half as common as tumors of the minor salivary glands. Fifteen percent of benign and 10 to 15 percent of malignant salivary gland tumors occur in the submandibular gland. Fifty to 70 percent of submandibular tumors are benign, and of these benign tumors 95 percent are pleomorphic adenomas. An occasional adenolymphoma is encountered. Thirty percent to 50 percent of submandibular tumors are malignant;[6] the types are the same as in the parotid gland but in different frequencies. Adenoid cystic carcinoma is the most common malignancy, varying in reported frequency from 28 percent in Foote and Frazell's series[15] of 60 submandibular cancers to 41 percent in Simons, Beahrs, and Woolner's[29] series of 51 cancers and 31 percent in Conley, Myers, and Cole's series of 115 patients.[9]

In Simons, Beahrs, and Woolner's series,[29] mucoepidermoid tumor was the second most common cancer (19 percent), and acinic cell, squamous cell, and malignant

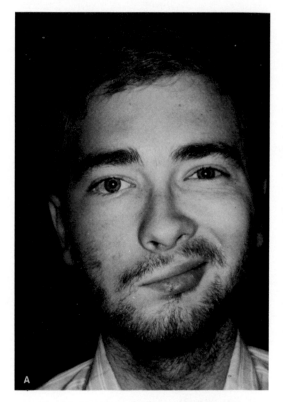
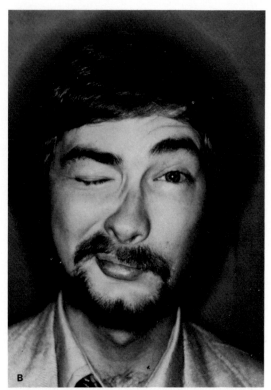
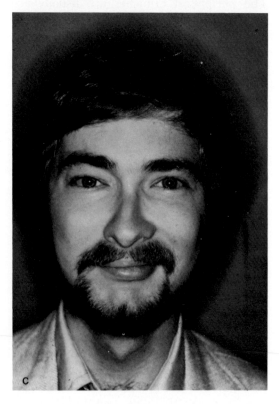

Fig. 20-10. (A) Facial paralysis following radical resection for carcinoma. (B) Free autogenous facial nerve graft functioning after 10 months. (C) Controlled smile after 10 months.

mixed tumors each accounted for about 8 percent of the malignant group. A rare fibrosarcoma and lymphosarcoma was found. Distant metastases occurred twice as frequently as with parotid cancer. Approximately one-half of patients with submandibular cancer lived 5 years without disease. Another 10 percent lived at least 5 years but with known recurrence of disease.

DIAGNOSIS

The principal distinction in diagnosis is the separation of the inflammatory lesions from the benign and malignant neoplasms. History and examination are essential primary steps.

Inflammatory lesions usually present with the characteristic signs of infection, such as pain, tenderness, redness, and purulent exudate from the duct. There may be stenosis of the duct, obvious or occult calculi, and intermittent swelling of the gland with meals. When the inflammatory process is subacute or chronic none of these criteria may be manifest. Dental occlusion x-rays are the most accurate for the diagnosis of gross calculi. Sialography of the submandibular gland has been disappointing as a diagnositc tool. A course of antibiotics frequently caused an improvement in the active inflammatory lesions, but the drugs do not affect the chronic fibrotic gland. The importance of attempting a diagnosis of inflammatory lesions in the submandibular region is highlighted by the fact that they comprise 80 to 90 percent of all swellings in the submandibular space.

The majority of submandibular gland tumors present as a painless, firm mass, which is best identified by bimanual palpation.

Biopsy is not indicated when there is a positive clinical diagnosis of inflammation. Incisional biopsy is rarely indicated in benign or malignant tumors of this gland. If the tumor is associated with either ulceration or near ulceration, this situation might be used to procure preoperative tissue for diagnostic purposes. Excision of the gland with frozen-section examination amounts to an excisional biopsy and offers the best opportunity for resolving the problem of management in a single-stage procedure. If the frozen section indicated a cancer, the surgeon should be prepared to proceed with an ablative procedure. This means that he should have discussed this possibility with the patient prior to operation and should have gained written consent for a radical procedure. Should the pathologist have any doubt about his position when apprised of the consequences of his diagnosis, the surgeon is obligated to wait for a firm diagnosis. Although the aspiration biopsy might seem ideal for these tumors, it is incorrect to plan an extensive ablative procedure on the basis of such a biopsy alone when it may present pleomorphic and, at times, obscure diagnostic patterns.

Primary lymphoma of the prevascular and postvascular lymph nodes and metastasis from an epithelial cancer to these nodes must be differentiated from primary cancer of the submandibular gland, since the management of each is quite specific and different. Lymphomas are usually treated by irradiation, and metastatic cancer by composite resection.

TREATMENT

The presence of a benign or malignant neoplasm in the submandibular gland presents the clinician with a multiple set of responsibilities. Differentiation of tumor from the more common conditions of calculi, ductal obstruction, chronic infection, and involvement of the lymph nodes adjacent to this gland must be made and this difficulty in diagnosis has posed problems that handicap the correct management of these tumors. In many instances, the concept of diagnosis and planning is absent. A lack of knowledge regarding the significant possibilities of cancer and the grave possibilities presented by the varieties of cancer of this gland can give a false sense of security that frequently proves disastrous. Management by local resection of the gland alone proves to be inadequate in the majority of cases of cancer.

The treatment of the malignant tumors has changed over the past three decades, evolving from resection of the gland only to augmented local resection and composite resection.

The well-differentiated mucoepidermoid carcinoma, some early malignant mixed tumors, and the rare acinic cell carcinoma may be treated by a monobloc resection of the primary lesion in the submandibular gland along with the associated muscles, nerves, and mucous membrane. The first criterion in planning the treatment is to establish the position of the neoplasm in the gland and its relationship to proximal structures.

These tumors may grow in any direction about the circumference of the gland, approximating the different structures in proximity with the gland in that position. The conservative operation includes resection of the submandibular gland; the floor of the mouth and sublingual glands; the periosteum of the mandible; the lingual, mylohyoid, and hypoglossal nerves; the platysma, mylohyoid, and digastric muscles; a small portion of the anterior tip of the parotid gland; and all areolar tissue about the submandibular and submental compartments. The prevascular and postvascular lymph nodes, the mylohyoid lymph node, and submental lymph nodes are included. A much more secure operation for recurrent tumors and all high grade and undifferentiated malignant neoplasms in this gland includes an extension of the perimeters into the tongue, including the lateral neck contents and horizontal ramus of the mandible.

Our experience has shown that irradiation plays an important role. It is indicated for all inadquate margins, recurrent cancers, tumors outside the capsule, nerve invasions, undifferentiated cancers, and adenoid cystic carcinomas.

One hundred and fifteen neoplasms of the submandibular gland were reviewed by Conley, Myers, and Cole.[9] Forty-seven per-cent were malignant and 53 percent benign. They proposed gland removal and frozen section. Because of the high incidence of malignancy in this series, permission should be obtained for composite resection. Any doubt regarding the validity of frozen section delays the procedure until the diagnosis is firm. The removal of only the submandibular gland was not considered an adequate cancer operation in most instances. Reoperation on uncontrolled local recurrence gives discouragingly low control rates.

Sublingual Gland

Sublingual gland tumors are rare. Rankow and Mignogna, in reviewing the literature in 1969,[25] found only 46 reported cases of primary sublingual tumors. Of these, 37 (80 percent) were malignant. Adenoid cystic carcinoma predominated, with well-differentiated mucoepidermoid carcinoma second. A small percentage of squamous cell cancers was also found. There was a slight female predominance, and the most common age group in the series was that of patients in the fourth to sixth decades. Statistically meaningful 5-year survival figures after surgery are not available because of the infrequency of sublingual gland cancer, but the smallness of the gland and its rich lymphatic drainage suggest a potential for local contiguous spread and early metastasis.

DIAGNOSIS

It is not always easy to determine whether a neoplasm located in the anterior floor of the mouth is of the minor salivary gland, the sublingual gland, or an anterior extension of the submandibular gland. Bimanual palpation helps to establish the position of this tumor in the sublingual compartment.

The diagnosis is made by the surgical removal of the entire gland and frozen-section examination. The surgeon must be aware of the fact that approximately 80 percent of the neoplasms arising in the sublingual gland are malignant. This startlingly high figure of malignancy stands in contrast to the relative infrequency of any type of neoplasia at this site.

TREATMENT

The well-differentiated mucoepidermoid carcinoma lends itself to local monobloc resection that includes the sublingual compartment and surrounding musculature, the periosteum, a portion of the submandibular gland, and undersurface of the tongue and adjacent mucosa. The approach may be intraoral or external. Metastasis to the lymph nodes is rare. The adenoid cystic carcinoma and other more aggressive malignant neoplasms undergo a more formidable type of local resection that includes a segment or margin of mandible, the sublingual gland on the opposite side, the ipsilateral sublingual and hypoglossal nerves in the area of the tumor, and a submental and submandibular dissection. Such composite resections in this anatomic site may cause gross aesthetic deformity and interference with functions, and thus, necessitate rehabilitative procedures. ·

TUMORS OF THE MINOR SALIVARY GLANDS

Chaudhry, Vickers, and Gorlin[4] reviewed the English language literature from 1927 to 1961 and found 1,320 cases of intraoral salivary gland tumors. Of these, 60 percent were benign and 40 percent malignant. The palate was the site of predilection for the majority of the tumors (46 percent) with the tongue being second (20 percent) and the cheek third (11 percent). The most common tumor was the pleomorphic adenoma which comprised 56 percent of all the tumors and 92 percent of the benign group. In the malignant group, adenoid cystic cancer was the most frequent tumor (37 percent). Because the mucoepidermoid tumor was not described until 1945,[33] its frequency could only be evaluated after that date, but it appeared to comprise about 20 percent of malignancies. Adenocarcinomas were the second most frequent type (33 percent) of malignancies.

Conley reviewed 200 cases of tumors of minor salivary gland origin in a personal series[5] and found 55.5 percent to be in females. Sixty-five percent of tumors were malignant with adenoid cystic carcinoma comprising 38.4 percent, mucoepidermoid carcinoma 26.2 percent, malignant mixed tumors 20.8 percent, and adenocarcinoma 14.6 percent. The most common site for both benign and malignant tumors was the palate (51 percent). Five percent of the patients who had a preoperative biopsy had a change in diagnosis when the entire specimen was examined. Thirty percent of the patients with malignant tumors did not have free margins and the majority of these were patients with adenoid cystic carcinoma. Twenty-seven percent of the malignant tumors metastasized with 51 percent of these

appearing in the lung and 31 percent in the cervical area. Actuarial statistics indicated 55 percent were free of tumor. The most pernicious tumor was adenoid cystic carcinoma with only 38 percent free of tumor at 5 years and only 6 percent at 20 years; 67 percent of those with mucoepidermoids, 66 percent with malignant mixed tumors, and 57 percent with adenocarcinomas survived over 5 years.

In a series of 80 cases reported by Stuteville and Corley[34] 89 percent of tumors were malignant, a figure at variance with the rest of the literature. In their group of cancers, 50 percent were adenoid cystic cancer, 24 percent were mucoepidermoid tumors, 20 percent were malignant mixed tumors, and only 3 percent were adenocarcinomas. The 5-year free-of-disease figure after surgery for adenoid cystic cancer was 58 percent, for mucoepidermoid carcinoma 73 percent, and for malignant mixed tumor 100 percent.

Treatment

The primary method of treatment is adequate monobloc resection, complemented in certain circumstances with neck dissection and irradiation. The surgical techniques are planned within the framework of the surgical anatomy of the involved region. The biologic fact that malignant tumors of the minor salivary glands originate within a small volume of glandular tissue and, within a short period of time, transgress the gland into the surrounding tissue mean that these tumors require astute planning and generous margins. Attaining this normal cuff in certain regions of the head and neck is anatomically and technically impossible.

PALATE

Malignant tumors of the palate are treated by a through-and-through excision into the nasal cavity and maxillary antrum. These specimens usually include portions of the hard and soft palates, alveolus, nasal septum, sinus, pterygoid plates, and muscles.

In the management of adenoid cystic carcinoma in this region all of the above perimeters are extended. The surrounding anatomy at this site is connected to the orbit and base of the skull by bony ridges and neurovascular pathways that facilitate tumor extension. Perimeters of the specimen frequently show neoplasm, even after generous preoperative planning, which is particularly pertinent in the adenoid cystic carcinoma. A full course of postoperative irradiation is given. The fenestrae in the palate are accommodated by prostheses and occasionally by local reconstruction.

In the treatment of benign tumors, an attempt is made to maintain the integrity of the palate. A small perforation resulting from the excision of a benign tumor may either close spontaneously or may be rehabilitated with a small regional flap.

NASAL CAVITY

Malignant tumors in the nasal and sinus cavities may be treated by local resection through degloving the middle third of the face or by lateral rhinotomy incisions. These neoplasms may compromise the orbit or cribriform area and are in intimate contact with foramina and neurovascular structures that lead directly into the intracranial cavity.

If the malignant tumor originates in the posterior portion of the nasal cavity, choanae, sphenoid, or nasopharynx, it presents the double handicap of being technically inaccessible and being in contact with the base of the skull. The advanced state of tumor development when the patient is first seen renders a grave outlook for patients with these tumors. Fortunately, incidence of this type of malignant neoplasia in this region is low. Irradiation is an essential part of the treatment, either as primary therapy or as a postoperative complement.

TONGUE, ALVEOLUS, FLOOR OF MOUTH

Malignant minor salivary gland tumors in the tongue, floor of the mouth, and alveolus are treated by local or composite resection. These tumors are technically accessible and lend themselves to ablative techniques. Although minor salivary gland tissue is abundant on the undersurface of the tip of the tongue, no tumors have been documented in this site. The lateral border and base of the tongue are infrequent sites for these tumors. It is difficult to separate some of these neoplasms in the floor of the mouth from primary growth in the sublingual and submandibular glands. Fortunately, the treatment is essentially the same. The surgical anatomy approximates these tumors with the mandible, the tongue, the upper neck, and the lingual, alveolar, hypoglossal, and mylohyoid nerves. Although there is a functional and aesthetic deficiency following the ablation of these areas, this can be ameliorated by appropriate skin grafts, flap transposition, and ultimately bone grafts.

LIPS, BUCCAL CAVITY

Malignant minor salivary gland tumors of the lips are discernible at an early stage of development and lend themselves readily to excision and cheiloplasty. The buccal area conceals the tumor for a much longer period of time, and there may be extensions into the buccal fat pads, under the malar compound, into the pyramidal lobe of the parotid, and into the retromolar space. Surgeons are tempted to underoperate these areas because of resultant deformities, and therefore may attempt the intraoral enucleation of the neoplasm. This is rarely successful and cannot be compared to the adequate exposure one attains from a lower lip-splitting and submandibular incision with elevation of the entire cheek. The more remote regional anatomy includes the infratemporal fossa, the maxilla, and the orbit. Skin grafting and regional flaps may ameliorate the local deficiency.

PHARYNX

Minor salivary gland tumors are very uncommon in occurrence in the supraglottis, glottis, hypopharynx, and trachea. Management is primarily by wide local resection.

The concept of the lateral neck dissection with respect to these tumors is selective. Primary malignant tumors of the minor salivary glands have a 5 percent incidence of metastasis to the neck on the first clinical examination. This rarely justifies a primary neck dissection unless the tumor is of such size and position as to compromise the neck. As these tumors mature, are unsuccessfully treated, and recur locally, the incidence of metastasis or direct extension to the neck rises to 31 percent.

Local Recurrence

Local recurrence was one of the dominant biologic features in the behavior of malignant minor salivary gland tumors.[5] In Conley's study[5], 40 percent of the patients presented with one or more recurrences. Forty-seven percent of the recurrences in the entire group occurred in the patients presenting with adenoid cystic carcinomas, 19 percent in the mucoepidermoid carcinomas, 17 percent in the malignant mixed tumors, and 17 percent in the adenocarcinomas. The recurrence rate of the specific tumors proved to be 50 percent for adenoid cystic carcinoma, 30 percent for mucoepidermoid carcinoma, 33 percent for malignant mixed tumor, and 47 percent for adenocarcinoma. This verifies the clinical impression that adenoid cystic carcinoma and adenocarcinoma are very difficult to control by local resection, and that the clinician must be prepared to deal with local recurrences in one-third to one-half of these cases. The average period of time for local recurrence with malignant tumors was approximately 48 months, thus establishing a rather protracted program in management. Several patients in this series underwent five to ten local operations in an unsuccessful attempt to control their neoplasm. The incidence of local recurrence proved to be almost 20 percent higher than the report of inadequate margins, thus establishing the pernicious and deceptive capacity of these tumors for occult extensions.

There were 7 recurrences in the 70 patients with benign tumors, and these were cured by reoperation.

Metastasis

Thirty-one percent of patients presented with metastasis to the lateral neck, and 51 percent had metastasis to the lung.[5] Adenoid cystic carcinoma was the chief offender. In addition to the lungs and neck, the minor salivary gland tumors metastasized to the bones, brain, breast, kidney, and chest. One-fifth of the malignant mixed tumors and the mucoepidermoid carcinomas presented metastases. In most instances, metastases appeared to be definitely associated with the biologic nature of the neoplasm and its chronicity and multiple recurrence rate and with the frequent unsuccessful attempts at local control. These disappointing situations emphasize the desirability of attempting to control these tumors at the first major ablative procedure.

FACTORS INFLUENCING PROGNOSIS AND TREATMENT

1. Biology
2. Surgical anatomy
3. Size
4. Capsule
5. Duration
6. Metastasis
7. Local recurrence
8. Extension beyond gland
9. Facial nerve involvement

The prognosis of malignant salivary gland tumors is governed primarily by the intrinsic biologic behavior of the neoplasm and by the adequacy of its management program. The spectrum of biologic potential extends from that of the very low grade, indolent neoplasm to that of a vicious, high grade type that overwhelms the patient. Although this range is in most instances, identifiable by the pathologist, it is not always possible for him to predict precisely how this tumor will behave in its host, and there are innumerable instances when the tumor boldly contradicts the prognostications derived from microscopic interpretation. This in no way nullifies the concept of microscopic identification, but alerts the clinician to some of the hidden imponderables intrinsic in the management program.

An analysis of the axiom of "adequate treatment" leaves much to be desired. At best, this concept incorporates a sincere attempt on the part of the physician to diagnose and take care of a neoplastic situation about which he may know very little, about which there is considerable disagreement of opinion among the various specialists treating the condition, and about which there is the eternal struggle in management between the use of ablative surgery (with possible mutilation), radiotherapy, and chemotherapy.

The *stage* in which the malignant neoplasm is first treated is obviously a significant determining factor in the prognosis. The early stages present great hope for cure in the low grade tumors, and some limited hope for cure in the high grade tumors. As the stage of the tumor proceeds to a much more advanced phase there is still oppor-

tunity for cure of patients with the low grade neoplasms, but rarely a chance for salvage of the patient with the high grade neoplasms.

NEOPLASIA OF THE SALIVARY GLANDS IN CHILDREN

Salivary gland tumors in children are uncommon, and the frequency of malignancy is different from that in adults. In a recent review of neoplasms in children by Schuller and McCabe,[28] 38 percent (149/428) were found to be malignant. They found that the distribution of various histologic types was consistent with that in the adult population (Table 20-7), with mucoepidermoid carcinoma being the most frequent and representing about 40 percent in the collective series.

The parotid gland is the most common

TABLE 20-7. SALIVARY GLAND NEOPLASMS IN
428 CHILDREN

Benign		Malignant	
Hemangioma	111	Mucoepidermoid carcinoma	73
Mixed tumor	94	Acinous cell carcinoma	18
"Vascular proliferative"	40	Undifferentiated carcinoma	14
Lymphangioma	18	Undifferentiated sarcoma	9
Lymphoepithelial tumor	3	Malignant mixed tumor	9
Cystadenoma	3	Adenocarcinoma	11
Warthin tumor	3	Adenoid cystic carcinoma	6
Plexiform neurofibroma	2	Squamous cell carcinoma	3
Xanthoma	2	Mesenchymal sarcoma	2
Neurilemmoma	1	Rhabdomyosarcoma	2
Adenoma	1	Malignant epithelial tumor	1
Lipoma	1	Ganglioneuroblastoma	1
Total	279	Total	149

(Schuller, D. E., and McCabe, B. F. 1977. Salivary gland neoplasms in children. Otolaryngolic Clinics of North America, 10:   399.)

site for neoplastic development in children, with a preponderance of benign soft tissue tumors of somatic tissue origin in the category of hemangioma and lymphangioma.

Children enjoy an appreciable immunity to neoplasia. The major salivary gland system participates in this phenomenon, and the minor salivary glands present an even higher immunity to both benign and malignant tumor development. The submandibular gland rarely manifests neoplasia. Fibrous tissue tumors and other benign mesenchymal derivatives, along with adenomas, are rare in occurrence. A not uncommon clinical entity occurring in childhood that must be differentiated from tumor of the parotid gland is chronic subacute parotitis and, lastly, foreign bodies. Differentiation is accomplished primarily by clinical examination.

The prognosis for malignant neoplasia of salivary gland origin in children is more favorable than in adults.

SUMMARY

Tumors of the salivary glands present a bewildering array of problems in diagnosis and management. A more rational approach to management of cancers of the parotid gland seems to be evolving, based upon careful retrospective analysis of the histopathology and biologic behaviour of these cancers, the incorporation of postoperative radiation therapy into the therapeutic program to complement radical surgery, and the appreciation of free-nerve grafting as an adjunctive procedure to improve quality of life for the patient. Improved success in the management of cancer arising in the submandibular and sublingual glands seems to be dependent upon an increased awareness of these conditions by surgeons operating in these areas and upon the application of aggressive surgical ablative procedures along with adjunctive radiation therapy. These principles apply as well to the ubiquitous cancers arising in the minor salivary glands.

REFERENCES

1. American Joint Committee for Cancer Staging and End Results Reporting. 1976. Manual for Staging of Cancer. American Joint Committee, Chicago.

2. Batsakis, J. G. 1974. Tumors of the Head and Neck. Clinical and Pathological Considerations. Williams, and Wilkins, Baltimore.

3. Beahrs, O. H., Woolner, L. B., Carveth, S. W., and Devine, K. D. 1960. Surgical management of parotid lesions. Review of 760 cases. American Medical Association Archives of Surgery, 80: 890.

4. Chaudhry, A. P., Vickers, R. A., and Gorlin, R. J. 1961. Intraoral minor salivary gland tumors. An analysis of 1,414 cases. Oral Surgery, Oral Medicine, and Oral Pathology, 14: 1194.

5. Conley, J. 1970. Concepts in Head and Neck Surgery. Georg Thieme, Stuttgart.

6. Conley, J. 1975. Salivary Glands and the Facial Nerve. Georg Thieme, Stuttgart.

7. Conley, J., and Dingman, D. L. 1974. Adenoid cystic carcinoma in the head and neck (cylindroma). Archives of Otolaryngology, 100: 81.

8. Conley, J., and Hamaker, R. C. 1975. Significance of facial paralysis in malignant tumors of the parotid gland. Archives of Otolaryngology, 101: 39.

9. Conley, J., Myers, E., and Cole, R. 1972. Analysis of 115 patients with tumors of the submandibular gland. Annals of Otology, Rhinology and Laryngology, 81: 323.

10. Davis, R. A., Anson, B. J., Budinger, J. M., and Kurth, L. 1956. Surgical anatomy of the facial nerve and parotid gland based upon a study of 350 cervicofacial halves. Surgery, Gynecology, and Obstetrics, 102: 384.

11. Dingman, R. O., and Grabb, W. C. 1962. Surgical anatomy of the mandibular ramus of the facial nerve based on the dissection of 100 facial halves. Plastic and Reconstroctive Surgery, 29: 266.

12. Eneroth, C. M. 1971. Salivary gland tumors in the parotid gland, submandibular gland, and the palate region. Cancer, 27: 1415.

13. Fletcher, G. H. 1976. Textbook of Radiotherapy. 2nd edn. Lea and Febinger, Philadelphia.

14. Fletcher, G. H., Tapley, N. du. V., and Patrico, M. B. 1975. Irradiation—Radiotherapists concept. In Conley, J., Ed.: Salivary Glands and the Facial Nerve, Georg Thieme, Stuttgart, 1975, 283.

15. Foote, F. W., Jr., and Frazell, E. L. 1953. Tumors of the major salivary glands. Cancer, 6: 1065.

16. Frazell, E. L. 1954. Clinical aspects of tumors of the major salivary glands. Cancer, 7: 637.

17. Gross, C. W., Nakamura, T., Maguda, T., et al. 1974. Malignant minor salivary gland tumors—a report of 32 cases. Canadian J Otolaryngology, 3: 56.

18. Hoopes, J. E. 1973. Primary tumors of the salivary glands and neck. In Grabb, W. C., and Smith J. W., Eds.: Plastic Surgery: A Concise Guide to Clinical Practice. 20th edn. Little Brown, Boston.

19. Johns, M. E. 1977. Salivary Gland Tumors: Therapy Based on Clinical-Pathologic Diagnosis. American Academy of Otolaryngology, Rochester, MN.

20. McCormack, L. J., Cauldwell, E. W., and Anson, B. J. 1945. The surgical anatomy of the facial nerve with special reference to the parotid gland. Surgery, Gynecology and Obstetrics, 80: 620.

21. McKenzie, J. 1948. The parotid gland in relation to the facial nerve. Journal of Anatomy 82: 183.

22. McWhorter, G. L. 1917. The relations of the superficial and deep lobes of the parotid gland to the ducts and to the facial nerve. Anatomical Record, 12: 149.

23. Mustard, R. A., and Anderson, W. 1964. Malignant tumors of the parotid. Annals of Surgery, 159: 291.

24. Perzin, K. H., Gullane, P., and Clairmont, A. C. 1978. Adenoid cystic carcinomas arising in salivary glands. A correlation of histologic features and clinical course. Cancer, 42: 265.

25. Rankow, R. M., and Mignogna, F. 1969. Cancer of the sublingual salivary gland. American Journal of Surgery, 118: 790.

26. Robinson, D. W., and Masters, F. W. 1977. Surgical treatment of disease of the salivary glands. In Converse, J. M., Ed.: Reconstructive Plastic Surgery, 2nd edn, W. B. Saunders Philadelphia, 2521.

27. Rosenfeld, L., Sessions, D. G., McSwain, B., and Graves, H. V., Jr. 1966. Malignant tumors of salivary gland origin: A 37-year review of 184 cases. Annals of Surgery, 163: 726.

28. Schuller, D. E., and McCabe, B. F. 1977. Salivary gland neoplasms in children. Otolaryngolic Clinics of North America 10: 399.

29. Simons, J. N., Beahrs, O. H., and Woolner, L. B. 1964. Tumors of the submaxillary gland. American Journal of Surgery, 108: 485.

30. Spiro, R. H., Huvos, A. G., and Strong, E. W. 1975. Cancer of the parotid gland. A clincopathologic study of 289 primary cases. American Journal of Surgery, 130: 452.

31. Spiro, R. H., Huvos, A. G., Berk, R., and Strong, E. W. 1978. Mucoepidermoid carcinoma of salivary gland origin. A clinicopathologic study of 367 cases. American Journal of Surgery, 136: 461.

32. State, D., and Grage, T. B. 1966 Surgical treatment of parotid tumors. In Current Problems in Surgery. Year Book Medical Publishers, Chicago, 1.

33. Stewart, F. W., Foote, F. W., and Becker, W. F. 1945. Mucoepidermoid tumors of salivary glands. Annals of Surgery 6, 122: 820.

34. Stuteville, O. H., and Corley, R. D. 1967. Surgical management of tumors of intraoral minor salivary glands. Report of eighty cases. Cancer, 20: 1578.

35. Thackray, A. C., and Lucas, R. B. 1974. Atlas of Tumor Pathology. Second Series Fascicle 10. Tumors of the Major Salivary Glands. Armed Forces Institute of Pathology, Washington, D.C.

36. Thackray, A. C., and Sobin, L. H. 1972. Histological Typing of Salivary Gland Tumours. World Health Organization, Geneva.

21 | Cancer of the External Auditory Canal, Middle Ear, and Mastoid

John S. Lewis, M.D.

INTRODUCTION

Cancers of the external auditory meatus, middle ear, and mastoid are quite rare. This is fortunate, since most are diagnosed late in the course of the disease. It has been noted that many of the patients with tumors in this anatomic area have a long history of purulent otitis media and have become accustomed to the discomfort, inconvenience, and occasional pain that characterizes chronic infection. Only when the symptoms become more pronounced or a new symptom, such as facial paralysis, supervenes do the patients present for treatment.

A lack of awareness on the part of the general physician that cancer can occur in the ear may further delay diagnosis. Even otolaryngologists who have an awareness of the disease may have never seen cancer in this area and may not maintain a high index of suspicion about the possibility that their patient may have malignant, rather than chronic inflammatory, disease.

The anatomic location of the temporal bone with respect to its relationships to major arterial and venous structures and the central nervous system may be somewhat intimidating to the surgeon. The substantial degree of cosmetic and functional crippling expected from the surgical procedure may add a negative emotional factor to the choice of management of the disease. However, with a chance for cure in the patient with moderately advanced cancer and with adequate rehabilitation possible, an aggressive approach to the management of cancer

of the temporal bone should be considered. The author's personal experience with the management of more than 150 patients with primary carcinoma of the ear forms the basis of this chapter.

ANATOMY

The human ear consists of three parts: the external ear, the middle ear, and the inner ear. The external ear, or pinna, is the ear's sound-collecting organ, directing sound into the external auditory canal to the tympanic membrane. In the middle ear, sound is magnified on its way to the inner ear. The latter is confined to the temporal bone and contains the cochlea (the neuroreceptor of the sound waves), and the semicircular canals, which help to control the balance of the body. Except for the auricle and soft-tissue portion of the external auditory canal, the ear is enclosed within the confines of the temporal bone of the skull.

Temporal Bone

The temporal bone forms part of the middle and posterior fossae of the skull and contributes to the base of the skull and its lateral wall. It is divided into four parts: squamous, mastoid, petrous, and tympanic.

The squamous portion has attached to it laterally the temporalis muscle and the masseter muscle, and its medial surface is directed towards the middle cranial fossa with a deep sulcus for the middle meningeal artery. The mastoid process has attached to it the auricular and occipital muscles. The principle bone is the downward-directed mastoid process, which contains air cells (Fig. 21-1). On the medial surface, there is a deep groove for the sigmoid (transverse) venous sinus (Fig. 21-2).

The petrous portion of the temporal bone, or petrous pyramid, contains the sensory organs of the inner ear, and its base is united with the mastoid. The 7th and 8th cranial nerves enter the petrous portion through the internal auditory canal; the facial nerve exits via the stylomastoid foramen of the mastoid (Fig. 21-2). The internal carotid artery traverses the foramen lacerum at its apex. The internal jugular vein enters the skull at its base, its bony canal forming part of the anterior-inferior wall of the middle ear (Fig. 21-2). The anterior surface of the petrous pyramid forms part of the middle cranial fossa, and in the middle of this surface is the arcuate eminence, which is formed chiefly by the underlying superior semicircular canal. The arcuate eminence is a key landmark, and in temporal bone resection the deepest cut is carried out just medial to it, with transection of the petrous pyramid at this point. Just lateral and anterior to this eminence is the tegmen tympani, which forms the roof of the tympanic cavity. The posterior surface of the petrous pyramid faces the posterior cranial fossa and is bounded above by the sulcus of the superior petrosal sinus. The inferior portion of the petrous pyramid forms—with the occipital bone—the jugular foramen. The lateral part of the foramen contains the

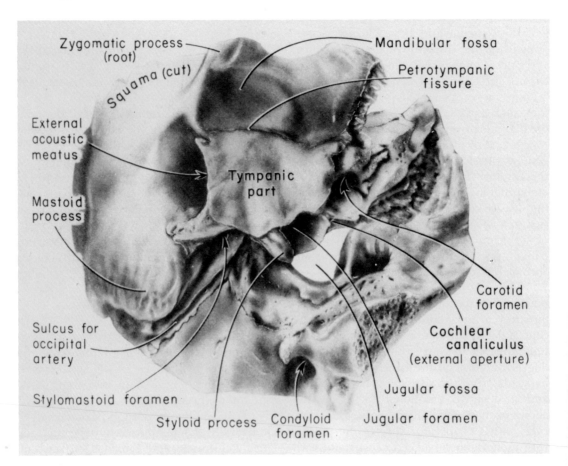

Fig. 21-1. Right temporal bone, inferior surface, with related occipital bone. (Anson, B. J., and Donaldson, J. A. 1973. Surgical Anatomy of the Temporal Bone and Ear. W. B. Saunders, Philadelphia.)

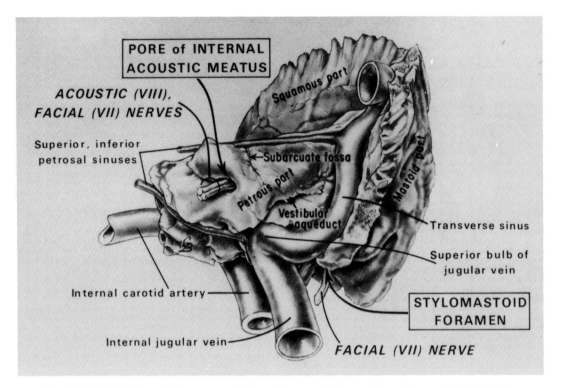

Fig. 21-2. Medial view of the temporal bone. (Anson, B. J., and Donaldson, J. A. 1973. Surgical Anatomy of the Temporal Bone and Ear. W. B. Saunders, Philadelphia.)

sigmoid portion of the lateral sinus, which joins with the jugular vein; the medial part is occupied by the inferior petrosal sinus, the glossopharyngeal nerve, and the vagus nerve.

The tympanic portion of the temporal bone is the smallest part and forms the anterior, inferior, and a part of the posterior wall of the external auditory canal. A coronal section of the temporal bone (Fig. 21-3) illustrates the relationship between the external ear, the external auditory canal, the middle ear, and the inner ear. The relationships are important in that tumor arising from the external ear may involve the auditory canal and mastoid. Cancer arising from the auditory canal usually involves the middle ear and may extend up through the tegmen into the middle cranial fossa. Cancer arising in the middle ear may involve the mastoid as well as the intracranial structures.

The eustachian tube extends from the tympanic orifice on the anterior wall of the tympanic cavity inferiorly to the pharynx. In the adult, the tube is usually 37 mm long, its lateral one-third is bony, and its medial two-thirds consists of cartilage. The tube terminates in the nasopharynx just anterior to the fossa of Rosenmüller. Cancer arising in the fossa of Rosenmüller in the nasopharynx may extend up the eustachian tube to involve the middle ear and auditory canal. Rarely does cancer migrate from the middle ear down the eustachian tube to the nasopharynx.

Although primary carcinoma of the eustachian tube has been described in the medical literature, it is most likely that carcinoma involving the eustachian tube arises either in the nasopharynx or in the middle ear, with direct extension into the eustachian tube.

External Ear

The external ear, also known as the auricle or pinna, consists of fibrocartilage closely invested by an adherent layer of skin. The lobule is the only site of subcutaneous tissue.

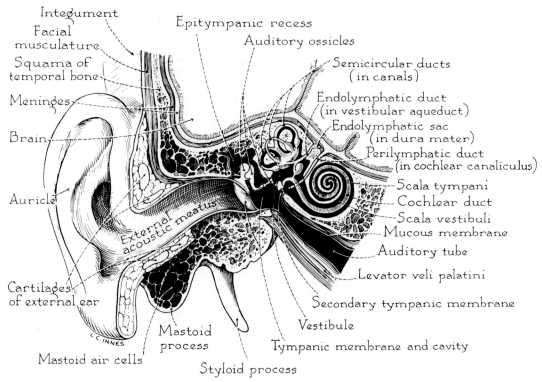

Integument
Facial
musculature.
Squama of
temporal bone
Meninges
Brain
Auricle
External
acoustic meatus
Cartilages
of external ear
L.C.INNES
Mastoid air cells
Mastoid
process
Styloid process

Epitympanic recess
Auditory ossicles
Semicircular ducts
(in canals)
Endolymphatic duct
(in vestibular aqueduct)
Endolymphatic sac
(in dura mater)
Perilymphatic duct
(in cochlear canaliculus)
Scala tympani
Cochlear duct
Scala vestibuli
Mucous membrane
Auditory tube
Levator veli palatini
Secondary tympanic membrane
Vestibule
Tympanic membrane and cavity

PARTS OF THE EAR. A VERTICAL SECTION IN THE PLANE OF THE EXTERNAL ACOUSTIC MEATUS AND THE AUDITORY TUBE. SEMISCHEMATIC.

Fig. 21-3. Cross section of the ear. (Anson, B. J., and Donaldson, J. A. 1973. Surgical Anatomy of the Temporal Bone and Ear. W. B. Saunders, Philadelphia.)

Three extrinsic muscles arise from the galea aponeurotica and insert into the pinna. The external ear has six intrinsic muscles, which are very rudimentary. A deep concavity, the cavum conchae, leads into the external auditory meatus.

The external auditory meatus, or external auditory canal, measures about 3.5 cm in length. The medial two-thirds has a complete bony wall lying within the temporal bone; the outer one-third of the canal is composed of fibrocartilage, which is continuous laterally with that of the auricle. The canal is lined by skin, which is closely adherent to the perichondrium and periosteum of the auditory canal. Laterally, the skin contains hair follicles, sebaceous glands, and ceruminous glands. The external auditory canal is related anteriorly to the temporomandibular joint. The inferior wall is related to the parotid gland, and the posterior wall

separates the canal from the mastoid air cells. The squamous portion of the temporal bone forms the superior wall and separates the canal from the middle cranial fossa. The skin of the external auditory canal is supplied by the auriculotemporal branch of the mandibular nerve, along with branches from the glossopharyngeal and vagus nerves. Lymphatics from the external auditory canal drain anteriorly to the preauricular nodes, posteriorly to the mastoid lymph nodes, and inferiorly to the subdigastric lymph nodes. Metastasis from cancer involving the auricle or the external auditory canal may involve any of these lymph nodes, particularly the subdigastric lymph nodes.

Middle Ear

The middle ear or tympanic cavity has a roof, a floor, and anterior, posterior, medial, and lateral walls, all of which may be invaded by cancer arising in the middle ear. The tympanic cavity communicates with the nasopharynx by means of the eustachian tube; in the opposite direction, the epitympanic recess passes from the middle ear to the tympanic antrum, which communicates with the mastoid portion of the temporal bone. The middle ear is lined with mucous membrane and is shaped like a very short cylinder with concave ends, the lateral aspect being formed by the tympanic membrane and the medial aspect by the lateral wall of the labyrinth. The roof of the middle ear (or tegmen) is a thin plate of bone, which separates the middle ear from the middle cranial fossa and which can be destroyed by cancer, resulting in intracranial invasion. The floor is intimately associated with the fossa of the internal jugular vein and it also gives rise to the styloid process, which is a key landmark in temporal bone resection. Deep to the styloid process lies the internal carotid artery, which should be avoided during temporal bone resection. The fallopian canal, containing the facial nerve, is located in the posterior or mastoid wall. Invasion of the facial nerve by cancer in the middle ear or in the mastoid can produce facial paralysis as an early sign of cancer. The facial nerve can also be the pathway for perineural invasion and spread of tumor into the posterior cranial fossa. Openings from the canal transmit the chorda tympani nerve, which traverses the tympanic cavity and is related to the tympanic membrane. The chorda tympani nerve contains autonomic fibers to the submaxillary gland and sensory fibers from the anterior two-thirds of the tongue.

The anterior, or carotid, wall of the middle ear communicates by the eustachian tube with the nasopharynx. This wall consists of a thin plate of bone, which is pierced by the carotidotympanic nerve, and separates the tympanic cavity from the carotid artery. More laterally, the anterior wall is related to the parotid gland and the temporomandibular joint. The medial wall is related to the inner ear, and inferiorly there is a promontory produced by the bulging basal turn of the cochlea. The tympanic plexus lies upon this surface. Below and behind the promontory is the oval window closed by the footplate of the stapes.

Traversing the tympanic cavity and extending from the tympanic membrane (which is the lateral boundary of the middle ear) to the medial wall are the auditory ossicles: the malleus, incus, and stapes. The malleus is firmly attached to the tympanic membrane and the stapes to the vestibular window, and both articulate with the incus. Sound waves are transmitted from the tympanic membrane through the ossicles to the perilymph of the inner ear. Destruction of the tympanic membrane and ossicles by cancer will result in a conductive hearing loss.

The main sensory supply of the middle ear is Jacobson's nerve, a branch of the glossopharyngeal nerve. It is not known whether lymphatic channels actually exist in the middle ear, and cancer in this region usually spreads by direct extension rather than by lymphatics.

EPIDEMIOLOGY AND ETIOLOGY

According to all published reports, cancer of the ear is a very rare condition. Towson and Shofstall[19] have pointed out that the proportion of cancer of the middle ear and mastoid to all otologic pathologic conditions is 1:5,000 to 1:20,000. Tod,[18] quoting from the records of the London Hospital, where 200,000 cases are seen annually, found only one case of cancer of the ear. Lodge[11] and his co-workers found six cases of cancer of the temporal bone in a population of 1 million people and estimated that 0.006 percent of living persons suffer from aural cancer at a given time. Schall[17] found only 15 patients with neoplasms in a 12-year period at the Massachusetts Eye and Ear Infirmary out of 90,040 patients seen with pathologic conditions of the ear. Furstenberg[8] found cancer of the middle ear in only 2 out of 40,000 patients treated by the Department of Otolaryngology at the University of Michigan Medical School. Among 212,000 cases of aural disease seen between 1905 and 1924 at the Manhattan Eye, Ear and Throat Hospital in New York, Robinson[15] found a diagnosis of tumor in only 48, or a ratio of 1:4,000.

Cancer of the middle ear and mastoid has approximately the same sex incidence, although cancer of the auditory canal is twice as common in females as in males. In the author's experience[10a] with 100 reported cases, the median age for carcinoma of the external auditory canal, middle ear, and mastoid was 55 years, the age span being 9 months to 75 years.

Cancer of the external ear is associated with thermal trauma, especially exposure to the actinic rays of the sun and frostbite. As a result, the most common carcinoma of the external ear is basal cell carcinoma, which can erode into the external auditory meatus and mastoid process. Although cancer of the external auditory meatus is often associated with chronic otitis media, there is no hard data to support the theory that the chronic drainage is the etiologic factor. Lodge and his associates[11] consider that cancer of the middle ear, mastoid, and auditory canal are comparable to Marjolin's ulcer with its chronic discharge producing cellular irritation that develops into cancer. Coachman[5] has reported a patient with squamous carcinoma of the middle ear secondary to cholesteatoma. I have found four cases of cholesteatoma of the middle ear associated with cancer.

In 1952, Aub[1] reported a case of epidermoid carcinoma of the middle ear, which appeared in a radium dial painter 31 years following exposure. Beal[2] in 1965 discovered another case of epidermoid carcinoma of the middle ear and mastoid in a radium dial painter and mentioned that there have been eight similar cases. Ruben[16] in 1977 reported a case of temporal bone carcinoma following radiation therapy to the head and neck area. He stated that the U.S. Armed Forces Institute of Pathology reported at least one case in which a malignant tumor occurring in the temporal bone was probably radiation-induced.

I have treated three primary carcinomas of the mastoid bone, two epidermoid carcinomas, and one angiosarcoma. Clairmont and Conley[4] reported only one case of a carcinoma primary in the mastoid bone, as compared to 61 cases of malignancy of the external auditory canal and 25 cases of cancer of the middle ear.

CLASSIFICATION

Zizmor and Noyek[20] have attempted to present a serviceable classification of the tumors and other osseous disorders of the temporal bone, and I have added additional tumors to the classification (Table 21-1).

Epithelial Cancers

Cancer of the auditory canal, middle ear, and mastoid is almost invariably squamous cell carcinoma, with some 86 percent of cancers being of the epidermoid type. Basal cell carcinomas constitute 8 percent, with adenocarcinomas and malignant melanomas comprising 2 percent. Spindle cell sarcomas and embryonal rhabdomyosarcomas each comprise 1 percent of the total. The gross features of squamous carcinoma are a large granulomatous mass filling the auditory canal and middle ear, and ulceration, bleeding, and secondary infection. Cervical metastases are present in approximately 10 percent of cases and usually involve the parotid node or the subdigastric lymph node.

Basal cell carcinoma may present as a rodent ulcer on the external ear, with erosion into the auditory canal or mastoid process. Rarely, basal cell carcinomas may arise in the external auditory meatus. Once bone is invaded by basal cell carcinoma, the behavior of the cancer is similar to that of a squamous cell carcinoma. Metastases from basal cell carcinoma are rare, and management consists of radical surgery and postoperative radiation therapy.

Malignant melanoma most commonly

TABLE 21-1. TUMORS OF THE TEMPORAL BONE

BENIGN TUMORS

   Epithelial-primary cholesteatoma

   Mesenchymal

      Jugulotympanic paraganglioma (glomus tumor, chemodectoma)

      Osteoma

      Hemangioma

      Neurogenic tumors

      Xanthoma

      Giant cell tumor

      Benign osteoblastoma

      Ceruminoma

MALIGNANT TUMORS

   Primary

      Epithelial

         Squamous cell carcinoma

         Basal cell carcinoma

         Adenocarcinoma (usually of ceruminous gland origin)

         Melanoma

      Mesenchymal

         Sarcoma

         Multiple myeloma

         Malignant xanthoma

         Angiosarcoma (hemangioendothelioma)

   Secondary

      Direct extension from:

         Nasopharynx

         External ear

         Parotid

         Temporomandibular joint

         Meningioma

      Distant metastasis from:

         Kidney

         Lung

         Prostate

         Breast

         Uterus

(Based on data in Zizmor, J., and Noyek, A. 1969. Tumors and other disorders of the temporal bone. Seminars in Roentgenology, 4: 2.)

occurs on the external ear, usually on the posterior surface. It has a great propensity to metastasize early to cervical nodes, so management must include radical excision of the primary tumor as well as radical neck dissection. I have had a case of malignant melanoma in a newborn whose mother had malignant melanomatosis. It is postulated that transplacental transportation of melanoma cells occurred, with implant into the middle ear.

Ceruminomas arise anywhere in the external auditory canal and generally present as firm, yellow, smooth tumors with dilated blood vessels on the surface. These may fill the external auditory meatus. Pulec, et al.[14] in 1963 reported a series of 21 cases from the Mayo Clinic and added an additional 15 cases in their report in 1977.[13a] Five types of ceruminoma have been described: adenoma, adenocarcinoma, adenocystic carcinoma, mixed tumor, and mucoepidermoid carcinoma. Malignant tumors outnumber benign tumors by about 2.5 to 2, and adenocystic carcinoma is by far the most common tumor. Men and women are affected about equally, and the median age is 48 years, although those with benign tumors average 57 years of age when first diagnosed. The presenting symptom of those with malignant tumors is ear pain, which becomes more severe as the disease progresses. Patients also present with a mass in the auditory canal, hearing loss, occasional discharge, tinnitus, and facial paralysis. Radiographic evidence of bony erosion of the auditory canal, mastoid, and petrous apex is present only in the far-advanced cases. Most reported cases have been treated by local excision, irradiation, or both. Local recurrence is a rule in these malignant tumors. Radical surgery, therefore, is mandatory. Pulec has pointed out that a 5-year cure is not a valid yardstick, and a 20-year cure is perhaps the only measure of success in eradicating this disease because of the indolent nature of the adenoid cystic carcinoma. In his series, from the onset of symptoms to death from disease, the patients lived an average of 16.5 years.

Malignant Mesenchymal Tumors

Primary sarcomas of the temporal bone are rare. A comprehensive review of the literature by Naufal[13] revealed only 211 reported cases. In 89 cases, the histologic picture was that of undifferentiated sarcoma including spindle cell, round cell, and anaplastic types. Sixty-four cases, all occurring in young children, were reported as embryonal rhabdomyosarcomas. There were 17 cases of fibrosarcoma, 7 of which originated in the nerve sheath. Tumors of the bone included 12 osteogenic sarcomas and 7 Ewing sarcomas. There were 8 tumors of vascular origin, 6 primary lymphomas, 5 myxosarcomas, 1 chondrosarcoma, 1 liposarcoma, and 1 meningeal sarcoma. I have reported[10a] an additional case of chondromyxosarcoma of the middle ear, osteogenic sarcoma of the temporal bone, and 2 cases of early aural rhabdomyosarcoma. Sarcomas other than the embryonal rhabdomyosarcomas are best handled by temporal bone resection. Radiation has little or no effect on the progression of this type of tumor.

Angiosarcoma, or hemangioendothelioma, is a rare malignant neoplasm of blood vessels; it consists of diffuse proliferation of atypical anastomosing capillaries and hyperplastic endothelial cells. I have recently treated a case of angiosarcoma of the mastoid. Attempts to differentiate angiosarcoma and hemangioendothelioma in the literature have led to confusion and have not satisfactorily produced a classification with prognostic value. In this regard, classification of hemangioendothelioma by grade of anaplasia, as formulated by Unni, et al.,[19a] seems the most reasonable indicator of prognosis.

Embryonal rhabdomyosarcoma usually arises in the middle ear and rapidly invades the middle cranial fossa through the facial nerve, tegmen tympani, and the mastoid process. Distant metastases are common, especially to bone and lung. Treatment of this variety of cancer must be by aggressive radiation therapy and chemotherapy. Cancer arising in this area has a propensity to extend intracranially through the tegmen tympani or inferiorly into the base of the skull or to migrate down the eustachian tube into the nasopharynx. Rarely does it extend medially into the petrous portion of the temporal bone. Preauricular extension can also occur through the external auditory meatus to involve the parotid gland.

Multiple myeloma is a disease of the hemopoietic cells of the bone marrow, and small translucent areas are frequently seen on radiographs of the skull and mastoid. Diagnosis is made on the basis of increased levels of serum protein and globulin and the appearance of Bence-Jones protein in the urine. The bone marrow is diagnostic with the appearance of plasmacytes, myelocytes, and erythroblasts. Chemotherapy and radiotherapy to discrete lesions is the treatment of choice.

Secondary Tumors of the Mastoid and Middle Ear

Secondary tumors may reach the temporal bone either by direct extension or by distant metastases. Direct extension of cancer of the deep lobe of the parotid gland into the auditory canal and middle ear is not unusual. The patient may present with Bell's palsy, which may not be properly investigated. The deep lobe of the parotid gland is palpated and if a mass is felt, a needle biopsy may identify the tumor. Cancer of the nasopharynx may extend up the eustachian tube into the middle ear and present as a friable, bleeding tumor that ruptures through the tympanic membrane. Radiotherapy is the treatment of choice but is usually only palliative at this stage of disease. Extensive cancer of the external ear frequently invades the mastoid and offers a poor prognosis for cure even using surgery and radiotherapy. Rarely do malignant tumors of the temporomandibular joint invade the middle ear and mastoid. They are usually malignant synoviomas.

The most common cancer to metastasize through the blood stream to the temporal bone is the hypernephroma. Other temporal bone metastases are from long bone, breast, prostate, uterus, and colon. Ear pain is a common first symptom and may present before the primary lesion is discovered. Neurologic symptoms rapidly follow because of the involvement of cranial nerves. Radiotherapy may relieve pain and give palliation to the patient.

PATIENT EVALUATION

Cancer of the ear has an insidious onset. Cancer of the external auditory canal and middle ear is usually associated with chronic inflammatory disease. The patient usually presents with a chronically infected auditory canal that fails to respond to antibiotics and local medication. Bleeding frequently supervenes, with a bloody discharge mixed with the mucopurulent material. Hearing loss occurs with the appearance of otorrhea and is one of the earlier signs. Pain is frequently associated with infection and bone erosion. When the middle and inner ear is involved, vertigo and facial paralysis may occur, and these symptoms usually indicate advanced cancer. Occasionally, however, cancer of the parotid gland may invade the external auditory canal and middle ear and present initially as facial paralysis. Many patients are diagnosed initially as having chronic inflammatory disease or choleastoma on routine x-ray examinations. Occasionally, middle ear and mastoid malignant tumors are associated with choleastomas. These cases are frequently subjected to mastoidectomy, and at the time of surgery the middle ear and mastoid are found to be filled with friable, bleeding tumor tissue and the pathologic confirmation of cancer is returned after the surgery.

On physical examination, the external auditory canal may be filled with a friable, bleeding mass that prevents further examination of the ear. The mass may represent either tumor or secondary infection with granulation tissue. Biopsy of the mass in the external auditory canal must be carried out early in order to establish the diagnosis in a timely manner.

External swelling in the preauricular region due to invasion from the parotid gland and associated lymph nodes may be noted. Cervical metastases may occur in the postauricular nodes and upper jugular nodes as well as in the parotid nodes. Rarely do the lymph node metastases appear before the primary site is detected. If nodes present in the posterior triangle associated with a tumor in the middle ear and auditory canal, one must suspect a primary tumor in the nasopharynx that may have migrated up the eustachian tube. The nasopharynx must be carefully examined in all cases.

Routine mastoid x-rays are helpful, since approximately 40 percent of cases demonstrate bone destruction. Polytomography is a much more valuable technique in detecting bone destruction and the extent of disease in the auditory canal and middle ear. If signs and symptoms suggest intracranial extension, CT scans are of inestimable value in determining the extent of intracranial disease. Carotid angiography, with the venous phase, is helpful in determining involvement of the sigmoid sinus. A patient presenting with a boring pain in the ear without any clinical findings should have the benefit of an x-ray examination. Metastatic carcinoma from the kidney, breast, lung, or prostate may be detected as an osteolytic process in the temporal bone. Rarely does a patient with lymphoma present with a bleeding mass in the auditory canal.

TREATMENT

Radical surgery and radiation therapy are the accepted methods of treatment of cancer of the middle ear, mastoid, and external auditory canal. There are advantages of using radiation therapy along with surgery, but the timing is important. Because the cancer involves a bony box at the base of the skull and extends intracranially readily, early radical treatment holds the only chance of curing the patient. Subsequent treatment when cancer extends beyond the middle ear and mastoid is strictly palliative.

Surgical Treatment

The surgical procedure carried out will depend on clinical and roentgenographic evidence of the extent of tumor involvement (Fig. 21-4).

Excision of the auditory canal is the procedure of choice if the tumor is confined to the membranous auditory canal and external auditory meatus. There should be at least a 0.5 cm margin between the lesion and the tympanic membrane with no x-ray evidence of invasion of the mastoid. A U-shaped incision is carried out, with the base above (Fig. 21-5). Skin, superficial fascia, temporalis muscle, and the superficial lobe of the parotid gland are transected, and the

flap is elevated from below. The external auditory canal is transected at the level of the external meatus, and the flap is elevated for a distance of 4 cm above the external auditory canal. A simple mastoidectomy is carried out, with exposure of the facial canal. The external auditory canal is excised with preservation of the facial nerve and in close proximity to the temporomandibular joint anteriorly and inferiorly to the level of the tympanic membrane (Figs. 21-6 and 21-7). A split-thickness skin graft of .016 inch is taken from the thigh, sutured circumferentially, and inverted into the auditory canal so as to form the lining of a new auditory canal (Fig. 21-8). Vaseline gauze immersed in bacitracin ointment is packed

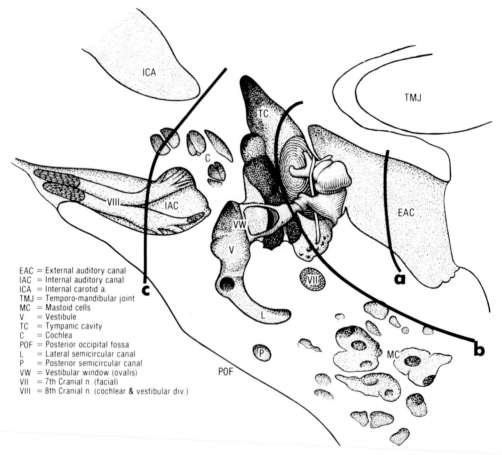

EAC = External auditory canal
IAC = Internal auditory canal
ICA = Internal carotid a.
TMJ = Temporo-mandibular joint
MC = Mastoid cells
V = Vestibule
TC = Tympanic cavity
C = Cochlea
POF = Posterior occipital fossa
L = Lateral semicircular canal
P = Posterior semicircular canal
VW = Vestibular window (ovalis)
VII = 7th Cranial n. (facial)
VIII = 8th Cranial n. (cochlear & vestibular div.)

Fig. 21-4. Cross section of temporal bone showing extent of resection: a, excision of auditory canal; b, partial temporal bone resection; c, subtotal resection of temporal bone (after Gacek, R. R. and Goodman, M. 1977. Management of malignancy of the temporal bone. Laryngoscope, 87: 1622).

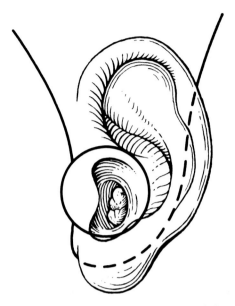

Fig. 21-5. Incisions for resection of the external auditory canal. (Reprinted by permission of the publisher, from Ballantyne, J. Ear. 3rd edn. In Rob, C., and Smith, R., Eds.: Operative Surgery Series. London: Butterworths (Publishers) Ltd. 1976.)

into the canal and is left in place 4 to 6 weeks.

Partial temporal bone resection may be used in the rare case in which the cancer involves the bony auditory canal and impinges on the tympanic membrane but does not involve the middle ear and mastoid. A similar incision to that described above is carried out and a simple mastoidectomy is performed with exposure and mobilization of the facial nerve from its canal. The auditory canal, tympanic membrane, malleus, and incus are removed along with the temporomandibular joint, and the defect grafted with a split-thickness skin graft.

Subtotal resection of the temporal bone is necessary when the cancer involves the middle ear and mastoid. The petrous process of the temporal bone lies in a venous lake surrounded (1) posteriorly and inferiorly by the lateral sinus including its sigmoid portion, which extends downward to the jugular bulb at the base of the skull; (2) superiorly and inferiorly by the petrosal venous sinuses; and (3) medially by the cavernous sinus. The carotid artery courses through the anteromedial aspect of the petrous tip and is seldom encountered in the resection. The facial nerve is sectioned both in the temporal bone and in the parotid gland. Occasionally the vagus nerve is traumatized at the skull base during the resection. In transection of the petrous process, the cochlea and semicircular canals are usually removed.

Temporal bone resection is a combination of intracranial and extracranial surgical en bloc resection of bone infiltrated by cancer (Fig. 21-9). This includes resection of the involved portions of the external auditory canal, middle ear, mastoid, and petrous process along with the temporomandibular joint, parotid gland, and base of zygoma. The initial exposure of dura and petrous pyramid is through a temporal craniotomy. The external ear and external auditory meatus are displaced superiorly through a U-shaped incision that exposes the squamous portion of the temporal bone, the base of the zygoma, and the temporomandibular joint. The muscular attachments to the mastoid are transected and a partial parotidectomy is performed to give clear definition to the styloid process and the temporomandibular joint. The inclusion of a cuff of parotid gland is especially important in anteriorly placed lesions. The facial nerve in the parotid gland may be tagged in its distal portion in order that facial-hypoglossal anastomosis may be performed either at the termination of the resection or at another sitting. The styloid process is a key landmark, for deep to it lies the internal carotid artery. The styloid process is transected along with its muscular attachments. The base of the zygoma is sectioned, and the neck of the mandible severed with a Gigli saw. The temporal muscle is preserved for coverage of dura. A temporal craniectomy is carried out. A high-speed air drill with a large cutting burr is utilized to expose the lateral sinus through the mastoid process and to trace it to the jugular bulb level. Between 60 and 100 ml of cerebrospinal fluid is withdrawn from previously placed malle-

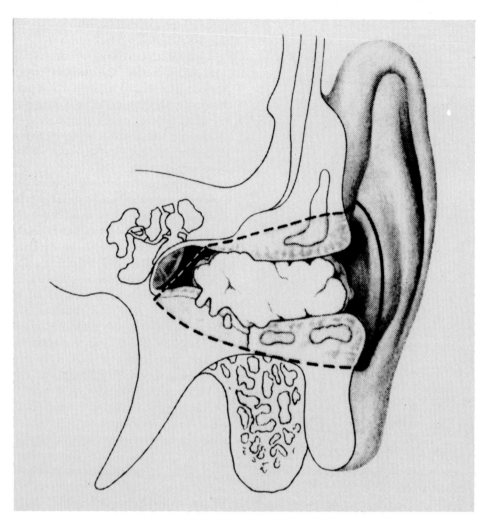

Fig. 21-6. Extent of resection of the external auditory canal. (Reprinted by permission of the publisher, from Ballantyne, J. Ear. 3rd edn. In Rob, C., and Smith, R., Eds.: Operative Surgery Series. London: Butterworths (Publishers) Ltd. 1976.)

able spinal needles to allow the dura to be separated from the underlying petrous bone. The path of least resistance for cancer extending from the middle ear is through the thin roof of the tegmen tympani into the middle cranial fossa. If dura is involved, it should be freed from the petrous roof with electrocautery and subsequently resected as a separate specimen. The dural defect is repaired with temporalis fascia. Occasionally the tumor has extended into the base of the skull or into the brain and is unresectable; this area should be marked with silver clips for postoperative radiotherapy. The Stryker saw is then utilized to cut through the petrosa lateral to the carotid

canal and medial to the arcuate eminence. The transection is completed with a curved chisel. Bleeding is controlled, and the dura is carefully scrutinized for tears. Temporal muscle is mobilized and rotated over the dura. The defect is covered either with a split-thickness skin graft or a posterior based scalp flap rotated into the defect. A lateral tarsorrhaphy is then carried out to protect the cornea.

In cases in which the entire external ear must be sacrificed or because of extensive preoperative radiotherapy the vitality of the external ear is jeopardized, either of two methods of wound closure is recommended: a posterior based scalp flap (Fig. 21-10)

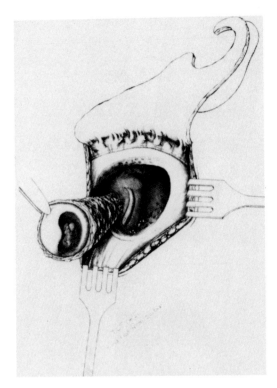

Fig. 21-7. Mobilized auditory canal, mastoid defect with exposed facial nerve before transection. (Reprinted by permission of the publisher, from Ballantyne, J. Ear. 3rd edn. In Rob, C., and Smith, R., Eds.: Operative Surgery Series. London: Butterworths (Publishers) Ltd. 1976.)

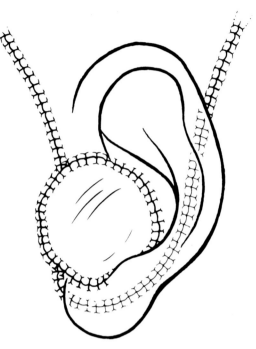

Fig. 21-8. Split-thickness skin graft lining ear canal defect. (Reprinted by permission of the publisher, from Ballantyne, J. Ear. 3rd edn. In Rob, C., and Smith, R., Eds.: Operative Surgery Series. London: Butterworths (Publishers) Ltd. 1976.)

with a split-thickness graft from the thigh covering the posterior donor defect, or a bipedicle scalp flap (Fig. 21-11). Either method has given satisfactory coverage and is particularly useful in control or prevention of cerebrospinal fluid leaks. In the event that the external ear must be amputated with the specimen, a prosthetic ear may be utilized (see Ch. 9).

LIMITATIONS OF SURGERY

The judgment of the surgeon as to the surgical procedure to be selected for an individual case must be based on clinical findings, biopsy results, x-ray studies (including mastoid films, tomograms, angiogram, and CT scan) plus the age and medical condition of the patient. The dura in the geriatric patient is likely to be more adherent to overlying bone and thinner and to have vessels more likely to rupture.

The decision to operate an early lesion confined to the auditory canal is relatively simple, except that a special effort should be made to preserve the facial nerve. In my group of 100 cases,[10a] it was found that preoperatively the tumor had extended beyond the temporal bone in 20 percent of the cases and that the margins were not free of disease even with the sacrifice of dura and lateral sinus and rarely temporal lobe; in addition, postoperative radiotherapy did little to control the disease in this 20 percent of cases. An additional 10 percent had x-ray evidence of confinement of the cancer to the temporal bone, but at surgery the cancer was found not to be resectable because of extension to the base of the skull. Even with approximately a 70 percent resectability, the local recurrence rate was 40 percent. The use of postoperative radiotherapy, there-

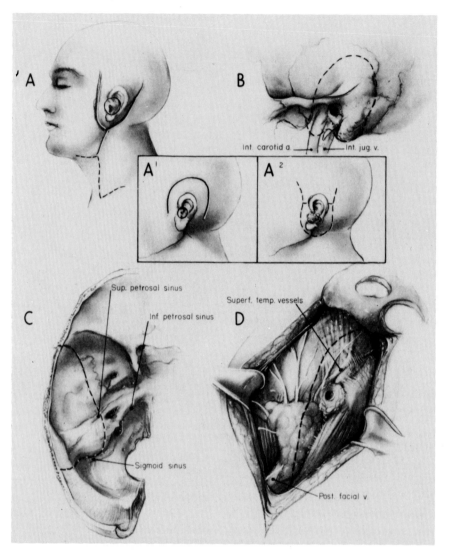

Fig. 21-9. Subtotal resection of the temporal bone. (A) U-shaped incision with extension for neck dissection; (A¹) original incision, (A²) incision when pinna is sacrificed. (B) Extent of bone resection. (C) Extent of petrosectomy. (D) Skin flap elevated superiorly, with excision of parotid. (Lore, J. M., Jr. 1973. An Atlas of Head and Neck Surgery. Vol. 1. 2nd edn. W. B. Saunders, Philadelphia.)

fore, has become a valuable adjunct to surgery.

If the patient has had a previous mastoidectomy for biopsy purposes, I use a sandwich type of radiotherapy program wherein the patient receives 3,000 rads preoperative radiotherapy and then 4 to 6 weeks later undergoes a temporal bone resection. When the wound has healed, a postoperative course of 3,000 to 3,500 rads is administered. If only a biopsy has been taken, then the definitive surgery is carried out followed by a therapeutic dose of 6,500 rads of supravoltage radiation postoperatively.

COMPLICATIONS OF SURGERY

Hemorrhage. Hypotensive agents contribute greatly to the reduction of blood loss;

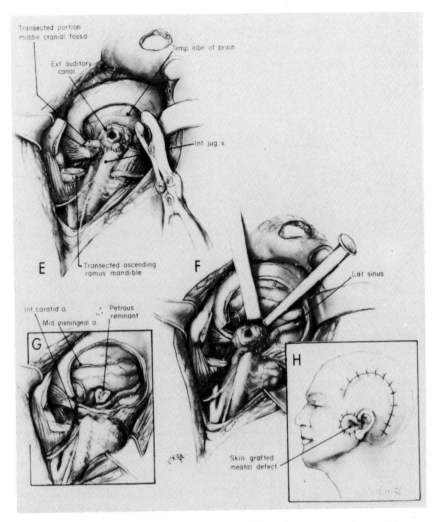

Fig. 21-9 continued. (E) Craniectomy with transection of zygoma and ascending ramus of mandible. (F) Transection through petrous apex. (G) Defect following temporal bone resection. (H) Closure of defect and skin graft to meatal defect. (Lore, J. M., Jr. 1973. An Atlas of Head and Neck Surgery, Vol 1. 2nd edn. W. B. Saunders, Philadelphia.)

the systolic blood pressure is kept at 80 to 90 mm Hg throughout the procedure. Surgical procedures in this area result in considerable bleeding, with the median blood loss between 2,500 to 3,000 ml. Fortunately, hemorrhage is chiefly of venous origin and can be controlled by local suture. The site of bleeding is usually the sigmoid sinus, and the use of vascular silk with a tampon of temporal muscle or Surgicel controls the bleeding. The smaller petrosal sinuses may be electrocoagulated. On the rare occasion

when the jugular bulb is transected in chiseling towards the skull base, a large pack can be inserted, left in place for 5 days and then removed. Upon removal, secondary skin grafting can be carried out.

Infection. The excision site is always covered by a split-thickness skin graft. The graft is prone to infection, especially when patients have received preoperative radiation. The most common organism is *Pseudomonas aeruginosa*. Adequate administration of carbenicillin and gentamycin is

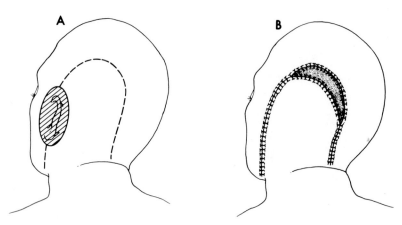

Fig. 21-10. Closure of ear defect with posterior based skin flap. (Lewis, J. 1975. Temporal bone resection. Archives of Otolaryngology, 101:23. Copyright 1975, American Medical Association.)

indicated when such infection is present. Occasionally portions of the skin graft are lost and must be replaced by secondary skin grafts.

Loss of Facial Nerve Function. During temporal bone resection, the facial nerve is severed both in the temporal bone and in the parotid gland. The cosmetic and functional handicap caused by the resultant facial paralysis is both demoralizing and debilitating to the patient. At the time of cutting across the extratemporal portion of the facial nerve, black silk sutures should be applied as markers. The hypoglossal nerve is easy to identify in the neck. If there is residual main trunk or upper division of facial nerve, then the hypoglossal nerve can be sutured directly to the facial nerve. If only peripheral branches of the facial nerve are available, the end of the hypoglossal nerve can be split or dissected far anterior to the

level where it branches in order to create the proper anastomosis. This may be accomplished by the use of fine (8-0) silk suture and the operating microscope.

The healing of these nerves seems not to be hindered by postoperative radiation therapy. Tonus and facial expression can be expected to return in 3 to 6 months following surgery. There should be no reluctance on the surgeon's part to do a hypoglossal-facial anastomosis at the time of temporal bone resection, as it not only produces reliable results in the relief of facial paralysis but does not produce any serious permanent deficits in speaking or deglutition. A lateral tarsorrhapy should be carried out at the end of the procedure in order to prevent corneal ulceration and to improve the cosmetic appearance.

Deafness and Vertigo. Hearing loss is complete following radical temporal bone

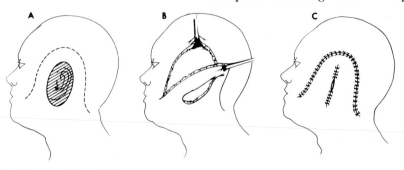

Fig. 21-11. Closure of ear defect with bipedicle scalp flap. (Lewis, J. 1975. Temporal bone resection. Archives of Otolaryngology, 101:23. Copyright 1975, American Medical Association.)

resection. Vertigo may last from 5 to 15 days and there may be a period of unsteadiness for several months.

Carotid Artery Thrombosis. Carotid artery thrombosis resulting in unilateral hemiplegia occurred in one of my patients due to trauma to the carotid vessel during surgery. Cerebral herniation may be prevented by rotating both a temporal muscle flap and scalp flap into the defect.

Radiation Therapy

Radiation therapy may be used as palliation for unresectable or recurrent lesions or as an adjunct to surgery. Either preoperative or postoperative irradiation can be used depending on the preference of the treating physician. Irradiation prior to any surgery has the advantage of an intact blood supply with well-oxygenated tumor cells, which are more readily killed by radiation than anoxic cells. The other advantage of radiation therapy over radical surgery is that no deformity, such as facial paralysis, is likely to result from the treatment.

Radiation therapy has disadvantages. The extent of disease cannot always be accurately defined, although tomography and a CT scan are of great assistance. In a small number of cases, although the cancer appears to be confined to the temporal bone, extension to the base of the skull does occur without evidence of bone destruction. Therefore, the radiotherapist must cover a much larger field in order to obtain proper tumor dose into all areas of possible extension. The brain and brain stem are irradiated, and some damage to them may occur. Boland and Patterson[3] have reported a 25 percent incidence of injury to the brain with the use of radiation for cancer of the ear. Osteoradionecrosis of the mastoid bone associated with pain and secondary infection almost always occurs.

Megavoltage irradiation preceding temporal bone resection would seem to be the optimal method of treatment, particularly for those patients who have had a mastoidectomy with cancer discovered at the time of operation or perhaps reported

a day to two postoperatively. Seeding of the wound with cancer cells at the time of surgery theoretically would be prevented, since the involved bone is removed surgically. Following preoperative irradiation, split-thickness skin grafts may not take and frequently will slough. Rotated scalp flaps are used to cover denuded bone, but even these flaps are in jeopardy. Radiation necrosis, with secondary infection and meningitis, is frequent.

There are many advantages to postoperative radiation: (1) The surgical procedure has removed the involved bone, allowing the radiotherapist to deliver accurately the necessary dosage of radiation and to spare uninvolved areas. (2) The wound is well healed, and the radiation is directed to an uninfected bed with less chance of radiation osteoradionecrosis. (3) The residual disease, if any, has been marked by surgical clips, thus allowing the radiotherapist to cone down on residual disease. Even though full-dose radiation may not be able to be administered, an adequate amount to cover any residual disease can be delivered.

Chemotherapy

Chemotherapy is used primarily for embryonal rhabdomyosarcoma of the middle ear. It is used in combination with local resection and radiation therapy.

Cryosurgery

Miller[12] reported six patients who had cryosurgical treatment to palliate primary or recurrent carcinomas of the ear. Two patients were treated primarily with cryosurgery after debulking the tumor. Three patients had recurrent tumor following subtotal temporal bone resection and radiotherapy. One patient had recurrent tumor following a full-course of irradiation for basal cell carcinoma. Although the healing was slow in each patient (up to 18 months), four of six were free of disease at 21 to 32 months after treatment.

END RESULTS

With the use of hypotensive anesthesia, high-speed air drills, and careful surgical dissection, the mortality from temporal bone resection has dropped in the last 10 years from 10 percent to under 5 percent. In my experience with a total of over 100 cases, the 5-year cure rate is 28 percent for all cases, and 25 percent for those with squamous carcinoma.[10a]

Conley and Schuller[6] have claimed a 5-year cure rate of 36.8 percent utilizing temporal bone resection followed by supervoltage radiation therapy carried to 6,000 rads.

Lederman,[10] in a group of 19 patients with middle ear malignancy, reported a 5-year survival rate of 30.7 percent for petromastoid malignancies treated by radiation therapy alone. Holmes[9] and Figi and Weisman[7] have reported a 5-year survival rate of 30 percent. My experience in a series of 51 cases of cancer involving the middle ear and mastoid treated by mastoidectomy and radiation therapy has given a 5-year cure rate of 6 percent. In my opinion, radical surgery combined with radiation therapy given postoperatively 6 weeks following surgery gives a patient the best chance of cure.

SUMMARY

The cancers of the auricle, external auditory meatus, middle ear, and mastoid are rare. Their anatomic location and rarity and their association with symptoms of chronic suppurative otitis media and otorrhea and the latter's anatomic location have mitigated against early diagnosis and effective treatment of these lesions. The advent of polytomography and CT scanning has given us the opportunity to better define the extent of these lesions preoperatively. The development of hypotensive anesthesia, high-speed air drills, and the routine use of antibiotics has decreased the mortality and improved the cure rate. The inclusion of postoperative radiation therapy as an adjunct to aggressive surgical resection has also helped to decrease the morbidity and increase the cure rate.

REFERENCES

1. Aub, J. C., Evans, R. D., Hempleman, L. H., and Mortland, H. S. 1952. Late effects of internally deposited radioactive materials in man. Medicine, 31: 221.

2. Beal, D., Lindsay, J. R., and Ward, D. H. 1965. Radiation-induced carcinoma of the mastoid. Archives of Otolaryngology 8: 9.

3. Boland, J., and Patterson, R. 1955. Cancer of the middle ear and external auditory meatus. Journal of Laryngology and Otology, 69: 468.

4. Clairmont, C., and Conley, J. J. 1977. Primary carcinoma of the mastoid bone. Annals of Otology, Rhinology and Laryngology, 86: 306.

5. Coachman, E. H. 1951. Carcinoma secondary to cholesteatoma. Archives of Otolaryngology, 54: 187.

6. Conley, J. J., and Schuller, D. E. 1977. Reconstruction following temporal bone resection. Archives of Otolaryngology, 103: 34.

7. Figi, F. A., and Weisman, P. A. 1964. Cancer and chemodectoma of the middle ear and mastoid. JAMA, 156: 1157.

8. Furstenberg, A. C. 1924. Primary adenocarcinoma of the middle ear and mastoid. Annals of Otology, Rhinology and Laryngology, 33: 677.

9. Holmes, K. S. 1965. Carcinoma of the middle ear. Journal of Faculty Radiology, 16: 400.

10. Lederman, J. 1965. Malignant tumors of the ear. Journal of Laryngology and Otology, 79: 85.

10a. Lewis, J. S. 1966. Cancer of the ear: A report of 100 cases. Laryngoscope, 70: 551.

11. Lodge, W. O., Jones, H. W., and Smith, M. N. 1955. Malignant tumors of the temporal bone. Archives of Otolaryngology, 61: 535.

12. Miller, D., Silverstein, H., and Gacek, R. 1971. Cryosurgical treatment of carcinoma of the ear. Transactions of the American Academy of Ophthalmology and Otolaryngology, 76: 1363.

13. Naufal, P. E., 1973. Primary sarcomas of the temporal bone. Archives of Otolaryngology, 98: 44.

13a. Pulec, J. L. 1977. Glandular tumors of the external auditory canal. Laryngoscope, 87: 1601.

14. Pulec, J. L., Parkhill, F. M., and Devine, K. D. 1963. Adenoid cystic carcinoma of the external auditory canal. Transactions of the American Academy of Ophthalmology and Otolaryngology, 67: 673.

15. Robinson, G. A. 1931. Malignant tumors of the ear. Laryngoscope, 41: 407.

16. Ruben, R. J., Thaler, S. U., and Holzer, N. 1977. Radiation-induced carcinoma of the temporal bone. Laryngoscope, 87: 1613.

17. Schall, L. A. 1934. Neoplasms involving the middle ear. Archives of Otolaryngology, 32: 548.

18. Tod, A. I., in discussion on Whitehead. 1907. A case of primary epithelioma of the tympanum following chronic otitis media. Proceedings of the Royal Society of Medicine (Section on Otology) 1: 34.

19. Towson, C. E., and Shofstall, W. H. 1950. Carcinoma of the ear. Archives of Otolaryngology, 51: 724.

19a. Unni, K. K., Ivine, J. C., Beabout, J. W., and Dahlin, D. C. 1971. Hemangioma, hemangiopericytoma, and hemangioendothelioma (angiosarcoma) of bone. Cancer, 27: 1043.

20. Zizmor, J., and Noyek, A. 1969. Tumors and other disorders of the temporal bone. Seminars in Roentgenology, 4: 2.

22 | Cancer of the Eye and Orbit

John E. Wright, M.D.

INTRODUCTION

Primary cancers in the eye and orbit are quite uncommon. This group of tumors presents a wide spectrum of histologic types, each with its own unique biologic behavior, ranging in intensity from those that are indolent and locally symptomatic to those with a marked propensity for local destruction as well as the tendency for wide-spread distant metastasis. These tumors also span all of the age groups. Rhabdomyosarcoma and retinoblastomas occur predominantly in infancy and childhood. Lymphomas and malignant tumors of the lacrimal gland tend to occur more frequently later in life.

New diagnostic modalities and treatment protocols that have been introduced in recent years have made a dramatic impact upon the diagnosis, methods of management, and end results in tumors affecting the eye and orbit. Computerized axial tomography (CT) has helped to refine the locating of such tumors as gliomas and meningiomas of the optic nerve. Management of lacrimal gland tumors is now carried out by a multidisciplinary team including ophthalmologists, head and neck surgeons, neurosurgeons, and plastic and reconstructive surgeons to insure both adequate resection of tumors and reconstruction of the orbit. Most dramatic, however, has been the introduction of a combination of chemotherapy and radiation therapy in the management of rhabdomyosarcomas. Whereas formerly these tumors were almost uniformly lethal, extremely high disease-free intervals and cure rates are now being reported.

ANATOMY

The orbit is a pyramidal space enclosed within bony walls (Fig. 22-1). The medial walls of the orbits lie anteroposterior parallel with each other. They separate the orbit from the ethmoid air cells on the lateral walls of the nose. The medial wall extends from the anterior lacrimal crest on the frontal process of the maxilla across the lacrimal bone and the orbital plate of the ethmoid to the body of the sphenoid and the optic foramen. The posterior lacrimal crest is a vertical ridge in the lacrimal bone. The fossa for the lacrimal sac lies between the anterior and posterior lacrimal crests and leads down into the nasolacrimal canal. At the junction of the medial wall and the roof, the anterior and posterior ethmoidal foraminae lie between the ethmoid and frontal bones. The orbital floor consists of the orbital process of the palatine bone at its apex. In front of this lies the orbital plate of the maxilla; the plate is usually grooved by the infraorbital nerve. The zygomatic bone extends into the orbital floor on its lateral aspect. The lateral wall of the orbit is composed of the greater wing of the sphenoid and the zygomatic bone.

Between the lateral orbital wall and the floor is the inferior orbital fissure, which leads into the pterygopalatine and infratemporal fossae. The roof of the orbit is the orbital plate of the frontal bone with the lesser wing of the sphenoid. There is a gap at the posterior part of the orbit between the greater wing and the lesser wings of the sphenoid; this is the superior orbital fissure leading into the middle cranial fossa. The

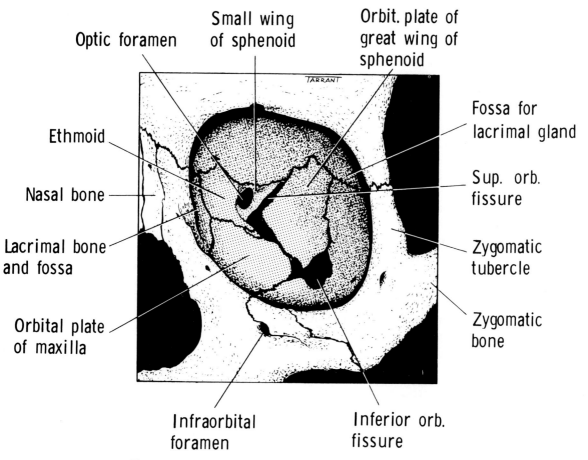

Optic foramen

Small wing of sphenoid

Orbit. plate of great wing of sphenoid

Ethmoid

Nasal bone

Lacrimal bone and fossa

Orbital plate of maxilla

Fossa for lacrimal gland

Sup. orb. fissure

Zygomatic tubercle

Zygomatic bone

Infraorbital foramen

Inferior orb. fissure

Fig. 22-1. Drawing of the bones comprising the orbital walls.

optic canal starts at the apex of the orbit and lies within the body of the sphenoid. The approximate dimensions of the adult male orbit are 34 mm (height), 41 mm (width), and 53 mm (length of floor). The volume of the orbital cavity is approximately 30 cc.

Periosteum covers the bones that form the orbital walls; the periosteum is attached firmly to the margins of the orbit and to the edges of the optic canal and the inferior and superior orbital fissures. Elsewhere, the periosteum is relatively free.

The orbit contains the eyeball, the optic nerve, the extrinsic muscles of the globe, and their vessels and nerves. The eyelids are covered in front with loose skin and behind with conjunctiva. The tarsal plates, which provide some rigidity to the lids, are part of

the orbital septum. The orbital septum is attached to the margins of the orbit and to the posterior lacrimal crest. Elsewhere it is attached to the upper margin of the superior tarsal plate and to the lower margin of the inferior tarsal plate.

At the margins of the orbit there is a wide aperture in the septum, i.e., the palpebral fissure between the eyelids. The septum is not of equal density; it is greatly thickened in the upper margin of the aperture to form the crescent-shaped superior tarsal plate and similarly in the lower margin to form the inferior tarsal plate. The septum is also thickened medially to form the medial palpebral ligament. Temporally the thickening is less marked; together with the lateral horn of the levator aponeurosis and the lateral canthal tendon the septum is attached to the periosteum overlying the orbital tubercule. The tarsal plates are crescent-shaped structures of dense fibrous tissue and contain the tarsal (meibomian) glands. The palpebral conjunctiva is firmly adherent to the deep surface of each tarsal plate and the eye lashes are anchored to the distal edge of the tarsal plate. Anterior to the orbital septum and tarsal plates is the palpebral part of the orbicularis muscle. The blood supply of the eyelids is derived from the palpebral branches of the ophthalmic artery. The lymphatic drainage is to the preauricular glands. It should be noted that behind the level of the orbital septum there are no lymph vessels or lymphatic glands within the orbit.

At the medial end of each lid margin is a low elevation surmounted by the lacrimal punctum. The latter opens into the lacrimal canaliculus, which leads from the punctum to the lacrimal sac. The lacrimal sac lies in the lacrimal groove. Some of the palpebral fibers of the orbicularis oculi are inserted into fascia surrounding the sac and, by squeezing the sac, aid the passage of tears through the canaliculi into the sac and onwards down the nasolacrimal duct; this duct is ¾ inch long and slopes downwards and laterally to open into the inferior meatus of the nose.

The conjunctiva is a transparent membrane that is attached to the margin of the cornea and loosely attached over the anterior part of the sclera and thence reflected to the inner surfaces of the eyelids where it is firmly attached to the tarsal plates. It is a firm membrane of fibrous tissue covered with stratified squamous epithelium except for a few scattered islands of columnar epithelium located behind the upper tarsal plate. The columnar cells are goblet cells secreting mucus.

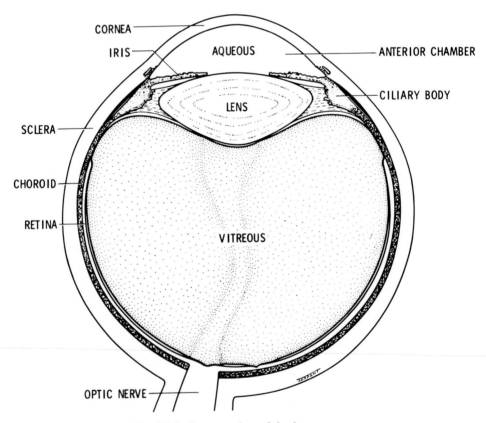

Fig. 22-2. Cross section of the human eye.

The structure of the eye can be readily appreciated in Figure 22-2, which shows a cross section of the adult eye. From the point of view of malignancy, the corneal epithelium is a continuation of the conjunctival epithelium and consists of squamous stratified cells. The uveal tract comprises the choroid, the ciliary body, and the iris. The ciliary muscle consists of unstriped muscle. The various layers of the retina can be seen in Figure 22-3. It should be noted that the retina is developed from a hollow outgrowth that protrudes from the cerebral vesicle, i.e. the optic vesicle. The optic vesicle becomes invaginated to form the optic cup, which consists of two layers of cells. The outer layer differentiates to form the pigment layer. The inner layer forms the remaining layers of the retina, with rods and cones outermost next to the pigment cells. The ganglion cells and their axons are innermost.

The optic nerve extends into the orbit from the optic canal. Its orbital length is approximately 3 cm. It is surrounded by pia mater, arachnoid, and dura. It is important to note that the subarachnoid space around the optic nerve extends up to the attachment of the nerve to the sclera.

The four rectus muscles arise from a fibrous ring surrounding the optic canal and the medial third of the superior orbital fis-

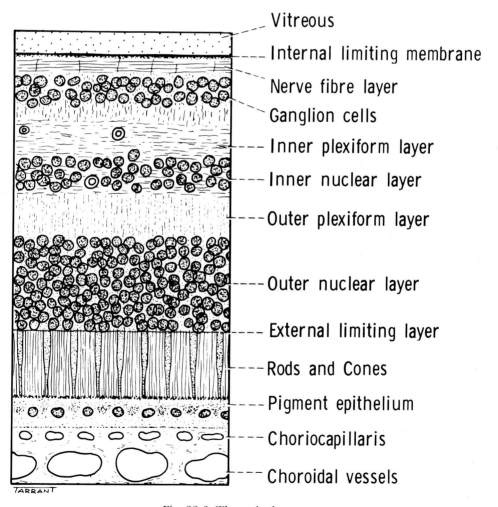

- Vitreous
- Internal limiting membrane
- Nerve fibre layer
- Ganglion cells
- Inner plexiform layer
- Inner nuclear layer
- Outer plexiform layer
- Outer nuclear layer
- External limiting layer
- Rods and Cones
- Pigment epithelium
- Choriocapillaris
- Choroidal vessels

Fig. 22-3. The retinal anatomy.

sure. The superior oblique and the levator palpebrae superioris muscles take origin from the bone above the ring. The muscles pass forward from the apex of the orbit to form a cone of muscles around the eyeball. However, the levator palpebrae superioris passes forwards beneath the roof of the orbit, and at the anterior end the muscle broadens into a tendon. This tendon passes through the orbital septum and is attached to the anterior surface of the tarsal plate and the skin of the eyelid. The inferior oblique muscle arises from the floor of the orbit just lateral to the lacrimal sac, and the muscle passes laterally below the globe to insert near the macula.

The 3rd, 4th, and 6th nerves supply the muscles that control eye movements. The sensory nerves within the orbit are branches of the first two divisions of the 5th cranial nerve. All these nerves enter the orbit through the superior orbital fissure. The ophthalmic artery is a branch of the internal carotid and is given off as the latter vessel emerges from the roof of the cavernous sinus. The ophthalmic artery passes through the optic foramen and enters the orbit, piercing the dura surrounding the optic nerve and spiraling around the lateral side of the nerve to pass forward above the nerve and medial to the nasociliary nerve. The main vein of the orbit is the superior ophthalmic vein, which passes backward through the orbit in the region of the trochlea, enters the muscle cone to run on the under surface of the superior rectus muscle and then runs across the upper surface of the optic nerve to exit from the orbit through the superior orbital fissure. The inferior orbital vein is much smaller and is of less importance.

There are four surgical spaces within the orbit: the subperiosteal space, which is a potential space between the walls and the lining periosteum; the peripheral surgical space, which lies between the muscle cone with its fascia and the orbital periosteum; the inner surgical space, which lies within the muscle cone; and the episcleral space,

which lies between the tenons capsule and the globe.

Recent work by Korneef[8] has cast doubt on this four space concept. However, for practical purposes the broad division into four spaces holds true. In addition, the connective tissue supports the globe so that it maintains its position within the orbit. Lockwood's ligament, which is a thickening of the connective tissue, forms a hammock below the globe and is attached medially to the posterior lacrimal crest and laterally to a prominence on the orbital surface of the zygomatic bone (Whitnall's tubercule).

There are a number of malignant tumors that occur in the eye and orbit. They will be discussed separately.

RHABDOMYOSARCOMA

Rhabdomyosarcoma is a tumor of children and adolescents occurring from infancy up to the age of about 16, with peak occurrence between 6 and 8 years. Although rare in adults,[7, 10] the neoplasm has been observed in all age groups. Indeed, several patients in their eighth decade have been observed to have this tumor. Rhabdomyosarcoma occurs more often in males than females (ratio 3:2).[7]

Clinical Features

These tumors usually grow rapidly within the orbit. This rapidity of onset is a particularly significant feature of the disease process, as is the marked local response to the vascular, rapidly enlarging tumor. The signs and symptoms, to a great extent, depend on the site of origin of the neoplasm. Anteriorly situated lesions produce localized swelling and redness of the eyelids often associated with chemosis. Children with this swelling are frequently regarded as having orbital cellulitis and are initially treated with antibiotics. However, the diagnosis soon becomes obvious, for despite antibiotic therapy, the mass continues to expand and there is no elevation of the white cell count. Lesions further back in the orbit will produce generalized swelling and proptosis (Fig. 22-4), often accompanied by edema of the optic disc with deterioration in the visual acuity secondary to the pressure of the tumor on the optic nerve. Essential initial investigations are roentgenograms of the skull, orbit, and sinuses, ultrasonic scans of the orbit, and chest roentgenogram. CT scanning of the orbit is rarely required, as the need to obtain a biopsy from the mass becomes imperative.

Pathology

These neoplasms are usually diffuse and friable; occasionally, they may be encapsulated and the inexperienced surgeon may think he is dealing with an odd dermoid

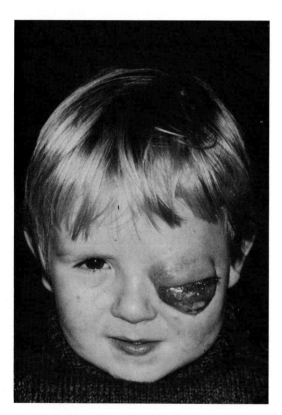

Fig. 22-4. Three-year-old child with full, rapidly developing proptosis.

cyst. However, in the majority of cases the lesion is diffuse and bleeds readily when sectioned. The mass is usually dull white or grey.

The histologic features of these tumors are somewhat variable. The more differentiated lesions are termed pleomorphic, whereas the more undifferentiated lesions are called embryonal; the latter are the most common. It is important that the diagnosis is supported by the recognition of cross striations in the cytoplasm of some of the cells. However, in some of the highly undifferentiated embryonal tumors this can be extremely difficult and may require electronmicroscopy of fresh specimens so that primitive myofilamentous cells and more differentiated myofibrillorhabdomyoblasts can be readily recognized. The histologic type does not appear to influence the prognosis. What does undoubtedly influence the prognosis is the speed with which the appropriate therapy is commenced.

Therapy

Once the histologic diagnosis has been made, it is most important that the patient be admitted to an oncology unit and a multidisciplinary approach to the problem be instigated. In addition to the initial investigations, bone scan and bone marrow aspiration studies should be performed. The clinician then has a choice of treatment. In the past, orbital exenteration was in many centers advocated as the best primary treatment for this condition.[7, 17] However, the use of radiotherapy as a primary procedure was advised by Lederman.[9, 10] Supervoltage radiotherapy can be given to the orbit in doses in excess of 5,000 rads in 6 weeks and has produced high local control rates as good as those obtained by surgery. Furthermore, radiotherapy produces less deformity than surgery does and, in those patients in whom the disease does not recur, useful vision is normally preserved in the eye on the affected side.

Of patients treated by surgery or radiotherapy alone, over 50 percent succumb to the disease, some with local recurrence but the majority with distant metastases. The prognosis was particularly poor for children below the age of 6. Nearly all local recurrences and metastases appeared within the first year after treatment; thus, a 2-year survival could be equated with cure.

The addition of chemotherapy has markedly improved the early prognosis so that the 2-year survival rate has now risen to over 80 percent. The tumors of younger children are particularly chemosensitive so that the poorer results in the younger children are no longer seen.

It is too early to know the long-term survival and complication rates of patients treated with combined chemotherapy and radiotherapy, but there is as yet no evidence of later recurrences or increased morbidity.

RADIOTHERAPY TECHNIQUE

Each case must be individually planned so that the high dose volume covers the tumor, and the cornea and lens are shielded as much as possible. It is of course important to avoid any irradiation to the other eye. Most cases can be treated by anterior and lateral fields. When there is a large protruding tumor, superior and inferior fields are preferable. An intraconal tumor should be treated mainly by a lateral field, and if necessary, the dose should be supplemented anteriorly by an orthovoltage field with corneal shielding.

Acute skin and conjunctival reactions to the radiotherapy occur, but subside rapidly and are rarely troublesome. After radiotherapy there is usually permanent loss of lashes, but in children dryness of the eye is rarely a problem. Some degree of posterior cortical cataract is seen in most cases. Progressive cataract is uncommon, but if it occurs it is readily amenable to operation. When the patient is a young child, there is some degree of impairment of growth of the irradiated orbit with consequent facial asymmetry.

CHEMOTHERAPY

The most effective drugs are actinomycin-D, doxorubicin (Adriamycin), vincristine, and cyclophosphamide (Cytoxan). The following scheme is recommended for those patients in whom investigations show no evidence of blood-borne metastases: vincristine, 1.5 mg/m^2; actinomycin-D, 1.0 mg/m^2; and cyclophosphamide, 300 mg/m^2.

These drugs can be given intravenously on the first day of chemotherapy and repeated 7 days later. After a further 7 days, radiotherapy is begun and a 5,000 rads tumor dose is administered in 5 to 6 weeks. During radiotherapy, vincristine, 1.5 mg/m^2, and cyclophosphamide, 200 mg/m^2, are administered intravenously once a week. Two weeks after the end of radiotherapy, vincristine, 1.5 mg/m^2; doxorubicin, 40 mg/m^2; and cyclophosphamide, 400 mg/m^2, are administered once every 3 weeks until the total dose of doxorubicin reaches 400 mg, at which time actinomycin-D, 1.0 mg/m^2, is substituted for doxorubicin. This regime is continued until 1 year has elapsed from the start of drug treatment.

SURGERY

Exenteration of the orbit should be reserved for those patients in whom there is a recurrence of the tumor or obvious failure of the combined chemotherapy and radiotherapy to control the growth of the tumor. This procedure is highly disfiguring.

The initial incision is down to the orbital margin through 360° using cutting diathermy. Once the orbital margin has been reached, the periosteum of the orbit can be elevated, the nasolacrimal duct cauterized, the anterior and posterior ethmoidal arteries diathermied, and the whole of the orbital contents removed. Following transection of the structures in the orbit, it is essential that the orbit be thoroughly cleaned and no tissue remain in the orbital apex at the end of the procedure. The orbit can be left to granulate but a much more satisfactory arrangement is to use a split-skin graft and apply it to the bare bone of the orbital walls. In the majority of patients, there is a 90 percent take of this type of graft, which speeds the healing process considerably.

ADVANCED CASES

More aggressive chemotherapy is recommended for patients with evidence of distant metastasis at presentation; the regime consists of the following: vincristine, 1.5 mg/m²; doxorubicin, 40 mg/m²; and cyclophosphamide, 300 mg/m², administered weekly for 6 weeks, provided the bone marrow will tolerate this.

Radiotherapy is started as soon as possible during this period of intensive chemotherapy. During radiotherapy, weekly injections of vincristine and cyclophosphamide are given as above. If a complete remission of the disease is obtained, vincristine, doxorubicin, and cyclophosphamide are given until the total dose of doxorubicin reaches 400 mg/m², at which time actinomycin-D, 1.0 mg/m², is substituted. This regime is continued for at least 18 months.

LACRIMAL GLAND TUMORS

Classification

Lacrimal gland tumors are relatively rare. The histologic features of this group of neoplasms are essentially the same as those

TABLE 22-1. WORLD HEALTH ORGANIZATION CLASSIFICATION FOR SALIVARY GLAND TUMORS

1. *Epithelial Tumors*
   a. Adenomas
      (1) Pleomorphic adenoma (mixed tumor)
      (2) Monomorphic adenoma
         (a) Adenolymphoma
         (b) Oxyphilic adenoma
         (c) Other types
   b. Mucoepidermoid tumors
   c. Acinic cell tumors
   d. Carcinoma
      (1) Adenoid cystic carcinoma
      (2) Adenocarcinoma
      (3) Epidermoid carcinoma
      (4) Undifferentiated carcinoma
      (5) Carcinoma in pleomorphic adenoma (malignant mixed tumor)

2. *Nonepithelial tumors*

3. *Unclassified tumors*

4. *Allied conditions*

seen in the salivary gland neoplasms. In 1953, Foote and Frazell reviewed the Memorial Hospital experience with 877 salivary gland tumors over a 20-year period.[4] The World Health Organization refined their classification into the categories shown in Table 21-1.

The incidence of the various groups of lacrimal gland tumors has been reviewed in a number of papers. In 1971 Forrest[5] re-

TABLE 22-2. DISTRIBUTION OF TUMOR TYPE AMONG 54 PATIENTS WITH LACRIMAL GLAND EPITHELIAL NEOPLASMS IN A 25-YEAR PERIOD AT THE UNIVERSITY OF LONDON INSTITUTE OF OPHTHALMOLOGY[1].

Type of tumor	Percentage	Number of Patients
Pleomorphic adenoma (mixed tumor)	55.5	30
Pleomorphic adenocarcinoma	3.7	2
Adenoid cystic carcinoma	24.1	13
Carcinomas (including adenocarcinomas, mucoepidermoid carcinomas, squamous cell carcinomas, and anaplastic carcinomas)	16.6	9

TABLE 22-3. HISTOLOGIC DIAGNOSIS
OF 265 EPITHELIAL TUMORS[3]

Diagnosis	Percentage	Number of Cases
Pleomorphic adenomas (mixed tumor)	51	136
Carcinoma in pleomorphic adenoma	12	34
Adenoid cystic carcinoma	27	70
Adenocarcinoma	7	19
Mucoepidermoid carcinoma	2	4
Miscellaneous carcinoma	1	2

viewed epithelial tumors of the lacrimal gland seen at the Harkness Eye Institute. He reported that 26 patients had benign mixed tumors, 20 patients had adenoid cystic carcinoma, and 10 patients had adenocarcinoma, undifferentiated carcinoma, or malignant mixed tumor. Ashton[1] reviewed the series of epithelial tumors of the lacrimal gland from the University of London Institute of Ophthalmology. In a 25-year period, there were 54 patients with lacrimal gland epithelial neoplasms. The tumors were distributed as shown in Table 22-2.

Font and Gammel[3] have reevaluated the Armed Forces Institute of Pathology series of epithelial tumors of the lacrimal gland. They found 265 lesions, of which the histologic diagnoses are shown in Table 22-3. Similar statistics have been obtained by Wright, et al.[16] who observed that 50 percent of all tumors arising from the lacrimal gland epithelium were pleomorphic adenomas. The remainder were carcinomas of varying degrees of malignancy.

Clinical Presentation

It is essential when dealing with lesions of the lacrimal gland that a neoplasm arising from the epithelium of the gland be recognized as soon as possible. The survival of the patient depends on the choice of treatment appropriate to the lesion. Carcinomas of the lacrimal gland cannot be distinguished from other rapidly expanding lesions in this region other than by histologic examination. However, benign mixed tumors can be readily recognized on clinical grounds.

The pattern of presentation of benign mixed lacrimal gland tumors is characteristic. They present in patients—who are in their late 20s to early 60s—as a slowly progressive, painless upper-lid swelling without inflammatory symptoms or signs. There is often a palpable mass in the outer temporal quadrant of the orbit. A careful detailed history will reveal that the duration of symptoms is longer than 12 months (Fig. 22-5). Radiographs usually reveal enlargement of the lacrimal fossa without invasion of overlying bone. Careful tomographic study may reveal this characteristic change when plain radiographs are negative. Occasionally, a benign mixed lacrimal gland tumor may present in a different way: the patient has had symptoms of short duration, there is a readily palpable mass, and radiographs are normal. The tumor in this situation arises from the palpebral lobe of the lacrimal gland and produces a slowly enlarging mass in the outer third of the upper eyelid. This mass is noticed at an early stage, and because it lies anterior to the lacrimal fossa there is no bone erosion. Inevitably the mass is either biopsied or removed and the true nature of the lesion discovered by frozen-section or routine histology.

The importance of recognizing this tumor cannot be overemphasized. The temptation to biopsy the lesion should be avoided, and total removal of the whole of the lacrimal gland through a lateral orbitotomy can be planned. Rupture of the capsule of a benign mixed tumor affects the prognosis adversely because of seeding of the tumor cells into the surrounding tissues. Recurrences are thus inevitable; and in many cases, although such recurrences are histologically nonmalignant, malignant change can occur. In patients in whom the recur-

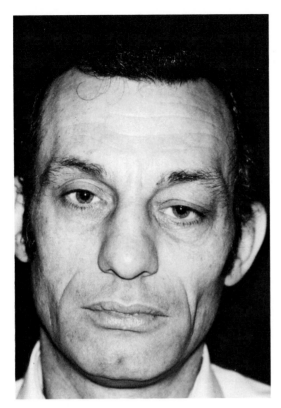

Fig. 22-5. Patient with a mass above the left eye for several years—benign mixed cell lacrimal tumor.

calcification within the malignant tumor can be demonstrated. In patients with such tumors it is important that both axial and coronal tomograms are obtained so that the structure of the bones in relation to the tumor can be examined in some detail. This type of assessment has now been supplemented by coronal and axial CT scans (Fig. 22-6).

Other lesions affecting the lacrimal fossa must be considered in the differential diagnosis. Acute dacryoadenitis, unless caused by a viral infection, usually responds to systemic antibiotic therapy. However, if there is a failure to respond to antibiotics over a period of 2 weeks, a tissue diagnosis should be made. Unfortunately, a good proportion of carcinomas involving the lacrimal gland are initially treated as cases of acute dacryoadenitis refractory to antibiotic therapy. Inflammatory pseudotumors are relatively common, as are lymphomatous lesions, the latter particularly in patients over 65 years old. Again, tissue must be obtained so that the appropriate treatment can be instigated. All these patients have a short history of lacrimal fossa swelling with or without associated inflammatory signs. In all these patients a biopsy should be obtained

rences remain benign, the prognosis is often indistinguishable from that seen in a true carcinoma. The tumor cells invade the apex of the orbit as well as the surrounding bone. Following a painful and lingering course death ensues, for in most cases the tumor spreads beyond the line of surgical resection; and although radiotherapy may be used as a palliative measure, benign mixed tumors are relatively radioresistant.

Malignant tumors arising from the lacrimal gland have two characteristic features: a short history with a rapidly worsening course, and pain. Radiographic findings may also be helpful in distinguishing between the malignant and benign lacrimal tumor. Carcinomatous lesions often enlarge so rapidly that radiographs in the early stages are normal. Later enlargement of the lacrimal fossa with or without demonstrable invasion of bone may be seen. Occasionally

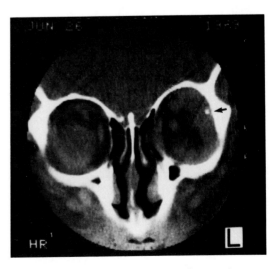

Fig. 22-6. Coronal CT scan of extensive adenoid cystic carcinoma of lacrimal gland. Note the calcification within the tumor (arrow).

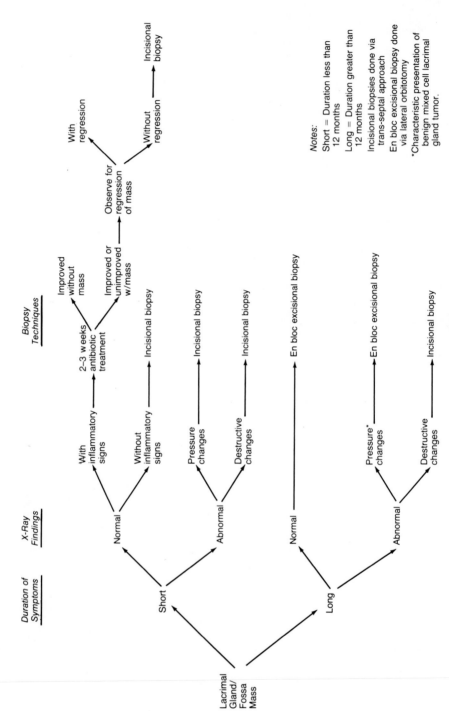

Fig. 22-7. Flowsheet of management of lacrimal gland/fossa masses based on duration of symptoms and radiographic findings.

through a transseptal incision. The extraperiosteal approach should never be used, because the integrity of the periosteal barrier must be maintained to prevent possible seeding of the extraperiosteal space by malignant cells.

Figure 22-7 describes a useful method of management of lacrimal gland/fossa masses. By following this flowsheet, a definite diagnosis can be reached at an early stage in clinical evaluation. Such diverse lesions as inflammatory masses, lymphomas, and carcinomas will be accurately identified.

Treatment

The choice of approach to the tumors is of prime importance, for the exposure should be such that the palpebral lobe and the structures of the eyelid can be dissected out using an operating microscope. It is essential in removing the lacrimal gland, plus tumor, that the capsule of the tumor is not touched and the periosteum overlying the tumor is removed at the same time. The modified lateral orbitotomy approach[16] offers the only way to achieve adequate removal of the tumor. A transcranial, anterior orbitotomy or the Burke lateral orbitotomy make it extremely difficult or impossible to avoid a subtotal, piecemeal removal of the gland and tumor.

Patients found to have adenoid cystic carcinomas and other malignant epithelial neoplasms should be evaluated to determine the extent of the tumor. When there is evidence of restriction of the tumor mass within the periosteal barrier without involvement of the orbital apex, a radical resection of the area can be undertaken. The skills of a neurosurgeon, head and neck surgeon, and plastic surgeon, as well as that of an ophthalmic surgeon should be united for such a surgical approach. Surgical resection in these cases should include portions of the lateral and superior orbital walls as well as removal of the lids and orbital contents. Radiotherapy and chemotherapy may be considered for those cases in which spread has occurred beyond even these wide surgical margins. The outlook for these patients is extremely poor.

LYMPHOMA

The orbit may be the site of a primary lymphoma or the presenting site of a generalized lymphoma. It may also become involved at a later stage in a patient under treatment for a systemic lymphoma. Orbital lymphoma occurs at all ages, but is most common in the middle-aged and elderly. In children, the Burkitts tumor predominates; whereas in the elderly, the well-differentiated lymphocytic form is the most common. The sex incidence is approximately equal—except in the elderly, among whom the disease is more common in females.

Lymphomatous tumors within the orbit vary from the well-differentiated lymphocytic type of lesions, sometimes called reactive lymphoid hyperplasia, through frank malignancy. Histologic interpretation of orbital biopsy material can be very difficult. Many specimens show a lymphocytic lesion in which there are no clear features of benign hyperplasia or of malignancy and are reported as lymphocytic tumors of indeterminate nature.[11]

Of those patients with a histologically definite malignant lymphoma but with no evidence of dissemination on full investigation, approximately 50 percent develop systemic lymphoma within 5 years. The remainder appear to be cured by local radiotherapy alone. There seems to be no need to give chemotherapy unless or until dissemination is found.

The malignant types of lymphomatous disease are often seen in the orbit as part of the generalized disease process. In a high proportion of patients in whom the biopsy shows frank malignancy, evidence of systemic lymphoma is found at the time of presentation or subsequently. On the other hand, disseminated lymphoma or chronic lymphatic leukemia occurs in only 25 percent of patients whose biopsy specimens are reported as indeterminate lymphocytic lesions.

Clinical Features

The majority of lymphomatous lesions occur in the anterior part of the orbit. In most cases, the mass is noticed by the patient at an early stage. There is usually a swelling of the eyelid with or without displacement of the eye (Fig. 22-8). A rubbery mass which has a characteristic reddish-pink appearance, is usually palpable and visible beneath the conjunctiva. Pain or signs of an inflammatory reaction are usually absent, a most important point in distinguishing this type of lesion from a pseudotumor. A tissue diagnosis is essential and can be readily obtained either by a transconjunctival or transseptal approach. It is advisable to perform full investigations for evidence of systemic spread, regardless of the histologic appearances. An exception can be made in the case of an elderly patient with an indeterminate tumor or a well-differentiated lymphocytic lymphoma, since the results of investigations are rarely positive.

Treatment and Prognosis

Those patients discovered to have systemic lymphoma are treated with a combination of chemotherapy and radiotherapy. In the majority of patients, however, investigations are negative, and these patients are treated by radiotherapy. A tumor dose of 3,000 rads in 3 weeks achieves virtually 100 percent local control regardless of the histologic type of tumor. Rapid regression occurs, and there are rarely any local complications of treatment.

The prognosis depends on the histologic type. The majority of well-differentiated lymphocytic lymphomata and indeterminate lymphocytic tumors do not disseminate; those that do, often run a protracted and relatively benign course as chronic lymphatic leukemia or cutaneous lymphoma.

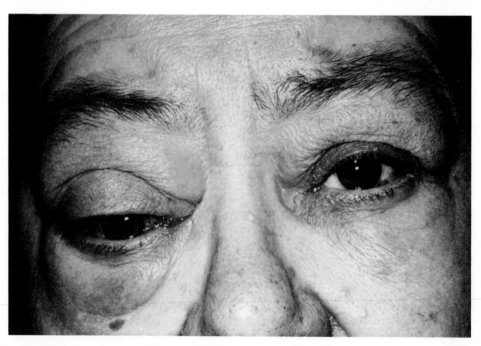

Fig. 22-8. Fifty-seven-year-old patient with 6-month history of progressive proptosis. Biopsy showed lymphocytic hyperplasia.

MELANOMA

Intraocular Melanoma

Primary melanoma of the uveal tract is the most common malignant tumor of the eye. In Europe and the United States, the incidence is approximately six cases per million people each year. The sexes are equally affected. Nearly all the cases occur after the age of 30, with a peak incidence in the sixth decade. Although the majority of malignant melanomas arise in the choroid, approximately 9 percent arise in the ciliary body and 6 percent in the iris.

CLINICAL FEATURES

The signs and symptoms produced by a choroidal melanoma depend on its site. A relatively small lesion at the macula will cause an early deterioration in vision, whereas a more peripheral melanoma may be present for some time before the patient notices a field defect. Pain is not normally a feature unless an anteriorly placed lesion causes secondary glaucoma. Ophthalmoscopy usually reveals the presence of an elevated, mottled brown mass in the fundus with an associated retinal detachment in the lower part of the fundus (Fig. 22-9). If there is no associated retinal detachment, the diagnosis becomes much more difficult because disciform macular degeneration, benign melanoma, or an area of low grade choroiditis can be confused with a malignant melanoma. Fluorescein angiography and ultrasonic scans may help to distinguish these different lesions.

TREATMENT

The approach to the management of uveal melanoma has changed considerably in recent years. Formerly, enucleation was performed immediately in nearly all patients with a clinical diagnosis of melanoma because of the belief that it gave the best chance of survival. It is now realized that many smaller melanomas can be safely watched for many years especially in elderly patients and that others can be managed by

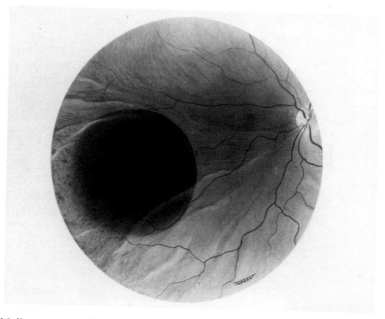

Fig. 22-9. Malignant choroidal melanoma. Note the retinal detachment associated with this tumor.

conservative measures with preservation of the eye. It has even been suggested that enucleation may shorten survival time because of dissemination of tumor cells during the operation.[18] However, the timing of the enucleation may coincide with a period of maximal symptomatology caused by a rapid growth phase of the melanoma. Thus the peak incidence of metastases could well occur whether the eye was enucleated or not.

Small tumors of less then 3 disc diameters can be observed carefully and need not be treated until there is definite evidence of growth. When growth is evident, the tumors may then be suitable for photocoagulation. Larger lesions that are remote from the macula and do not involve the optic nerve can be treated by radioactive cobalt applicators in a similar manner to retinoblastoma. Recommended dose is 8,000 rads in 2 weeks at the apex of the tumor—a much higher dose than that used for retinoblastoma. Some ophthalmologists have advocated using cryotherapy to destroy melanomas. However, this type of treatment can only be applied to fairly small melanomas and when using this type of therapy or photocoagulation there is always a danger that the spread of malignant cells into the vitreous may be encouraged. The site and size of melanomas within the globe will determine the most suitable type of therapy.

Enucleation remains the treatment of choice for those patients with large lesions and poor vision caused by involvement of the macula or the optic nerve or an extensive retinal detachment. It is also indicated when there is pain, secondary glaucoma, or possible involvement of extrascleral structures. If extraocular extension is found at enucleation, the orbit should be exenterated with preservation of the eyelids. Some clinicians subsequently treat the patient with chemotherapeutic agents in an attempt to reduce the chances of the patient developing metastatic disease. In several centers, extraocular extension of a melanoma is treated with radiotherapy. A high dose is required, so 6,000 rads in 6 weeks is usually given. The relative radioresistance of melanoma is probably due to a high capacity for intracellular repair of radiation damage, and thus, an equivalent biologic dose in fewer fractions, for example 3,000 rads in 6 fractions, may give better results.

Tumors of the iris present early and can usually be removed by iridectomy, with excellent long-term results.

RESULTS AND PROGNOSIS

The overall survival for choroidal melanoma is 70 percent at 5 years and declines to 50 percent at 10 years. Survival rates from melanoma of the ciliary body appear to be similar in the small number of cases available for review. Malignant melanoma of the iris has a much better prognosis with only about 5 percent of patients succumbing from the disease. The prognosis for uveal melanoma is related to histologic type, the spindle type having a better prognosis than the epitheloid and mixed cell types.

The prognosis for small lesions treated by photocoagulation or local irradiation is excellent, with less than 10 percent of patients developing metastatic disease. Of patients requiring enucleation, approximately half eventually die of metastases. Zimmerman et al.[18] estimate that the death rate from choroidal melanomas is approximately 1 percent a year, while the mortality curves of surgically treated melanoma patients show an abrupt rise in mortality after a hiatus of 3 months. During the second year after enucleation, the mortality in their series was 8 percent; this rate declined progressively over several years, and returned to the pretreatment rate of 1 percent. They concluded that their evidence suggests that the current enucleation technique reduces survival by the blood-borne spread of tumor cells at the time of surgery.

Local recurrence in the orbit is not common, occurring in about 20 percent of patients in whom extraocular extension was found at enucleation. It is very rare when no extraocular extension was found. Postoperative radiotherapy to the orbit probably reduces the incidence of local recurrence, but as no controlled clinical trials have been performed, clear evidence as to the value of radiotherapy is lacking. All patients who develop blood-borne spread eventually die of the disease. The mean duration of survival after presentation of metastases is 1 year.

Primary Orbital Melanoma

Such melanomas are extremely rare. They may occur de novo or may arise in association with preexisting pigmentation such as the nevus of Ota. The patients usually present with proptosis—evidence of an expanding mass within the orbit. The diagnosis is usually made at orbitotomy. Subsequent treatment is determined by whether there is any evidence of systemic dissemination. Therefore, patients with primary orbital melanoma should be evaluated by an oncologist so that a complete physical evaluation can be performed. Exenteration of the orbit is usually the most appropriate treatment and is sometimes combined with chemotherapy and radiotherapy.

OPTIC NERVE GLIOMA

The optic nerve is not a true nerve because it possesses neither Schwann cells nor a true sheath. It is surrounded by the same covering as the brain, and the intrinsic supporting structures are true neuroglial cells. It is, therefore, a tract of the central nervous system comparable to the white matter of the brain. However, there is one important difference—the nerve fibers of the tract are separated by vascular connective tissue septa extending into the tract from surrounding pia. It is to the abnormal proliferation of supporting neuroglial cells that the term glioma has been applied. Gliomas arise throughout the central nervous system. However, those arising within the optic nerve chiasm or tract are usually extremely slow growing to such an extent that in the analysis of one particular series,[6] they appeared to show many of the characteristics of congenital hamartomas. This group of tumors are called optic nerve gliomas.

Optic nerve gliomas are fairly rare. The majority of cases have been encountered in children and only occasionally does the lesion become apparent in anyone over 20 years of age. There is a strong association between neurofibromatosis and optic nerve glioma. In some series, up to 30 percent of the children with gliomas had evidence of neurofibromatosis.

The presence of an enlarging tumor within the optic nerve produces a deterioration in vision usually associated with increasing proptosis. In some cases, there may be no proptosis and the child may present to the ophthalmologist with an "amblyopic" squinting eye. Sometimes these children are subjected to prolonged occlusion of the good eye in a vain attempt to improve the vision in the eye that is incapable of improving. Examination of the fundus will reveal optic atrophy in certain anteriorly placed gliomas, and there may be associated optic disc edema. An afferent pupillary defect can be demonstrated in nearly all cases. Investigation of the tumor should include CT scans, both axial and coronal; axial polytomography of the orbit and particularly optic canals; and if the child is old enough to coop-

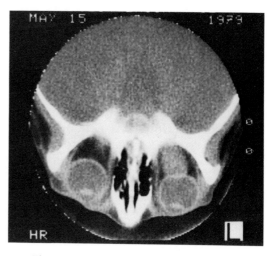

Fig. 22-10. Optic nerve glioma. Axial CT scan showing diffuse enlargement of the optic nerve within the left orbit.

erate, an accurate assessment of the visual fields. Ultrasonic scans of the optic nerve may be of some help in assessing the position and size of the optic nerve tumor; but undoubtedly the most useful investigation is CT scanning, which will accurately delineate the position and size of the glioma (Fig. 22-10).

Management

The management of these tumors is dependent on the size and extent of the tumor and its histologic type. The diagnosis cannot rest on clinical grounds alone, and a biopsy of the tumor should be obtained. The vast majority of the gliomas seen in children have an extremely slow growth rate. A simple proliferation of astrocytes will produce an increase in the number of glial cells compared to the number present in a normal section of the optic nerve. Some cells undergo vacuolization producing a mucoid substance that may accumulate in certain areas of the tumor. An associated arachnoid hyperplasia, which has been described by a number of authors, may account for a considerable portion of the enlargement of the nerve.

Because of the slow rate of growth of these tumors, some clinicians have advocated an extremely conservative approach and think that surgical intervention plays no part in the management.[6] However, while a good proportion of the children with optic nerve glioma show no deterioration over a long period of time, some children undoubtedly exhibit progression of the tumor. The protocol which I have adopted at Moorfields Eye Hospital in London is to observe gliomas that are confined to the orbit with no evidence of enlargement of the optic canal. However, if there is evidence—either at the time of initial presentation or at a later date—of enlargement of the optic canal, then the optic chiasm is approached through a transcranial exposure. The nerve is transected at the chiasm, and the intracanalicular and intraorbital portion of the optic nerve removed. If at the initial presentation there is evidence of involvement of the chiasm, a transcranial approach is used and the extent of the tumor in relation to the chiasm assessed. It the tumor is resectable, the tumor together with the involved optic nerve is removed.

The technique used for removal of the optic nerve from the globe to the chiasm is a two-stage procedure, with the first stage being the transcranial approach using a frontal flap. The nerve is transected at the chiasm, the optic canal is unroofed, and the nerve resected at the posterior part of the orbit. The orbital roof is not transgressed. The second stage is to remove the orbital portion of the optic nerve; this time the approach is through a lateral canthotomy incision. The nerve is transected at the posterior part of the globe, which is rotated nasally. The optic nerve containing the tumor is transected out of the orbit, and the globe, together with the attached muscles, is restored to its former position. In a relatively large series of cases, no case of phthisis bulbi has been encountered and the cosmetic results are quite excellent.

Some authors have advocated radiotherapy for optic nerve glioma. One of the problems in dealing with such a low grade tumor is that the lethal dose for the surrounding tissue is approximately the same as for the tumor so that effective radiotherapy to the region of the chiasm is precluded. Again, one is in the same dilemma as in dealing with tumors confined to the orbit, and on balance—although the therapeutic effect of radiotherapy is somewhat dubious—it is probably worthwhile treating the lesion, since then the relatives and friends of the patient feel that everything possible has been done.

Optic nerve gliomas in adults are extremely rare and are usually malignant. In these patients there develops within a short period of time rapid loss of vision with progressive proptosis and evidence of invasion of the intracranial structures. Sometimes malignant cells appear in the vitreous body. In these patients once the diagnosis has been established through examination of a biopsy, subsequent treatment depends on the extent of the spread of what is a highly malignant tumor. In the vast majority of cases, the tumor has extended beyond the bounds of surgical resection and the primary treatment is radiotherapy. Occasionally the tumor may be resected surgically, but in the main the outlook for these patients is extremely poor.

PRIMARY OPTIC NERVE MENINGIOMA

Meningiomas arising primarily from the optic nerve sheath are comparatively rare. They are most commonly seen in women between the ages of 35 and 60. Analysis of a large series of patients seen at Moorfields Eye Hospital showed that the predominant feature of optic nerve sheath meningiomas is early visual loss.[15] Proptosis occurred later and was never of a great degree unless the lesion was long standing, which is in contrast to tumors that arise elsehwere in the orbit. A slowly enlarging cavernous hemangioma or neurilemmoma will usually produce marked proptosis before there is evidence of any compression of the optic nerve; the exception is a small lesion expanding within the bony confines of the orbital apex. This course of events is explicable when one considers the site of origin of a meningioma of the optic nerve sheath. Meningiomas arise from the meningocytes of the arachnoid within the fibrous capsule provided by the

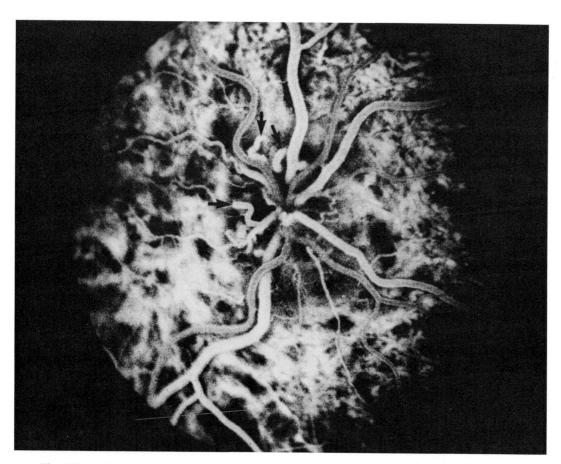

Fig. 22-11. Primary optic nerve meningioma. Optic nerve head demonstrating gross disc edema, with opticociliary shunt vessels arrowed.

surrounding dura. The enlarging tumor is thus initially confined by the dura and compresses the optic nerve causing visual deterioratioh. Proptosis occurs later when the tumor bursts out through the dura into the orbit and forms an enlarging space-occupying lesion within the muscle cone. Occasionally, visual loss is absent initially and the patient develops proptosis at an early stage. It is likely that the meningiomatous tissue in these cases extended through the dura fairly quickly and failed to compress the optic nerve to any great extent.

Edema and atrophy of the optic disc together with the development of opticociliary shunt vessels give some indication of the effect of the pressure of the enlarging tumor within the dural sheath (Fig. 22-11). The pressure is such that invasion of the optic nerve head by tumor tissue has been recorded.[12] These shunt vessels allow egress of blood from the retinal veins to the choroidal vessels. This is probably caused by meningiomatous tissue pressing on the central retinal vein immediately behind the globe.

Routine plain radiographs with optic canal views should be performed on all patients suspected of having a primary optic nerve tumor. Routine plain radiographs are almost invariably negative in retrobulbar sheath meningioma as opposed to the foraminal type of meningioma, which usually presents obvious radiographic signs. Computerized tomography can reveal fairly small tumors of the optic nerve. These new high resolution scanners, which provide axial and coronal views of the orbital content, have provided extremely valuable methods of assessing the size and extent of optic nerve tumors.

It is particularly important that all patients are thoroughly examined by a neurologist. Visual fields must be accurately assessed, and a general medical examination including biochemical and hematologic evaluation must be performed.

Management

The outlook for vision in this group of patients is extremely poor. However, in a few patients some restoration of vision may be achieved if the tumor is located anterior to the entry of the central retinal artery or it has burst through the dural sheath at an early stage to form a pedunculated mass within the orbit. Resection of such tumors with preservation of vision has been recorded. In the majority of patients, however, treatment is directed towards preventing potential extention of the meningioma up the optic canal to the middle fossa and secondarily towards relieving disfiguring proptosis. The prime consideration in reaching a decision about removal of such tumors is the level of vision. These tumors are not aggressive and they behave in a similar way to intracranial meningiomas, which are slow growing; thus, the patients often survive for many years with or without surgical intervention.

There are actually two schools of thought. One group favors surgical removal of the intraorbital portion of the optic nerve, together with the meningioma, once vision has been completely lost. The other group favors conservative management of the patient and the avoidance of surgical removal. Henderson (in an unpublished study) has reported a series, at the Mayo Clinic, of nine patients with primary orbital meningiomas and with survival of up to 19 years after the initial diagnosis. Only one patient of the nine had died, and this death was suicide. When there is progressive proptosis, both groups feel that surgical intervention is justified in order to remove the bulk of the tumor. The third method of treatment is to use radiotherapy. This will certainly reduce the size of the mass, and some reduction in the proptosis will follow.

RETINOBLASTOMA

This malignant growth is predominantly a disease of infancy and childhood. It occurs about once in 34,000 live births either as a somatic mutation or as an inherited, autosomal dominant characteristic due to germinal mutation. Hereditary cases are 70 percent bilateral, and in unilateral cases the unaffected eye must be watched for possible later involvement. Five percent of cases have demonstrable deletions of the long arm of chromosome 13, and children with this deletion commonly have other abnormalities including mental retardation.

Retinoblastomas arise from the photoreceptive cells of the retina. These tumors are of a "small round cell type" with their cells having dense nuclei and scant cytoplasm and are arranged in solid sheets of pseudorosettes.

Of the clinical features present during the early stages of the disease, the most common presenting sign is a white reflex that is seen through the child's pupil. Occasionally, the parents may observe a squint and in older children a deterioration in vision may be noted. The most important investigation is the examination of both eyes under general anesthesia by an experienced ophthalmologist using a binocular indirect ophthalmoscope. Examination of the fundus commonly shows small whitish or yellowish plaques covered by detached retina (Fig. 22-12). In some cases, extension of the tumor into the vitreous can be observed. In more advanced cases the tumor may grow to such a size that it causes a secondary glaucoma.

sometimes with an increase in the size of the globe. The differential diagnosis of retinoblastoma is between larval granulomatosis due to *Toxocara canis*, Coats disease, and primary hyperplastic vitreous. Helpful investigative techniques include ultrasonic scanning of the globe and CT scans. If there is a suspicion of central nervous system involvement by the tumor, then an examination of the cerebrospinal fluid, including the use of cytology tests, should be performed. In all cases of retinoblastoma, chest x-ray and bone scan studies should be obtained. The classification of retinoblastoma suggested by Reese and Ellsworth[13] is an attempt to relate tumor extent in the eye to treatment alternatives and prognostic criteria and thus to aid in comparison of results. The stages according to their classification are as follow:

I   Single or multiple tumors of less than 4 disc diameters, at or behind the equator.

II   Single or multiple tumors of 4 to 10 disc diameters, at or behind the equator.

III   Tumors anterior to the equator or a single tumor larger than 10 disc diameters, at or behind the equator.

IV   Mutliple lesions, some greater

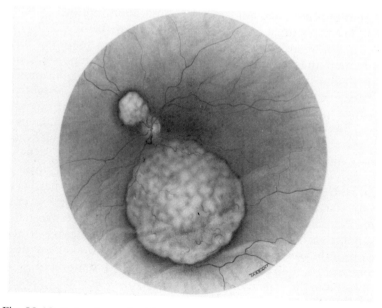

Fig. 22-12. Extensive retinoblastoma with associated retinal detachment.

than 10 disc diameters. Any lesion extending anterior to the ora serrata.

V   Large lesions involving more than half the retina. The presence of vitreous seedings.

In later stages, there may be extraocular extension when the tumor passes backwards in the optic nerve to the brain. There may be extension of this tumor into the orbit producing a massive proptosis, sometimes with perforation of the globe.

Treatment

The treatment of retinoblastoma has moved away from the earlier policy of enucleation of the worse or affected eye and conservative treatment of the remaining eye. The aim now is twofold: to eradicate tumor and to maintain maximum vision.

Tumors smaller than 3 mm in diameter that are anteriorly situated can be effectively treated with cryotherapy; more posteriorly situated lesions can be treated with photocoagulation. However, when the small tumors are adjacent to the optic disc or macula, external beam irradiation by a single lateral field is more appropriate. A tumor of 3 to 10 mm in size can be treated with a radioactive cobalt plaque. Again, should the lesion be near the macula or optic disc lateral beam irradiation is preferable. For a tumor larger than 10 mm, irradiation to the whole of the eye is recommended.

If there are more than two tumors present in one eye, radiation should be given to the whole eye by external beam. With only two tumors it may be possible to treat both tumors by those methods previously described.

When tumors have involved a major portion of the vitreous cavity, then the whole eye should be treated with radiotherapy. The eye should be enucleated if the optic nerve is obviously infiltrated. When there are bilateral tumors, each eye should be treated based on its individual condition. If enucleation of one eye is required, then efforts to preserve vision in the remaining eye are all the more important. Postoperative

radiation to the orbit and optic foramen should be given if there is evidence of extrascleral extension or optic nerve infiltration. When such extension or infiltration exists, the risk of tumor dissemination into the blood stream or into the central nervous system via the subarachnoid space is very high, and consideration should be given to chemotherapy and irradiation of the central nervous system.

The presence of metastases is a grave prognostic sign, since the chances of long-term survival are minimal. Patients in stage V are now being treated with chemotherapy, and the effect of this treatment is currently being evaluated in a number of centers. The most commonly used combination of drugs is cyclophosphamide, vincristine, and actinomycin-D, given intravenously every 2 or 3 weeks. When the risk of central nervous system involvement is high, consideration should be given to the use of irradiation of the whole central nervous system as well as to intrathecal methotrexate and systemic combination chemotherapy.

In specialized centers where experience with these rare tumors has been obtained, a cure rate of 85 to 90 percent is usual if the methods of treatment outlined above are used. Fortunately, a dose of 3,500 rads is adequate to control most retinoblastomas; a complication rate of less than 10 percent is expected at this level. Occasionally, a cataract may form following the radiotherapy, but the lens changes may be minimal and usually do not significantly impair vision. In young children, reduced growth of the orbital bones following radiotherapy may result in deformity; but this effect is much less marked with megavoltage than with orthovoltage therapy. The occurrence of sarcomas around the orbit and especially osteogenic sarcomas has been reported following irradiation in several series. Most cases, however, were treated with high dosage using orthodosage irradiation with its higher bone absorption dose. It must be remembered that there is a genetic tendency for osteogenic sarcoma to form in a proportion of retinoblastoma patients.

The overall results of treating these rare malignant tumors are good; Bedford[2] has reported a cure rate of 100 percent for stages I and II, and 75 percent for the less common stages IV and V, with an overall cure rate of 90 percent.

ORBITAL AND INTRAOCULAR METASTASES

The orbit is an uncommon but well-recognized site for metastases from malignancy arising elsewhere in the body. Frequently such tumors arise from the breast, lung, prostate, or gastrointestinal tract. No particular part of the orbit is more frequently affected than another. In some cases the tumor mass rapidly expands and displaces the globe and the diagnosis is made from tissue obtained at biopsy. A schirrous carcinoma of the breast does, however, produce a typical clinical picture—a metastasis produces a fibrosing mass within the orbit and this mass causes retraction of the globe and a relative enophthalmos; the initial complaint, in most patients, is of double vision. A female patient with no history of trauma and with normal radiographs who experiences double vision accompanied by enophthalmos invariably has a primary schirrous carcinoma of the breast.

An uncommon but well-recognized metastasis encountered in infants and young children is a neuroblastoma. These tumors originate in the sympathetic nervous system; usually the primary tumor is well advanced and has evidence of metastases to other sites, but occasionally the orbital tumor is the first sign of the disease. The child is noticed to have swelling of the eyelids, chemosis, and proptosis, with rapid progression of these signs often with an associated inflammatory reaction within the orbit. Tissue should be obtained from the orbit in those cases in which the diagnosis is in doubt so that radiotherapy and chemotherapy can be started.

The majority of intraocular metastases

occur in the choroid of the posterior pole. Metastases in other parts of the uveal tract and the retina and in the conjunctiva have been described but are exceedingly rare. More than half of all choroidal metastases arise from carcinoma of the breast. Patients developing choroidal metastases from carcinoma of the breast usually have other soft tissue metastases, especially in the lungs. Occasionally the choroidal metastasis is the presenting sign of dissemination, but in such a patient other unsuspected metastases can usually be detected at the same time. About one-third of choroidal metastases arise from carcinoma of the bronchus. Metastases from most other types of malignant tumor have been reported from time to time, but all are very rare. The patient with choroidal metastases complains of defective vision and sometimes pain in the affected eye. Examination reveals a solid-looking retinal detachment in the posterior pole, with the elevated area appearing pale in color and often having hemorrhagic areas. The lesion must be distinguished from primary malignant melanoma and other causes of retinal detachment. Usually this is quite easy because of the history of malignancy elsewhere.

The prognosis for all patients with choroidal or orbital metastases is grave. Few survive more than a few years. Nevertheless, palliative treatment is indicated to relieve symptoms and maintain morale. Nearly all cases respond to radiotherapy with regression of the tumor leading to relief of pain if present, and preservation of the remaining useful vision in the affected eye. In a few cases there can be quite marked improvement of vision. When there are bilateral lesions, treatment can be given by a single lateral field or by opposed lateral fields, taking care to avoid both lenses. A fairly high dose should be given to avoid regrowth of the tumor during the patient's remaining lifespan, so a 3,500-rad to 4,000-rad tumor dose in 3 weeks is recommended.

When a patient has a secondary tumor arising from a prostatic carcinoma, treatment with estrogen will often produce a quite dramatic resolution of the primary and secondary tumors.

SUMMARY

Cancers affecting the eye and orbit encompass a variety of tumor types ranging from small, locally aggressive indolent tumors to locally very aggressive tumors with a propensity for distant metastasis. Early diagnosis of these tumors by improved diagnostic modalities including computerized axial tomography as well as by new treatment protocols including radiation and chemotherapy have led to the preservation of vision as well as to the much improved cure rate of many of these tumors.

REFERENCES

1. Ashton, N. 1975. Epithelial tumours of the lacrimal gland. Modern Problems in Ophthalmology, 14: 306.

2. Bedford, M. A., Bedotto, C., and Macfaul, P.A. 1971. Retinoblastoma: A study of 139 cases. British Journal of Ophthalmology, 55: 19.

3. Font, R. L., and Gamel, J. W. 1978. Epithelial tumours of the lacrimal gland. An analysis of 265 cases. In Jakobiec, F., Ed.: Ocular and Adnexal Tumours. Aesculapius Press, Birmingham, AL, 787.

4. Foote, F. W., and Frazell, E. L. 1953. Tumors of the major salivary glands. Cancer, 6: 1065.

5. Forrest, A. W. 1971. Pathologic criteria for effective management of epithelial lacrimal gland tumors. American Journal of Ophthalmology, suppl., 71: 178.

6. Hoyt, W. F., and Baghdassarian, S. A. 1969. Optic glioma of childhood. Natural history and rationale for conservative management. British Journal of Ophthalmology, 53: 793.

7. Jones, I. S., Reese, A. B., and Kraut, J. 1966. Orbital rhabdomyosarcoma: An analysis of sixty-two cases. American Journal of Ophthalmology, 61: 721.

8. Koorneef, L. 1976. Spatial Aspects of Orbital Musculofibrous Tissue in Man. Swets and Zeitlinger BV, Amsterdam and Lisse.

9. Lederman, M. 1964. Radiation treatment of primary malignant tumours of the orbit. In Bonivk, M., Ed.: Ocular and Adnexal Tumors: New and Controversial Aspects. C. V. Mosby, St. Louis, 477.

10. Lederman, M., and Wybar, K. 1976. Ocular malignant diseases. Proceedings of the Royal Society of Medicine, 69: 895.

11. Morgan, G., and Harry, J. 1978. Lymphocytic tumours of indeterminate nature: A 5-year follow-up of 98 conjunctival and orbital lesions. British Journal of Ophthalmology, 62: 381.

12. Newell, F. W., and Beaman, T. C. 1958. Ocular signs of meningioma. American Journal of Ophthalmology, 45: 30.

13. Reese, A. B., and Ellsworth, R. M. 1964. Management of retinoblastoma. Annals of the New York Academy of Sciences, 114: 958.

14. Wright, J. E. 1976. Surgery on the orbit. In Miller, S. J. H., Ed.: Operative Surgery. Butterworth, London, 131.

15. Wright, J. E. 1977. Primary optic nerve meningiomas: Clinical presentation and management. Transactions of the American Academy of Ophthalmology and Otolaryngology, 83: 617.

16. Wright, J. E., Stewart, W., and Krohel, G. 1979. Clinical presentation and management of lacrimal gland tumours. British Journal of Ophthalmology, 64: 600.

17. Zimmerman, L. E. 1964. New concepts regarding certain orbital and lacrimal gland tumors. In Boniuk, M., Ed.: Ocular and Adnexal Tumors: New and Controversial Aspects, C. V. Mosby, St. Louis, 395.

18. Zimmerman, L. E., and McLean, I. W. 1979. An evaluation of enucleation in the management of uveal melanomas. American Journal of Ophthalmology, 87: 741.

23 | Cancer of the Thyroid Gland

Oliver H. Beahrs, M.D.
Paul D. Kiernan, M.D.
John P. Hubert, Jr., M.D.

INTRODUCTION

The incidence of thyroid cancer in the population at large is very low and difficult to determine. In 1978, approximately 16 percent of deaths in the United States were caused by cancer (roughly 390,000).[1] Because the thyroid gland ranks about 25th in frequency among the anatomic sites that develop malignant tumors, only 1,100 deaths will be due to thyroid cancer (compared with 92,400 for lung cancer and 42,000 for colon cancer).

The United States Public Health Service has estimated the number of new cases of thyroid cancer per year at 25 per 1 million population. Sokal[58] has calculated a similar rate from the medical literature. Annual mortality from thyroid cancer is five deaths per 1 million men and eight deaths per 1 million women, the disparity between case rate and mortality being attributed to the excellent prognosis for most patients. If these numbers are accepted, one must conclude that, even when present, thyroid cancer is an infrequent cause of death.[63] Thus, the proposal that all goiters and all nodules should be excised to prevent death from cancer probably is indefensible.

The geographic distribution of thyroid cancer has been linked to the distribution of nodular goiter. There seems to be a high incidence of thyroid cancer in the so-called endemic areas, such as Switzerland and the Great Lakes region of the United States. However, Cuello and associates[19] have disagreed with this hypothesis. For example,

Iceland and Hawaii are two areas in which a high incidence of thyroid cancer is associated with a low incidence of nodular goiter. In the United States, the incidence of carcinoma of the thyroid is the same in Chicago and Detroit (Great Lakes region) as it is in Birmingham and Dallas, where nodular goiter is much less common.[15]

Similarly, racial factors bear no relationship to the incidence of thyroid cancer; however, ethnic differences in diet, customs, or areas of residence may. In Israel, a country with one of the highest incidences of thyroid neoplasia, cancer of the thyroid is more common among Jews of European origin than among Jews born in Asia.[52] In South Africa, Bantus have a much higher incidence of thyroid cancer than do blacks from other regions.

At the Mayo Clinic, 10 to 20 percent of patients with nodular goiters diagnosed clinically are treated surgically. The incidence of cancer in these patients has been 5 percent over a period of several decades. However, in recent years, the incidence has increased somewhat, the data being based on a more critical selection of patients for operation. Currently, malignancies are present in 12 to 14 percent of patients undergoing thyroid surgery because of suspicion of cancer. For those with nodular goiters that are asymptomatic and not suspected of being cancerous, the incidence of cancer remains at about 4 percent (Table 23-1). Papillary cancer has been found incidentally in 0.5 to 2.0 percent of patients with parenchymatous hypertrophy (Graves

TABLE 23-1. INCIDENCE OF CARCINOMA OF
THYROID GLAND IN CASES IN WHICH
OPERATION FOR EXOPHTHALMIC GOITER OR
ADENOMATOUS GOITER WAS PERFORMED
1938 TO 1947, INCLUSIVE

Clinical Diagnosis	Total	Ca Present No.	%
Exophthalmic goiter	3,029	14	0.5
Carcinoma not suspected	3,027	13	0.4
Adenomatous goiter			
With hyperthyroidism	2,229	26	1.2
Carcinoma not suspected	2,222	19	0.9
Without hyperthyroidism	3,247	244	7.5
Carcinoma not suspected	3,121	118	3.8

(Beahrs, O.H., Pemberton, J. deJ., and Black, B.M. 1951. Nodular goiter and
malignant lesions of the thyroid gland. Journal of Clinical Endocrinology and
Metabolism 11:1157, © (1951) The Endocrine Society.)

disease).[5] The occurrence of cancer in patients with adenomatous goiter and hyperthyroidism (Plummer disease) who are treated surgically is 1 percent or less.

In an autopsy series, Mortensen and coworkers[45] found primary cancer of the thyroid in 2.8 percent of the cases, this representing 5.3 percent of cases involving multinodular goiter and 9.2 percent of cases involving single-nodule goiter (Table 23-2). They also found cancer metastatic to the thyroid in 1.8 percent of the cases, this representing 3.4 percent of cases involving nodular glands.

Although cancer of the thyroid may occur in a person of any age, the incidence of cancer in nodular goiters is much higher in children than in adults. Hayles and associates[33] noted an incidence of 50 to 70 percent in children. Thus, even though the true incidence for children may be somewhat less than this, a pediatric patient with nodular goiter should undergo thyroidectomy.

Thyroid disease is seen more frequently in women, although malignancy presenting in nodular goiters is more frequent in men.[50] Overall, the incidence of thyroid cancer is higher in women than in men, with ratios ranging from 2:1[15, 45] to 8:3[3] (Table 23-3).

Cancer is seen more frequently in a thyroid gland that is considered clinically to be

TABLE 23-2. MALIGNANT INVOLVEMENT OF
THYROID GLANDS REMOVED AT 1,000 CONSECUTIVE
ROUTINE AUTOPSIES

Type of Malignancy	No.	Incidence (%) In All 1,000 Glands	In 525 Nodular Glands
Primary carcinoma	28	2.8	5.3
Metastatic involvement	18	1.8	3.4
Total	46	4.6	8.7

(Mortensen, J.D., Bennett, W. A., and Woolner, L.B. 1954. Incidence of carcinoma in
thyroid glands removed at 1000 consecutive routine necropsies. Surgical Forum, 5:
659.)

TABLE 23-3. SEX RATIO OF DIFFERENT
TYPES OF THYROID CANCER

Type of Cancer	Male	Female
Papillary	1.0	2.3
Follicular	1.4	1.0
Medullary (solid)	4.0	1.0
Anaplastic	1.0	1.3

(Beahrs, O.H., and Kubista, T.P. 1968. Diagnosis of thyroid
cancer. In Cancer Management: A Special Graduate Course on
Cancer. J. B. Lippincott, Philadelphia, 573.)

a single nodule than to be multinodular. In
reviewing our cases, we elected not to separate these two groups, because a nodule that
is considered to be single at clinical examination frequently is found to be multiple at
surgery. Therefore, we prefer to use the
term "discrete nodule" for what seems to be
a solitary nodule on palpation.

ETIOLOGY

The cause of thyroid cancer is unknown.
Evidence suggests that previous radiation
therapy to the thyroid region may be one of
the contributing factors.[17, 21, 24, 60, 64, 67] This
is especially true in children and adolescents—a group in which many have had irradiation of the head and neck for lymphadenitis, tonsillar hypertrophy, enlarged
thymus, or acne. Wood and associates[69]
found an increased incidence of thyroid
cancer in persons exposed to radioactive fall-
out in Nagasaki and Hiroshima, irrespective of their age at the time of exposure.
Therapeutic doses of interstitial irradiation
of the thyroid tissue, as in the treatment of
thyroid disease with ^{131}I, have not been
shown to cause cancer.

Crile[16] suggested that some cancers are
hormone-dependent. Clark et al.[15] noted an
increased occurrence of thyroid cancer in
endemic goiter areas and attributed it to excessive and long-standing stimulation of the
gland by thyrotropic hormone in the pres-

ence of some other factors. This hypothesis
can be analyzed in terms of the initiator-
promoter theory for the mechanism of carcinogenesis, with the injurious factors (either hereditary or acquired) being the initi-
ator and the prolonged action of thyrotropin on the gland serving as the promoter.
This hypothesis is supported by the finding
that the administration of antithyroid drugs,
which induces increased secretion of thyrotropin, can experimentally produce thyroid
cancer in certain strains of animals that are
at high risk of developing cancer. However,
the opposite is suggested by the high incidence of thyroid cancer in Iceland and Hawaii, where the incidence of nodular goiter
is low and the thyrotropin secretion is not
increased among the population.

EMBRYOLOGY AND ANATOMY

Thyroid Embryology

About the fourth week of embryonic life, a
median diverticulum arises from the pharyngeal floor between the first and the second branchial pouch.[47] A solid cord of cells
becomes canalized to form the thyroglossal
duct and grows downward, ventral to the
pharynx. This tubular duct subsequently divides into a series of cellular cords to form
the isthmus and the lateral lobes of the thyroid.

The thyroglossal duct normally undergoes degeneration, leaving behind the foramen cecum at its upper end, and in nearly
50 percent of cases, leaving the pyramidal
lobe of the thyroid gland at its lower end.
Failure of the duct to degenerate entirely
results in thyroglossal duct cyst formation or
accessory thyroid-tissue residuals, most commonly lingual thyroid at the foramen cecum.

Rather late in fetal life, the capsule of
the gland is formed from adjacent mesenchymal tissue. Consequently, tissues foreign
to the thyroid, such as parathyroids, may be
enclosed in its capsule.

Anatomy

The thyroid is the largest endocrine gland of the body, weighing approximately 30 g.[36] It is located in the anterior and lower part of the neck and is composed of a smaller central part, the isthmus, with two larger lateral structures, the lobes. In nearly half of the cases, a third lobe—the pyramidal lobe—arises from the upper border of the isthmus[38] (more often from the left than the right side of it) and ascends sometimes as high as the hyoid bone. The isthmus covers the second, third, and fourth tracheal rings. The lateral lobes usually extend from the middle of the thyroid cartilage superiorly to the sixth tracheal ring inferiorly. Anteriorly, the lobes are covered by the skin, subcutaneous tissue, and muscles—platysma, sternocleidomastoid, superior belly of the omohyoid, sternohyoid, and sternothyroid. The deep surface of the gland is related to the first five or six tracheal rings, the cricoid cartilage, and the lower half of the thyroid cartilage. The thyroid is related medially to the esophagus and recurrent laryngeal

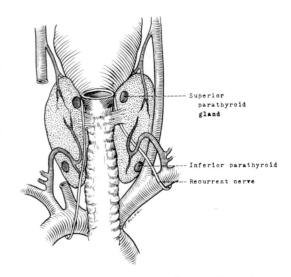

Fig. 23-2. Anatomy of the thyroid gland, from behind. (Hollinshead, W.H. 1952. Anatomy of the endocrine glands. Surgical Clinics of North America, 32: 1115.)

nerve and laterally to the carotid sheath, containing the carotid artery, internal jugular vein, and vagus nerve. The postero-medial and posteroinferior portions of the lateral lobes are related to the superior and inferior parathyroid glands, respectively.

Blood Supply

The thyroid is a highly vascular organ, with a normal flow rate of 5 ml/g per minute. Knowledge of its blood supply facilitates any related surgical procedure and minimizes hemorrhage. The thyroid gland is served by two pairs of arteries (superior and inferior thyroid arteries), two pairs of veins (superior and inferior thyroid veins), and an inconstant artery (thyroidea ima) and vein (middle thyroid).[49]

The superior thyroid artery is the first branch of the external carotid artery, arising from its lower anterior part (just below the tip of the greater horn of the hyoid bone), turning caudad to the apex of the corresponding lobe of the thyroid, and dividing into glandular branches. Medially, the superior thyroid artery is in relation to the inferior constrictor muscle and the ex-

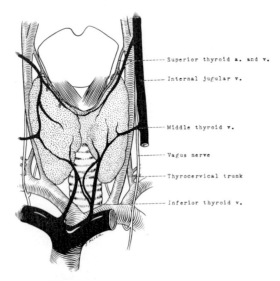

Fig. 23-1. Anatomy of the thyroid gland, from the front. Note pyramidal lobe not illustrated; middle thyroid veins (illustrated) present variably. (Hollinshead, W.H. 1952. Anatomy of the endocrine glands. Surgical Clinics of North America, 32: 1115.)

ternal laryngeal branch of the superior laryngeal nerve. Details of the anatomic relationship between the external branch of the superior laryngeal nerve and the superior thyroid vessels will be discussed under "Innervation." Superficially, the superior thyroid artery is covered at its origin by the anterior border of the sternomastoid muscle, for a short distance thereafter by fascia, platysma, and skin, and caudad by omohyoid, sternohyoid, and sternothyroid muscles.[20]

The superior thyroid artery gives rise to infrahyoid, sternocleidomastoid, and laryngeal branches. The laryngeal branches enter the larynx with the internal branch of the superior laryngeal nerve. As the superior thyroid artery reaches the upper pole of the lateral lobe, it trifurcates into an anterior branch that supplies the gland anteriorly, a posterior branch that courses behind and supplies the gland posteriorly, and an isthmic branch that crosses medially along the upper border of the isthmus to the opposite side.[61]

The superior thyroid vein accompanies the superior thyroid artery and ends in the internal jugular vein. On the anterior surface of the thyroid gland are prominent connections between the superior and the inferior thyroid veins.

A middle thyroid vein, which has no corresponding artery, is often present; this vein leaves the gland in its midportion to follow the outer border of the omohyoid muscle, cross the common carotid artery, and terminate in the internal jugular vein.[31]

The inferior thyroid artery is a branch of the thyrocervical trunk, which arises from the subclavian artery. It ascends along the anterior border of the anterior scalenus muscle and, opposite the cricoid cartilage, turns medially, traversing deep to the common carotid artery and to the middle of the posterior border of the corresponding lobe of the thyroid. It then curves medially and downward and descends to the lower half of the lobe.[20] The inferior thyroid artery provides the major blood supply to the upper half of the trachea, usually through three branches, of which the first and lowermost is the largest.[42] The branch near the lower pole of the thyroid gland is the third and uppermost and is the smallest. Division of that branch during surgical removal of the thyroid should not impair tracheal vascularization. As the inferior thyroid artery passes medially behind the gland, it crosses the recurrent laryngeal nerves—in front, behind, or on both sides of them.[36] It is covered anteriorly by a carotid sheath, which contains the common carotid artery, the internal jugular vein, and the vagus nerve. Usually, the inferior thyroid artery closely approximates the middle cervical sympathetic ganglion.[36] In a detailed analysis of the anatomy of the thyroid as seen in 100 consecutive cases, Hunt and associates[38] found that the inferior thyroid artery was absent from the left side in 5 cases and absent from the right side in 2.

The inferior thyroid veins originate on the anterior surface of the gland and descend anterior to the trachea. Both may terminate in the left innominate vein or the left may end in the left and the right in the right innominate vein. Both inferior thyroid veins may have numerous connections and form a plexus in front of the trachea beneath the isthmus.

In 10 percent of cases,[20] a fifth artery normally present in the embryo (the thyroidea ima) arises from the aortic arch innominate artery or lower common carotid artery and reaches the inferior border of the isthmus after running upward on the anterior surface of the trachea.

Innervation

The thyroid gland receives its innervation from the sympathetic and parasympathetic divisions of the autonomic nervous system. The sympathetic fibers arise from the cervical ganglion and enter with the blood vessels. The parasympathetic fibers are derived from the vagus nerve and reach the gland via branches of the laryngeal nerves. The relationship of the thyroid gland to the recurrent laryngeal nerve, the external laryngeal nerve, and the cervical sympathetic system is of major surgical importance.

Embryologically, the recurrent laryngeal nerves (inferior laryngeal nerves) originate from the vagus nerves near the fourth branchial arches. These arches later become the aortic arch on the left and the subclavian artery on the right, and as these structures descend in the upper thorax, they "pull" the recurrent laryngeal nerves with them.[46]

On the right side, the recurrent laryngeal nerve leaves the vagus nerve as the latter crosses the first portion of the subclavian artery; the recurrent laryngeal nerve then turns upward and medially behind that artery and the common carotid artery, and (most often but not always) travels upward in the groove between the trachea and the esophagus. This nerve ascends toward the right lobe of the thyroid gland and crosses or is crossed by the inferior thyroid artery or passes between its branches. On reaching the lower border of the inferior constrictor muscle, the recurrent laryngeal nerve passes deep to the muscle and gains access to the laryngeal muscles.

On the left side, the recurrent laryngeal nerve turns under the arch of the aorta and ascends into the neck, most often in the tracheoesophageal groove. At the level of the inferior border of the thyroid lobe, the left recurrent laryngeal nerve, like its counterpart, may be in front of, behind, or between the terminal branches of the inferior thyroid artery. Hunt and associates[38] reported that the right recurrent laryngeal nerve was located in the tracheoesophageal groove in 64 percent of cases and lateral to the trachea in 33 percent, and that the left nerve was thus located in 77 percent and 22 percent of cases, respectively. The right nerve was anterolateral to the trachea in 6 percent as was the left in 4 percent, thus being in increased danger of division during subtotal lobectomy.

A few patients (0.3 to 0.6 percent) have a "nonrecurrent" laryngeal nerve on the right side, originating from the cervical trunk of the vagus at the level of the thyroid cartilage and passing directly into the cricothyroid membrane.[46, 49, 51, 59] Unawareness of this anomaly may result in damage to the nerve by dissection lateral and posterior to the thyroid gland.

The recurrent laryngeal nerve supplies all of the intrinsic muscles of the larynx except the cricothyroid and is sensory for the mucous membrane of the larynx below the vocal cord folds. Damage to one nerve will result in ipsilateral vocal cord paralysis, and the vocal cord subsequently will assume a fixed position near the midline. Such a patient will be afflicted by hoarseness, but the airway will not be compromised. Bilateral injury will result in postoperative respiratory difficulties that may necessitate tracheostomy.

The superior laryngeal nerve arises from the nodose ganglion of the vagus nerve near the latter's exit from the jugular foramen in the skull. The nerve divides high in the neck into a large internal laryngeal nerve and a small external laryngeal nerve. The latter descends on the fascia of the inferior constrictor muscle and courses below the oblique attachment of the sternothyroid muscle which is on the thyroid cartilage to innervate the cricothyroid muscle.[44] Durham and Harrison[28] found that the external branch of the superior laryngeal nerve was intimately related to the superior thyroid vessels at the superior pole of the thyroid gland in 85 percent of their cases. So only in 15 percent does the nerve penetrate the cricopharyngeal muscle before reaching the region of the superior pole of the thyroid gland, and in these cases would be protected from trauma during ligation of the superior thyroid vessels.

Change in voice after thyroid surgery may be due to nerve injury or laryngeal edema. Unilateral damage of the external laryngeal nerve may result in variable huskiness or weakness of the voice, and bilateral injury may add easy fatigability in speaking or a decrease in range, volume, or pitch.[44] Such effects may last from 1 week to a few months.

Another vulnerable structure, the cervical sympathetic chain, is near the inferior thyroid artery, where the latter arches medially from the thyrocervical trunk. This is the usual location of the middle cervical ganglion. Damage to the chain may occur, and this can result in Horner syndrome. Beahrs and Vandertoll[7] reported two such instances among 584 patients who had more than one thyroid operation. In each patient, the clinical signs of Horner syndrome were transient. Damage usually occurs during attempts to ligate the inferior thyroid artery as far laterally as possible in order to avoid damaging the recurrent laryngeal nerve.[57] De Quervain[22] showed experimentally that slight trauma could result in such a syndrome. He also postulated that stretching the chain with lateral retraction of the carotid sheath to expose the inferior thyroid artery or compressing the chain itself between the retractor tip and the transverse vertebral process would cause damage. Such damage may explain the transient effects that were noted in both patients.[7]

Lymphatic System

The lymphatic drainage of the thyroid gland is mainly by lymphatic vessels (Fig. 23-3) that accompany the arterial blood supply. The superior border of the isthmus, the medial surface of the lateral lobes, and the ventral and dorsal surfaces of the upper part of the lateral lobes drain into the superior lymphatic channels that empty into the superior pretracheal or Delphian node(s) and the upper deep cervical nodes.[36] The inferior channels drain most of the isthmus and lower portions of the lateral lobes into the lower deep cervical nodes and into the inferior pretracheal nodes.

CLASSIFICATION

Hazard and Smith[34] established a simplified classification of primary thyroid adenocarcinoma in 1964. It was subsequently accepted by the American Thyroid Association. There are four classes: papillary

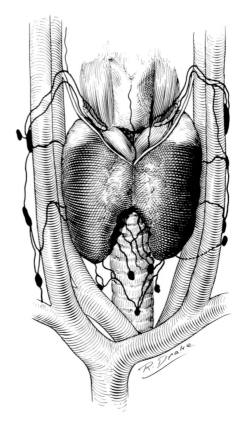

Fig. 23-3. Usual lymphatic drainage of the thyroid gland. Deep cervical and anterior cervical nodes are shown. (Mahorner, H.R., Caylor, H.D., Schlotthauer, C.F., and Pemberton, J. de J. 1927. Observations on the lymphatic connections of the thyroid gland in man. Anatomical Record, 36: 341.)

adenocarcinoma, follicular adenocarcinoma, medullary carcinoma, and anaplastic carcinoma. The relative incidences of the various types are shown in Table 23-4. The papillary group includes all lesions that have any papillary component, even though the lesion may be only 10 percent papillary. In our experience, all of these lesions have the same biologic behavior, and, for this reason, we have not considered subdivisions of the groups.

In addition to the primary carcinomas, there are two other groups of malignant neoplasms that must be considered in any discussion on cancer of the thyroid gland: lymphoma and metastatic carcinoma.

TABLE 23-4. CLASSIFICATION AND INCIDENCE OF CARCINOMA OF THE THYROID (MAYO CLINIC: 1926–1960)

Type	Cases No.	%
Papillary	736	62
Follicular	208	18
Medullary (solid) with amyloid	77	6
Anaplastic	160	14
Total	1,181	100

(Modified from Woolner, L.B., Beahrs, O.H., Black, B.M., McConahey, W.M., and Keating, F.R., Jr. 1968. Thyroid carcinoma: General considerations and follow-up data on 1181 cases. In Young. S., and Inman, D.R., Eds.: Thyroid Neoplasia, Proceedings of the Second Imperial Cancer Research Fund Symposium. Academic Press, London, 51.)

Papillary Adenocarcinoma

The most common cancer of the thyroid is papillary adenocarcinoma. It has a varied histologic architecture, being composed mainly of papillary excrescences, follicles, so-called psammoma bodies, and ground-glass nuclei. The term replaces such compound titles as "papillary and follicular," "mixed follicular and papillary," and "papillary and alveolar," all of which have appeared in the literature, apparently as synonyms. Although histologic subdivision of these synonyms is not useful, the exact or approximate microscopic architecture of a given papillary adenocarcinoma may be appended to the diagnosis, if desired (for example, papillary adenocarcinoma, predominantly papillary in structure; or papillary adenocarcinoma, mixed papillary and follicular in structure). Certain well-encapsulated tumors of completely papilliferous architecture sometimes have been described as "papillary cystadenoma." In some classifications, papillary carcinomas with a mixed pattern but a follicular structure greatly predominating have been removed from the general group of papillary carcinoma and designated "follicular carcinoma" or "follicular adenocarcinoma"—in effect, tending to make two subdivisions of one family of tumors in which no apparent difference in behavior exists.

Papillary adenocarcinoma, a slowly growing tumor that is often multicentric in the thyroid gland, spreads by regional lymphatic vessels to the tracheoesophageal or cervical lymph nodes, or both, in 50 percent or more of cases. It spreads to distant sites infrequently. The primary lesion may be small and not palpable, and the first evidence of the lesion can be the occurrence of lymphadenopathy in the lateral region of the neck (22 percent of malignant cervical nodes with occult lesions).

Small papillary tumors, with or without bulky metastatic deposits in cervical lymph nodes, are described under the term "occult papillary carcinoma," because the primary lesion is usually not appreciated on physical palpation. Synonyms for this lesion have included the terms "occult sclerosing carcinoma" and "unencapsulated sclerosing tumor." In the older literature, before the true nature of the condition was recognized, the term "lateral aberrant thyroid was frequently used to describe the metastatic deposits. The unusually benign behavior of these small carcinomas is now well established. They are slow-growing and readily curable. They may occur at any age but are most frequently seen in children or young adults. Microscopically, the tumor is composed of papillary projections and of neoplastic but well-differentiated follicles in varied proportions. A "solid" component is seen in some tumors, especially in those seen in younger persons. In other lesions, psammoma bodies are present.

Papillary adenocarcinomas occur as occult papillary carcinoma, intrathyroidal papillary carcinoma, and extrathyroidal carcinoma (Table 23-5). Occult papillary adenocarcinoma is defined arbitrarily as a tumor 1.5 cm or less in greatest diameter, with or without regional nodal metastasis. The primary tumor itself is usually not palpable on clinical examination. Intrathyroidal papillary adenocarcinoma, although larger than

TABLE 23-5. PAPILLARY CARCINOMA
(MAYO CLINIC: 1926–1960)

Category	Cases No.	%
Occult	244	35
Intrathyroid	354	50
Extrathyroid	68	10
Biopsy only*	38	5
Total	704	100

*No inoperable cases after 1950.
(Modified from Woolner, L.B., Beahrs, O.H., Black, B.M., McConahey, W.M., and Keating, F.R., Jr. 1968. Thyroid carcinoma: General considerations and follow-up data on 1181 cases. In Young, S., and Inman, D.R., Eds.: Thyroid Neoplasia, Proceedings of the Second Imperial Cancer Research Fund Symposium. Academic Press, London, 51.)

that of the occult type, refers to primary lesions confined essentially within the thyroid gland. In extrathyroidal papillary carcinoma, the primary lesion extends well beyond the capsule of the thyroid to involve such structures as the larynx, trachea, or esophagus. In any case, the terms "occult," "intrathyroidal," or "extrathyroidal" refer only to the primary lesion and not to the presence or absence of lymph node metastasis, which may or may not occur.

Follicular Adenocarcinoma

This heading includes a subgroup of thyroid neoplasms. Follicular carcinoma grows slowly, generally occurring in a somewhat older age group than papillary adenocarcinoma. The tumors tend toward gross encapsulation and especially toward vascular invasion. The most frequent sites of metastasis are the bones and lungs. Unlike tumors of the papillary type, these lesions seldom spread to regional nodes. Histologically, a papillary structure is virtually absent. Among the group, there is a wide diversity of architecture, varying from small follicles to solid sheets of cells. The term "follicular carcinoma" is used because the follicle is the most frequently observed feature.

The follicular pattern may be reminiscent of "fetal" adenomatous growth. Previously used terminology includes such terms as "metastasizing adenoma," "localized carcinoma in follicular adenoma," "benign metastasizing goiter," "wucherende struma," "encapsulated angioinvasive carcinoma," "malignant adenoma,"[31] "adenocarcinoma in an adenoma,"[48] or "atypical adenoma."

Also included as follicular carcinomas are variants whose pattern is largely solid or even similar to that of Hürthle cell tumors. Although some classifications include Hürthle cell carcinoma as a separate histologic entity, some difficulties are encountered in such an approach. The main problem is one of definition in that many tumors show slight or partial Hürthle cell transformation; the change may be extensive in one portion of the tumor and absent in another. Although the basic nature of this change is unknown, a secondary phenomenon probably superimposes on a preexisting adenoma or carcinoma.

Medullary Carcinoma

Medullary thyroid carcinomas are circumscribed, encapsulated, and slow-growing. Distant hematogenous metastasis, especially to the lungs, liver, and other parts of the body, is common. While they may spread hematogenously, the lesions have a propensity to involve regional lymph nodes in a way similar to (or even greater than) that of their papillary counterpart.

Medullary carcinoma (a neoplasm of the calcitonin-secreting or C cells of the thyroid) was rarely mentioned in the earlier literature on thyroid carcinoma, being first described by Hazard and co-workers[35] in 1959. Histologically, the tumor is distinctive, being composed of small round or spindle cells without pattern and with an abundant hyaline stroma that usually gives the staining reaction for amyloid. Some medullary carcinomas contain zones that are histologically identical with those of carcinoid tumor of the bowel; a spindle cell component is frequently prominent. The distribution of amyloid-staining material may be spotty; nevertheless, the tumor is readily distinguished microscopically from the rapidly growing anaplastic type.

Medullary carcinoma of the thyroid gland may occur as an isolated entity or may be associated with pheochromocytoma or parathyroid disease or both.[10, 68] Block and associates[11] have described other lesions and symptoms that are associated with medullary thyroid carcinoma (Fig. 23-4). Of 139 patients with medullary thyroid carcinoma surgically treated at our institution between January 1926 and December 1973[13], 29 (20.9 percent) had a familial form. The familial forms (multiple endocrine neoplasia, types 2A and 2B) have been well described in the literature and differ on the basis of phenotype (type 2B characterized by multiple, mucosal neuromas). In this series of 139 patients the median age of the group was 51 years (range 2 to 73), whereas the median age of the 29 patients with a familial form of medullary thyroid carcinoma was 21 years (range 2 to 60), 13 of 16 patients with the familial form were less than 20 years old.

Anaplastic Carcinoma

The term "anaplastic" is used to encompass a group of rapidly growing and lethal thyroid carcinomas of varied histologic structure. It is preferred to "undifferentiated carcinoma," a term that could equally apply to slowly growing neoplasms—for example, solid tumors with amyloid stroma.

Anaplastic carcinoma occurs in the usual cancer age group (those in the fifth and sixth decade of life). Histologically, the tumor exhibits various undifferentiated patterns characterized by rapid growth and extension into contiguous structures. The most common histologic type is a variant featuring spindle and giant cells, although there is a small cell type. Some of the small cell varieties may be difficult to distinguish from the more anaplastic varieties of lymphoma. The anaplastic carcinomas are aggressive and usually result in death within a few months.

Lymphoma

Primary lymphoma of the thyroid is a localized lymphoma comparable to that seen in other extranodal sites.[71] The disease is uncommon but is being reported with increasing frequency. Most patients are elderly women with a huge mass of recent development. Obstructive symptoms are common in advanced disease.

The pathologic changes may be varied and perplexing. Given a lymphoma-like lesion in the thyroid, the pathologist has no difficulty in the microscopic diagnosis if the cells appear to be anaplastic and if the sur-

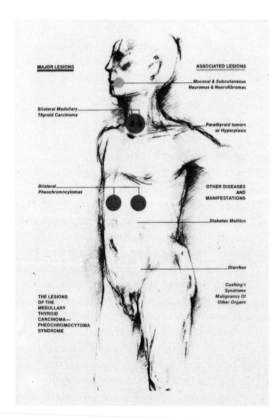

Fig. 23-4. Lesions of the medullary thyroid carcinoma—pheochromocytoma syndrome. (Block, M.A. 1969. Medullary thyroid carcinoma: a component of an interesting endocrine syndrome. CA, Cancer Journal for Clinicians, 19: 74.)

rounding structures are invaded. However, when there is no extension beyond the capsule, and particularly when the infiltrating cells in the thyroid appear as mature lymphocytes or plasma cells as seen in thyroiditis, the diagnosis may be difficult.

Although the prognosis is generally considered to be poor, the natural course of the disease may be unpredictable. However, the presence or absence of local invasion appears to be the determining factor affecting the prognosis of primary thyroid lymphoma.[12, 53, 55] The treatment, in general, is subtotal or total resection of the thyroid, followed by external irradiation.

Carcinoma Metastatic to Thyroid

The thyroid gland usually is considered to be an infrequent site of metastatic involvement from primary carcinoma of other organs. This is peculiar because the thyroid is one of the most richly arterialized tissues in the body. Mortensen and associates[45] found metastatic cancer to the thyroid in 3.4 percent of 1,000 routine autopsies, while Wychulis and colleagues[73] found that only 14 of 20,262 patients who underwent surgery on the thyroid at the Mayo Clinic from 1940 through 1962 had metastatic cancer to the thyroid. The primary lesion was hypernephroma in eight patients, adenocarcinoma of the breast in four, transitional cell tumor of the bladder in one, and adenocarcinoma of the rectum in one. A vigorous attack on such metastatic lesions may be warranted in patients who are getting along satisfactorily after the tumor at the primary site and elsewhere is considered controlled.

PATIENT EVALUATION

General Considerations

The diagnosis of cancer is firmly established only by histologic study of the thyroid and tumor tissue. If symptoms and findings are suggestive of cancer, operation is indicated. Although needle biopsy may be used in place of open surgical exploration, we do not recommend it. If the specimen obtained by needle biopsy is negative for cancer, one cannot be certain that the tissue is representative of the tumor or has been obtained from it. However, if the tissue is cancerous, the procedure may have an adverse effect, such as disturbing the cancer or permitting implantation of tumor cells in other tissues along the needle tract. Generally, the only thyroids for which we routinely use needle biopsy are those suspected of having Hashimoto thyroiditis.

Because excision of all abnormalities of the thyroid gland is not feasible, patients must be selected carefully for operation. The decision must be based on an evaluation of the history, physical findings and results of laboratory studies. The experience of the examiners also is an important factor in determining whether or not cancer will be recognized.

Differential Diagnosis

The differential diagnosis of cancer of the thyroid gland includes other lesions of the thyroid that may present as nodular goiter. The various types of thyroiditis are included because physical examination frequently reveals them to be nodular goiter, and they may be confused with true tumors.

Hashimoto thyroiditis occurs most frequently in women. Such a goiter is most often rubbery, firm, and bilaterally symmetric. Basal metabolic rate is eventually low (-10 to -30 percent). Clinically evident myxedema may be present, as well as circulating antithyroid antibodies. Diagnosis can be confirmed by needle biopsy of the gland. If treatment is medical, close observation is essential for 3 to 6 months to ensure that cancer (occurring in 3 percent) is not coexistent.[70]

Subacute granulomatous (de Quervain) thyroiditis generally can be diagnosed if there is a typical prodrome of upper respiratory infection with neck pain (for example, pain extending to the mandible and ear) and exquisite tenderness in the region of the thyroid gland. The sedimentation rate also may be increased, and a thyroid that has been discretely nodular may be diffusely enlarged. Frequently, there is no radioactive iodine uptake. When the clinical diagnosis is established, conservative treatment is indicated. In about one-third of patients with subacute thyroiditis, however, the clinical and physical findings are atypical. In these, an operation may be necessary to establish the diagnosis and to rule out cancer. Cancer is infrequently seen with this type of goiter.

Riedel struma (fibrous) thyroiditis is infrequently seen, occurring in about 1 of 1,000 to 2,000 thyroidectomies. In these situations, the lesion presents as a discrete nodule or a diffuse, indurated, and extremely fixed lesion that may compromise the tracheal lumen. Goiters of this type may need to be removed to rule out cancer and to free the airway. After the diagnosis is established, the lesion need not always be totally resected because of the technical difficulties associated with removal. Occasionally, mediastinal or retroperitoneal fibrosis and sclerosing cholangitis are coexistent. Cancer rarely coexists.

Adenomas comprise the largest number of neoplastic nodular goiters. Only those with a reasonable likelihood of being cancerous should be operated on in order to establish a definitive diagnosis and to carry out the appropriate surgical procedure.

Other masses in the midline of the neck—dermoid cysts, thyroglossal duct remnants and cysts, lymphadenopathy of the Delphian lymph node, and some laryngeal and esophageal tumors and lipomas—must be considered and may require exploration to establish the correct diagnosis.

Symptoms

Commonly, the patient with a malignancy of the thyroid is asymptomatic and the mass is found incidentally during a general examination. Some patients have a lump in the neck as their only complaint. A history of the sudden appearance or rapid enlarge-

ment of a thyroid mass can be interpreted as being merely suggestive of malignancy, since hemorrhage into an adenoma or cyst or thyroiditis may be responsible for a similar course of events. In a 1968 review,[3] more than half of the patients with thyroid cancer gave no history of a preexisting thyroid nodule or goiter (Table 23-6). All of the patients with the medullary or anaplastic type either had no history of a nodule or had a nodule for less than 1 year. Thirty percent of patients had noted an increase in the size of the thyroid nodule or mass.

Usually, the more undifferentiated the tumor, the more symptomatic are patients at the time of their presentation (Table 23-7). Pain is present in the thyroid region most often in patients with anaplastic carcinoma but is not a typical symptom of malignant thyroid disease. In general, pain, particularly pain referred to the mandible or ear, is indicative of thyroiditis rather than cancer. Similarly, hemorrhage into a cyst or adenoma may cause severe neck pain. A sensation of fullness or pressure in the neck, associated with a history of recent increased size of a goiter, is suggestive of malignancy. Hoarseness usually results from infiltration and destruction of the recurrent laryngeal or vagus nerve. According to Pemberton and Black,[50] associated dysphagia is usually due to malignant infiltration of the esophagus. Dyspnea and stridor may result from distortion, compression, or invasion of the trachea by tumor.

If a cancer develops in a hyperfunctioning gland, then symptoms of thyrotoxicosis may be present. It is rare to see a thyroid cancer that is hormonally active (except medullary). In this respect, thyroid gland malignancies differ from those of most of the other endocrine glands, since the latter usually exhibit overt symptoms and signs of hormonal activity. Tests of thyroid function (with the exception of those performed on thyrocalcitonin-producing medullary carcinomas and thyroxine-producing follicular carcinomas) have no practical application in the diagnosis of tumors of the thyroid because the functional status of the gland is

TABLE 23-6. DURATION OF THYROID NODULE OR GOITER
IN PATIENTS WITH THYROID CANCER, BY TYPE

| Duration (yr) | Papillary | Percentage of Patients | | Anaplastic |
		Follicular	Medullary	
No history	52	42	75	70
<1	30	10	25	30
1–2	8	5		
2–3	2	20		
3–4	4	5		
4–5	0	0		
>5	4	18		
Total	100	100		

(Beahrs, O.H., and Kubista, T.P. 1968. Diagnosis of thyroid cancer. In Cancer Management:
A Special Graduate Course on Cancer. J. B. Lippincott, Philadelphia, 573.)

TABLE 23-7. CLINICAL SYMPTOMS IN PATIENTS WITH THYROID CANCER

| Clinical symptoms | Percentage of Patients* With Symptoms | | | |
	Papillary	Follicular	Medullary	Anaplastic
None	73	63	50	28
Neck pain	10	5	0	72
Tightness, fullness increased size of neck	8	11	25	15
Hoarseness	6	0	25	43
Dysphagia	6	16	50	25
Dyspnea	2	0	0	43

*Some patients had more than one significant symptom.
(Beahrs, O.H., and Kubista, T.P. 1968. Diagnosis of thyroid cancer. In Cancer Management: A Special Graduate Course on Cancer.
J. B. Lippincott, Philadelphia, 573.)

not usually affected by the malignant lesion. In advanced malignancy, when most of the active thyroid tissue is replaced by tumor, thyroid function tests may indicate progressively increasing myxedema, a nonspecific finding.

Metastatic deposits of thyroid cancer may be responsible for a multitude of symptoms. The finding of pulmonary metastasis in a patient with a goiter or thyroid mass suspected of being cancerous increases the accuracy of the clinical diagnosis. Pulmonary metastasis may present as chest pain, cough, or dyspnea. Bone metastasis may be manifested by bone pain or pathologic fractures. In the rare instance of functioning metastasis, there are symptoms of thyrotoxicosis even after removal of the entire gland.

Pulmonary lesions have been present at initial presentation in 8 percent of patients with the papillary type, 16 percent with the follicular type, and 28 percent with the anaplastic type. Occasionally, osteolytic lesions are present and may aid in the clinical diagnosis of cancer of the thyroid gland.[4]

The syndrome of coexisting medullary

carcinoma, parathyroid disease, and pheo-chromocytoma (multiple endocrine neo-plasms—MEN) may produce symptoms related to the excessive production of cate-cholamine. Similarly, medullary carcinoma can be associated with the clinical pattern of overproduction of corticotropin (Cush-ing syndrome) and with symptoms and signs identical to those of the carcinoid syn-drome[43] (diarrhea, flushing, and asthma).

Signs

Generally, tenderness indicates a focus of thyroiditis or an intrinsic hemorrhage.

Vocal cord paralysis usually is due to in-filtration of the recurrent laryngeal or vagus nerve by malignant tissue. Clark and associ-ates[15] reported that 10 percent of their pa-tients with papillary carcinoma had associ-ated vocal cord palsy, whereas 36 percent with anaplastic tumors had vocal cord paral-ysis. It is very unusual for even a large be-nign goiter to produce vocal cord paralysis by compressing or stretching the recurrent nerve. Mediastinal tumors, aneurysms of the aortic arch, or an enlarged left atrium may affect the intrathoracic portion of the nerve and cause vocal cord palsy. One study[3] noted vocal cord paralysis before op-eration in 8.5 percent of patients. In this group, the tumor was considered to be fixed to the adjacent trachea in 20 percent of pa-tients and to the larynx or overlying soft tis-sues less frequently. Fifteen percent of pa-tients with papillary carcinoma in that series had cervical lymphadenopathy but no pal-pable nodule.

Deviation or compression of the tra-chea may be confirmed by roentgeno-graphic examination of the thoracic inlet. In far-advanced disease, carcinoma of the thy-roid may infiltrate the tracheal wall, giving rise to hemoptysis and respiratory obstruc-tion. Fixation of a goiter results from infil-tration of the adjacent structures and is present in many patients with thyroiditis (es-pecially Riedel fibrous thyroiditis). Fixation may occasionally be noted when a large be-nign goiter becomes wedged in the thoracic inlet. Invasion or compression of vessels of the neck is a relatively infrequent finding. However, obstruction of the veins may oc-cur, precipitating venous congestion and edema of the head and neck. In a patient with a large cervical goiter, the examiner may precipitate suffusion of the patient's face, giddiness, or syncopal episodes by hav-ing the patient raise his hands above his head—this is known as Pemberton's sign. Encroachment on the carotid sheath may render it impossible to detect the carotid ar-tery pulse; this sign, one associated with thy-roid carcinoma, was described by Sir James Berry[9] and is known as Berry's sign. In-volvement of the cervical sympathetic nerve is manifested as Horner's syndrome.

Physical Examination and Characteristics

A comprehensive outline for examination of the thyroid gland has been reported by Do-byns.[25] Only the essentials are repeated here. Proper evaluation of the thyroid gland demands a thorough visual and palpatory examination. The most thorough and effi-cient assessment is conducted with the ex-aminer facing the patient (Fig. 23-5). A nod-ule may frequently be seen with the patient in slight hyperextension and swallowing on request.

The examination begins with palpatory identification of the thyroid notch. Next, the examiner palpates the thyrocricoid mem-brane and cricoid, realizing that the isthmus is usually inferior to the cricoid. After pal-pating the isthmus (Fig. 23-5), one then pro-ceeds laterally to the thyroid lobes.

Having placed the four fingers of one hand at the nape of the patient's neck to reinforce a verbal request for the patient to flex the neck, the examiner uses the thumb of his same hand to push the trachea contra-laterally, thereby immobilizing it while facil-itating palpation of the contralateral thyroid lobe. Using his other hand, the examiner palpates the thyroid lobe, pinching it be-tween thumb and index and middle fingers. As the patient swallows, the examiner re-laxes his pinch-like grip, allowing the thy-roid to rise with the larynx until the inferior

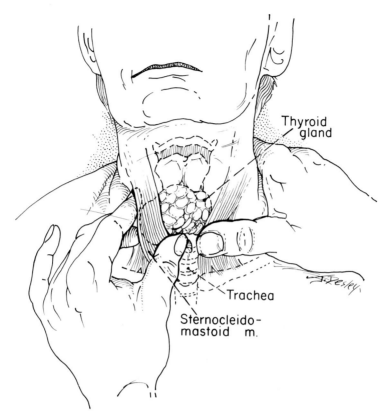

Fig. 23-5. Physical examination of the thyroid gland.

pole of the lobe moves above thumb and finger; pressure may then be reapplied (Fig. 23-5). Progressive relaxation allows further palpation of the gland as it slides back to its former position. The examination is not complete until both sides have been evaluated and until the presence or absence of cervical adenopathy has been assessed. During swallowing, a nodule within the thyroid moves with the thyroid, while nodes of the cervical chain do not.

The physical character of the nodule is the most important diagnostic clue of malignancy. Features such as size, consistency, margins, surface of the gland, fixation, presence of tenderness, and number of nodules should be noted. In our experience the great majority of malignant lesions have been 5 cm or less in diameter. Most malignant nodules are harder than benign lesions or normal thyroid tissue, although malignant nodules may be softer than benign nodules. For example, granulomatous or fi-

brous thyroiditis may be rock-hard, whereas papillary or follicular tumors may be only firm. In multinodular goiter, that part of the gland occupied by malignant tissue will usually differ on palpation from the other nodules and from surrounding normal thyroid tissue. This difference in consistency is usually obvious to the examiner if tumor develops in the anterolateral aspects of the gland, but may be difficult or even impossible to appreciate if the tumor is deep within the gland or close to its posterior surface.

In our operative experience, physical examination of a thyroid carcinoma revealed a discrete (single) nodule in 50 percent of patients, multinodular enlargement in 25 percent, and diffuse enlargement in 15 percent.[3] The right lobe was involved in 40 percent, the left in 30 percent, and both lobes in 30 percent.

If tumor extends beyond the thyroid capsule, the margins of the gland may become vague or impossible to determine.

Roentgenographic examination may reveal the extent of a goiter that is difficult to palpate, especially if the goiter projects substernally. However, the roentgenogram does not contribute to the differentiation of type of goiter, unless such a lesion appears to be calcified; then the chance of cancer being present is greatly reduced.

LABORATORY STUDIES

Thyroid Scannings

The scanning techniques using radioactive tracers may supply important information but the scans should not be considered diagnostic. Such techniques should not be the sole basis for management. Nonfunctioning thyroid tissue, whether the nodule is cancerous or represents thyroiditis, frequently is seen as a "cold" spot on a gammagram, especially if the nodule is large enough to be identified clinically. If the tumor is functioning, the lesion might show up as a "hot" spot, which reduces but does not rule out the chance of cancer being present. In a series of thyroid carcinomas that were radioactively scanned, 61 percent showed cold nodules, 29 percent showed normal scans, and 10 percent showed hot spots at or near the site of malignant lesions.[3] Robinson and associates[52] noted carcinoma in 22 percent of cold nodules and in 4.4 percent of hot nodules, while Jackson and Thomson[39] found carcinoma in 20 and 8 percent, respectively. Croll and Brady[18] stated that, for all practical purposes, hot nodules are essentially benign. Similarly, McCormack and Sheline[40] did not find any patient with malignancy among their patients with hot nodules.

Cold areas on a scan may be due to carcinoma, but they also may be due to hemorrhage into an adenoma, a nonfunctioning adenoma, cystic changes, thyroiditis, or surgical excision of part of the gland. Similarly, a small cold area may be covered by adjacent normal or hyperfunctioning thyroid tissue (begnign or malignant), thus rendering the scan deceptively negative. When a cold area is not noted on a repeat scan and the patient has been given thyrotropin, it is usually due to resumption of normal ^{131}I concentration indicating the presence of functional (thyroid) tissue, and excluding malignancy.

In practice, if a nodule in the thyroid gland warrants removal on the basis of history and physical findings, a radioactive iodine study need not be done. When the choice of treatment of a lesion is not obvious, a scan should be obtained to aid in deciding what should be done. Studies using radioactive iodine are useful in detecting ectopic-functioning thyroid tissue. Thoracic goiters and metastatic thyroid deposits (usually of the follicular type) are particularly likely to concentrate ^{131}I, especially in the absence of a normal competing thyroid gland.

Calcitonin Screening for Medullary Carcinoma

In patients with medullary carcinoma the presentation varies. In one series,[13] a painless lump in the thyroid gland was found in 50 percent of patients; about 80 percent had palpable tumor of the thyroid gland at clinical examination; 25 percent had concomitant or preceding cervical adenopathy; and 10 percent had vocal cord paralysis.

Initially in our experience,[13] 13 (9.3 percent) asymptomatic family members at high risk had medullary thyroid carcinoma diagnosed solely on the basis of a family screening procedure using the measurement of immunoreactive plasma calcitonin. These patients, siblings and children of patients with proved medullary carcinoma, were unaware of any symptoms or signs.

The annual incidence of disease recognized at our institution has tripled during the past 5 years because of our use of screening procedures based on the measurement of calcitonin to identify persons at high familial risk.[67] In 5 years, plasma immunoreactive calcitonin was measured in 219 primary relatives of 36 patients who had histologically proved medullary thyroid carcinoma and no family history of thyroid tumor, pheochromocytomas, or hyperparathyroidism.[56] This screening identified 57 new affected members in seven families. In effect, at least 19 percent of patients presumed to have sporadic medullary thyroid carcinoma were actually index cases to kindreds having familial medullary thyroid carcinoma.

Twelve of twenty-nine patients (41.4 percent) with familial medullary thyroid carcinoma had pheochromocytoma and one other had bilateral adrenal medullary hyperplasia. All pheochromocytomas were located in the adrenals. Ten of these thirteen patients had bilateral tumors, and three had multicentric tumors in either one or both adrenal glands. Five patients had hypertension, three having the paroxysmal type. The levels of urinary metanephrines and vanillylmandelic acid were elevated in six patients. Three of the thirteen patients had recurrences after surgical treatment of the pheochromocytoma. By definition, these were malignant pheochromocytomas.

Parathyroid disease was found only in the 15 patients with MEN type 2A syndrome. In 13 patients, hyperplastic parathyroid tissue was found at operation, yet the serum calcium level was abnormally elevated in only 7 of 10 patients in whom it was measured.

TREATMENT

General Remarks

The most effective treatment for cancer of the thyroid gland is thyroidectomy. However, distant metastasis from follicular carcinoma or inoperable follicular lesions in the neck can be treated, sometimes very effectively, with radioactive iodine. This is also true of some papillary carcinomas that have a follicular component. External radiation is of value for a few inoperable anaplastic cancers, but cure of these by any method is infrequent. Radiation also may be valuable in the management of lymphoma of the thyroid.

Because the behaviors of thyroid cancer vary, each type should be discussed separately. Opinions have differed as to the extent of surgical procedure required to control each type. Crile[16] and others favored conservative measures, but Tollefsen and DeCosse[62] and, more recently, Clark and colleagues[14] advocated radical surgical treatment. Woolner and associates[72] reviewed the experience at the Mayo Clinic in the management of two groups (885 and 1,181 patients) with thyroid cancer who were followed up for as long as 40 years. Treatment was primarily by conservative surgical measures. These reports and one by Beahrs and Tachovsky[6] form the basis for the following discussion.

If thyroidectomy is to be justified for diagnosing cancer or for managing most papillary lesions, the mortality risk of surgery should be near zero. At the Mayo Clinic the overall mortality rate for thyroidectomies is 0.1 percent. For elective primary thyroidectomy, the mortality rate has been zero during the last two decades. Similar mortality rates have been reported by others.[23, 32] When secondary thyroidectomy is done, complications occur with increased frequency (for example, about twice those after primary thyroidectomy).[7]

Surgery

PREOPERATIVE CONSIDERATIONS

Prior to thyroid or parathyroid surgery, the vocal cords should be examined for normal function. Preoperative preparation of patients with thyrotoxicosis is important if an operative or a postoperative thyroid storm is to be avoided. Such patients may be made euthyroid by the administration of an antithyroid drug or, as we prefer, Lugol's solution (10 drops three times a day) for 7 to 10 days prior to operation. Even if euthyroidism is not attained, the surgery will be safer; and the use of Lugol's solution may decrease the vascularity of the gland and reduce its size.

AT OPERATION

For surgery, the head-up position is used. The patient is placed on the operating table with a folded towel between his shoulder blades so that the occiput rests on the edge of the upper end of the table and his neck can be maximally hyperextended. A footboard is placed flat against his feet to prevent the patient from sliding downward. The head of the table is elevated 30° during surgery.

Although some surgeons use superficial cervical local anesthesia for thyroid surgery, we prefer general anesthesia—and endotracheal intubation. Sodium thiopental is usually the anesthetic used. With the patient asleep and reliably immobile, the surgeon can give greater attention to the technical details of the operation.

The skin of the neck and upper thorax is cleansed with soap, alcohol, and Freon. After a colorless solution of thimerosal (Merthiolate) is applied to the operative site, the patient is ready for draping. Two sterile towels are placed beneath his head. The bottom towel is left so, and the top towel is draped about the head, completely covering the ears. Two sterile towels are then placed longitudinally so as to overlap the towel about the head and extend down over the chest. Two towels are placed across the chest, with the upper towel lying just below the clavicle. A rectangular "thyroid screen" is then positioned at the head of the table by an assistant. A sterile sheet, fitting the screen, is placed under the patient's chin, separating the neck in the operative field from the patient's face. This sheet is attached to the head towel and the longitudinally placed towels by a towel clip on each side. Then two sheets are placed full length so that they extend from just below the clavicles down over the patient and the instrument stand.

OPERATIVE TECHNIQUE

A transverse (collar) incision is made in the line of a natural skin crease, approximately 3 cm above the suprasternal notch and midportion of the clavicle on each side (Fig. 23-6). The incision is carried through the skin, subcutaneous tissue, and platysma and can be extended laterally as far as necessary for removal of the goiter. Two rake retractors are placed under the platysma of the upper flap and held upward with tension by the assistant. The upper flap is developed by sharp dissection of the areolar tissue with the scalpel, in a plane of cleavage between the platysma and the fascia overlying the strap muscles. Then the retractors are removed, and the surgeon pulls the upper flap upward with his left hand (using a sponge between his thumb and index finger) while he completes the dissection between the platysma and overlying tissue to the level of the notch of the thyroid cartilage. The lower flap is similarly developed downward to the suprasternal notch. A transversely placed towel is secured to the

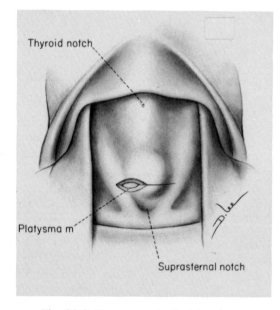

Fig. 23-6. Transverse (collar) incision in neck at about one-third the distance from suprasternal notch to thyroid notch. Incision should be long enough to expose thyroid area and be symmetrical. (Beahrs, O.H., and Tachovsky, T.J. 1969. Surgery of the thyroid gland. In Goldsmith, H.S., Ed.: Practice of Surgery. Vol. 4. Harper and Row, Hagerstown, MD, Ch. 11.)

margins of the skin incision with towel clips. A self-retaining retractor is positioned to hold the edges of both the upper and lower flaps apart, thus exposing the cervical fascia covering the prethyroid strap muscles (sternohyoid and sternothyroid).

Exposure and Examination of the Thyroid Gland. The cervical fascia is incised with a scalpel or small scissors along the midline (the latter recognized by its whitish raphe) between the prethyroid muscles, which runs from the upper margin of the thyroid cartilage to the sternal notch. There is usually a transverse cervical vein in the lower part of this incision, and this vein should be clamped, divided, and ligated to avoid bleeding into the operative field. The prethyroid muscles are freed from the surface of the gland by the surgeon's right index finger and retracted laterally. This retraction facilitates separation of tissues in normal planes and aids in hemostasis. We do not find it necessary to cut the strap muscles at any time. Of course, a thyroid carcinoma locally invading the muscles will necessitate en bloc excision of the thyroid gland with the overlying involved muscles. Retracting the muscles laterally helps define the cleavage plane to identify structures lateral and posterior to the thyroid lobes (Fig. 23-7). The entire gland is carefully examined and explored by the surgeon's right index finger, and a decision is made about the extent of the thyroid resection to be carried out.

Exposure of Trachea and Section of Isthmus. The portion of trachea below the isthmus is exposed by use of a toothed forceps to strip any loose connective tissue away from its surface. Usually, venous connections form a plexus in front of the trachea. A Kocher clamp is placed across the upper part of these vessels, close to the isthmus, and another one is placed distally above the sternal notch. The vessels are divided between these two clamps, and the inferior bundle is ligated. If a thyroidea ima artery is present, it is also clamped, divided, and ligated at this time. The upper clamp is used to elevate the isthmus, which is undermined with scissors freeing it from the tra-

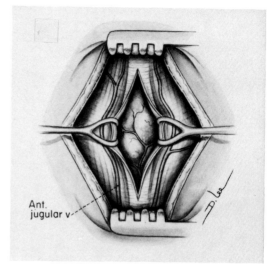

Ant. jugular v.

Fig. 23-7. Strap muscles (sternothyroid and sternohyoid) are separated in midline and retracted laterally. (It is not necessary to transect these and best not to do so.) Exposure and separation of tissues in normal cleavage plane are facilitated, as is hemostasis. (Beahrs. O.H., and Tachovsky, T.J. 1969. Surgery of the thyroid gland. In Goldsmith, H.S., Ed.: Practice of Surgery, Vol. 4, Harper and Row, Hagerstown, MD, Ch. 11.)

chea. The portion of the trachea above the isthmus or cricoid cartilage is exposed by peeling away from it any loose connective tissue. Vessels that may be present are ligated. The pyramidal lobe, if present, is freed from surrounding tissues and retracted downward (Fig. 23-8). Between the clamps, the thyroid isthmus is divided with the scalpel and is ligated.

Identification of Recurrent Laryngeal Nerves and Parathyroids. Two Kocher clamps are used to grasp the thyroid lobe to be excised. The prethyroid muscles and the carotid sheath are retracted laterally by the second assistant while the first assistant exerts upward and medial traction on the clamps placed on the thyroid lobe. The surgeon—while pushing the lobe medially with his left thumb over a sponge—gently dissects, with toothed forceps held closed in his right hand, the loose connective tissue posterolateral to the lobe in search of the recurrent laryngeal nerve. If a middle thyroid

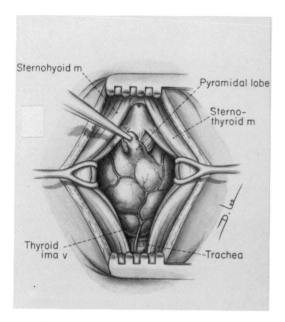

Sternohyoid m.

Pyramidal lobe

Sterno-
thyroid m

Thyroid
ima v

Trachea

Fig. 23-8. Trachea is exposed and pyra-
midal lobe is freed. (Beahrs, O.H., and
Tachovsky, T.J. 1969. Surgery of the
thyroid gland. In Goldsmith, H.S., Ed.:
Practice of Surgery. Vol. 4. Harper and
Row, Hagerstown, MD, Ch. 11.)

vein is present, it is clamped, divided, and
ligated.

The inferior thyroid artery is identified, and this aids in locating the recurrent
laryngeal nerve. This artery passes medially
behind the thyroid gland and crosses the recurrent laryngeal nerve—in front, behind,
or on both sides of it (Fig. 23-9). Often a triangle is formed by the common carotid artery posteriorly, the inferior thyroid artery
superiorly, and the recurrent laryngeal
nerve anteroinferiorly. Once identified, the
nerve can be followed in its upward course,
first close to the posterior surface of the
gland, but then plunging away from it as it
reaches the lower border of the inferior
constrictor muscle. If the right recurrent laryngeal nerve on the right side cannot be
identified, the possibility of a nonrecurrent
laryngeal nerve should be considered.

The inferior parathyroid gland is often
found below the terminal branch of the inferior thyroid artery or along its course on
the posterior aspect of the thyroid (Fig. 23-

9). The upper parathyroid gland is usually
found above the upper terminal branch of
the inferior thyroid artery. When both the
parathyroid glands and the recurrent laryngeal nerve have been definitely identified,
the inferior thyroid artery can be ligated if
desired (not necessarily divided) as far laterally as possible to avoid injury to the recurrent laryngeal nerve. One should remember that the artery occasionally is
absent and one should be aware of the
possibility of traumatizing the cervical sympathetic chain during this procedure.

Division of Superior Thyroid Vessels.
While anterior and lateral traction of the
lobe by the first assistant's left hand pulls
the superior thyroid vessels away from the
medially located external laryngeal nerve
three Kocher hemostats are applied—at the
end of the superior pole—across the vessels.
The hemostats are applied just deep enough
to include only the superior thyroid vessels,
avoiding the external branch of the superior
laryngeal nerve. The first assistant holds the
two upper clamps with his right hand as the
surgeon, holding the lower clamp with his
left hand, divides the superior thyroid vessels between the middle and lowermost
clamps.

**Excision of Lobe and Ligation of Superior
Thyroid Vessels.** With the first assistant
still holding the two clamps on the superior
thyroid pedicle, the surgeon holds, with his
left hand, the two Kocher clamps previously
placed on the thyroid lobe and the lowermost clamp on the superior thyroid pedicle
as he places additional Kocher clamps
around the lobe in a horizontal plane,
catching the capsule and outlining that portion to be excised. The second assistant takes
the two cephalad clamps (on the superior
thyroid vessels) from the first assistant. The
surgeon, while applying upward traction on
the clamps in his left hand, excises that portion of the lobe isolated by the newly placed
clamps. If proper tension is applied on the
clamps elevating the lobe, minimal use of
the scalpel is required. A cuff of tissue
should be left above each clamp to facilitate
ligation later. When both lobes must be ex-

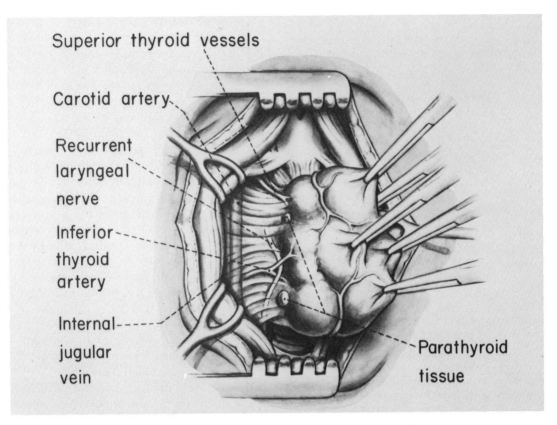

Superior thyroid vessels

Carotid artery

Recurrent laryngeal nerve

Inferior thyroid artery

Internal jugular vein

Parathyroid tissue

Fig. 23-9. Thyroid lobe is retracted outward and lateral from its bed, and tension on its tissues exposes adjacent anatomy. (Modified from Beahrs, O.H., and Tachovsky, T.J. 1969. Surgery of the thyroid gland. In Goldsmith, H.S., Ed.: Practice of Surgery. Vol. 4. Harper and Row, Hagerstown, MD, Ch. 11.)

cised, usually 2 to 3 g of tissue are left behind, if feasible, to avoid hypothyroidism.

Preferably, tissue removed should be studied immediately by frozen-section techniques to determine the type of disease that is present. If further removal of remaining tissue is warranted by the type of pathologic process encountered, this is done while the neck is still open.

The clamped vessels are then ligated. Two suture ligatures are placed around the superior thyroid vessels. The first one is placed around the uppermost clamp—not too deeply, thus avoiding trauma to the external branch of the superior laryngeal nerve. After the second suture is tied, the long end is used to approximate the capsule of the gland to the pretracheal fascia over the remnant of the gland. This is accomplished by using a running suture from the

upper portion of the remaining lobe to its lower part, locking the suture, and further reapproximating the capsule with a running locked suture (Fig. 23-10). The recurrent laryngeal nerve (laterally) must not be included in the running suture. The other lobe is checked again to ensure the absence of a pathologic process. If extensive surgery has been done, or if there is some concern regarding the airway postoperatively, a silk suture is attached to the third tracheal ring and brought to the outside through the wound. If tracheostomy should be required suddenly during the postoperative period, simple traction on this suture would bring the trachea anteriorly into view immediately, thus facilitating the operation. If serious respiratory difficulty is anticipated postoperatively, a tracheostomy is performed during the operation.

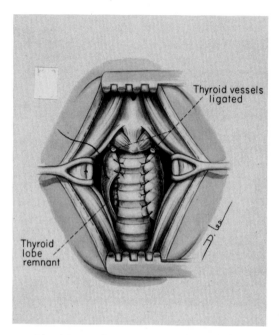

Fig. 23-10. If partial lobectomy or subtotal thyroidectomy is done, remnants of thyroid lobe are anchored to adjacent trachea to keep anatomy of neck organized and to aid in controlling hemorrhage from remaining thyroid tissue. (Beahrs, O.H., and Tachovsky, T.J. 1969. Surgery of the thyroid gland. In Goldsmith, H.S., Ed.: Practice of Surgery. Vol. 4. Harper and Row, Hagerstown, MD, Ch. 11.)

If bilateral benign disease is present, a similar procedure is carried out on the opposite side. If cancer is present, a subtotal thyroidectomy, as described above, or a total thyroidectomy is done, removing thyroid tissue consistent with the type of disease present—but with care to protect nerves and parathyroid tissue.

Closure. After careful examination of the operative site to ensure that there is no bleeding, the wound is closed. A small Penrose drain is placed laterally (on both sides if both lobes have been operated on) and brought to the outside through the wound in the midline. The strap muscles are reapproximated with interrupted sutures, as is the platysma muscle. The skin is closed with interrupted 4-0 silk sutures. A loose wrap dressing is applied to the wound.

Postoperative Care

Postoperative care includes the intravenous administration of fluids and mild sedation on the day of the operation. The patient will often resume oral alimentation on the night of the operative day and nearly always on the following day. Close attention is given to excess bloody drainage and airway patency. If hematoma occurs and there is any hint of impending airway embarrassment, the patient is immediately returned to the operating room for exploration of the wound. If any significant stridor or respiratory embarrassment occurs, the wound should be opened immediately. If there is a hematoma, it should be immediately evacuated. The wound should always be thoroughly washed and reclosed in the operating room.

If dissection during thyroid surgery has been extensive, the signs of hypoparathyroidism are looked for and the serum calcium level is determined daily while the patient remains in the hospital. Calcium replacement therapy is undertaken only if signs of hypocalcemia are present.

The drain is usually shortened the day after surgery and is removed the following day (the third day) unless continuing drainage is excessive. The vocal cords should be examined after the operation. The dermal sutures are removed on the fourth postoperative day, and the patient usually can be dismissed from the hospital at that time.

FACTORS INFLUENCING EXTENT OF SURGERY

Papillary Carcinoma

Papillary carcinoma usually is treated by total lobectomy on the side of the lesion, and because of the high incidence of multicentric lesions, subtotal lobectomy is done on the opposite side. Because the lesion may not be a carcinoma, total lobectomy need not be an en bloc resection. Subtotal lobectomy, on the side of and including the site of the lesion, may be the first step. If frozen-section study confirms the presence of a papillary carcinoma, then resection of the residual lobe should be done. Part of the thyroid tissue on the contralateral side can be saved, maximizing protection of the recurrent laryngeal nerve and preserving the parathyroid glands.[54]

When both lobes of the thyroid gland are grossly involved by cancer, total thyroidectomy should be done. Although some surgeons recommend unilateral or even bilateral radical neck dissection for these patients, we recommend a conservative surgical approach. In the absence of cervical metastasis on clinical examination and gross examination at thyroidectomy, lymphadenectomy of the neck is not advised. However, when lymph nodes appear to be involved, a modified or sometimes a radical dissection of the neck is done. Nodes in the tracheoesophageal region should always be examined, because these nodes generally are the first to be involved with metastatic spread of papillary lesions. If nodal metastasis to the lateral neck is extensive, radical neck dissection is done, but this is necessary in only about 10 percent of patients.[8]

Occult papillary carcinomas (lesions ≤1.5 cm in diameter), with or without cervical nodal metastasis, seem to be completely curable and rarely if ever result in distant metastasis or death of the patient.[37] Follow-up data through 1966 on 244 patients (240 traced) with occult papillary carcinoma revealed that the survival curve for patients with or without positive nodes is essentially identical with that for normal persons of comparable age and sex (Fig. 23-11). Of 137 patients with occult carcinoma of the thyroid, followed a mean time period of 25.3 years, possibly 1 (0.73 percent) has died of thyroid cancer.[37] We hasten to add that cause of death in this one patient remains in question. Thus, the true incidence of death related to thyroid cancer in this group of occult papillary carcinomas of the thyroid may well be zero.

As was anticipated by the senior author in 1960, a long follow-up period has demonstrated that occult papillary carcinoma (with or without metastasis) is a curable disease when treated by rather conservative surgical means. As such, no longer need patients be subjected to unnecessarily radical surgery on the basis of theoretical considerations. Needless morbidity, whether that of tetany, laryngeal nerve dysfunction, or cosmetic deformity, should be averted where radical surgery can be replaced by a reasonable conservative operation. It is suggested that occult papillary adenocarcinoma of thyroid origin be treated by total ipsilateral lobectomy and, almost always, a partial lobectomy contralaterally (to remove unknown small concomitant lesions) or a total lobectomy when there are gross multilobar lesions involving both lobes. Neck dissection is not indicated in the absence of clinical or gross adenopathy. If metastatic nodes are present, these should be removed by a modified neck dissection. Rarely is a radical neck dissection indicated. Similarly unnecessary are medical attempts to ablate residual thyroid. Such attempts are expensive and meddlesome and, we suspect, add nothing to the effectiveness of surgery in the eradication of this disease.

By accepting the conservative surgical approach in the management of cervical metastasis, an occasional patient will be subjected to secondary operation(s). This does not alter that patient's long-term prognosis.

Follicular Carcinoma

Because spread from follicular carcinoma via lymphatic vessels to the cervical lymph nodes occurs infrequently, modified or radical neck dissection is practically never indicated. The primary lesion is almost always single; therefore, treatment is total lobectomy with removal of the isthmus. Even though the opposite lobe is usually not involved, partial removal ensures a wider margin around the lesion.

Follicular carcinomas do "function" and take up significant amounts of radioactive iodine. This is particularly true in the absence of normal thyroid tissue. Therefore,

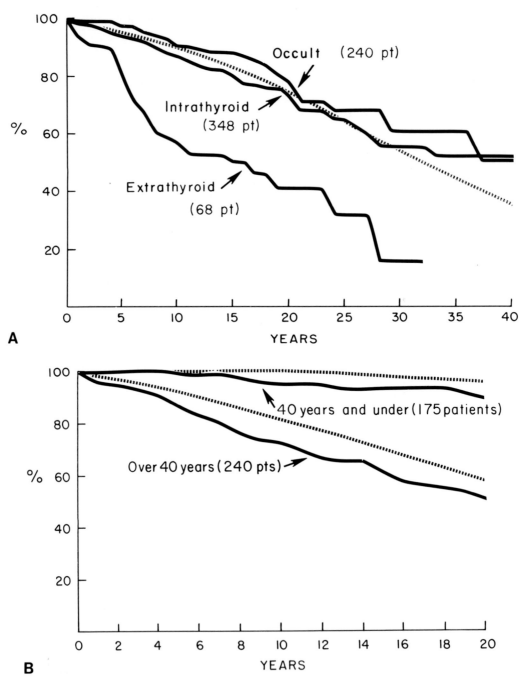

Fig. 23-11. Papillary carcinoma. (A) Survival curves for patients with occult, intrathyroidal, and extrathyroidal lesions and for normal persons (dotted line) of comparable age and sex. (B) Survival curves, excluding occult papillary carcinoma. Normal curves (dotted lines) are for comparable age and sex. (Woolner, L.B., Beahrs, O.H., Black, B.M., McConahey, W.M., and Keating, F.R., Jr. 1968. Thyroid carcinoma: General considerations and follow-up data on 1181 cases. In Young, S., and Inman, D.R., Eds.: Thyroid Neoplasia, Proceedings of the Second Imperial Cancer Research Fund Symposium, p. 51. Copyright by Academic Press Inc. (London) Ltd. Reprinted with permission.)

when distant metastasis is known or is believed to have occurred, total thyroidectomy is advisable. This would eliminate normal tissue that would compete for radioactive iodine. Surgical removal of all normal tissue at the initial resection, or at a second operation after metastasis has been found, will facilitate subsequent treatment with radioactive iodine. Surgical removal of normal thyroid tissue is preferable to the use of radioactive iodine, because a maximal dose of radioactive iodine can then be given to treat the metastatic deposits.

Medullary Adenocarcinoma

These tumors are somewhat more aggressive and spread, as do the papillary carcinomas, via the regional lymphatic system. Because of the high incidence of bilaterality and multicentricity of lesions, total thyroidectomy usually should be performed. Frozen-section examination of the nodes in the tracheoesophageal grooves, the upper mediastinum, and the internal jugular chain should be routinely performed. If metastatic disease is present, upper mediastinal nodes should be cleared and radical neck dissection(s) performed on the side(s) of proven metastatic disease.

The incidence of clinical recurrence was noted by Chong and associates[13] to be 23 percent in patients with adequate initial surgical treatment. The incidence of recurrence may actually be higher, because 12 of the patients without clinical recurrence have had persistently elevated concentrations of calcitonin after surgery.

After surgery, patients should be reassessed using periodic measurements of calcitonin, stimulation tests with infusion of calcium or pentagastrin, or both when appropriate.[27, 30, 66] If the level of immunoreactive plasma calcitonin is still abnormally high, selective venous catheterization may assist in locating metastatic sites. If such identification is achieved, the surgeon may be better guided in the management of residual or recurrent disease.

Anaplastic Carcinoma

Most of these lesions grow rapidly, infiltrate into the lateral and midline structures of the neck, and spread to distant sites early. Unfortunately, there is no satisfactory treatment for these lesions. Surgical removal may be possible, but usually the surgeon has to be content with removal of only some portion of the bulk of the tumor to ensure an adequate airway. External radiation therapy may be of some help in providing palliation and delaying the progress of the tumor. However, in some instances, tracheostomy is the only palliative measure indicated.

Cervical Metastases

For regional cervical metastasis, either a radical or a modified radical neck dissection should be done. Both can be accomplished safely—radical neck dissection with a mortality rate of 1.5 percent and the modified procedure with a lesser rate. For certain lesions with extensive metastasis, radical neck dissection is the most effective technical procedure for removing regional spread. However, for most papillary lesions, when regional nodes are involved by metastasis, a modified dissection can adequately remove the nodal groups involved in the adjacent fascia and fat. The primary advantage of the modified procedure is that the sternocleidomastoid muscle and spinal accessory nerve are preserved (all other tissues sacrificed in a radical neck dissection may be removed in a modified neck dissection), and thus the anatomic contour of the neck is preserved. The cosmetic result is important, because most of these patients are women. Attention to cosmesis seems justified as long as the future well-being of the patient is not jeopardized.

COMPLICATIONS

Vocal cord paralysis due to accidental injury of a recurrent laryngeal nerve is a significant complication of thyroid surgery. As far as the airway is concerned, a patient can tolerate the functional loss of one vocal cord but not of both. With paralysis of one cord, the voice is hoarse at first, but it frequently returns to near-normal because the opposite cord may compensate and cross the midline to touch the paralyzed cord.

Iatrogenic, permanent vocal cord paralysis should not occur if the surgeon is careful during exposure of the recurrent laryngeal nerves. In our overall experience with many surgeons using several techniques for thyroidectomy, the incidence of unexpected unilateral cord paralysis is 1 percent (there have been no permanent bilateral cord paralyses).[4] If injury to the nerve from clamping or ligature is recognized immediately and corrected, vocal cord function usually will return. Doyle and associates[26] reported the return of nerve function after suture of severed nerves and also after implantation of proximal recurrent laryngeal or vagal fibers into posterior cricoarytenoid muscle. Such measures failing, Arnold,[2] Goff,[29] and others have shown that significant improvement in phonation may be achieved by vocal cord injection with Teflon paste.

Superior laryngeal nerves can be injured. Fortunately, the consequences usually are not serious. Some voice fatigue seems to be about the only notable consequence. Rarely is the cervical sympathetic nerve injured. When this happens, injury usually occurs during ligation of the inferior thyroid artery. After such an injury, Horner syndrome develops.[57]

Hypoparathyroidism is another serious complication. During thyroidectomy, one should attempt to identify and preserve parathyroid tissue. One should consider permanent tetany acceptable only when bilateral "wide-field" total thyroidectomy is necessary. In our experience, the incidence of permanent hypoparathyroidism is 0.3 percent after conservative surgical procedures, 4 percent after total thyroidectomy, and 40 percent or more after extensive radical thyroidectomy.[4] The respective inci-

dences of temporary hypocalcemia are somewhat higher. Parathyroid function returns to normal within a few weeks to several months if it is going to return.

When parathyroid tissue has been accidentally removed, various suggestions have been made, such as inserting it into muscle or emulsifying it and injecting it into a vein so that it will implant into lung tissue. The success of such measures has been increasing.[65] Currently, research is in progress on the transplantation of parathyroid tissue in patients with permanent hypocalcemia. When tetany occurs acutely after thyroidectomy, calcium gluconate should be given intravenously to relieve symptoms, after which calcium lactate (usually 4 to 6 g per day) may be administered orally, in suspension or tablet form . Vitamin D, 50,000 to 100,000 units per day, should also be given for hypocalcemia.

Airway complications can be prevented by the use of tracheostomy when the adequacy of the airway is questionable, either immediately after operation or during the postoperative period. A Penrose drain or a suction catheter should always be used for drainage of the operative site to prevent hematoma formation or the collection of fluid in the operative site. However, before the wound is closed, the operative site should always be dry.

Myxedema may occur after total or subtotal thyroidectomy if the patient is not given replacement therapy postoperatively. Therefore, we give selected patients either desiccated thyroid (180 mg per day) or a synthetic preparation such as sodium levothyroxine (Synthroid, 0.15 to 0.2 mg per day) to pervent myxedema and as further treatment in patients whose cancer may be hormone-dependent.[16, 41]

PROGNOSIS

Papillary Carcinoma

The prognosis of papillary carcinoma appears to vary according to the extent of the primary tumor when first treated.[41] Survival curves and the number of known deaths from these lesions indicate a more serious outlook for patients with extension of the primary papillary carcinoma beyond the thyroid capsule (Fig. 23-11)—the respective 40-year mortality rates for intrathyroidal and extrathyroidal lesions being 3 and 16 percent.

Whether or not cervical lymph nodes are involved has no apparent bearing on prognosis, as shown by the excellent results in children, nearly all of whom have metastatic involvement of such nodes.[33] Moreover, in our experience with 136 adults with papillary carcinoma, none has had an unresectable recurrence because of inadequate initial treatment of cervical metastatic lesions.

For patients 40 years old or less, the 5-year survival rate is 98.8 percent and the 10-year rate is 94.9 percent; these are 99 and 96 percent, respectively, of rates expected in a normal group of the same age distribution. Only the 10-year rate is significantly less than normal. For patients more than 40 years old, the 5-year survival rate is 86.8 and the 10-year rate is 72.8 percent; these are 95 and 90 percent, respectively, of the rates expected in a normal group with the same age distribution. Both rates are significantly less than normal. Comparison of known deaths from thyroid carcinoma in the two age groups provides evidence that papillary carcinoma of the thyroid is more serious in patients more than 40 years old.

Variation in histologic pattern in papillary carcinoma was studied by Woolner and colleagues[72] to determine whether the behavior of a papillary tumor with predominantly papillary architecture was comparable to that of one predominantly (80 to 100 percent) follicular. On the basis of a 15-year follow-up of patients 40 years old or less at operation, the survival rate for the 34 with predominantly papillary carcinoma was 7 percent lower than that for the 62 with predominantly follicular tumor. Among patients more than 40 years old at operation, the survival rate for the 61 with pre-dominantly papillary tumor was 17 percent lower than that for the 54 with predominantly follicular tumor. None of these differences is statistically significant. However, one subtype of papillary carcinoma—those rare instances when papillary carcinoma coexists with anaplastic carcinoma—is associated with a dreadful prognosis.[74]

Follicular Carcinoma

The two most important prognostic factors in follicular carcinoma are the degree of vascular invasion (Fig. 23-12) and the histologic grade of the tumor. The majority of such tumors are grade 2 (Broders' classification), in contrast to the predominance of grade 1 tumors in the papillary group. In a series of 208 follicular carcinomas of the thyroid studied, half had slight or equivocal vascular invasion and half had moderate-to-marked invasion. The survival rate for patients with tumors having slight vascular invasion or none closely approximates that for normal persons of comparable age and sex. The survival rates (34 percent at 10 years and 16 percent at 20 years) for patients whose tumors had moderate-to-marked invasion were much lower than for patients whose tumors were noted to be less invasive.

Of 104 patients with tumors having none-to-slight vascular invasion, only 3 died from follicular carcinoma. Death as a result of persistent tumor occurred 17, 21, and 22 years after the original surgery. In striking contrast to the good results of treatment in that group is the very serious outcome of tumors that were moderately or markedly invasive. Of 104 patients in this category, 61 died from thyroid carcinoma. The mean survival time from surgery to death for these patients was 6 years. Local recurrence was a frequent complication, as were bone and pulmonary metastases. Long-term follow-up data on patients with follicular carcinoma and moderate or extensive vascular invasion indicated a poorer prognosis than those patients with none-to-slight vascular invasion.

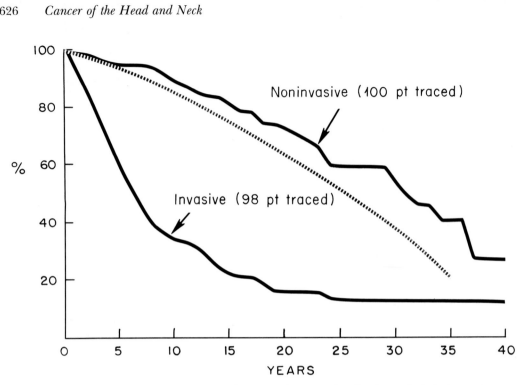

Fig. 23-12. Follicular carcinoma. Survival curves (six operative deaths excluded) for patients with slight or equivocal capsular invasion and patients with moderate or marked invasion (including recurrent and inoperable tumors); also shown is curve (dotted line) for normal persons of comparable age and sex. (Woolner, L.B., Beahrs, O.H., Black, B.M., McConahey, W.M., and Keating, F.R., Jr. 1968. Thyroid carcinoma: General considerations and follow-up data on 1181 cases. In Young, S., and Inman, D.R., Eds.: Thyroid Neoplasia, Proceedings of the Second Imperial Cancer Research Fund Symposium, p. 51. Copyright by Academic Press Inc. (London) Ltd. Reprinted with permission.)

Medullary Carcinoma

In patients with medullary carcinoma, the prognosis seems to be affected significantly by the grade of malignancy and the presence or absence of cervical node metastasis at operation (Fig. 23-13). The survival of patients with medullary carcinoma and negative cervical lymph nodes at initial surgery (65 traced patients) was compared with survival of patients with medullary carcinoma and nodal metastasis (74 traced patients). The 5-year and 10-year survival rates for the patients without nodal metastasis were not significantly different from the rates for normal persons of comparable age and sex. The 10-year survival rate of patients whose nodes were positive was 40 percent. This was approximately 45 percent below the rate for normal persons of comparable age

and sex. Lymph node metastasis was associated with rapid deterioration and a grave prognosis.

Initially, it was somewhat difficult for us to understand that patients with bilateral medullary thyroid carcinoma survived longer than patients with unilateral medullary tumor. It is significant that 82 percent of patients with bilateral disease had familial disease, and their mean age at diagnosis was 21 years versus 51 years for the whole group.

In our recent experience, nodal metastasis was found in 23 percent of patients with familial disease (and primarily diagnosed at this institution).[56] This contrasts with an incidence of 53 percent for patients with presumed sporadic disease seen at this institution.[13] We attribute the difference in nodal metastasis to family screening and

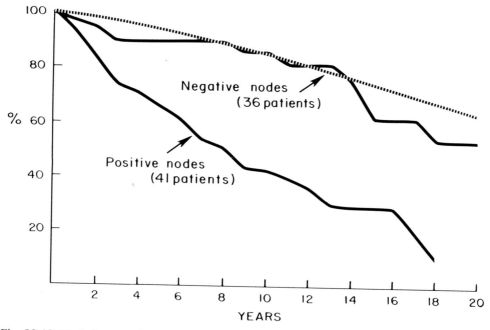

Fig. 23-13. Medullary carcinoma. Survival curves for patients with metastatic involvement of cervical lymph nodes at initial operation, for patients without such involvement, and for normal persons of comparable age and sex (dotted line). (Woolner, L.B., Beahrs, O.H., Black, B.M., McConahey, W.M., and Keating, F.R., Jr. 1968. Thyroid carcinoma: General Considerations and follow-up data on 1181 cases. Young, S., and Inman, D.R., Eds.: Thyroid Neoplasia, Proceedings of the Second Imperial Cancer Research Fund Symposium, p. 51. Copyright by Academic Press Inc. (London) Ltd. Reprinted with permission.)

earlier diagnosis in those familial disease.

A recent publication[56] from the Mayo Clinic cited factors that may influence the persistence or recurrence of medullary thyroid carcinoma:

They are: age at diagnosis of primary tumor, the neuroma phenotype, inadequacy of primary surgery, and the presence of regional metastasis at primary surgery, and the presence of regional metastasis at primary surgery. Fig. [23-14] shows the incidence of MTC [familial medullary thyroid carcinoma] persistence or recurrence as a function of patient age at diagnosis of the primary tumor. No patient under age 10 has had persistence or recurrence. Diagnosis from the second to seventh decades was associated with a progressively increasing incidence of persistence or recurrence, from 31% to 67%. Of the nine patients with the neuroma phenotype,

six (67%) have recurrence. Of the seven with inadequate primary surgery, four (57%) have recurrence. Of the 17 who had regional metastasis at the time of primary surgery, 14 (82%) have persistence or recurrence. . . . 9 of the 11 patients who underwent secondary surgery have had persistence or recurrence subsequent to that.

Anaplastic Carcinoma

With current methods of treatment for anaplastic carcinoma, few survivors can be expected (Fig. 23-15). Usually the course of the disease is measured in months, although it has been prolonged in the few cases in which papillary and squamous carcinoma have been associated. In these cases, it is likely that a papillary adenocarcinoma, after existing for a long time, has undergone anaplastic transformation.

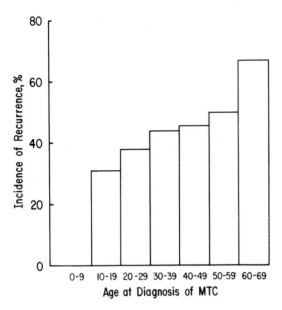

Fig. 23-14. Incidence of persistence or recurrence of familial medullary carcinoma of thyroid as function of age at initial diagnosis. (Sizemore, G.W., Carney, J.A., and Heath, H., III. 1977. Epidemiology of medullary carcinoma of the thyroid gland: A 5-year experience (1971-1976). Surgical Clinics of North America, 57: 633.)

SUMMARY

Cancer of the thyroid gland occurs uncommonly. Though most lesions are well-differentiated and have a benign course, some patients do die of the disease. Because mortality and morbidity for thyroidectomy are low, operation should be advised for selected patients who have nodular goiters that might be cancerous or who have goiters that are suspected of being cancerous.

Cognizant that thyroid carcinomas are often noninvasive, localized, and slow growing and that a number of vital structures are located near or course nearby the thyroid, our group recommends reasonably conservative surgery, always individualizing the surgery according to the nature and extent of the patient's disease. In this respect, we follow the teaching of Johann von Mikulicz in protecting and preserving the recurrent laryngeal nerves and the parathyroid glands.

Recognition of the different biologic behavior of the various types of thyroid carcinoma is paramount to the appropriate selection of surgical procedure. For example, while some cancers histologically appear to be a mixture of papillary and follicular components, in our experience such lesions behave as though they were purely papillary even though the papillary component may be only 10 percent of the total.

Papillary Carcinoma

Only when lymphatic channels are involved do we advocate complementary modified neck dissection(s), in addition to ipsilateral total lobectomy, isthmectomy, and contralateral subtotal thyroidectomy. Prognosis is related to the extent of the primary lesion relative to the thyroid gland rather than to the presence or absence of regional lymphatic metastasis. Patients with intrathyroidal lesions (those not involving structures outside the thyroid capsule) fare better than do patients with extrathyroidal lesions.

Follicular Adenocarcinoma

Like papillary lesions, follicular adenocarcinomas are usually low-grade, yet unlike them, they spread primarily via the bloodstream. Presence or absence of encapsulation and vascular invasion are important prognostic features. In more than 40 years of follow-up, the mortality rate associated with moderate-to-severe vascular invasion was approximately 17 times that when lesions had none-to-slight invasion. Ipsilateral total lobectomy with contralateral subtotal lobectomy and isthmectomy is advised in the absence of metastatic disease. Modified radical neck dissection may be added when there is lymphatic involvement, and because follicular lesions typically are functional (that is, take up radioactive iodine), we advise careful total thyroidectomy if distant

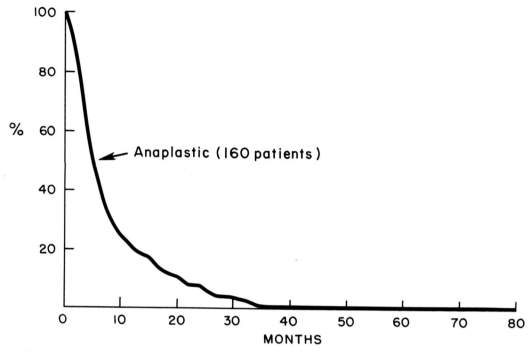

Fig. 23-15. Anaplastic carcinoma. Survival curve by month. (Woolner, L.B., Beahrs, O.H., Black, B.M., McConahey, W.M., and Keating, F.R., Jr. 1968. Thryoid carcinoma: General considerations and follow-up data on 1181 cases. In Young, S., and Inman, D.R., Eds.: Thyroid Neoplasia, Proceedings of the Second Imperial Cancer Research Fund Symposium, p. 51. Copyright by Academic Press Inc. (London) Ltd. Reprinted with permission.)

metastasis or vascular invasion is evident. Subsequent doses of ^{131}I are then fully concentrated upon residual malignancy.

Medullary Carcinoma

Often multicentric, medullary carcinoma has a clinical course that can be most accurately prognosticated by the presence or absence of involvement of regional lymph nodes. Twenty years of follow-up on patients with and without positive nodes showed that 46 and 6 percent, respectively, died of their disease. We advocate total thyroidectomy with concomitant radical neck dissection if there is lymphatic involvement.

Twenty percent of patients have familial disease. In these, the lesions may be detected early, even in a premalignant phase. Other potentially concomitant familial disorders may be detected if affected persons and their families are properly screened.

Anaplastic Carcinoma

The undifferentiated nature of this neoplasm obviates radioactive iodine as realistic therapy and gives a good clue to the tumor's propensity for rapid growth, widespread metastasis, and early death. Seventy-five percent of patients with anaplastic disease are dead of their disease within 12 months of the histologic diagnosis. Surgery involves debulking the tumor, ensuring an adequate airway, and planning for postoperative irradiation, with hope for but little expectation of significant effect.

REFERENCES

1. American Cancer Society. 1978. Cancer Facts and Figures Based on Rates from NCI Third National Cancer Survey. Government Printing Office, Washington, D. C.

2. Arnold, G.E. 1963. Alleviation of aphonia or

dysphonia through intracordal injection of Teflon paste. Annals of Otology, Rhinology and Laryngology, 72:   384.

3. Beahrs, O.H., and Kubista, T.P. 1968. Diagnosis of thyroid cancer. In Cancer Management: A Special Graduate Course on Cancer. J. B. Lippincott, Philadelphia, 573.

4. Beahrs, O.H., and Pasternak, B.M. 1969. Cancer of the thyroid gland. Current Problems in Surger, December, 1-38.

5. Beahrs, O.H., and Sakulsky, S.B. 1968. Surgical thyroidectomy in the management of exophthalmic goiter. Archives of Surgery, 96:   512.

6. Beahrs, O.H., and Tachovsky, T.J. 1969. Surgery of the thyroid gland. In Goldsmith, H.S., Ed. Lewis' Practice of Surgery. Vol. 4. Harper and Row, Hagersstown, MD, 1.

7. Beahrs, O.H., and Vandertoll, D. J. 1963. Complications of secondary thyroidectomy. Surgery, Gynecology and Obstetrics, 117: 535.

8. Beahrs, O.H., and Woolner, L.B. 1959. The treatment of papillary carcinoma of the thyroid gland. Surgery, Gynecology and Obstetrics, 108:   43.

9. Berry, J.: Cited by Bailey, H. 1960. Demonstrations of Physical Signs in Clinical Surgery. 13th edn. John Wright and Sons, Bristol, England.

10. Block, M.A. 1969. Medullary thyroid carcinoma: A component of an interesting endocrine syndrome. CA, Cancer Journal for Clinicians, 19:   74.

11. Block, M.A., Horn, R.C., Jr., Miller J.M., Barrett, J.L., and Brush, B.E. 1967. Familial medullary carcinoma of the thyroid. Annals of Surgery, 166:   403.

12. Burke, J.S., Butler, J.J., and Fuller, L.M. 1977. Malignant lymphomas of the thyroid: A clinical pathologic study of 35 patients including ultrastructural observations. Cancer, 39:   1587.

13. Chong, G.C., Beahrs, O.H., Sizemore, G.W., and Woolner, L.H. 1975. Medullary carcinoma of the thyroid gland. Cancer, 35:   695.

14. Clark, R.L., Ibanez, M.L., and White, E.C. 1966. What constitutes an adequate operation for carcinoma of the thyroid? Archives of Surgery, 92:   23.

15. Clark, R.L., Cole, V.W., Fuller, L.M., Healey, J.E., Jr., Hill, C.S., Jr., Ibanez, M.L., Macdonald, E.J., and White, E.C. 1967. Thyroid. In MacComb, W.S., and Fletcher, G.H., Eds.: Cancer of the Head and Neck.

Williams and Wilkins Company, Baltimore, 293.

16. Crile, G., Jr. 1964. Survival of patients with papillary carcinoma of the thyroid after conservative operations. American Journal of Surgery, 108:   862.

17. Crile, G., Jr., and Wilson, D.H. 1959. Transformation of a low grade papillary carcinoma of the thyroid to an anaplastic carcinoma after treatment with radioiodine. Surgery, Gynecology and Obstetrics, 108:   357.

18. Croll, M.N., and Brady, L.W. 1963. Thyroid scintillation scanning: Methodology and interpretation. New York State Journal of Medicine, 63:   211.

19. Cuello, C., Correa, P., and Eisenberg, H. 1969. Geographic pathology of thyroid carcinoma. Cancer, 23:   230.

20. Cunningham, D.J. 1951. In Brash, J.C., Ed.: Cunningham's Text-Book of Anatomy. 9th edn. Parts 1 and 2. Oxford University Press, London.

21. DeGroot, L., and Paloyan, E. 1973. Thyroid carcinoma and radiation: A Chicago endemic. JAMA, 225:   487.

22. De Quervain, F., cited by Smith, I., and Murley, R. S. 1965. Damage to the cervical sympathetic system during operations on the thyroid gland. British Journal of Surgery, 52:   673.

23. De Quervain, F., and Giordanengo, G. 1935-1937. Die akute and subakute nichteitrige Thyreoiditis. Mitteilungen aus den Grenzge bieten der Medizin and Chirurgie, 44:   538.

24. Division of Cancer Control and Rehabilitation, National Cancer Institute. 1977. Irradiation-Related Thyroid Cancer (Publication no. [NIH] 77-1120). United States Department of Health, Education, and Welfare, National Institutes of Health.

25. Dobyns, B.M. 1969. Goiter. Current Problems in Surgery, January, 2-60.

26. Doyle, P.J., Everts, E.C., and Brummett, R.E. 1968. Treatment of recurrent laryngeal nerve injury. Archives of Surgery, 96:   517.

27. Dunn, E.L., Nishiyama, R.H., and Thompson, N.W. 1973. Medullary carcinoma of the thyroid gland. Surgery, 73:   848.

28. Durham, C.F., and Harrison, T.S. 1964. The surgical anatomy of the superior laryngeal nerve. Surgery, Gynecology and Obstetrics, 118:   38.

29. Goff, W.F. 1969. Teflon injection for vocal

cord paralysis. Archives of Otolaryngology, 90: 98.

30. Goltzman, D., Potts, J.T., Jr., Ridgway, E.C., and Maloof, F. 1974. Calcitonin as a tumor marker: Use of the radioimmunoassay for calcitonin in the postoperative evaluation of patients with medullary thyroid carcinoma. New England Journal of Medicine, 290: 1035.

31. Graham, A. 1924. Malignant epithelial tumors of the thyroid: With special reference to invasion of blood vessels. Surgery, Gynecology and Obstetrics, 39: 781.

32. Hawe, P., and Lothian, K.R. 1960. Recurrent laryngeal nerve injury during thyroidectomy. Surgery, Gynecology and Obstetrics, 110: 488.

33. Hayles, A.B., Johnson, L.M., Beahrs, O.H., and Woolner, L.B. 1963. Carcinoma of the thyroid in children. American Journal of Surgery, 106: 735.

34. Hazard, J.B., and Smith, D.E. 1964. The thyroid. Monographs in Pathology, 5: 1.

35. Hazard, J.B., Hawk, W.A., and Crile, G., Jr. 1959. Medullary (solid) carcinoma of the thyroid: A clinicopathologic entity. Journal of Clinical Endocrinology and Metabolism, 19: 152.

36. Hollinshead, W.H. 1954. Anatomy for Surgeons. Vol. 1. The Head and Neck. Paul B. Hoeber, New York.

37. Hubert, J.P., Jr., Kiernan, P.D., and Beahrs, O.H. Unpublished data.

38. Hunt, P.S., Poole, M., and Reeve, T.S. 1968. A reappraisal of the surgical anatomy of the thyroid and parathyroid glands. British Journal of Surgery, 55: 63.

39. Jackson, I.M.D., and Thomson, J.A. 1967. The relationship of carcinoma to the single thyroid nodule. British Journal of Surgery, 54: 1007.

40. McCormack, K.R., and Sheline, G.E. 1967. Long-term studies of solitary autonomous thyroid nodules. Journal of Nuclear Medicine, 8: 701.

41. Mazzaferri, E.L., Young, R.L., Oertel, J.E., Kemmerer, W.T., and Page, C.P. 1977. Papillary thyroid carcinoma: The impact of therapy in 576 patients. Medicine (Baltimore), 56: 171.

42. Miura, T., and Grillo, H.C. 1966. The contribution of the inferior thyroid artery to the blood supply of the human trachea. Surgery, Gynecology and Obstetrics, 123: 99.

43. Moertel, C.G., Beahrs, O.H., Woolner, L.B., and Tyce, G.M. 1965. "Malignant carcinoid syndrome" associated with noncarcinoid tumors. New England Journal of Medicine, 273: 244.

44. Mosoman, D.A., and DeWeese, M.S. 1968. The external laryngeal nerve as related to thyroidectomy. Surgery, Gynecology and Obstetrics, 127: 1011.

45. Mortensen, J.D., Bennett, W.A., and Woolner, L.B. 1954. Incidence of carcinoma in thyroid glands removed at 1000 consecutive routine necropsies. Surgical Forum, 5: 659.

46. Nobles, E.R., Jr. 1970. Nonrecurrent laryngeal nerve. Archives of Surgery, 100: 741.

47. Patten, B.M. 1968. Human Embryology. 3rd edn. McGraw-Hill, New York 432.

48. Pemberton, J. deJ. 1939. Malignant lesions of the thyroid gland: A review of 774 cases. Surgery, Gynecology and Obstetrics, 69: 417.

49. Pemberton, J. deJ., and Beaver, M. G. 1932. Anomaly of right recurrent laryngeal nerve. Surgery, Gynecology and Obstetrics, 54: 594.

50. Pemberton, J. deJ., and Black, B.M. 1954. Cancer of the Thyroid. American Cancer Society, New York.

51. Reeve, T.S. Coupland, G.A.E., Johnson, D.C., and Buddee, F.W. 1969. The recurrent and external laryngeal nerves in thyroidectomy. Medical Journal of Australia, 1: 380.

52. Robinson, E., Horn, Y., and Hochmann, A. 1966. Incidence of cancer in thyroid nodules. Surgery, Gynecology and Obstetrics, 123: 1024.

53. Rossi, R., Cady, B., Meissner, W.A., Sedgwick, C.E., and Werber, J. 1978. Prognosis of undifferentiated carcinoma and lymphoma of the thyroid. American Journal of Surgery, 135: 589.

54. Rustad, W.H., Lindsay, S., and Dailey, M.E. 1963. Comparison of the incidence of complications following total and subtotal thyroidectomy for thyroid carcinoma. Surgery, Gynecology and Obstetrics, 116: 109.

55. Shimkin, P.M., and Sagerman, R.H. 1969. Lymphoma of the thyroid gland. Radiology, 92: 812.

56. Sizemore, G.W., Carney, J.A., and Heath, H., III. 1977. Epidemiology of medullary carcinoma of the thyroid gland: A 5-year experience (1971–1976). Surgical Clinics of North America, 57: 633.

57. Smith, I., and Murley, R.S. 1965. Damage to the cervical sympathetic system during operations on the thyroid gland. British Journal of Surgery, 52:   673.

58. Sokal, J.E. 1959. The problem of malignancy in nodular goiter—recapitulation and a challenge. JAMA, 170:   405.

59. Stewart, G.R., Mountain, J.C., and Colcock, B.P. 1972. Non-recurrent laryngeal nerve. British Journal of Surgery, 59:   379.

60. Swelstad, J., Scanlon, E. F., Murphy, E.D., Garces, R., and Khandekar, J.D. 1977. Thyroid disease following irradiation for benign conditions. Archives of Surgery, 112:   380.

61. Thorek, P. 1962. Anatomy in Surgery. 2nd edn. J. B. Lippincott, Philadelphia, 166.

62. Tollefsen, H.R., and DeCosse, J.J. 1963. Papillary carcinoma of the thyroid: Recurrence in the thyroid gland after initial surgical treatment. American Journal of Surgery, 106:   728.

63. VanderLaan, W.P. 1947. The occurrence of carcinoma of the thyroid gland in autopsy material. New England Journal of Medicine, 237:   221.

64. Wagner, D.H., Recant W.M., and Evans, R.H. 1978. A review of one hundred and fifty thyroidectomies following prior irradiation to the head, neck and upper part of the chest. Surgery, Gynecology and Obstetrics, 147:   903.

65. Wells, S.A., Jr., Gunnells, J.C., Shelburne, J.D., Schneider, A.B., and Sherwood, L.M. 1975. Transplantation of the parathyroid glands in man: Clinical indications and results. Surgery, 78:   34.

66. Wells, S.A., Jr., Baylin, S.B., Linehan, W.M., Farrell, R.E., Cox, E.B., and Cooper, C.W. 1978. Provocative agents and the diagnosis of medullary carcinoma of the thyroid gland. Annals of Surgery, 188:   139.

67. Wells, S.A., Jr., Baylin, S.B., Gann, D.S., Farrell, R.E., Dilley, W.G., Preissig, S.H., Linehan, W.M., and Cooper, C.W. 1978. Medullary thyroid carcinoma: Relationship of method of diagnosis to pathologic staging. Annals of Surgery, 188:   377.

68. Williams, E.D., Brown, D.L., and Doniach, I. 1966. Pathological and clinical findings in a series of 67 cases of medullary carcinoma of the thyroid. Journal of Clinical Pathology, 19:   103.

69. Wood, J.W., Tamagaki, H., Neriishi, S., Sato, T., Sheldon, W.F., Archer, P.G., Hamilton, H.B., and Johnson, K.G. 1969. Thyroid carcinoma in atomic bomb survivors: Hiroshima and Nagasaki. American Journal of Epidemiology, 89:   4.

70. Woolner, L.B., McConahey, W.M., and Beahrs, O.H. 1959. Struma lymphomatosa (Hashimoto's thyroiditis) and related thyroidal disorders. Journal of Clinical Endocrinology and Metabolism, 19:   53.

71. Woolner, L.B., McConahey, W.M., Beahrs, O.H., and Black, B.M. 1966. Primary malignant lymphoma of the thyroid: Review of forty-six cases. American Journal of Surgery, 111:   502.

72. Woolner, L.B., Beahrs, O.H., Black, B.M., McConahey, W.M., and Keating, F.R., Fr. 1968. Thyroid carcinoma: General considerations and follow-up data on 1181 cases. In Yung, S., and Inman, D.R., Eds.: Thyroid Neoplasia, Proceedings of the Second Imperial Cancer Research Fund Symposium. Academic Press, London, 51.

73. Wychulis, A.R., Beahrs, O.H., and Woolner, L.B. 1964. Metastasis of carcinoma to the thyroid gland. Annals of Surgery, 160:   169.

74. Wychulis, A.R., Beahrs, O.H., and Woolner, L.B. 1965. Papillary carcinoma with associated anaplastic carcinoma in the thyroid gland. Surgery, Gynecology and Obstetrics, 120:   28.

24 | Cancer of the Parathyroid

Paul D. Kiernan, M.D.
John P. Hubert, Jr., M.D.
Oliver H. Beahrs, M.D.

INTRODUCTION

Sir Richard Owen (cited by Taylor)[80] first described what are now known as the parathyroid glands. The Swedish anatomist Sandström[65] further clarified the anatomy of the parathyroid glands, but fruitful pathophysiologic breakthroughs awaited von Recklinghausen's description[84] of osteitis fibrosa cystica and Schlagenhaufer's[68] suggestion that parathyroid gland abnormality might be the cause of such bone disease.

In 1925, Collip[15] reported the isolation of parathyroid hormone and showed how it could, by affecting serum and urinary calcium and phosphorus levels, cause the bone changes that von Recklinghausen had described. Within the year, Mandl[53] cured a patient who had osteitis fibrosa cystica by removing the offending parathyroid adenoma. Recognizing that more than 75 percent of all patients with osteitis fibrosa cystica had renal stones. Albright et al.[1] reviewed all of the cases involving renal stones at the Massachusetts General Hospital. Within a decade hyperparathyroidism had been diagnosed in 67 patients with renal stones at that institution.[16]

Primary hyperparathyroidism is an uncommon but not rare entity, with a reported incidence of approximately 0.1 percent in the patient population of one large clinic.[13] Despite reports citing incidences of parathyroid carcinoma of as much as 5.3 percent in patients with primary hyperparathyroidism,[16, 28, 43, 49, 51, 56, 63, 67, 78] studies from the Mayo Clinic revealed that the incidence was between 0.5 and 1.5 percent.[82, 83, 86] Since 1939, when Meyer et al.[55] first described malignant primary hyperparathyroidism, carcinoma of the parathyroid glands has been found to occur uncommonly.

CLASSIFICATION

Theoretically, parathyroid malignancy may be primary or secondary and functioning or nonfunctioning.[41] In an autopsy study of other primary malignancies, Horwitz et al.[42] cited an incidence of 5.3 to 11.9 percent of secondary (metastatic) involvement of one or more parathyroid glands. The primary malignant lesions that most frequently were metastatic to the parathyroid were of the breast, blood (leukemia), and skin (malignant melanoma).

Generally, malignant lesions metastatic to the parathyroid glands do not affect endocrine function, though instances of hypofunction and hyperfunction have been cited.[42, 47] While extensive metastatic replacement of parathyroid tissue might be expected to reduce the level of endocrine function by an amount proportional to the percentage of gland replaced or destroyed, hyperfunction is probably an unusual effect—more theoretic than real. Hypercalcemia in these situations is more often than not the result of bony metastasis.

In an extensive review, Holmes et al.[41] found that the ratio of functioning to nonfunctioning primary malignant parathyroid neoplasms is more than 10 to 1. In this chapter, all primary (malignant) parathyroid lesions will be considered hormonally hyperactive. This assumption allows for an accurate and dependable differentiation of malignant lesions that are of similar cell type and close anatomic proximity (for example, malignancies of the thymus, thyroid, and parathyroid).

EMBRYOLOGY AND ANATOMY

A thorough knowledge of normal parathyroid embryology, anatomy, and physiology is fundamental to the understanding and recognition of parathyroid carcinoma.

Embryology[23]

Ordinarily, two pairs of parathyroid glands develop, one from the third branchial pouch and the other from the fourth. Subsequently, both pairs of glands move caudally—those originating from the fourth branchial pouch, the superior parathyroids, traveling the least—assuming a position posterior to the midthyroid level.

The inferior parathyroids usually migrate farther. These glands tend to descend beyond their superior counterparts and, with the thymus gland (also originating from the third branchial pouch), usually assume a position near the lower pole of each thyroid lobe. It is believed that, because the inferior glands migrate relatively farther, they tend to be more variably located than the superior glands.

Anatomy[23]

Parathyroid glands vary greatly in size, shape, number, and location. Whereas the inferior parathyroids are generally heavier than the superior glands, normal individual glands usually weigh between 30 and 35 mg. Parathyroid carcinomas are typically much larger. Characteristically, glands vary from yellowish-tan to reddish-brown and have a fine texture that distinguishes them from the surrounding lymph nodes, fat, thymus, and thyroid. Each gland is often tongue-shaped, the base of which composes the vascular hilus. The fine vascular supply of each gland is apparent on critical inspection of the hilus; this also allows their differentiation from nearby structures.

Typically, only four parathyroid glands exist. In 354 autopsies, Alveryd[2] found 1,405 parathyroid glands (histologically verified), noting 4 in 90.6 percent of cases, 5 in 3.7 percent, and 3 in 5.7 percent. In a series of 428 autopsies. Gilmour[33] found four parathyroids in 87 percent of cases studied, five glands in 6.0 percent, and three glands in 6.1 percent. Beahrs had found seven parathyroids in a patient with benign primary hyperparathyroidism.

Sometimes found within the thyroid (3.0 percent of instances),[81] the parathyroids more often lie immediately adjacent posteriorly. The superior parathyroids are found most often at the level of the upper two-thirds of the thyroid. The inferior parathyroids are usually found on the inferior surface of the lower pole of the thyroid gland, near the intersection of the recurrent laryngeal nerve and the inferior thyroid artery. The inferior parathyroids are rarely found above the midthyroid level, are occasionally found caudad to the lower lobe, and may even extend into the anterior mediastinum. Vail and Coller[81] found parathyroids within thymic tissue in 3.4 percent of cases studied.

Alveryd[2] found superior parathyroids located typically cephalad to the inferior thyroid artery, while the inferior parathyroids were more often than not located caudad. Such was true in his experience in 58.5 percent of cases on the right and 71.5 percent of cases on the left. Gilmour[33] found superior and inferior parathyroid glands cephalad and caudad to the inferior thyroid artery in 92 percent and 99 percent of cases, respectively (Fig. 24-1).

When parathyroid glands are difficult to locate, it may be helpful to trace the inferior thyroid vasculature[77] because the inferior thyroid artery serves as the major blood supply to the parathyroids in more than 95 percent of cases. In less than 10 percent of

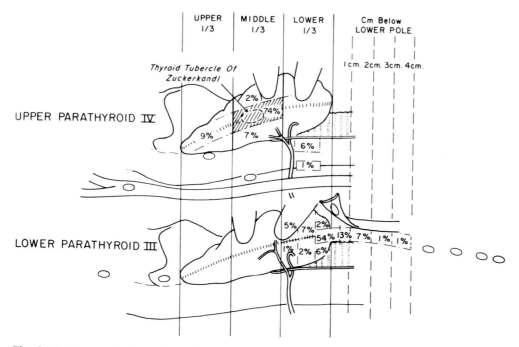

Fig. 24-1. Schematic view of lateral aspect of reflected thyroid gland, illustrating location of parathyroid glands found by anatomic dissection. (Data from Gilmour.[33])

cases, the superior thyroid artery supplies either superior gland or supplies both glands. Rarely does the thyroidea ima or another vessel, normally supplying the larynx, trachea, esophagus, or mediastinum, supply any of the parathyroid glands.

Parathyroid tissue may be found anywhere from the level of the hyoid bone to the inferior mediastinum (Fig. 24-2). Ectopically located glands are found most often in the mediastinum.[57] In the mediastinum, superior parathyroids, after having traversed the tracheoesophageal groove caudad are most often found in the posterosuperior mediastinum. When inferiorly displaced, inferior parathyroid tissue is most often found in the anterosuperior mediastinum.

PHYSIOLOGY

To preserve homeostasis with regard to mineral metabolism, parathyroid and thyroid gland hormones act on vitamin D—a product of 7-dihydrocholesterol and sunlight (Figs. 24-3 A and B).[7]

The chief cells of the parathyroid glands, via a classic, negative feedback system, secrete parathyroid hormone in direct response and possibly in indirect response to abnormally low and high serum concentrations of calcium and phosphorus, respectively. Parathyroid hormone appears to affect the calcium-phosphorus balance at three major sites[48]: bone, gastrointestinal tract, and kidney. In the hyperparathyroid state, parathyroid hormone, with vitamin D, increases calcium resorption and absorption.[29] At the kidney, it indirectly allows increased phosphate excretion.

Thyrocalcitonin, elaborated by the thyroid parafollicular or "C" cells, lowers abnormally elevated calcium levels by decreasing the resorption of calcium by bone.[48] Thyrocalcitonin acts directly on bone and is not known to have any direct effect on parathyroid hormone.

ETIOLOGY

The incidence of malignancy of the thyroid and salivary glands has increased among

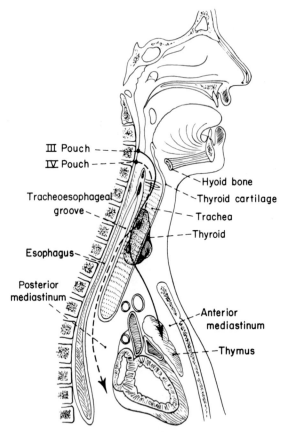

III Pouch

IV Pouch

Tracheoesophageal groove

Esophagus

Posterior mediastinum

Hyoid bone

Thyroid cartilage

Trachea

Thyroid

Anterior mediastinum

Thymus

Fig. 24-2. Diagnostic line of descent of parathyroid glands from branchial pouches III and IV, indicating structures and spaces that the glands are closely related to as well as their most usual locations adjacent to lateral and posterior capsule of thyroid gland. (Beahrs, O.H., Edis, A.J., and Purnell, D.C. 1977. Unusual problems in parathyroid surgery. American Journal of Surgery 134: 502.)

persons previously exposed to irradiation of the head and neck.[79] Similar influences may likewise affect parathyroid tissue. While some authors have documented an increased incidence of parathyroid adenomas among persons with previous exposure of the head and neck to irradiation, we know of no existing data referable to parathyroid carcinomas.

An entity of familial parathyroid carcinoma occurring in two forms has been documented:[21, 31, 53] one associated with a history of benign familial hyperparathyroidism and the other associated with a history of malignant familial hyperparathyroidism.

PATIENT EVALUATION

Symptoms and Signs

Although benign primary hyperparathyroidism is predominantly (3:1) a disease affecting women, the male-to-female ratio among patients with parathyroid carcinoma is approximately 1:1.[61] A neck mass is palpable in 31 to 45 percent of patients who have parathyroid carcinoma, compared with less than 1 percent of patients who have benign primary hyperparathyroidism. Additional features that should arouse suspicion of malignant disease are unilateral vocal cord paralysis without prior neck surgery[8] and recurrence of hypercalcemia after surgical treatment for primary hyperparathyroidism.[37, 41, 85]

Patients with benign primary hyperparathyroidism may have any combination of symptoms and signs relative to hypercalcemia (Table 24-1).[67] Although the symptoms and signs referable to malignant primary hyperparathyroidism (Table 24-2) vary somewhat from its benign counterpart (Table 24-3), skeletal, renal, and gastrointestinal manifestations of disease predominate.

We believe that nonspecific changes in mood and behavior probably occur in almost every patient who has significant and abnormal hypercalcemia. Such alterations are difficult to define precisely. Nevertheless, many hyperparathyroid patients, after correction of their hypercalcemia, show significant improvement in their general well-being.

Roentgenographic Features

The most extreme skeletal manifestations are the "brown" tumors (Fig. 24-4 A, B, C, and D), which von Recklinghausen[84] first described and which occur as bone resorp-

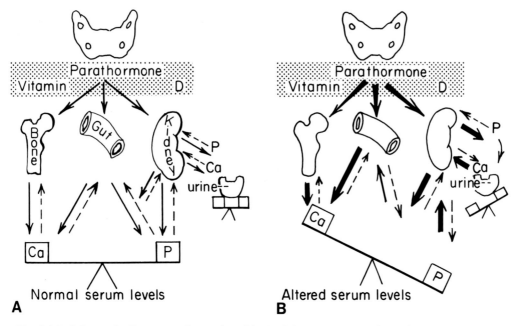

Fig. 24-3. Schematic diagrams of parathyroid physiology. (A) normal; (B) hyperparathyroidism. (Modified from Harrold, C.C., and Wright, J. 1966. Management of surgical hypoparathyroidism. American Journal of Surgery, 112: 482.)

tion yields cystic spaces that fill with fibrous tissue. This entity is seen less frequently now because of the earlier detection of hypercalcemia. Presently, vague aches and pains or roentgenographic changes (Fig. 24-4B and C, and D) unassociated with symptoms predominate.

In the past, many of the patients were found to have renal stones, probably because the mean concentrations of serum calcium tended to be higher in patients with malignant primary hyperparathyroidism (14.5 to 15.9 mg/dl) than in patients with the benign form (12 mg/dl).[53, 61, 83] The incidence of patients afflicted with significant renal disease should decrease as broader biochemical screening allows earlier detection of the hypercalcemic state.

Serum Profile

Primary hyperparathyroidism can be diagnosed on the basis of four serum tests: calcium, phosphorus, creatinine, and protein. The widespread use of multichannel, biochemical screening (including that of serum calcium level) should result in the earlier detection of hypercalcemia. This in turn should greatly improve the prognosis if definitive surgical treatment is promptly undertaken.[46] At the Mayo Clinic, the serum calcium level is measured by atomic absorption spectrophotometry, with normal levels ranging between 8.9 and 10.1 mg/dl. Because the serum concentration of calcium is related to the serum concentration of protein, the calcium level may increase or decrease as much as 0.8 mg/dl for every 1 g/dl of serum albumin or globulin gained or lost. In the presence of normal renal function, decreased serum phosphorus, and a normal serum protein, hypercalcemia documented on three separate occasions differentiates primary hyperparathyroidism from numerous other possible causes of hypercalcemia.[70] (See Table 24-4 for other possible causes of hypercalcemia.)

Parathyroid hormone immunoassay may have an important role in the diagnostic differentiation.[4, 5, 10, 60, 64, 73] Because parathyroid carcinoma, by definition, must demonstrate hormonal hyperfunction and

TABLE 24-1. SYMPTOMS AND SIGNS ASSOCIATED WITH HYPERPARATHYROIDISM

Skeletal
  Bone pain, bone cysts (brown tumor), chondrocalcinosis, osteitis fibrosa cystica, osteoporosis, pathologic fractures

Urologic
  Polyuria, polydipsia, calculi, nephrocalcinosis, renal insufficiency

Neuropsychiatric
  Fatigue, apathy, depression, muscle weakness, depressed tendon reflexes, disorientation, psychotic behavior, stupor, coma, death

Gastrointestinal
  Anorexia, nausea, vomiting, abdominal discomfort, duodenal or gastric ulcer, pancreatitis

Multiple endocrine adenomatosis syndromes
  Adrenal, pancreas, pituitary, thyroid, APUD cell system

Metastatic calcification
  Ocular keratopathy, nephrocalcinosis, vascular calcification, periarticular calcification, chondrocalcinosis

Serendipity syndrome
  Asymptomatic and uncomplicated hypercalcemia usually detected by biochemical screening procedures

(Modified from Scholz, D.A., Purnell, D.C., Goldsmith, R.S., Smith, L.H., Riggs, B.L., and Arnoud, C.D. 1972. Diagnostic considerations in hypercalcemia syndromes. Medical Clinics of North America, 56: 941.)

because normocalcemia hyperparathyroidism and nonfunctioning parathyroid malignancy can occur,[41] parathyroid hormone immunoassay may be used to confirm the histologic criteria.

In recent years, radioimmunoassay of parathyroid hormone has been valuable for the diagnosis and accurate characterization of primary hyperparathyroidism. Patients with hypercalcemia unrelated to primary hyperparathyroidism in whom the normal negative feedback mechanisms are intact will have depressed levels of parathyroid hormone. In patients with primary hyper-

TABLE 24-2. SYMPTOMS AND SIGNS IN 61 CASES OF PARATHYROID CARCINOMA

Symptom/sign	No.	%
Bone disease	39	64
Palpable neck mass	19	31
Urolithiasis	18	30
Renal disease	13	21
Pancreatitis	6	10
Weakness	5	8
Peptic ulcer	5	8
Nausea and vomiting	3	5

(Schantz, A., and Castleman, B. 1973. Parathyroid carcinoma: A study of 70 cases. Cancer, 31: 600.)

TABLE 24-3. CLUES TO DIAGNOSIS OF HYPERPARATHYROIDISM IN FIRST 343 CASES AT THE MASSACHUSETTS GENERAL HOSPITAL

Clue	Cases	
	No.	%
Renal stones	195	56.9
Bone disease	80	23.3
Peptic ulcer	27	7.9
Fatigue	10	2.9
Pancreatitis	9	2.6
Central nervous system signs	7	2.0
Hypertension	6	1.7
Mental disturbance	3	0.9
Multiple endocrine abnormalities	3	0.9
No symptoms	2	0.6
Lump in neck	1	0.3

(Modified from Cope, O. 1966. The story of hyperparathyroidism at the Massachusetts General Hospital. Reprinted by permission from The New England Journal of Medicine 274: 1174. Modified to include percentages.)

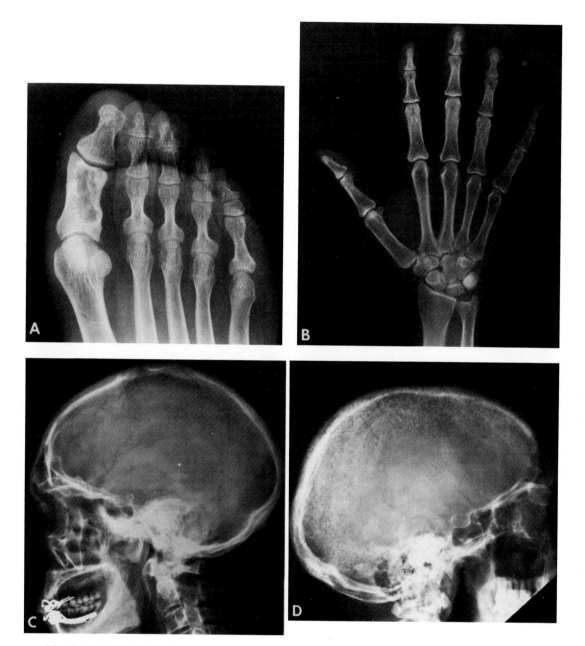

Fig. 24-4. (A) Multiple bone cysts (brown tumors). (B) Subperiosteal cortical erosion of distal phalanges, as well as generalized demineralization of bones. (C) and (D) Roentgenograms of skull. Figure C is normal, Figure D shows generalized demineralization, as well as the classic salt-and-pepper configuration.

parathyroidism related to adenoma, hyperplasia, or carcinoma, the normal negative feedback inhibition system is destroyed, thus accounting for elevated levels of parathyroid hormone in the presence of elevated levels of serum calcium.

Of special note is the discovery that parathyroid hormone exists as several immunologically distinct fragments (NH_2-terminal and COOH-terminal).[5] Arnaud,[4] Arnaud et al.,[5] and Silverman and Yalow[73] showed that serum assays that are high in

TABLE 24-4. CAUSES OF HYPERCALCEMIA

Common	Uncommon
Malignancy	Leukemia
With metastases	
Without metastases	Hyperthyroidism
Hyperparathyroidism	Myxedema
Primary	Hyperparathyroidism
Thiazide therapy	"Tertiary"
Myeloma	Addisonian crisis
Sarcoidosis	Immobilization
	Young adults and children
Hypervitaminosis D	Paget's disease
Milk-alkali syndrome	Diruetic phase of renal tubular damage
	Idiopathic hypercalcemia of infancy
	Acromegaly

(Scholz, D.A., Purnell, D.C., Goldsmith, R.S., Smith, L.H., Riggs, B.L., and Arnaud, C.D. 1972. Diagnostic considerations in hypercalcemic syndromes. Medical Clinics of North America, 56: 941.)

specificity for COOH-terminal fragments are superior to those with NH_2-terminal specificity in distinguishing normal from hyperparathyroid patients. In approximately 90 percent of cases, the primary hyperparathyroidism can be diagnosed on the basis of a COOH-terminal fragment assay system. The remaining 10 percent, who have normal levels of parathyroid hormone, have inappropriately elevated levels of serum calcium, thus allowing the diagnosis to be made.[87]

TREATMENT

At Initial Diagnosis

At least 20 percent of asymptomatic patients with benign primary hyperparathyroidism will require parathyroidectomy within 4 years of follow-up from the date of biochemical diagnosis.[62] Therefore, once primary hyperparathyroidism has been diagnosed, we advocate immediately proceeding with cervical exploration.

TABLE 24-5. A RECOMMENDED SCHEDULE FOR EMERGENCY TREATMENT OF HYPERCALCEMIA

1. Begin electrocardiographic monitoring
2. Institute appropriate supportive measures:
    a. Intravenous infusion of saline
    b. Potassium replacement as needed
    c. Vasopressor agents as needed
3. Furosemide (100 mg/h) intravenously
4. If response is inadequate, proceed with one of the following measures:
    a. EDTA infusion—do not continue beyond 24 h
    b. Phosphate infusion (1.5 g of phosphorus infused over 6 to 8 h) may be repeated daily, but more than two infusions usually are not required; follow with phosphate given orally
    c. Mithramycin (25 μg/kg) intravenously
5. If renal failure is unresponsive to diuretics, calcitonin may be used safely
6. Prepare for earliest surgical intervention

(Modified from Goldsmith, R.S. 1972. Treatment of hypercalcemia. Medical Clinics of North America, 56: 951.)

Antecedent surgery occasionally involves some delay in operation. Associated conditions, such as renal impairment, cardiac dysrhythmias, and congestive heart failure, mandate the individualization of treatment. Nevertheless, a fundamental plan, which may be instituted on an emergency basis in any situation of life-threatening hypercalcemia, is also necessary.[52, 76] Such a plan, along with pertinent pharmacologic recommendations, has been reported (Tables 24-5 and 24-6).[36]

It is unusual that coincident conditions mandate undue delay in neck exploration. Renal stones may be observed for spontaneous passage or may be removed after parathyroidectomy, unless a true urologic emergency exists, as for a septic patient with a completely obstructed ureter(s). Similarly, parathyroidectomy during pregnancy should precede delivery in order to prevent possible neonatal tetany.[22] Functioning islet cell tumors and pheochromocytomas should usually be removed before parathyroidectomy. Other conditions, myocardial infarction and renal failure among them, may delay the neck exploration. If complications that necessitate procrastination of general anesthesia develop, operation can be performed using a combination of cervical block and intravenously administered diazepam or a similar amnesic; rarely should such circumstances occur, however.

Operative exploration for hyperpara-

TABLE 24-6. USUAL DOSES OF HYPOCALCEMIC AGENTS

Drug	Route	Dosage	Reported Complications	Contraindications
Sodium chloride solution (isotonic)	Intravenous	1 liter every 3-4 h	Pulmonary edema	Congestive heart failure, renal insufficiency, hypertension
Furosemide	Intravenous	100 mg/h	Volume depletion, hypokalemia	Renal insufficiency
EDTA	Intravenous	50 mg/kg body weight over 4-6 h	Renal failure, hypotension	Renal insufficiency
Mithramycin	Intravenous	25 μg/kg body weight	Hemorrhage, thrombocytopenia, nausea, vomiting	Bleeding disorder, renal insufficiency, liver impairment
Phosphate	Intravenous	1 mmol/kg body weight over 6-8 h*	Extraskeletal calcification, hypocalcemia	Renal insufficiency, hyperphosphatemia
	Oral	1-2 mmol/kg body weight daily*	—	—
Calcitonin	Intravenous	1-5 MRC units/kg body weight/day	Nausea, vomiting	Thrombotic disorders

*One millimole of phosphate is equivalent to 31 mg of phosphorus.
(Modified from Goldsmith, R. S. 1972. Treatment of hypercalcemia. Medical Clinics of North America, 56: 951.)

thyroidism serves a diagnostic as well as a therapeutic role, because it identifies the number and size of glands, clarifies the type of disease, and effects treatment. Special tests for the localization of parathyroid glands, such as arteriography and selective venography, are seldom necessary. Arteriography, effective in 70 to 90 percent of instances applied,[25, 28] is associated with considerable morbidity. Both venography and arteriography are expensive and time-consuming and are not as accurate in defining the anatomic location of tumor as is the surgeon who is familiar with parathyroid embryology and anatomy.[18]

Black[11] has shown that the location of primary parathyroid carcinomas correlates well with the location of parathyroid adenomas. Beahrs has demonstrated that adenomas are readily found at primary explorations in more than 98 percent of cases. Similarly, Beahrs, et al.[9] and others[66, 85] have successfully localized tumors in 62 to 88 percent of secondary explorations.

At Initial Exploration

SURGICAL TECHNIQUES

After the usual transverse cervical (collar) incision, the thyroid is exposed. The strap muscles are not transected because traction and countertraction on these muscles helps expose the underlying anatomy.

All four parathyroid glands should be visualized systematically to ensure that no disease is overlooked. Superior parathyroids are found most easily because of their more constant position (most often at the level of the upper two-thirds of the posterior thyroid capsule). The inferior parathyroids are more variable in location—below the inferior thyroid artery in most instances—and in some, they are caudad to the inferior margin of the thyroid pole and even into the anterior mediastinum.

The inferior thyroid artery or its branches should lead to the inferior glands. The characteristic color of a normal para-

thyroid gland usually contrasts with that of surrounding tissues; however, in diseased states, sharp contrast may not always be apparent. Lymph nodes, lobules of fat, and thymic and thyroid tissue may be confused with parathyroid tissue.

Caution is urged when biopsy of normal-appearing parathyroid tissue is considered. If a biopsy specimen is to be taken, the antihilar area of the gland should be chosen, and its surface merely shaved with small scissors, so as not to disturb the fragile blood supply of the gland. If four normal-appearing glands are found and histologically confirmed, a diligent search should be made for accessory parathyroid tissue.

In the Mayo Clinic experience, as well as that of others, parathyroid glands will be found in "abnormal" position in approximately 19 percent of patients.[66] In two-thirds of this 19 percent, the parathyroid tumors will be found in the tracheoesophageal groove.[66] As previously stated, between 1 and 3 percent of patients will have parathyroid tissue within the thymus or the thyroid gland.[81]

If parathyroid disease is not found after a thorough search of the usual locations, the tracheoesophageal groove should be scrupulously inspected. Vascular pedicles descending to the mediastinum, as well as to the thymus gland itself, may be retrieved via a cervical approach. If parathyroid disease is still not evident, the pretracheal and prevertebral fascia should be thoroughly dissected from the level of the hyoid bone to the superior mediastinum. If disease is not identified and the operating surgeon feels confident he has not overlooked the lesion in the usual places, subtotal thyroidectomy may be a reasonable next step.

Still failing to discover parathyroid disease and confident that diffuse glandular hyperplasia is present (especially true if fewer than four glands have been identified), the surgeon should immediately search the mediastinum. Although we have performed mediastinal exploration mostly as a secondary procedure (6 to 12 weeks after initial surgery and after demonstrating persistent hypercalcemia), scarification at the site of the previous dissection of the neck and superior mediastinum has been troublesome. Therefore, before the first operation, we stress the possibility (1.4 per cent in the Mayo Clinic experience)[69] of extending the cervical exploration into the mediastinum.

Mediastinal exploration may be performed via routine median sternotomy or by using Clagett's modification.[14] In addition to removal of all thymic tissue, pericardium may need to be incised. In 65 percent of patients requiring median sternotomy, the parathyroids are located anteriorly; in the remaining 35 percent, they lie posterosuperiorly.[9]

If no parathyroid lesions are found, then preparations should be made to facilitate possible, subsequent reexploration. All identified parathyroid tissue should be carefully marked with long silk sutures or silver clips. The operation is terminated, and the sternal edges are reapproximated with interrupted wire. A retrosternal catheter is left attached for suction during the first few postoperative days. The cervical incision is closed (see Ch. 23).

RECOGNITION OF MALIGNANT PRIMARY HYPERPARATHYROIDISM

Parathyroid carcinoma may have been suspected on the basis of preoperative information, for example, a male patient with serum calcium levels exceeding 14 mg/dl or a palpable neck mass or both.[53] At the operation, gross findings that should arouse suspicion of malignancy, in increasing order of diagnostic usefulness, are (1) glandular induration, (2) capsular thickening, (3) evidence of dense fibrous reaction about a gland, (4) adherence or frank invasion of surrounding nerves, vessels, muscles, or thyroid gland, and (5) evidence of lymphatic metastasis.

As with any surgery, close alliance between surgeon and surgical pathologist enhances the precise recognition and identification of diseased tissue. Even experienced surgeons occasionally mistake lymph node for parathyroid tissue or the reverse. An expeditious operation is facilitated by frozen-section identification of carefully excised tissue; however, exact definition may be delayed, pending interpretation of permanent sections.

Histologic criteria as defined by Schantz and Castleman (Table 24-7),[67] coupled with the aforementioned observations, are helpful in the diagnosis of parathyroid malignancy but, short of absolute identification of local invasion or distant metastases, are not 100 percent reliable.[45] For example, tumor cells may be seen within capsules or blood vessels in benign adenomatous parathyroid disease.[11, 12]

If one encounters local extension or invasion of parathyroid tissue into contiguous tissues or regional lymph nodes, or recognizes any of the factors that Cope,[16] and Schantz and Castleman[67] have delineated as being suggestive of a malignancy, then a diagnosis of carcinoma must be considered. Local invasion or evidence of distant spread should influence the type of operation undertaken. Extent of operation for noninvasive and minimally invasive parathyroid carcinoma should include generous resection of thyroid gland, as well as adjacent muscle, fat, and nodal tissue. If the tumor invades the recurrent laryngeal nerve or ipsilateral jugular chain, sacrifice of the nerve is appropriate and neck dissection should be considered.[40, 51] Because of the typical low grade,

TABLE 24-7. HISTOLOGIC CRITERIA FOR PARATHYROID CARCINOMA (67 CASES)

Finding	No.	%
Fibrous trabeculae	60	90
Mitotic figures	54	81
Capsular invasion	45	67
Blood vessel invasion	8	12

(Schantz, A., and Castleman, B. 1973. Parathyroid carcinoma: A study of 70 cases. Cancer, 31: 600.)

slow growth, and late occurrence of distant metastasis (usually lymphatic) with parathyroid carcinoma, a most aggressive attack on the disease should be pursued at the earliest opportunity.

Schantz and Castleman noted 26 percent and Holmes et al.[41] noted 52 percent of patients with parathyroid carcinoma as having metastatic disease at the initial operation. Because in 32 to 50 percent of the cases of metastases the lesions are localized to regional lymph nodes and the morbidity and mortality of parathyroid carcinoma generally are related to the systemic effects of hypercalcemia, radical excision seems desirable for palliation as well as for hope of cure.[17, 18, 41, 67]

At Reoperation

Reoperation usually implies an inadequate initial surgical treatment—a malignant lesion may not have been recognized, was not properly resected, or had advanced beyond the bounds of curative surgery. While reoperation may be considered for hope of cure, more likely it will have been performed for palliation of recalcitrant disease.

Because of the hazards of reoperative neck surgery, a thorough preoperative evaluation of the need for further surgery, as well as meticulous dissection at reoperation, are absolute mandates to the surgeon. Before reoperation, all previous operative notes and all histologic slides should be reviewed. Because parathyroid carcinomas have been detected on routine roentgenograms of the chest[50] and have been detected in 70 percent of cases when ultrasonography[3] or selenomethionine scanning[32] was used, we agree with others[18] that such noninvasive techniques are sometimes useful and therefore on occasion may be performed preliminary to reoperations in the neck or mediastinum (or both). Only after dissection has proved to our satisfaction that local recurrence does not exist in the neck or in the mediastinum do we consider expensive, time-consuming, as well as hazardous arteriography-venography for localization of metastatic disease preliminary to extirpation.

Recrudescence of disease has been noted in 30 to 70 percent of patients surgically treated.[61, 67] In instances when patients refuse the surgical intervention that has been advised or when metastasis is so widespread as to be beyond judicious resection, chronic medical therapy has been used. If persistent or recurrent lesions cannot be excised, the use of medications such as calcitonin[6, 39, 58, 75] and hexestrol[35] has been advocated, as well as the more common modalities such as phosphates,[19, 20, 44, 58, 72] sulfate, EDTA,[24, 30] mithramycin,[74] and other agents (Tables 24-5 and 24-6), along with oncologic radiation or chemotherapy.

COMPLICATIONS

The complications of parathyroid surgery are essentially those of thyroid surgery (see Ch. 23). In recent experience with 327 cervical explorations performed for predominantly benign parathyroid disease,[66] one patient (0.3 percent) suffered permanent, unilateral vocal cord paralysis and eight other patients (2.4 percent) suffered transient, unilateral vocal cord paralysis. No bilateral recurrent laryngeal nerve injuries occurred. All 327 patients had vocal cord examinations performed by otolaryngologists both before and after operation.

Acute exacerbation of gout or pseudogout was noted in 2.7 percent of the above series of 327 patients. Three patients (0.9 percent) had pneumothorax after extensive cervical exploration of the anterior mediastinum. Two patients (0.6 percent) hemorrhaged postoperatively, with one (0.3 percent) hemorrhaging so significantly as to require reoperation for control of bleeding. One patient (0.3 percent) incurred transient renal failure with pancreatitis, and another (0.3 percent) suffered a wound infection. In the Mayo Clinic experience with the surgical treatment of benign and malignant parathyroid disease, operative mortality is rare (0.1 percent).[40, 66]

Complications of medical therapy may occur (for example, ectopic deposition of calcium, hypotension, renovascular thrombosis, nephrotoxic changes, hypocalcemia, and hypomagnesemia, among others).[20, 27, 38, 71, 72] One other problem with medical therapy may be the spreading of disease while the physician is procrastinating with regard to surgical intervention. The Mayo Clinic's experience with the surgical treatment of all too often advanced parathyroid malignancy would seem to reinforce the general observation that early diagnosis of malignancy, followed by prompt and appropriate surgery, should improve the prognosis.[46] Of the patients seen at the Mayo Clinic who had metastatic disease noted at operation, the 5-year survival is 35.7 percent. None is known to have been cured.[83]

END RESULTS

Less than 50 percent of the patients who were surgically treated for parathyroid carcinoma and were followed for 5 years (Schantz and Castleman)[67] died of parathyroid disease. However, only 29 percent of the patients followed for 5 years were alive and without residual malignancy. The 10-year survival rate was approximately 13 percent.[67] Neither the presence of vascular invasion nor the relative number of mitotic figures was a reliable predictor of prognosis.[67] Hypercalcemia or metastases (or both) have recurred as early as 3 weeks and as late as 19 years after operation.[26, 41]

The interval between the time of initial operation and the recurrence of hypercalcemia is important; longer intervals are associated with better prognosis.[67] Cures from reoperation for parathyroid carcinoma occur rarely; as Holmes et al.[41] noted, 90 percent of patients reoperated on for recurrent tumor died within 2 years of reoperation. In the Mayo Clinic's experience, no patient who had local or distant metastasis at the initial operation or who underwent reopera-

tion for recurrent disease is known to have been cured.[83]

SUMMARY

Parathyroid carcinoma may occur as a primary or as a secondary malignancy. Primary malignancies are more frequent and herein have been defined as necessarily exhibiting hyperfunction in order to facilitate differentiation from histologically similar tumors that may occur in anatomic proximity.

Surgical treatment must be on the basis of precise knowledge of pertinent embryology, anatomy, and physiology. Because of the desirability of early diagnosis and intervention for localized disease, surgery serves a diagnostic as well as a therapeutic function.

Diagnostic arteriography and venography should rarely be resorted to, because they are expensive, time-consuming, and hazardous procedures. Instead, cervical exploration may be expeditiously and safely conducted by a surgeon experienced in the identification of parathyroid glands and knowledgeable in parathyroid pathophysiology and embryology. The mediastinum does not commonly require exploration.

One cannot emphasize too strongly the need to recognize and treat parathyroid malignancy at the earliest opportunity. The extent of operation for noninvasive and minimally invasive parathyroid carcinoma should include generous resection of adjacent thyroid gland, muscle, fat, and nodal tissue. If tumors invade the recurrent laryngeal nerve or ipsilateral jugular chain (or both), sacrifice of nerve is appropriate and neck dissection should be considered.

Medical therapy may under emergency circumstances be employed before operation or as a terminal effort to palliate the morbid consequences of recalcitrant hypercalcemia. Although morbidity may be incurred with either medical or surgical intervention, early and aggressive surgical intervention offers the only chance for cure.

REFERENCES

1. Albright, F., Baird, P. C., Cope, O., and Bloomberg, E. 1934. Studies on the physiology of the parathyroid glands. IV. Renal complications of hyperparathyroidism. American Journal of the Medical Sciences, 187: 49.

2. Alveryd, A. 1968. Parathyroid glands in thyroid surgery. I. Anatomy of parathyroid glands. II. Postoperative hypoparathyroidism—identification and autotransplantation of parathyroid glands. Acta Chirurgica Scandinavica, suppl., 389: 1.

3. Arima, M., Yokoi, H., and Sonoda, T. 1975. Preoperative identification of tumor of the parathyroid by ultrasonotomography. Surgery, Gynecology and Obstetrics, 141: 242.

4. Arnaud, C. D. 1973. Parathyroid hormone: Coming of age in clinical medicine (editorial). American Journal of Medicine, 55: 577.

5. Arnaud, C. D., Goldsmith, R. S., Bordier, P. J., and Sizemore, G. W. 1974. Influence of immunoheterogeneity of circulating parathyroid hormone on results of radioimmunoassays of serum in man. American Journal of Medicine, 56: 785.

6. Au, W. Y. W. 1975. Calcitonin treatment of hypercalcemia due to parathyroid carcinoma: Synergistic effect of prednisone on long-term treatment of hypercalcemia. Archives of Internal Medicine, 135: 1594.

7. Avioli, L. V., and Haddad, J. G. 1975. Vitamin D: Current concepts. Metabolism, 22: 507.

8. Beahrs, O. H., Angelos, S. P., and Woolner, L. B. 1963. Carcinoma of the parathyroid gland: Report of a case. Surgical Clinics of North America, 43: 1123.

9. Beahrs, O. H., Edis, A. J., and Purnell, D. C. 1977. Unusual problems in parathyroid surgery. American Journal of Surgery, 134: 502.

10. Benson, R. C., Jr., Riggs, B. L., Pickard, B. M., and Arnaud, C. D. 1974. Immunoreactive forms of circulating parathyroid hormone in primary and ectopic hyperparathyroidism. Journal of Clinical Investigation, 54: 175.

11. Black, B. K. 1954. Carcinoma of the parathyroid. Annals of Surgery, 139: 355.

12. Black, B. K., and Ackerman, L. V. 1950. Tumors of the parathyroid: A review of twenty-three cases. Cancer, 3: 415.

13. Boonstra, C. E., and Jackson, C. E. 1971. Serum calcium survey for hyperparathyroidism: Results in 50,000 clinic patients. American Journal of Clinical Pathology, 55: 523.

14. Clagett, O. T., and Root, G. T. 1944. Surgical approach for tumors of the thymus. Surgery Gynecology and Obstetrics, 78: 397.

15. Collip, J. B. 1925. The extraction of a parathyroid hormone which will prevent or control parathyroid tetany and which regulates the level of blood calcium. Journal of Biological Chemistry, 63: 395.

16. Cope, O. 1966. The story of hyperparathyroidism at the Massachusetts General Hospital. New England Journal of Medicine, 274: 1174.

17. Davies, D. R., Dent, C. E., and Ives, D. R. 1973. Successful removal of single metastasis in recurrent parathyroid carcinoma. British Medical Journal 1: 397.

18. Davies, D. R., Shaw, D. G., Ives, D. R., Thomas, B. M., and Watson, L. 1973. Selective venous catheterisation and radioimmunoassay of parathyroid hormone in the diagnosis and localisation of parathyroid tumours. Lancet, 1: 1079.

19. Dean, A. C. B., Lambie, A. T., and Shivas, A. A. 1969. Hypercalcaemic crisis and squamous carcinoma of the renal pelvis. British Journal of Surgery, 56: 375.

20. Dent, C. E. 1962. Some problems of hyperparathyroidism. British Medical Journal, 2: 1495.

21. Dinnen, J. S., Greenwood, R. H., Jones, J. H., Walker, D. A., and Williams, E. D. 1977. Parathyroid carcinoma in familial hyperparathyroidism. Journal of Clinical Pathology, 30: 966.

22. Dorey, L. G., and Gell, J. W. 1975. Primary hyperparathyroidism during the third trimester of pregnancy. Obstetrics and Gynecology, 45: 469.

23. Dozois, R. R., and Beahrs, O. H. 1977. Surgical anatomy and technique of thyroid and parathyroid surgery. Surgical Clinics of North America, 57: 647 (Aug.).

24. Dudley, F. J., and Blackburn, C. R. B. 1970. Extraskeletal calcification complicating oral neutral-phosphate therapy. Lancet, 2: 628.

25. Eisenberg, H., Pallotta, J., and Sherwood, L. M. 1974. Selective arteriography, venography and venous hormone assay in diagnosis and localization of parathyroid lesions. American Journal of Medicine, 56: 810.

26. Ellis, H. A., Floyd, M., and Herbert, F. K. 1971. Recurrent hyperparathyroidism due

to parathyroid carcinoma. Journal of Clinical Pathology, 24: 596.

27. Fhraeus, B., Andersson, L., Bergdahl, L., and Westling, P. 1973. Postoperative hypoparathyroidism: hazards from vitamin D therapy. Acta Chirurgica Scandinavica, 139: 437.

28. Farr, H. W., Fahey, T. J., Jr., Nash, A. G., and Farr, C. M. 1973. Primary hyperparathyroidism and cancer. American Journal of Surgery, 126: 539.

29. Favus, M. J. 1978. Vitamin D physiology and some clinical aspects of the vitamin D endocrine system. Medical Clinics of North America, 62: 1291.

30. Foreman, H., Finnegan, C., and Lushbaugh, C. C. 1956. Nephrotoxic hazard from uncontrolled edathamil calcium-disodium therapy. JAMA, 160: 1042.

31. Frayha, R. A., Nassar, V. H., Dagher, F., and Salti, I. S. 1972. Familial parathyroid carcinoma. Journal Medical Libanais, 25: 299.

32. Garrow, J. S., and Smith, R. 1968. The detection of parathyroid tumours by selenomethionine scanning. British Journal of Radiology, 41: 307.

33. Gilmour, J. R. 1938. The gross anatomy of the parathyroid glands. Journal of Pathology and Bacteriology, 46: 133.

34. Gilmour, J. R., and Martin, W. J. 1937. The weight of the parathyroid glands. Journal of Pathology and Bacteriology, 44: 431.

35. Goepfert, H., Smart, C. R., and Rochlin, D. B. 1966. Metastatic parathyroid carcinoma and hormonal chemotherapy: Case report and response to hexestrol. Annals of Surgery, 164: 917.

36. Goldsmith, R. S. 1972. Treatment of hypercalcemia. Medical Clinics of North America, 56: 951.

37. Haff, R. C., and Ballinger, W. F. 1971. Causes of recurrent hypercalcemia after parathyroidectomy for primary hyperparathyroidism. Annals of Surgery, 173: 884.

38. Harrold, C. C., and Wright, J. 1966. Management of surgical hypoparathyroidism. American Journal of Surgery, 112: 482.

39. Hill, C. S., Jr., Ouais, S. G., and Leiser, A. E. 1972. Long-term administration of calcitonin for hypercalcemia secondary to recurrent parathyroid carcinoma. Cancer, 29: 1016.

40. Hoehn, J. G., Beahrs, O. H., and Woolner, L. B. 1969. Unusual surgical lesions of the parathyroid gland. American Journal of Surgery, 118: 770.

41. Holmes, E. C., Morton, D. L., and Ketcham, A. S. 1969. Parathyroid carcinoma: A collective review. Annals of Surgery, 169: 631.

42. Horwitz, C. A., Myers, W. P. L., and Foote, F. W., Jr. 1972. Secondary malignant tumors of the parathyroid glands: Report of two cases with associated hypoparathyroidism. American Journal of Medicine, 52: 797.

43. Jarman, W. T., Myers, R. T., and Marshall, R. B. 1978. Carcinoma of the parathyroid. Archives of Surgery, 113: 123.

44. Kahil, M., Orman, B., Gyorkey, F., and Brown, H. 1967. Hypercalcemia: Experience with phosphate and sulfate therapy. JAMA, 201: 721.

45. Kay, S., and Hume, D. M. 1973. Carcinoma of the parathyroid gland: How reliable are the clinical and histologic features? Archives of Pathology and Laboratory Medicine, 96: 316.

46. Kiernan, P. D., and Beahrs, O. H. 1979. Perspectives on the surgical treatment of cancer. International Advances in Surgery and Oncology, 2: 99.

47. King, E. S. J., and Wood, B. 1950. Parathyroid tumour with visceral metastases. Journal of Pathology and Bacteriology, 62: 29.

48. Krane, S. M., and Potts, J. T., Jr. 1977. Skeletal remodeling and factors influencing bone and bone mineral metabolism. In Thorn, G. W., Adams, R. D., Braunwald, E., Isselbacher, K. J., and Petersdorf, R. G., Eds.: Harrison's Principles of Internal Medicine. 8th edn. McGraw-Hill, New York, 2005.

49. Krementz, E. T., Yeager, R., Hawley, W., and Weichert, R. 1971. The first 100 cases of parathyroid tumor from Charity Hospital of Louisiana. Annals of Surgery, 173: 872.

50. Lee, Y. T., and Hutcheson, J. K. 1974. Mediastinal parathyroid carcinoma detected on routine chest films. Chest, 65: 354.

51. McGarity, W. C., and Boehm, G. 1975. Carcinoma of the parathyroid. Southern Medical Journal, 68: 166.

52. Macleod, W. A. J., and Holloway, C. K. 1967. Hyperparathyroid crisis: A collective review. Annals of Surgery, 166: 1012.

53. Mallette, L. E., Bilezikian, J. P., Ketcham, A. S., and Aurbach, G. D. 1974. Parathyroid carcinoma in familial hyperparathyroidism. American Journal of Medicine, 57: 642.

54. Mandl, F. 1925. Therapeutischer Versuch bei Ostitis fibrosa generalisata mittels Exstirpation eines Epithelkörperchentumors. Wiener Klinische Wochenschrift, 38: 1343.

55. Meyer, K. A., Rosi, P. A., and Ragins, A. B.

1939. Carcinoma of the parathyroid gland. Surgery, 6: 190.

56. Myers, R. T. 1974. Followup study of surgically-treated primary hyperparathyroidism. Annals of Surgery, 179: 729.

57. Nathaniels, E. K., Nathaniels, A. M., and Wang, C.-A. 1970. Mediastinal parathyroid tumors: A clinical and pathological study of 84 cases. Annals of Surgery, 171: 165.

58. Pak, C. Y. C., Wills, M. R., Smith, G. W., and Bartter, F. C. 1968. Treatment with thyrocalcitonin of the hypercalcemia of parathyroid carcinoma (letter to the editor). Journal of Clinical Endocrinology and Metabolism, 28: 1657.

59. Pak, C. Y. C., Wortsman, J., Bennett, J. E., Delea, C. S., and Bartter, F. C. 1968. Control of hypercalcemia with cellulose phosphate (letter to the editor). Journal of Clinical Endocrinology and Metabolism, 28: 1829.

60. Palmieri, G. M. A., Nordquist, R. E., and Omenn, G. S. 1974. Immunochemical localization of parathyroid hormone in cancer tissue from patients with ectopic hyperparathyroidism. Journal of Clinical Investigation, 53: 1726.

61. Pollack, S., Goldin, R. R., and Cohen, M. 1961. Parathyroid carcinoma: A report of two cases and a review of the literature. Archives of Internal Medicine, 108: 583.

62. Purnell, D. C., Scholz, D. A., Smith, L. H., Sizemore, G. W., Black, B. M., Goldsmith, R. S., and Arnaud, C. D. 1974. Treatment of primary hyperparathyroidism. American Journal of Medicine, 56: 800.

63. Pyrah, L. N., Hodgkinson, A., and Anderson, C. K. 1966. Primary hyperparathyroidism. British Journal of Surgery, 53: 245.

64. Riggs, B. L., Arnaud, C. D., Reynolds, J. C., and Smith, L. H. 1971. Immunologic differentiation of primary hyperparathyroidism from hyperparathyroidism due to nonparathyroid cancer. Journal of Clinical Investigation, 50: 2079.

65. Sandström, I. 1880. Om en ny körtel hos menniskan och ttskilliga däggdjur. Ups Läkaref. Förh., 15: 441.

66. Satava, R. M., Jr., Beahrs, O. H., and Scholz, D. A. 1975. Success rate of cervical exploration for hyperparathyroidism. Archives of Surgery, 110: 625.

67. Schantz, A., and Castleman, B. 1973. Parathyroid carcinoma: A study of 70 cases. Cancer, 31: 600.

68. Schlagenhaufer. 1915. Zwei Fälle von Parathyreoideatumoren. Wiener Klinische Wochenschrift, 28: 1362.

69. Scholz, D. A., Purnell, D. C., Woolner, L. B., and Clagett, O. T. 1973. Mediastinal hyperfunctioning parathyroid tumors: Review of 14 cases. Annals of Surgery, 178: 173.

70. Scholz, D. A., Purnell, D. C., Goldsmith, R. S., Smith, L. H., Riggs, B. L., and Arnaud, C. D. 1972. Diagnostic considerations in hypercalcemic syndromes. Medical Clinics of North America, 56: 941.

71. Scott, R. D. M., Falconer, C. W. A., Fitzpatrick, K., and Proter, G. M. L. 1976. Magnesium depletion and hypocalcaemia after removal of a parathyroid carcinoma. Scottish Medical Journal, 21: 37.

72. Shackney, S., and Hasson, J. 1967. Precipitous fall in serum calcium, hypotension, and acute renal failure after intravenous phosphate therapy for hypercalcemia: Report of two cases. Annals of Internal Medicine, 66: 906.

73. Silverman, R., and Yalow, R. S. 1973. Heterogeneity of parathyroid hormone: Clinical and physiologic implications. Journal of Clinical Investigation, 52: 1958.

74. Singer, F. R., Neer, R. M., Murray, T. M., Keutmann, H. T., Deftos, L. J., and Potts, J. T., Jr. 1970. Mithramycin treatment of intractable hypercalcemia due to parathyroid carcinoma. New England Journal of Medicine, 283: 634.

75. Sjöberg, H. E., and Hjern, B. 1975. Acute treatment with calcitonin in primary hyperparathyroidism and severe hypercalcaemia of other origin. Acta Chirurgica Scandinavica, 141: 90.

76. Smith, L. C., Bradshaw, H. H., and Holleman, I. L., Jr. 1963. Hyperparathyroid crisis: A surgical emergency. American Surgeon, 29: 761.

77. State, D. 1964. The enlarged inferior thyroid artery, a valuable guide in surgery of parathyroid adenomas. Surgery, 56: 461.

78. Straus, F. H., II, and Paloyan, E. 1969. The pathology of hyperparathyroidism. Surgical Clinics of North America, 49: 27.

79. Swelstad, J. A., Scanlon, E. F., Oviedo, M. A., and Hugo, N. E. 1978. Irradiation-induced polyglandular neoplasia of the head and neck. American Journal of Surgery, 135: 820.

80. Taylor, S. 1976. Hyperparathyroidism: Retrospect and prospect. Annals of the Royal College of Surgeons of England, 58: 255.

81. Vail, A. D., and Coller, F. C. 1966. The number and location of parathyroid glands recovered from 202 routine autopsies. Missouri Medicine, 63: 347.

82. van Heerden, J. A., Beahrs, O. H., and Woolner, L. B. 1977. The pathology and surgical management of primary hyperparathyroidism. Surgical Clinics of North America, 57: 557.

83. van Heerden, J. A., Weiland, L. H., ReMine, W. H., Walls, J. T., and Purnell, D. C. 1979. Cancer of the parathyroid glands. Archives of Surgery, 114: 475.

84. von Recklinghausen, F 1891. Die fibröse oder deformirende Ostitis, die Osteomalacie und die osteoplastische Carcinose, in ihren gegenseitigen Beziehungen. Festschr. Rudolf Virchow, (Berlin), pp. 1-89.

85. Wang, C.-A. 1977. Parathyroid re-exploration: A clinical and pathological study of 112 cases. Annals of Surgery, 186: 140.

86. Woolner, L. B., Keating, F. R., Jr., and Black, B. M. 1952. Tumors and hyperplasia of the parathyroid glands: A review of the pathological findings in 140 cases of primary hyperparathyroidism. Cancer, 5: 1069.

87. Yendt, E. R., and Gagne, R. J. A. 1968. Detection of primary hyperparathyroidism, with special reference to its occurrence in hypercalciuric females with "normal" or borderline serum calcium. Canadian Medical Association Journal, 98: 331.

25 | Unusual Tumors

Donald F.N. Harrison, M.D.

To the oncologist dealing with breast or bronchial carcinomas, all head and neck tumors are uncommon! The rarity with which specific neoplasms occur is, however, related not only to individual experience but also to ethnic and geographic factors—which play such an important but often neglected role in disease incidence. Over the past 15 years, my work at the Royal National Throat, Nose and Ear Hospital, in London, has offered a unique opportunity of seeing and treating patients from many parts of the world as well as from our own indigenous and racially mixed population. However, such unusual experience does not allow me to quantify the actual numbers of patients seen in any precise or meaningful manner. It is not possible to quote accurate incidence rates for such varied populations and in selecting conditions considered unusual enough for inclusion in this chapter I have been guided both by previous published reports and the frequency with which I have personally encountered these conditions.

Table 25-1 gives a list of selected tumors seen by me between 1962 and 1977 and provides one way of comparing the relative rarity of each condition. This is certainly more reliable than quoting spurious, unqualified incidence rates although it must be appreciated that these patients have come from a total population far exceeding those resident within the British Isles.

All tumors can destroy normal tissue, whether by pressure or invasion and I have interpreted this part of my chapter in the most general terms. However, not all destructive lesions are tumors and when diagnosis may be in doubt or the lesion behaves in a manner similar to a neoplasm it has seemed reasonable to include it among other more clearly defined neoplasms.

Although epithelial tumors are the most common tumors within the head and neck, they are effectively dealt with elsewhere; and thus I have confined myself to unusual destructive lesions arising from mesenchyme or neuroectoderm. To avoid overcomplicating a complex subject the various conditions have been grouped under general headings, since this permits flexibility without suggesting close correlation.

VASCULAR TUMORS

Although vasoformative tumors arising within the soft tissues of the head and neck are clearly recognized, they represent a source of controversy to the histopathologist. Many occur at or shortly after birth (hamartomas) and can reach considerable size untreated. Hemangiomas are frequently classified according to their histologic characteristics although these may be confusing and unrelated to rate of growth or tendency to invade. True malignancy is found in both angiosarcoma and hemangiopericytoma; however, the multicentric variety of the former (Kaposi sarcoma) is probably seen and diagnosed more frequently than the somewhat obscure and highly lethal local condition.

Juvenile Postnasal Angiofibroma

Despite its probable existence since the time of Hippocrates in the 4th century B.C.[32] and its universal occurrence around the world, it

TABLE 25-1. RELATIVE INCIDENCE OF
SOME COMMON AND UNCOMMON
TUMORS IN AN UNSELECTED GROUP
OF 1,185 PATIENTS SEEN BY THE
PROFESSORIAL UNIT, ROYAL
NATIONAL THROAT, NOSE AND EAR
HOSPITAL, LONDON, 1962–1977

Location and/or Type of Tumor	Number of Patients
Laryngeal cancer	
Glottic	183
Supraglottic	227
Pyriform fossa	82
Postcricoid—cervical esophagus	71
External and middle ear carcinoma	42
Glomus jugulare tumors	15
Nasopharynx—carcinoma and	
lymphoma	49
Chordoma	6
Paranasal sinus	
Carcinoma	162
Osteoma	35
Maxilla	
Osteogenic sarcoma	8
Ameloblastoma	3
Palate—all tumors	48
Tongue—all tumors	52
Tonsils—all tumors	45
Salivary glands	40
Nose	
Malignant melanoma	42
Olfactory neuroblastoma	7
Angiofibroma	20
Malignant granuloma	18
Wegener granulomatosis	30

is surprising that so much confusion and difference of opinion continues regarding this uncommon and unusual tumor. Occurring primarily in adolescent males, this highly vascular and locally destructive tumor has been reported in a baby aged 5 weeks and a man aged 49 years, who incidentally was receiving testosterone therapy. Osborn and Sokolovski[55] and Fitzpatrick[20] have reported the occurrence of this tumor in females. The supposition that spontaneous regression always occurs during early adult life has been long disproved. The natural evolution following diagnosis is one of increasing growth, although the rate may be primarily related to the relative amounts of angiomatous and collagenous tissue present. These amounts are found to be variable in excised tumors, and a preponderance of fibrous stroma may explain the occasional trouble-free removal of a previously unsuspected and undiagnosed lesion. Certainly, some tumors grow more rapidly and aggressively than others, but only the occasional instance of a nonirradiated sarcomatous degeneration in an adult has been reported.[17]

Friedberg in 1940[21] published his recognition of the important vascular element in this tumor and coined the term angiofibroma, although the site of origin was then thought to be the nasopharynx. The concepts of Bensch and Erving in 1971 of an origin from embryologic chondrocartilage between basiocciput and sphenoid was really a search for accessible fibrous tissue in the roof of the nasopharynx.

Other etiologic proposals were related to the concept of a nasopharyngeal origin until less restricted surgical exposure and sophisticated radiologic examination revealed that the site of origin is usually broadly based and situated on the posterolateral wall of the nasal cavity where the sphenoidal process of the palatine bone meets the horizontal ala of the vomer and the root of the pterygoid process. This area includes the superior margin of the sphenopalatine foramen and the posterior end of the middle turbinate, thus explaining the ease with which spread occurs to sphenoid, nasopharynx, pterygomaxillary fissure, and infratemporal fossa. Secondary attachments frequently occur providing the tumor with additional blood supply.

Intracranial spread may occur from infratemporal fossa to middle cranial fossa or from pterygomaxillary fissure via inferior and superior orbital fissure. Rarely, involvement of the anterior cranial fossa may occur by tumor extension through the sinus or extension lateral to the cavernous sinus. The frequency of intracranial extension has been reported as 20 percent by Ward et al.[78] This, however, has not been my own experience in a thorough evaluation of 20 patients: I and most surgeons have experienced a relative absence of severe intracranial complications when removing these tumors. It is now suggested that these tumors are most probably hamartomas or persistent aberrant erectile tissue, which under hormonal influence expand and fill with blood. Since no reliable evidence exists to substantiate a theory that the predominantly male patients suffer from endocrine abnormality or that the rare female cases have defective genetic patterns, it must be assumed that this is primarily a vascular abnormality occurring in a restricted age and sex-linked population.

Angiography invariably shows a dilated internal maxillary artery particularly with angiofibromas extending into the pterygopalatine fossa. This probably reflects the increased blood flow to this lesion, and the vessel is clipped or tied as part of the surgical excision. Histologic examination of ten arteries in our department has shown no abnormality of the vessel wall.

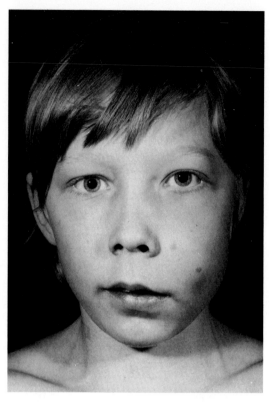

Fig. 25-1. Twelve-year-old boy with left facial swelling and slight proptosis from postnasal angiofibroma.

SYMPTOMS AND DIAGNOSIS

With such clearly defined symptoms in young males as nasal obstruction and epistaxis, it is surprising that over half of my own patients had significant symptoms for over a year before definitive diagnosis. Although histologic diagnosis presents no difficulty, biopsy is not invariably indicated, since in well vascularized tumors bleeding may be severe and uncontrollable. The clinical picture is usually distinctive enough to permit diagnosis. Presumptive diagnosis from the typical angiographic appearance may be preferable to the risk of obtaining a biopsy. Proptosis or facial swelling indicates

extension through the inferior orbital fissure or pterygomaxillary fossa (Fig. 25-1). Extension of the tumor into the palate may produce a submucosal swelling (Fig. 25-2).

Apart from the soft tissue mass seen in the nasopharynx on radiography, Holman and Miller[38] described a classical radiologic feature related to the tumor's origin close to the pterygomaxillary groove. As the tumor grows laterally behind the maxilla, it produces an anterior bowing of the posterior wall of the maxilla (Fig. 25-3). Opacification and expansion of the sphenoid is common but fortunately no case has yet been reported of attachment of angiofibroma to pituitary or cavernous sinus. Enlargement of the superior orbital fissure in patients with proptosis is characteristic, and many surgeons feel that coronal and axial tomography can provide all necessary information regarding tumor extension.

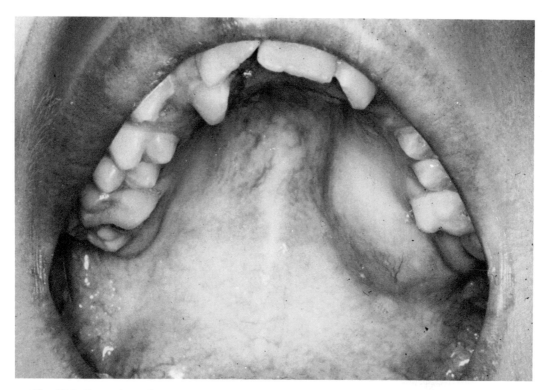

Fig. 25-2. Extension of postnasal angiofibroma into palate producing a large soft submucosal swelling.

More recently, both radiologists and surgeons have advocated angiography for all patients with suspected or proven angiofibroma in order to delineate feeding vessels for possible embolization, and also to detect unsuspected intracranial extension. Subtraction studies give excellent visualization of these tumors (Fig. 25-4) but this investigation is not without hazard, and computerized axial tomography (CT) may well prove to be both safer and more efficient in providing this information (Fig. 25-5).

TREATMENT

Although theoretically attractive there is no reliable evidence to suggest that cryosurgery is of real value in the treatment of the primary lesion; cryosurgery may be useful, however, to treat small accessible recurrences. High blood flow and relative inaccessibility makes the effective application of

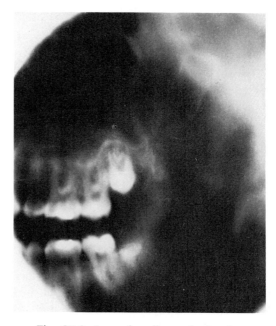

Fig. 25-3. Lateral radiograph showing anterior bowing of posterior wall maxillary antrum secondary to angiofibroma in the pterygomaxillary fossa.

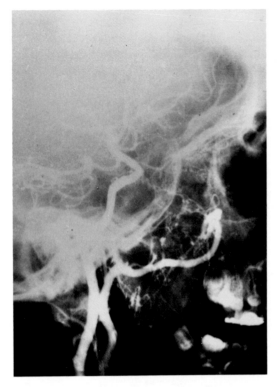

Fig. 25-4. Subtraction studies after carotid angiography showing large internal maxillary artery feeding a postnasal angiofibroma.

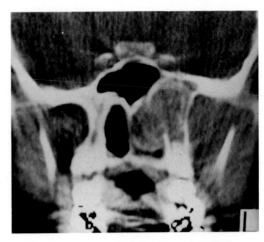

Fig. 25-5. CT scan showing destruction of left pterygoid plates from a large postnasal angiofibroma.

the cryoprobe virtually impossible. Arguments in favor of preoperative estrogen therapy—testosterone now being thought to increase the size of the lesion rather than hasten involution—are based on varied and imaginative speculation. Schiff[66] in 1959 advocated the use of both estrogen and androgen therapy basing his opinion on random biopsies from four patients. His evidence was flimsy, and in fact, systemic estrogen is a vasodilator and a large dose will produce unwelcome side effects in the male. Systemic usage of estrogen is employed by a few clinicians, usually as Stilbestrol 5 mg a day for a month. This dosage is almost homeopathic, and there is as yet no published evidence to support the administration of this drug in larger, more therapeutic dosages.

There has been general agreement for over a century that every effort should be made to remove this tumor surgically. Although it seems likely that small remnants of tumor undergo natural resolution, this is by no means certain and a thorough removal should be attempted when possible. Unfortunately, regrowth of residual tumor, high blood loss, and even an occasional death have followed inadequate or ill-prepared surgery. Briant et al.[9] have reported a follow-up of 45 patients with juvenile angiofibroma who had been treated with 3,000 to 3,500 rads of supervoltage radiotherapy; ten of the patients had previously had surgery. Long-term control, ranging from 2 to 20 years was obtained in 80 percent of the patients in this series. Seven of the nine failures had further radiotherapy with eventual control. Briant and co-workers stressed the need for adequate pretreatment evaluation of tumor extent to prevent "geographic misses" and the need for long term observation, since complete resolution may take many months. They have seen no patient with a radiation-induced tumor, but there remains a general consensus among others that irradiating young patients with nonmalignant tumors using high dosage radiotherapy is undesirable.

Many surgeons reserve radiation treatment for surgically inaccessible tumors or for cases in which adequate surgery would lead to severe disability. Gill et al.[27] described the surgical management of two patients with intracranial extension of angiofibroma and stressed the value of a multidisciplinary approach. Combined craniofacial approach allows control of intracranial feeding vessels with mobilization of tumor adherent to middle fossa dura. However, they reported no details of follow-up and the efficacy of radiotherapy in such cases cannot be denied.

Surgical Approach. Assuming that the tumor is surgically accessible, then the most serious hazard to the patient and to the effective removal is blood loss. Attempts at reducing blood flow to the tumor by hypotensive anesthesia, ligation of the internal maxillary artery, or selective embolization are all advocated, but these techniques are difficult to evaluate because blood loss is variable and may be deceptive unless related to estimated blood volume. Provided that adequate access is obtained before the surface of the tumor is traumatized, blood loss should be restricted to the short period during which the tumor is actually removed. The limited view provided by the transpalatal approach may result in increased hemorrhage and residual tumor in inaccessible sites such as the sphenoid or the pterygomaxillary groove. Lateral rhinotomy[34] has the advantage of allowing excellent assessment prior to traumatizing the tumor and, if necessary, tumor involving the maxillary antrum or orbital floor can be removed via this approach. Most extensive tumors will require a Weber-Fergusson incision with preservation of the teeth-bearing alveolus, which allows tumor extension into the pterygomaxillary fossa to be removed. Long-term follow-up has shown that there is no cosmetic deformity nor interference with the eruption of secondary dentition.

END RESULTS

Despite an assumption that juvenile angiofibromas undergo spontaneous involution after puberty as a result of an increase in the amount of tumor collagen, reliable evidence suggests that in most patients tumor growth persists and regression, if it occurs, may take many years. As with many other tumors, the larger they are the more difficult is effective therapy. When possible, these tumors should be removed surgically after thorough radiologic evaluation. Even so, small amounts may well be left, since they are not encapsulated and may be attached to muscle, bone, or even dura. Some appear to be unusually active and may regrow rapidly requiring further surgery or radiotherapy. However, 2 years free from tumor usually signifies cure.

Analysis of 20 patients with previously untreated angiofibromas treated by surgical excision gives a recurrence rate of 15 percent (3 patients) within a minimum follow-up period of 2 years. One of these 3 patients had a lesion involving the superior constrictor muscle; this lesion was impossible to resect with any certainty. In one other patient I failed to appreciate the true extent of the involvement of the pterygopalatine fossa and attempted clearance via lateral rhinotomy rather than by a more extensive exposure. Further surgical removal in each of the 3 patients resulted in long-term cure.

Hamartomas and Hemangiomas

The term hamartoma has been used for over 70 years for these tumorlike malformations resulting from inborn errors of tissue development. Since they can be derived from any germinal layer, they may be found throughout the body. It has been suggested that the term should be applied only to lesions for which there is definite evidence of developmental anomaly, either actual malformation present at birth or an inborn tissue anomaly that manifests itself by excessive growth until the age of puberty, rather like the juvenile angiofibroma.

The nomenclature depends on the tissue type that predominates; thus in vascular predominance it is angiomatous. It is now generally considered that hemangiomas are in fact hamartomas rather than true neoplasms and as such probably comprise the most common single tumor in the head and neck in infancy.

In the adult they are uncommon but may be exceedingly troublesome. Most vascular lesions are clinically obvious by being pulsatile, by having a bruit, or at the very least by being visibly discolored. Occasionally their firm consistency may mimic a solid neoplasm but rate of growth is usually slow. Clinical appearance and size will vary, and lesions may be superficial or deeply placed. Histologically, most are composed of dilated vascular spaces lined with endothelium, and may contain phleboliths. Cavernous hemangiomas may undergo spontaneous thrombosis and involution. Spontaneous hemorrhage is surprisingly uncommon. Although lesions that are present at or soon after birth may involute, those presenting in adulthood tend to increase in size.

TREATMENT

Unless causing physical or psychological symptoms, small lesions can be left undisturbed. Obvious increase in size, bleeding, or obstructive symptoms will indicate the need for local excision as reported by Weimert and Gilmore[80] and many others (Fig. 25-6). This should present little difficulty although Jarzab[40] recommends cryosurgery for lesions involving the face, lips, tongue, and oral cavity. Regression is slow with cryosurgery, but the cosmetic result is excellent and certainly in multiple superficial lesions this technique may be eminently practicable. The larger and more deeply situated malformations seen in adult life present greater difficulties. Arteriography is mandatory, although it does not necessarily convey an accurate picture of the true extent and vascularity of the lesion. Attempts at radical excision of lesions involving the floor of the mouth or the tongue are rarely feasible and would inevitably lead to loss of tongue bulk. Mucosal involvement can be successfully treated with cryosurgery to minimize dangers of trauma from food or laryngeal obstruction. The considerably increased blood flow requires repeated applications of the nitrogen probe but is certainly worthwhile. When vascular lesions arise within or involve the maxilla, the danger of hemorrhage is greater, particularly after dental extraction.

Although hemangiomas and hamartomas are no longer considered true neoplasms, sudden accelerated growth does occur, possibly secondary to alteration in the hemodynamics of the feeding and draining vessels. However, it is agreed that few cases have been reported in which a diagnosis of hemangiosarcoma has been substantiated. Recognition and diagnosis of maxillary hemangioma may be difficult and must follow an episode of hemorrhage.

Radiologic appearances are variable, particularly in the young, and confusion with osteogenic sarcoma is likely. Discoloration in the alveolar buccal sulcus or palate is significant, but arteriography provides substantive evidence. Surgical resection is the treatment of choice, since neither radiotherapy, injection of sclerosing fluids, corticosteroids, or embolization is likely to produce other than temporary palliation.[75]

CASE REPORT

Mrs. Rose N., aged 72 years, had been seen in a neurosurgical unit in October 1977 with a history of 10 years of right-sided proptosis. Carotid angiography showed an intraorbital vascular lesion, and transcranial exploration of the orbit was performed January 1978. A hemangioma was found and partially removed with some reduction in proptosis, although vision remained poor. When I saw her in September 1978 there was some degree of proptosis, and a huge nonpulsatile swelling of the cheek with a blue mass filled the right alveolar buccal sulcus, nasal passage, and the palatal mucosa on the right side. Tomography, carotid angiography, and CT scan (Figs. 25-7, 25-8) confirmed the vascular nature of the mass and its destruction of the entire orbital floor and ethmoidal labyrinth. The internal maxillary appeared to be the main arterial

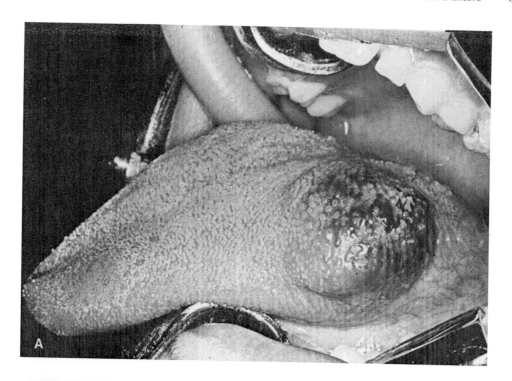

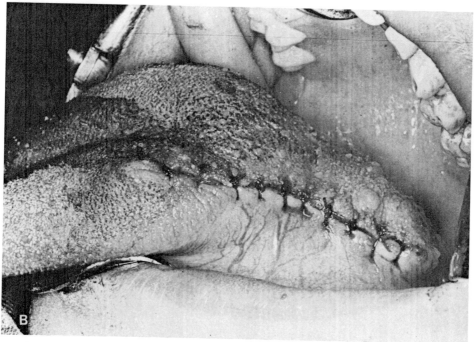

Fig. 25-6. (A and B) Hamartoma on lateral surface of the tongue in an 8-year-old girl.

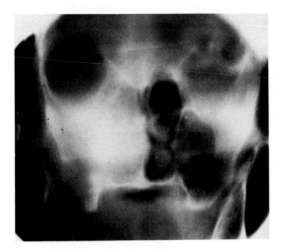

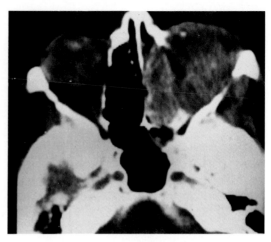

Fig. 25-7. Woman aged 72 years with swelling right face. Vertical tomography showing tumor of right maxilla destroying orbital floor, lateral wall of nose, and inferior part of posterolateral wall of maxillary antrum.

Fig. 25-8. CT scan shows involvement of right orbit and nasal passages as well as extension into infratemporal fossa.

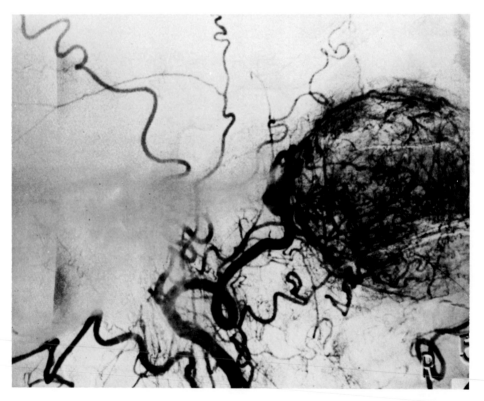

Fig. 25-9. Common carotid angiogram showing extreme vascularity of tumor shown in Figure 25-8.

supply (Fig. 25-9), and utilizing an extended Weber-Fergusson incision and resection of the zygoma and coronoid process of the mandible, this vessel was exposed and ligated. It appeared of normal size in fact! The maxilla and eye was then removed with total blood loss of four units for the entire operation.

Histologically, the tumor was a hemangioma but comparison with the angiograms of October 1977 confirmed that considerable growth had occurred during a period of 9 months, probably from residual orbital hemangioma.

COMMENT

My conclusion from the study of 18 large adult lesions is that when technically possible they should be removed surgically. A small amount of residual tumor may well involute secondary to surgical destruction of its blood supply but an unexpected increase in growth may lead to surgical inaccessibility.

Angiosarcoma and Hemangiopericytomas

Although uncommon, angiosarcomas are rapidly growing neoplasms affecting skin, soft tissues, and underlying bone and arising from the vascular endothelial cell. The scalp is said to be the most common site for angiosarcomas involving the skin, and here they present as a diffuse discolored blush. Erosion of adjacent bone is common as is speckled calcification in the soft tissue swelling, although the latter is more typically seen in hemangiopericytoma. Extension through the dermis, together with a propensity for regional and systemic metastasis, gives 3-year survival figures of no more than 50 percent. The combination of radical surgery and radiotherapy is the treatment of choice, with radiotherapy alone reserved for inoperable or inaccessible lesions.

Hemangiopericytoma is a well-recognized though uncommon tumor, first described by Stout and Murray in 1942.[72] The tumor arises from the pericytes of Zimmermann, which are unique cells found spiralling around the outside of blood capillaries and postcapillary venules. The function of these cells is unknown but they may control the caliber of the vessel. Because the pericyte is found around almost all capillaries and venules, hemangiopericytomas have been found in most parts of the body. Hollman and associates in 1971[37] reported on 276 cases with a 16 percent occurrence in the head and neck region. More recent papers, which attempt to classify these tumors into benign, border line malignancy, and malignancy on the basis of histologic evaluation, give a metastatic rate of 37.5 percent for borderline tumors and 78 percent for frankly malignant lesions.[50]

The most common sites for this tumor are the extremities and the retroperitoneal space, but small numbers of cases have been reported of occurrences in the nasal cavity, maxilla, and larynx. The site of origin can be anywhere, and symptoms include obstruction, epistaxis, or simple discomfort. Diagnosis is from biopsy, and treatment is usually surgical excision because radiotherapy has been considered ineffective. However, Mira, Chu, and Fortner[52] reported on 29 tumors (12 in the head and neck) presenting in 11 patients, who were treated with primary radiotherapy using a variety of techniques. Although their results are difficult to evaluate, a response rate of 96 percent was obtained, suggesting that these tumors were radiosensitive. However, regression was slow and the patients still died from systemic metastasis. Local recurrence of tumor in 24 percent suggested inadequate dosage. In those cases involving the nose, resection via a lateral rhinotomy followed by radiotherapy is probably the most effective form of treatment.

Since the inherent malignancy of individual tumors is difficult to estimate prior to surgical excision, local cryosurgery or systemic chemotherapy should be reserved for inoperable lesions. Congenital hemangiopericytomas behave quite differently from those found in older children or adults. Infantile tumors occur more superficially in the subcutaneous tissues and are often multilobulated. With the exception of isolated reports of tumors localized in the brain, most behave in a benign manner without metastasis or recurrence after local excision.

Chemodectomas

This term was first used around 1950 for a group of tumors histologically similar to each other and arising from the chemoreceptive tissue in the head and neck. They are found in the carotid body (at the bifurcation of the carotid artery), in the ganglion nodosum of the vagus, in the aortic arch, and within the glomus jugulare. However, chemoreceptor tissue is widely dispersed throughout the body, and rarely tumors may be found in the orbit, nose, and larynx.[45]

Chemodectomas resemble the paragangliomas of the sympathetic nervous system, but the chromatin reaction is negative and they are occasionally called "nonchromatin paragangliomas." Carotid body tumors are more common in people living at high altitudes, presumably because chemoreceptive tissues react to changes in blood pH and oxygen tension. Chemodectomas may, in addition, secrete norepinephrine or epinephrine, producing symptoms not dissimilar to a pheochromocytoma of the adrenal medulla. Such catecholamines are rapidly inactivated, and their urinary metabolites vanillylmandelic acid (VMA), methoxyhydroxyphenylethylene glycol (MHPG), and metanephrines can be measured. Preoperative consideration of problems arising from release of these substances forms an important part of the surgical management of these tumors.

Carotid Body Tumors

The carotid body is the largest of the paraganglia and tumors arising in this site are the most common of the extremely uncommon chemodectoma tumors. Measuring approximately $5 \times 3 \times 2$ mm, the carotid body is situated within the adventitia of the common carotid artery but extends to the bifurcation. Actual size of these tumors is difficult to estimate since growth tends to take place preferentially in two directions —superiorly towards the skull base and medially towards the pharynx where in large tumors an intraoral swelling may be present. The most common presenting symptom is of a slow-growing painless cervical mass of several years' duration, located in the region of the carotid bifurcation. There may be a history of a sudden unexplained increase in the size of the mass. Although firm, the swelling may be compressible, pulsate, be accompanied by a bruit, and feel warm. Movement of the mass is free from side to side but not inferiorly and superiorly. Occasionally, pain is complained of and extension to the skull base may produce cranial nerve palsies.

Diagnosis is reached by means of carotid angiography, which demonstrates a circumscribed vascular blush at the carotid bifurcation with separation of the internal and external carotid arteries (Fig. 25-10). The extent of the tumor and feeding vessels and also the condition of the contralateral carotid system can be estimated at this time—information essential if surgery is contemplated. Instances of familial occurrence of carotid body tumors are reported as are multiple chemodectomas in single individuals, e.g., bilateral carotid body with bilateral glomus jugulare tumors.

Management.   Characteristically, these tumors grow slowly with minimal symptoms. The average duration of symptoms before definitive diagnosis is about 4 years. Histology retains a constant benign appearance, and malignancy is only diagnosed in the presence of cervical or systemic metastasis. The occurrence of metastasis is uncommon, occurring in between only 2 and 9 percent of all carotid body tumors.

Embolization of carotid body tumors is hazardous because of the risk of emboli entering the brain through the internal carotid artery. Effective usage of this therapy has not been reported in any large series of patients. There is little evidence to suggest that radiotherapy is of value in treating ca-

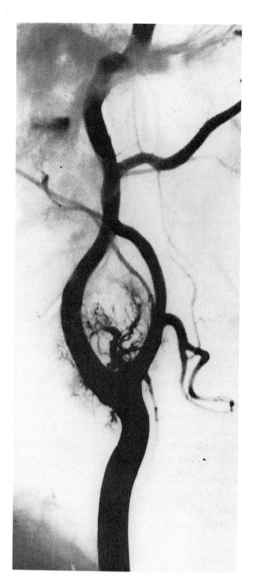

Fig. 25-10. Common carotid angiogram illustrating separation of internal and external carotid vessels by a carotid body tumor.

rotid body tumors, and the alternative thus lies between no treatment and surgical excision. The high morbidity and mortality rates associated with attempts at removal and related to ligation of the common or internal carotid arteries can be minimized by planned hypothermia and the services of a vascular surgeon skilled in the art of vessel grafting. Subadventitial dissection is essential, since the tumor arises from this layer rather than from the media. However, this may be difficult and in large tumors planned carotid bypass with arterial grafting is preferable to the dangers of unexpected carotid ligation. Even so, an operative mortality rate of five percent may occur, with a higher figure for nonfatal hemiplegia.

Conley[13] has succinctly summarized his indications for surgical resection: (a) histologically malignant but resectable, (b) aggressive growth patterns, (c) small tumors occurring in a patient under 50 years of age, and (d) interference with swallowing or breathing. Unfortunately, such an analysis is not always possible, and thus patients are best treated in centers possessing facilities for vascular replacement.

GLOMUS JUGULARE

Some 4 years after Guild[31] described chemoreceptor tissue in relationship to the jugular bulb, the first case of a highly vascular tumor arising from this area was recognized by Rosenwasser.[63] Similar tissue, and tumors, are found along the course of the tympanic nerve (glomus tympanicum), in the middle ear, and in the auricular branch of the vagus. Although rarely malignant, these tumors have a variable rate of growth and a long natural history. If untreated, most patients eventually develop neurologic or other serious deficits. In general, behavior of the tumor is related to local invasion from the site of origin although there is no reliable evidence to show that this is related to specific histologic features. Glomus tumors grow along pathways of least resistance, extending intracranially, destroying the middle or inner ear, and producing damage to the facial nerve or within the jugular foramen. Analysis of clinical and radiologic findings provides an indication of tumor extent and assists in determining management and, possibly, prognosis.

Bickerstaff and Howell[6] attempted to correlate symptomatology with prognosis by relating aural symptoms to neurologic signs.

Their classification, although practicable, implies that there is a measurable differential rate of growth. Attempts to apply their criteria to clinical experience have proven unhelpful. Spector, Ciralsky, and Ogura[71] have provided a more realistic analysis of the importance of clinical findings. They found as follows:

1. Otologic findings, excluding labyrinthine invasion, have no prognostic significance nor do they denote the feasibility of tumor resectability.

2. No single sign or symptom indicates tumor extent.

3. Facial nerve paralysis has no prognostic significance.

4. Cranial nerve involvement assists in localizing tumor extent but not suitability for resection.

5. Invasion of the labyrinth is associated with a 75 percent incidence of intracranial extension.

Diagnosis and Management. Chemodectomas are the most commonly found neoplasm in the middle ear, and almost every patient presents with some aural symptoms. Tumors growing from paraganglionic tissue related to the tympanic branch of the glossopharyngeal nerve and glomus tympanicum are confined to the middle ear and can be effectively removed by surgery. The large and more serious lesions grow from glomus tissue in the adventitia of the jugular bulb and about half of these cases present with cranial nerve involvement. Aural symptoms depend upon tumor bulk producing conductive hearing loss, bulging and discoloration of the tympanic membrane, or an aural polyp. Extension from the middle ear space produces pain, sensorineural deafness, and vertigo—symptoms found in about 25 percent of glomus jugulare lesions. Pulsatile tinnitus or other subjective sensations are present in over 60 percent of these patients. Expansion of the jugular foramen may be associated with a variety of cranial nerve defects, such as 10th and 11th nerve paresis; the paresis may occur after approximately 8 years in patients with glomus jugulare or vagale tumors if it is not present initially at diagnosis.

Intracranial extension is common with glomus jugulare tumors and may extend to middle or posterior fossa producing headache, pain, papilledema, or even hydrocephalus. Diagnosis is made from the otologic appearance and biopsy, supplemented by tomography and carotid angiography. Retrograde jugularography may show extension into the internal jugular vein, but it is doubtful if any investigation can give a wholly accurate impression of the true extent of this tumor.

Differential diagnosis includes hemotympanum, high jugular bulb, and extension of other tumors arising within the area of the jugular bulb.

The long natural history of these tumors renders it difficult to assess and compare the results of the present forms of therapy—surgical excision, irradiation, and combination of the two. Surgical excision is preferable for small tumors localized to the middle ear (glomus tympanicum), but these represent only a small proportion of cases diagnosed. Because of their location and vascular nature, radical excision of large lesions is difficult, dangerous, and accompanied by a recurrence rate that varies from series to series but is probably never less than 30 percent.[74] Most recurrences occur within 3 years and can be treated with radiotherapy instead of second operations, which are rarely feasible. There have been highly divergent views concerning the efficacy of primary radiotherapy, since most of these tumors are not very radiosensitive. However, following radiotherapy an increase in stromal fibrosis occurs and there appears to be at least inhibition of growth if not marked regression in tumor size. Preoperative radiotherapy may possibly reduce bleeding, thus leading to more effective surgical resection. A tumor dose of 4,000 to 5,000 rads is recommended, and an analysis of 15 of my own patients with large glomus jugulare lesions treated primarily with radiotherapy and followed up for an average of 8 years showed 13 to be alive and well. One other patient had received subsequent surgery and was well 14 years later. Combination of radiotherapy and surgery may prove to be the best treatment for accessible large tumors, while radiotherapy alone may be the best treatment for inoperable cases. However, the absence of long-term controlled trials makes realistic evaluation of most published reports difficult and major surgical resection is not for the inexperienced.

Patients with vagal body tumors present with a painless mass, usually behind the angle of the mandible in the lateral pharyngeal space. Delay in diagnosis may be as long as 4 years, and there may be neurologic deficits involving the 9th, 10th, 11th, and 12th cranial nerves or the cervical sympathetic chain. Ipsilateral vocal cord paresis was the most common defect in my own series of 7 patients, although Specter, Ciralsky, and Ogura[71] found the glossopharyngeal nerve the most frequently involved—but this nerve is not easy to test! Surgical excision of these tumors is effective, but invariably it is accompanied by a need to sacrifice the 10th and 12th cranial nerves. Local recurrence rates of 25 percent are quoted.

GLOMUS OF THE LARYNX

Although extremely uncommon, chemodectomas arising within the larynx present many unusual features among which is a high incidence of malignancy.[2] A paired laryngeal glomus is found in each plica ventricularis just above the anterior end of the vocal cord. A second glomus, glomus laryngicum inferior, is situated cranial to the division of the recurrent laryngeal nerve into anterior and posterior branches. These two areas are the sites of tumor growth. Hoarseness, dysphagia, and sometimes severe pain are the common features of this condition; a biopsy confirms the diagnosis. Catecholamine excretion may be increased, as in the illustrative case history below, and this tumor should be treated by radical surgery to minimize the risk of metastasis.[30]

Case Report

The patient, a white male aged 70 years, was seen in July 1977 with a history of dysphagia and left neck pain for the

past 13 years. He was found to have a vascular-looking swelling occupying the posterior half of the left aryepiglottic fold. Biopsy showed this to be a chemodectoma and at this time urinary catecholamines were raised: VMA level was 50 μmol/24 hour (normal 35 μmol/24 hours) and total metanephrine level was 8.3 μmol/24 hours (normal 5.5 μmol/24 hours). Blood pressure varied between normal and mild hypertension. Four days later, the tumor was resected via a transthyroid lamina approach. The arytenoid was removed with the specimen. The tumor did not reach the ventricle. Frozen-section biopsy showed tumor margins to be free. Postoperatively there was immediate relief of pain and the catecholamine levels returned to normal.

By January 1978, the pain had returned together with a small swelling related to the region of the operation scar. Catecholamine levels were slightly raised, but a positive biopsy from the larynx was not obtained until March

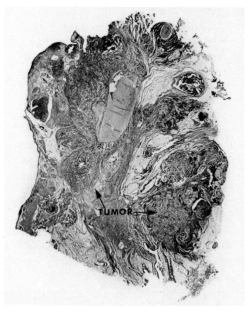

Fig. 25-11. Serial section through laryngectomy specimen showing extension of chemodectoma through previous thyroid window produced during partial laryngectomy operation (magnification × 2).

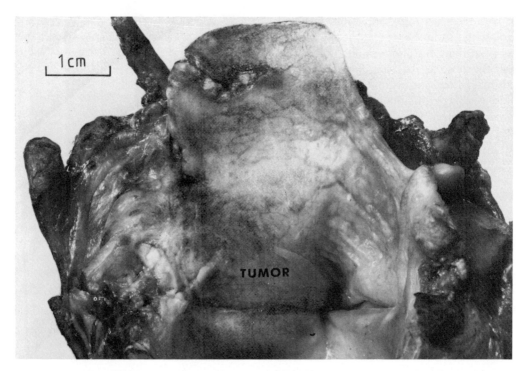

Fig. 25-12. View of laryngectomy specimen showing regrowth of chemodectoma in the region of left supraglottis and now extending to involve left vocal cord.

1978, by which time obvious recurrence was present within the larynx (Fig. 25-11). Total laryngectomy (Fig. 25-12) again relieved the pain, but multiple subcutaneous metastases developed within 1 month. These were painful and presented over the scalp, axilla, trunk, and right shoulder. Removal of these circumscribed deposits produced pain relief, but new deposits appeared within days. Over 20 deposits were removed on one occasion (Fig. 25-13). Radiotherapy to the metastases was ineffective. The patient died under narcosis in June 1978, 1 year after diagnosis. Evidence of raised catecholamine levels was present during this period and may be related to clinical malignancy.

Development of the multiple, painful dermal deposits is typical of malignant laryngeal glomus tumors, and in general this lesion should be treated by horizontal supraglottic laryngectomy if feasible as a primary procedure.

NONHEALING GRANULOMAS OF THE UPPER RESPIRATORY TRACT

For many years, nonspecific locally destructive granulomatous conditions have been recognized clinically as affecting the nose and occasionally other parts of the respiratory tract. Their natural history differs significantly from lesions produced by syphilis or tuberculosis, and until recently most patients died within 18 months. Histopathologists, faced with small, possibly nonrepresentative biopsy specimens, contributed to clinical confusion by elaborating hypotheses that conveniently ignored clinical behavior. Not surprisingly, these world-wide lesions received a bewildering variety of names including malignant nasal granuloma, sacrolupus pernio, lethal granulomatous ulceration of midline facial tissues, granulomatous ulcer of the nose and face, osteomyelitis necroticans, mutilating granuloma, and Wege-

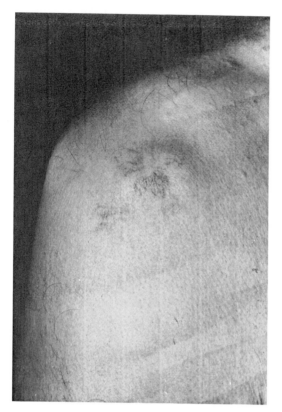

Fig. 25-13. Deposit from laryngeal glomus tumor in skin of right shoulder.

ner granulomatosis. Whatever the terminology, these varied conditions are rare. Clinical and pathologic clarification depended upon accumulation of sufficient personal experience emphasizing that there are certainly two (possibly three) completely different conditions. Appropriately treated, these conditions can be controlled or possibly cured; I[33] have emphasized the need to attain a clinical diagnosis rather than to await a histopathologic confirmation.

Wegener Granulomatosis

The most clearly defined and recognized syndrome is the necrotizing granuloma described by Wegener in 1939.[79] Although occasionally affecting the nose, the *lethal* lesions occurred in the lungs and kidneys. Goodman and Churg in 1954[29] described the pathologic features and diagnostic criteria of this condition in seven patients. Without demonstrable lesions in kidneys or lungs, it is debatable whether this diagnosis should be made. The criteria are as follow:

1. Necrotizing granulomatous lesions in the respiratory tract (nose, paranasal sinuses, larynx, trachea, or lungs).

2. Generalized focal necrotizing vasculitis involving arteries and veins almost always in lungs and usually widely disseminated in other sites.

3. Glomerulitis characterized by necrosis and thrombosis of loops of the capillary tuft, capsular adhesion, and evolution as a granulomatous lesion.

The etiology is obscure. Infection has been suggested, though no single organism has been isolated. The resemblance of the pathologic lesions to systemic lupus erythematosis has been noted, and autoimmunity secondary to hypersensitivity to an unknown agent is a favored theory. Cell-mediated immune studies have shown dissociation between an intact macrophage migration inhibition function, impaired skin delayed hypersensitivity, and lymphocyte transformation to a number of antigens. It has been suggested therefore that Wegener granulomatosis may be associated with a partial cell-mediated immunodeficiency.

Wegener originally thought that this syndrome was a variant of polyarteritis nodosa, and upper respiratory tract lesions are certainly found in this condition. The prime cause for confusion resulted from failure to appreciate that lesions may occur in the nose, or indeed elsewhere, without immediate severe pulmonary or renal disease. Failure to adequately examine the lungs and kidneys delays diagnosis and effective therapy, for death in this disease is invariably from renal failure.

Clinical features are well recognized, the onset being insidious with nonspecific symptoms of infection in some part of the respiratory tract. The disease occurs typically in a previously healthy young to middle-age adult of either sex. However, the constitutional upset is quite out of proportion to the severity of the local lesion, and the patient usually seeks attention because of severe malaise, fever, or progressive weakness. If untreated, death from renal failure occurs within 6 months.

Biopsy from granulomatous lesions within the nose, middle ear (Fig. 25-14), or elsewhere show giant-cell granulomas, but there is never the degree of local destruction seen with the more confusing "malignant" granulomas. The former progress slowly, never becoming neoplastic, and after effective systemic therapy there is only minimal tissue loss. Chest radiographs show areas of infarction that have undergone necrosis and liquefaction with cavity formation (Fig. 25-15). Some patients may present with hemoptysis. Although nasal biopsy may suggest a

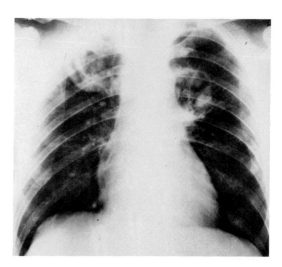

Fig. 25-15. Chest radiograph of patient with Wegener granulomatosis showing cavitation in both upper lobes.

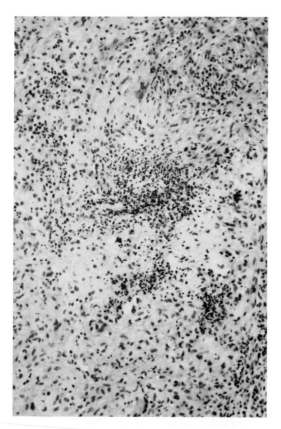

Fig. 25-14. Section of Wegener granulomatosis affecting nose (magnification × 160). Three vessels show necrosis and acute inflammation of their walls. There are granulomatous changes with giant cells and some necrosis.

diagnosis of Wegener granulomatosis, the complete syndrome requires evidence of renal involvement. Red cells or casts will be present in the urine; renal biopsy may be justified in some cases, since early diagnosis is essential to institute early treatment in an effort to minimize permanent renal damage.

TREATMENT

In my experience, delay in diagnosis and the relative ineffectiveness of local radiotherapy or systemic steroids resulted in a mortality rate of over 85 percent. However, about 1965 a number of reports appeared suggesting that addition of a variety of cytotoxic drugs to the steroid regime might halt renal destruction. Methotrexate, 5-fluorouracil, cyclophosphamide, chlorambucil, and many other drugs were used and proved to be effective but with unacceptable side effects preventing long-term usage. My own experience with azathioprine has shown this drug to be both effective and virtually free from undesirable complications.[33]

The dramatic change in prognosis for patients with Wegener granulomatosis produced by the addition of cytotoxic drugs to the treatment regime is not due to increased immunosuppression or an antiinflammatory action. Both antimetabolites and alkylating agents appear to be effective, and it seems possible that they have an unspecified direct action of their own. Azathioprine and the steroid prednisolone are powerful drugs with potentially serious side effects. They may act synergistically inducing some side-effects, such as the risk of infection.

Controlled trials have suggested that daily addition of azathioprine in a dosage of 2.5 mg/kg body weight reduced the total maintenance dose of prednisolone needed by about 45 percent with no increase in serious side effects. Immediately after diagnosis, treatment is started with azathioprine as described above, rising to a maximum daily dosage of 200 mg. Prednisolone is then added until the erythrocyte sedimentation rate (ESR) has returned to near normal limits. The ESR is always markedly raised and may be the first indication to the clinician that the patient is seriously ill. Within 48 hours of beginning treatment, most patients experience dramatic subjective improvement in their condition; however, long-term prognosis is almost entirely dependent upon the degree of permanent renal damage. A creatinine clearance level of less than 10 ml/min, a plasma creatinine level greater than 884 μmol/l, and a plasma urea level exceeding 42 mmol/l is certain to indicate severe renal damage. Such patients may be salvaged, but in my own experience I have found that they will eventually die from ascending pyelonephritis. Removal of circulating immune complexes by plasma exchange and immune suppression is certainly possible and may improve both pulmonary and renal function. Clearance of such immune complexes may not only take out supposed pathogenic material but may possibly enable the reticuloendothelial system to recover its own capacity for immune-complex clearance. In my experience, renal dialysis alone has been less satisfactory.

Most drugs are eliminated from the body, wholly or in part, by renal excretion.

If given in standard dosage to patients with reduced renal function, they will accumulate in body fluids and may reach toxic concentrations. Many patients with Wegener granulomatosis have levels of creatinine clearance, plasma creatinine, and urea that reveal moderate to severe renal failure. Care must therefore be taken when prescribing drugs. Tetracycline, cephaloridine, chloramphenicol, nitrofurantoin, and chlorpropamide should be avoided completely.[68]

With this regime of combined azathioprine and prednisolone (occasionally cyclophosphamide may be added for a short period to gain initial control), the nasal lesions disappear and pulmonary infarction areas become necrotic and liquify, and then fibrose. Similar fibrosis occurs in the kidneys, and the final degree of renal impairment can then be assessed. Such patients are now considered candidates for renal transplantation. Since the toxic effects of both azathioprine and prednisolone are closely related, every attempt must be made to reduce the dosage as much as possible. Unfortunately, the most reliable guide to dosage appears to be the ESR, and when elevated this estimation has been taken by me to indicate that dosage is too low. As yet only one patient has been successfully weaned off all therapy, but most are now completely off azathioprine and being maintained on relatively low doses of prednisolone.

Although perivasculitis may present in any region of the body, including the nose, a diagnosis of Wegener granulomatosis can only be made if findings relate to the syndrome described by Wegener in 1939. This requires evidence of renal involvement. The presence of red cells or casts in the urine is sufficient indication for diagnosis, although this can be substantiated by renal biopsy. Early diagnosis should be an indication for immediate therapy with combined azathioprine and prednisolone and with the ESR being used for guidance as to drug dosage. Providing renal damage is moderate, long-term survival should be excellent; in cases of more severely damaged kidneys, transplantation is feasible. Examination of over 30 patients with nasal lesions has shown residual tissue loss following treatment to be restricted to septal perforations except in those patients receiving radiotherapy. The latter treatment has no place in the management of this condition.

Nonhealing Nasal Granuloma (Malignant Granuloma)

It has long been recognized that a granulomatous condition exists that slowly destroys the tissues of the face but whose natural history is completely different from that seen in the nasal lesions of Wegener granulomatosis. Nonhealing granuloma is a slowly progressive destructive ulceration of the tissues of the nose, sinuses, and occasionally pharynx. Soft tissues, bone, and cartilage are all eventually destroyed by what has been described as a "wave of granulation tissue advancing irregularly into healthy parts, breaking down behind as it advances in front." On December 9, 1896, Dr. Peter McBride[49] showed photographs of a "case of rapid destruction of the nose and face" in a young house painter who gave a history of gonorrhea but not syphilis. This demonstration was before the Laryngological Society of London, England, under its President, Felix Semon. The patient suffered gross destruction of the nose and upper lip culminating in his death 18 months later. The pathologists at that time failed to recognize the underlying pathology, but it has since been suggested that this was in fact a case of "malignant granuloma."

The first clear account of the condition was published by Dr. Robert Woods of Dublin in 1921,[82] the term malignant granuloma being proposed by his colleague Dr. O'Sullivan. Unfortunately, succeeding researchers, usually reporting small numbers of patients, have successfully confused the issue by relating this condition to Wegener granulomatosis or by including patients with disseminated malignancy. The local tissue destruction, necrosis, and infection seen with malignant granuloma makes histologic evaluation of biopsy material difficult, but

Michaels and Gregory[51]—who have probably had the most experience with the pathologic features of this condition—described the constant presence of widespread necrosis and atypical cells, collectively termed NACE (necrosis with atypical cellular exudate). The cytologic features of these cells are such as to suggest malignancy, and they believe that this is a histiocytic lymphoma.

Personal experience with a considerable number of these patients has revealed that the natural history is variable in relation to time and that the prodromal stage, consisting of nasal obstruction with discharge, may last several years or as short as a few weeks. Local necrosis then occurs with crusting, bleeding, and a purulent smelly discharge. Tissue destruction extends to in-

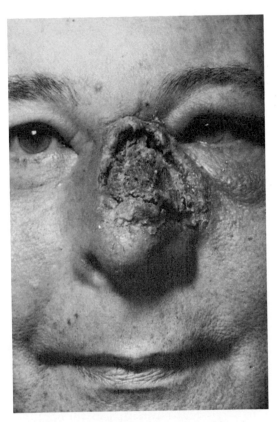

Fig. 25-16. Man aged 54 years with a 1 year history of nasal bleeding and crusting over dorsum of nose. Biopsy suggested nonhealing granuloma and patient was given 5,000 rads radiotherapy.

volve surrounding skin (Figs. 25-16 and 25-17) and may involve the face, palate, and pharynx. Death usually occurs from cachexia, and there is little pain.

There is no doubt that patients with similar natural histories are seen with pathologic evidence of metastatic spread to regional lymph nodes, lungs, or elsewhere. This has been shown to be a malignant lymphoma, and I have seen 3 patients who developed nasal malignant lymphomas 1 to 2 years after a noncurative dose of radiotherapy was administered for a "nonhealing nasal granuloma." The clinician, ignoring the patient's clinical history while waiting for histopathologic classification, may delay

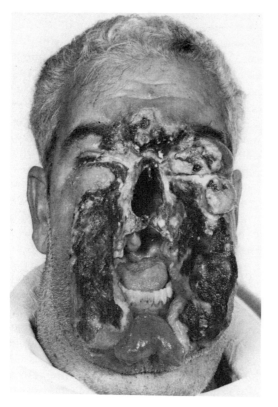

Fig. 25-17. For 4 years this man had received treatment for an undiagnosed increasing destruction of facial tissues. At various times this had been called "carcinoma-syphilis-rodent ulcer and tuberculosis." The features are typical of a midline destructive process that has been uncontrolled.

too long or even worse embark on an inadequate program of therapy.[22] To the experienced clinician, there is no resemblance between malignant granuloma and the nasal or systemic lesions of Wegener. Nasal biopsy will eliminate other possible granulomatous conditions thus allowing a diagnosis to be made and therapy to commence. Steroid therapy is of no value; and except for the use of antibiotics, treatment is confined to the use of radiotherapy. Dosage relates to individual preference: if the physician believes the condition to be definitely malignant, then a curative regime must be employed.

My own opinion based on 18 patients is that the lesion is a malignant lymphoma under unusually effective immunologic control. Many patients will be cured with 1,000 rads of cobalt 60, though eventually local regrowth in 4 of my 18 patients demonstrated a malignant lymphoma. However, the argument that these patients should receive primary curative dosage to avoid the risk of regional or systemic metastasis is not illogical and there may yet be a place for systemic chemotherapy. This has not been employed by me on the grounds of possible immunologic suppression.

Local excision is limited to the removal of necrotic tissue, because attempts at wide removal of actively growing granulation tissue simply result in a larger defect with regrowth of the original tissue. Radiotherapeutic control is followed by a rapid fall in the elevated ESR, but no attempt should be made to repair the resulting defect for at least 2 years. Prosthetic devices should be used for cosmetic purposes (Fig. 25-18).

Evolution of effective means of curing or prolonging the life of patients with malignant granuloma or Wegener granulomatosis has clearly demonstrated that these are two quite separate conditions. However, an occasional patient presents with features common to both conditions, although never in my experience has a malignant granuloma patient presented with the renal lesions necessary for a diagnosis of Wegener granulomatosis. Whether patients with fea-

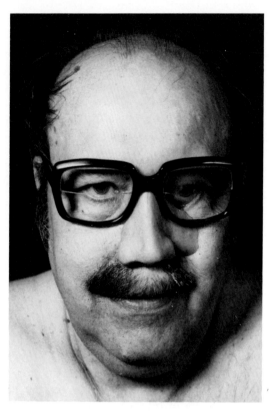

Fig. 25-18. Custom-made prosthesis to cover defect produced by a radiotherapeutically controlled midline granuloma from which dead tissue had been surgically removed.

tures of both conditions suffer from a new, unrecognized disease or some bizarre variation of the conditions I have described is debatable. There are, however, no reasons for continuing a policy of confusion that has resulted in patients with clearly defined malignant granuloma or Wegener granulomatosis receiving inadequate therapy. Despite the rarity of these two conditions, much interest and confusion has been generated in an attempt to classify what are, in effect, different clinical entities. Representative biopsy material may be almost impossible to obtain because of necrosis and secondary infection. Although biopsies are obviously essential to eliminate other diagnoses, most histopathologists are inexperienced in the examination of even classical cases; in the past, however, this inexperience has been of

little importance because most patients died. My personal experience, and that of our specialist pathologists, has provided an opportunity to evaluate both clinical behavior and histopathologic changes in a relatively large group of patients. The suggestions outlined in this section are based therefore on personal experience rather than on evaluation of the somewhat confusing literature on this subject.

NEUROGENIC TUMORS OF THE HEAD AND NECK

The most common of the neurogenic tumors arise from proliferation of the neurolemmal or Schwann cells of myelinated nerves. Two types of tumor are recognized pathologically: schwannoma and neurofibroma, both of which develop from the same parent cell. Malignant schwannomas occasionally occur and probably arise from perineural fibroblasts; they are more properly termed neurogenous sarcomas.

The neurilemmoma (or schwannoma) was first described in 1910, when it was called a neurinoma. Its true cell of origin was not recognized until 1935, when it was correctly called a neurilemmoma. A slow-growing, well-encapsulated tumor, it is found in all parts of the head and neck. Unremoved, it can become exceedingly large and may undergo hemorrhage and cystic degeneration. Histologically, the tumor cells are elongated and spindle-shaped, in places producing palisading of nuclei—this is the Antoni A type appearance. Antoni B type tumors show a considerable degree of cell, pleomorphism, with irregular cell types scattered in loose connective tissue, but do not show definable palisading. However, both features—cell pleomorphism and palisading—may be found in individual tumors and probably bear no relation to frequency of local recurrence or malignant change.

Neurofibromas are nonencapsulated and often multiple, as in von Recklinghausen disease for which the risk of malignant change is said to vary between 10 and 30 percent. Ghosh et al.[26] reported 5-year survival rates of 65.7 percent for patients with malignant schwannomas, with rates falling to 30 percent when the condition was associated with multiple neurofibromas.

Analysis of large numbers of patients with neurilemmomas shows that at least 65 percent of lesions occur in the central nervous system and that of the remainder occurring in the peripheral nerves at least one-third are found in the head and neck. Here they present as problems in differential diagnosis and in certain sites, mechanically interfere with function. True incidence and site distribution are difficult to assess because only the unusual or bizarre tumor is reported and many small, insignificant lesions remain untreated or unrecorded.

Laryngeal Tumors

All neurogenic laryngeal tumors are uncommon. In 1969, Cummings, Montgomery, and Balogh[16] reviewed the literature bringing the total number of reported cases to 89. Between 1968 and 1977, 150 benign laryngeal tumors were seen in my own hospital—of these only 2 were neurofibromas. However, the size of the tumors and the origin from the internal branch of the superior laryngeal nerve produces severe supraglottic obstruction. Sudden hemorrhage or cystic degeneration may lead to acute airway problems.

Pain is rarely a significant symptom, and patients complain of progressive dyspnea, hoarseness, dysphagia, or a feeling of fullness or a lump in the throat.

The tumor is seen as a smooth submucosal swelling confined to the false cord or aryepiglottic fold—the true cord being usually spared. Biopsy—and thus, differentiation from other laryngeal tumors or cysts—is often difficult because of the firm consistency of most neurogenic tumors.

There is general agreement that these intralaryngeal lesions should be removed completely. This is rarely possible by endoscopic excision unless the lesion is very small.

The most effective means is by a lateral pharyngotomy approach with removal of part of the thyroid lamina if necessary. Preliminary tracheostomy is indicated and the approach then allows even large tumors to be removed without damage to the laryngeal mucosa or risk of uncontrolled bleeding.[53] Laryngofissure has the disadvantage of inadequate exposure of the upper and posterior aspect of the larynx—the usual site of origin.

CASE REPORT

A 13-year-old boy was discovered to have an obstructive laryngeal swelling, during induction of anesthesia for correction of strabismus. The swelling was located in the left vallecula and occupied most of the left aryepiglottic fold. Biopsy showed this to be a neurofibroma, and it was removed via a lateral pharyngotomy. Seven years later he was seen again with hoarseness and dyspnea secondary to local recurrence of the tumor. Again it was removed via a lateral pharyngotomy, and it has not recurred. However, 14 years after initial diagnosis this patient has now developed clinical evidence of von Recklinghausen disease.

Most of the reported cases of laryngeal neurilemmomas (or neurofibromas, as authors do not always differentiate between these tumors) suggest that the lesions arise from the vallecula, vestibule, or pyriform fossa, that is, above the true cords. The most common nerve of origin is therefore the internal branch of the superior laryngeal nerve after it has passed through the thyrohyoid membrane.

Neurogenous tumors are the most common primary neoplasms developing within the lateral (or parapharyngeal) space and may arise from any of the last four cranial nerves or, indeed, from sympathetic or parasympathetic tissue. The nerve sheath tumors most frequently affect the vagus nerve, but there are no specific clinical features that allow accurate preoperative diagnosis. Presenting symptoms are related to both tumor mass and pressure on surrounding cranial nerves. Involvement of 9th, 10th, and 11th cranial nerves may cause pain, hoarseness, or dysphagia. Dysarthria with atrophy of the ipsilateral half of the tongue occurs when the hypoglossal nerve is involved.

Although surgical excision via a lateral approach confirms the diagnosis and is effective therapy, preoperative angiography is essential to differentiate the mass from a carotid body tumor or vagal chemodectoma and to establish the position of the internal carotid artery (Fig. 25-19). Transoral removal is never indicated as it is both hazardous and ineffective, leading to inadequate removal and regrowth of tumor. Although Horner syndrome may result from pressure of the tumor on the superior cervical ganglion, it most frequently results from operative trauma. Rapid increase in size of these usually slow-growing lesions suggests malignant change. The latter results in early nerve deficit, skin ulceration, and local re-

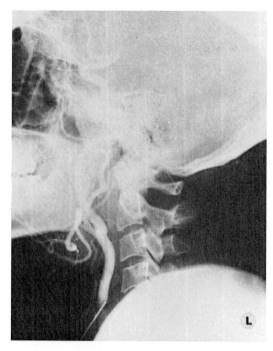

Fig. 25-19. Common carotid angiogram of a lateral pharyngeal space neurilemmoma showing anterior displacement of the internal carotid artery.

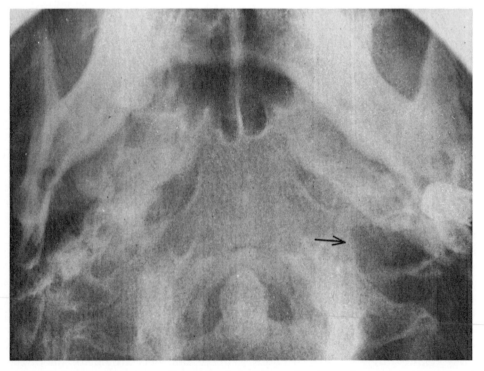

Fig. 25-20. Submento-vertex radiograph of skull base showing enlargement of left jugular foramen.

currence with possibly systemic metastasis. Regional lymph node metastases do not appear to be common, and since there is frequently difference of opinion regarding the diagnosis of malignancy in these tumors, the preferred treatment is still radical excision with possibly postoperative radiotherapy.[14]

Difficulty in differential diagnosis and treatment is more challenging in less accessible sites such as the jugular foramen. Clinical similarity to glomus body tumors is considerable, as both neurogenous tumors and glomus body tumors are more common in females, can produce both tinnitus and hearing loss, show as a reddish mass in the hypotympanum, which is well vascularized, and involve the cranial nerves in the jugular foramen as well as produce radiologically noted enlargement of this foramen (Fig. 25-20).[23] Since definitive diagnosis cannot be made clinically, surgical exploration and biopsy is essential. Radiotherapy has no demonstrable effect upon neurogenic tumors, and once diagnosis of schwannoma is established, surgical removal—preferably by an otologic approach—should be attempted. These tumors are slow-growing and even subtotal removal, when achieved by the development of a decompression cavity, is effective in preventing increase in symptoms.

Primary neurogenic tumors are also found in the nasal cavity and paranasal sinuses. When arising from the nasal septum, they are best removed by lateral rhinotomy (Fig. 25-21); there are more difficulties in removal when the paranasal sinuses are also involved. Robitaille, Seemayer, and El Deiry[62] analyzed 15 cases from the world literature; the majority of the 15 cases were schwannomas. Epistaxis was common in ethmoidal lesions, while pain was a feature when the maxillary sinus was involved. The importance of early diagnosis and radical surgical excision is emphasized, particularly for those tumors associated with von Recklinghausen disease. Cure rates were good and only those patients whose lesions were part of von Recklinghausen disease showed local recurrence of tumor.

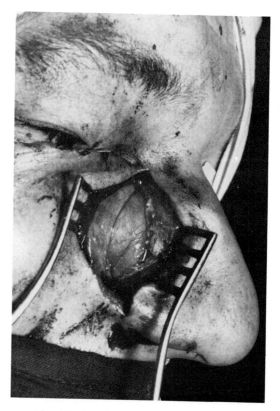

Fig. 25-21. Right lateral rhinotomy exposing primary intranasal schwannoma.

Olfactory Neuroblastoma

With the exception of benign neurofibromas and schwannomas, tumors arising from neuroectoderm are extremely uncommon. Neurogenous tumors arising within the nasal passages and paranasal sinuses make up less than 3 percent of all true neoplasms in this area. By far the rarest of such lesions are the olfactory neuroblastomas, originally called "esthesioneuroepitheliome olfactif" by Berger, Luc, and Richard in 1924.[5] In man, the olfactory neuroepithelium covers the superior nasal turbinate and upper part of the nasal septum terminating in nerve filaments that pass through the cribriform plate of the ethmoid to synapse with neuronal processes of the olfactory bulb. It is generally agreed that malignant tumors in this region arise from the basal layer of the olfactory mucosa, and the term "esthesis" refers rather nonspecifically to sensation or sensory perception. "Olfactory" is in many ways a better topographic designation, since it refers more specifically to the site of origin. In the past there were doubts as to the exact site of origin, but now it is known that the Organ of Jacobson, sphenoplatine ganglion, and ganglion of Loci do not relate to clinical experience and that the olfactory placode does not persist into the postnatal period.

By 1972 only 130 cases had been reported; but the incidence seems to be increasing, probably because of better differential diagnosis. I have personally treated 7 new cases within the last 4 years, but no one has yet published a large personal series and most series that have been published were gathered together over many years during which time treatment modalities will have changed considerably.

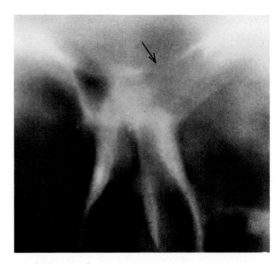

Fig. 25-22. Coronal tomogram showing defects in left cribriform plate produced by an olfactory neuroblastoma.

PROBLEMS IN DIAGNOSIS

No racial or true sexual predominance has been shown for this tumor; moreover, this tumor has been reported in patients from 8 to 80 years old, though never in the newborn. However, over 60 percent of these patients are aged between 15 and 35 years, which is much younger than the peak incidence for anaplastic carcinoma, malignant lymphoma, or melanoma—all conditions that may cause confusion in histologic diagnosis. The etiology is unknown; however, Herrold[36] showed that it was possible to produce in hamsters by systemic administration of nitrosodiethylamine nasal malignant neuroepithelial tumors that looked and behaved like human olfactory neuroblastomas.

Clinical presentation is similar to most malignant nasal tumors: obstruction, anosmia, and especially epistaxis because this is an extremely vascular tumor. Expansion of the nasal framework, proptosis, or even cerebral infection indicates extension of the lesion outside the site of origin; and tomography together with CT scanning is of great importance in planning surgical excision (Fig. 25-22). Examination reveals a fleshy, pinkish-grey polypoidal mass that bleeds easily; diagnosis is made by biopsy.

Kadish, Goodman, and Wang[42] suggested that staging could be made on clinical grounds including presenting symptoms, physical findings, and roentgenographic changes. Their suggested stages were group A, tumor confined to nasal cavity; group B, tumor involving nasal cavity and paranasal sinuses; and group C, tumor spreading beyond nasal cavity and sinuses. Their report was based upon 17 patients and they suggested that the more extensive tumors occurred in the youngest age group; however, in view of the small number of patients involved such conclusions are probably conjectural.

Attempts to classify cellular patterns and thus relate the histologic appearance to clinical malignancy have been unsuccessful if not frankly misleading. Histologic criteria used to identify these tumors from other intranasal malignancies include the occurrence of neuroepithelial cells arranged in pseudorosettes; a surrounding stroma composed of undifferentiated nuclei; and marked microvascularity with palisading of neuroepithelial cells around blood vessels with a basic similarity to adrenal or sympathetic ganglionic neuroblastoma. Although originally thought to arise from the esthesioneuroblast, these tumors are now consid-

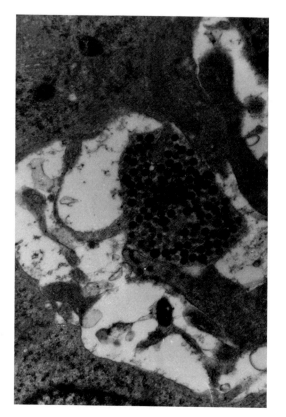

Fig. 25-23. Electron microscopic section of an olfactory neuroblastoma showing tumor cells with slender cytoplasmic processes blown out into bulbous endings filled with abundant membrane bound electron-dense catecholamine granules; magnification × 30,000 (Siemens Elmskop).

ered to arise from cells of neural crest origin. Similar cells produce secretory tumors, such as pheochromocytomas and neuroblastomas, elsewhere in the body. Electron microscopic studies have shown bags of catecholamines in the cytoplasm (Fig. 25-23) of material taken from these tumors. Touch preparations of fresh tumor tissue shows typical greenish-yellow catecholamine fluorescence induced by ultraviolet light after exposure to paraformaldehyde vapor.[41] We have employed such techniques in diagnosing all our patients and considering the variability of the appearance of this tumor under light microscopy, it may be thought that reliable diagnosis of this tumor cannot be made without these new techniques. Because catecholamines are present in the tumor, assays of urinary vanillylmandelic acid (VMA), dopamine, and homovanillic acid (HVA) are essential in monitoring the success of subsequent therapy (Fig. 25-24). Such estimations have been performed in my own patients and indicate that even after all macroscopic tumor has been removed levels may remain elevated for many months (Fig. 25-25).

TREATMENT AND PROGNOSIS

The best results in treatment have been obtained by a combination of surgery and radiotherapy. Possible errors in histopatholog-

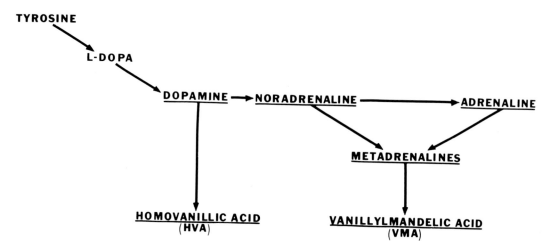

Fig. 25-24. Schematic and simplified catecholamine profile.

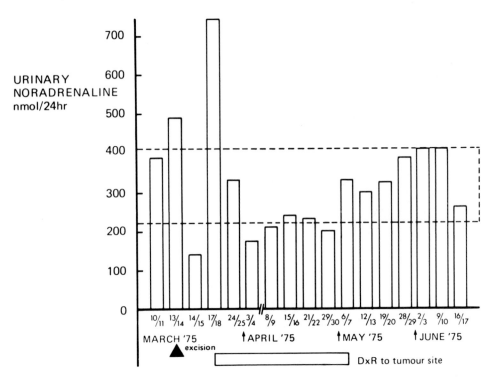

Fig. 25-25. Variations in urinary norepinephrine (noradrenaline) in a patient whose olfactory neuroblastoma was excised on March 13, 1975.

ic diagnosis—for not all reported cases have confirmed diagnosis by electron microscopy—absence of clinical staging, and virtually no information regarding levels of catecholamine secretion, make it impossible to compare the efficacy of radiotherapeutic dosage or the relationship between surgery and radiotherapy. Regional or systemic metastases occurred in about 20 percent of patients, but the most common cause of death was failure to control local disease.

Although the 5-year survival rate can be 50 percent, many of these patients will have local disease at that time and a more realistic 5-year cure rate is 30 percent. A detailed analysis of life expectancy and its relationship to the natural history of this disease has been recorded by Bailey and Barton.[3] Their studies of the literature suggest that surgery alone is rarely adequate and that the best 5-year cure rates have been obtained by combinations of surgery and radiotherapy. Response to radiotherapy is variable, and it would appear logical to carry

out as radical a removal of the neoplasm as technically possible—by lateral rhinotomy or craniofacial resection—prior to irradiation. With this combination a 5-year cure rate of at least 50 percent can be expected, and for more localized tumors this may be considerably exceeded.

Close examination of the site of origin of the tumor in my own cases showed that in two instances it grew not from the cribriform plate area but from the lateral nasal wall, closely mimicking anaplastic carcinoma of the ethmoid. Awareness of the existence of this tumor together with more efficient and sophisticated means of histologic diagnosis and catecholamine estimation should lead to earlier diagnosis. Radical excision of all tumor followed by curative dosage of radiotherapy and careful long-term follow-up should improve the prognosis, but local recurrence following adequate initial therapy is difficult to treat. Cryosurgery and possibly chemotherapy may have some effect in curing recurrences, but as with so many tumors the best opportunity of cure is in the initial management program.

Meningioma

Approximately 15 percent of all intracranial tumors are meningiomas; however, the true incidence is probably greater, since small asymptomatic tumors are occasional incidental findings at autopsy. Meningiomas arising or presenting outside the cranial cavity or spinal canal are most uncommon, and most of these reported cases represent local extension of an intracranial lesion. Review of the literature revealed that the most frequent sites in which extracranial meningiomas are found are the paranasal sinuses, frontal and temporal bone, orbit, nasal cavity, and pharynx. Extracranial presentation of an intracranial tumor is said by Farr, Gray, and Vrana[18] to occur in 18 percent of cases with 3 percent involving the nasal cavity, nasopharynx, or paranasal sinuses. However, other reports quote a much lower incidence of extracranial presentation, but all agree that primary extracranial meningiomas are exceedingly uncommon.

It is generally accepted that meningiomas arise from the same cells that give origin to the arachnoid villi and endothelium. Such cells develop from the neural crest and are neuroectodermal in origin. Direct extension of what is usually a slow-growing tumor may occur by erosion of bony structures. Malignant meningioma is most uncommon, diagnosis being based on unusual cellular activity, local infiltration, and the development of systemic metastases; incidence figures of less than 1 percent are quoted for malignant meningioma. The remaining explanation for extracranial meningioma is primary extracranial development, a diagnosis only possible when no evidence of an intracranial connection can be obtained. Such cases have been clearly documented and various theories have been advanced to explain their origin:

a. Histologically both intracranial and extracranial meningiomas are identical. Possibly, arachnoid-cell nests may be pinched off and left during embryonal development. Tumor may then develop later.

b. Displacement of undifferentiated cells—a mixture of neuroectodermal and mesodermal tissue—may occur during the complex embryologic development of the skull base and tumors might be expected to arise along the lines of fusion of embryonic bones. This "cell nest" theory has received much attention as a possible explanation for many other unusual tumors but is probably not relevant. Perhaps the unusual relationship of meningiothelium and endoneurium in the nose merits further consideration. Meanwhile the favored explanation is "embryologic arachnoid nests".[43]

Diagnosis of this tumor is substantiated by biopsy of an intranasal or intrasinus mass; the tumor may show the classical features of concentrically lamellated whorls of fibroblasts and psammoma bodies. Clinical history is usually lengthy; one patient of mine had slowly increasing proptosis for almost 3 years, the true extent of bony destruction being shown on routine paranasal sinus roentgenograms and by tomography (Fig. 25-26).

Characteristic findings include sclerosis of adjacent bone and occasional tumor calcification. Olfactory groove meningiomas may show hyperostosis of the planum sphenoidal and inferior displacement of the cribriform plate.

Intracranial extension can be shown by technetium flow studies and by brain scan assisted by carotid angiography; however, CT studies have probably replaced such investigations in providing the necessary information[59] (Fig. 25-27).

Displacement of normal soft tissue, bony erosion, tumor vascularity, and the presence or absence of intracranial tumor must all be determined prior to the planning of therapy. Despite its usual benign histologic appearance, however, meningioma sometimes demonstrates marked invasive properties. Extension, particularly from the anterior cranial fossa, through cribriform plate or orbital roof does not necessarily indicate malignancy because

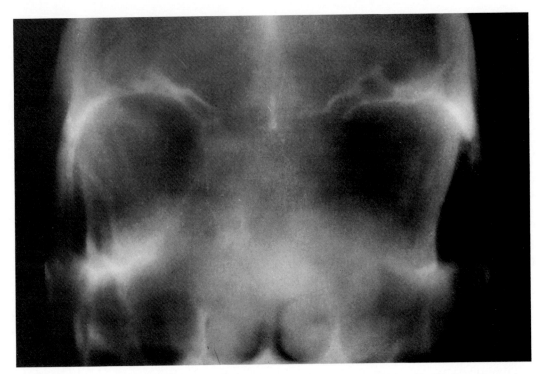

Fig. 25-26. Tomogram shows extensive bone destruction of the medial wall of both orbits and of the ethmoids from extracranial meningioma.

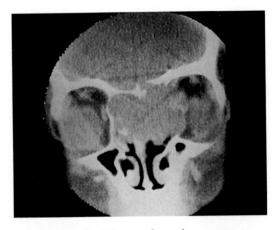

Fig. 25-27. CT scan shows large tumor involving sphenoid and ethmoid, with invasion of posterior orbit on left and soft tissue invasion on right. Floor of anterior cranial fossa is breached with erosion of wing of sphenoid on left. Irregular calcification suggests meningioma or chondrosarcoma.

variations in growth rate are not uncommon in other slow-growing tumors (such as osteomas) and the presence of congenital or acquired bony dehiscences in the floor of the cranial fossa or indeed the naturally occurring bony foramina—such as the cribriform apertures and orbital formina—may assist in the extracranial spread.

Radiotherapy has no part to play in the management of this tumor, and treatment is designed to eradicate the tumor surgically. Extracranial extension or involvement of the olfactory groove demands a multidisciplinary approach, the latter being successfully achieved by the combination of frontal craniotomy and lateral rhinotomy. Meningiocytes have been shown within the sheath of the optic nerve, and intraorbital meningiomas may arise from the sheath of the optic nerve although extension through the optic foramen may be difficult to differentiate from enlargement produced by posterior growth of a primary intraorbital tumor.

Granular Cell Tumor

Despite continuing confusion regarding the cell of origin, the frequency with which this tumor is found within the oral cavity (at least 40 percent of all reported cases) requires inclusion of this tumor within this chapter.

When originally described in 1926 by Abrikossoff,[1] the tumor was thought to originate from embryonic muscle fibers, hence the term myoblastoma. Such an explanation as to its origin is now less favored because electron microscopy has shown inconsistent association with muscle; more popular now is a neuroectodermal theory based on derivation from the Schwann cell. This does not, however, detract from the possibility that the cell component may be reactive, representing a nonneoplastic response to a variety of stimuli.

This tumor may be either pedunculated or sessile and may occur in any age group, although 70 percent of patients are within their fourth to sixth decade. In children it predominantly involves the skin, with a tendency to multiple lesions. There is no significant sex difference, but a black to white ratio of about 4:1 is reported. Although tumors have been found in almost every part of the body, approximately 30 percent occur within the tongue (Fig. 25-28). As a solitary nonulcerated nodular mass arising from dermis or submucosal tissue, a clinical diagnosis is difficult. Tumor size varies and is dependent largely on site of origin. Small lesions on the vocal cord will attract attention long before much larger tumors on the tongue because the tumor itself is painless and causes only symptoms related to its presence. Overlying pseudoepitheliomatous hyperplasia is frequently found in biopsy material and if found particularly in the larynx may lead to an erroneous diagnosis of "pseudocarcinoma," with the granular cells being dismissed as merely histiocytes.

Most lesions are circumscribed or even pseudoencapsulated, and the remainder are poorly demarcated. All should be treated

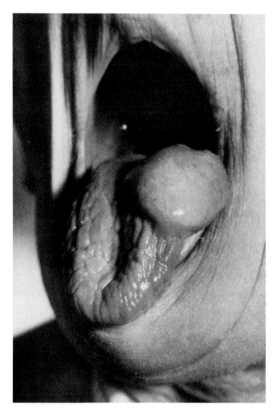

Fig. 25-28. Granular cell tumor producing a large pedunculated mass on the dorsum of the tongue.

by adequate surgical excision, as radiotherapy has no part to play except in the very occasional malignant variety. Local recurrence may occur after as long as 10 years following surgery[73] and is more likely where adequate local excision is difficult.

Apart from the tongue, the most frequent—and often most troublesome—site for this tumor within the head and neck is the larynx. In 1970, Booth and Osborn[7] reported 5 patients with granular cell myoblastoma of the larynx seen at our own institution between the years 1948 and 1970. Further patients with this lesion have been treated at this institution since that time but Booth and Osborn's findings remain relevant. The peak incidence of occurrence is the fourth decade. Approximately 10 percent of granular cell tumors occur within the larynx, and most tumors are situated on the posterior third of the vocal cord. The

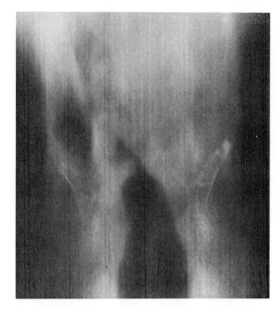

Fig. 25-29. Woman aged 42 years. Laryngeal tomography showing a left transglottic mass that on biopsy proved to be a granular cell tumor. Fixation of left vocal cord together with obstruction from tumor mass required tracheostomy; symptoms had been present for 2 years. Treatment was total laryngectomy.

most common presenting symptom therefore is hoarseness. Size and rate of growth is variable. Treatment is uniformly local removal, which may require procedures varying from endoscopic removal to total laryngectomy (Fig. 25-29).[56] Inadequate removal leads to a slow regrowth in the tongue, but the natural history of laryngeal myoblastoma may be dissimilar because patients with histologically proved inadequate surgical excision have shown no clinically detectable regrowth.

TUMORS INVOLVING BONE

All forms of tumor arising from mesenchymal tissue are relatively uncommon, particularly those arising from the bones of the craniofacial region. The most common benign tumor is the osteoma, which is said to occur in the frontal sinuses of at least 1 per-

cent of the population, with an unusually high incidence among the Arab population. The osteoma, described as a slow-growing, benign osteogenic tumor containing mature bone, is also found on the lingual surface of the mandible. Small osteomas at this site are usually asymptomatic and are discovered as an incidental finding during a routine radiographic examination. However, when large they protrude from the mandible and require surgical removal. Such endosteal osteomas must be differentiated from reactive bone sclerosis or the gigantic type of cementoma. The osteomas, which are usually bilateral, are easily removed by burr or chisel.

Of rather more clinical significance, and frequently growing to a large size thereby producing considerable deformity, are the peripheral osteomas of the paranasal sinuses. These tumors occur most frequently in the frontal sinus, but the site of origin is frequently undetected and reports vary as to tumor classification: some authors classify these tumors according to the space occupied, others according to the probable site of origin.[66] Most authors place the ethmoidal labyrinth before the maxillary sinus as a more frequent site of origin of the osteoma, with the sphenoidal sinus as a very rare place of origin.[66] Although frequently described as slow growing, the rate of growth may vary unexpectedly, because although diagnosis is usually made between the second and fourth decades these tumors may enlarge quite quickly in the younger patient. Most series show a male to female ratio of 2:1. Depending upon site of origin, symptoms vary from severe external deformity (Fig. 25-30) to headaches, facial pain, and sinus infection. Radiologic examination (Fig. 25-31) shows a sharply defined radiopaque calcified mass, but does not always show the site of attachment. Biopsy is rarely technically feasible because of the hardness of the tumor, but postoperative histologic examination shows them to be composed either of hard, compact bone (a composition termed "ivory") or of peripheral compact bone surrounding a cancellous center ("spongy") (Fig. 25-32). Sometimes

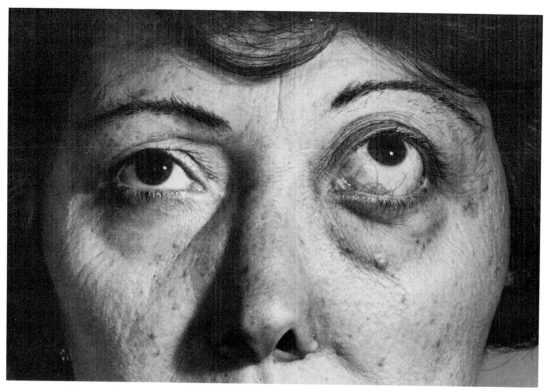

Fig. 25-30. Woman aged 42 years with osteoma of maxilla producing gradually increasing left facial deformity and left proptosis since age 11.

there is a mixture of both types. This variation in structure is explained by the differing development of the facial bones and has been used by some authors as a means of determining the true site of origin, as well as an explanation of development.

When in the course of development two different tissues of different embryonic origin come in contact, tumor growth is likely. The individual facial bones are developed either from membrane, cartilage, or from both elements. The skull vault is membrane, ethmoid is cartilage, and maxilla is membrane and cartilage, as are the temporal, occipital, and sphenoid bones. Membrane bone gives rise to compact osteomas, and cartilage to cancellous, while bones of mixed origin can be expected to produce "mixed" osteomas. The areas where membrane and cartilage come together are between the lesser wing of the sphenoid bone and the orbital plate of the frontal bone. These might be expected to be areas of predilec-

tion for osteoma formation. It is doubtful whether trauma or infection play any part in the occurrence of the osteomas.

Symptoms produced by enlargement of this tumor will depend upon the site of origin. If the frontal sinus is the site of origin, the interfrontal septum will atrophy and the sinus will slowly fill with osteoma before erosion of one or more surrounding walls occurs. Within the ethmoidal labyrinth individual cells may be filled, giving the tumor an unusual lobulated appearance. When growing into the orbit from the orbital plate of the ethmoid, gradual proptosis will occur (Fig. 25-30) and subsequent infection may result in blindness. Osteomas of the maxillary antrum may be of compact or cancellous bone and are usually attached to one bony wall by a pedicle, which is usually narrow and composed of vascular cancellous bone. Occasionally, the mass may fill the cavity displacing the orbital floor and producing diplopia and facial deformity (Fig.

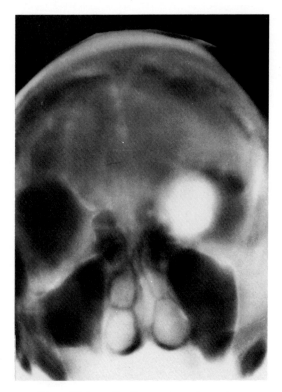

Fig. 25-31. Radiograph of patient shown in Figure 25-30.

25-33); it has been suggested that such rarities are in fact cases of leontiasis ossea. If this tumor is in fact a developmental anomaly, rather than a true neoplasm, then it may bear some relationship to the odonto-

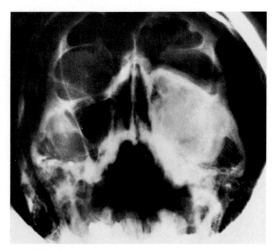

Fig. 25-33. Large osteoma filling left maxillary antrum and producing swelling of face and proptosis secondary to displacement of orbital floor.

genic keratocyst, which develops at the same period of time and in the same anatomical area.

Treatment is only indicated if the patient has symptoms that can be clearly attributed to the tumor, although the smaller the osteoma the easier it is to remove. When attachment is by a narrow pedicle, a sharp blow on the mass frequently produces release. However, when the frontal sinus is completely filled, removal may require wider exposure by osteoplastic flap or exter-

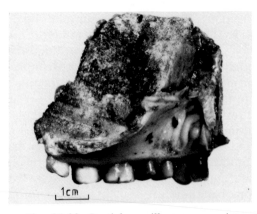

Fig. 25-32. Partial maxillectomy specimen cut to show cancellous nature of the bone. This was extremely vascular and despite hypotensive anesthesia blood loss was six units.

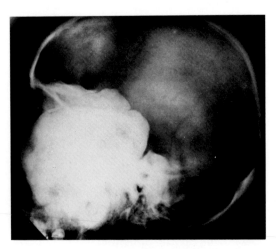

Fig. 25-34. Huge osteoma of the maxillary sinus.

nal frontal procedure. With ethmoidal lesions, lateral rhinotomy may be necessary. Total maxillectomy may be necessary with the large maxillary osteomas; this technique proved to be technically impossible, however, in the patient shown in Fig. 25-34 because of the extreme vascularity of the cancellous bone and the tremendous size of the tumor, which was present since the age of 10 years. Slow regrowth may occur if the site of attachment is not completely removed, and regrowth frequently proves to be in the vicinity of centers of primary or secondary ossification.

In 1943 Fitzgerald[19] reported the case of a woman with multiple osteomas, dermoids, and multiple colonic polyposis. Gardener[24] described a family with osteomas of facial bones, sebaceous cysts, and skin fibromas together with colonic polyposis. This syndrome is now considered an autosomal dominant disorder of connective tissue. The osteomas usually occur at puberty, particularly in the skull and facial bones, and are followed by epithelial anomalies such as polyps, sebaceous cysts, adenocarcinomas, and odontomas. If untreated, the colonic polyps become malignant. The osteomas rarely regrow after local removal.

Osteogenic Sarcoma

Despite being the most common primary malignant tumor of bone, osteogenic sarcomas are rare, with an incidence of about one case per 100,000 population. Most tumors occur in the long bones; and only 6 percent occur in the jaws, with the mandible being more common than the maxilla.

Age of diagnosis for osteogenic sarcoma of the jaws is older than for that of long bones; the former is within the third and fourth decades, although the span ranges from 14 to 72 years in recorded cases. It has been suggested that osteogenic sarcoma of the jaws has a lesser tendency to metastasize than that of the long bones and that death is more often due to local recurrence and inanition. Overall prognosis appears to be more favorable, but the total number of patients is small for this rare condition. Five-year survival figures of 5 to 25 percent are given for long bones, but Garrington et al.[25] and Caron, Hajdu, and Strong[11] quote figures of 33 to 35 percent when the jaws are involved.

ETIOLOGY

Trauma, preexisting bone conditions, and previous irradiation have all been implicated in the development of this tumor. Occasionally, a significant history of previous trauma is given by patients but the exposed situation of the jaws makes the significance of this debatable. Development of osteogenic sarcoma in bones affected by Paget disease is well established but only a few patients have developed osteogenic sarcoma of the jaw in association with this condition. Caron et al.[4] cited two cases of the latter, and one of my own cases has been reported by Windle-Taylor.[81] My patient gave a 10-year history of polyostotic Paget disease and presented with facial swelling and proptosis (Fig. 25-35). Radiographs showed gross Paget disease with destruction of orbital floor and a mass filling the nasal passage. Treatment with intra-arterial chemotherapy was ineffective, and the patient died within 3 months.

Criteria for confirming radiation induced osteogenic sarcomas include histologic proof, development of the tumor within the area of previous radiotherapy, and a long symptom-free latent period. Radiation to the orbit for retinoblastoma certainly brings with it a risk of subsequent osteogenic sarcoma, but there is no evidence of any relationship between total dosage and either the incidence or the induction period of osteogenic sarcoma.

Previous radiotherapy for retinoblastoma, fibrous dysplasia, or squamous carcinoma remains the most common determinable factor in the development of osteogenic sarcoma of the jaw and was found by Li-Volsi[48] in 14 patients; the time-delay ranged from 7 to 42 years. In my own 8 cases of

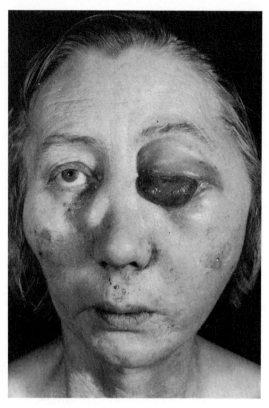

Fig. 25-35. Woman aged 58 years with polyostotic Paget disease and osteogenic sarcoma of the left maxilla involving the orbit.

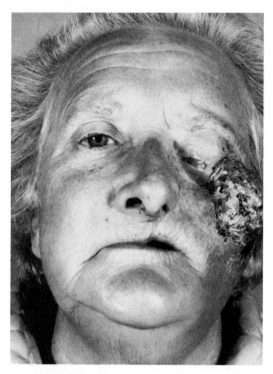

Fig. 25-36. Woman aged 60 years with radiation-induced fibrosarcoma of the left maxilla 12 years after radiotherapy for squamous carcinoma of the left maxillary antrum.

osteogenic sarcoma of the upper jaw, one woman aged 60 years had received 5,000 rads of superficial radiotherapy for a squamous carcinoma of the maxillary antrum 12 years previously (Fig. 25-36). A fibrosarcoma developed in the same maxilla, and she died 3 years later following combination of surgery and chemotherapy.

DIAGNOSIS

Patients presenting with painful enlargement of the mandible and evidence of nerve involvement will show radiologic evidence of bone destruction. Differential diagnosis may be difficult and includes osteoid osteoma, fibrous dysplasia, metastatic carcinoma, osteogenic sarcoma and other sarcomatous conditions. Subtotal mandibulectomy is the treatment of choice with ex-

pectation of a 5-year survival rate of 30 percent. In the upper jaw, rapidly enlarging facial or palatal swelling (Fig. 25-37) together with loosening of teeth, epistaxis, and pain, lead to suspicion of malignancy.

Radiology shows extensive bony loss, and the diagnosis is based on biopsy. Histologic appearances vary particularly in the amount of osteoid and chondroid tissue, but these variations appear to be unrelated to prognosis.

It is doubtful if radiotherapy is of any real value in the management of this condition, and radical excision is essential. Unfortunately, this disease is rarely localized to the maxilla, and adjuvant chemotherapy is recommended to minimize risk of local recurrence as well as to combat pulmonary metastases. I have used doxorubicin hydrochloride (Adriamycin), since this has had

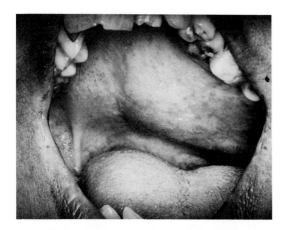

Fig. 25-37. Swelling of the left palate in a 30-year-old man who had symptoms of epistaxis and left facial swelling for only 2 months. Diagnosis was osteogenic sarcoma of the maxilla.

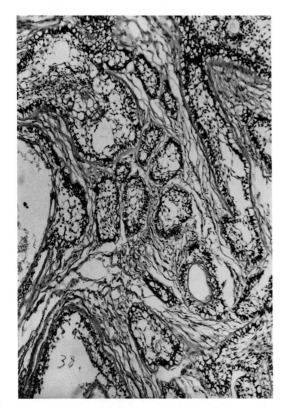

Fig. 25-38. Histologic section of ameloblastoma showing tumor follicles of variable size and shape, with central degenerative changes and cyst formation and a moderate amount of connective tissue stroma.

some effect on long-bone osteogenic sarcoma.

Osteogenic sarcoma is a rare tumor, growing rapidly in relatively young patients. At the time of diagnosis, the tumor is usually extensive and rarely completely resectable by even the most radical surgical procedure. Combination of surgery, radiotherapy, and chemotherapy rarely prevents local recurrence, and many patients die from local recurrence before pulmonary metastases have time to develop. Prognosis is unrelated to histologic differentiation; and although two of my own patients have survived for over 3 years, it appears probable that the overall prognosis is no better than for osteogenic sarcoma elsewhere in the body.

Ameloblastoma

The pathology of this tumor has been recognized, though not necessarily unanimously, since 1868. Originally called adamantinoma because of its resemblance to the enamel organ of the tooth germ, the term ameloblastoma was suggested around 1930.[39] It is a rare form of locally invasive epithelial tumor arising from the odontogenic apparatus and represents less than 1 percent of all neoplasms and cysts of the jaws. The incidence in the mandible is at least five times greater than in the maxilla, and this ratio is maintained even in Africans, for whom it is a common tumor of mandible and is seen at an unusually young age.[54]

Controversy continues regarding histopathologic differentiation and site of origin,[44] and the following proposals as to origin are still considered: malformed and supernumerary tooth germs, cell nests of the epithelial sheath of Hertwig, odontogenic cysts, and surface epithelium.

Symptomatically, this tumor usually presents as a painless swelling without ulceration, and in the maxilla particularly there may be considerable facial deformity. Toothache, looseness of teeth, or the production of an oroantral fistula leads to suspicion of overt malignancy, and the tumor may feel cystic or give a sensation of egg-shell crackling. Typical radiologic appearance is of multilocular radiolucent defects showing a honeycomb appearance. Unilocular bone cysts may resemble a dentigerous cyst, but there is frequently some erosion of related teeth or destruction of surrounding bone.

There appears to be no sex predominance either for the maxilla or mandible occurrences and except for Africans most patients are diagnosed between the age of 20 and 50 years. Slow growth of the tumor results in delay in diagnosis, which in my experience is 6 months and matches that of paranasal sinus carcinoma.

PATHOLOGY AND NATURAL HISTORY

In 1937 Robinson[61] surveyed the histopathology of 311 patients who had a diagnosis of ameloblastoma. Apart from confirming known characteristics related to age and sex, he concluded that the tumor was "anatomically benign and clinically persistent." However, in his series, 4.5 percent of the patients developed systemic metastases that were diagnosed as malignant ameloblastomas. Other reports have given an incidence of 2 percent for malignancy and have shown ameloblastoma to metastasize to lymph nodes and lungs. Robinson divided his cases into solid and cystic varieties together with a group showing a mixed pattern. Most solid tumors in fact show some cystic areas (Fig. 25-38), and further division of ameloblastoma on a histologic basis into follicular (resembling the dental follicle) and plexiform (resembling the stellate reticulum) is possible. There is a varying degree of vascularity, and variations, such as melanoameloblastoma and adenoameloblastoma, are recognized but behave somewhat differently from ameloblastoma. Histologic confusion with basal cell carcinoma or adenoid cystic carcinoma is possible and adequate biopsy is essential for diagnosis. Most reports confirm the radio-resistance of the ameloblastoma, but criteria for surgical management of these tumors have yet to be agreed upon.

No prospective studies have been undertaken to determine the amount of surgery necessary to completely remove or control this tumor while preserving function and appearance. Crawley and Levin[15] have discussed this matter in detail and stress the following:

1. Compact bone is eroded rather than invaded by tumor. The Haversian system of compact bone at the inferior border of the mandible is not invaded beyond clinical and radiographic margins. Consequently, the lateral and medial cortical plates of the mandible, being compact bone, need only be removed for surgical access.

2. Medullary bone is invaded by tumor although this may not be detected radiologically unless the cortical plate is eroded. This explains local recurrence after wide resection—the true extent of medullary bone invasion was underestimated. Although residual tumor cells may not always be viable, medullary bone should be removed beyond macroscopical evidence of tumor.

TREATMENT

The early treatment was conservative, being simple enucleation and curettage. Local recurrence was high, but it has been suggested by Waldron[77] that this does not necessarily imply failure because recurrence is often limited to a small area, which can be treated more conservatively than the original large lesion. Figures of between 50 and 90 percent recurrence rate following curettage have been reported; however, the thoroughness of curettage, size of original tumor, and length of time before recurrence are rarely quoted. It is now suggested that in the mandible wide excision without sacrificing the lower border should be attempted. If segmental resection is needed, then reconstruction,—using iliac crest bone, rib graft, or Kirschner wire—is usually possible. Postoperative radiotherapy is indicated for patients with malignant ameloblastomas who have some prospect of long-term control.[70]

Although there appears to be no histologic difference between ameloblastomas occurring in the maxilla and mandible, the former appear to be more aggressive—this may be related to structural differences in bone as well as to the close relationship of nasal cavity, orbit, and skull base. Certainly, small maxillary tumors may be effectively removed surgically, while larger ameloblastomas require total maxillectomy and possibly radiotherapy. In my limited experience of 3 patients with this tumor in the maxilla, partial maxillectomy was effective in 1 and total maxillectomy in the remaining 2. Although there is no indication for removal of the eye, total maxillectomy together with exploration of the infratemporal fossa can no longer be considered a mutilating procedure if adequate prosthetic help is available. However, if local excision is considered, then postoperative radiotherapy is advisable.

FIBROUS DYSPLASIA

Much of the confusion in the literature concerning fibrous dysplasia stems from the multiplicity of titles under which cases have been described—Lichtenstein and Jaffe[47] have reported no fewer than 37 synonyms.

A range of benign fibro-osseous lesions occur in the jaws. Although conditions such as fibrous dysplasia, ossifying fibroma, and giant cementoma are recognized, clinical and histologic differentiation is not always possible even though specific features have been described for each entity.[67]

In the case of fibrous dysplasia, the normal bony architecture of fiber bone is replaced by collagen, fibroblasts, and varying amounts of osteoid or calcified tissue. In this woven immature bone, there is random birefringence under polarized light and there is no maturation to lamellar bone. Although the fibrous stromal background may become more collagenous, the ground-glass pattern is seen radiologically to merge gradually into normal bone. Unlike the ossifying fibroma, the fibrous lesion cannot be enucleated. However, with fracture, and in cortical areas, lamellar bone may be present. Pepler[58] has shown that in both fibrous dysplasia and ossifying fibroma the stromal cells are rich in alkaline phosphatase, suggesting that they are osteoblasts and not fibroblasts. Certainly the gross appearance of the lesions is unhelpful, since they both feel fibrous with gritty or bony areas.

Theories relating to the etiology of fibrous dysplasia vary from failure of bone formation in the embryonic mesenchyme, to microhemorrhage, and the ever popular trauma, but yet no specific etiologic factor has been conclusively proven. It is known, however, that the disease usually occurs in early childhood. Although a polyostotic form, associated with café-au-lait pigmentation and sexual precocity, is recognized as Albright syndrome, fibrous dysplasia of the jaws is usually seen in the monostotic form. The monostotic form is first diagnosed in infancy or childhood, affects the maxilla rather more than the mandible, and occurs slightly more often in females; presentation is usually as a painless swelling of the affected part. Growth is usually slow, but occasionally may be so rapid as to cause clinical confusion with osteogenic sarcoma.

Any bone may be involved but skull and vertebrae are usually spared. Although the facial bones are said to be involved in over half of reported cases, this may reflect a clinician's special interst. However, the jaws are invariably involved in all polyostotic cases.

Most lesions in the jaws appear within the first two decades, and it is at this time that growth is most active. Although small lesions may produce little in the way of symptoms, larger tumors cause considerable asymmetry and distortion and in the maxilla pronounced bulging in the canine fossa (Fig. 25-39) or over the zygoma is observed. Extensive involvement of the maxilla may cause proptosis. Pain is uncommon in the jaws, and pathologic fracture—although occurring in long bones—appears not to occur in the mandible where the lesion is usually seen in the region of the angle. In

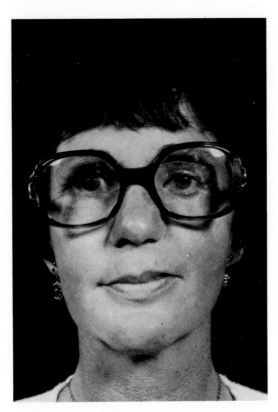

Fig. 25-39. Distortion (L) upper alveolus from fibrous dysplasia.

children, teeth in the affected part may fail to erupt and if present may be displaced but not loosened.

Fibrous dysplasia can be diagnosed radiologically from an early age. The affected area usually appears translucent, but as the patient grows the area increases in size and becomes more opaque as the fibrous tissue calcifies. At the calcification stage the area appears uniformly dense and is often described as having a "ground-glass" appearance. With increasing age the lesion may become more calcified showing a sclerotic appearance although calcification is often interspersed with radiolucent cystlike areas suggesting multiloculation. None of these appearances are pathognomonic, and radiologic changes must be related to histopathologic appearances and clinical behavior.

Treatment

Because these tumors are not painful and produce little disturbance of function, most patients seek treatment for cosmetic reasons. Since areas of fibrous dysplasia usually continue to enlarge during the period of general growth, remodeling operations are best deferred until growth has ceased. This may not be until the third decade and even then some regrowth may follow surgery.

Hormone therapy is ineffective and radiotherapy has been reported as producing sarcomatous change. Malignant change in nonirradiated fibrous dysplasia has been reported, but the true incidence is difficult to determine. Sudden increase in growth of long-standing areas of dysplasia must be viewed with suspicion and emphasizes the need to follow up these patients for long periods of time. Occasionally, the deformity may be so cosmetically unacceptable that early operation is necessary but in such cases the patient or parents must be warned that regrowth is likely. In the young, the affected bone is soft and may be curetted away; hemorrhage, however, is brisk because the bone is well vascularized. Older patients will have harder, sclerotic bone, and the area is relatively avascular. Trimming is carried out with gouge or cutting burr.

Some mention should be made of the condition commonly called cherubism, as some researchers consider this a variant of polyostotic fibrous dysplasia. Although this disorder is classified as a developmental disorder of bone-forming mesenchyme, the natural history differs from fibrous dysplasia. In cherubism, there is a definite hereditary tendency and the changes appear earlier than in dysplasia; growth ceases between 12 and 15 years of age at which time there may be regression. Although the maxillae may be involved, the most common sites are the angles of the mandible—producing an appearance similar to that seen in paintings of Renaissance angels!

There is seldom pain or functional disability, and the lesions are usually bilateral in contradistinction to fibrous dysplasia. Bilateral cervical lymphadenopathy is described, the nodes showing reactive hyperplasia. Since the possibility of regression or even complete resolution at puberty exists, treatment of cherubism must be individualized. Curettage for diagnostic purposes is indicated, but further surgical correction should be left until the disease is quiescent (which may not be until after 20 years of age). Lymphadenopathy has not been recorded in adults, since it usually regresses after the age of 5 years.

SOFT-TISSUE SARCOMA

These arise from poorly differentiated or undifferentiated mesenchymal cells of supporting connective tissue. Consequently, a wide variety of tumors are recognized and named according to the supposed cell of origin. They make up a diverse and complex group of neoplasms with rhabdomyosarcoma and malignant schwannoma the two most common tumors to be found in the head and neck. Russell et al.[64] analyzed 1,215 cases of soft tissue sarcomas from all sites in an attempt to produce a practical and effective system of staging. Sixty-four percent of cases occurred after the age of 35 years and the average age of the patients was 43 years. The male to female ratio was 1.1 to 1; and it was noted that each individual tumor had one or two sites of notable predilection. As with other malignancies, the size of the primary lesion and the presence of lymph node involvement or systemic metastases all influenced prognosis and were used in staging. However, the additional parameter—grade of malignancy—was considered and, although difficult to apply, was closely correlated with prognosis and survival. Highly malignant tumors such as rhabdomyosarcoma or angiosarcoma were lethal at all grades of malignancy, whereas close correlation was shown for fibrosarcoma and liposarcoma.

With the exception of the embryonal rhabdomyosarcoma, soft-tissue sarcomas are uncommon in the head and neck and only small numbers of patients have been recorded in the literature. Twenty-three adolescents and adults with a variety of soft tissue sarcoma of the head and neck area were reported in 1977 by Goepfert et al.[28] Prognosis was again related to the histologic and cytologic features of the tumor as well as to the size and the occurrence of metastases or invasion of bone, blood vessels, or nerves. These cases represented the total experience from the M.D. Anderson Hospital, Houston, between 1960 and 1974, thus indicating the relative rarity of these lesions within the head and neck. Combined surgery and radiotherapy had improved otherwise poor cure rates, and Goepfert and co-workers suggested that long-term chemotherapy may lessen recurrence after apparent disappearance of the primary tumor. My own experience with 6 patients with fibrosarcoma involving the nasal cavity or paranasal sinuses treated by combination radiotherapy and radical surgery has given no better results than for other malignant tumors within this region. Confusion between fibrous dysplasia and ossifying fibroma may explain the occasional surprisingly good result. However, in comparison with osteogenic sarcoma and rhabdomyosarcoma, fibrosarcomas appear to grow more slowly and metastasize less frequently.

Alveolar Soft-Part Sarcoma

In 1952 Christopherson, Foote, and Steward[12] reported 12 cases of a tumor which because of its obscure histogenesis and characteristic alveolar or organoid arrangement of cells they called "alveolar soft-part sarcoma." Histologic pattern is not dissimilar to the carotid body tumor and confusion is occasionally reported. It has been suggested that the source of origin might be chemoreceptor tissue, and in the past this tumor was confused with both granular cell tumor and metastatic adenocarcinoma.

These tumors are uncommon but are

found most usually in the lower extremities, anterior abdominal wall, retroperitoneal region, and floor of the mouth. Buchanan[10] analyzed 10 cases presenting within the head and neck (including the patient described below) concluding that this tumor is highly malignant with a pronounced tendency for systemic metastases even after radical excision of primary lesion.

CASE REPORT

In June 1972, a 17-year-old white female was seen by me because of a swelling of the right mandible (Fig. 25-40). This had been present for 2 years and was slowly increasing in size. Involving the ramus from angle to zygmomatic arch, it was visible beneath the buccal mucosa although there was no ulceration or pain. Biopsy and right carotid angiogram suggested a chemodectoma,

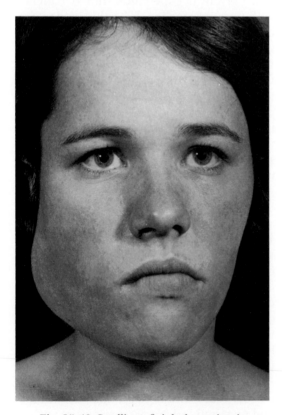

Fig. 25-40. Swelling of right lower jaw in a 17-year-old girl with an alveolar soft-part sarcoma.

but review of these studies eventually led to a diagnosis of alveolar soft-part sarcoma. Plasmacytoma, chemodectoma, and adenocarcinoma were all considered at some time in the differential diagnosis. Radical excision of the affected bone was performed in September 1972 without undue difficulty, since the internal carotid artery was displaced but not obviously involved. Despite the absence of preoperative radiotherapy, primary reconstruction of the bony defect was considered unwise until histologic confirmation of surgical clearance was available. However, for social reasons this repair was delayed. One year later metastatic deposits appeared in the lungs and vertebrae producing paraplegia. Death occurred May 1974, 4 years after the tumor first appeared.

Cumulative survival rates for this tumor have been given as 82 percent for 2 years, 60 percent for 5 years, and 50 percent for 10 years. However, this is undoubtedly influenced by tumor site and thus ease of local infiltration. Although responding to radiotherapy, local recurrence is rapid; and as with most other soft tissue sarcomas the combination of radiotherapy, surgery, and possibly chemotherapy may offer the best chance of long-term survival.

CHORDOMA

This is one of the few malignant tumors that arise from vestigial embryonic tissue yet retain primitive histologic features. It is now realized that the tumor develops from the notochord, an axial structure found in all chordates. Although retained as the sole axial structure in lower chordates, such as Amphioxus, it is replaced by the vertebral column and part of the skull base in higher forms such as man.

The most comprehensive review of these unusual tumors was written by Wright;[83] in his paper he described the early discussions by Kirchow and Müller in 1858 regarding the origin of tumors related to the region of the clivus of Blemenbach.

Controversy continued until the end of the 19th century, and the first authenticated case of chordoma was reported around 1910 in the German literature. Although unusual, an increasing number of cases have been reported and in 1955, Utne and Puch[76] reviewed 505 patients.

In man, the notochord plate develops cranial to the primitive streak, early in the third week of intrauterine life. During the fifth week, the notochord becomes enclosed within the bodies of the primitive vertebra. Passing through the mesenchymatous tissue that later forms the bodies of the atlas and odontoid processes it enters the basiocciput before coming to lie directly in contact with the endothelium of the primitive pharynx. Because it cannot proceed further cranially than Rathke's pouch, it comes to lie within the body of the sphenoid, and thus terminates caudal to the pituitary fossa (Fig. 25-41). As the vertebral column develops, the notochord bar divides into segments and finally disappears as a recognizable entity except for its representation as the nucleus pulposus.

Notochordal remnants have been found in the region of the clivus and nasopharyngeal and pharyngeal submucosa, and in the bodies of cervical vertebra. However, true neoplasms are thought to arise from detached remnants of notochord rather than from the original root of its adult counterpart. Approximately half of all reported chordomas are found in the craniocervical region. Richter, Batsakis and Boles[60] (Fig. 25-42) and Wright[83] suggest that this predominance, together with the high incidence in the sacral region, may be related to the complex development of the upper occipital somites in the 8-week-old embryo. The upper three myotomes descend to form the musculature of the tongue; the corresponding sclerotomes fuse with the parachordal cartilage to form the basal plate from which the basiocciput and basisphenoid develop. Eventually, the dermatomes of the region degenerate and there is great developmental upheaval. It is quite possible that small derivatives of the disintegrating notochord become separated from the true notochord and form ectopic remnants. A similar process of disintegration and activity occurs in the caudal region, where the tail fold is being formed. Again, primitive tissue may be left, thus explaining the high inci-

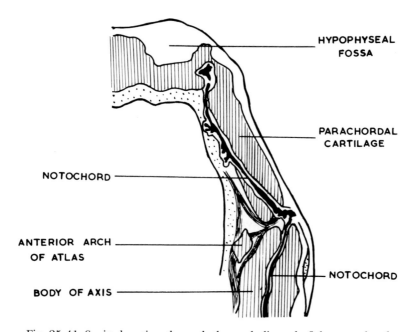

Fig. 25-41. Sagittal section through the cephalic end of the notochord.

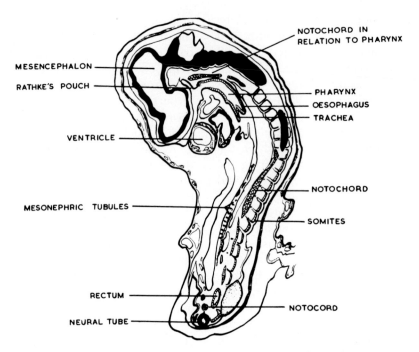

Fig. 25-42. Chick embryo: 36 somite stage showing the relation of notochord to pharynx and vertebral bodies.

dence of such tumors as chordoma and teratoma and those associated with spina bifida.

In the cervical, thoracic, and lumbar regions of the vertebral column there is not the same degree of activity and degeneration, and chordal ectopia is less likely to be found. Although notochordal remnants have been found in cadavers along the whole of the notochordal tract, there is no information regarding the frequency of these remnants or the likely incidence of tumor formation. Since the topographic distribution of chordal vestiges correspond closely to the sites of occurrence of clinical chordoma, a reason has been sought to explain this malignant change. Although trauma has been postulated, it has not been significantly substantiated, and it may well be that most remnants have malignant potential.

Diagnosis and Natural History

With an incidence of less than 1 percent of all neoplasms affecting the central nervous system, chordomas are rare. Consequently, most reports are based on small personal series or cases collected from various sources and thus carry the inevitable risk of inbuilt errors. My own experience is limited to 6 patients with cranio-occipital or cervical lesions. There is general acceptance that chordomas arising from the upper end of the notochord develop at an earlier age than those from the sacrococcygeal region, and most cranial or cervical vertebral tumors are found in the 30- to 40-year-old age group. They have been reported at all ages although the difficulty of both clinical and histologic diagnosis imposes some doubt as to the authenticity of some of the older reports. Sex predominance is said to favor males, particularly in the sacrococcygeal group; but total numbers may be too small to allow accurate assessment.

The natural history of chordoma is a slowly growing, locally invasive tumor that causes bone destruction and extension into soft tissues. In the vertebral region it may infiltrate the vertebral bodies and grow anteriorly into the paraspinal tissues or posteriorly to surround the spinal cord. Within the spinal canal it can readily grow up or down the lumen. Bone at the site of origin may show variable amounts of destruction, depending upon both the site of origin and the subsequent direction of extension. The true extent of bone destruction can only be revealed by tomography or CT scanning and as with other tumors is invariably more extensive than expected. The tumor appears to break through the cortex and form a soft tissue mass extending out from the bone. Calcification has been described within the tumor, and some bony changes are found in over 80 percent of all cranio-vertebral lesions. Regional or systemic metastases are extremely rare and since radical excision of the tumor is invariably impossible, the natural history is primarily one of repeated local regrowth following attempts at local removal. Few patients survive longer than 5 years although isolated instances of long-term survival have been reported.[60, 83]

Clinical diagnosis of chordoma is unlikely, since the symptoms are largely those of an invasive bone destroying tumor localized to the cranio-occipital or cervical vertebral region. Severe pain is a constant feature of this tumor and is either fronto-orbital or distributed along the cervical nerves. When the chordoma originates close to the clivus, visual disturbance, paresis of ocular muscles, or involvement of the trigeminal nerve may cause the patient to seek the help of a neurologist or ophthalmologist. Involvement of the hypophyseal region causes disturbance of endocrine function. If the chordoma arises within or extends to the nasopharynx, symptoms will be indistinguishable from those produced by an invasive nasopharyngeal carcinoma.

Cervical chordoma may be ignored by the patient for many months, since symptoms of dysphagia, hoarseness, or dyspnea may occur slowly. However, pain is an early feature of chordoma in this region, and this pain is difficult to control by most analgesics. The protrusion of a cervical chordoma into the lumen of the pharynx in a way that displaces the esophagus or larynx will be covered by intact mucosa and will rarely ulcerate except after biopsy. Such swellings are firm and lobulated often leading to a provisional diagnosis of osteoma.

Most chordomas seen by the otolaryngologist present within the nasopharynx; however, these are probably extensions either from a cranio-occipital tumor or upward from a high cervical neoplasm.

The difficulty or near impossiblity of diagnosis before bone involvement makes complete surgical excision of this tumor impossible. Histologic diagnosis from biopsy material often presents problems because there are no absolute or entirely specific features in this tumor. Heffelfinger et al.[35] have, however, suggested that it is possible to differentiate chordoma from a more benign chondroid chordoma. The latter may contain such an abundant cartilaginous component that a diagnosis of chondroma or even chondrosarcoma is suggested. More often there seems to be a mixture of chondroid and chordoma elements, and the identification of syncytial chordoma cells in a cartilaginous matrix confirms the neoplasm as a chondroid chordoma. The importance of this differentiation is that it has been suggested that the average survival time for the chondroid chordoma is over 15 years, while that for the typical chordoma is only 4 years.

Treatment

Although the chordoma appears as a lobulated, firm mass with occasionally an apparent capsule, bone invasion and soft tissue extension make radical excision impossible except perhaps for tumors localized to the nasopharynx or for those lying prevertebrally and not invading the vertebral body.

Despite the very high local recurrence rate following attempts at surgical excision, regrowth is often slow and repeated surgical excisions may prolong the patient's life for many years. In my own experience, however, such procedures become increasingly difficult because of intense fibrosis, and it has been suggested that initial resection should be followed by radiotherapy. Dosage levels vary, since no radiotherapist has treated more than a few patients; but levels would appear to be related to the site of residual tumor to avoid serious bone necrosis or damage to the brain or spinal cord. Pain relief may be obtained in this way, and combination therapy may offer the patient with extensive disease the best prospect of long-term palliation.

PLASMACYTOMA

Although plasmacytomas may present as medullary or extramedullary tumors and in single or multiple forms, it has been suggested that all are manifestations of the same disease. Each exhibits characteristic histologic features of monomorphism: sheets of plasma cells on a delicate reticular stroma and a scarcity of Russell bodies. Although the cells become bigger with increasing immaturity and there may be an increase in nuclear size, it has not been proven that specific histologic features can be related to tumor aggressiveness. Prognosis is possibly related to site and marrow involvement, as a 5-year survival rate of 60 percent for extramedullary tumors has been quoted by Pahor[57] but only 5.7 percent for multiple myeloma. Multiple myeloma or generalized myeloma almost always begins in the bone marrow; however, it may manifest itself as a solitary bone or extramedullary soft tissue tumor. Some patients will develop generalized disease, while others die from local invasion of tumor. Although variance in sex ratio (male to female 3:1 for extramedullary tumors but 1:1 for multiple myeloma), and a lower age incidence in the more benign tumors is recognized, patients with solitary lesions must have lengthy follow-up because the risk of multiple myeloma developing eventually is quoted as between 30 and 70 percent.

The first case of extramedullary plasmacytoma was reported at the beginning of this century, and by 1973[8] over 250 cases had been recorded. At least 85 percent occur within the head and neck primarily in the nose, sinuses, and nasopharynx. Ten percent of these tumors in the head and neck are said to be in multiple sites. All are rare, and the incidence of extramedullary tumors compared with multiple myeloma is about 1:40.

Nasal and paranasal sinus tumors present with symptoms common to other tumors in this region—nasal obstruction, rhinorrhea, epistaxis, and headaches. Bone erosion is common. In appearance the lesion may be polypoid or sessile and frequently becomes lobulated as it increases in size. The color is dependent upon the capillary network within the tumor stroma, but in my own experience of 14 patients the color was always red or pink. Ulceration is uncommon except after biopsy; involvement of the cervical lymph nodes, said to be present in 25 percent of patients, is not necessarily a bad prognostic sign, although it may indicate systemic disease.

Involvement of the jaws certainly occurs in multiple myeloma—although the disease usually affects the mandible, particularly posteriorly where the marrow spaces are larger. Solitary plasmacytoma of the jaws or other bones has been described as a clinical entity, but it is probably part of a single spectrum of plasma cell disorders. Rarely will these lesions be diagnosed clinically in the absence of previously established marrow disease. After histologic diagnosis, and this may require electron microscopy or the use of special techniques, each case of extramedullary plasmacytoma requires intensive radiologic, hematologic, and biochemical investigation to exclude the diagnosis of myeloma. Radiology detects the presence of local bone erosion and a skeletal survey is necessary to exclude intramedullar lesions.

Although there are no characteristic hematologic features of extramedullary plasmacytoma; elevated ESR, myeloma cells in bone marrow, lymphocytosis, and anemia are common with multiple myeloma. Myeloma protein is demonstrated in serum proteins, and serum electrophoresis shows changes in levels of IgA, IgD, IgG, and IgM. This will require the use of immunoglobulin diffusion techniques because of the low protein concentrations. An increased titer does not necessarily indicate multiple myeloma but when associated with isolated plasmacytoma suspicion of the presence of multiple myeloma is aroused. Examination of the urine for Bence Jones protein is also indicated.

Unfortunately, no single test is sufficient for diagnosis in the early case of extramedullary myeloma and the risk of subsequent development of systemic disease probably exists in all patients. However, the rational selection of initial treatment is dependent upon the extent of local disease and the presence or absence of systemic involvement. Extramedullary plasmacytoma is a rare condition and published reports are insufficient to substantiate the definite effectiveness of any single treatment regime. Long-term survival has been reported for patients treated with radiotherapy, surgery, combinations of both, and more recently, additional chemotherapy. Dosage of radiotherapy has varied from 3,500 rads to 7,500 rads; but my own experience has convinced me that, as with many other tumors, radical resection followed by a curative dosage of radiotherapy offers most patients the best chance of local tumor control. Melphalan (or other favored drugs) is given for systemic disease or for multiple lesions. Successful treatment of localized lesions still warrants routine screening for systemic disease, although this may not always be practical. Local recurrence may occur many years after treatment, and multiple myeloma has been recorded as developing 36 years after treatment of an extramedullary plasmacytoma.

Increase in the number of marrow plasma cells (6 to 8 percent or more) with increased level of serum immunoglobulins (especially IgA and IgG) have been suggested as early signs of developing multiple myeloma—this has certainly been my own experience.

It is clear that a multidisciplinary approach is important for diagnosis, treatment, and follow-up. Multiple myeloma must be excluded in every patient with a diagnosis of extramedullary plasmacytoma; and in every patient with effective local control, a long-term survey is essential. Although not all plasmacytomas are radiosensitive, combination of radiation and radical surgery is probably the most effective means of obtaining local tumor control.

SUMMARY

In deciding which tumors should be included in this chapter I have been influenced by my own experience as well as by quoted incidence rates. Inevitably, many interesting and rare conditions have been omitted, because I have written from my own personal knowledge of each neoplasm rather than only distilling the recorded wisdom of others. The unique opportunity of working in a large specialty hospital draining a population far exceeding its own nationals provides facilities for treating unusual conditions. Some are so rare that only an occasional patient will be seen, thus minimizing the value of any didactic comment —these tumors I have omitted. Rarity is of course relative, and obviously the frequency with which any tumor is seen will vary with the size and status of the institution, draining population, and other factors. Diagnosis may be difficult and even experienced histopathologists differ in their interpretation of biopsy material. Availability of specialized academic departments and national tumor panels increase the likelihood of accurate diagnosis and may well lead to more frequent diagnosis of unusual conditions.

REFERENCES

1. Abrikossof, A. 1926. Verber Myome ausgehend von der guergestreiften willkürlichen Muskulatur. Virchow's Archiv Für Pathologische Anatomie und Physiologie und für Klinische Medizin, 240: 215.

2. Adlington, P. and Woodhouse, M. A. 1972.

larynx. Journal of Laryngology and Otology, 86: 1219.

3. Bailey, B. J., and Barton, S. 1975. Olfactory neuroblastoma; management and prognosis. Archives of Otolaryngology, 101: 1.

4. Benson, H. and Ewing, J. 1940. Neoplastic Disease; a Treatise on Tumors. 4th ed. W. B. Saunders, Philadelphia.

5. Berger, L., Luc, H. and Richard, A. 1924. L'esthesioneuroepitheliome olfactif. Bulletin de l'Association Française Pour l'étude du cancer, par., 13: 410.

6. Bickerstaff, E. R., and Howell, J. S. 1953. The neurological importance of tumors of the glomus jugulare. Brain, 76: 576.

7. Booth, J. B., and Osborn, D. A. 1970. Granular cell myoblastoma of the larynx. Acta Otolaryngologica, 70: 279.

8. Booth, J. B., Cheesman, A. D., and Vincenti, N. H. 1973. Extramedullary plasmacytoma of the upper respiratory tract. Annals of Otology, Rhinology and Laryngology, 82: 709.

9. Briant, T. D. R., Fitzpatrick, P. J. and Berman, J. 1978. Nasopharyngeal angiofibroma; a twenty year study. Laryngoscope, 88: 1247.

10. Buchanan, G. 1975. Two rare tumours involving the infratemporal fossa; alveolar soft part sarcoma and haemangiopericytoma. Journal of Laryngology and Otology, 89: 375.

11. Caron, A. S., Hajdu, S. I., and Strong, E. W. 1971. Osteogenic sarcoma of the facial and cranial bones; a review of forty-three cases. American Journal of Surgery, 122: 719.

12. Christopherson, W. M., Foote, F. W., Jr., and Stewart, F. W. 1952. Alveolar soft-part sarcomas; structurally characteristic tumors of uncertain histogenesis. Cancer, 5: 100.

13. Conley, J. 1965. The carotid body tumor. A review of 29 cases. Archives of Otolaryngology. 81: 187.

14. Conley, J. 1972. Neurogenic tumors of the head and neck. Journal of the Otolaryngology Society of Australia, 3: 362

15. Crawley, W. A., and Levin, L. S. 1978. Treatment of the ameloblastoma; a controversy. Cancer, 42: 357.

16. Cummings, C. W., Montgomery, W. W., and Balogh, K., Jr. 1969. Neurogenic tumors of the larynx. Annals of Otology, Rhinology and Laryngology, 78: 76.

17. Donald, P. J. 1978. Sarcomatous degeneration in a nasopharyngeal angiofibroma. Otolaryngology, 86: 216.

18. Farr, H. W., Gray, G. F. Jr., Vrana, M, and Panio, M. 1973. Extracranial meningioma. Journal of Surgical Oncology, 5: 411.

19. Fitzgerald, G. M. 1943. Multiple composite odontomes coincidental with other tumorous conditions; report of case. Journal of the American Dental Association, 30: 1408.

20. Fitzpatrick, P. J. 1970. The nasopharyngeal angiofibroma. Canadian Journal of Surgery, 13: 228.

21. Friedberg, S. A. 1940. Vascular fibroma of nasopharynx (nasopharyngeal fibroma). Archives of Otolaryngology, 31: 313.

22. Friedmann, I., Sando, I., and Balkany, T. 1978. Idiopathic pleomorphic midfacial granuloma (Stewart's type). Journal of Laryngology and Otology, 92: 601.

23. Gacek, R. R. 1976. Schwannoma of the jugular foramen. Annals of Otology, Rhinology and Laryngology, 85: 215.

24. Gardener, E. J. 1962. Follow-up study of a family group exhibiting dominant inheritance for a syndrome including intestinal polyps, osteomas, fibromas and epidermal cysts. American Journal of Human Genetics, 14: 376.

25. Garrington, G. E., Schofield, H. H., Cornyn, J., and Hooker, S. P. 1967. Osteosarcoma of the jaws. Analysis of 56 cases. Cancer, 20: 377.

26. Ghosh, B. C., Ghosh, L., Huvos, A. G., and Fortner, J. G. 1973. Malignant schwannoma. A clinicopathologic study. Cancer, 31: 184.

27. Gill, G., Rice, D. H., Ritter, F. N., Kindt, G., and Russo, H. R. 1976. Intracranial and extracranial nasopharyngeal angiofibroma. A surgical approach. Archives of Otolaryngology, 102: 371.

28. Goepfert, H., Lindberg, R. D., Sinkovics, J. G., and Ayala, A. G. 1977. Soft-tissue sarcoma of the head and neck after puberty. Archives of Otolaryngology, 103: 365.

29. Goodman, G. C., and Churg, J. 1954. Wegener's granulomatosis, pathology and review of the literature. Archives of Pathology and Laboratory Medicine, 58: 533.

30. Greenway, R. E., and Heeneman, H. 1975. Chemodectoma of the larynx. Canadian Journal of Otolaryngology, 4: 499.

31. Guild, S. R. 1941. A hitherto unrecognized structure, the glomus jugularis. Anatomical Record, 79: suppl. 3, 28.

32. Harma, R. A. 1958. Nasopharyngeal angiofibroma. Acta Otolaryngologica, suppl., 146: 1.

33. Harrison, D. F. N. 1974. Non-healing gran-

ulomata of the upper respiratory tract. British Medical Journal. 4: 205.

34. Harrison, D. F. N. 1977. Lateral rhinotomy; a neglected operation. Annals of Otology, Rhinology and Laryngology, 86: 756.

35. Heffelfinger, M. J., Dahlin, D. C., MacCarty, C. S., and Beabout, J. W. et al. 1973. Chordomas and cartilaginous tumors of the skull base. Cancer, 32: 410.

36. Herrold, K. M. 1964. Induction of olfactory neuroepithelial tumors in Syrian hamsters by diethylnitrosamine. Cancer, 17: 114.

37. Hollman, G., Horner, F., and Daum, R. 1927. Beitrag zur klink des Himangiopericytoma. Langenbecks Archiv Für chirurgie, 330: 128.

38. Holman, C. B., and Miller, W. E. 1965. Juvenile nasopharyngeal fibroma. Roentgenologic characteristics. American Journal of Roentgenology, 94: 292.

39. Ivy, R. H., and Curtiss, L. 1937. Adamantinoma of jaw. Annals of Surgery, 105: 125.

40. Jarzab, G. 1975. Clinical experience in the cryosurgery of hemangioma. Journal of Maxillofacial Surgery 3: 146.

41. Judge, D. M., McGavran, M. H., and Trapukdi, S. 1976. Fume-induced fluorescence in diagnosis of nasal neuroblastoma. Archives of Otolaryngology, 102: 97.

42. Kadish, S., Goodman, M., and Wang, C. C. 1976. Olfactory neuroblastoma. A clinical analysis of 17 cases. Cancer, 37: 1571.

43. Kjeldsberg, C. R., and Minckler, J. 1972. Meningiomas presenting as nasal polyps. Cancer, 29: 153.

44. Kramer, I. R. 1963. Ameloblastoma: A clinicopathological appraisal. British Journal of Oral Surgery, 1: 13.

45. Lack, E., Cubilla, A. L., Woodruff, J. M., and Farr, H. W. 1977. Paragangliomas of the head.and neck region: A clinical study of 69 patients. Cancer, 39: 397.

46. Leopard, P. J. 1972. Osteoma of the maxillary antrum. British Journal of Oral Surgery, 10: 73.

47. Lichtenstein, L., and Jaffe, H. L. 1942. Fibrous dysplasia of bone. Archives of Pathology and Laboratory Medicine, 33: 777.

48. LiVolsi, V. A. 1977. Osteogenic sarcoma of the maxilla. Archives of Otolaryngology, 103: 485.

49. McBride, P. 1897. Case of rapid destruction of the nose and face. Medical Press and Circular, (London), 43: 32.

50. McMaster, M. J., Soule, E. H., and Ivins, J. C. 1975. Hemangiopericytoma: A clinico-

pathologic study and long-term follow-up of 60 patients. Cancer, 36: 2232.

51. Michaels, L., and Gregory, M. M. 1977. Pathology of "non-healing (midline) granuloma." Journal of Clinical Pathology, 30: 317.

52. Mira, J. C., Chu, F. C. H., and Fortner, J. G. 1977. The role of radiotherapy in the management of malignant hemangiopericytoma. Report of eleven new cases and review of the literature. Cancer, 39: 1254.

53. Nanson, E. M. 1978. Neurilemmoma of the larynx: A case study. Head and Neck Surgery, 1: 69.

54. Onuigbo, W. I. 1978. Jaw tumours in Nigerian Igboa. British Journal of Oral Surgery, 15: 1223.

55. Osborn, D. A., and Sokolovski, A. 1965. Juvenile nasopharyngeal angiofibroma in a female. Report of a case. Archives of Otolaryngology, 82: 629.

56. Ottosson, B. G. 1964. Myoblastoma of the larynx. Acta Otolaryngologica. 58: 87.

57. Pahor, A. L. 1977. Extramedullary plasmacytoma of the head and neck, parotid and submandibular salivary glands. Journal of Laryngology and Otology, 91: 241.

58. Pepler, W. J. 1966. Ossifying fibromas and their relation to fibrous dysplasia and other tumours. Journal of Pathology and Bacteriology, 79: 408.

59. Persky, M. S., and Som, M. L. 1978. Olfactory groove meningioma with paranasal sinus and nasal cavity extension; a combined approach. Otolaryngology, 86: 714.

60. Richter, H. J., Jr., Batsakis, J. G., and Boles, R. 1975. Chordomas; nasopharyngeal presentation and atypical long survival. Annals of Otology, Rhinology and Laryngology, 84: 327.

61. Robinson, H. B. G. 1937. Ameloblastoma; a survey of 379 cases from literature. Archives of Pathology and Laboratory Medicine, 23: 831.

62. Robitaille, Y., Seemayer, T. A., and El Deiry, A. 1975. Peripheral nerve tumors involving paranasal sinuses: a case report and review of the literature. Cancer, 35: 1254.

63. Rosenwasser, H. 1945. Carotid body tumor of middle ear and mastoid. Archives of Otolaryngology, 41: 64.

64. Russell, W. O., Cohen, J., Enzinger, F., Hajdu, S. I., Heise, H., Martin, R. G., Meissner, W., Miller, W. T., Schmitz, R. L., and Suit, H. D. 1977. A clinical and pathological staging system for soft tissue sarcomas. Cancer, 40: 1562.

The ultrastructure of chemodectoma of the

65. Samy, L. L., and Mostafa, H. 1971. Osteomata of the nose and paranasal sinuses with a report of twenty one cases. Journal of Laryngology and Otology, 85: 449.

66. Schiff, M. 1959. Juvenile nasopharyngeal angiofibroma. Laryngoscope, 69: 981.

67. Schmaman, A., Smith, I., and Ackerman, L. 1970. Benign fibro-osseous lesions of the mandible and maxilla. Cancer, 26: 303.

68. Sharpstone, P. 1977. Diseases of the urinary system. Prescribing for patients with renal failure. British Medical Journal, 2: 36.

69. Shuangshoti, S., and Panyathanya, R. 1943. Ectopic meningiomas. Archives of Otolaryngology, 98: 102.

70. Singleton, J. 1970. Malignant ameloblastoma. British Journal of Oral Surgery, 8: 154.

71. Spector G. J., Ciralsky, R. J., and Ogura, J. H. 1975. Glomus tumors in the head and neck: III. Analysis of clinical manifestations. Annals of Otology, Rhinology and Laryngology, 84: 73.

72. Stout, A. P., and Murray, M. R. 1942. Hemangiopericytoma, vascular tumor featuring Zimmermann's pericytes. Annals of Surgery, 116: 26.

73. Strong, E. W., McDivitt, R. W., and Brasfield, R. D. 1970. Granular cell myoblastoma. Cancer, 25: 415.

74. Thomsen, K. Elbrond, O., and Andersen, A. P. 1975. Glomus jugulare tumours (a series of 21 cases). Journal of Laryngology and Otology, 89: 1113.

75. Tyldesley, W. R., and Littlewood, A. H. M. 1975. Haemangioma of the maxilla: A case report. British Journal of Oral Surgery, 13: 56.

76. Utne, J. R. and Pugh, D. G. 1955. Roentgenologic aspects of chordoma. American Journal of Roentgenology, 74: 593.

77. Waldron, C. A. 1966. Ameloblastoma in perspective. Journal of Oral Surgery, 24: 331.

78. Ward, P. H., Thompson, R., Calcaterra, T., and Kadin, M. R. 1974. Juvenile angiofibroma: A more rational therapeutic approach based upon clinical and experimental evidence. Laryngoscope, 84: 2181.

79. Wegener, F. 1939. Über eine eigenartige rhinogene Granulomatose mit besonderer Beteiligung des Arteriensystems und der Nieren. Beitraege zur Pathologischen Anatomie und zur Allgemeinen Pathologie, 102: 36.

80. Weimert, T. A., and Gilmore, B. B. 1978. Multiple head and neck hemangiomas in the adult. A case report and review of the literature. Journal of Laryngology and Otology, 92: 937.

81. Windle-Taylor, P. C. 1977. Osteosarcoma of the upper jaw. Journal of Maxillofacial Surgery, 5: 62.

82. Woods, R. 1921. Observations on malignant granuloma of the nose. British Medical Journal 2: 65.

83. Wright, D. 1967. Nasopharyngeal and cervical chordoma—some aspects of their development and treatment. Journal of Laryngology and Otology, 81: 1337.

26 | Hodgkin and Non-Hodgkin Lymphoma Presenting in the Head and Neck

Gianni Bonadonna, M.D.
Roberto Molinari, M.D.
Alberto Banfi, M.D.

INTRODUCTION

Most malignant lymphomas and some leukemias are essentially proliferative diseases of immunologically active cells; hence, the increasingly popular term "immunoproliferative disease" used to describe them collectively. During the past two decades important advances have been made particularly in terms of histopathology, natural history, staging, and therapeutic approach.[5, 12, 15] Much of the progress achieved in the control of this complex group of diseases was derived from accurate staging procedures and from aggressive treatment modalities designed specifically with curative intent. Modern treatment of lymphomas requires experience in the field of clinical oncology and a particular skill in the use of available therapeutic modalities. Although treatment can be successfully coordinated by a practicing physician, patients usually achieve maximum benefit from the improved staging procedures and treatment plans offered at specialized centers. There, medical oncologists, pathologists, and radiation therapists can provide facilities for proper staging, intensive therapy, and adequate supportive treatment. More important, since long-term disease-free survival or cure in given subgroups depends on the initial treatment selection, prospective treatment plans derived from an integrated interdisciplinary approach are more easily performed in specialized institutions.

This chapter will briefly condense the essential information concerning the natural history, the histopathology and staging classification as well as treatment strategy of Hodgkin disease and the non-Hodgkin lymphomas with special reference to the involvement of lymphatic tissue of the head and neck. Physicians should be aware that the enormous impact on current practice for these diseases was built on the fundamental concept that although all types of lymphomas often present with involvement of the head and neck structures, other lesions are frequently concomitant in distant occult sites or rapidly developed in other organs and tissues.

TOPOGRAPHY OF LYMPHATIC TISSUE IN THE HEAD AND NECK AREA

Although lymphoid cells are almost ubiquitous, lymphoid follicles are particularly concentrated in some specific organs such as thymus, spleen, and lymph nodes and in such anatomic sites as the submucosa of the upper respiratory and digestive tract. A certain amount of lymphoid tissue is also present in other structures such as bone, testicle, and salivary glands. Such a distribution is to be borne in mind in the study of lymphomas of the head and neck, since in this region they often arise in extranodal sites. Moreover, an interesting association was recently

699

documented between non-Hodgkin lymphoma in the Waldeyer's ring and in the gastrointestinal tract.

The largest amount of lymphoid tissue in the head and neck region is concentrated in the cervical lymph nodes. A considerable portion of the lymphoid tissue is also concentrated within the pharynx, where nasopharyngeal, palatine, and lingual tonsils constitute real lymphoid organs. Together with very numerous lymphoid follicles distributed in the pharyngeal submucosa, they form the so-called Waldeyer's ring. In addition, ethmoid and nasomaxillary mucosa, salivary glands (especially parotid, submaxillary, and sublingual), and lacrimal glands are sites wherein lymphoid tissue is abundant. Lymphoid follicles are scattered almost everywhere, with a relative preference for oral cavity, bone, and thyroid gland.

HISTOLOGICAL CLASSIFICATION

The malignant lymphomas comprise a broad spectrum of cell types and histopathologic patterns. Accurate diagnosis and classification constitutes one of the most difficult topics in morphologic examination of one or more tissue specimens. Prerequisites include adequate biopsies and technical excellence in the preparation of tissue slides. Without benefit of the normal architecture of an intact lymph node, the pathologist frequently cannot differentiate a lymphoma from a benign process. In recent years, the examination of imprints and smears of fresh lymph node biopsy material as well as the use of electron microscopy morphology and the study of immunologic membrane markers has greatly improved the classification of human lymphoid malignancies.

Currently, lymphoma is classified into Hodgkin disease and non-Hodgkin lymphoma. This oversimplified terminology attempts not only to overcome decades of controversy and confusion, but to facilitate communication among clinicians. While research and conceptual disputes continue,

physicians should be aware of the important achievements that were found to be reproducible and to bear clinical relevance.

In 1965 at an International Symposium held in Rye, New York, the classification originally proposed for Hodgkin disease by Lukes and Butler was modified by a Nomenclature Committee into four groups: nodular sclerosis, lymphocytic predominance, mixed cellularity and lymphocytic depletion.[10a] The Rye classification was widely accepted by clinicians not only because of its simplicity and reproducibility but because it gives a crude correlation with prognosis and is therefore useful in management. The separation of cases of Hodgkin disease into the four histologic types is subjective; no clear-cut rules exist that permit unquestionable classification of every case into one of the four categories. Admittedly, the mixed cellularity group is a less clearly defined category and includes a range of cases. The cell population in Hodgkin disease is heterogenous. The precise nature of neoplastic cells, i.e., Reed-Sternberg cells and their mononuclear counterparts, has not yet been established. Recent studies have strongly suggested derivation from the monocyte-macrophage system.[3]

The term non-Hodgkin lymphoma comprises a group of primary neoplasms of the lymphoreticular tissue which involves stem cells and lymphocytes or histiocytes in varying degrees of differentiation. These neoplasms occur essentially in a homogenous population of a single cell type. The term itself and the many classifications proposed reflect the difficulties encountered in the morphologic characterization of these proliferative processes. The tendency of different authors to apply the same terms to different entities has compounded the problem of communicating the diagnosis and of comparing the results of therapy.

A detailed discussion on new experimental classifications is beyond the scope of this chapter. Clinicians should first be aware that the terminology of lymphosarcoma, reticulum cell sarcoma, and giant follicular lymphoma that was widely used in the past is no longer considered adequate to characterize various processes morphologically. About a decade ago the histologic classification that Rappaport proposed in 1956 was rediscovered and gradually applied to clinicopathologic as well as to treatment studies, both retrospective and prospective.[12] The original Rappaport classification, although not up to date with the understanding of modern immunology, was found by clinicians to be an effective tool, identifying important distinctions in prognosis between the generally indolent nodular (or follicular) lymphomas and the more aggressive diffuse lymphomas. In addition to architectural patterns of growth, the Rappaport scheme describes the malignant cell population as either lymphocytic, histiocytic, or mixed lymphocytic-histiocytic. Again, there is a prognostic value, in that lymphocytic cytology is more favorable than a histiocytic one in both the nodular and diffuse lymphomas. For prognostic and therapeutic purposes, most clinicians have termed as *favorable* histology the nodular lymphocytic, nodular mixed lymphocytic-histiocytic, and diffuse lymphocytic well-differentiated lymphomas, and as *unfavorable* histology all diffuse lymphomas as well as those with nodular histiocytic lymphoma.[12, 15]

Most dissatisfaction with the Rappaport scheme resulted from the recognition that many lymphomas, termed histiocytic by Rappaport on morphologic grounds alone, have recently been shown by ultrastructural and immunologic techniques to be neoplasms of large or transformed lymphocytes. Therefore, the term "histiocytic" is a misnomer and the true histiocytic tumors are very rare.[3, 12, 15] New classification systems have been recently proposed based on functional studies (e.g. the Lukes and Collins classification and the Lennert classification subsequently modified into the Kiel classification).[12, 15] However, none of the newer classification systems have yet been established as superior to the Rappaport scheme, especially in terms of reproducibility and clinicopathologic correlations.

Today, the classification of Rappaport is utilized by most hemopathologists with some modifications[3, 12] as reproduced in Table 26-1. With new immunologic and cytochemical techniques, it is now widely acknowledged that all nodular lymphomas are composed of monoclonal neoplastic follicular B-lymphocytes. Non-Hodgkin lymphomas with a diffuse pattern of growth are heterogeneous clinically and morphologically. Biopsy specimens cannot distinguish between lymphocytic well-differentiated lymphoma and chronic lymphocytic leukemia. These diseases bear identical monoclonal B-cell markers, and this strongly supports the concept that both processes are

TABLE 26-1. HISTOLOGICAL CLASSIFICATION OF NON-HODGKIN LYMPHOMAS

Type	Marker
Nodular (follicular) pattern	
Lymphocytic, well differentiated	B-cell
Lymphocytic, poorly differentiated	
Mixed lymphocytic— "histiocytic"	Heterogeneous
"Histiocytic"	
Diffuse pattern	
Lymphocytic, well differentiated	B-cell
Lymphocytic, intermediate differentiation	
Lymphocytic, poorly differentiated	
Mixed lymphocytic— "histiocytic"	
"Histiocytic"	Heterogeneous
Undifferentiated, pleomorphic (non-Burkitt)	
Undifferentiated, Burkitt type	B-cell
Lymphoblastic (with and without convoluted cells)	T-cell
Unclassified	

clinicopathologic variants of a single neoplastic disorder. The large cell lymphomas ("histiocytic," mixed lymphocytic-"histiocytic," and undifferentiated non-Burkitt) are often difficult to classify on histologic grounds. Approximately 50 to 60 percent of non-Hodgkin lymphoma cases have B-cell features, while far fewer have T-cell markers (5 to 10 percent) or a monocytic-histiocytic origin (5 percent). In about one-third of the cases the cells lack detectable markers ("undefined" or "null"). In Burkitt lymphoma of African and non-African patients, the monotonous population of morphologically "primitive" cells may be related to some B-lymphocytes of normal germinal centers. In about 50 percent of lymphoblastic lymphomas, there are distinctive convoluted nuclear configurations (convoluted lymphoblastic lymphoma). Lymphoblastic lymphomas occur most commonly in the adolescent age group. The clinical and immunologic features indicate that lymphoblastic lymphomas are tumors essentially identical to acute lymphoblastic leukemia of T-cell type. Other lymphoreticular neoplasms in which T-cell markers have been detected in most cases are mycosis fungoides and Sezary syndrome.[3]

In children, only a limited number of known histologic types of non-Hodgkin lymphoma are encountered. The nodular pattern is almost universally absent and all subgroups show histologically a high-grade malignancy. The histologic types include lymphoblastic lymphoma (with or without convoluted cells), Burkitt lymphoma, and "histiocytic" lymphoma.

CLINICAL MANIFESTATIONS

Incidence of Primary Involvement

Nearly 80 percent of all malignant lymphomas arise in the lymph nodes, and the neck represents the primary clinical localization in approximately half of the cases. The occurrence in cervical lymph nodes is predominant in Hodgkin disease (65 to 70 percent) compared with non-Hodgkin lymphoma (about 30 percent). When only the cervical nodes are involved, the age and sex distribution is similar to the well-known general pattern of lymphomas, even if striking differences emerge from studies on geographic distribution. In general, the incidence of Hodgkin disease is prevalent in patients aged less than 30 years, while the opposite occurs for non-Hodgkin lymphoma. The male to female ratio is 3:2 for Hodgkin disease and 5:3 for non-Hodgkin lymphoma.

Primary extranodal presentation is exceptional in Hodgkin disease (1 percent); whereas, this occurs in 20 percent of patients with non-Hodgkin lymphoma. Within the latter group, the most commonly involved site is the head and neck area (38 percent), followed by the gastrointestinal tract (30 percent). The remaining primary extranodal sites are distributed among different organs and tissues in the body. The distribution shows a wide geographic variability. In the head and neck, the most commonly involved extranodal sites (Fig. 26-1) are those forming Waldeyer's ring.[2, 9, 14] This prevalence greatly varies from series to series (44 percent up to 81 percent) according to reports from different countries. The remaining extranodal non-Hodgkin lymphomas are distributed in a wider range of sites in the head and neck, such as the nasal cavities, ethmoidal and maxillary sinuses (15 percent), orbit (8 percent), salivary glands (8 percent), oral cavity (5 percent), and thyroid (3 percent). The majority of extranodal non-Hodgkin lymphomas show a diffuse histologic pattern, and diffuse histiocytic lymphoma represents the single largest subgroup.[14] Burkitt lymphoma is nearly always extranodal. Extranodal non-Hodgkin lymphomas of the head and neck can occur in every age group. However, they are more frequently observed in younger patients (third to fifth decade). Localization other than Waldeyer's ring seems to be slightly predominant in children and adolescents, while in elderly patients the most frequent primary site is the tonsil. In general, no pre-

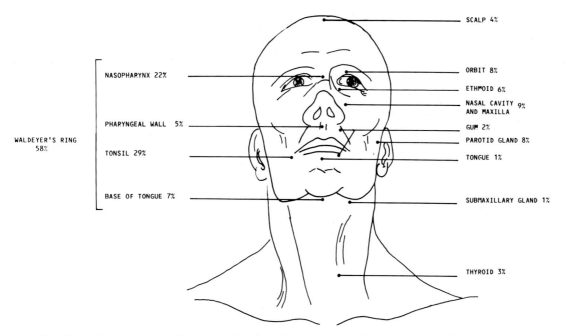

Fig. 26-1. Most commonly involved sites in primary extranodal lymphomas of the head and neck.

dilection of site is demonstrable in either sex.

Clinical Presentations

CERVICAL NODES

Cervical adenopathy is frequently the initial sign of malignant lymphomas. Since it can also represent the only first sign of many other illnesses, ranging from a benign extranodal lump to a metastasis of malignant tumors located either within the head and neck area or in distant organs below the clavicle, the knowledge of some semeiologic features can strongly help in the diagnostic approach.

When the largest diameter of the node is less than 2 cm, no firm semeiologic rules are available for a differential diagnosis even between benign inflammation or malignancy. If the size is greater, the node should always be considered suspicious. Therefore, every effort should be made in order to first exclude or confirm the concomitance of an extranodal malignancy.

The single lymphomatous node is generally firm, but softer and more elastic than a metastasis from epidermoid cancer; the former is mobile and its surface is smooth. The adenopathy of Hodgkin disease is frequently more firm than that of non-Hodgkin lymphoma. Multiple nodes are more frequently seen in the latter illness, wherein they can also be bilateral (one-fourth of cases) and confluent. Mobility can be maintained also in very large isolated nodes, but frequently two or three nodes conglomerate in one polycyclic mass. Non-Hodgkin lymphoma preferentially presents in the upper cervical nodes; whereas, Hodgkin disease can be detected in every site of the cervical region, with a slight prevalence in supraclavicular nodes. In the presence of a single supraclavicular lymphomatous node, pathology nearly always reveals Hodgkin disease (Fig. 26-2). The evolution of the adenopathy is also important in differential diagnosis. A rapidly progressive growth is more frequently seen in non-Hodgkin lymphoma, while in Hodgkin disease the lymph node or nodes usually grow slowly and often fluctuate. However, the most important diag-

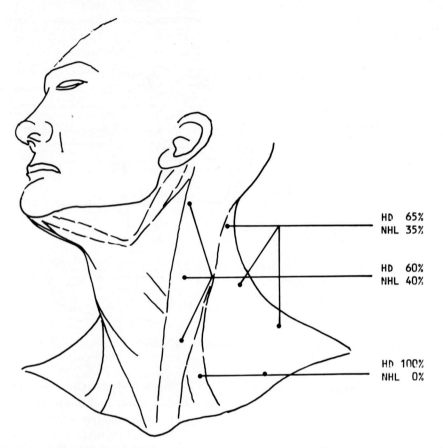

HD   65%
NHL 35%

HD   60%
NHL 40%

HD 100%
NHL 0%

Fig. 26-2. Relative incidence of Hodgkin Disease (HD) and non-Hodgkin lymphoma (NHL) with primary cervical presentation.

nostic problem is to differentiate a lymphoma from neck metastases of epidermoid cancer.

WALDEYER'S RING

Palatine Tonsil.   The most frequently involved site within the pharynx is the palatine tonsil, where non-Hodgkin lymphoma represents 25 percent of all malignant tumors. Early symptoms are few. Frequently, the first sign is only a feeling of obstruction even in the presence of a very large mass. Pain is rare and occurs when the tumor ulcerates. Three clinical presentations are possible:

1. Hypertrophic tonsil, wherein the covering mucosa is reddish, and smooth and the crypts are levelled; this is the most com-

mon aspect revealed by an ENT routine examination performed in the presence of a lymphomatous neck node.

2. The tonsil is very large (filling the soft palate and the pharyngeal wall), with no ulceration; the appearance is that of a painless phlegmon.

3. The tonsil is replaced by frank neoplastic tissue, widely ulcerated; the ulcer can involve soft palate, pillars, and pharyngeal wall.

Concomitant neck adenopathy is very frequent (75 to 80 percent of cases), mainly in the third type of presentation. Bilateral involvement is not exceptional, and sometimes clinical examination or biopsy samples reveal multiple localizations within Waldeyer's ring. When the lesion is locally advanced, especially if associated with cervical adenopathy, the diagnosis of malignancy is easy and histology can solve a clinical doubt between epithelial or lymphoproliferative tumor. In earlier phases, i.e., when the tumor is ulcerated, a correct diagnosis (particularly of young patients) can be difficult if the physician is not aware of the possible neoplastic nature of the illness. The most common mistakes are represented by protracted treatment with antibiotics, incision of a hypothetic phlegmon, and tonsillectomy without histopathologic documentation. A unilateral enlarged tonsil in a young man or woman is to be considered suspicious and requires biopsy, with the sample taken deeply from the tonsillar tissue. It should be remembered that this procedure is almost painless even without anesthesia.

Nasopharynx. This localization of lymphoma is less frequent than that of the palatine tonsil. Again, early symptoms are very few and consist of hearing loss, mainly unilateral, and of respiratory obstruction. Pain, bleeding, and neurologic signs are rare compared with their occurrence in epidermoid or undifferentiated cancer. Radiologic signs of bone involvement are also rare (<10 percent). Nasopharyngeal lymphoma presents almost always as a fungating tumor and can completely fill the cavity. Nasal cavities or ethmoid cells can be involved by the tumor, and in this case the real primary site can remain doubtful. Neck adenopathies are generally concomitant in 90 percent of the cases. In children, cervical adenopathy is the only sign that may arouse suspicion of malignancy, since adenoiditis is a common illness in this age group. In adults the differential diagnosis between lymphoma and nasopharyngeal carcinoma can be difficult clinically and histopathologically.

Base of Tongue and Pharyngeal Walls. Like the nasopharyngeal tonsil, if not more so, the lymphoid tissue of the base of the tongue undergoes a progressive involution after puberty. Consequently, this localization of lymphoma is rare (less than 15 percent of all malignant tumors of this region). The same incidence is estimated for the other oropharyngeal regions, wherein the soft palate is the most frequently involved

site. The most frequent symptom in both the base of the tongue and the pharyngeal walls, is the appearance of a guttural voice, often associated with dysphagia. The lymphomatous lesion presents the same features as described for the other pharyngeal sites, that is, soft, fungating, and not ulcerated. Deep infiltration is exceptional.

OTHER EXTRANODAL SITES

Nasal and Paranasal Cavities. Lymphomas represent 3 to 8 percent of all malignant tumors occurring in the nasomaxillary region. The incidence of different localizations varies from series to series with the lateral wall of the nasal cavity prevailing. The upper gingiva and the hard palate are rarely affected. Symptoms are not early and consist of serous-hemorrhagic discharge, nasal obstruction, bleeding, and, sometimes, pain. The lymphomatous tissue fills the cavity and can be visible through the nostril or through posterior rhinoscopy. Quite often, a concomitant sinusitis makes the diagnosis difficult. When the tumor is located in the ethmoid, the most common objective sign is represented by a swelling of the internal contour of the orbit or by a levelling of the sulcus between nose and cheek. Cervical adenopathy is present in about one-fourth of all the cases.

Orbit. Primary lymphoma of the orbit frequently occurs as a growing mass displacing the eyeball and is mainly localized in the upper external part of the cavity. Like other orbital malignancies, tumor progression can cause a number of physical signs that are typical for this region (Fig. 26-3).

Salivary Glands. The incidence of lymphoma in salivary glands (Fig. 26-4) is controversial, since it is often difficult to establish whether the primary site of origin is the salivary parenchyma or an adjacent lymph node. Early symptoms and signs are not different from those of benign salivary tumors, and the histologic diagnosis of lymphoma often represents an unpleasant surprise after parotidectomy.

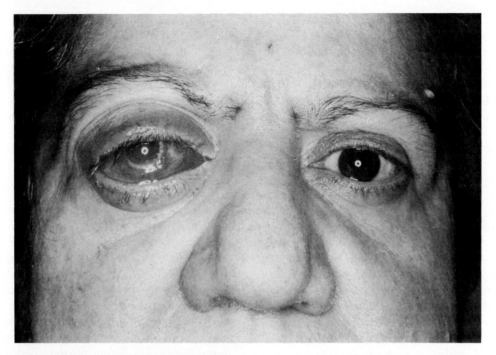

Fig. 26-3. Diffuse lymphocytic poorly-differentiated primary lymphoma in the orbital cavity.

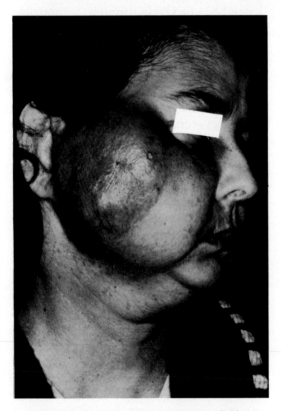

Fig. 26-4. Voluminous non-Hodgkin lymphoma of the parotid gland with infiltration of the skin.

BURKITT LYMPHOMA

In tropical Africa, this type of lymphoma constitutes approximately 50 percent of all malignancies occurring in children and affects males more than females. In the United States and in Europe this type of lymphoma is very rare and presents a different clinical pattern.[16] In African children the tumor shows a striking predilection for one or more parts of the jaw (50 percent of the cases). The first sign is loosening of teeth, and the tumor develops mainly intraorally. The maxilla is involved three times more frequently than the mandible. The tumor grows rapidly, causing a progressive enlargement of the jaw and producing a marked deformity (Figs. 26-5 A and B). In one-third of the patients a concomitant abdominal involvement (ovary, kidney, retroperitoneal lymph nodes) is present. Pain is almost absent and is due only to tumor bulk. In nonendemic areas, the onset in the jaw is infrequent and abdominal involvement predominates. Neck adenopathy, which is very rare in Africa, is more frequently present in non-African children

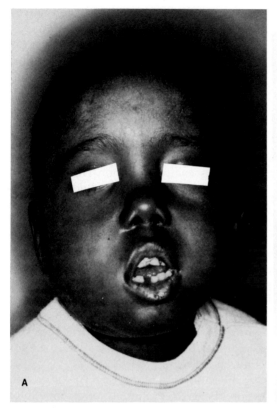
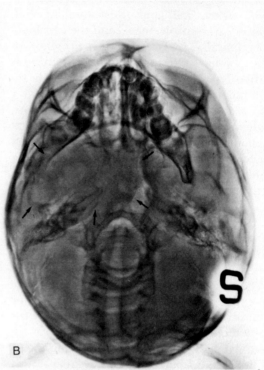

Fig. 26-5. (A) Burkitt lymphoma in a 5-year-old Somalian child. Clinically the tumor involves the maxilla, the mandible, and the pterygomaxillary fossa. (B) Roentgenogram (axial view) of the same patient showing involvement by tumor of the mandible and the base of the skull.

and can represent in these patients the first sign of the illness.

Other clinical presentations of head and neck lymphomas are very seldom reported.[9, 14] A relatively high incidence is found in the thyroid, internal ear and temporal bone, scalp, skin of the face, and mandible. Finally, simultaneous involvement of multiple sites is rather frequent, mainly within Waldeyer's ring.

DIAGNOSIS AND STAGING

Initial Diagnosis

Proper rules for correct initial diagnosis can be summarized as follows:

1. In the presence of extranodal disease, the first biopsy should be performed on the primary tumor, even if cervical ad-

enopathies are present. Once the diagnosis of lymphoma is established, the removal of one or more lymph nodes is recommended for a more precise histologic classification. When repeated punch biopsies are histologically negative or inconclusive, whatever type of surgical approach necessary for diagnosis should be performed, e.g., tonsillectomy with serial microscopic examination in suspicious cases. It should be remembered that primary aggressive surgical treatment of extranodal lymphoma is rarely indicated.

2. In cases of cervical nodal presentation, the clinician should first rule out the presence of a primary carcinoma in order not to reduce the chance of success of subsequent radical treatment by an untimely node biopsy. A thorough head and neck examination is mandatory even when the diagnosis of lymphoma is already known from a previous cervical biopsy. In either case, two op-

posite semeiologic features must be remembered: a cervical mass can displace the pharyngeal wall and thus simulate Waldeyer's ring involvement; and the capability of clinically appreciating the presence of lymphoma within the lymphoid structures is often limited so biopsies are frequently required.

3. A correct cervical biopsy consists, whenever possible, of the removal by excisional biopsy of one or more deeply situated lymph nodes in their entirety. Needle and frozen-sections biopsies are not helpful in diagnosing lymphomas.

Proper Staging

During the past 15 years, different efforts were made to properly stage lymphomas. The intent was always that of improving the method of selecting patients suitable for curative radiotherapy and those suitable for a systemic treatment program with or without irradiation. Over the years, lymphography, needle-marrow biopsy, laparotomy, and laparoscopy have become important

steps in the clinical accuracy for staging lymphomas of both adults and children. The systematic use of available procedures to determine the extent of disease led first to the Rye (1965)[10a] and then to the Ann Arbor (1971)[7a] International Staging Classifications for Hodgkin disease. The latter staging system has also been adopted for the group of non-Hodgkin lymphomas. At present, the clinical utility of the Ann Arbor staging system is less evident for non-Hodgkin lymphoma, and especially for childhood non-Hodgkin lymphoma. In fact, besides the frequent difficulty in the assignment of all types of extranodal presentation to the four established stage designations the survival of most patients with *nodular* lymphoma is prolonged even when bone marrow disease is evident at presentation and the survival of patients with *diffuse* lymphomas tends to be comparatively short even with nodal disease alone. The latter is particularly true for children.

The adoption of the Ann Arbor classification (Table 26-2) implies a dual system of stage designation: clinical staging (CS) and

TABLE 26-2. THE ANN ARBOR STAGING CLASSIFICATION[7a]

Stage I
   Involvement of a single lymph node region or of a single extralymphatic organ or site (IE)

Stage II
   Involvement of two or more lymph node regions on the same side of the diaphragm, or localized involvement of an extranodal organ or site (IIE) and of one or more lymph node regions on the same side of the diaphragm

Stage III
   Involvement of lymph node regions on both sides of the diaphragm, which may also be accompanied by localized involvement of an extranodal organ or site (IIIE) or spleen (IIIS) or both (IIISE)

Stage IV
   Diffuse or disseminated involvement of one or more distant extranodal organs with or without associated lymph node involvement

In addition
   Fever > 38° C (100.5° F), night sweats, and/or weight loss > 10 percent of body weight in the 6 months preceeding admission are defined as systemic symptoms, and denoted by the suffix letter B. Asymptomatic patients are denoted by the suffix letter A.
   Biopsy-documented involvement of stage IV sites is identified by the following symbols: marrow = M+; liver = H+; lung = L+; pleura = P+; bone = O+; skin = D+.

pathologic staging (PS). Clinical staging is decided on the basis of the history, physical examination, initial diagnostic biopsy, laboratory tests, and radiographic studies of the patient. Pathologic staging adds definitive additional histopathologic information obtained through biopsy of strategic sites (bone marrow, liver, spleen, abdominal nodes) as well as other clinically involved tissue (bone, skin, lung,). The classification also incorporates the concept that certain selected patients with localized extranodal "E" disease (Waldeyer's ring, bone, skin) have a more favorable prognosis than patients with clearly disseminated (stage IV) involvement.

Table 26-3 outlines the procedures deemed necessary to carry out correct CS and PS. Most of the studies should be repeated once the initial treatment is completed; this repetition is needed to properly assess the status of complete remission or to restage the presence of a single recurrence. One of the major differences at presentation between patients with Hodgkin disease and those with other malignant lymphomas is the marked tendency for extranodal involvement in non-Hodgkin lymphoma. As a result, in non-Hodgkin lymphoma much more attention must be paid to such areas as bone, liver, gastrointestinal tract, Waldeyer's ring, and bone marrow. The last is undoubtedly the most important single organ to evaluate thoroughly prior to the initiation of treatment. Bone marrow biopsy, with or without aspiration, is an essential part of the staging procedures.

Due to the high incidence of primary site in Waldeyer's ring in non-Hodgkin lymphoma, physical examination should include a systematic exploration of the pharynx with biopsy on any evident or suspicious growth. Since about 20 percent of all patients with lesions in Waldeyer's ring also show involvement of the stomach either at the time of initial presentation or within 2 years of diagnosis,[2] gastroscopy is strongly recommended in cases with pharyngeal lymphoma.

More aggressive staging techniques, including exploratory laparotomy and laparoscopy, have been advocated in recent years.[6] Laparotomy has provided an unparalleled contribution to staging accuracy and knowledge of the natural history of all lymphomas. In fact in adult Hodgkin disease that is CS I or II because of cervical adenopathy, laparotomy can detect occult abdominal disease in about 20 percent of patients (liver 1 to 4 percent, spleen 15 to 20 percent, abdominal nodes 5 to 10 percent). In comparative patients with CS I or II non-Hodgkin lymphoma, the occult findings are in 30 to 40 percent of patients (liver 15 to 20 percent, spleen 20 to 25 percent, abdominal nodes 20 to 40 percent). Among adult patients with nodal and extranodal presentation, the lowest risk of occult distant disease exists for cases classified as diffuse histiocytic lymphoma (<10 percent) and the highest risk for cases classified as nodular lymphoma (up to 40 percent).[6, 8, 12, 15]

Today the role of routine laparotomy as a staging procedure should be critically reevaluated for lymphoma patients in general.[6] However, staging laparotomy remains a necessary procedure for those patients in whom treatment continues to be based on radiotherapy alone such as those with CS I and II Hodgkin disease. In patients with localized non-Hodgkin lymphoma for whom combined radiotherapy-chemotherapy appears indicated, recent sequential studies[6, 8] have shown that laparoscopy with four to six hepatic biopsies can substitute for laparotomy to detect or rule out stage IV diseases. The advantages of laparoscopy over laparotomy are represented by the fact that the first can be easily repeated to restage patients, can be performed under local anesthesia, produces minimal morbidity and reduces costs and stay in the hospital. Laparotomy may be necessary as a final procedure for CS I and II patients who have diffuse histiocytic lymphoma. In fact, once this type of surgical staging rules out the presence of occult abdominal disease, a high relapse-free survival can be obtained with extensive radiotherapy alone.[4]

In children with head and neck lymphomas, staging procedures for Hodgkin

TABLE 26-3. DIAGNOSTIC WORKUPS

Necessary Procedures for Proper Staging

CS
1. Detailed history with special attention to the presence or absence of systemic symptoms.
2. Careful physical examination, emphasizing peripheral node chains, size of liver and spleen, Waldeyer's ring, and bony tenderness.
3. Adequate surgical biopsy reviewed by an experienced hemopathologist. In primary extranodal lymphomas, biopsy should also include a lymph node when palpable.
4. Routine laboratory tests: complete blood count, erythrosedimentation rate, liver function tests, serum uric acid, serum copper.
5. Chest roentgenogram (anteroposterior and lateral) and bilateral lower extremity lymphography.
6. Roentgenologic examination of the gastrointestinal tract in non-Hodgkin lymphoma. Gastroscopy should be added in the presence of Waldeyer's ring involvement.

PS
7. Core needle biopsy of bone marrow from posterior iliac crest. Biopsy should be bilateral especially in non-Hodgkin lymphoma.
8. Laparoscopy with multiple liver biopsies if procedure 7 is normal and no other distant extranodal lesions are present. In Hodgkin disease, laparoscopy is indicated in CS IB, IIB, IIIA and IIIB if the treatment program consists of combined radiotherapy-chemotherapy; in CS IA with involvement of upper cervical nodes and lymphocytic predominance histology; in obese, elderly, and emotionally unstable patients; and in cases with other systemic diseases. Laparoscopy is indicated in all adult patients with non-Hodgkin lymphoma.
9. Exploratory laparotomy with splenectomy, needle and wedge biopsy of liver, and biopsies of para-aortic, mesenteric, portal, and splenic hilar lymph nodes is indicated in Hodgkin disease with CS I and II (A and B) and IIIA if therapeutic decisions will depend on the identification of splenic involvement. In non-Hodgkin lymphoma, laparotomy remains an investigational tool for research centers. It may be necessary as a final procedure for CS I and II diffuse histiocytic lymphoma.
10. Lumbar puncture with cytologic examination of cerebrospinal fluid in all children with non-Hodgkin lymphoma.
11. Cytologic examination of any effusions.

Useful Procedures in Certain Patients

1. Additional laboratory tests: Coombs test, serum protein electrophoresis, and quantitative immunoglobulins.
2. Mediastinal tomograms and chest tomograms.
3. Intravenous pyelogram if bulky retroperitoneal nodes are present or if abdominal radiation therapy is planned.
4. Skeletal survey (thoracolumbar vertebrae, pelvis, proximal extremities) in the presence of areas of bone tenderness or pain. Roentgenogram of the base of skull in non-Hodgkin lymphoma with nasopharyngeal involvement.
5. Radioisotopic evaluation as needed of liver, spleen, bone and brain; tumor scan with gallium-67-citrate or indium-111-labeled bleomycin when the results of other conventional diagnostic procedures are not conclusive.
6. Abdominal sonography or computed tomography.
7. Immunologic evaluation: skin tests (Varidase, mumps, *Candida*), immunization with neoantigens (DNCB, KLH), peripheral blood lymphocyte typing.

disease are practically identical to those used in adults. Pediatric patients usually show a comparative lesser incidence of liver infiltration and a higher incidence of splenic involvement. In children with non-Hodgkin lymphoma, excessive staging procedures do not appear to be worthwhile in devising a therapeutic strategy. However, CS (whenever possible with lymphography) must be supplemented by marrow biopsy (with or without aspiration) and cytologic examination of spinal fluid.

NATURAL HISTORY

Hodgkin Disease

The clinical course of patients with disease limited to head and neck structures is not substantially different than that of patients with stage I and II (A and B) disease in whom the disease originated in other sites. In practically all patients the disease involves the lymph nodes. The rare cases (1 percent) with Waldeyer's ring involvement show a clinical course similar to that seen in cases with primary onset in the cervical lymph nodes.

The most significant information on the mode of spread is derived from the retrospective evaluation of older series in which radiotherapy was the only therapeutic tool and the irradiation was not systematically extended to adjacent uninvolved lymphatic sites. Through this evaluation it can be established that patients do exist who are definitely cured after irradiation delivered only to the involved site where the disease, in accordance with the theory of unicentric origin, was really localized. Usually, these types of patients are few (4 to 5 percent) and are mostly young males presenting with a single adenopathy located in the upper cervical area or in the Waldeyer's ring and with lymphocytic predominance histologically.

In all other patients the clinical course is well known for Hodgkin disease. When there is progressive disease, aside from the cases with true or marginal recurrence, initial new manifestations occur in about 80 percent of cases in nodal sites; there is a predilection for those sites that are anatomically contiguous (subclavicular, axillary, mediastinal) or functionally related (para-aortic). In about 20 percent of patients the disease recurs in distant nodal chains (iliac and inguinal) or in extranodal sites (liver, lung, bone marrow). In particular, one should remember that the presence of adenopathy in the supraclavicular fossa can represent an indirect manifestation of occult disease that is either in the mediastinum or in the retroperitoneal node chains in spite of negative chest roentgenogram or lymphography or even exploratory laparotomy.

The majority of treatment failures occur within 4 years from initial therapy. However, relapse can be observed even after several years and diagnosis can often be delayed when the disease is localized in deep sites (e.g. mediastinum and abdomen).

Non-Hodgkin Lymphomas

EXTRANODAL PRESENTATION

The involvement of an extranodal site often represents the only clinical manifestation of non-Hodgkin lymphoma.[2, 9, 14] This has been demonstrated by the possibility of achieving cure in a certain number of cases by delivering radiotherapy only to the involved area. Diffuse histiocytic lymphoma is the most frequent histologic subgroup. Disease progression can occur along three main pathways:[4] local progression with invasion of surrounding structures, involvement of regional lymph nodes, dissemination to noncontiguous lymph nodes, and/or distant extranodal sites.

Local progression can represent, even for a long period of time, the only type of growth. In particular, this occurs for non-Hodgkin lymphoma arising from the orbit and paranasal sinuses, as well as that from the parotid gland. In these cases the lymphoma tends to overcome the anatomic confines of the involved region by invading the surrounding tissues, with extensive destruction of the adjacent bone structures.

The early involvement of regional lymph nodes is the most common mode of spread from Waldeyer's ring lymphomas.[2, 14] This is demonstrated by the subsequent course of the disease and by the high incidence of patients (40 to 50 percent) presenting with cervical adenopathy as the first sign of disease or by patients with CS II who, at the time of diagnosis, show unilateral or bilateral cervical adenopathy as the only apparent sign of disease besides the Waldeyer's ring involvement (over 90 percent). The tendency to early involvement of regional nodes is only evident for other extranodal primary sites.[9, 14] However, primary non-Hodgkin lymphoma in the nasopharyngeal space can present with concomitant involvement of regional nodes and local invasion of surrounding structures such as the base of the skull.[2]

The third mode of spread is represented by involvement of distant node chains (retroperitoneal, mesenteric, inguinal) or viscera (liver, lung) and distant extranodal sites (bone marrow and skin). Subsequent mediastinal involvement occurs rarely in patients with non-Hodgkin lymphoma compared with its occurrence in those with Hodgkin disease. This type of spread is similar to the metastatic dissemination observed with carcinomas and is a prognostically unfavorable sign, since the lymphoma cannot be controlled by radiotherapy alone. The results obtained in recent series studied with lymphography, laparoscopy, and exploratory laparotomy,[6, 8, 12, 15] and, therefore selected from the point of view of staging, have indicated that occult dissemination is present in a considerable number (30 to 40 percent) of patients with CS I and II and particularly in patients with nodular histology. New clinical manifestations can develop early during the course of radiotherapy (about 10 percent of patients). In the majority of patients (70 to 80 percent) relapses are documented within the first 2 years from the end of primary treatment. In children with primary extranodal non-Hodgkin lymphoma of the head and neck, the invasion of bone marrow and the central nervous system is frequent and early.

The association between Waldeyer's ring and gastrointestinal (in particular, the stomach) involvement is not unusual. It can be seen both initially and as the first and often the sole sign of relapse in 10 to 15 percent of patients with CS I and II. This association should receive more attention from epidemiologic studies, and is important for staging and therapeutic decisions.[2, 14]

NODAL PRESENTATION

The course of non-Hodgkin lymphoma presenting with unilateral or bilateral cervical adenopathy is markedly influenced by the histologic type (favorable and unfavorable histology).[11, 12, 15]

Diffuse lymphomas, and especially the diffuse histiocyte type, show a spread that is similar to that of primary extranodal lymphomas. In fact, there is the possibility that patients classified as PS I have a true localized disease and can therefore be cured with limited radiotherapy alone. There is also the tendency to spread initially to contiguous lymphatic sites or, occasionally, to extranodal sites of the head and neck (e.g. Waldeyer's ring and the salivary glands). More often, the disease rapidly spreads to distant nodal and extranodal sites. The involvement of mediastinal nodes and of the gastrointestinal tract is rare. In the presence of nodular lymphomas, the disease is rarely localized.[12, 15] The lymphoma is often occult in distant sites such as the mesenteric nodes, bone marrow, and liver. In most patients with initial "localized" nodular lymphoma, the disease shows an indolent course with subsequent recurrences that can be documented even after many years from primary therapy.

Burkitt Lymphoma

The clinical course of this type of lymphoma as observed in Europe and in North America is not substantially different from that of patients described in Africa.[16] When the disease is localized to head and neck structures, extranodal tissues are preferentially involved, namely maxilla, orbit, mandible, and thyroid. The tendency to invade the surrounding tissues and to involve more extranodal structures is characteristic.

In patients with involvement of head and neck structures, disease progression occurs in 40 to 50 percent of the patients. In about half of the patients relapsing after complete remission induced by chemotherapy, there is a rapid regrowth of tumor in the initial site(s) within 10 weeks from the first dose of chemotherapy. In patients with this early relapse, there is a concomitant spread to the central nervous system (about 50 percent of cases) and the prognosis is poor. In the remaining relapsing patients, new disease manifestations occur late and preferentially in distant uninvolved sites. The late relapses rarely involve the central nervous system. In these patients the tumor can again respond to retreatment with chemotherapy and prognosis is definitely better compared to that of the first group.

TREATMENT STRATEGY AND CURRENT RESULTS

General Principles

Treatment for all types of lymphomas should be built upon a strategically designed approach for each histologic subgroup and stage. It is highly recommended that both primary therapy as well as treatment for recurrent disease result from a prior agreement between radiation therapists and medical oncologists. Treatment can be individualized in the presence of emergency situations, involvement of strategic site(s), and old age.

Whenever possible, for the majority of untreated patients, the approach must have curative intent regardless of stage. Physicians must be aware of current concepts concerning complete remission, restaging procedures, disease-free survival, supportive therapy, and acute and late treatment morbidity.

It is essential that certain features be available for optimal modern radiotherapeutic techniques: megavoltage beam energies of a linear acclerator or ^{60}Co teletherapy unit, with a capability of treatment distances of 100 to 140 cm; the capability of treating large fields to encompass multiple node chains both anteriorly and posteriorly; and the employment of doses in the tumoricidal dose range for malignant lymphomas, i.e. approximately 3,500 rads over 3.5 to 4 weeks to 4,500 rads over 4 to 6 weeks. To properly shape a large field, a simulator is essential to permit special individualization for a given patient.

As far as chemotherapy is concerned, physicians must be familiar with the use of modern effective combination regimens, with the concepts of prolonged cyclical therapy and dose reduction schedule in the presence of temporary toxicity, as well as with the technique of treating patients on an ambulatory basis. In general, single agent chemotherapy is employed only in a few circumstances, such as for elderly patients with concomitant severe illnesses, those living in isolated areas, and patients with psychological disturbances. In certain nodular lymphomas, good results may be obtained with single agents.

Hodgkin Disease

During the past decade, the treatment of Hodgkin disease has evolved into a fairly established strategic approach based primarily upon pathologic stage and presence or absence of systemic symptoms. The majority of patients in whom after pathologic staging with laparotomy the disease appears limited to one or both cervical regions present with no systemic symptoms (PS IA and IEA, and

IIA and IIEA). For these patients the recommended primary treatment is radiotherapy including the mantle (bilateral neck, axillae, mediastinal and bilateral hilar structures in-continuity) and a "spade" field (para-aortic, common iliac, and splenic pedicle in-continuity) to tumoricidal dose levels. Whenever cervical involvement is detected in the upper cervical region (i.e. above the level of the thyroid notch), a matching Waldeyer's field is added to include the preauricular nodes. The results of aggressive radiotherapy yield a 5-year disease-free survival rate of 75 to 80 percent and a total survival rate in excess of 90 percent. For patients with PS IB or IEB or IIB or IIEB, the most often utilized treatment is total nodal irradiation with mantle and full inverted Y fields that include pelvic and iliofemoral lymph nodes. Again, a 75 to 80 percent disease-free survival rate is obtained.

The use in both A and B groups of adjuvant chemotherapy with six cycles of MOPP (nitrogen mustard, vincristine, procarbazine, and prednisone) significantly improves the initial freedom from relapse duration but improvement in the total survival rate is only minimal and not yet significant. Therefore, adjuvant MOPP cannot yet be recommended as a routine addition to the radiation management of PS I and II Hodgkin disease.[13] Furthermore, there are reports showing an increased risk of second neoplasms (e.g. acute myeloblastic leukemia) in patients who receive both radiotherapy and MOPP chemotherapy.[1]

The major side effects during the course of radiotherapy include hair loss over the occipital area, dryness of the mouth and throat, and dysphagia. Nausea and vomiting are often seen during the abdominal field treatment. Bone marrow depression may occur during the abdominal-pelvic irradiation, and this may require interruption of treatment. Of more significance are the long-term side effects. They are usually related to the volume of normal tissue that has been irradiated, the total dose given, and the size of the daily dose or fraction. Their prevention is far more important than their treatment, and no technical and medical effort should be spared to minimize the radiation sequelae. The long-term side effects may include radiation pneumonitis (frequent and transient), radiation carditis and pericarditis, hypothyroidism, spinal cord damage (transient), growth retardation in children (e.g. shoulders and clavicle), and reduction or suppression in fertility when the pelvis is being irradiated.

Non-Hodgkin Lymphoma

Compared to Hodgkin disease, less firm guidelines for the routine primary treatment approach can be provided for stage I and II non-Hodgkin lymphoma of the head and neck area. In general, megavoltage irradiation utilizing tumoricidal doses remains the treatment of choice for the majority of adult patients presenting with nodal and extranodal disease, regardless of histologic subgroup. If such therapy is delivered in adequate volumes, the cure rate can be maximized. In cases with extranodal localizations of diffuse histiocytic lymphomas, a tumor dose of at least 5,000 rads must be delivered, as local (true) recurrence is not infrequent. At least the proximal adjacent lymph node-bearing region(s) should always be included in the radiation field (regional extended radiotherapy). Besides primary site (nodal or extranodal), stage and histology have a major impact on survival. With all techniques employed, the 5-year survival rate achieved with radiotherapy as primary treatment ranges from 33 to 50 percent for the group of patients with nodal and extranodal disease classified as CS I and II (CS I rate = 40 to 79 percent, CS II = 18 to 56 percent). Fifty-five percent to 83 percent of patients with nodular histology survive 5 years compared with 26 to 50 percent of those with diffuse patterns.[5] Whether radiotherapy should be supplemented with some forms of systemic therapy is an important question, since the main reason for treatment failure is not local recurrence, but rather disease outside the irradiated area.[11]

Modern treatment strategy for adults

with localized non-Hodgkin lymphoma also takes into consideration the prognostic value of histologic subgroups. PS I and IE and II and IIE are usually established after marrow biopsy combined with laparoscopy.

FAVORABLE HISTOLOGY

The recommended primary treatment is regional extended radiotherapy to a tumor dose of about 4,500 rads. The relapse-free survival rate at 5 years is about 80 percent; the total survival rate is in the excess of 90 percent. There is little evidence to support the use of total nodal radiotherapy for patients whose PS was carried out with exploratory laparotomy. Since occult mesenteric lymphadenopathy can be present in as many as 40 percent of patients with negative lymphogram, if radiation therapy is to be administered with curative intent and surgical staging has not been performed, it would be advisable to encompass the entire abdominal contents. Adjuvant chemotherapy following radiotherapy (involved field, regional extended, total nodal) utilizing six cycles of CVP (cyclophosphamide, vincristine and prednisone) failed to improve the relapse-free survival rate.[10, 11]

UNFAVORABLE HISTOLOGY

In patients treated with regional extended radiotherapy, treatment must be supplemented with adjuvant chemotherapy. In fact, combined therapy statistically improved both relapse-free and total survival rates at 5 years.[11] Figure 26-6 shows the relapse-free and overall survival rates at 5 years for patients with Waldeyer's ring lymphomas who were randomly treated with regional extended radiotherapy alone or radiotherapy plus six cycles of CVP.[11] In adult patients with diffuse histiocytic, diffuse mixed lymphocytic-histiocytic, or diffuse undifferentiated non-Burkitt lymphoma a more aggressive form of adjuvant chemotherapy with an Adriamycin containing regimen such as BACOP (bleomycin, Adria-

mycin, cyclophosphamide, vincristine, and prednisone) or CHOP-Bleo (cyclophosphamide, Adriamycin, vincristine, prednisone and bleomycin)[7] appears more indicated in an adjuvant situation[11] and theoretically could yield better results. CVP still remains indicated for diffuse lymphocytic poorly differentiated lymphoma. In patients staged with laparotomy, a more extensive irradiation program (total nodal radiotherapy) yielded a 65 to 70 percent relapse-free survival rate at 5 years for PS I and II (A or B with or without E). With this program, no advantage in survival rate was demonstrated by adjuvant CVP.[10] Extensive radiotherapy alone was found particularly useful to obtain a high relapse-free survival rate for PS I and II patients who had diffuse histiocytic lymphoma and staging with exploratory laparotomy.[4] In conclusion, for adult patients with unfavorable histology and disease localized in the head and neck, the extent of surgical staging as well as the treatment of choice remain to be further defined.

In children with head and neck lymphomas, treatment must be aggressive and should utilize early combination chemotherapy and central nervous system prophylaxis in all histologic subgroups.[12, 15] Treatment is complex and cannot be summarized in a few words. Therefore, once the histologic diagnosis is established, it is always advisable to refer the child to a qualified pediatric oncologic team. Burkitt lymphoma is perhaps the ultimate in tumor sensitivity to chemotherapy. High intravenous doses of cyclophosphamide (40 to 75 mg/kg every 4 weeks) have been the standard approach and have resulted in long-term cure in the majority of patients with stage I Burkitt lymphomas in the head and neck area.[7, 16]

In general, radiotherapy for non-Hodgkin lymphomas of the head and neck, in particular for those involving the extranodal sites such as the orbital region and the paranasal sinuses, requires a very accurate technical approach to avoid severe post-irradiation complications. The use of inter-

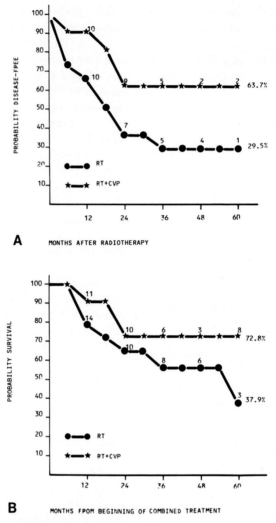

Fig. 26-6. Actuarial (A) relapse-free and (B) overall survival curves of pathologic stage I and II non-Hodgkin lymphoma with primary tumor in the Waldeyer's ring. Comparison between irradiation followed by adjuvant combination chemotherapy (CVP).

posed lead shields, an accurate beam collimation and direction, and a complete fixation of the patient are the most important means for protecting the eye, the spinal cord, the thyroid gland and for reducing xerostomia and dysphagia. In fact, although for non-Hodgkin lymphoma the dose level is generally significantly lower compared to that used for epidermoid cancer, larger fields must always be employed to broadly encompass both the extranodal sites and the entire cervical region.

PROGNOSTIC FACTORS

Hodgkin Disease

The prognosis of patients with disease localized to cervical nodes is not substantially different from that of disease localized to other anatomic sites. Favorable prognostic signs are—besides localized disease (PS I and II)—the absence of systemic symptoms (A) and the presence of certain histologic subgroups (lymphocytic predominance and nodular sclerosis). Patients with these characteristics have a 90 to 95 percent 5-year survival rate. Prognosis also seems to be related to age and sex, i.e. more favorable in young patients and in females. However, the importance of age and sex cannot be easily separated from the above mentioned factors.

A different prognostic value can also be attributed to the site of adenopathy within the cervical region. In fact the most favorable results can be expected in patients with PS IA, lymphocytic predominance histology and involvement of upper cervical region or Waldeyer's ring. For this particular type of patient, most clinicians believe that a conservative treatment, i.e., irradiation limited to the neck and Waldeyer's ring, can provide the same results as subtotal nodal radiotherapy. On the contrary, the presence of supraclavicular adenopathy per se may be associated with less favorable prognosis, since it could indicate the presence of occult disease in less accessible sites such as mediastinal and/or retroperitoneal lymph nodes.

Finally, other important, though less easy to evaluate, prognostic factors are represented by the number and the volume of the involved lymph nodes as well as by the invasion of the surrounding tissues (stage IE and IIE).

Non-Hodgkin Lymphomas

EXTRANODAL PRESENTATION

The evaluation of prognostic factors is related in part to the involved anatomic site. In fact, even though stage and histology are the most relevant prognostic elements, the characteristics of the involved site and of the local growth (volume, relation with surrounding structures) should not be neglected. These characteristics can represent a limiting factor to the performance of effective radiotherapy and, therefore, affect prognosis.

As far as stage is concerned, it has been largely documented that the most favorable prognosis is related to patients with disease limited to one extranodal site (stage IE).[5] In general, stage IIE shows better prognosis than nodal stage II because in most patients stage IIE lymphoma has a tendency to develop initially as local-regional disease (primary extranodal site plus regional adenopathy) and, therefore, is more easily controlled with regional extended radiotherapy.

The histologic types and patterns are known important prognostic factors. As already mentioned, the long survival of nodular lymphoma does not necessarily mean cure. Rather, this survival is often the result of an indolent course of the disease, which frequently recurs in nodal and/or extranodal sites.[5, 12, 15] Unfavorable prognosis is usually associated with the presence of diffuse histology with the exception of diffuse well-differentiated lymphocytic lymphoma (5-year survival rate in excess of 80 percent). The cause of treatment failure in diffuse histiocytic lymphoma can be attributed to both true local recurrence after irradiation as well as to new distant manifestations. Diffuse lymphocytic poorly differentiated lymphomas show tendency to early recurrence in the bone marrow with abnormal lymphoid cells in the peripheral blood.[12, 15]

As far as prognosis related to the primary anatomic site of involvement is concerned, the following considerations can be made. The involvement of *Waldeyer's ring* is usually associated with less favorable prognosis compared with other extranodal sites.[9, 11, 14] Prognosis is also related to the specifically involved site and is more severe in patients with *nasopharyngeal* lymphoma because of the possible extension to the base of the skull or to nasal fossae and/or paranasal sinuses (10 percent of cases). In primary lymphomas of the *orbit*, prognosis can be aggravated by the technical difficulty in delivering adequate doses of irradiation without producing irreversible damage to the involved eye or a decreased visual function of the contralateral eye. Because primary lymphomas of *paranasal sinuses* are often clinically recognized only when they have invaded the surrounding osseous structures (maxilla, orbit) the prognosis is poorer. The primary involvement of the *parotid* gland seems to be associated with a relatively favorable prognosis. In primary *thyroid* lymphoma, prognosis is inversely correlated with the volume of the infiltrated gland as well as with the degree of infiltration of surrounding tissues.

Correlation between age and sex and survival cannot be fully appreciated without consideration of the above-mentioned prognostic factors. For instance, in childhood non-Hodgkin lymphoma, the well known early invasion of the bone marrow and central nervous system is attributable to the occurrence in this age group of very aggressive disease, i.e., large cell lymphomas.

Finally, the presence of systemic symptoms, which is prognostically very significant in Hodgkin disease, is a rare event in non-Hodgkin lymphoma in general and particularly in that of the head and neck. Furthermore, fever and loss of weight frequently are related to complications due to local tumor growth and not necessarily to the presence of distant occult disease.

Nodal Presentation

Similarly to extranodal presentation, stage and histology represent the most important prognostic factors in the nodal group also.[12, 15] The possibility of cure for patients with nodal PS I is similar to that for those with extranodal PS I.[5] Stage II lymphomas, especially in the presence of supraclavicular adenopathy, have more tendency to spread to distant nodal and extranodal sites. Nodular lymphomas have better prognosis than diffuse lymphomas with the exception of the diffuse lymphocytic well-differentiated type. In patients with diffuse histiocytic lymphoma a relapse-free survival in excess of 2 years almost always signifies permanent cure.[4, 5, 11, 12]

REFERENCES

1. Arseneau, J. C., Sponzo, R. W., Levin, D. L., Schnipper, L. E., Bonner, H., Young, R. C., Canellos, G. P., Johnson, R. E., and De Vita, V. T. 1972. Non-lymphomatous malignant tumors complicating Hodgkin's disease. New England Journal of Medicine, 287: 1119.

2. Banfi, A., Bonadonna, G., Basso Ricci, S., Milani, F., Molinari, R., Monfardini, S., and Zucali, R. 1972. Malignant lymphomas of Waldeyer's ring: Natural history and survival after radiotherapy. British Medical Journal, 600: 140.

3. Berard, C. W. Jaffe, E. S., Braylan, R. C., Mann, R. B., and Nanba, K. 1978. Immunologic aspects and pathology of the malignant lymphomas. Cancer, 42: 911.

4. Bitran, J. D., Kinzie, J., Sweet, D. L., Variokojis, D., Griem, M. L., Golomb, H. M., Miller, J. B., Oetzel, N., and Ultmann, J. E. 1977. Survival of patients with localized histiocytic lymphoma. Cancer, 39: 342.

5. Bonadonna, G., Lattuada, A., and Banfi, A. 1976. Recent trends in the treatment of Non-Hodgkin's lymphomas. European Journal of Cancer, 12: 661.

6. Bonadonna, G., Beretta, G., Castellani, R., Canetta, R., Spinelli, P., Gennari, L., Rilke, F., and Veronesi, U. 1977. Current views on surgical staging in planning the treatment of malignant lymphomas. In Tagnon, H. J., and Staquet, M. L., Eds.: Recent Advances in Cancer Treatment. Raven Press, New York, 55.

7. Canellos, G. P., Lister, T. A., and Skarin, A. T. 1978. Chemotherapy of the Non-Hodgkin's lymphomas. Cancer, 42: 932.

7a. Carbone, P. P., Kaplan, H. S., Smithers, D. W., and Tubiana, M. 1971. Report of the committee on Hodgkin's disease staging classification. Cancer Research, 31: 1860.

8. Chabner, B. A., Johnson, R. E., Young, R. C., Canellos, G. P., Hubbard, S. P., Johnson, S. K., and De Vita, V. T. 1978. Sequential nonsurgical and surgical staging of non-Hodgkin's lymphoma. Cancer, 42: 922.

9. Fierstein, J. T., and Thawley, S. E. 1978. Lymphoma of head and neck. Laryngoscope, 88: 582.

10. Glatstein, E., Donaldson, S. S., Rosenberg, S. A., and Kaplan, H. S. 1977. Combined modality therapy in malignant lymphomas. Cancer Treatment Reports, 61: 1199.

10a. Lukes, R. J., Craver, L. F., Hall, T. C., Rappaport, H., and Rubin, P. 1966. Report of the nomenclature committee. Cancer Research 26: 1311.

11. Monfardini, S., Banfi, A., Bonadonna, G., Milani, F., Valagussa, P., and Lattuada, A. 1979. Improved five year results after combined radiotherapy-chemotherapy in stage I-II non-Hodgkin's lymphomas. International Journal of Radiation, Oncology, Biology, Physics. (In Press).

12. Proceedings of the Conference on non-Hodgkin's Lymphomas. 1977. Cancer Treatment Reports, 61: 935.

13. Rosenberg, S. A., Kaplan, H. S., Glatstein, E. J., and Portlock, C. S. 1978. Combined modality therapy of Hodgkin's disease. A report on the Stanford Trials. Cancer, 42: 991.

14. Rudders, R. A., Ross, M. E., and De Lellis, R. A. 1978. Primary extranodal lymphoma. Response to treatment and factors influencing prognosis. Cancer, 42: 406.

15. Symposium on non-Hodgkin's lymphomata. 1975. British Journal of Cancer, 31: suppl. II, 1.

16. Ziegler, J. L. 1977. Treatment results of 45 American patients with Burkitt's lymphoma are similar to the African experience? New England Journal of Medicine 297: 75.

27 | Reconstructive Procedures

Alando J. Ballantyne, M.D.

The ideal treatment of head and neck cancer is to effect a cure without functional, cosmetic, or psychological impairment. All of the present treatment modalities leave some kind of defect except in the case of very small cancers. Surgical treatment always necessitates removal or destruction of tissue, and extensive surgical procedures may seriously disrupt the normal functioning of the individual even when reconstruction is carried out.

Restoration of function and aesthetic acceptability should be the primary goals of reconstruction. After the creation of extensive defects involving the skull, face, neck, upper alimentary tract, and trachea, a primary reconstruction in a single stage may not be feasible. The priorities in the timing of reconstructive procedures may be divided into several categories:

I. Obligatory—To preserve life and to avoid catastrophic postoperative course
   A. Cover the brain and dura
   B. Provide protection for the carotid artery and other vessels
   C. Seal off the mediastinum
   D. Provide protection for the eye
II. Immediately Desirable—To restore function and cosmetic sufficiency as rapidly as possible
   A. Resurfacing of skin or mucosal defects
      1. Skin grafts
      2. Tongue or cheek flaps
      3. Local or regional flaps
   B. Reestablish oral competence and alimentary continuity
   C. Support of the mandible following resection of the anterior arch
   D. Support of the hyoid bone following resection of the anterior arch of the mandible
   E. Support of the eye following removal of the floor of the orbit
   F. Graft of the spinal accessory, facial or other nerves that are sacrificed during the surgical procedure
III. Optional Immediate—This category includes those reconstructive procedures that are of less urgency and largely cosmetic in nature such as reconstruction of the nose or ear or reconstruction of the mandible.
IV. Mandatory Delayed—The defects in this category are such that reconstruction has to be delayed, either because of the magnitude of the defect or because the physiological condition of the patient would not support a prolonged procedure. When there is any question about whether a complete reconstruction should be done and a lesser procedure would be safer, the lesser procedure should be the one of choice.

OBLIGATORY RECONSTRUCTIVE PROCEDURES

Coverage of the Brain and Dura

Although the unirradiated brain can be covered with a split-thickness skin graft, it is much safer to cover exposed brain with a fascia lata graft and a scalp flap. Any portion of the undersurface of the brain in which the dura has been sacrificed must be covered with a substitute for the dura and a skin flap, otherwise herniation of the brain may take place. A case that illustrates coverage of a large defect in the skull and dura utilizing a fascia lata graft and scalp flap is illustrated in Figures 27-1 A–D.

Coverage of the Carotid Artery and Other Major Vessels

No particular problems should be encountered in a neck dissection done in nonirradiated fields if the carotid artery is left intact and the skin does not have to be sacrificed. Even if the skin is sacrificed, coverage of the carotid artery can be done with a simple skin graft. However, once the neck has been irradiated, the risk of exposure of the carotid artery increases. To avoid this problem, the incision for a neck dissection should be placed so that there is no junction of incisions over the carotid artery itself. If it is necessary to sacrifice skin over the carotid artery, the safest procedure is to use nonirradiated flaps to cover the vessels. The

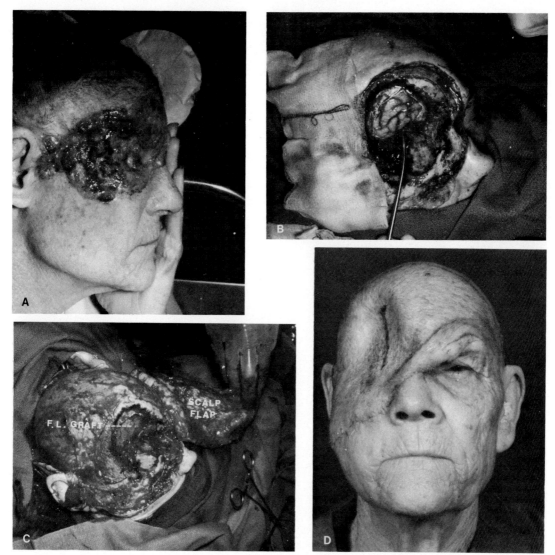

Fig. 27-1. (A) Extensive basal cell carcinoma that had destroyed eye and bone and had invaded dura. (B) Defect in bone and dura after resection. (C) Closure of dural defect with fascia lata graft and mobilization of scalp flap. (D) Defect covered with scalp flap.

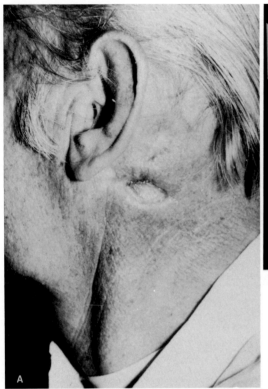

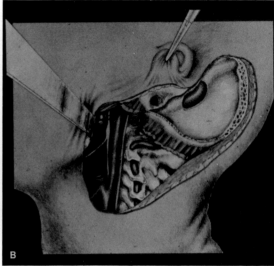

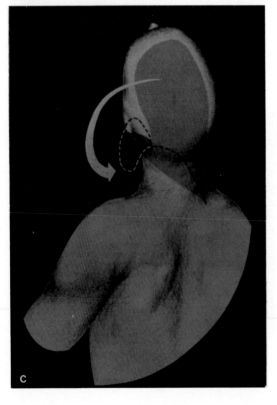

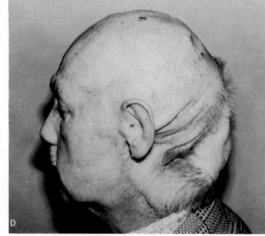

Fig. 27-2. (A) Recurrent metastatic squamous cell carcinoma, after irradiation, involving postauricular nodes, underlying skull, transverse processes of vertebrae, parotid, and surrounding tissues. (B) Diagrammatic representation of structures exposed after resection of tumor. (C) Diagrammatic representation of transposition of scalp flap. (D) Scalp flap in position.

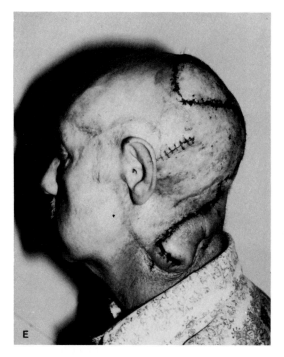
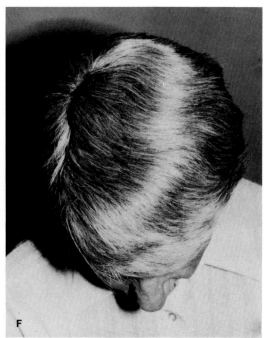

Fig. 27-2 continued. (E) After return of unused portion of flap. (F) Coverage of scalp defect with hairpiece.

most commonly used flap for this purpose is the medially based deltopectoral flap. In complex cases in which many vessels are exposed, such as the internal carotid artery, the vertebral artery, the transverse sinus, and the stump of the internal jugular vein, a deltopectoral flap may be utilized. In certain cases in which the deltopectoral flap should have been delayed but was not, a safer procedure is to use the entire scalp (Figs. 27-2 A–F). The patient in this figure had received radiation therapy for a postauricular metastasis from a primary scalp cancer and required a surgical procedure that created a defect exposing the vertebral artery, the transverse sinus, the jugular foramen, and the internal carotid artery. The external carotid artery also had to be sacrificed. Since the skin defect extended high over the occipital area of the scalp, we felt that it was safer to use an entire scalp flap rather than a nondelayed deltopectoral flap. The primary wound coverage was satisfactorily achieved and the excess scalp subsequently returned to its usual position. The

patient has been without evidence of recurrence in the ensuing 5 years.

Should wound breakdown occur following radical neck dissection, there is much less danger of carotid artery rupture if the entire vessel has been left intact than if the external or any of the smaller branches of the carotid has been sacrificed. If the carotid artery becomes exposed, it is sometimes feasible to excise all of the radiated skin of the neck, clean off the carotid artery, and cover the defect with a deltopectoral flap (Figs. 27-3 A and B). When it is necessary to sacrifice skin and external carotid in the heavily irradiated neck, the point of ligation of the external carotid can be protected by a pedicled dermal graft (Figs. 27-4 A–D).

If the external carotid artery is sacrificed in the performance of a pharyngectomy and the pharyngeal defect is repaired with a skin graft over the point of ligation, postoperative irradiation will almost certainly lead to perforation of the artery. When the carotid artery is exposed on the mucosal side after resection of the pharynx

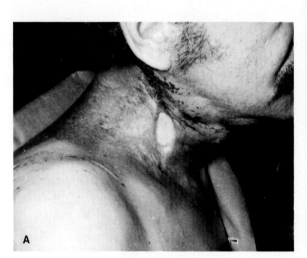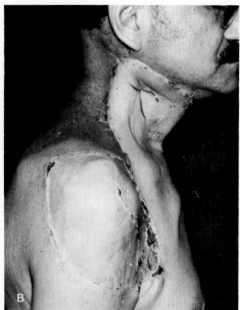

Fig. 27-3. (A) Wound breakdown over carotid artery following limited neck dissection in an irradiated field that had received 7,500 rads, half of which was given in twice daily increments. (B) After excision of skin of entire neck, cleaning of carotid artery and replacement with deltopectoral flap. No recurrence in 7 years.

or cervical esophagus, it is necessary to provide protection to seal off the carotid artery from the pharyngeal secretions. The flaps most commonly used for this purpose are the forehead and deltopectoral. The use of a deltopectoral flap for such coverage is illustrated in Figures 27-5 A–C. This patient presented with recurrent cancer of the base of the tongue following radiation therapy. A modified neck dissection and resection of the base of the tongue and pharynx was done and the defect was closed with a deltopectoral flap, the lower portion of which was tubed to leave a temporary fistula. Subsequently, the unused portion of the flap was returned to the donor site and the fistula was closed. The patient later required a modified neck dissection on the left side but is currently living, 7 years after surgery, without evidence of recurrence.

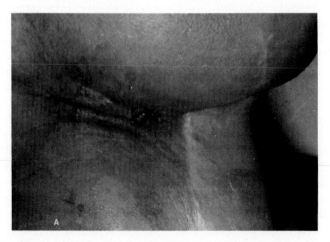

Fig. 27-4. (A) Extensive recurrent cancer in right upper neck following irradiation.

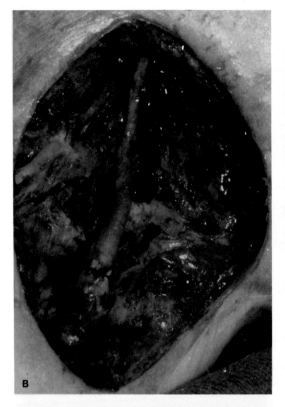

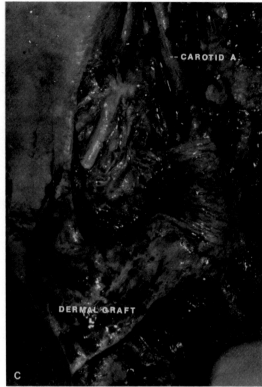

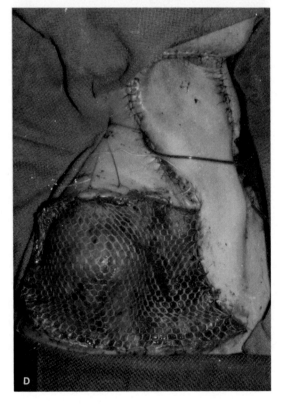

Fig. 27-4 continued. (B) Operative defect after resection of recurrent cancer. Resection of external carotid and stripping internal carotid to base of skull. (C) Pedicled dermal graft used to cover site of external carotid artery. (D) Coverage of defect with deltopectoral flap. No recurrence in 4 years.

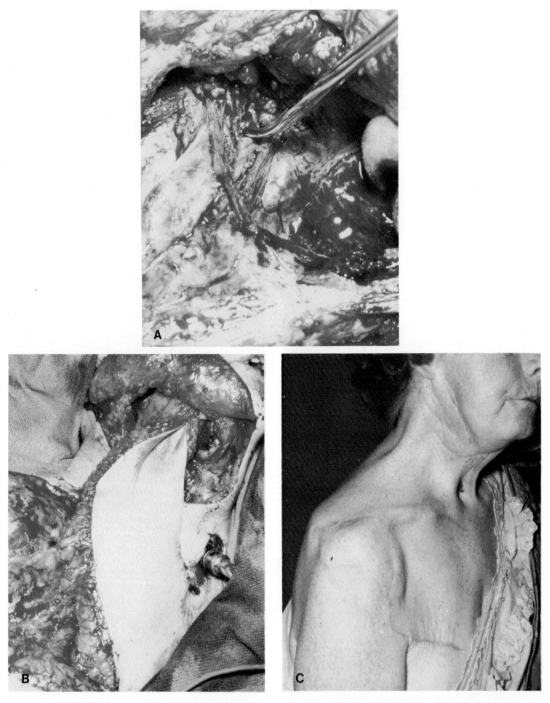

Fig. 27-5. (A) Defect left after resecting recurrent cancer of base of tongue, pharyngeal wall, and soft palate. Hemostat points to a histologically positive retropharyngeal lymph node on medial side of internal carotid artery. (B) Use of deltopectoral flap to cover carotid artery. (C) After closure of fistula and return of unused portion of flap to donor site.

Seal Off the Mediastinum and Cover the Innominate Artery

If the cervical esophagus and trachea have been resected leaving the innominate artery, the pleura, and other structures in this area exposed, it is mandatory that these be covered in order to avoid a catastrophe. If adequate local skin exists, this can be utilized, but if the defect goes well down into the mediastinum, it will be necessary to use adjacent skin such as laterally or medially based deltopectoral flap or a flap of skin from the area of the posterior neck based on the transverse cervical artery. If the trachea has been resected low in the mediastinum, it should never be brought up to the skin, for such a maneuver will create pressure on the innominate artery and result in erosion of this vessel. A skin flap from the chest should be fashioned and brought down into the mediastinum and sewn around the trachea. Such a flap will seal off the mediastinum, cover the vessels and pleura, and will adequately support the trachea and cover the adjacent structures (Figs. 27-6 A–C).

Provide Protection for the Eye

Resection of only the lower lid in the course of an ablative cancer procedure creates a relatively simple defect that can be corrected by use of a full-thickness skin graft, a portion of upper lid, or a flap to which the upper lid can be sutured. Resection

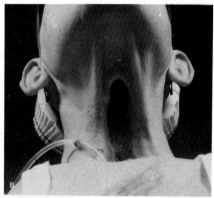

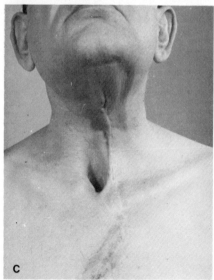

Fig. 27-6. (A) Operative defect after resection with modified bilateral neck dissection for cancer of cervical esophagus. (B) After rotation of chest flap to cover vessels and trachea. Pharyngeal defect was partially repaired with split-thickness skin graft. (C) Following closure of defect with local tissues. No recurrence in 14 years.

of both lids, conjunctiva, and lacrimal gland creates a challenging problem, since provision must be made for creation of conjunctival sac, secretion to bathe the cornea, and some form of covering to place over the newly created conjunctival sac. Such a problem is fortunately uncommon, but Figures 27-7 A–E illustrate that this can be accomplished with conservation of vision. This patient, who had a basal cell nevus syndrome, had neglected her multiple skin cancers until the right eye had been destroyed. Subsequently, both lids, the conjunctiva, the lacrimal gland and part of the extraocular muscles of the left eye were invaded. The surgical procedure necessitated removal of the skin of the nose, portions of the extraocular muscles, and all of the conjunctival sac. Stensen's duct and the mucosa of the cheek adjacent to the opening of the duct were mobilized to create a conjunctival sac and provide lubrication for the eye, and a flap of skin from the lower face and upper neck was used to cover the newly created conjunctival sac. Although the cosmetic and functional result was undesirable, the patient has had useful vision for the 11 years since the surgical procedure was performed.

IMMEDIATELY DESIRABLE RECONSTRUCTIVE PROCEDURES

Resurfacing of Skin or Mucosal Defects

SKIN COVERAGE

Many patients with skin cancers have multiple lesions, particularly those with fair skin who have been exposed to the sun for many years. These patients are likely to

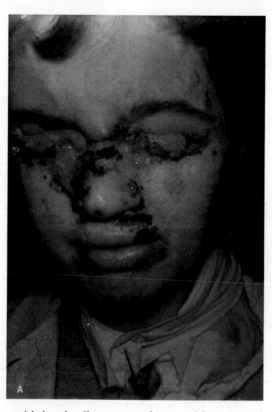

Fig. 27-7. (A) Patient with basal cell nevus syndrome with cancers destroying right eye and lids and surrounding structures on left.

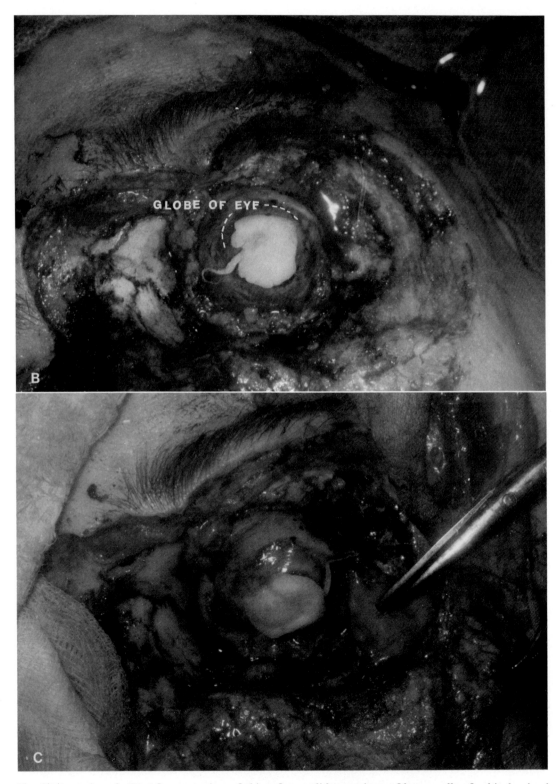

Fig. 27-7 continued. (B) After resection of skin of nose, lids, portions of bony walls of orbit, lacrimal gland, conjunctiva, and portions of extraocular muscles. (C) Stenson's duct and surrounding mucosa are migrated to form conjunctival sac and to provide lubrication for eye.

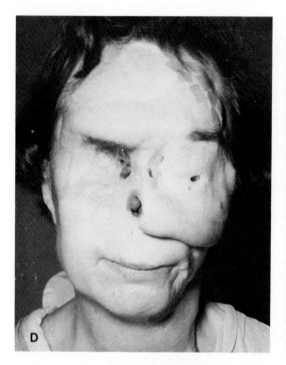
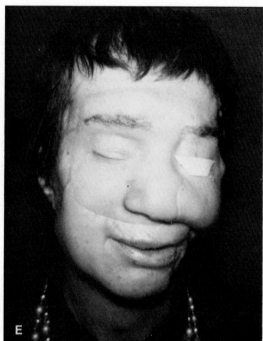

Fig. 27-7 continued. (D) Conjunctival sac and surrounding structures covered with skin flap from lower face and upper neck. Slit present for eye. (E) Appearance with prosthesis used after exenteration of left orbit. Useful vision after 11 years.

have numerous keratoses as well as invasive cancers. Such problems are best treated by total excision of the abnormal skin and resurfacing with full-thickness or split-thickness skin grafts as indicated. The infraclavicular area provides a large amount of skin that can be used to resurface the entire midportion of the face. This gives both a good texture and color match. Multiple lesions of the skin of the nose create a problem that is best managed by total resection of the abnormal skin with preservation of the bony and cartilaginous structures; this procedure leaves a surface that can be readily covered with full-thickness skin taken from the infraclavicular area. The best cosmetic result for the nose is secured by making the incision at the edge of the free margin of the ala nasi, up along the side of the nose and across the bridge (Figs. 27-8 A–E). Small defects in the skin of the nose or cheek can be resurfaced using local tissue flaps. Large defects, if they involve considerable loss of tissue other than skin, can be covered using either forehead flaps, deltopectoral flaps, or skin of the neck flap.

MUCOSAL COVERAGE

The simplest means of covering a mucosal defect is by use of local tissues. However, unless the lesion excised is small, local tissues may not be sufficient unless one elects to use either a flap from the tongue, hard palate, or buccal mucosa. In many patients, the mucosa adjacent to the primary cancer is abnormal with dysplastic changes and it is unwise to use tongue or mucosal flaps to cover the primary defect. A split-thickness skin graft can be satisfactorily employed, although there is considerable hesitancy among many surgeons to use this technique because of the possibility of contracture. If the split-thickness graft is made large enough and is stented properly, the entire mucosa of the tongue and/or the mouth can be removed and satisfactory coverage obtained with a good functional result (Figs.

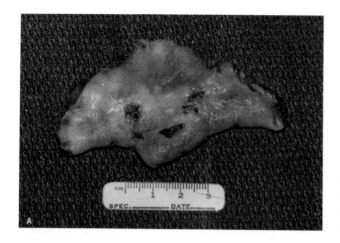

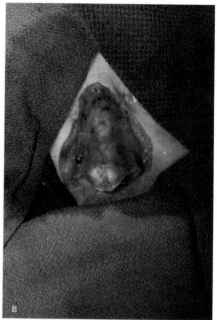

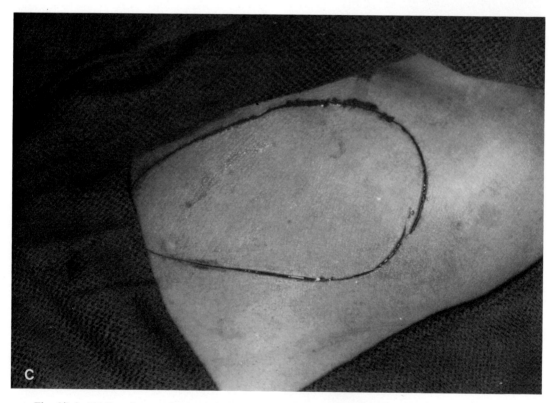

Fig. 27-8. (A) Specimen of resected skin from nose containing multiple basal cell carcinomas. (B) Defect after removal of skin of entire nose. (C) Full-thickness skin graft being taken from infraclavicular area by free-hand knife method.

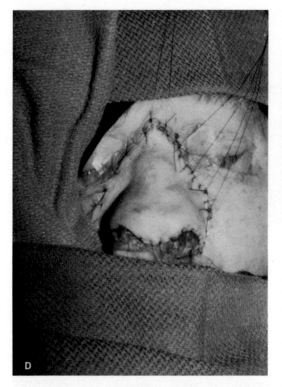

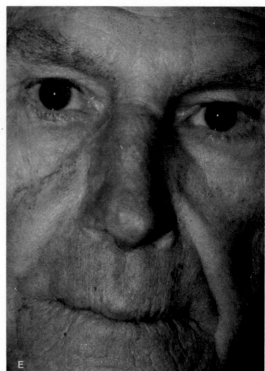

Fig. 27-8 continued. (D) Skin graft in place. (E) Postoperative appearance after replacement of entire skin of nose with full-thickness graft.

27-9 A and B). In defects of the floor of the mouth, even if a marginal resection of the mandible has been done, the defect can be covered with a split-thickness skin graft. The graft should be large enough so that any contracture that takes place will not result in limitation of motion of the tongue.

Reestablishment of Oral Competence

When all or a portion of the upper and lower lips have been excised, it is highly desirable to accomplish primary reconstruction so as to avoid interference with eating

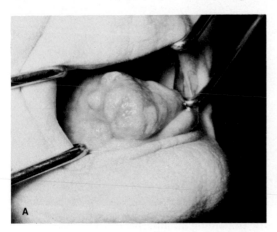

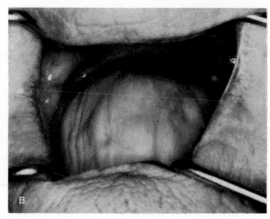

Fig. 27-9. (A) Patient with long history of multiple squamous cell carcinomas of the tongue. (B) Appearance after resection of all of mucosa of oral tongue and replacement with split-thickness skin graft. No further cancers in 6 years.

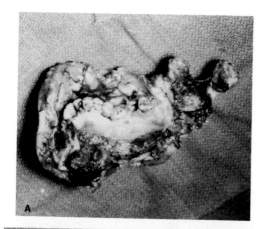

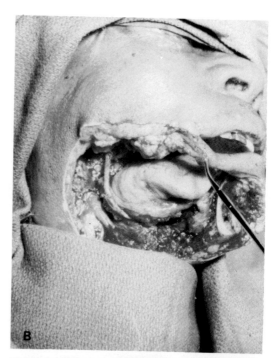

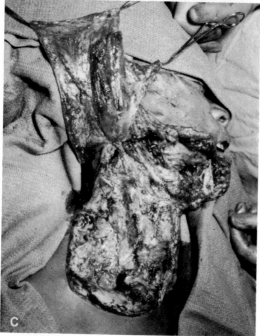

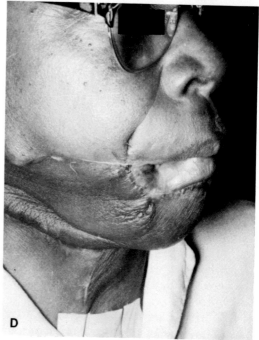

Fig. 27-10. (A) Operative specimen of extensive cancer involving buccal mucosa, gum, and skin. (B) Operative defect. (C) Skin of neck flap with underlying sternocleidomastoid muscle elevated to provide closure. (D) Immediate postoperative result.

and speaking. Small defects of the lower lip can be closed by primary approximation. Larger defects involving more than a third of the lip can be closed with an Abbe-Estlander or reverse Abbe-Estlander flap or with Bernard flaps. The entire lower lip can be removed and reconstructed using either a single or, if necessary, a bilateral composite cheek and buccal mucosa flap.

When it is necessary to resect the entire upper lip, reconstruction is somewhat more complicated but can be done using either a lined neck flap or forehead flap. Full-thickness defects involving skin and buccal mucosa can be immediately repaired in a variety of ways:

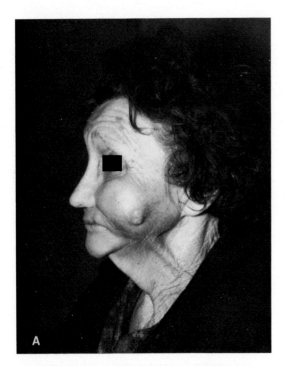

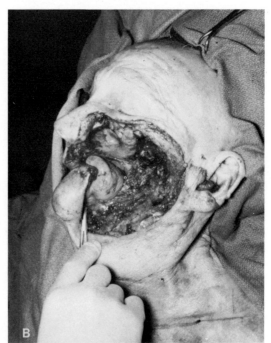

Fig. 27-11. (A) Extensive spindle cell squamous carcinoma recurrent after irradiation. (B) Operative defect. (C) Nine days postoperative when patient was ready to leave the hospital after repair with three flaps.

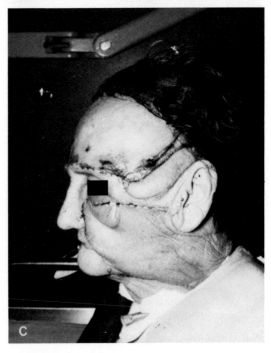

1. If sufficient tongue and upper buccal sulcus mucosa remain, the mucosal defect can be closed by primary approximation of remaining tongue and buccal mucosa, or if necessary, by using a tongue flap. The external coverage can then be provided by using either a deltopectoral flap or simple skin of the neck flap or a composite flap of sternocleidomastoid muscle with its overlying skin, with secondary coverage of the defect in the skin of the neck with a deltopectoral flap (Figs. 27-10 A–D).

2. In cases in which it is necessary to remove a portion of the lips, the buccal mucosa, mandible, and skin, it is possible to use three flaps to effect immediate primary closure. This technique requires a forehead flap for the reconstruction of the mucosal defect, a neck flap to cover the external surface, and a deltopectoral flap to resurface the neck (Figs. 27-11 A–C).

3. When the entire mandible, buccal mucosa, and skin of the chin and upper neck have been removed, primary reconstruction in one stage can be done by using a combination of a neck flap for the mucosal surface and to cover the prosthesis and a

deltopectoral flap to cover the neck defect and chin defect (Figs. 27-12 A–F). The patient in this figure had a huge osteogenic sarcoma that had grown out through the skin of the chin. In order to resect the tumor, it was necessary to remove the entire mandible and the skin of the chin and upper neck, leaving only a small remnant of mucosa of the lower lip. An immediate total

mandibular prosthesis composed of acrylic was placed in the defect. The prosthesis was wrapped with a flap of skin from the neck to line the remaining buccal mucosa and floor of the mouth. Part of the flap was de-epithelialized where it joined the floor of the mouth so that primary approximation could be done and again deepithelialized externally so that the deltopectoral flap could be

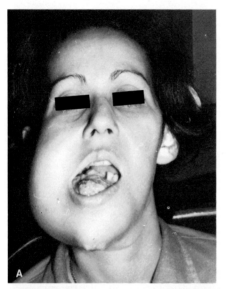
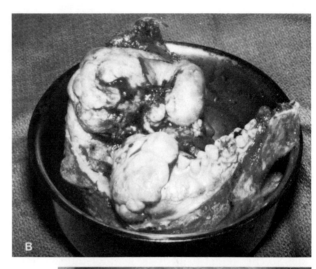
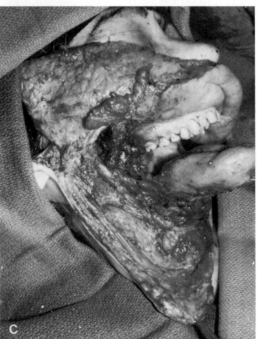
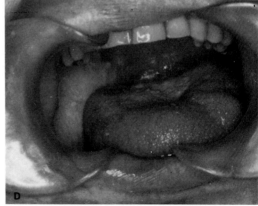

Fig. 27-12. (A) Extensive osteogenic sarcoma involving mandible, buccal mucosa, and skin. (B) Operative specimen. (C) Operative defect. (D) After insertion of acrylic prosthesis for entire mandible and reconstruction of buccal mucosa with flap from skin of neck.

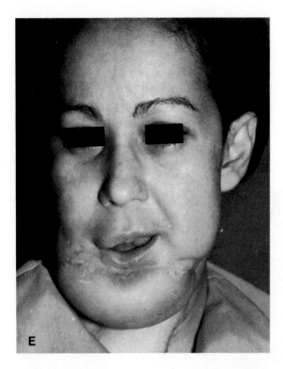
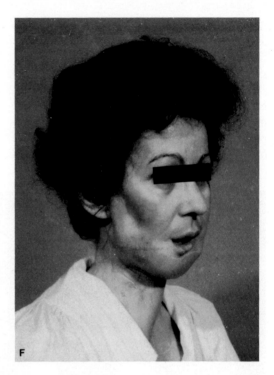

Fig. 27-12 continued. (E) Immediate postoperative result. (F) After insertion of second prosthesis and cosmetic procedures to chin.

sewn to the defect to provide a water-tight seal. This resulted in immediate reconstruction of oral competence so that the patient was able to take food by mouth and speak. One year later, the temporary prosthesis was removed and replaced by a better-fitting prosthesis and revisions were made in the skin and cheek to improve cosmetic appearance.

Restoration of Alimentary Continuity

Surgical resection of cancer of the pharynx and cervical esophagus can produce crippling functional disabilities. In defects of the upper alimentary tract above the larynx, one sometimes has to choose between leaving the larynx with preservation of phonation, but some dysphagia, or removing the larynx and imposing some difficulty in communicating. Whether one elects to leave the larynx and risk aspiration and dysphagia depends to some extent upon the physical condition and the wishes of the patient. If the patient is elderly and has poor respiratory reserve, the larynx should be removed as a primary procedure. The method chosen to repair defects in the pharynx will depend upon the location and size of the primary tumor. Ordinarily, it is possible to leave the larynx in place with the expectation of recovery of swallowing function, if the tumor lies above the tip of the epiglottis. The pharyngeal wall defects created can be satisfactorily covered with a split-thickness skin graft providing that one is operating in an unirradiated field. If the patient has had prior irradiation, the chances of being able to swallow satisfactorily are poor, but if the patient is adamant about saving the larynx, the defect in the pharynx can be closed using a forehead flap, deltopectoral flap, or trapezius myocutaneous flap. When a total pharyngectomy has been done, there are several techniques that may be used for closure. Split-thickness skin grafts can be used for an entire circumferential replacement of the pharynx. These have the advantage of simplicity, but do tend to develop a stricture at the junction of the split-thickness skin graft and cervical esophagus. Reconstruction with a deltopectoral flap or trapezius myocutaneous flap provides better material for coverage of the carotid arteries and carries less risk of stricture formation at the junction of the skin flap and the cervical esophagus.

If it is necessary to resect the entire base of the tongue, primary reapproximation of the remaining tongue to the epiglottis or hyoid bone is a satisfactory means of effecting immediate reconstruction. Resection of the base of the tongue, pharyngeal wall, and soft palate produces a defect that cannot ordinarily be closed using local tissues. Repair can be done with a deltopectoral flap or trapezius myocutaneous flap to resurface the pharyngeal wall and base of the tongue. A deltopectoral flap cannot ordinarily be used in a single stage to reconstruct the base of the tongue, pharyngeal wall, and soft palate, but at a second stage the sternal end of the deltopectoral flap can be migrated into the defect and used to reconstruct the soft palate.

During the surgical treatment of postcricoid carcinomas, it is almost always necessary to resect the larynx. The choice of closure will then depend upon a number of factors. Skin grafts or local or regional flaps, such as a deltopectoral flap, can be used for closure. As one progresses further distally along the alimentary tract, the number of potential reconstructive techniques decreases. Here, again, the choice of closure will depend upon the anatomy of the patient and the availability of other tissues. A patient with a long neck is much easier to perform surgery in than is the patient with a very short, thick neck and a low-lying cervical esophagus. A patient with a long, thin neck in whom the cervical esophagus has been removed can have a repair effected by split-thickness skin grafts, by a laterally or medially based deltopectoral flap, or by another segment of the alimentary tract. In patients with short necks in whom the cervical esophagus has been resected and in whom it would be difficult to turn in a deltopectoral flap that is medially based, a laterally based flap can be used and can be satisfactorily turned well down into the superior mediastinum. A myocutaneous trapezius flap based on the transverse cervical artery can be used to reconstruct any defect in the pharynx or cervical esophagus well down into the mediastinum and has the advantage of not requiring a second procedure to close the stoma.

The alternative to the use of skin grafts or local or regional flaps in reconstruction of defects of the pharynx and esophagus is the use of another segment of the alimentary tract. Stomach or colon can be used providing there has been no previous disease in these areas and the vasculature is adequate. In recent years, the use of a free graft of a segment of small intestine using microvascular anastomoses has become more popular. As more surgeons become proficient in this technique, the necessity for the use of complicated flaps may diminish significantly. Flaps, however, may still be the preferred means of treatment if one elects to use postoperative radiation, since the gastrointestinal tract, except for the stomach, tolerates radiation therapy poorly.

The advantages of the stomach as a substitute for cervical esophagus are the use of single anastomosis, and that the stomach can be brought through the posterior mediastinum with total removal of the esophagus and paratracheal and paraesophageal lymph nodes and minimal interference with respiratory function.

The disadvantages of the use of the stomach include the frequency of gastric reflux and occasional difficulty in emptying as a result of the interruption of the vagus (this may be avoided, however, by pyloromyotomy) and the occasional occurrence of insufficient length to reach high enough into the neck for satisfactory anastomosis.

The colon can be used as a substitute for cervical esophagus providing there is no disease demonstrated by barium enema and providing the vasculature, as estimated by angiography, is adequate. Figures 27-13 A–D illustrate the use of colon for replacement of cervical esophagus. The disadvantages of colon bypass are that it requires three anastomoses and the colon must be placed retrosternally, which sometimes cre-

ates respiratory embarrassment in the patient who has poor functional reserve.

Split-thickness skin grafts to reconstruct the lower pharynx, the postcricoid area, and the cervical esophagus can be employed satisfactorily with the anastomoses

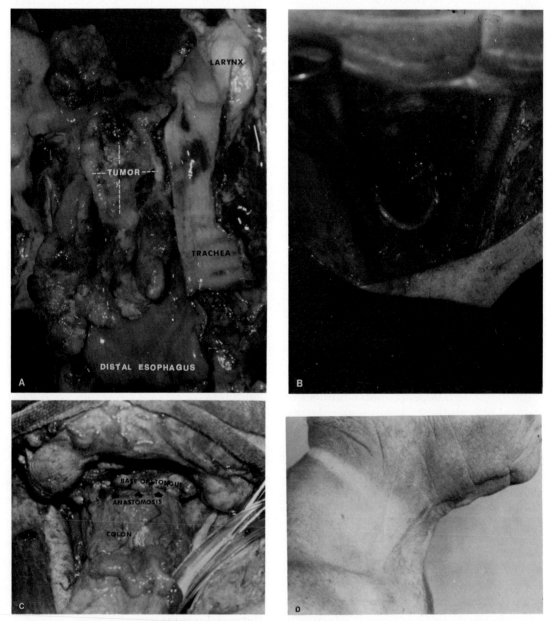

Fig. 27-13. (A) Operative specimen of cancer of cervical esophagus. Larynx and trachea divided in half to expose posterior pharynx and esophagus. The patient also had a bilateral modified neck dissection and paratracheal node dissection with positive nodes found in both sides of the neck and both paratracheal areas. (B) Operative defect. (C) Colon anastomosis to pharynx. (D) Postoperative result. No recurrence in 5 years.

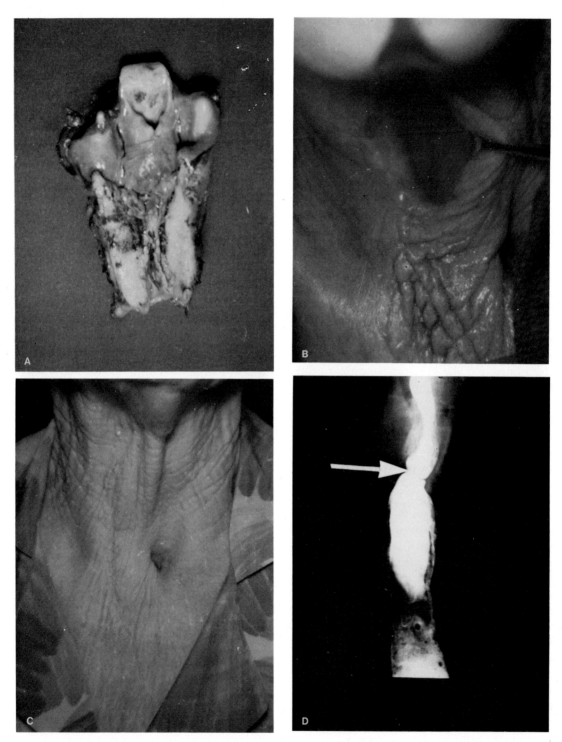

Fig. 27-14. (A) Operative specimen of cancer of cervical esophagus. (B) Esophagus reconstructed with split-thickness skin graft. Temporary fistula created through which packing used to keep skin graft in place was withdrawn. (C) Postoperative appearance. No recurrence in 7 years. (D) Esophagram showing point of anastomosis of skin graft to distal esophagus at level of aortic arch.

being made as low as the level of the aortic arch, with all the surgery being done through the neck (Figs. 27-14 A–D). The hazard of this type of procedure is that the skin graft must be held in place by a pack and if the patient should vomit and disrupt the pack, the skin graft would be dislodged, with catastrophic results. However, with the use of total parental hyperalimentation, it might be feasible to reevaluate this rapid method of reconstruction, which causes minimal operative trauma, since the stomach could be kept empty during the postoperative period and nutritional support given with hyperalimentation.

Support of the Mandible Following Resection of the Anterior Arch

The amount of disability following resection of the mandible will depend upon which portion is resected. Resection of the ascending ramus and the horizontal ramus to the level of the mental foramen ordinarily provides very little functional or cosmetic disability. However, removal of the anterior arch causes both severe cosmetic and functional disability due to the loss of support for the hyoid bone. Unless conditions are relatively ideal, immediate reconstruction of the mandible should not be done. The requirements for immediate reconstruction are adequate mucosal coverage, adequate soft tissue coverage, and secure fixation of prosthesis or bone to remaining mandible. Ameloblastomas and other relatively benign tumors of the mandible which usually do not involve much mucosa and seldom involve the soft tissues about the mandible can be resected with immediate reconstruction using one of a variety of prostheses. A prosthesis constructed of acrylic for the ascending ramus and either a tubular metal prosthesis or bar for the horizontal ramus is a very satisfactory device. If a segment of the horizontal ramus has been resected and the surgeon wishes to provide some support to keep the fragments in proper alignment, it is possible to use a Steinman pin placed in the mandibular canal. Proper placement of

the Steinman pin with sealing of the bone ends with methyl methacrylate to hold the pin in position results in good stabilization of the mandibular fragments.

Support of the Hyoid Bone Following Resection of the Anterior Arch of the Mandible

Removal of the suprahyoid muscles along with either a marginal or segmental resection of the anterior mandible allows the laryngeal complex to drift downward producing obstruction of the pharynx even though the mandible remains in place. Support for the hyoid can be obtained by drawing it up to the remaining mandible with appropriate sutures placed either through or around the mandible (Figs. 27-15 A–D). If the anterior arch of the mandible has been removed, it is possible to support the hyoid bone from the zygomatic arch with wires. Such a means of support maintained until fibrosis takes place will obviate additional procedures to free up the larynx when a definitive reconstructive procedure is done.

Support of the Eye Following Resection of the Floor of the Orbit

Surgical resection of the maxillary sinus for primary antral cancer or for cancer of the skin invading the maxilla and extending along the infraorbital nerve may require resection of the bony floor and lateral walls of the orbit. If it is elected to preserve the eye, the orbital contents should be supported by a properly placed skin graft (Figs. 27-16 A–D).

Grafting of the Spinal Accessory, Facial, or Other Nerves

The single most severe functional disability following radical neck dissection if the spinal accessory nerve is severed is shoulder drop. If it is not possible to save the spinal accessory nerve, it is highly desirable to interpose a nerve graft between the ends of the spinal accessory nerve at the time of the

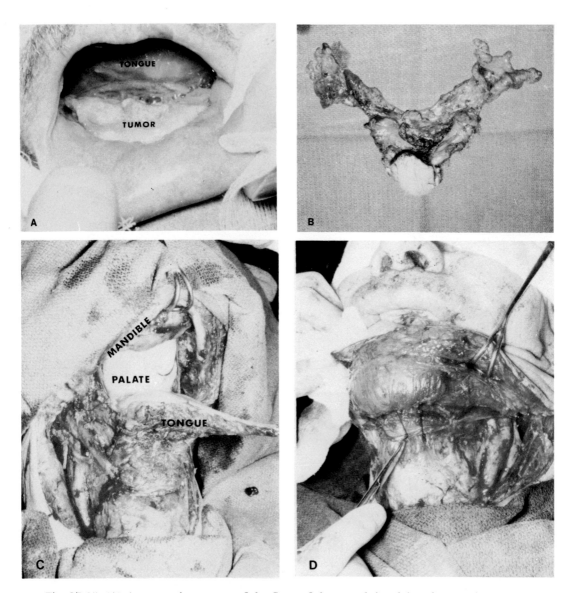

Fig. 27-15. (A) An extensive cancer of the floor of the mouth involving the anterior tongue. (B) Operative specimen of partial glossectomy, marginal resection of mandible, resection of the floor of the mouth and of the suprahyoid muscles, and bilateral modified neck dissection. (C) Operative defect. (D) After repositioning the tongue, the hyoid is supported from the mandible.

initial surgery. Such a nerve graft can be taken from the greater auricular nerve or the supraclavicular nerves. The success rate following this nerve grafting procedure should approximate 100 percent. Recovery ordinarily takes place within 6 months and the trapezius on the side of the nerve graft should be as strong as on the opposite side.

When the facial nerve is resected dur-

ing removal of parotid tumors or in the case of invasion of the parotid area by cancers of the skin or other sites, it is desirable at the time of the initial operative procedure to interpose a graft between the proximal and distal ends of the nerve. Such a graft can be secured from the greater auricular nerve. This nerve is usually of sufficient size so that it can be divided into a number of fascicles

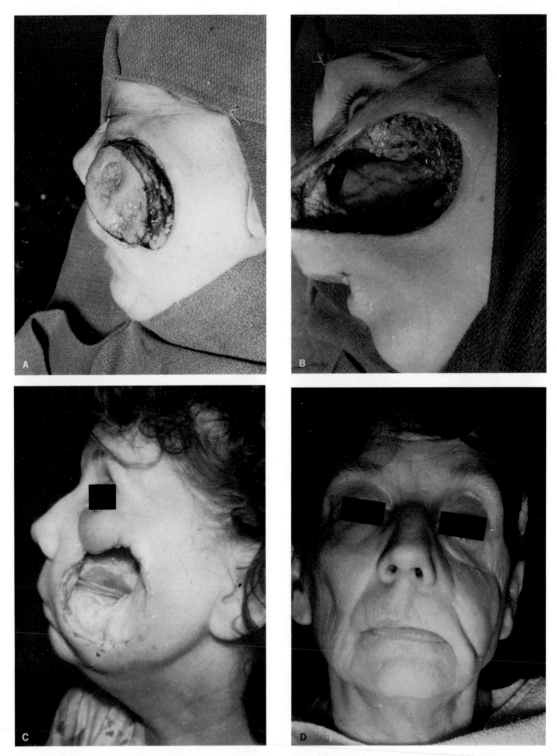

Fig. 27-16. (A) Extensive cancer of maxillary antrum invading skin. (B) Defect after removing maxilla and floor of the orbit. (C) Defect lined by split-thickness skin graft, which is used to support orbital contents. (D) After closure of cheek defect with tubed pedicle.

with the proximal end secured to the stump of the facial nerve and the fascicles anastomosed to the distal ends of the facial nerve branches. When necessary, the facial nerve can be traced up into the stylomastoid foramen as far as needed to secure free margins and nerve grafted at this point.

If the nerve graft is placed in a satisfactory bed and is covered with adequate soft tissue, the success rate should be very high. If only bone remains following resection of the facial nerve, the bed can be improved using either a portion of the sternocleidomastoid or posterior belly of the digastric or temporalis muscle to provide nutritional support for the nerve graft.

Following regeneration of the nerve, the face in repose should be symmetrical, and although there will always be some asymmetry as the patient grimaces or otherwise exercises the face, the functional result is certainly worth the time and effort to employ a nerve graft (Figs. 27-17 A–E).

OPTIONAL IMMEDIATE PROCEDURES

This category includes those reconstructive procedures that are largely cosmetic in nature and should not be done unless conditions are nearly ideal or unless the patient demands such a procedure. If the entire nose is resected, an immediate reconstruction can be done but this does not usually give a very pleasing cosmetic result unless the bony framework remains. If there is any question as to the adequacy of the surgical margins, it is far better to simply resurface the defect with a skin graft and have the maxillofacial prosthodontist construct a nasal prosthesis. The prosthetic noses have the disadvantage of changing color and can be a source of embarrassment to the patient if they should inadvertently be removed in public. However, the skilled maxillofacial prosthodontist can fashion an appliance that is much more aesthetically pleasing

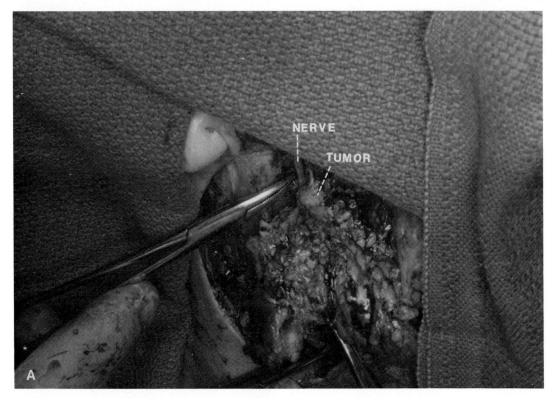

Fig. 27-17. (A) Adenoid cystic carcinoma of parotid invading and surrounding the facial nerve.

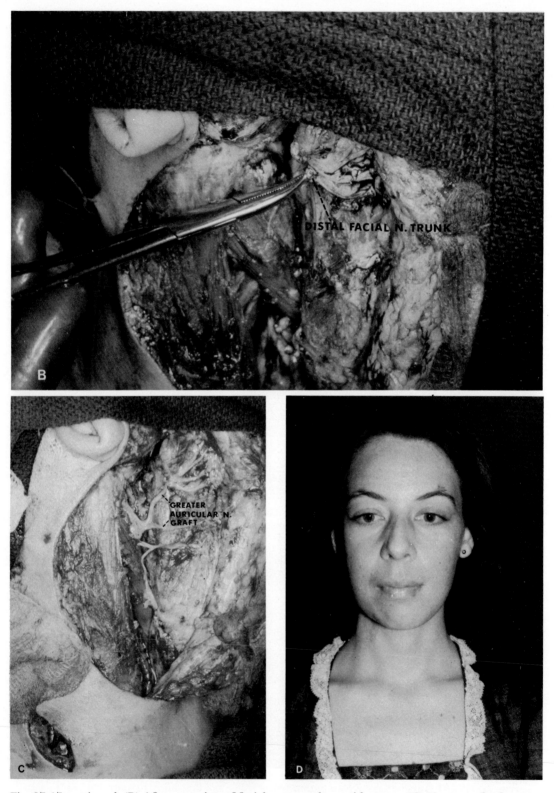

Fig. 27-17 continued. (B) After resection of facial nerve and parotidectomy. (C) Nerve graft of greater auricular nerve interposed. (D) Face in repose following recovery of function.

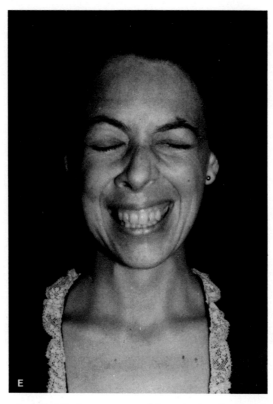

Fig. 27-17 continued. (E) Appearance of face during forced closure of eyes.

than most of the total nose reconstructions (Figs. 27-18 A and B). The same also applies to the immediate reconstruction of the ear. Although it is possible to reconstruct relatively small segments of the ear at the time of the initial surgical procedure, total ear reconstruction is, at best, difficult. It requires multiple staged procedures, so that it is more practical as well as aesthically acceptable to replace the missing part with a well-constructed prosthesis.

When considering immediate reconstruction of the mandible, the physician has to weigh the possible rate of failure against the functional result hoped to be achieved. The local condition of the tissues and the segment of the mandible resected are ordinarily determining factors that should be taken into consideration. Autogenous bone, either rib or iliac crest, should not be used unless conditions are ideal. It is preferable to use a prosthetic appliance constructed of perforated tubular tantalum or other mate-

rial rather than risk loss of an implanted segment of autogenous bone (Figs. 27-19 A–D). Should the prosthesis fail, it is ordinarily a simple matter to remove it through an incision made over the prosthesis.

MANDATORY DELAYED PROCEDURES

When one is dealing with elderly patients and those who have been irradiated, the safest procedure from the standpoint of risk of postoperative complications and local wound complications should be chosen. The patient who has received heavy radiation to both sides of the neck and pharyngeal area and who requires a total pharyngectomy presents a real challenge, and unless adequate nonirradiated tissue is available, the creation of pharyngeal fistulae should be considered. Such a wound ordinarily can be expected to heal satisfactorily and any time

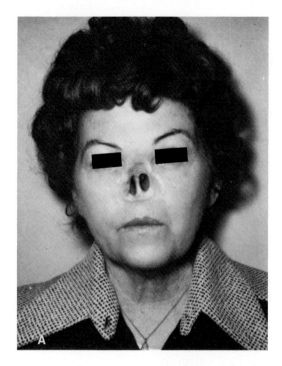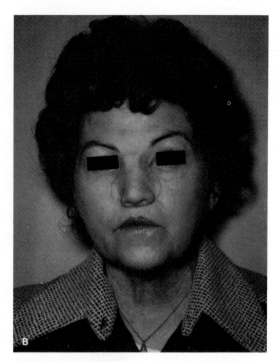

Fig. 27-18. (A) Operative defect following resection of nose. (B) With prosthesis in place.

lost in staging the reconstruction is more than made up by insuring the postoperative safety of the procedure. Any measures that will minimize the risk of carotid perforation or other disastrous complications are well worthwhile for the patient as well as for the peace of mind of the surgeon. In the aged individual who is poorly nourished, the simplest procedure that will get the patient through the immediate postoperative course is the one to be adopted (Figs. 27-20 A–C).

CHOICE OF RECONSTRUCTIVE MATERIALS

With the exception of prosthetic materials that can be used in defects of the skull, mandible, and facial bones, essentially all of the substances employed in reconstruction are autogenous. Skin grafts and skin flaps have been in use for centuries and their use in reconstructing head and neck defects is nothing new. However, new flaps are con-

stantly being devised, and new uses for old flaps are being advocated, providing the surgeon with a variety of techniques that can be employed. No dogmatic approach should be adopted for the reconstruction of all defects, but rather a number of options should be considered with the best one chosen to fit the magnitude of the defect, the age and nutritional condition of the patient, and the cosmetic result desired. The following brief summary of some of the uses, advantages, and disadvantages of the various materials and techniques that can be employed may provide a framework around which choices can be made.

Skin Grafts

Grafts vary in thickness, texture, and color, and care must be taken to select the graft that best fits the purpose. For restoration of function in the mouth or pharynx, a split-thickness graft is adequate. When the cosmetic result is more important, a full-thickness graft should be employed. The post-auricular skin provides a limited amount of

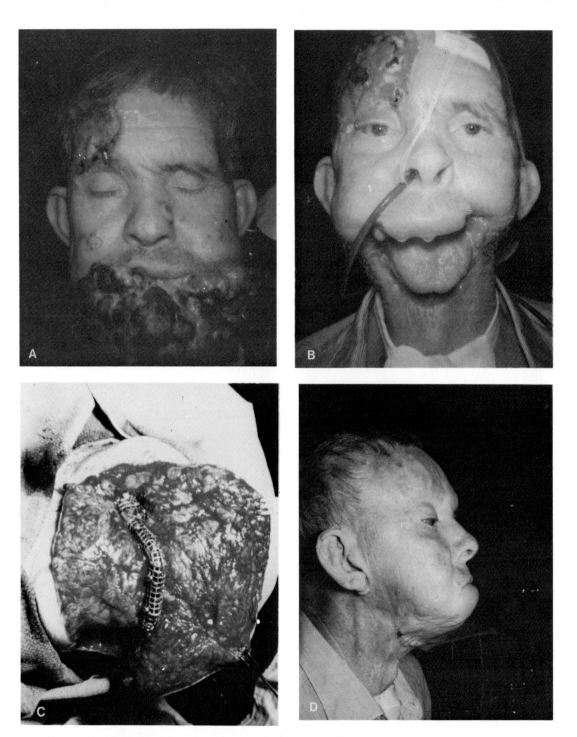

Fig. 27-19. (A) Extensive cancer of lower lip recurrent after irradiation. (B) Operative defect. (C) Prosthesis being inserted after repair of lip defect with pedicle graft. (D) Postoperative appearance. No recurrence in 12 years.

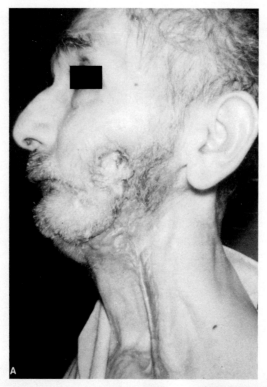

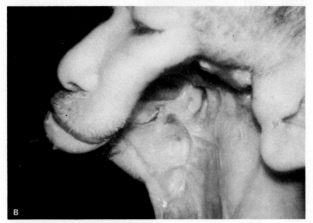

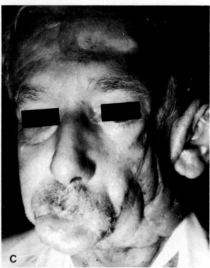

Fig. 27-20. (A) Extensive cancer of buccal mucosa, tongue, maxillae, and skin of neck recurrent after irradiation and surgery. (B) Postoperative defect. The carotid artery had to be sacrificed to the foramen lacerum. Reconstruction delayed. (C) After repair using a variety of flaps. Patient survived 10 years after the ablative procedure and died of other causes.

high quality skin that matches facial skin well in color and texture. A much larger amount of skin can be obtained from the infraclavicular area. Full-thickness grafts from this region provide good material for resurfacing the nose and face and can be used to reconstruct the entire lower lid if enough conjunctiva remains (Figs. 27-21 A and B). Much of the skin of the external ear can be resected along with the underlying carti-

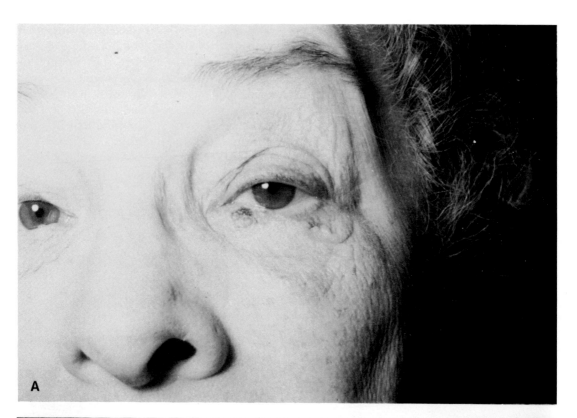

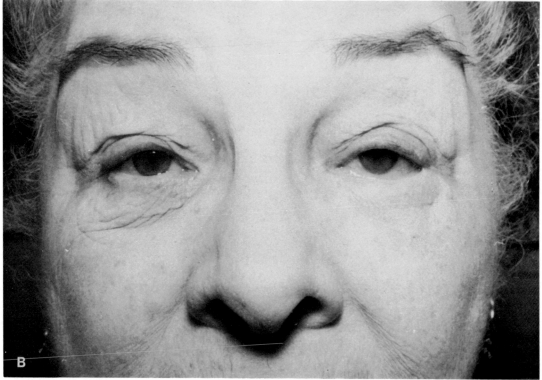

Fig. 27-21. (A) Melanoma of the lower lid. (B) Following resection of the entire lower lid and reconstruction with full-thickness graft.

lage, and a good cosmetic result can be obtained if a rim of cartilage is left around the helix and the defect is closed with a graft from the infraclavicular area.

Dermal Grafts

Dermal grafts are grafts taken from the dermal layer after a split-thickness epithelial graft has been raised (Figs. 27-22A-C). The primary use has been to cover the carotid artery when there is a chance for flap breakdown with fistula and exposure of the carotid. Dermal grafts are also used to cover mucosal defects because they are supposed to better simulate mucosa than do split-thickness skin grafts. The advantages of dermal grafts include the following: they can be bur-

ied under flaps; they can be used with either side up; they are thicker and easier to suture in place; if exposed to air, they will epithelialize over; and their use causes less pain than split-thickness skin grafts at the donor site. Disadvantages include the fact that the take rate is a little lower than that of split-thickness grafts; and that occasionally an epithelial cyst may form in the graft when it is buried and may present problems.

Mucosal Grafts and Flaps

Buccal mucosa grafts can be used to replace conjunctival mucosa. Mucosal flaps of the buccal mucosa, hard palate, and tongue can be used to resurface defects in the oral cavity or tonsillar region. The tongue can

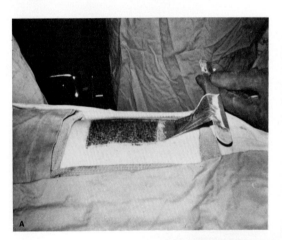
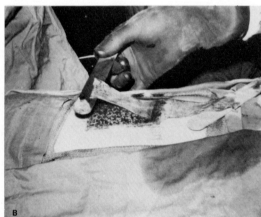
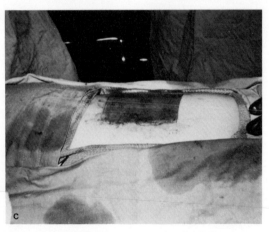

Fig. 27-22. (A) A split-thickness skin graft is raised and left attached. (B) A dermal graft is taken from the same site using a new dermatome blade. (C) The split-thickness skin graft is replaced after the dermal graft has been removed.

be used to provide a new vermilion border for a reconstructed lip. However, caution should be exercised in using mucosa for resurfacing purposes if there is associated leukoplakia or if the presence of multiple intraoral primary cancers suggests that another primary cancer might develop in the migrated mucosa.

Skin Flaps

A great variety of skin flaps are now in use, the most common being local flaps, skin of neck flaps, forehead and scalp flaps, deltopectoral flaps, posterior cervical flaps, and a variety of myocutaneous flaps. It is not within the province of this discussion to consider all of the flaps and their uses, and for this purpose the reader is referred to the references.

Local flaps of the cheek, forehead, and neck are ordinarily employed by transposition, advancement, or rotation to close facial or neck defects and give the best cosmetic result because texture and color match are excellent. They should not be employed unless the epithelial surface of the flap is normal and the defect into which they are migrated is microscopically free of cancer. Few problems are so distressing as the recurrence of cancer beneath an artistically constructed flap.

SKIN OF NECK FLAPS[2, 4, 11]

These flaps can be constructed in a variety of ways and used to resurface defects in the face or oral cavity. They have the advantage of being pliable and of having a reliable blood supply if the base is constructed adequately. They have the disadvantage of sometimes being hair-bearing in the male, and this would be disadvantageous if used in the oral cavity or pharynx. If skin of neck flaps are employed in the mouth or pharynx, a temporary fistula is necessary unless it is felt that the blood supply of the flap is sufficiently good to deepithelialize an area to provide primary approximation to mucosa.

FOREHEAD AND SCALP FLAPS[9, 10]

The principal advantage of these flaps is their usually very reliable blood supply. They can be used in various combinations to resurface oral or oropharyngeal defects and defects in the skull, face, orbits, or lips. Their main disadvantage is their lack of pliability and the production of a severe cosmetic defect at the donor site, particularly in males. A further disadvantage is the presence of hair in scalp and in some patients with narrow foreheads, their usefulness in resurfacing oral defects would be limited (Figs. 27-23 A–D).

DELTOPECTORAL FLAPS[3, 12]

These are remarkably versatile flaps that can be employed to reconstruct a variety of defects and, since they are taken below the clavicle, produce very little cosmetic and no functional deformity. Their viability can be improved, if necessary in the elderly, poorly nourished, or diabetic patient, by delaying procedures. Extensions of the flap to shoulder and upper arm can give a great quantity of pliable tissue for use in repair of complicated defects.

POSTERIOR CERVICAL FLAPS[2, 11]

The disadvantage of a relatively poor blood supply limits the use of posterior cervical skin flaps unless delayed. Their primary usefulness would seem to be in covering skin of neck defects or when other flaps are not available. The donor site is cosmetically acceptable.

COMPOSITE FLAPS

These flaps employ muscle and skin and may contain, in addition, bone or cartilage. They rely on well-vascularized muscle on a named arterial vessel supplying the muscle for their blood supply. Platysmal myocutaneous flaps,[6] and myocutaneous flaps of sternomastoid, pectoralis major,[13] trapezius,[5] and latissimus dorsi muscles all can be employed to advantage. The sternomastoid flap has a relatively unreliable blood

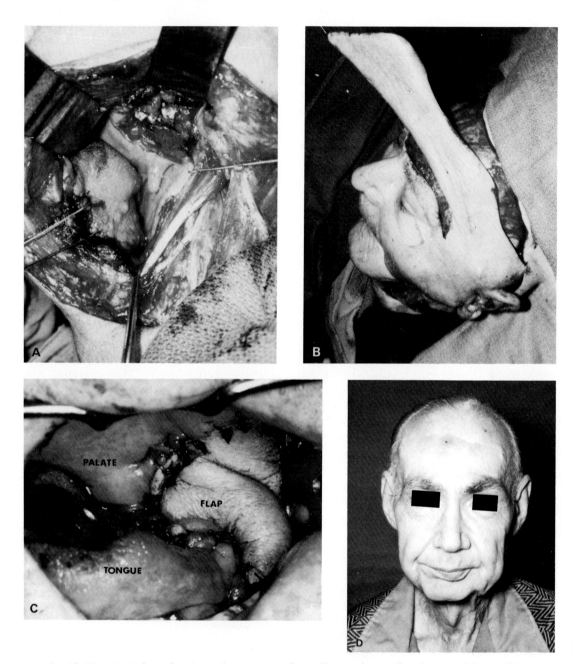

Fig. 27-23. (A) Defect after resecting cancer of tonsillar region, soft palate, and base of the tongue. (B) Forehead flap raised. (C) Forehead flap sutured in position. (D) Postoperative appearance.

supply unless the occipital artery is carefully preserved. The platysmal myocutaneous flap relies on a random blood supply that may be unreliable in some individuals. The other flaps with named vessels are ordinarily extremely reliable.

Free Grafts with Microvascular Anastomoses

A great variety of free grafts are possible and their number is constantly increasing.[1, 8] Among those currently in vogue are omen-

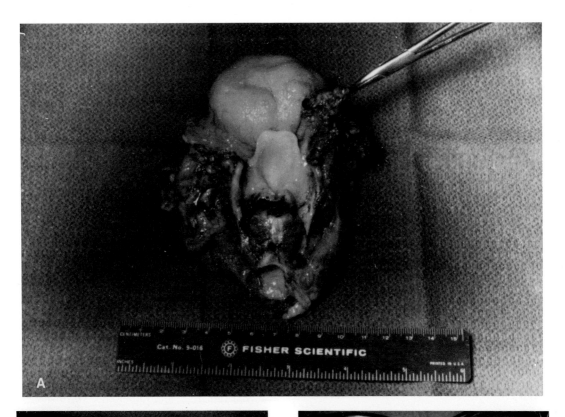

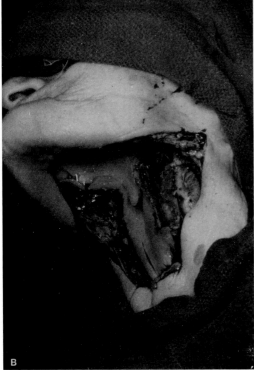

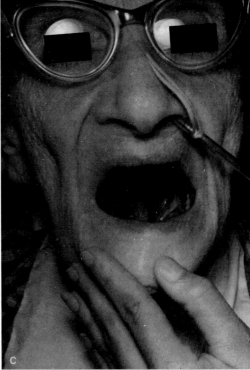

Fig. 27-24. (A) Operative specimen of adenocystic carcinoma involving entire tongue and tonsillar region. (B) Operative defect. (C) Postoperative appearance after repair with split-thickness skin graft.

tal grafts, segments of small or large intestine,[7] groin flaps, skin of foot grafts with dorsalis pedis and metatarsal, various muscle and skin grafts, and rib and intercostal muscle and vessel grafts. The disadvantage of the free grafts is the amount of time consumed during the operative procedure and the necessity for special training and instruments. The place of these grafts in the armamentarium of the reconstructive surgeon is still being developed.

Tube Pedicle Flaps

With all the present emphasis on immediate reconstruction in one stage, it is easy to lose sight of the fact that in some patients and with some defects, this might not be possible. Because of its pliability and versatility, the tubed pedicle flap will probably continue to be the method of choice for some of the complex defects involving lips, palate, cheeks, and nose.

Skin Grafts versus Skin Flaps

Despite the obvious advantages of flaps, one should not forget that a simple split-thickness skin graft can be used to resurface many of the intraoral defects with a very adequate functional result. In the aged and debilitated patient, a split-thickness skin graft may well be the method of choice for some complex defects such as that illustrated in Figures 27-24 A-C. Following total glossectomy, laryngectomy, and partial pharyngectomy, the defect in this figure was reconstructed in one stage with a split-thickness skin graft sewn to the remaining mucosa. No flap would have served as well in this aged and debilitated patient.

SUMMARY

In the surgical approach to any head and neck cancer problem, the satisfactory ablation of the primary cancer with its possible nodal metastases should be the primary objective of the surgeon. The possible magnitude of the defect should be kept in clear perspective and a variety of plans formulated for possible use depending upon the result at the time of the completed surgical resection. No reconstructive procedure, however elaborate and artistically conceived, should preempt the adequate surgical removal of the cancer, nor should such a plan be rigidly adhered to if events during the operative procedure dictate a safer course. All those reconstructive procedures which are mandatory should be accomplished and the other procedures as outlined can be done if the clinical situation permits.

REFERENCES

1. Acland, R. D., and Flynn, M. B. 1978. Immediate reconstruction of oral cavity and oropharyngeal defects using microvascular free flaps. American Journal of Surgery, 136: 419.

2. Bakamjian, B. and Littlewood, M. 1964. Cervical skin flaps for intraoral and pharyngeal repair. British Journal of Plastic Surgery, 17: 191.

3. Bakamjian, V. Y., Long, M., and Rigg, B. 1971. Experience with the medially based deltopectoral flap in reconstructive surgery of the head and neck. British Journal of Plastic Surgery, 24: 174.

4. Barbosa, J. F. 1974. Surgical Treatment of Head and Neck Tumors. Von Becker Froon, R. (trans). Grune & Stratton, New York.

5. Demergasso, F., and Piazza, M. 1979. Trapezius myocutaneous flap in reconstructive surgery for head and neck cancer: An original technique. American Journal of Surgery, 138: 533.

6. Futrell, J. W., Johns, M. E., Edgerton, M. T., Cantrell, R. W., and Fitz-Hugh, G. S. 1978. Platysma myocutaneous flap for intraoral reconstruction. American Journal of Surgery, 136: 504.

7. Grage, T. B., and Quick, C. A. 1978. The use of revascularized ileocolic autografts for primary repair after pharyngolaryngoesophagectomy. American Journal of Surgery, 136: 477.

8. Harii, K., Torii, S., and Seikguichi, J. 1978. The free lateral thoracic flap. Plastic and Reconstructive Surgery, 62: 212.

9. Lewis, M. B., and Remensnyder, J. P. 1978. Forehead flap for reconstruction after ablative surgery for oral and oropharyngeal malignancy. Plastic and Reconstructive Surgery, 62: 59.

10. Lore, J. M. 1973. An Atlas of Head and Neck Surgery. (2nd ed.) W. B. Saunders, Philadelphia.

11. Mathes, S. J., and Vasconez, L. O. 1978. The Cervicohumeral flap. Plastic and Reconstructive Surgery, 61: 7.

12. Montgomery, W. W. 1971. Surgery of the Upper Respiratory Tract. Lea and Febiger, Philadelphia.

13. Withers, E. H., Franklin, J. D., Madden, J. J., and Lynch, J. B. 1979. Pectoralis major musculocutaneous flap: A new flap in head and neck reconstruction. American Journal of Surgery, 138: 537.

28 | Management of Complications

Victor L. Schramm, Jr., M.D.
Eugene N. Myers, M.D.

"The only surgeon who has no complications is the one who doesn't operate."

INTRODUCTION

This maxim has stood the test of time but
should not be used as an excuse by the surgeon who has more than the usual number
of complications. Over the years physicians
and patients have viewed head and neck
surgery in a negative way, in part because of
the complications resulting from the therapeutic program.

Complications evolving from head and
neck surgery may range from very minimal
ones that can be easily corrected to life-
threatening or fatal situations, such as those
posed by rupture of the carotid artery system. In these contemporary times, maximum therapeutic programs, including chemotherapy, radiation therapy, and massive
surgical extirpative therapy, are being utilized particularly for patients with far advanced cancer. This increases the potential
for serious sequelae so that it is becoming
ever more essential to minimize complications.

The postoperative hospitalization of
the usual laryngectomy patient may change
from the routine 10 to 14 days to 2 or 3
months if the same patient develops a pharyngocutaneous fistula. Because of the enormous pressures on organized medicine to
examine the cost-benefit ratio of its health-
care efforts, it is incumbent upon us to make
every effort to reduce the complications of
head and neck surgery.

We are certain that most, though not
all, complications can be prevented. The
prevention of complications really begins
when the patient is first seen in the office

756

with careful preoperative evaluation and
with attention to the care of multisystem disease. Nutritional therapy in the malnourished patient and intensive nursing care are
combined with meticulous surgical technique to prevent complications. It is with
this thought in mind that we explore this
subject with an emphasis on prevention.

PSYCHOSOCIAL COMPLICATIONS

Psychological and social problems commonly antedate the appearance of the head
and neck tumor. Personality disorders, commonly of the passive-aggressive or passive-
dependent type, compound the difficulties
of recognizing and expressing emotion.
Denial of the presence or significance
of a malignancy is often an extension of
the patient's usual psychological defense
mechanisms, particularly as they relate to
the problems of alcohol abuse. It is estimated that 30 to 90 percent of patients with
head and neck cancer have a history of alcoholism.[15] Feelings of failure and guilt that
may have been present previously are highlighted by the thought of cancer and may
result in an unrecognized depression. Family support, which is essential for physical as
well as psychological rehabilitation, may be
poor or nonexistent because of prior alien-
ation most frequently related to alcoholism.
The financial costs related to therapy and
loss of income further complicate both psychological factors and family relationships.

Cognizance of, and an organized approach to, the management of psychosocial problems associated with head and neck cancer are essential parts of the overall management. The importance of these factors is underscored by the recognition that up to 30 percent of patients who have been treated for head and neck cancer die without evidence of malignant disease. In our patients the main noncardiovascular factors in these deaths were complications of psychological depression, alcoholism, and disinterest in self-preservation, leading to a "failure to thrive." The overall approach to these problems must be a positive one capitalizing on the patient's psychological, physical, and family strengths.

An organized preoperative evaluation and discussion by nursing staff, psychiatrist, social worker, speech therapist, and, in some cases, maxillofacial prosthodontist is essential. The degree of cosmetic and functional disability that the patient, family, and health care personnel expect to result from therapy should be determined, and unrealistic images should be countered by an honest discussion of the actual possibilities and modes of rehabilitation. The patient and, to an extent, the family must understand that they share with the health care team the responsibility for an uncomplicated recuperation. To avoid the assignation of blame for failure to eradicate disease, the therapy team must help the patient and family to understand that whereas an optimal plan for management of the cancer has been outlined and they may be hopeful regarding the outcome, complete biologic control of the tumor cannot be guaranteed.

ANESTHESIA-RELATED COMPLICATIONS

Complications related to anesthetic management may occur from the time of anesthesia induction through the postoperative period. Anesthesia considerations have been discussed in detail in Chapter 6, and only those situations requiring joint recognition and management will be presented here. The observations that follow are based on an analysis of 1,200 head and neck procedures performed at the Eye and Ear Hospital of Pittsburgh.

The most common problems were those related to intraoperative fluid management, particularly overhydration. Twelve percent of the patients in our series had radiographic and clinical signs of pulmonary edema and required fluid restriction and diuretic therapy in the early postoperative period. Those patients having intraoperative hypotension or early postoperative pulmonary congestion or edema were noted to have an eight times greater chance of pneumonia and wound complications, including necrosis of regional flaps, when compared to the other patients in this series. Blood and crystalloid replacement sufficient to prevent hypotension and maintain a urinary output between 30 and 50 ml per hour is associated with a markedly decreased postoperative pulmonary and wound complication rate.

Intraoperative airway complications are most commonly related to a misplaced endothracheal tube. This is recognized subjectively by a change in pulmonary compliance and objectively by blood-gas determinations indicating hypoxia and hypercarbia. The surgeon must allow the anesthetist to reposition the tube in order to correct endobronchial intubation or endotracheal tube obstruction caused by the bevel of the tube lying against the posterior wall of the trachea. We have been able to minimize such complications in our oral cavity and laryngopharyngeal resections by doing a preliminary tracheotomy under local anesthesia and inserting an armored, cuffed endotracheal tube after general anesthesia has been induced. Care is taken to insure that the cuff is just inside the trachea, and the tube is secured by suturing the tube to the skin of the chest. The tube is then marked with methylene blue at the level of the skin incision so that if the tube migrates, necessary adjustments can be made in a timely fashion.

Intraoperative aspiration of blood, salivary secretions, or gastric contents may also result in airway obstruction and bronchospasm. Such problems may be corrected by suction and saline lavage. Postoperative aspiration of blood or gastric contents results in a clinical picture of pulmonary edema that may be distinguished from aspiration primarily by the type of secretion that is suctioned from the tracheobronchial tree. The use of steroids, bronchodilators, and mechanical ventilation with positive end-expiratory pressure for 24 to 48 hours may also be necessary.

Pneumothorax may occur from pulmonary overinflation causing rupture of an emphysematous bleb or from extension of a pneumomediastinum. Distinction must be made between pneumothorax and a displaced endotracheal tube by repositioning of the tube and auscultation of the chest. If the cardiopulmonary compromise is severe, immediate aspiration of the air from the affected pleural cavity through the second intercostal space is indicated. A chest tube should be placed if persistent hypercarbia and hypoxia are noted, or if the radiographically estimated pneumothorax is greater than 15 percent.

Cardiac dysrhythmias, ischemia, and infarctions may occur at any time during a surgical procedure. These problems are most commonly encountered at the time of endoscopy.[30] Patients with a prior history of cardiac disease or evidence of electrocardiographic abnormality are most susceptible. Manipulation in and around the larynx triggers the reflex involving the afferent fibers of the superior laryngeal nerve and the cardioinhibitory fibers of the vagus nerve.[32] Simply removing the endoscope and ventilating the patient usually results in prompt cessation of the dysrhythmia. Occasionally the intravenous administration of lidocaine may be necessary.

Intraoperative bradycardia with hypotension or cardiac dysrhythmia requiring alteration of anesthesia management occurred in 8 percent of our series. Bradycardia and hypotension are nearly always associated with compression of the bifurcation of the carotid artery and may be alleviated simply by relieving the compression or by infiltration of 1 to 2 ml of lidocaine into the adventitia at the carotid bifurcation to block the carotid sinus reflex. Dysrhythmia and associated hypotension may also occur when the patient is in a relatively light plane of anesthesia and is stimulated by pain, laryngeal manipulation, or ocular pressure. The surgeon must immediately stop the inciting manipulation until the dyrhythmia has been corrected and the plane of anesthesia has been deepened.

The incidence of intraoperative or early postoperative myocardial infarction in our series was less than 1 percent. This complication occurred only in those patients with a previous history of severe cardiac disease. Postoperative cardiac monitoring is mandatory in any such patient who sustains an intraoperative dysrhythmia or hypotension. Any patient who has electrocardiographic evidence of ischemia should be managed by the medical consultant in the coronary care unit.

Intraoperative malignant hyperthermia is a rare complication in an elderly population and did not occur in our series. When intraoperative hyperthermia did occur it was related to intraoperative sepsis or, rarely, to transfusion reaction. Hyperthermia, in the absence of skeletal muscle rigidity, should therefore be considered to be a result of sepsis or a transfusion reaction and evaluation and management should be directed toward those etiologic factors. Symptomatic treatment with cooling using intravenous fluids below body temperature usually is adequate to allow completion of the operative procedure. Routine use of a cooling blanket to help regulate intraoperative temperature in major cases is recommended.

INTRAOPERATIVE COMPLICATIONS

Surgical complications specific to anatomic or regional sites are to be considered in each surgical chapter. Operative complications that may occur in association with any procedure include corneal abrasion, hemorrhage, and air embolus.

Corneal abrasions occur when the eye is exposed and may be injured by surgical drapes or direct trauma from surgical instruments. This complication is best prevented by instilling 1 percent methyl cellulose into the eye preoperatively and securing the eyelid with a temporary tarsorrhaphy suture. Taping the eyelids is a good second choice particularly if the eyes are not included in the sterile surgical field. Though ophthalmolic ointments are commonly used, if an abrasion does occur the presence of ointment delays epithelial migration and healing. Treatment of an abrasion includes irrigation of the eye with physiologic salt solution, covering the cornea with methyl cellulose, and patching the eye. Early intensive treatment of acute corneal abrasion by an ophthalmologist may prevent the problems encountered with chronic corneal erosion. Solutions such as pHisoHex may cause a severe chemical conjunctivitis and should be avoided.

Sudden intraoperative *hemorrhage* is an unusual and usually avoidable consequence of surgical resection. This is particularly true during maxillectomy and major oral cavity resection. When major bleeding is anticipated, the surgeon should complete that part of the operative procedure which is not usually associated with heavy bleeding and then inform the anesthesiologist of anticipated major blood loss so that the patient may be properly managed. The resection can then be completed in expeditious fashion without hypotension. If, however, uncontrolled hypotension results, bleeding should be controlled by pressure or packing while blood volume is replaced. The latter technique is also preferred when unanticipated bleeding occurs from the carotid system or from the upper or lower end of the jugular vein during a neck dissection. After blood replacement and correction of hypotension, definitive treatment of the hemorrhage may be safely instituted.

Air embolism occurs most commonly when the head of the operating table has been elevated 15° to 20° and when the pa-tient is breathing spontaneously. Both of these situations result in a relatively reduced thoracic-venous pressure, which increases the chance of the entry of air into the cervical venous system. Air embolism may be suspected if a sucking noise is heard during a surgical dissection; a diagnosis is made by the identification of a "mill wheel" murmur, Doplar ultrasound detection, electrocardiographic changes, and hypotension. Details on the management of this problem can be found in Chapter 6.

Radical Neck Dissection

The most serious complications of radical neck dissection are vascular in nature. The most dramatic of these is injury to the carotid artery system. This complication rarely occurs during an orderly neck dissection done by a surgeon with a 3-dimensional knowledge of the anatomy of the neck. Bleeding from a transected major branch, such as the superior thyroid artery, is prevented by double-tie or suture ligature. When massive bleeding does occur, local pressure is applied to the bleeding site while proximal-distal control of the artery is obtained. If bleeding is from the external carotid artery or one of its branches, the vessel may be safely ligated. If a laceration of the common or internal carotid artery has occurred, repair of the laceration with a 5-0 nylon suture is preferred. Prior to final closure of the laceration, distal arterial occlusion is temporarily released to promote back bleeding and removal of intraarterial air. During arterial repair, blood pressure may be supported by lightening the level of general anesthesia and replacing fluid and blood. If carotid artery rupture is associated with invasion of the arterial wall by metastatic carcinoma, ligation and resection of the artery are indicated.

Bleeding from the distal end of the internal jugular vein may be potentially more dangerous and more difficult to control than arterial bleeding. Bleeding may occur from laceration of the internal jugular vein during the dissection preliminary to ligation or may result from tearing of a venous tributary from the posterior aspect of the vein. A most dangerous injury is at the junction of the internal jugular and subclavian veins. To prevent air embolism, the patient must immediately be placed in a level or head-down position. Bleeding is temporarily controlled by pressure while distal dissection is completed. If the jugular is avulsed at the subclavian, it may be necessary to resect a portion of the clavicle to gain exposure. Blind grasping of the bleeding site with a hemostat is to be avoided not only because of further tearing of the vein but also because of the possibility of damage to other structures in that area.

Hemorrhage from the proximal aspect of the internal jugular vein is disconcerting but far less dangerous. Air embolism may be prevented by distal compression of the vein if it has not been previously ligated, and bleeding may be controlled by pressure. If proximal control cannot be obtained with clamps and ligature, then the jugular foramen may be packed with oxidized cellulose or muscle and oversewn with the posterior belly of the digastric muscle. Alternatively, the mastoid tip may be removed in an effort to gain direct control.

Chylous leak can usually be prevented by isolating the lymphatic pedicle found between the carotid artery and the phrenic nerve and clamping this pedicle prior to dividing and ligating it. Equal care should be taken on both sides of the neck. Intraoperative chylous leak should be recognized when opalescent fluid is noted in the posterior and inferior aspect of the dissected neck. The fluid is clear at surgery because the patient had nothing by mouth overnight, but would be chylous (milky) after feedings have begun. In order to establish the site of the leak the area of the lymphatic pedicle should be irrigated and closely investigated. This should be done with the patient in a supine position during a sustained hyperventilation. If there is difficulty in locating the exact site of the chyle leak, use of the operating microscope may be helpful. Also, central venous instillation of cardiac green, a dye used for cardiac output studies,

will result in a green discoloration of the chyle and make the site more easily identifiable. Once the chylous leak has been isolated, it should be clamped and secured with a tie rather than a suture ligature, as the needle will further tear the lymphatic channels.

Nerve injury during radical neck dissection may be either intentional or inadvertent. The spinal accessory, cervical cutaneous, and greater auricular nerves are intentionally sacrificed during the standard radical neck dissection. If the spinal accessory nerve is unintentionally injured during a modified neck dissection, some return of trapezius function can be anticipated if a neurorrhaphy is done at the time of neck dissection. An interposition graft of greater auricular nerve also results in decreased shoulder disability, but should be considered only if tumor clearance in the area of the nerves can be ensured.

A nerve injury that is not commonly recognized nor easily avoided is that to the motor branches of the cervical plexus that supply the deep muscles of the neck. Injury to these nerves may explain the variation in the degree of disability of the shoulder produced by sacrifice of the spinal accessory nerve. We refer particularly to injury to the nerve supply of the levator scapulae, which enters that muscle near its midpoint along with its vascular supply. This may be avoided by leaving the deep layer of the deep cervical fascia intact in that area.

Injury to the phrenic nerve may occur without its transection, and care must be exercised in identifying this nerve during dissection. If the phrenic nerve is transected it should be reapproximated, although this is of little benefit in the immediate postoperative period when the function of the diaphragm is most important. Injury to the cervical contributions to the phrenic nerve may be avoided by dissecting the neck from the posterior triangle anteriorly and transecting the cervical cutaneous nerves distal to their phrenic contributions. Hemostasis by electrocautery should also be avoided in the area of the phrenic nerve.

Injury to the brachial plexus is uncommon and may be avoided by undermining the posterior triangle of the neck and visualizing the entire brachial plexus prior to transection or to clamping of the posterior triangle fat. Transection of the brachial plexus to obtain tumor clearance is not indicated.

Injury to the vagus nerve will result in ipsilateral hypopharyngeal and vocal cord anesthesia and/or vocal cord paralysis. No cardiac or gastrointestinal dysfunction is known to result from transection of the vagus. Nerve repair or grafting will not result in successful return of function. In patients whose vagus nerve has definitely been transected, injection of the true vocal cord with Teflon may be indicated in the early postoperative period to provide rehabilitation of cough, voice, and deglutition.

Unilateral loss of hypoglossal nerve function results in little disability unless there is also other substantial crippling of the swallowing function such as that occurring in composite resection or supraglottic laryngectomy. If the nerve is cut inadvertantly, neurorrhaphy should result in reasonable return of function in 3 to 4 months. Bilateral loss of function may occur in laryngectomy with resection of a base of tongue cancer and would result in severe crippling of the swallowing function and impair the ability to learn esophageal speech.

Injury to the cervical sympathetic chain results in Horner syndrome. Swift[33] found this in 11 of 33 patients undergoing radical neck dissection. No patient complained of change in pupillary size, drooping of the eyelid, or change in facial sweating. Usually the only alteration was miosis, often with slight ptosis. In two patients there was anhydrosis and in two others there was decreased moisture on the side of the miosis. Such injury generally occurs in dissection around or posterior to the carotid sheath. Neurorrhaphy is of no value following sympathetic nerve transection.

Paralysis of the facial nerve system is an unusual complication of radical neck dissection. Special care should be exercised when the posterior belly of the digastric muscle is sacrificed to encompass nodal metastasis in the upper spinal accessory chain, since the stylomastoid foramen is located at the posterior superior aspect of the posterior belly. The facial nerve may be identified at the stylomastoid foramen, as is done in parotid surgery, and dissected free from the neck specimen. If facial nerve injury is recognized at the time of surgery, neurorrhaphy should be done. Blunt trauma to the area of the mastoid tip and the tail of the parotid from tissue retraction may produce this injury but the injury is not usually recognized until the early postoperative period. Immediate or delayed onset of facial nerve paralysis following radical neck dissection is unusually prolonged in its recovery and lateral tarsorrhaphy is indicated for eye protection. We have had three such patients in our series. The paralysis cleared in two patients in 3 to 4 months. The third has a partial residual paresis.

Unilateral sacrifice of the marginal mandibular branch of the facial nerve may be necessary when there is obvious nodal metastasis in the upper neck. This results in little disability and only minimal cosmetic deformity. However, loss of function of both marginal mandibular nerves, as may occur in dissections for anterior floor-of-mouth lesions or in bilateral neck dissections, does result in an incompetent oral commissure. This may be even more disabling when associated with sensory loss to the lower lip.

POSTOPERATIVE WOUND COMPLICATIONS

Neck Dissection Complications

Frequent and serious postoperative complications occur in patients who have undergone radical neck dissection. These patients usually have extensive tumor and frequently have multisystem medical problems and significant nutritional depletion. The addition of planned or unplanned preoperative radiation therapy, prolonged operative time and wound exposure, and frequently, more extensive primary resection all add to the likelihood of postoperative complications.

Hematoma is one of the more common complications and predisposes to wound infections, flap necrosis, carotid exposure, and fistula formation. An effort should be made to diagnose any coagulation defect prior to surgery. Because of the prevalence of alcholism and liver damage in this patient population, special attention to platelet count and prothrombin time is mandatory. Thrombocytopenia, especially after the use of greater than 5 units of transfused blood, and disseminated intravascular coagulation occur infrequently but predispose to hematoma formation. Meticulous hemostasis is by far the most important factor in preventing hematoma formation. It is our strong conviction that the occurrence of hematoma is directly related to how compulsive the surgeon is in obtaining hemostasis. Prior to closure at least two medium drainage catheters should be placed in the supraclavicular fossa and posterior triangle; two other catheters should be placed anterior to the carotid artery and adjacent to the pharyngeal or oral cavity closure in composite resections. Constant suction should be maintained during the early postoperative period and bulky external compression dressings applied to help coapt the skin to the underlying structures in the dissected neck.

Hematoma formation may be noticed as the patient is being moved off of the operating table or into the postanesthesia recovery room. The features that usually call attention to the presence of a hematoma are the presence of a ballotable mass in the supraclavicular fossa, eccymosis of the skin of the cervical and pectoral area, excessive blood in the suction drainage bottle, and upper airway distress in patients without tracheotomy.

When a hematoma is recognized the patient should be returned immediately to the operating room. The wound must be opened and the hematoma evacuated under sterile conditions. Adequate blood replacement must also be instituted, as it is not uncommon to lose 1 to 2 units of blood in such situations. A major bleeding point is usually not identified but all bleeding points must be ligated. The wound must be irrigated and new drains inserted. The pressure dressings are then reapplied and the patient returned to the recovery room for further observation. A patient without tracheotomy may develop upper airway obstruction from the hematoma, forced against the trachea by the pressure dressing. In such a situation, whether in the recovery room or on the ward, the sutures must be removed and the hematoma immediately evacuated to relieve airway obstruction. We reviewed 100 consecutive radical neck dissections performed by our Department from 1973 to 1977. There were two patients who developed a hematoma, both in the immediate postoperative period. One was diagnosed in the recovery room, the other as the last skin sutures were being placed. Both were treated as described above without untoward effects.

Seroma occurs infrequently and is usually diagnosed about the fifth postoperative day. It is noted as a ballotable mass in the supraclavicular fossa without eccymosis of the cervical flaps or a history of hematoma. The etiology of this complication is obscure, but seroma probably represents lysis of blood from a small hematoma which creates an osmotic gradient for serum collection. Seromas are usually managed by serial aspiration under sterile conditions, with or without pressure dressings, and resolve in several weeks. Opening of the cervical flap should be avoided, as bacterial contamination and wound infection frequently result.

Chylous fistula also occurs infrequently. The first indication of its presence may be excessive hemovac drainage, either immediately postoperatively, or at the time nasogastric feedings are begun. Occasionally a chyle leak will be noted as a bulge beneath the skin of the supraclavicular fossa.[5,21] In addition to elevation of skin flaps, the infiltration of chyle will also produce induration, edema, and erythema of the overlying skin. A chylous fistula may also lead secondarily to chylothorax[4] with signs mimicking a pleural effusion. The latter complication requires placement of chest tube drainage. The consequences of a chylous fistula may lead to fatality. Weakness and peripheral edema resulting from loss of fat, protein, lymphocytes, and electrolytes may occur.

The incidence of chylous fistula, as with hematoma, is directly proportional to meticulousness of surgical technique. In our series of neck dissections cited above, no chylous fistula occurred. Once a chylous fistula is recognized, treatment should begin immediately. Uncommonly, the amount of chyle recovered in the hemovac drains or by aspiration is under 100 ml per 24 hours, and rapidly decreases in amount with aspiration and pressure dressings. More commonly, the chyle is noted early in the postoperative period and the volume is great, possibly reaching 2,000 ml in 24 hours. Once the diagnosis of chylous fistula is made, the patient should be returned to the operating room as soon as possible, preferably before tissue induration occurs. The same method of identification and management of the chylous leak as mentioned above will usually be successful.

Late treatment of the chylous fistula is more complex. Fluid, electrolyte, and protein losses must be replaced. The electrolyte composition is the same as that of plasma, and the protein content of chyle is between 2 and 4.5 percent. Protein loss may be replaced by albumen. If chylous fistula persists despite attempts at closure, consideration should be given to total parenteral nutrition via a contralateral subclavian catheter. Should the initial attempt at closure be unsuccessful or if late local treatment is necessary, suturing of Gelfoam or Surgicel impregnated with thrombin and placement of flap over the leak may be successful. Iodoform gauze packing of an open wound and healing by second intention may ultimately be necessary if the chylous fistula is not corrected early in its course.

Bilateral neck dissection produces complications related to venous and lymphatic obstruction. At present there seems to be little difference in the rate of complications whether the second neck dissection is performed simultaneously or as a planned, staged procedure.[17,35] Airway obstruction, and facial and conjunctival edema occur frequently. Increased intracranial pressure occurs infrequently, but the possibility should be anticipated in each patient. The presence of marked facial edema does not necessarily indicate intracranial edema. When possible, sparing an internal jugular vein on the side of least tumor involvement decreases intracerebral complications to almost zero. Preservation of an external jugular vein has also been advised[35] and may decrease both facial venostasis and intracranial pressure. When either planned or unplanned staged bilateral neck dissection is performed, the presence of extensive tumor may preclude preservation of either the internal or external jugular vein.

A tracheostomy must be performed in all patients at the time of the staged second neck dissection or of a simultaneous bilateral neck dissection to avoid upper airway obstruction secondary to laryngeal edema. During and after surgery the patient should be kept in a semi-Fowler position avoiding the use of circumferential constricting dressings that may decrease venous return. If conjunctival edema is severe, a temporary suture tarsorrhaphy will aid in the prevention or treatment of conjunctival dryness and ulceration.

Measurement of jugular vein stump pressure, or lumbar spinal fluid pressure may demonstrate cerebral pressures approaching 60 cm of H_2O.[17] Pressure on the posterior neck or a rotation of the head of 45° causes a further increase in cerebral venous pressure. Increased intracranial venous pressure results in cerebral edema, which may cause impaired neurologic function, such as blindness, stroke, or coma, or death. In addition, there is a consistent antidiuretic effect.

Management of these complications in addition to avoidance of compression dressings and elevation of the head include diuretic therapy and careful monitoring of fluid balance, in addition, if lumbar spinal fluid pressure is 50 cm H_2O or greater or if the patient exhibits confusion or coma, a lumbar subarachnoid drain should be placed and small increment fluid removal continued until venous collateral drainage is established and intracranial pressure is decreased. The use of steroids, manitol, and subarachnoid-peritoneal shunt has also been recommended.

Sequelae of Radical Neck Dissection

Sequelae of radical neck dissection include shoulder dysfunction, sternoclavicular joint enlargement, stress fracture of the clavicle, gustatory sweating, sensory loss, neuroma, and cervical flap scar contracture. Weakness, deformity, and pain in the shoulder region are the disagreeable sequelae of classical radical neck dissection in almost every patient.[26,31] Normal function of the trapezius muscle is lost when the spinal accessory nerve is cut. Participating muscles that compensate for loss of trapezius function are the rhomboids and the levator scapula, although the latter may also be denervated by cutting its branch from the cervical plexus.

With paralysis of trapezius function, the vertebral border of the scapula becomes flared and this flaring is accentuated when the arm is abducted from the side against resistance. Abduction of the shoulder is limited. Patients with marked loss of shoulder abduction characteristically try to compensate by contralateral flexion of the trunk. Even though the trapezius is paralyzed, the forward flexors of the shoulder may elevate the arm, thus causing it to appear that the patient is abducting the arm, while in reality he is using forward flexors to raise the arm above the head.[26] Since rotation of the shoulder joint must accompany abduction, the extremes of external rotation generally are lost because of disuse. Pain associated with the surgery may also limit extremes of shoulder motion. The scapulohumoral joint

tends to lose motion and in some cases develops a condition known as periarthritis or adhesive capsulitis. The characteristic position of the scapulohumoral complex postoperatively is forward and downwards.

Functional limitations following radical neck dissection are due to pain on motion of the scapulohumoral joint and inability to fully abduct the shoulder due to loss of stability of the scapula. Cosmetic problems include forward and downward displacement of the shoulder complex and atrophy of the trapezius muscle. Saunders and Johnson[26] have devised a treatment program for these patients, the results of which are relief of pain, an improvement in posture, and functional improvement of the arm as shoulder motion increases. They describe a program that includes the use of an infrared luminous 250 watt lamp at home for pain, strengthening the scapular retractors and elevators using regressive resistance technique, range of motion exercises to increase scapulohumoral joint motion, and active stretch of the shortened scapular protractor (serratus anterior). Our own experience is similar, and we have had excellent success in preserving form and function in those few patients who are well enough motivated to persist with the treatment protocol (Fig. 28-1).

Occasionally following radical neck dissection, particularly bilateral radical neck dissection, there is both apparent and real enlargement of the sternoclavicular joint (Fig. 28-2A and B). This is partly due to the head of the clavicle becoming more prominent because of the removal of the sternomastoid muscle. The sternoclavicular joint is also stressed by the gravity from the weight of the arm on the clavicle, which is unsupported due to atrophy of the trapezius muscle. The result of this torque-like action is subluxation of the head of the clavicle in an upward and forward direction through the weakest part of the capsule.[12] With continued stress, periarticular fibrosis sets in followed by synovial proliferation as is seen in osteoarthritis of weight-bearing joints. Once a mass is recognized as the sternoclavicular

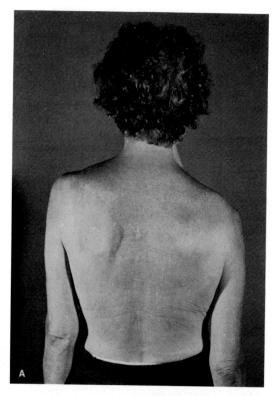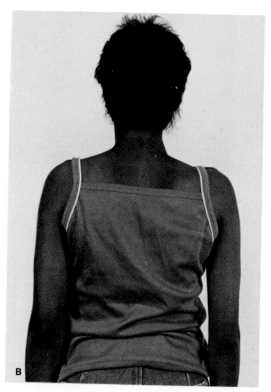

Fig. 28-1. (A) Deformities following a classical radical neck dissection : forward and downward displacement of shoulder, atrophy of trapezius. This patient does not participate in the prescribed exercise program. (B) Patient following radical neck dissection demonstrating atrophy of trapezius but no shoulder displacement. This patient participated enthusiastically in the prescribed exercise program.

head rather than metastatic cancer no treatment is necessary.

Stress fractures of the clavicle occur infrequently as a sequela of radical neck dissection. Pfeifle et al.[24] described three patients each of whom had developed a rapidly enlarging mass in the area of the clavicle a few months after radical neck dissection. Radiography revealed fractures of the clavicle, although there was no history of antecedent trauma. They referred to these as "pseudotumors" and attributed their development to stress fractures with luxuriant callus formation. Cummings and First[6] reported a stress fracture of the clavicle that occurred 15 months after radical neck dissection and deltopectoral flap reconstruction of a defect in the oral cavity. The patient had also received radiation therapy prior to surgery. The fracture in

this patient was confirmed by physical examination and radiographic appearance shortly after it occurred. This was substantiated by repeat radiography, which demonstrated complete healing of the fracture with normal callus 6 weeks later. We have had two cases similar to that of Cummings and First. One patient had received preoperative radiation therapy followed by radical neck dissection for metastatic squamous cell carcinoma with an unknown primary tumor. The fracture occurred 3 years after surgery, was diagnosed by radiography (Fig. 28-3) and healed promptly. The other patient had a fracture 9 months following neck dissection and radiation therapy that resulted in a nonunion. Biopsy of the site did not demonstrate tumor and secondary healing resulted.

The syndrome of *gustatory sweating* oc-

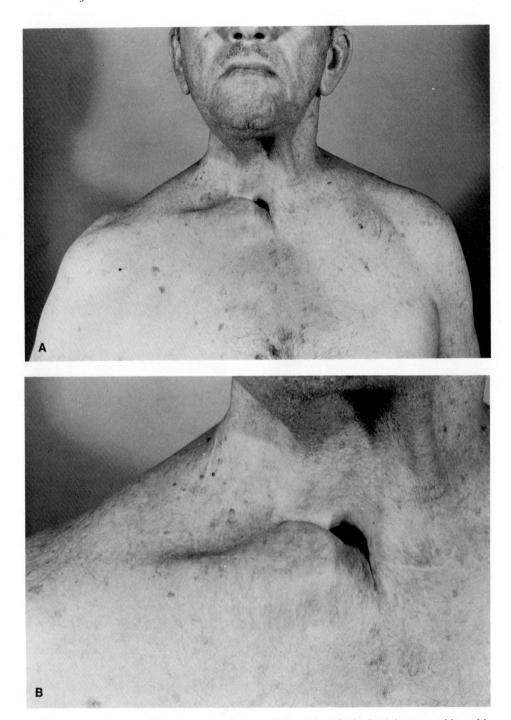

Fig. 28-2. (A and B) Demonstrates enlargement of the sternoclavicular joint caused by subluxation of the head of the clavicle in a patient following laryngectomy and radical neck dissection.

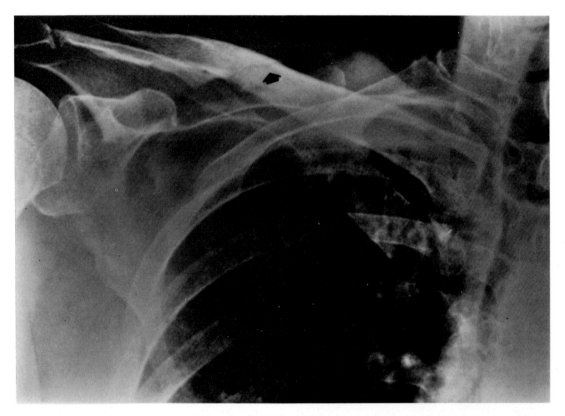

Fig. 28-3. Patient with stress fracture of midclavicle (arrow) following radiation therapy and radical neck dissection.

curred in six patients following radical neck dissection and was described in detail by Myers and Conley in 1970.[20] Five of these patients had sweating that occurred on the skin of the neck during eating. One patient had sweating on the skin of the face. The most typical location was in the submandibular area on the upper cervical flap (Fig. 28-4). The most interesting case was that of gustatory sweating in the deltopectoral flap; this flap had been transposed to completely replace the skin of the neck that had been excised at the time of radical neck dissection (Fig. 28-5). The aberrant regeneration of autonomic fibers following injury best explains the abnormal sweating. The fact that nerves to the sweat glands are functionally cholinergic but anatomically sympathetic is the critical factor in establishing this abnormal pathway and allowing neurohumoral transmission of nerve impulses (Fig. 28-6).

No patients in this series were treated, although the sweating could be blocked by injection of local anesthesia into the area of the lingual nerve, suggesting that section of this nerve might prove to be curative.

Sensory loss following radical neck dissection may be very bothersome to the patient. The anesthesia or hypesthesia is produced routinely by sectioning of the branches of the cervical plexus. The area of anesthesia or hypesthesia is predictable and involves the entire neck, the chest from midline to just below the insertion of the deltoid laterally and inferiorly to the nipple line (sparing the axilla), posteriorly across the scapular spine, superiorly to the occiput and including almost the entire ear.[33] The patients' complaints about sensory loss diminish with time.

Patients should be cautioned not to expose this denervated skin to extremes of

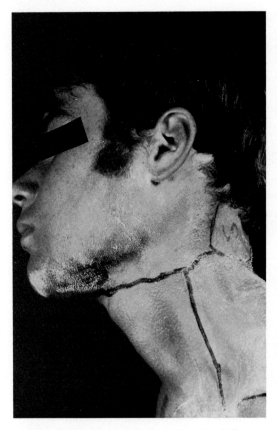

Fig. 28-4. Gustatory sweating in left submandibular area demonstrated by starch-iodine (Minor) reaction.

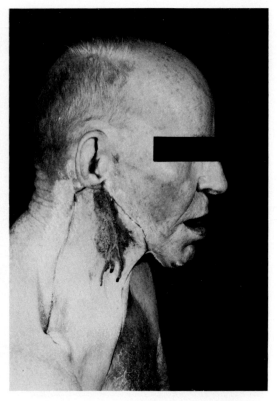

Fig. 28-5. Profuse gustatory sweating demonstrated on deltopectoral flap. Sweating is sharply limited to flap by scar (black lines). (Modified from Myers, E.N., and Conley, J. 1970. Gustatory sweating after radical neck dissection. Archives of Otolaryngology, 91:534-542. Copyright 1970, American Medical Association.)

temperature, as we have seen cases of severe burns of the ear from a hair dryer in a beauty shop and loss of cervical skin due to frost bite. These thermal injuries are probably due to lack of awareness of the agent because of loss of sensation and possibly due to loss of autonomic control in the area.

Neuromas of the cutaneous roots of the cervical nerves are relatively common and may cause pain, tenderness, or hyperesthesia. Since neuromas present as a mass in the upper cervical region, usually posterior to the carotid artery, recurrent cancer is suspected and must be ruled out. Simple tapping on the neuromas produces the typical paresthesia that is diagnostic. Graham in his review of 50 patients could find no correlation between the occurrence of neuroma and the use of preoperative or postoperative irradiation or a particular type of cervi-

cal flap or whether the nerve was simply cut or cut and ligated. He found no recurrence of neuromas after treatment by resection, high ligation, and local instillation of triamcinolone.[9]

Significant *scar contracture* of the cervical flap incisions may occur if wound dehiscence has occurred or if the vertical limb of a cervical incision is placed more than 4 cm anterior to the border of the trapezius muscle (Fig. 28-7). Multiple Z-plasty will remove the tension of the scar contracture but will not improve the cosmetic appearance, as rather large Z-plasty limbs are required and their use will leave additional scar in the neck.

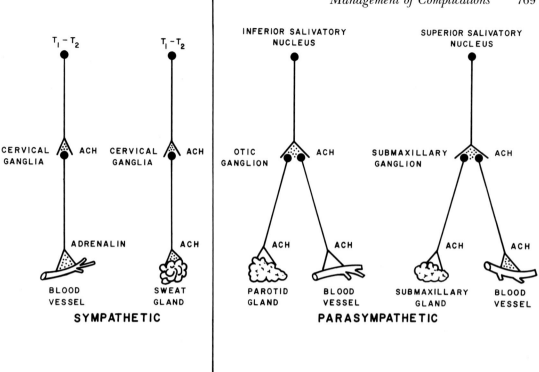

Fig. 28-6. Neurohumoral substances necessary for transmission of nerve impulses. Sweat glands are chemically cholinergic but anatomically sympathetic. (Modified from Myers, E.N., and Conley. J. 1970. Gustatory sweating after radical neck dissection. Archives of Otolaryngology, 91: 534-542. Copyright 1970, American Medical Association.)

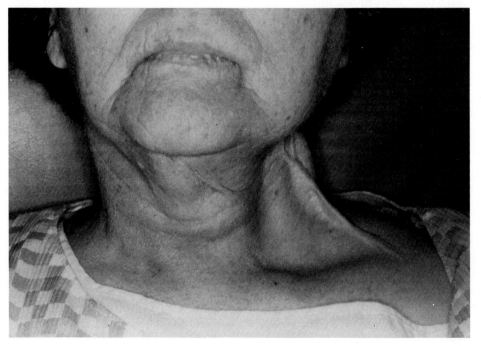

Fig. 28-7. Scar contracture in vertical limb of incision for radical neck dissection. This complication can be avoided by placing the incision more medial to trapezius.

Wound Infection

Wound complications such as infections, flap necrosis, salivary fistula, and carotid exposure or carotid rupture share interrelated causative factors. Predisposing factors to be considered include the patient's general status, the status of the local and regional tissues, and the tumor stage. The patient's nutritional status is of utmost importance. If the patient's weight loss has been greater than 10 percent of normal body weight, the possibility of a major complication should be anticipated and preventative measures taken. These patients should be treated preoperatively with hyperalimentation (see Ch. 5). During hyperalimentation, attempts should be made to optimize the patient's general medical condition.

There is disagreement as to the role played by planned preoperative radiation therapy in the frequency of postoperative complications. However, it is generally conceded that when complications do occur, the irradiated patients have more prolonged morbidity. The rate of complications for patients who have undergone primary radiation therapy and who require surgery for postradiation-persistent disease is significantly higher than for those who did not have this treatment.

The size of the tumor also has some influence on the rate of postoperative complications. Patients with large tumors requiring preoperative tracheostomy because of airway obstructions have a greater incidence of postoperative complications, particularly wound infections. These patients also more frequently require neck dissection for nodal metastasis and are more frequently treated with preoperative radiation therapy. The combination of these factors also influences the outcome of wound healing.

The location of the tumor as well as its size should be considered in that pyriform sinus and superior hypopharyngeal carcinomas have greater postoperative fistula rates than oral cavity or supraglottic carcinomas. This is probably due to attempting primary closure of the pharynx in the presence of inadequate pharyngeal mucosa. The lowest fistula rate occurs in those patients who have primary glottic tumors. Though weight loss may be the only factor that can be influenced directly, preoperative planning should consider the other factors and, as much as possible, compensate for them.

Specific technical factors that adversely affect the wound complication rate may not be readily identifiable for the individual patient, but certain general factors can be identified. The importance of surgical technique cannot be quantified; however, the variation in reported operative morbidity rates, ranging from 10 to 50 percent for unradiated patients and 25 to 75 percent for radiation-failure surgery patients, suggests that this indeed is an important factor. Tissue trauma and devitalization, applying excessive tension, crushing, and tissue strangulation all lead to breakdown of mucosal closure and wound infection. Closure of a wound under tension or failing to complete a water-tight closure, particularly in a patient who had prior radiation therapy, almost invariably leads to fistula formation. Development of postoperative wound hematomas are commonly complicated by wound abscess. Cervical skin incisions must be planned so as not to stress the vascular supply of the flap and so as to avoid placing a major portion of the suture line in such a manner that it crosses either the mucosal closure or the carotid artery.

Postoperative care also may influence wound complications. Maintenance of a postoperative hemoglobin level above 12.5 g percent, patent hemovac suction lines, and vigorous postoperative oral and pulmonary care decrease the degree of bacterial colonization of mucosal closure lines and decrease the chance of infection.

Wound infections may occur from direct inoculation at the time of surgery or from salivary leak through a mucosal closure. Antibiotic prophylaxis has now been generally accepted as appropriate. Timing of antibiotic administration appears to be important. An antibiotic in sufficient concentration at the time of bacterial contamination provides maximum effect. If the antibiotic is continued for only 24 to 48 hours postoperatively, secondary overgrowth of resistent bacteria is less likely. The choice of antibiotic for prophylaxis at present appears to be either one of the cephalosporins, penicillin, or, in penicillin-allergic patients, clindamycin.[2, 7, 29]

Unfortunately, preoperative wound and skin cultures do not correlate with organisms isolated from subsequent wound infections.[11] The bacterial flora encountered in wound infections varies with the reporting institution. In general, half of the isolated organisms may be expected to be gram positive. Roughly one-third of the infections are *Staphylococcus aureus,* one-third gram negative organisms, and one-third anaerobic organisms. Though *Bacteroides fragilis* had not previously been encountered with frequency in head and neck surgery, this organism has been responsible for 15 percent of infections in our institution in the past 3-year period. The majority of wound infections will also involve a mixed bacterial flora.

The treatment of wound infections depends upon the site and extent of infection. Open wounds such as those found in tracheostomy, skin graft donor or recipient sites, or maxillectomy cavities are best treated by cleansing and irrigation and application of antiseptic solutions. Cellulitis or abscess formation beneath skin flaps will routinely occur several days after the recommended prophylactic antibiotics have been discontinued. Wound culture for both aerobic and anaerobic organisms should precede administration of antibiotic therapy. Whatever antibiotic is chosen, it should be given in sufficiently large dosage by intravenous administration so that adequate tissue levels may be achieved. If an abscess is identified, drainage is mandatory and a compression dressing should be placed to minimize further elevation of the local flaps. Packing of an abscess cavity with gauze impregnated with Betadine solution is a helpful adjuvant to wound care.

Necrosis of a local skin flap may be re-lated to poor design of the flap with compromise of the blood supply, intraoperative trauma, excessive postoperative pressure, or wound infection. Flap necrosis is infrequent except in the cervical area related to neck dissection. We employ the utility or "hockey stick" type of cervical flap when neck dissection and laryngectomy or pharyngectomy are done and have had no significant flap necrosis. Incisions for in-continuity neck dissection and oral cavity or oropharyngeal resection should include a transverse incision located midway between the clavicle and mandible and a vertical posterior incision located 1 to 2 cm anterior to the trapezius. The incision should be angulated slightly toward the midline so that the junction of the vertical and transverse incisions leaves angles that are both greater than 90°. The anterior aspect of the transverse incision either may be carried across the midline or extended upward for division of the lower lip. A prior biopsy incision, usually in the jugular-digastric area, may be excised utilizing a MacFee flap. The disadvantage of the latter flap is that it is not appropriate for laryngeal surgery and the upper limb of the incision may closely approximate mucosal closure for oral cavity or oropharyngeal resections.

Skin necrosis is most common in the posterior-inferior aspect of the utility incision or at the angle of the trifurcation in a half-H type incision. These areas are well away from the carotid artery and, unless flap necrosis is extensive, will cause little problem. The eschar that forms should be left intact until epithelialization proceeds beneath it. If the area of skin flap necrosis is large but does not involve the area overlying the carotid artery and is not associated with a fistula, secondary skin grafting provides simple and effective reepithelialization.

An unplanned *salivary fistula* is the most common cause of prolonged postoperative morbidity and hospitalization. Salivary fistula may occur despite optimal preparation. However, fistula formation may be minimized by appropriate preoperative planning and good surgical technique, administration of postoperative radiation therapy when combined therapy is indicated, and elimination of tension on wound closures by the interposition of regional flaps or skin grafts.[28]

When a fistula is diagnosed either by recognizing saliva in the hemovac drains, by drainage through a skin incision, or by aspiration of pus and saliva from a fluctuant wound, further undermining of the cervical flaps should be minimized. This may be accomplished by inserting a suction catheter into the fistulous tract as a counter drain, debriding necrotic tissue, and maintaining cervical flap apposition by compression dressings or by exteriorizing the fistula by sewing pharyngeal mucosa to skin as far away as possible from the carotid artery. If the neck flaps have not been elevated over the carotid artery, diversion of saliva from the wound by pharyngeal suction, T-tube drain[34], or insertion of a Montgomery salivary by-pass tube is adequate for early management.

If the fistula is less than 1 cm in its greatest dimension, maintenance of a clean wound will usually allow for spontaneous closure. If skin necrosis has extended such that the carotid artery has been exposed, coverage of the carotid with an undelayed deltopectoral flap is indicated. The rotation of a flap is unnecessary if the carotid artery had previously been covered with a dermal graft. Once carotid protection has been assured, nutrition via nasogastric feeding or total parenteral nutrition and continued local wound care is maintained either until the fistula spontaneously closes or until the wound is clean and the edges of the fistula are mature and covered with epithelium. Small fistulas may close within 2 weeks, but larger fistulas may require wound care for as long as 6 weeks prior to secondary closure.

If secondary closure of a small fistula is necessary in a patient who has not had radiation therapy, a two-layer closure including a local trapdoor flap for inner lining and a cervical rotation flap for outer lining with skin grafting of the donor site frequently provides one-stage closure. Larger fistulas require regional skin flaps, usually the deltopectoral flap, for closure. For moderate-sized fistulas an inner epithelial lining may be obtained by transposing a local trapdoor flap based on the edges of the fistula and covering the raw surfaces with a nondelayed deltopectoral flap.[19] (Fig. 28-8 A–D) Sufficient skin surrounding the fistula must be removed in order to provide a recipient site with sufficient vascularity for inset of the flap. The deltopectoral flap may be returned after approximately 3 weeks or may be left as permanent flap by excising intervening cervical skin. A planned pharyngostome may be closed in the same manner.

Carotid artery exposure is the most common life-threatening complication of head and neck cancer surgery. The incidence of carotid artery exposure and necrosis ranges from less than 1 percent in patients who have not had radiation to 50 percent in patients who have had "unplanned" preoperative radiation.[10, 25] Incidence of death from carotid rupture and emergency ligation may be as high as 25 percent with one-half of the surviving patients sustaining a neurologic deficit. The complications result primarily from uncontrolled hypotension. Fortunately, major carotid artery bleeding is usually heralded by a minor "warning bleed." In these circumstances, more elective management with adequate blood pressure maintenance, even if ligation is necessary, will result in few deaths and less than 25 percent sequelae.

Prevention of carotid artery complications begins at the time of primary surgery. The carotid must be carefully protected from drying, and injury to the artery during dissection must be avoided. A dermal graft should be applied when the possibility of carotid artery exposure is high, such as in patients who have undergone unplanned preoperative radiation therapy or in those patients having extensive hypopharyngeal resections. The dermal graft must be free of perforations, must be large enough not only to cover the entire carotid but 1 to 2 cm on either side of the artery, and must be ap-

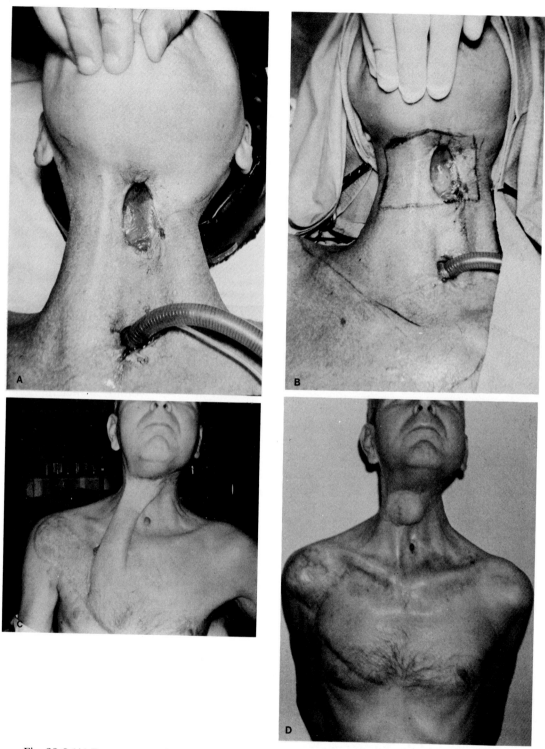

Fig. 28-8 (A) Demonstrates large matured pharyngocutaneous fistula that followed total laryn-gectomy and radical neck dissection in a patient who had not received radiation. (B) Trap door flap outlined on neck; (C) deltopectoral flap transposed to cover trapdoor flap and its donor site; (D) closed pharyngocutaneous fistula after release and return of deltopectoral flap.

plied on the anterior medial aspect of the artery so that the stumps of the transected superior thyroid and facial arteries are covered so that saliva cannot dissect beneath the dermal graft. If attention is paid to these technical factors, the incidence of carotid rupture, even though the dermal graft is exposed to saliva, or air or both, approaches zero.[25] If a dermal graft is utilized, care must be exercised to avoid inclusion of epithelium on the graft, or else an inclusion cyst will result. If the dermal graft has been exposed over the carotid because of necrosis of the cervical flap, epithelialization will occur promptly.

Patients who have not had a dermal graft who experience carotid artery exposure because of major wound complications are at great risk of carotid artery rupture. Recognition of this problem must be followed by diversion of the salivary stream away from the artery as well as by immediate transposition of a deltopectoral flap to provide coverage of the artery. This flap may later be utilized in reconstruction of the wound.

If the carotid artery rupture occurs while the patient has a tracheostomy, the tracheostomy cuff should be inflated. External pressure must be applied to the artery to control bleeding. The patient is then transported to the operating room and hypotension corrected by administration of intravenous fluids, colloid, and blood. The carotid artery is then exposed above and below the area of bleeding and temporarily ligated. If bleeding is from a branch of the external carotid, that artery may be ligated or the external carotid may be ligated proximally and distally to the site of bleeding. Rupture of the common carotid or the carotid bulb will require ligation and division of the artery, since oversewing the site of bleeding or patch grafting will only lead to secondary rupture. The proximal stump of the carotid should be oversewn with monofilament nylon, and the stump then buried in the muscle of the neck. If the external carotid system has been ligated, the remaining patent carotid should be covered by a nondelayed deltopectoral flap. If the carotid has

been sacrificed, cervical skin should be sutured to the remnant of pharyngeal or hypopharyngeal mucosa, leaving the fistula to be closed at a later time. Prevention of delayed neurologic sequelae by postligation administration of low dose heparin has been advocated but has not been universally accepted.[13]

Osteoradionecrosis occurs most commonly when the radiated bone has been partially devascularized by surgical resection or when exposed in a wound to air or saliva. It may also occur in patients with carious teeth or gingivitis or where postradiation extractions are done. If internal bone fixation is necessary and postoperative radiation therapy is anticipated, wire sutures or metal appliances should be avoided, since radiation "hot spots" will result, increasing the chance of local osteoradionecrosis. Removal of sequestered and exposed bone may be necessary to control the severe pain, foul odor, and disability that is related to the affected bone. When the mandible is exposed in an open wound, sufficient bone should be removed so that soft-tissue coverage may be accomplished.

Tracheostomy Complications

A tracheostomy placed for airway management in patients with head and neck tumors may result in intraoperative as well as early and delayed postoperative complications. Intraoperative complications are increased when the patient with a compromised airway undergoes tracheostomy under local anesthesia. For that reason whenever feasible in this circumstance, oral endotracheal intubation should first be accomplished. Intraoperative bleeding is usually from vessels around the isthmus of the thyroid or from the isthmus itself. These vessels may be identified and divided before ligating or cauterizing them. The tracheostomy should be inserted below the second tracheal ring and, if the thyroid isthmus cannot be retracted above this site, the isthmus should be isolated, divided, and suture ligated. Prior to insertion of the tracheostomy tube or endotracheal tube, the wound should be inspected for bleeding so as to prevent troublesome intraoperative or postoperative bleeding and tracheal aspiration of blood.

Air embolus and pneumothorax occur most commonly in struggling air-hungry patients. In patients with marked emphysema the apex of the lung may, with straining, extend into the lower neck. Dissection lateral to the trachea is, therefore, to be avoided. Packing of the tracheostomy wound or tight closure of skin around the tracheostomy tube should be avoided, as it leads to pneumomediastinum and subcutaneous emphysema. Laceration of the cricoid cartilage may occur rarely, usually when an urgent tracheostomy is performed. After the airway has been established, this should be recognized and tracheostomy done at a lower level and the cricoid cartilage and outer perichondrium repaired.

Postoperatively displaced or extruded tubes may be prevented by suturing the tracheostomy tube to the surrounding skin. Placing traction sutures in the cartilage above and below the tracheotomy opening is an excellent technique to facilitate repositioning of the tracheostomy tube or replacing the tube in the early postoperative period and is recommended for all head and neck surgery patients.[23] A low-pressure cuffed tracheostomy tube should always be used to avoid pressure necrosis of the tracheal wall from asymmetrical cuff inflation or malposition of the tip of the tracheostomy tube. The position of the tip of the tracheostomy tube should be checked by obtaining a chest radiograph immediately postoperatively, as unexpected bronchial intubation or low tracheal placement with the tip of the tube being obstructed by the tracheal wall or carina can be corrected easily by placement of a shorter tube.

The most dramatic complication of tracheotomy is bleeding from the innominate artery. This usually occurs 2 to 3 weeks following tracheostomy, but may occur earlier in previously irradiated patients or when a low tracheotomy has been done. The patient usually has a small amount of bright red blood from the tracheotomy tube as a warning sign. It should be assumed in these situations that rupture of the innominate artery has occurred. Inflation of the tracheostomy cuff or placement of a cuffed tube should be immediately accomplished, and pressure may be applied to the innominate artery by finger dissection between the trachea and the sternum through the tracheotomy wound. If this fails to control the bleeding immediately, an oral endotracheal tube should be placed with the cuff overinflated just distal to the tracheotomy opening. Packing of the wound and finger pressure will usually allow time for resuscitation and thoracotomy.

Airway obstruction at the level of the tracheostomy may occur from granuloma, tracheal cartilage necrosis, tracheomalacia, or in-fracturing of calcified tracheal rings. Granulomas should be removed endoscopically. The ultimate management of tracheal stenosis depends upon many factors and will not be discussed at this time. Prevention, however, includes excising the anterior third of the tracheal ring if the patient has calcified cartilage, and careful tracheal wound care to eliminate necrosing infection. Occasionally, a persistent tracheocutaneous fistula will require local wound cauterization or excision of an epithelial tract with secondary closure.

Tracheostomal stenosis, following total laryngectomy, results from circumferential scarring of stomal skin or retraction of the trachea. If low tracheal resection has been necessary, the trachea should be mobilized by anterior and posterior dissection to avoid vascular compromise and then secured to the undersurface of the clavicular heads with subperichondrial absorbable sutures. If a stomal stenosis occurs, it may be managed conservatively by continued use of a tracheostomy tube or the use of tracheal buttons. However, in patients who fail to respond to such conservative measures, Z-plasty reconstruction and secondary mobilization of the trachea will be necessary.

Regional Flap Complications

Successful reconstruction of defects by regional flaps depends on the arterial and venous supply of the flap, the condition of the patient and recipient bed, and technical factors of the reconstruction. The forehead flap is a dependable arterial flap. The deltopectoral flap is an arterial flap to the anterior axillary line and a random flap beyond that line. Other flaps used in head and neck reconstruction are of random vascular pattern and, because their viability is less predictable, should be used only when other flaps are unavailable or have failed.

A major complication rate of 10 to 15 percent and a total complication rate of 25 to 35 percent may be expected when either a deltopectoral flap or forehead flap reconstruction is utilized.[1, 3, 14, 18, 22] As is true of other complications, patients who are debilitated, who have had prior radiation therapy, particularly those with postradiation persistent disease, and those who develop early postoperative tumor persistence have a higher rate of flap complications. Technical factors that increase the likelihood of flap-related complications include folding of the distal portion of the flap to give external as well as internal coverage, kinking and angulation of the inset portion of the flap (particularly in combined tonsil and tongue reconstruction), traction or tension on the flap, constriction of the carrier portion of the flap (either under cervical skin flaps or under the zygomatic arch), and drying of the carrier portion of the flap.

Delay of a deltopectoral flap is of possible benefit only for the random part of the flap if the length-to-width ratio in that portion of the flap is extended beyond 1:1. Except for the delay necessitated by split-thickness skin graft lining of the undersurface of the flap, the delay may actually increase the possibility of flap complication. When using a forehead flap for an intraoral or pharyngeal defect, the zygomatic arch may be removed to avoid constriction of the carrier portion of the flap.

In our series of 117 deltopectoral and 20 forehead flaps, major flap necrosis occurred in 25 patients.[27] These complications occurred primarily in patients who had undergone planned or unplanned preoperative radiation therapy. An associated factor in these patients, although unrecognizable at the time of surgery, was a high incidence of regional or distant tumor recurrence within 3 years of surgical therapy. When major flap necrosis becomes evident, the necrotic portion of the flap should be debrided and the remaining portion of the flap used to provide coverage for the carotid artery, or, if the carotid artery is protected, should be returned to the donor site. Though a portion of the remaining flap may be utilized in subsequent reconstruction, a contralateral deltopectoral flap is also required for secondary closure of the fistula. Major bleeding may occur if a salivary fistula develops beneath a pedicle flap. The management of carotid artery rupture has been previously discussed. Bleeding from the temporal artery at the time of division of a forehead flap may be difficult to control because the bleeding originates deep within the wound. The area may be temporarily packed while better exposure is obtained for direct identification of the bleeding site.

Minor complications of regional flap reconstruction are defined as those prolonging hospitalization or requiring minor secondary operative procedures. Separation of the flap anastomosis or delay in fistula closure following return of the flap, but with spontaneous healing, are most common. The small areas of flap necrosis, when they occur in this circumstance, should be debrided to prevent further flap loss from necrotizing infection. Loss of the skin graft placed over the donor site may require secondary skin grafting of the shoulder defect when a deltopectoral flap is returned. Elevation of the periosteum over the forehead will result in loss of overlying skin graft and will require removal of the outer table of bone and often secondary rotation of a local scalp flap for resurfacing.

A partial or total facial paralysis may also result from trauma when a forehead flap is rotated over the zygomatic arch. Return of facial function in these situations is usually poor, so that identification of the area of the facial nerve branches with a nerve stimulator at the time of surgery is mandatory. A hair-bearing flap transposed into the area of the oral cavity or pharynx produces annoying difficulty with hygiene. Periodic trimming of the hair or excision of the hair-bearing skin, and secondary skin grafting, may be necessary.

Simultaneous reconstruction of a mandibular defect in a previously radiated patient will nearly inevitably lead to exposure of the graft, whether bone or metal. This complication is best avoided by utilizing secondary reconstruction if it is indicated. If graft exposure does not occur, removal of the graft will be necessary.

Deglutition

Some derangement of swallowing is common following many of the surgical procedures done for head and neck cancer. Aspiration and chronic malnutrition are major obstacles in the patient's rehabilitation. The etiology of swallowing dysfunction in postoperative patients is outlined in Table 28-1. A combination of factors is usually recognizable in individual patient situations, and rehabilitation requires the coordinated efforts of the physician and nursing staff, swallowing therapist, maxillofacial prosthodontist, and the patient.

Attempts at oral nutrition should not begin until wound healing is adequate, pain resulting from oral and laryngeal movement is minimal, the airway is good, and the tracheostomy tube has been removed and the tracheostomy wound healed. The disabilities in deglutition experienced by patients with supraglottic laryngectomy and those with major pharyngeal resections are similar in that the net result is difficulty swallowing the bolus of food with resultant aspiration. An organized approach to swallowing rehabilitation is most successful. Training should begin several days prior to the time the patient is expected to eat with a discussion of swallowing function, what difficulties might

TABLE 28-1. ETIOLOGY OF POSTOPERATIVE SWALLOWING DYSFUNCTION

I. Neurologic
  A. Central
    1. Borderline intelligence and/or motivation
    2. Neuromuscular incoordination
  B. Peripheral
    1. Sensory (anesthesia or pain)
      a. Glossopharyngeal
      b. Superior laryngeal
      c. Lingual
    2. Motor
      a. Facial
      b. Pharyngeal plexus
      c. Recurrent laryngeal
      d. Hypoglossal

II. Mechanical
  A. Oral
    1. Oronasal communication
    2. Resection of oral tongue and/or mandible
  B. Pharyngeal
    1. Velopharyngeal incompetence
      a. Palate
      b. Lateral pharyngeal wall
      c. Base of tongue
    2. Obstruction
      a. Arytenoid and hypopharyngeal edema
      b. Pharyngeal stenosis
      c. Cricopharyngeal spasm
      d. Recurrent cancer
  C. Laryngeal
    1. Fixation—tracheostomy, partial resection
    2. Open incompetence

III. Respiratory
  A. Aerodigestive separation
    1. Laryngectomy
    2. Tracheostomy
  B. Airway obstruction
  C. Inadequate expiratory volume and velocity

be encountered for the particular patient, and what techniques might be used to compensate for the surgically created dysfunction.

The patient should be instructed to practice pharyngotracheal separation by grunting or straining with the mouth open. If the patient is able to feel his abdominal muscles tense while the mouth is open, glottic closure and increased subglottic pressure will be achieved. Second, the patient should be instructed to grunt and follow this with a cough, without a second inspiration. A "dry swallow" should then be practiced until this can be done comfortably and efficiently. The dry swallow should begin with a moderate inspiration followed by conscious glottic closure, swallow, and cough prior to subsequent inspiration. A physician or specially trained swallowing therapist should be in attendance to provide instruction at the time of the first meal and frequently thereafter. A choice of foods should be available depending on the type of prior surgical therapy. For the patient with total laryngectomy liquids or pureed foods are easiest to swallow. For most other patients, pureed or semisolid foods such as scrambled eggs, hot cereals, and other foods of mashed potato consistency are most easily swallowed. Liquids should be either hot or cold, and preferably carbonated. Milk products are best avoided initially, except for patients with a total laryngectomy, because of the tendency to thicken the oral secretions. Intravenous fluid supplementation may be necessary but should be given intermittently so that the patient is not hampered while eating by the attachment of IV fluid tubing.

Frequently, reteaching is necessary, and a degree of privacy should be initially provided so that the patient may cough and expectorate any residual unswallowed food. If aspiration is too great, or caloric intake is inadequate, postponing further eating for several hours or several days should be considered. Some patients may not even accomplish this rehabilitation of the swallowing act in the hospital. They may be discharged with a nasogastric tube in place to practice and usually return within a month able to swallow well.

Specific correction of many of the factors responsible for swallowing dysfunction may be possible. Open glottic incompetence due to recurrent laryngeal nerve paralysis may be corrected temporarily by injection of Gelfoam into the involved true vocal cord, or permanently by Teflon injection. Open glottic incompetence following hemilaryngectomy may also be improved at times by Teflon injection, but may require thyrotomy and interposition of a muscle pedicle graft. Disability resulting from major resection of the oral tongue or tongue base should be anticipated at the time of surgery and reconstructed by a regional pedicle flap.

An oral-nasal communication is relatively easily corrected with a prosthesis. Velopharyngeal incompetence due to soft palate resection may also be improved or completely corrected by a speech-aid type prosthesis. The importance of preoperative planning in conjunction with the maxillofacial prosthodontist cannot be overemphasized.

Edema of arytenoid mucosa, seen commonly after combined radiation and surgical therapy, may produce both airway obstruction and obstruction to the esophageal inlet. Careful resection of redundant mucosa is often helpful. Use of the laser in this circumstance is beneficial in that it allows more precise resection and minimizes further postoperative edema and scarring. Adynamic segments of hypopharyngeal musculature or redundant pedicle flap reconstruction may require secondary excision.

Incoordination of pharyngeal movement and altered synchrony with the cricopharyngeal muscle result more commonly than is recognized following oral cavity and hypopharyngeal resection. Though cricopharyngeal myotomy is done routinely following supraglottic or partial laryngopharyngectomy resections, primary or secondary cricopharyngeal myotomy may be necessary in other circumstances as well. Hypopharyngeal or esophageal stenosis following laryngectomy can usually be alleviated by dilatation. If the stenosis can be managed satisfactorily by dilatation but is recurrent, the patient may be taught to dilate the hypopharyngeal area himself two or three times per week with a mercury-filled dilator.

Many of the other factors listed in Table 28-1 cannot be corrected, though they may be modified by practice and compassionate instruction. Pain associated with swallowing may be partially alleviated by administration of an analgesic 30 to 45 minutes prior to meals. If the physical and psychological difficulties produced by malnutrition and surgical and radiation therapy are too great, temporary intravenous hyperalimentation or tube feeding by a nasogastric tube, esophagostomy or gastrostomy is indicated. It is not surprising that when patients are in better physical and mental condition following supplemental feedings, they will learn to eat with little or no instruction.

General Complications

Deep vein thrombosis following head and neck surgery is uncommon considering the length of surgery and the age of the patient population. Deep vein thrombosis has been demonstrated by ^{125}I fibrinogen uptake to be as high as 27 percent.[8] However, only one-third of the patients who have deep vein thrombosis demonstrated by this technique have clinical evidence of thrombosis. Clinically significant thrombosis usually develops between the third and sixth postoperative days, either with classic signs of edema, erythema, and cyanosis in the lower extremity or with pulmonary embolus. In all patients, including head and neck surgery patients, administration of intravenous fluids through ankle veins is associated with an increased evidence of postoperative thrombophlebitis and should be avoided. Elevation of the legs by as little as 10° during the intraoperative and postoperative period and early postoperative ambulation reduces these complications significantly.

Pulmonary complications such as atelectasis and pneumonia occur commonly in patients who have undergone head and neck surgery. The patient's underlying chronic pulmonary disease, as well as aspiration of blood, saliva, and gastric contents, should be anticipated in every patient. Post-operative tracheostomy care must include humidification and 40 percent oxygen administration, frequent sterile suctioning, intermittent pulmonary hyperventilation, and Ambu bag or mechanical positive-pressure ventilation. A cuffed tracheostomy tube should be mandatory in all patients. Prolonged use of mechanical intermittent positive-pressure breathing is not cost effective and may promote bacterial cross contamination. The exception is the patient who develops postoperative respiratory insufficiency and must be managed by constant mechanical ventilation.

Patients who develop atelectasis or pneumonia frequently benefit from rigid or flexible fiberoptic bronchoscopy with direct removal of inspissated secretions and saline lavage of the tracheobronchial tree. Ambu bag hyperventilation held for 10 seconds following suctioning will decrease the incidence of atelectasis and help to expand atelectatic segments of lung. Major pleural effusions occasionally occur in association with pulmonary embolus or with pneumonia and should be managed by aspiration. In the patients under treatment for advanced disease, the presence of pleural effusion should be viewed with suspicion. Thoracentesis should be performed and cytology obtained to evaluate the possible presence of metastatic disease.

Central Nervous System Complications

Central nervous system complications not related to increased venous pressure are primarily due to exposure or transection of dura. A cerebral spinal fluid (CSF) leak following temporal bone resection or maxillectomy may not be recognized until the secondary complication of meningitis occurs. If a CSF leak is recognized, the patient's head should be elevated 20° to 30° and a lumbar-subarachnoid drainage catheter inserted. If spinal fluid examination obtained by lumbar puncture indicates secondary bacterial meningitis, the need for high dose intravenous penicillin and chloramphenicol therapy is established. Subsequent management should be planned with neurologic or neurosurgical consultation. If the CSF leak is not diminishing or meningitis not improving within 48 hours, consideration should be given to reexploration of the wound to identify and close the dural defect if the patient's condition permits.

In the presence of meningitis, or when confusion or somnolence occur, the possibility of a subdural, epidural, or brain abscess should be evaluated with computerized tomography. Presence of an abscess dictates the need for surgical drainage. Occasionally, diffuse cerebritis will result from either meningitis or any of the intracranial abscesses. Increased intracranial pressure in these circumstances should be controlled by spinal fluid drainage and mannitol, and subsequently, when infection has been controlled, with steroids. *Pseudomonas* meningitis is relatively more common than other types of infection following temporal bone resection and should be managed by intrathecal gentamycin with monitoring of serum creatinine levels and blood and spinal fluid levels of gentamycin. In addition, if infectious complications result, packing should be removed from the maxillectomy or temporal bone cavity in most instances.

SUMMARY

Complications in head and neck surgery may be anticipated and minimized by good preoperative evaluation, nutritional therapy, careful planning of surgical and radiation therapy, and by intensive nursing care. We believe that in the past, too much attention has been paid to the postoperative care and the struggle with complications that occurred and too little attention paid to prevention: bringing the patient to optimum condition for surgery with respect to his general medical problems and advanced state of malnutrition. We feel that, in the future, if the use of nutritional therapy and postoperative radiation therapy become more widespread, and meticulous surgical technique is emphasized, that the number of complications of head and neck surgery will diminish.

REFERENCES

1. Bakamjian, V. Y. 1965. A two-stage method for pharyngoesophageal reconstruction with a primary pectoral skin flap. Plastic and Reconstructive Surgery, 36: 173.

2. Becker, G. D., Parell, G. J., Busch, D. F. Finegold, S. M., and Acquarelli, M. J. 1978. Anaerobic and aerobic bacteriology in head and neck cancer surgery. Archives of Otolaryngology, 104: 591.

3. Biller, H. F., Ogura, J. H., and Brownson, R. J. 1973. The forehead flap: Technique and complications. Archives of Otolaryngology, 97: 316.

4. Coates, H. L., and DeSanto, L. W. 1976. Bilateral chylothorax as a complication of radical neck dissection. Journal of Laryngology and Otology, 90: 966.

5. Crumley, R. L., and Smith, J. D. 1976. Postoperative chylous fistula prevention and management. Laryngoscope, 86: 804.

6. Cummings, C. W., and First, R. 1975. Stress fractures of the clavicle after a radical neck dissection. Plastic and Reconstructive Surgery, 55: 366.

7. Dor, P., and Klastersky, J. 1973. Prophylactic antibiotics in oral, pharyngeal and laryngeal surgery for cancer (a double blind study). Laryngoscope, 83: 1992.

8. Graham, J. M., Robinson, J. M. P., Ashcroft, P. B., and Glennie, R. 1976. Deep vein thrombosis in ear, nose and throat surgery. Journal of Laryngology and Otology, 90: 427.

9. Graham, W. P. III. 1973. Cervical neuromas following extensive maxillofacial surgery. Journal of Surgical Oncology, 5: 485.

10. Joseph, D. L., and Shumrick, D. L. 1973. Risks of head and neck surgery in previously irradiated patients. Archives of Otolaryngology, 97: 381.

11. Ketcham, A. S., Lieberman, J. E., and West, J. T. 1963. Antibiotic prophylaxis in cancer surgery and its value in staphylococcal carrier patients. Surgery, Gynecology and Obstetrics, 117: 1.

12. Lamb, C. E. M. 1976. Sternoclavicular joint enlargement following block dissection. British Journal of Surgery, 63: 488.

13. Leikensohn, J., Milko, D., and Cotton, R. 1978. Carotid artery rupture. Management and prevention of delayed neurologic sequelae with low-dose heparin. Archives of Otolaryngology, 104: 307.

14. Lewis, M. B., and Remensnyder, J. P. 1978. Forehead flap for reconstruction after ablative surgery for oral and oropharyngeal malignancy. Plastic and Reconstructive Surgery, 62: 59.

15. Lowry, W. S. 1975. Alcoholism in cancer of the head and neck. Laryngoscope, 85: 1275.

16. McGuirt, W. F., McCabe, B. F., and Krause, C. J. 1979. Complications of radical neck dissection: A survey of 788 patients. Head and Neck Surgery, 1: 481.

17. McQuarrie, D. G., Mayberg, M., Ferguson, M., and Shons, A. R. 1977. A physiologic approach to the problems of simultaneous bilateral neck dissection. American Journal of Surgery, 134: 455.

18. Mendelson, B. C., Woods, J. E., and Masson, J. K. 1977. Experience with the deltopectoral flap. Plastic and Reconstructive Surgery, 59: 360.

19. Myers, E. N. 1972. The management of pharyngocutaneous fistula. Archives of Otolaryngology, 95: 10.

20. Myers, E. N., and Conley, J. 1970. Gustatory sweating after radical neck dissection. Archives of Otolaryngology, 91: 534.

21. Myers, E. N., and Dinerman, W. S. 1975. Management of chylous fistulas. Laryngoscope, 85: 835.

22. Park, J. S., Sako, K., and Marchetta, F. C. 1974. Reconstructive experience with the medially based deltopectoral flap. American Journal of Surgery, 128: 548.

23. Parnes, S. M., and Myers, E. N. 1976. Traction sutures in a tracheostomy using a ligature passer. Transactions of the American Academy of Ophthalmology and Otolaryngology, 82: ORL 479.

24. Pfeifle, K., Koch, H., Rehrmann, A., and Nwoku, A. L. 1974. Pseudotumors of the clavicle following neck dissection. Journal of Maxillofacial Surgery, 2: 14.

25. Reed, G. F., and Halsey, W. S. 1975. Protection of the carotid artery in radical neck dissection. Laryngoscope, 85: 1353.

26. Saunders, W. H., and Johnson, E. W. 1975. Rehabilitation of the shoulder after radical neck dissection. Annals of Otology, Rhinology and Laryngology, 84: 812.

27. Schramm, V. L., and Myers, E. N. Skin grafts vs. flaps. Plastic and Reconstructive Surgery, in preparation.

28. Schramm, V. L., and Myers, E. N. Skin grafts in oral cavity reconstruction. Archives of Otolaryngology, In press.

29. Seagle, M. B., Duberstein, L. E., Gross, C. W., Fletcher, J. L., and Mustafa, A. Q. 1978. Efficacy of Cefazolin as a prophylactic antibiotic in head and neck surgery. Otolaryngology, 86: ORL568.

30. Strong, M. S., Vaughan, C. W., Mahler, D. L., Jaffe, D. R., and Sullivan, R. C. 1974. Cardiac complications of microsurgery of the larynx: Etiology, incidence and prevention. Laryngoscope, 84: 908.

31. Summers, G. W. 1974. Physiological problems following ablative surgery of the head and neck. Otolaryngologic Clinics of North America, 7: 217.

32. Suzuki, M., and Kirchner, J. A. 1967. Laryngeal reflex pathways related to rate and rhythm of the heart. Annals of Otology, Rhinology and Laryngology, 76: 774.

33. Swift, T. R. 1970. Involvement of peripheral nerves in radical neck dissection. American Journal of Surgery, 119: 694.

34. Vogel, H., and Strong, M. S. 1978. Use of a T-tube in management of a pharyngeal fistula after laryngectomy. Plastic and Reconstructive Surgery, 62: 573.

35. Weingarten, C. Z. 1973. Simultaneous bilateral radical neck dissection. Peservation of the external jugular vein. Archives of Otolaryngology, 97: 309.

29 | The Chemotherapy and Immunotherapy of Head and Neck Cancer

Gregory T. Wolf, M.D.
Paul B. Chretien, M.D.

CHEMOTHERAPY OF HEAD AND NECK SQUAMOUS CARCINOMA

Current Concepts

The current ongoing trials of chemotherapy in head and neck cancer constitute the most clinically important investigations of the effectiveness of chemotherapy because of the emphasis on the adjuvant effects of chemotherapeutic drugs in combination with conventional therapy on localized and potentially curable tumors. If this approach reduces the high recurrence rates associated with conventional treatment for advanced head and neck squamous carcinomas, it will provide rationale for determination of the effects of adjuvant chemotherapy in other solid malignancies that are associated with high local recurrence rates after conventional local therapy and for which effective therapeutic agents are available. This new use of chemotherapy in the treatment of head and neck cancer began in 1975 with the report of investigations conducted at the National Cancer Institute that showed that methotrexate in dose regimens sufficiently high to require leucovorin rescue could be given preoperatively to patients with head and neck cancer without affecting perioperative morbidity.[109] Furthermore, significant tumor regressions were observed during the brief interval between administration of the

drug and operation. These findings led to the institution by the NCI of a prospective controlled trial to determine the long-term results of this unique application of systemic chemotherapy. The perceived importance of these investigations led to a rapid proliferation of studies designed to assess the effect of adjuvant chemotherapy in potentially curable tumors by head and neck oncologists at individual institutions and by collaborating head and neck cancer treatment centers. Because these trials are so recently initiated they cannot yet be evaluated for the long-term effects of the regimens; however, the results to date allow an analysis of the immediate effects on the tumor and the patient, i.e., the feasibility of this application of chemotherapy.

These intensive and widespread investigations constitute a new frontier in the treatment of head and neck cancer. Unfortunately for us, the authors of this chapter, the task of delineating the current role of chemotherapy in the treatment of head and neck cancer is a most difficult one. This is not so much because of the plethora of recent data available on the activity of drugs in patients with previously untreated and potentially curable tumors but because of the tenuous nature of the so recently made observations and the uncertainty of the significance of these observations.

Despite the apparent uniqueness of these ongoing trials, in truth, they are but

782

logical extensions of the first studies of the effects of chemotherapeutic agents in head and neck cancer.[29, 34, 53, 94] These early studies were conducted by surgeons confronted with inoperable tumors which either were not amenable to radiotherapy or which had been previously treated with radiation therapy. In attempts at palliation, surgeons derived methods of infusing the tumors with drugs introduced into the arterial system supplying the tumor. In these anecdotal clinical experiments, they observed that certain drugs led to dramatic reductions in tumor size, healing of ulcerating lesions, and cessation of local bleeding. Subsequently, the most active drugs were employed in attempts at palliation of incurable tumors, using intermittent systemic drug administration in long-term low dosage regimens. These larger trials allowed a more precise determination of the relative efficacy of the available drugs and of the identification of inactive drugs.

The results of these studies, which of necessity were usually uncontrolled, provide a basis for current recommendations for the use of chemotherapy in the palliation of incurable tumors and in part provide guidelines for the design of trials to evaluate the adjuvant effect of chemotherapy combined with conventional treatment. These data are summarized in this chapter and are organized into the following sections:

1. Chemotherapeutic drugs that have a relatively high level of activity in head and neck squamous carcinoma.

2. Practical considerations and guidelines for the use of these drugs for the palliation of incurable tumors.

3. The current results of trials of chemotherapy in combination with surgery or radiotherapy in patients with advanced but clinically localized tumors.

4. Guidelines for the use of chemotherapy as an adjuvant to conventional treatment.

The major goal of this chapter is to present data and guidelines critical for decision making in the use of chemotherapy for these tumors. It constitutes neither a handbook of chemotherapy nor an atlas for the design of trials. The pertinent medical literature is succinctly presented in tables with references to exhaustive reviews of published data on most drugs that have been evaluated in head and neck cancer. Response rates cited in the text correspond to tumor regression of 50 percent or greater. The application of the principles or guidelines for the design of adjuvant trials and the multiple variables affecting the results of clinical evaluations of chemotherapeutic agents in patients with head and neck carcinoma are presented in published data from centers conducting such trials.

Active Chemotherapeutic Drugs

Although the number of chemotherapeutic agents that have been evaluated in head and neck squamous carcinoma equals or exceeds that of most solid malignancies, three agents—methotrexate, bleomycin, and cisplatinum—have consistently led to relatively high tumor regression rates compared to other drugs tested. Thus, these agents are the first choice for either palliation of advanced tumors or for incorporation into adjuvant treatment regimens. Other agents also active in these tumors are listed in Table 29-1 and are mentioned in the descriptions of combination chemotherapy regimens in which they were used.

Important in the evaluation of the efficacy cited for these agents is the assumption that the tumor regression rates reported for these drugs are probably less than maximal, since the primary factor that reduces drug activity—prior treatment—has occurred in most patients. In general, the patients entered in these trials either had incurable primary tumors or tumors recurrent after radiation therapy or surgery. These factors frequently were associated with malnutrition and compromised function of liver, lung, or other central organs and overall poor performance status, which are also factors known to adversely affect tumor regression rates and durations of tumor response. Thus, in selected patients in good health

TABLE 29-1. TOXICITY OF CHEMOTHERAPEUTIC DRUGS COMMONLY USED
IN PATIENTS WITH HEAD AND NECK SQUAMOUS CARCINOMA

Drug	Precautions	Dose Limiting Toxicity	Other Toxicity
Methotrexate	Adequate renal function Excretion facilitated by urinary alkalinization	Hematologic	Stomatitis Diarrhea Hepatic toxicity Renal toxicity
Bleomycin	Adequate renal and pulmonary function Limit total dose to 300–400 mg	Pulmonary fibrosis Stomatitis	Hyperpyrexia Nausea, vomiting Alopecia Allergic reactions Dermatologic
Cis-platinum	Adequate renal function Adequate hydration Avoid nephrotoxic antibiotics Avoid aluminum containing administration equipment	Renal	Ototoxicity Nausea, vomiting Alopecia Neuropathy Anaphylaxis (rare)
Cyclophosphamide	Adequate hydration	Hematologic	Nausea, vomiting Hemorrhagic cystitis Alopecia
Adriamycin	Heart disease Adequate hepatic function Limit total dose to 500 mg/m^2	Hematologic	Cardiomyopathy Alopecia Diarrhea Stomatitis
Vincristine	Adequate hepatic function	Neuropathy	Mild hematologic Alopecia
5-fluorouracil	Adequate hepatic and renal function	Hematologic Diarrhea	Nausea, vomiting Stomatitis Alopecia Neurologic (rare)

with curable tumors previously untreated, drug activity may be greater than that observed in these previous trials.

Several additional considerations limit interpretation of the historical data concerning drug activity in head and neck squamous carcinoma. In current trials, tumor responses are defined as complete (CR) meaning 90 to 100 percent regression of clinically apparent tumor, or partial (PR), usually defined as at least 50 percent reduction in the size of the tumor as derived by the product of the two maximal linear dimensions at right angles to each other. In present assessments of drug activity, these data are provided because of the association that is now apparent between extent of tumor regression and the duration of tumor response. It is because this relationship was not appreciated during the period of accumulation of most of the data on drug activity for palliation of head and neck squamous carcinoma that extent of tumor regression was not recorded. Also, tumor regression by site was rarely reported, yet current trials show differing responses of the primary tumor, nodal and distant metastases in individual patients. Nor was tumor regression by site of the primary tumor usually recorded, a factor that more recent data show to vary when regression rates at various head and neck primary tumor sites are determined for individual drug regimens. Investigations now in progress will provide the information needed for selection of appropriate regimens for palliation of tumors at differing primary and metastatic sites. Other factors that may influence tumor regression rates include histologic grade of tumor and type of previous therapy, i.e., whether the tumor is recurrent after surgical treatment or radiation therapy or both and if chemotherapy has been administered prior to the regimen being assessed. It is important to emphasize, however, that none of these now apparent deficiencies in data collection are perceived as significant impediments in the utilization of these data for treating individual patients or in the design of prospective trials, primarily because of the repeated demonstration of similar relative activities of the drugs tested.

METHOTREXATE

Methotrexate is the most extensively studied chemotherapeutic drug in patients with head and neck squamous carcinoma and represents the standard to which other drugs are compared. Methotrexate acts by tight but reversible binding to dihydrofolate reductase, thereby inhibiting the conversion of folic acid to tetrahydrofolate, a necessary precursor for thymidylic acid biosynthesis. The resulting inhibition of DNA, RNA, and protein synthesis can be avoided by administering citrovorum factor (leucovorin), which is converted directly to tetrahydrofolate, thereby bypassing the methotrexate-induced enzymatic block. Leukopenia and thrombocytopenia are dose-limiting toxicities (Table 29-1). The cumulative experience with systemic methotrexate indicates an overall response rate of 40 percent to 50 percent in patients with recurrent or metastatic cancer (Table 29-2). Intermittent weekly or biweekly schedules of 40 to 60 mg/m² achieve better response rates and less toxicity than either daily low dose regimens or intermittent 5-day courses of 5 to 25 mg/day each month (Table 29-3). The cytotoxic specificity of methotrexate for the S-phase of the cell cycle and the effectiveness of leucovorin in limiting methotrexate toxicity led to trials of continuous 24 to 42 hour infusions of moderate dose (240 to 320 mg/m²)

TABLE 29-2. CUMULATIVE RESPONSE RATES WITH SINGLE DRUG CHEMOTHERAPY IN HEAD AND NECK SQUAMOUS CARCINOMA

Drug	Evaluable Patients	Response Rate (%)
Methotrexate[11]	1038	43
Hydroxyurea[21]	18	39
Cyclophosphamide[21]	77	36
Cisplatinum[44, 97, 122, 123]	159	30
Vinblastine[21]	35	29
Adriamycin[21]	34	23
Bleomycin[72]	346	21
5-fluorouracil[21]	118	15
Chlorambucil[21]	34	15
Procarbazine[21]	31	10

TABLE 29-3. EFFECT OF METHOTREXATE SCHEDULE ON TUMOR RESPONSE IN ADVANCED HEAD AND NECK SQUAMOUS CARCINOMA

Dose and Schedule*	Evaluable Patients	Response Rate (%)
40–60 mg/m² IV, weekly or biweekly[21]	100	50
5–25 mg/day × 5 IV, monthly[21]	107	29
50 mg/day IA with L.R.[21]	308	55
240 mg/m² IV, 24 hr. infusion, q 4 days with L.R.[21]	51†	70
360–1080 mg/m² IV, 36–42 hr. infusion, biweekly with L.R.[12, 125]	53	40
>1 g/m² IV, infusion or bolus, weekly with L.R.[52, 58, 81, 125]	48†	62

*Abbreviations Used: IV, Intravenous: IA, Intra-arterial; L. R., Leucovorin rescue.
†Most patients were previously untreated.

and high dose (> 1 g/m²) methotrexate followed by leucovorin "rescue." In a randomized prospective comparison of weekly low dose methotrexate (40 to 60 mg/m²) to biweekly moderate dose infusions, better survival and response durations were demonstrated with the weekly dose regimen compared with the biweekly infusion when all prognostic factors were considered.[27] Other recent studies have suggested very high response rates to high dose regimens;[58, 81, 125] however, a randomized comparison of twice-weekly conventional dose methotrexate (40 to 200 mg/m² and leucovorin) with weekly high dose (1 to 7.5 g/m² and leucovorin) failed to demonstrate a significant difference in response rates or duration of response between these regimens.[52] In addition, toxicity was less with the low dose regimen. Patients failing to respond to

low dose methotrexate did not subsequently respond to high dose therapy. At the present time, the additional cost, risk of toxicity, and the complexity of high dose methotrexate regimens do not justify their routine use.

Methotrexate administration by intra-arterial infusion has been extensively studied because of the tendency for head and neck carcinomas to remain localized for long periods of time and the possibility of delivering high concentrations of the drug to the primary site while avoiding major systemic toxicity. An overall response rate of 55 percent in 308 cases (Table 29-3), however, has not indicated a distinct therapeutic advantage over the systemic route, since patients selected for intra-arterial therapy in these studies often had localized disease and frequently experienced serious complications from intra-arterial cannulation and drug administration. The results of other single drug and combination intra-arterial chemotherapy trials are summarized in Table 29-4.

BLEOMYCIN

Bleomycin represents the second most extensively studied chemotherapeutic drug in head and neck squamous carcinoma. The presumed mechanism of action of bleomycin is primarily through DNA-strand scission. Important characteristics of bleomycin include a natural affinity for epidermoid cells, a relative lack of hematologic toxicity, a potential cell-cycle synchronizing effect with low dose continuous infusions, and a potential synergism with radiotherapy. Mucositis and irreversible pulmonary fibrosis are dose limiting toxicities (Table 29-1). Response rates for bleomycin vary from 6 percent to 45 percent, although route of administration and schedule do not appear to influence response rates (Table 29-5). Response rates by tumor site are highly variable and response durations are generally less than 3 months. The potential synchronizing effect of bleomycin infusions, lack of hematologic toxicity, and short response duration that are associated with single agent

TABLE 29-4. INTRA-ARTERIAL SINGLE DRUG AND COMBINATION CHEMOTHERAPY IN ADVANCED HEAD AND NECK SQUAMOUS CARCINOMA

Investigator	Drugs*	Evaluable Patients	Response Rate (%)
Donegan and Harris[31]	5 FU	71	45
	MTX	18	39
	BLM	10	30
	MTX-5FU-BLM	15	87
Freckman[34]	MTX-5FU-CTX-VBL-DAC†	159	45
Demard et al.[28]	VCR-BLM	36‡	33
Auersperg et al.[6]	MTX-BLM-VBL†	36	78
Rogers[94]	MTX-5FU-5FUDR-HN₂-TSPA†	152	62

*Abbreviations used: BLM, bleomycin; CTX, Cytoxan; DAC, dactinomycin; 5FU, 5-fluorouracil; HN₂, nitrogen mustard; MTX, methotrexate; TSPA, thiotepa; VBL, vinblastine; VCR, vincristine.
†Drugs were used singly or in combination.
‡Patients were previously untreated.

bleomycin administration suggest that the optimal benefit from bleomycin should be attained in combination chemotherapy regimens.

CIS-PLATINUM (CIS-DIAMINEDICHLOROPLATINUM-II)

Cis-platinum is the most recently introduced chemotherapeutic drug with significant activity in head and neck squamous carcinoma. The postulated mechanism of action of cis-platinum is related to its alkylating properties, whereby complementary strands of DNA are cross-linked and DNA replication prevented. Dose limiting renal toxicity has been minimized by vigorous hydration and diuresis, thereby allowing dose escalation and augmentation of the therapeutic index of cis-platinum. Hematologic toxicity is usually moderate and transient. Data from trials of single agent cis-platinum indicate a response rate of 25 percent to 30 percent in heavily pretreated subjects (Ta-

TABLE 29-5. EFFECT OF BLEOMYCIN SCHEDULE ON TUMOR RESPONSE IN ADVANCED HEAD AND NECK SQUAMOUS CARCINOMA

Dose and Schedule	Evaluable Patients	Response Rate (%)
20 mg/m² IV or IM, twice weekly[39]	53	45
10–30 mg/m² IV, twice weekly[13]	48	38
10 mg/m² IV, twice weekly[38]	64	19
9.25 mg/m² IV, daily to toxicity[126]	46	13
10 mg/m² IV or IM, twice weekly[32]	81	6

ble 29-6); however, the significant activity of cis-platinum is substantiated by a high rate of clinically complete responses, particularly in previously untreated patients. Both high dose (120 mg/m² IV bolus) and low dose (20 mg/m² IV bolus daily × 5 days) regimens appear to achieve similar overall response rates, rates of complete responses, and median durations of response.[99] In a randomized comparison in heavily pretreated patients, biweekly high dose cis-platinum administration resulted in a similar response rate to that achieved with weekly high dose methotrexate.[82] The significant activity of cis-platinum, along with its minimal hematologic toxicity, has led to the rapid introduction of cis-platinum into combination chemotherapy regimens.

OTHER SINGLE AGENTS

Adriamycin, cyclophosphamide, hydroxyurea, and the vinca alkaloids represent other drugs with significant chemotherapeutic activity in head and neck squamous carcinoma. These drugs have been utilized primarily in combination regimens. In particular, vincristine has been frequently incorporated in combination regimens because of its cell-synchronizing characteristics and minimal hematologic toxicity. Newer drugs, such as mitomycin C, PALA (L-aspartic acid

N-(phosphonoacetyl) disodium salt), m-AMSA (acridinyl anisidide), vindesine, dibromodulcitol, and gallium nitrate are currently being evaluated in head and neck cancer and may prove useful as single agents or in combination with established drugs.

Chemotherapy for Palliation

In general, incurable head and neck cancers are symptomatic, so the term chemotherapy for palliation is appropriate. Not infrequently, however, patients present with local recurrences or distant metastases that are asymptomatic. In these patients the use of chemotherapy would best be described as prophylactic in anticipation of symptoms, but for practical purposes the treatment of these patients is included in this discussion.

Advanced, recurrent, or metastatic squamous carcinoma of the head and neck is associated with a dismal prognosis. Few therapeutic options are available to the clinician faced with a situation of disseminated disease or massive recurrence following unsuccessful combined therapy. The administration of systemic chemotherapy to selected patients not amenable to other forms of palliation has resulted in significant tumor regressions and subjective improvements without appreciable increases in overall sur-

TABLE 29-6. EFFECT OF CIS-PLATINUM SCHEDULE ON TUMOR RESPONSE IN ADVANCED HEAD AND NECK SQUAMOUS CARCINOMA

Dose and Schedule	Evaluable Patients	Response Rate (%)
50 mg/m² bolus, day 1 + 8, monthly*	65	25
3 mg/kg short infusion, q 3–4 weeks[122]	26	30
120 mg/m² short infusion, q 3 weeks[97, 123]	37†	38
80 mg/m² 24 hr. infusion, q 3 weeks[44]	16‡	38
20 mg/m² bolus, daily × 5, q 3 weeks[97]	15	27

*Panettiere, F. J. (personal communication).
†22 patients were previously untreated.
‡6 patients were previously untreated.

vival rates. The goals of such therapy have been prolongation of disease-free survival and enhancement of quality of life.

SINGLE DRUG REGIMENS

From a practical standpoint, single drug regimens are the least complicated, least toxic, and most readily available form of palliative chemotherapy. Of the commercially available drugs approved for use in patients with head and neck cancer, methotrexate and bleomycin are the most active drugs for recurrent cancer. Reported response rates for systemic methotrexate are consistently higher than those for bleomycin; however, it is difficult to make meaningful comparisons among nonrandomized studies of these drugs. Furthermore, many bleomycin studies have included patients previously treated with methotrexate.[72] In previously treated patients, single drug chemotherapy is associated with short response durations. However, prolonged survival and response duration have been observed in individual patients who achieve a clinical complete tumor response. Significant tumor responses are more frequently noted in previously untreated patients, which indicates that palliative chemotherapy may be most effective in such patients. Despite a lack of evidence that proves that multidrug chemotherapy is more effective than single drug chemotherapy in patients with recurrent cancer, recent studies indicate that multidrug regimens may result in more frequent complete responses. This, in turn, suggests that multidrug treatment would also be associated with longer survival and response durations.

MULTIDRUG REGIMENS

The efficacy of combination chemotherapy in hematologic and a variety of solid malignancies led to the testing of this approach in head and neck squamous carcinoma. Initially, most regimens were adapted from experiences in the treatment of other tumors. Recently, however, combinations incorporating the most active drugs in head and neck squamous cancer have been specifically designed and tested in patients with recurrent or metastatic disease (Table 29-7). A

TABLE 29-7. SYSTEMIC COMBINATION CHEMOTHERAPY IN ADVANCED HEAD AND NECK SQUAMOUS CARCINOMA

Investigator	Regimen*	No. Patients			Response Rate (%)	Median Response Duration (Months)
		Evaluable	CR*	PR*		
Holoye et al.[41]	BLM-CTX-MTX-5FU	22	4	9	59	†
Cortes et al.[25]	BLM-CTX-MTX-5FU	26	7	8	62	3–12
Ratkin et al.[89]	BLM-VCR-MTX	14	0	6	43	4.7
Livingston et al.[61]	BLM-VCR-CTX/MTX/ ADR-MeCCNU‡	28	5	12	61	6
Price et al.[85]	BLM-VCR-MTX-HC- 5FU±ADR	85	†	†	67	†
Wheeler et al.[121]	BLM-VCR-MITO±MTX	13	3	8	85	3
Presant et al.[84]	CTX-BCNU-ADR	31	1	10	35	5.4

*Abbreviations Used: ADR, Adriamycin; BCNU, bis chloroethyl nitrosourea; BLM, bleomycin; CTX, Cytoxan; 5FU, 5-fluorouracil; MeCCNU, methyl-chloroethyl cyclohexyl nitrosourea; MTX, methotrexate; MITO, mitomycin C; VCR, vincristine; HC, hydrocortisone; CR, complete response; PR, partial response.
†Not reported.
‡Sequential cycles.

number of trials combining methotrexate and bleomycin yielded a cumulative response rate of 47 percent in 81 evaluable patients.[72] The addition of other drugs such as Cytoxan, 5-fluorouracil, vincristine, Adriamycin, or mitomycin-C to methotrexate or bleomycin has achieved response rates ranging from 43 percent to 85 percent (Table 29-7). Two important observations made with combination regimens in previously treated patients have been the higher response rates and increased frequency of clinical complete responses compared with single drug regimens. This has been particularly evident with combinations incorporating cis-platinum (Table 29-8). Most studies of combination chemotherapy demonstrated a longer median survival in responding patients compared to patients who did not respond to chemotherapy; however, the duration of response has not been significantly longer than that achieved with the best single agents. Some studies of combination regimens also showed longer median survivals in patients experiencing a complete response compared to partial responders.[49, 61, 115] The observation that combination chemotherapy regimens are associated

with higher complete response rates and that complete responders survived longer than partial responders would suggest that multiagent regimens may be more effective than single drugs as palliative therapy. The morbidity associated with intensive multi-drug chemotherapy, however, must be carefully weighed against any expected improvement in the patient's quality of life and survival.

With the possible exception of cis-platinum based regimens, combination chemotherapy has not been demonstrated to be clearly superior to the best single agents. In a single small randomized trial, weekly conventional dose methotrexate proved as effective as the combination of cis-platinum, bleomycin, and vincristine.[8] A number of additional randomized trials are currently underway comparing single drug with multidrug combination therapy. Until the results of these studies are available, the added cost, toxicity, complexity, and frequent need for hospitalization associated with combination chemotherapy suggests that the routine use of multidrug regimens for palliation is not warranted at present.

TABLE 29-8. SYSTEMIC COMBINATION CHEMOTHERAPY INCORPORATING CIS-PLATINUM IN ADVANCED HEAD AND NECK SQUAMOUS CARCINOMA

| Investigator | Regimen* | No. Patients | | | Response Rate (%) | Median Response Duration (Months) |
		Evaluable	CR*	PR*		
Bonomi et al.[15]	DDP-ADR	16	1	5	37	4.5
Lyman[63]	DDP-BLM	9	2	4	67	3.8
Caradonna et al.[20]	DDP-BLM-MTX	14	2	9	79	3
Kaplan et al.[49]	DDP-BLM-MTX	46	8	21	63	11 (CR) 5 (PR)
Elias et al.[33]	DDP-BLM-HDMTX	11	0	6	54	2–3
Leone and Ohnuma[56]	DDP-BLM-HDMTX	24	1	5	25	2
Amer et al.[3]	DDP-BLM-VCR	27	0	13	48	6
Baker and Al-Sarraf[8]	DDP-BLM-VCR	8	1	4	63	†

*Abbreviations used: ADR, Adriamycin; BLM, bleomycin; DDP, cis-platinum; HDMTX, High dose methotrexate; MTX, methotrexate; VCR, vincristine; CR, complete response; PR, partial response.
†Not reported.

PRACTICAL CONSIDERATIONS AND GUIDELINES

The failure of most palliative single drug and combination chemotherapy trials to demonstrate significant prolongation of patient survival may be due in part to the extremely poor prognosis of most patients entered in these early trials. The higher response rates recently achieved in less debilitated and less heavily pretreated patients and the significant survival durations noted in patients achieving a complete response provide rationale for palliative chemotherapy in selected patients who have a sufficiently long expected survival and adequate medical status to warrant administration of toxic and debilitating drugs.

Decision making in the treatment of patients with incurable tumors requires consideration of both tumor and patient factors. Of major concern are the following factors, many of which are interrelated.

1. *The status of the tumor region:*

a. Previous therapy and residual effects on the tumor and adjacent tissues. Fibrosis, scarring, and loss of supporting tissues is accompanied by reduced tumor vascularity, thereby limiting access of systemic drugs to the neoplasm.

b. Tumor size and local changes such as ulceration, infection, bleeding. Large tumors with proportionally fewer cells in growth phase may respond poorly to drugs. Local ulceration and infection may lead to serious bleeding or sepsis when drugs are added.

c. Obstruction or interference with the function of the digestive or respiratory passageway. These factors contribute to central organ dysfunction, toxicity of chemotherapeutic drugs, and the ability of the patient to tolerate therapy.

d. Obstruction of major blood vessels such as the carotid artery or superior vena cava. Regression of tumors involving major vascular structures may lead to serious or fatal hemorrhage or tumor embolization.

e. Involvement of bone, nerves, sinuses, and severity of associated symptoms. Extensive tumors involving these structures are frequently resistant to palliation by chemotherapy. They are often so painful that large frequent doses of narcotics are necessary to obtain relief of symptoms. This leads to loss of appetite, poor food intake, and rapid weight loss which reduces tolerance to chemotherapy.

2. *The status of the patient:*

a. General health and nutritional status, body weight in relation to ideal and usual weight, and, if present, cause and rate of weight loss are important factors in determining the ability of the patient to tolerate therapy and in predicting potential tumor response.

b. Functional level of central organs, especially the liver, kidneys, heart, and lungs; status of the hematopoietic system and etiology of deficiencies, if present. Organ system dysfunction frequently limits maximal application of drug regimens and reduces the chances of achieving effective therapy.

c. Performance status or general level of activity; ability to comprehend and adhere to outpatient therapy regimens.

d. Life expectancy due to the tumor as well as to concomitant diseases. Expected survival that is markedly shorter than that which might be achieved with the addition of chemotherapy is generally associated with such severe debilitation as to preclude a beneficial result from the administration of highly toxic drugs.

After assessing the patient by these broad guidelines, the primary decisions for treatment of individual patients are whether to use single or multiple drug regimens and whether the patient requires hospitalization for treatment. Patient preference should be determined after consideration of the morbidity of the regimens and the required aggressiveness of the treatment. As with chemotherapy for other malignancies, the previous experience and expertise of the treatment team is critical, particularly if the morbidity of intensive multiple drug chemotherapy is to be kept at a minimum. For Phase I and II clinical trials, these considerations are usually an integral part of the clinical protocols but may be modified by the goals of the trial and the experience of the investigators with the specific treatment regimen.

Outpatient single drug, low dose chemotherapy regimens are usually selected for patients with incurable, relatively asymptomatic, previously untreated tumors. Such therapy is also considered for patients with local recurrences after unsuccessful surgery or radiation therapy who are relatively asymptomatic, and for patients with distant metastases that are either asymptomatic or associated with pain as a primary complaint.

Multiple drug regimens should be considered for patients with recurrent tumors that are associated with interference with swallowing or severe pain, but who have good hematopoietic and central organ function, minimal weight loss and good performance status. Similar patients who have had previous treatment with chemotherapy should also be considered for multiple drug regimens because of the reduced response rates to single agents in patients previously treated with chemotherapy. In such patients, the most critical factor limiting aggressive multiple drug chemotherapy regimens is the residual toxic effects of the first regimen. For example, residual renal toxicity from previous administration of methotrexate would usually interdict the use of regimens employing cis-platinum. The cumulative toxicity of drugs such as Adriamycin or bleomycin may limit their utilization in long-term palliative regimens, in addition to the limitations imposed by preexisting cardiac or pulmonary disease. Patients with recurrent tumors who have a grave prognosis because of obstruction of the digestive or respiratory pathways, local bleeding, obstruction of major blood vessels, marked debility, compromise of central organ and hematopoietic function, or other factors associated with high morbidity with the use of chemotherapy should be treated on an inpatient basis with multiple drug regimens. This treatment should be undertaken only by experienced investigators in institutions with facilities for the management of complications associated with the use of chemotherapy in such patients.

In addition to the possible therapeutic benefit of chemotherapy for patients with incurable tumors, there are utilitarian reasons for the use of chemotherapy in these patients. The derivation of more effective and less toxic chemotherapeutic regimens depends on Phase I and Phase II studies that utilize the population of patients with recurrent and metastatic carcinoma. These investigations are best carried out in institutions having experienced medical oncologists and support personnel where first and second line therapy would be determined and randomized comparisons made with single drug regimens. Such studies have already identified a number of combination regimens with significant activity, particularly in previously untreated patients. These preliminary data have led to the recent incorporation of combination chemotherapy into adjuvant strategies for patients with high risk but potentially curable head and neck squamous carcinoma.

Chemotherapy as an Adjuvant to Radiation Therapy and Surgery

RATIONALE OF ADJUVANT CHEMOTHERAPY

The effectiveness of conventional surgery or radiation therapy in curing patients with squamous carcinoma of the head and neck is well established. Single modality treatment strategies employing surgery or radiotherapy for small, locally confined tumors have resulted in 5-year survival rates of 70 to 90 percent. In patients with extensive primary tumors or regional metastases, however, 5-year survival rates range from 0 to 60 percent. Combinations of surgery and radiation therapy in patients with advanced tumors have not significantly improved the generally poor overall survival rates achieved with either modality alone. This has been attributed to failures in the control or prevention of distant metastases despite occasional reductions in local recurrence rates and prolongation of disease-free intervals.[9, 18, 48, 86]

A significant proportion of head and neck cancer patients have advanced tumors when first diagnosed and although most patients may have all clinically detectable tumor ablated by resection or irradiation, many will develop local or distant recurrence within 2 years. The primary reasons for these failures may be the failure to eradicate local or regional microscopic tumor within or adjacent to the area encompassed by surgery or radiation therapy and the growth of preexisting occult metastases.

The effectiveness of conventional surgery and radiation therapy is limited to the treatment of localized cancers. The rationale for combining radiation therapy with surgery is to decrease the incidence of local recurrences, and thus this combination offers no curative benefit for patients with occult distant metastases or neoplastic extension outside the perimeter of local therapy. Chemotherapy, however, is effective systemically and limited primarily by gross tumor mass rather than by the anatomic distribution of tumor. Most cytotoxic drugs act by first-order kinetics and kill that portion of the tumor cell population which is actively growing and susceptible. Since the growth fraction of a tumor is inversely proportional to the size of its cell population, a reduction in tumor mass through effective local modalities should enhance the ability of chemotherapy to either eradicate residual microscopic tumor deposits[101] or reduce the number of tumor cells to a point where immunologic mechanisms may be effective. Numerous animal studies show that chemotherapy given in maximum tolerated doses is effective in eradicating small tumor deposits and preventing death if given with, or shortly after, small but normally fatal inoculi of viable tumor cells. In animal models of metastasizing neoplasms, the protective effect of chemotherapy following surgical tumor resection can also be demonstrated.[99] The goal of adjuvant therapy is to destroy residual local-regional tumor cells and systemically disseminated cells that are not eradicated by local modalities. Future therapies for advanced head and neck cancer must be directed at both local and systemic tumor control if improved cure rates are to be achieved.

The initial clinical trials of adjuvant chemotherapy were based on the once popular hypothesis that recurrences following tumor resections were due to vascular and lymphatic spread of viable tumor cells at the time of surgical manipulation. The fact that many patients with locally advanced cancer who were cured of local or regional tumor relapsed at distant sites indicated that subclinical foci of disease were present at the time of potentially curative local-regional treatment. The small number of residual circulating tumor cells at the time of local therapy and the low probability that a residual cell will result in a metastasis suggests that elimination of these cells would not affect overall survival.[59] Therefore, adjuvant treatment is directed at established micrometastases. The early studies utilizing brief, perioperative chemotherapy at less than maximal doses showed no benefit from the adjuvant treatment. Animal studies with a variety of transplantable, metastasizing solid tumors, however, showed best results when intensive, frequently multidrug, chemotherapy was used following surgical resections. Subsequent clinical success in treating leukemias and lymphomas with chemotherapy alone or in combination with radiation therapy indicated the potential of cytotoxic drugs for eradicating disseminated tumor cells. A basis was thus provided for adjuvant chemotherapy in patients with solid malignancies who were at high risk of developing distant metastases.

Adjuvant chemotherapy has been most successful in the pediatric malignancies of Wilms tumor, Ewing sarcoma, and rhabdomyosarcoma.[40, 96] Despite aggressive local therapies, these usually fatal malignancies were found to be curable in 60 to 90 percent of cases when combination chemotherapy was added to surgical resection and irradiation. The application of adjuvant chemotherapy strategies to the treatment of breast cancer and osteosarcoma also yielded encouraging results.[14, 70] A large number of chemotherapeutic drugs active in recurrent or metastatic head and neck cancer produce regression rates of local-regional tumors approaching those achieved with palliative radiation therapy. When viewed with the encouraging results of adjuvant regimens in other solid tumors, these data suggest that adjuvant chemotherapy should be beneficial in advanced, potentially curable head and neck cancer patients and provide justification for such clinical trials.

The major rationale for the use of chemotherapy as an adjuvant prior to surgery and prior to or during radiation therapy in patients with local-regional head and neck carcinoma is derived from the effects of palliative chemotherapy regimens in patients with incurable tumors. These data were reviewed in the preceding sections. In these studies, the higher response rates and the longer duration of responses achieved with chemotherapy in previously untreated patients when compared to the effects in patients with tumors recurrent after surgery or radiation therapy provide rationale for the administration of chemotherapy prior to surgery and prior to or during radiation therapy for local-regional tumors. This strategy, based on the observation of the greater effectiveness of chemotherapy in previously untreated patients, is utilized in an attempt to reduce local tumor extent with the anticipation that this will in turn reduce the incidence of local-regional tumor recurrence after surgery. It is hypothesized that the incidence of such recurrences will be lower than that achieved with chemotherapy administered after local therapy because of the reduced effectiveness of chemotherapy on residual tumor following local therapy. A second hypothesis is that chemotherapy administered at this early interval in the treatment program may also reduce the incidence of eventual distant metastases by eradication of occult metastases when these foci are relatively small and that attempts at eradication will be less successful when adjuvant chemotherapy is given at an interval after local therapy, since these foci would likely be larger in size.

In trials in which chemotherapy is being evaluated as an adjuvant after local therapy in patients without clinically manifest residual tumor but who are at high risk for local-regional recurrence and distant metastases, the hypothesis postulated is similar to that in evaluations of the effect of postoperative chemotherapy in patients with other solid malignancies; namely, that eradication of residual and metastatic tumor is more likely to be achieved by chemotherapy when these foci are microscopic than when they are clinically apparent.

These theoretic considerations suggesting a potential benefit of chemotherapy in combination with local therapy for patients with potentially curable head and neck squamous carcinoma have not been adequately tested. Few adjuvant studies have been designed as controlled prospective randomized trials comparing chemotherapy as an adjuvant to conventional therapy with conventional treatment alone. Most of the completed randomized studies of adjuvant chemotherapy have been trials in which single drug chemotherapy was used prior to or concurrent with radiation therapy. The results of these studies are summarized in Table 29-9 and reviewed in the subsequent sections in which the individual drugs utilized

TABLE 29-9. RANDOMIZED CLINICAL TRIALS COMPARING CHEMOTHERAPY AND RADIATION TO RADIATION ALONE IN PATIENTS WITH ADVANCED HEAD AND NECK SQUAMOUS CARCINOMA

Investigator	Drug	Schedule	Evaluable Patients	Results		Comments
				RT	RT + CT	
Kramer[55]	MTX	25 mg q 3 days × 5 then RT	631	23.1	23.4 (mos. mean survival)	Marginal increase in 4-year survival for oral cavity-hypopharynx sites.

TABLE 29-9. CONTINUED

Investigator	Drug	Schedule	Evaluable Patients	Results RT	Results RT + CT	Comments
Knowlton et al.[54]	MTX	0.2 mg/kg/day × 5 or 240 mg/m² × 3 then RT	96	10% (5-yr. survival)	9%	No difference in local control, survival or distant metastases.
Condit[24]	MTX	1–4 mg/kg biweekly during RT	40	3.4 (mos. remission duration)	5.1	No significant difference.
Cachin et al.[19]	BLM	15 mg twice weekly during RT	186 (oropharynx)	≈67% CR rate both groups.		Higher early death rate in BLM group due to higher rate of major complications.
Kapstad et al.[50]	BLM	15 mg three times/ wk, weeks 1 + 2, 4 + 5 during preoperative RT (3,000 rads)	29	43% (mean 2-yr. disease-free survival)	93%	No difference in morbidity. Increased 2-yr disease-free survival in BLM group.
Stefani et al.[106]	HYD	80 mg/kg twice weekly during orthovoltage RT	126	47% (CR rate)	42%	No difference in local tumor response, distant metastases or survival
Richards and Chambers[92]	HYD	80 mg/kg q 3 days during RT then maintenance (some surgery)	40	14% (CR rate)	77%	Difference in response rates not significant, more distant metastasis in RT alone group.
Gollin et al.[37]	5FU	10 mg/kg/day × 3, then 5 mg/kg/ day × 4, then 5 mg/kg 3 times/ wk during RT	155	19.8 (mos. mean survival)	28.3	No difference in 3-yr survival. Significant increase 5-yr survival for oral cavity.
Petrovich et al.[80]	MTX-VCR	50–100 mg/kg MTX, .015 mg/ kg VCR, 2 courses prior to RT	23	8 (mos. median survival)	12	More responses, increased survival (*P* = .09) in combined therapy group.

Abbreviations used: MTX, methotrexate; BLM, bleomycin; HYD, hydroxyurea; 5FU, 5-fluorouracil; VCR, vincristine; RT, radiotherapy; CT, chemotherapy; CR, complete response.

are discussed. Other studies on which a current appraisal of adjuvant chemotherapy must rely include nonrandomized trials of multidrug chemotherapy combined with radiotherapy and single or multidrug regimens prior to or following surgery and radiation therapy. Recently, however, several randomized trials have been initiated that are designed to test the efficacy of chemotherapy as initial treatment or as maintenance therapy in patients undergoing potentially curative surgery and radiotherapy. The regimens used and response rates to the initial chemotherapy are summarized in Table 29-10.

TRIALS OF ADJUVANT CHEMOTHERAPY AND RADIATION THERAPY

The effect of single drug chemotherapy combined with radiation therapy in the treatment of patients with head and neck carcinoma has been extensively investigated. The initial regimens were designed empirically with chemotherapy administered as preliminary treatment or in conjunction with standard radiation fractionation schemes. The stated rationale for these studies was derived from experimental observations of the potential radiosensitizing effects of specific drugs as well as of the relative effectiveness of chemotherapy in reducing the bulk of untreated and therefore relatively large well-vascularized tumors as discussed above. These investigations also postulated that the addition of systemic chemotherapy may result in a therapeutic or prophylactic effect on subclinical distant metastases. However, the results of randomized trials of single or multidrug chemotherapy and radiation therapy have not consistently shown benefit from this approach.

Methotrexate.   The largest experience with chemotherapy as an adjuvant to radiation therapy has been reported in studies in which methotrexate was used.[24, 54, 55] Experimentally, methotrexate in vitro kills cells in the S phase of the cell cycle, thereby arresting cells at the G_1-S transition which is a relatively radiosensitive phase of the cell cycle.

This effect was particularly evident in cultured Hela cells that were in the exponential growth phase.[105] The results of randomized clinical trials utilizing methotrexate and radiation, however, have not been encouraging. The largest trial, with 631 evaluable patients, showed no overall differences in the 3-year survival rate with methotrexate administered prior to full course radiotherapy compared with radiotherapy alone.[55, 62] When the results of this study were analyzed by tumor site, a marginal increase in 4-year survival was suggested for patients with oral cavity or hypopharyngeal tumors treated with the adjuvant regimen. No differences were noted in the frequency of distant metastatic relapse among the treatment groups. Similarly, other randomized trials in which higher doses of methotrexate,[34] intra-arterial methotrexate,[7, 91] or simultaneous methotrexate and radiotherapy[24] were used failed to demonstrate a definite therapeutic advantage for methotrexate combined with radiotherapy over radiotherapy alone.

Bleomycin.   Trials in which bleomycin was administered during radiotherapy attempted to exploit the potential radiosensitizing effects of that drug. In a large randomized European trial in patients with oropharyngeal cancers, no significant differences in tumor response or patient survival were noted with bleomycin (15 mg twice weekly) during radiotherapy compared to radiotherapy alone.[19] Provocative preliminary results, however, were reported in a small trial in which a similar bleomycin regimen (15 mg three times per week) was combined with radiation (3,000 rads) as preoperative therapy for patients with resectable head and neck cancers.[50] An increased 2-year disease-free survival rate was reported in the patients receiving adjuvant bleomycin compared with those receiving low dose preoperative radiotherapy and placebo. No differences in morbidity were noted between the two treatment groups. Unfortunately, this trial consisted of only 29 evaluable patients, most with laryngeal sites of primary tumor and with no clinical lymph node metastases. Both advanced T and N

TABLE 29-10. ADJUVANT CHEMOTHERAPY PRIOR TO SURGERY OR RADIOTHERAPY IN PREVIOUSLY UNTREATED PATIENTS WITH HEAD AND NECK SQUAMOUS CARCINOMA

Investigator	Regimen	Evaluable Patients	Response Rate to Chemotherapy (%)	Comments
Tarpley et al.[109]	MTX 240 mg/m² day 1 + 5, surgery day 12–15.	30 (resectable)	77	Demonstrated feasibility of this approach, delayed recurrences compared with historical controls.
Kirkwood et al.[52]	MTX 1–7.5 g/m² weekly × 5, then definitive surg. + / or RT, repeat MTX for responders after S/RT.	23 (III–IV)	52	No difference in recurrence or distant metastases in responders vs. non-responders but longer disease-free interval in responders.
Taylor et al.[110]	MTX 60 mg/m² days 1, 5, 9 in 2 wks prior to surg. + / or RT. Escalated to mucosal toxicity.	10 (III–IV)	80	Acceptable toxicity, 76% 2-year survival.
Hong et al.[42]	DDP 120 mg/m² day 1, BLM 15 mg/m² infusion days 3–10, DDP repeat day 22, then surgery (19 patients) or RT.	38 (some unresectable)	76	High rate of clinical CR's (20%).
Al-Sarraf et al.[2]	DDP 100 mg/m² day 1, BLM 30 mg/day day 2–5, VCR 1 mg days 2+ 5. Surg. +/ or RT after 2 courses of chemo.	27 (III–IV)	86	59% response rate after one course chemo. Acceptable toxicity.
Tejada[112]	MTX 50 mg/m² at 0 hrs, DDP 20 mg/m² at 17–24 hrs, repeat weekly × 4 then surg.	66 (III–IV)	63	Minimal toxicity.
Randolph et al.[88]	DDP 120 mg/m² day 1 + 22, BLM 10 mg/m²/day, infusion days 3–10, then RT.	21 (IV, unresectable)	71	Two year disease-free survival of 9%, acceptable toxicity.

Abbreviations used: MTX, methotrexate; RT, radiotherapy; S, surgery; DDP, cis-platinum; BLM, bleomycin; VCR, vincristine; CR, complete response.

class tumor stages were more prevalent in the patients who received radiation therapy alone preoperatively.

Hydroxyurea and 5-Fluorouracil. Randomized trials of hydroxyurea concurrent with radiotherapy demonstrated increased tumor reduction and acceptable toxicity with combined therapy but did not conclusively show increased survival benefit for patients treated with the adjuvant chemotherapy.[43, 92, 106] The results of two trials in which adjuvant 5-fluorouracil during radiation therapy was compared to radiation therapy alone suggested that improved disease-free survival with this adjuvant may depend on tumor site. Paralleling the results achieved with methotrexate and radiation in patients with oral cavity tumors,[55] Gollin and associates[37] reported a statistically significant improvement in the 5-year survival rate for patients with advanced oral cavity tumors treated with 5-fluorouracil preceding and during radiotherapy. The higher apparent susceptibility of oral cavity tumors to chemotherapeutic drugs has also been reported by others.[10] A significant improvement in the short-term disease-free interval was also observed in patients with maxillary sinus carcinomas treated with intra-arterial 5-fluorouracil during radiation therapy; however, the overall 2-year survival rate did not differ between the treatment regimens and the toxicity of the adjuvant chemotherapy was excessive.[100]

From the available data, it can be concluded that systemic methotrexate, bleomycin, hydroxyurea, or 5-fluorouracil administered as single drug adjuvants with radiation therapy achieved enhanced tumor regressions without significant improvement in the overall survival rate, disease-free interval, or rate of distant metastases. Depending on the chemotherapeutic drug utilized, moderate to severe morbidity was encountered that frequently necessitated interrupted or incomplete radiotherapy schedules. Trials of intra-arterial chemotherapy combined with radiation therapy generally resulted in significant toxicity and morbidity with no documented clinical benefit over that achieved with radiation therapy alone.

Multidrug Regimens.   The increased tumor response rates observed with multidrug versus single drug chemotherapy in other neoplasms also stimulated investigations of combination chemotherapy as an adjunct to radiation therapy in patients with head and neck carcinoma. Data from randomized trials of multidrug regimens is limited; however, encouraging results have been reported from several randomized and nonrandomized prospective trials.[23, 80, 102] Compared with randomized single drug adjuvant chemotherapy trials, nonrandomized clinical trials of multidrug chemotherapy combined with radiation therapy demonstrated increased tumor response rates and were associated with increased toxicity.[35, 102] Significantly improved patient survival was suggested in a study in which the combination of vincristine, bleomycin, and methotrexate was administered in four cycles, one before and one after radiotherapy with two courses given during radiation therapy. In this trial, radiation therapy was interrupted for drug administration. The reported 4-year survival rate of 56 percent was significantly better than the survival of matched historical controls treated with radiation therapy alone.[23] Excluded from the combined therapy analysis, however, was a significant percentage of patients who were felt to be generally unfit for combined therapy. The addition of chemotherapy resulted in frequent interruption of radiation therapy treatment because of mucosal toxicity, even though overall toxicity was considered acceptable. Another trial in which a similar treatment strategy, drug selection, and schedule were employed reported excessive toxicity that was felt to more than offset any modest improvement in tumor control achieved with the combined therapy.[35] The only randomized trial of multidrug chemotherapy combined with radiotherapy compared the addition of two courses of a vincristine-methotrexate regimen prior to radiation therapy to radiation therapy alone.[80] Preliminary results of that trial suggested significantly longer median survival for the combined therapy group. Based on these preliminary data suggesting improved response rates and survival with adjuvant multidrug regimens, a number of nonrandomized trials have been initiated recently to evaluate the efficacy and toxicity of bleomycin-based combinations combined with radiation therapy. The impact that the combination of chemotherapy and radiation therapy might have on the subsequent development of distant metastases in treated patients has not been determined. Some reports suggested lower rates of distant metastases after combined therapy,[62, 71, 80, 92] while others found either no differences[37, 54] or higher rates of metastases.[106]

TRIALS OF ADJUVANT CHEMOTHERAPY AND SURGERY

At present, minimal data are available to delineate the role of chemotherapy as an adjunct to conventional surgery or to combined surgery and radiotherapy in patients with head and neck cancer. The results of early studies involving preoperative intra-arterial chemotherapy (primarily methotrexate) were derived from small numbers of patients with tumors at various anatomic sites and lacked comparable control populations, thereby making interpretation of the contribution of the chemotherapy to tumor control difficult. Recently, trials of systemic adjuvant chemotherapy as initial therapy in patients with potentially curable head and neck carcinoma have been initiated. The results of the preliminary trials are summarized in Table 29–10. Interest in this innovative treatment strategy followed the provocative study by Tarpley and his associates, which demonstrated that preoperative moderate dose methotrexate achieved a high tumor response rate in previously untreated patients and could be combined with planned surgical resections without significant toxicity.[109] Short-term follow-up of these patients suggested a significant increase in disease-free interval compared with matched historical controls, but no dif-

ference in overall recurrence rates. A similar conclusion was reached in the analysis of a trial in which much higher doses of methotrexate were used preoperatively.[52] In this study, a high rate of serious complications was associated with the combined treatment regimen. Taylor and associates[111] reported provocative preliminary results from a trial in which three courses of conventional dose methotrexate and leucovorin were administered prior to surgery and radiotherapy. A 2-year survival rate of 75 percent was achieved in 17 patients with advanced cancers, 7 of whom had been previously treated. The authors attributed the encouraging results of this trial to the fact that chemotherapy was escalated in each course to levels that produced mucocutaneous toxicity.[111]

Multidrug chemotherapy combining cis-platinum with either bleomycin or methotrexate as a preoperative regimen has been investigated in several recent trials.[2, 42, 112, 122, 123] These studies reported major response rates from 63 percent to 86 percent, frequent complete clinical responses, and acceptable toxicity. Based on these results, a number of prospective, randomized studies were designed to determine the efficacy of adjuvant chemotherapy as initial treatment or maintenance therapy in previously untreated patients with potentially curable Stage III and IV squamous carcinoma of the head and neck (Table 29–11).

The multi-institutional trial sponsored by the National Cancer Institute represents the most carefully controlled current study of adjuvant chemotherapy in combination with local therapy for potentially curable tumors. In this study, a preoperative regimen of cis-platinum (100 mg/m²) followed by a 5-day bleomycin infusion (15 mg/m² bolus, then 15 mg/m²/day) is utilized. Two weeks after completion of chemotherapy, the response to chemotherapy of the primary tumor and regional metastases is assessed. Surgical resection is done 3 weeks after the start of the induction of chemotherapy and is followed by conventional radiotherapy.

TABLE 29-11. CURRENT RANDOMIZED CLINICAL TRIALS OF ADJUVANT
CHEMOTHERAPY FOR UNTREATED PATIENTS WITH STAGE III AND IV
RESECTABLE HEAD AND NECK SQUAMOUS CARCINOMA

Protocol	Drug	Conventional Modalities	No. of Arms	Schema
EST-1375	MTX	S, RT, S + RT	2	Maintenance MTX (40 mg/m²) biweekly × 1 yr vs. observation only
RTOG-7914	DDP	S, RT, S + RT	2	Maintenance DDP (80 mg/m²) monthly × 6 mos. vs. observation only
SEG 79-356	MTX-BLM-DDP	S+ RT	2	Preoperative MTX (70 mg/m² q 6 hr × 4, days 1 + 21), DDP (2 mg/kg, days 3 + 24), BLM (30 mg weekly × 6) then S + RT vs. S + RT
NCI-HNCP-178	DDP-BLM	S + RT	3	DDP (100 mg/m², day 1), BLM (15 mg/m²/ day infusion, days 3–7) then S + RT vs. same pre-op. chemo., S + RT, then DDP (80 mg/m² monthly × 6 vs. S + RT
Olivari[75]	MTX-HDMTX-DDP	S + RT	3	MTX (40 mg/m², days 1 + 8), S + RT vs. HDMTX (1.5 gm/m², days 1 + 8), S + RT vs. DDP (50 mg/m², days 1 + 2), S + RT

Abbreviations used: MTX, methotrexate; HDMTX, High dose methotrexate; DDP, Cis-platinum; BLM, bleomycin; S, surgery; RT, radiotherapy; EST, Eastern Cooperative Oncology Group; RTOG, Radiation Therapy Oncology Group; SEG, Southeastern Oncology Group; NCI, National Cancer Institute.

After stratification for site, stage, and participating institution, patients are randomly assigned to one of three treatment policies: conventional surgery and radiotherapy; induction chemotherapy, surgery, and radio- therapy; or induction chemotherapy, surgery, and radiotherapy followed by monthly maintenance chemotherapy for 6 months using cis-platinum (80 mg/m²/course). This study incorporates all of the major considerations critical for assessment of the efficacy of adjuvant chemotherapy. A highly active regimen was chosen that is minimally immunosuppressive and that can be administered during a brief period immediately prior to conventional therapy. Adjuvant regimens prior to and following local treatment are studied and concurrent randomized controls are included. Tumors arising from six commonly encountered head and neck tumor sites are specifically selected for which accrual of a large number of patients with tumors at each site could be expected. Conventional modalities of surgery and radiotherapy are standardized among the treatment regimens, and quality control of each therapeutic modality is an integral part of the trial. Data on patient performance and nutritional status are collected throughout the trial with specific guidelines for ancillary patient care such as nutritional support and dental care. Early and late toxicity resulting from the various modalities is assessed and follow-up is standardized among all patient groups. The results of this study and others like it should delineate the role of adjuvant chemotherapy in combination with local therapy in the treatment of patients with local-regional head and neck cancer.

GUIDELINES FOR THE USE OF CHEMOTHERAPY AS AN ADJUVANT

The high incidence of complete and partial regressions of previously untreated local-regional head and neck squamous carcinomas achieved with short intensive courses of chemotherapy in recent trials argue for its use in individual patients with advanced tumors that historically have been associated with high rates of local recurrence and distant metastases after local therapies. At this point, it is important to summarize that which can be concluded from the current trials in such situations and to emphasize the information sought from these studies that is not yet available.

From the completed and ongoing studies of the effects of chemotherapy adminis-

tered prior to local treatment it can be concluded thus far that regimens employing cis-platinum are associated with high levels of immediate tumor regression and that in previously untreated patients, frequent and major tumor regressions can be achieved with regimens that are well tolerated in patients having good nutritional status and otherwise good health. In previously treated patients, regression rates are markedly less with such regimens; however, there is some evidence suggesting that more intensive multidrug regimens associated with high incidences of systemic toxicity and occasional drug-related deaths yield higher regression rates. In consideration of the use of such regimens, it is important to realize that this associated morbidity was reported in patients treated by oncologists skilled in the use of toxic multidrug regimens and that this treatment was undertaken in centers having the capacity for managing severe complications of chemotherapy. These results argue strongly that attempts at achieving local-regional tumor regression in previously treated patients by using intensive chemotherapy as an adjunct to subsequent local therapy be undertaken only by highly experienced therapists and in cancer treatment centers.

For decision making concerning the use of relatively well-tolerated chemotherapy regimens in previously untreated patients, it must be emphasized that although sufficiently high levels of tumor regression are achieved to allow evaluation of the usefulness of chemotherapy in tumors associated with a high incidence of local recurrences, sufficiently long follow-up of patients so treated has not been achieved to conclude whether the incidence of local-regional recurrences will be reduced by use of adjuvant chemotherapy. If fewer recurrences are observed after the conventional follow-up interval of 2 to 3 years, longer follow-up will be necessary to determine whether local recurrence will subsequently become manifest, suggesting that the adjuvant chemotherapy merely prolonged the interval to local recurrence. Such results would be important, not only because of this effect, but because they would raise the speculation whether a postoperative adjuvant chemotherapy regimen would reduce the incidence or further delay the development of local-regional recurrence.

Critical data concerning the effects of adjuvant chemotherapy prior to local therapy that are not yet available are the impact on distant metastases and second primaries. Theoretically, it is possible that immunologic functions and other host mechanisms important in the control of established tumors may be sufficiently depressed by the chemotherapy regimen or that the delay of local therapy associated with the administration of chemotherapy may lead to the establishment of micrometastases that would eventually result in greater numbers of clinical metastases after adjuvant therapy than would be obtained with treatment by local therapy alone. The impact of adjuvant chemotherapy on second primary tumors is a remote concern at this time, considering the low cure rates achieved in primary tumors with local therapies alone. Nonetheless, it is theoretically possible that adjuvant chemotherapy may lead to an increased incidence of second primaries if the regimens are immunosuppressive and influence the transformation of occult preneoplastic cells into foci of invasive cancer. On the other hand, effective regimens may eradicate these foci and reduce the incidence of second primaries.

The effect of adjuvant chemotherapy after local therapy is also not sufficiently tested to allow its use with predictable results in individual patients. In patients with advanced tumors, the greater impact is more likely to be in eradicating or delaying the growth of micrometastases. It is also possible that such regimens may increase the incidence and shorten the time to the appearance of not only distant metastases but also of local-regional recurrences. Furthermore, the results obtained may vary with the drugs used and depend on the effect of the drug on the residual tumor and the host-tumor defense mechanisms.

From the foregoing, it is apparent that conclusive data regarding the effects of adjuvant chemotherapy in head and neck squamous carcinoma must be derived before active drugs can be routinely used in the treatment of individual patients with sufficient reliability to predict the effects that may ensue, both immediate and long term, and both beneficial and possibly detrimental to the patient's status.

At present, a number of controlled clinical trials are in progress that attempt to define the effects of chemotherapy in combination with local therapy for these tumors (Table 29-11). The trials vary in design according to the precise information sought. The schemata for several current induction chemotherapy regimens are presented in Figures 29-1 and 29-2.

The trial being conducted by the National Cancer Institute (NCI) is an important model for adjuvant trials, since it evaluates the effect of adjuvant chemotherapy given before and after conventional therapy. A number of critical factors were considered in the design of this trial to ensure that the trial would yield interpretable results. These factors, however, would also be important in the design of trials with differing regimens and objectives.

A most important factor in the design of the NCI and similar adjuvant trials is the limitation of eligible tumor sites to those commonly encountered in head and neck cancer treatment centers and among those sites, limited eligibility to those tumors that can be easily staged and monitored clinically. Study of commonly encountered sites ensures relatively rapid patient accrual and completion of patient entry in the shortest possible time. Study of tumor sites that are easily staged and monitored ensures minimal variation in the assessment of the effects of therapy among the investigators participating in the trial.

The importance of the determination of the effects of the chemotherapy regimens on tumors arising from differing anatomic sites is derived from data of previous trials that show varying responses to chemother-

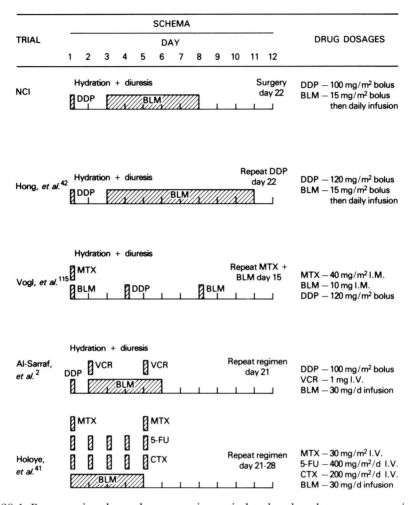

Fig. 29-1. Preoperative chemotherapy regimens in head and neck squamous carcinoma.

apy depending on individual tumor site. In the determination of end results, the variability in the effects of the drug regimen on tumors at individual sites is accounted for by initial stratification of patients by tumor site. Equally important are the differing results of treatment by TNM stage, and therefore, tumor stage represents another variable by which the patients are stratified. Because of the potential for an adverse effect of the drug regimen, ethical considerations dictate that only patients with tumor stages associated with low cure rates after local therapy are selected for study. However, only patients having clinically resectable tumors without distant metastases are entered, since the goal of the trial is to evaluate the effects

of chemotherapy as an adjuvant to local therapy in patients with potentially curable tumors. Other patient entry criteria that may affect end results and for which comparability among treatment groups must be ensured include nutritional status, activity or performance status, absence of associated serious diseases or compromise of function of central organs, and no prior or concomitant malignancy.

Imperative in the NCI and similar trials is that the conventional therapy be easily standardized and that the trials include a control group that receives conventional therapy only. Standardization of conventional therapy, both surgery and radiation therapy, is achieved by agreement of all par-

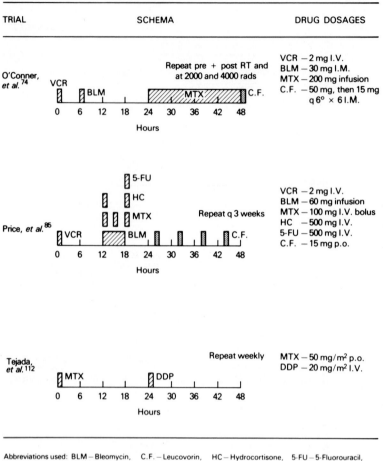

TRIAL	SCHEMA	DRUG DOSAGES

Fig. 29-2. Kinetically based adjuvant chemotherapy regimens.

ticipating investigators to a detailed treatment routine. In a further attempt to achieve uniformity in treatment among participating institutions, participation is limited to as few investigators as is consistent with a reasonable rate of patient accrual and to centers in which patients with eligible tumors are treated at a frequency sufficient to ensure completion of patient entry in a predetermined interval of time.

The drug regimen in such trials should be tested in pilot studies to determine the associated toxicity. Such preliminary investigations should include evaluation of the overall toxicity of the drug regimen in combination with the local therapy regimen. Regimens with excessive toxicity should not

be considered in these initial trials because of their limited usefulness. In second generation protocols, more intensive and toxic regimens that are initially evaluated in major treatment centers may be considered for multi-institutional trials in patients with advanced tumors if the current trials show a significant benefit of adjuvant chemotherapy.

Chemotherapy for Head and Neck Squamous Carcinoma: A Summary

A large number of chemotherapeutic agents with differing mechanisms of action induce significant regressions of head and neck squamous carcinomas. Extensive trials with methotrexate, bleomycin, and more recently cis-platinum delineate these as the most active drugs tested. For palliation of incurable, previously untreated tumors and for treatment of metastases in patients who have not previously received chemotherapy, low dose single drug regimens that have minimal toxicity and can be administered on an outpatient basis appear to be as effective as more intensive and multidrug regimens. Paralleling the results with treatment of other tumors by chemotherapy, the duration of tumor regression is related to the extent of regression achieved, i.e., head and neck tumors that regress completely are associated with longer disease-free intervals than tumors that only regress partially. For palliation of patients with previously treated carcinomas, complete tumor regressions are infrequently achieved with single drug regimens. In several trials, multidrug regimens, which in some instances are associated with notable toxicity, appear to have achieved greater complete response rates and longer response durations than achieved with single drug regimens. Additional studies are needed to delineate the patient populations in which the morbidity of high dose multidrug regimens would be justified by the potential for clinical benefit.

The effects of chemotherapy as an adjuvant with local therapy have been most extensively studied in patients receiving radiation therapy. Single drug adjuvant regimens offered no advantage over radiation therapy alone, but several multidrug adjuvant regimens increased the response durations over those achieved with radiation therapy alone. Short-term high dose regimens associated with significant rates of partial and complete tumor regression (within 1 to 3 weeks) have been administered prior to surgery and radiation therapy without significantly increasing the morbidity associated with local therapy. However, randomized trials designed to determine the clinical effects of the adjuvant chemotherapy on potentially curable tumors have not been in progress sufficiently long to ascertain the ultimate effects of these adjuvant regimens.

At this time, it is not known whether the incidence of local and regional recurrences, the tumor-free interval, or the incidence of distant metastases are increased or decreased by adjuvant chemotherapy, regardless of whether the drugs are administered before, after, or both before and after local therapy.

THE CHEMOTHERAPY OF SALIVARY GLAND MALIGNANCIES

The poor prognosis associated with recurrent or disseminated salivary gland malignancy has emphasized the need for more effective palliative treatment regimens and for the development of effective adjuvant therapies using radiation or chemotherapy in the primary treatment of advanced localized tumors. Cancers of salivary gland origin include a variety of histologic tumor types that are associated with differing biologic behavior and clinical outcome after primary treatment. Five-year survival rates vary from 80 percent for mucoepidermoid carcinomas to 40 percent for squamous cell carcinomas.[73] Tumor recurrence after primary treatment occurs in 40 to 50 percent of patients. These recurrences are frequently multiple with distant metastases occurring in 20 to 40 percent of the patients.[47, 87, 103, 104] In the majority of patients with tumor recurrence, survival is short and surgery or radiotherapy ineffective.

Recently, adjuvant radiotherapy has been used after the primary surgical treatment of selected advanced cancers having tumor characteristics that are associated with high recurrence rates. However, the potential role of chemotherapy in the management of these patients or in the treatment of tumor recurrences and distant metastases is not clear. This lack of information on the potential benefit of chemotherapy is partially due to the relative rarity of these neoplasms, the small numbers of patients with recurrent tumors treated with chemotherapy, and the conflicting reports of single drug efficacy. The limited experiences with single drug or combination chemotherapy have not allowed identification of consistently active regimens for patients with advanced salivary gland carcinoma. In addition, the interpretation of existing chemotherapy data is limited further by the variety of histologic tumor types arising from major and minor salivary glands.

The most extensive experience with chemotherapy for salivary gland malignancy was reported by Rentschler and associates in which 36 evaluable patients received one or more of 30 different drugs.[90] The number of adequate trials for any single drug or combination was insufficient for conclusions to be drawn, but activity was suggested for Adriamycin particularly in metastatic adenoid cystic carcinoma. Other investigators have suggested that alkylating agents and antimetabolites may also be effective drugs.[30,45,68]

With the limited data available, it is difficult to recommend guidelines for use of chemotherapy in patients with recurrent salivary gland malignancy. A number of drugs are probably active. Drug selection should be guided by tumor histology and depend on whether the tumor is predominantly of epithelial or glandular origin. Agents known to be effective against tumors of a particular cell type would be logical primary choices. Combination regimens incorporating Adriamycin should be considered in tumors of mixed cell type or in adenoid cystic carcinomas. Combinations proven effective for cancers of other organs such as lung, in which a variety of histologic tumor types are seen, would be reasonable choices for initial trials in salivary gland malignancy.

It is obvious that the data needed to better define the role of chemotherapy can only be achieved through collaborative studies in which a reasonable number of patients with these relatively rare tumors can be treated and evaluated in a uniform manner. The future development of adjuvant regimens for localized salivary gland carcinomas will depend on the data derived from these studies. It is reasonable to project that the design of adjuvant regimens will build on previously identified active regimens and will base patient selection on tumor histology, the defined patterns of local extension, and the frequency and site of metastases.

THE IMMUNOTHERAPY OF HEAD AND NECK SQUAMOUS CARCINOMA

Considerable evidence has emerged indicating the existence of an immunologic response to neoplasia in man. Furthermore, the demonstrations of correlations among immune reactivity, tumor extent, and prognosis in cancer patients suggest that the administration of agents that modify host immunity by enhancing or restoring immune reactivity may result in objective benefit to the patient in terms of increased cure rate, prolonged survival, or increased disease-free interval. Thus far, however, the clinical applicability of this approach has been limited despite identification of a large number of substances capable of affecting immune reactivity and the derivation of data defining some of the immunologic mechanisms operative in animal tumor systems. The demonstration of effective immunotherapy in man has been hampered by a limited understanding of (1) the in vivo effects of the agents utilized, (2) the complexity of the cellular interactions involved, (3) the parameters necessary to monitor the results of therapy, and (4) the critical relationship between host tumor burden and immune reactivity. It is not surprising that at present the current results of trials that might substantiate the theoretic basis for immunotherapy in man are inconclusive.

Immunotherapy can be considered as the administration of any agent or treatment which stimulates, modifies, or restores in a specific or nonspecific fashion, host immune reactivity and results in the regression or prophylaxis of tumors. This broad definition encompasses all forms of conventional cytoreductive therapy, since the ablation of a tumor mass alone is known to produce immunologic reverberations in the host. However, for the purposes of conciseness, this discussion will be limited to only those chemical and biologic agents capable of affecting systemic immune reactivity that have been used clinically as adjuvants to conventional therapy in patients with head and neck cancer.

The in Vitro and in Vivo Effects of Immunotherapeutic Agents

The traditional classification of immunotherapeutic agents used in systemic approaches to immunotherapy is based on their postulated in vivo effects. The agents are arbitrarily divided into two categories: those that actively increase host immune reactivity specifically through vaccination with tumor cells or cell extracts or nonspecifically through administration of agents having this effect, such as bacterial organisms or their products, and those that passively augment immune reactivity. Passive immunotherapy consists of the administration or removal of serum containing either tumor specific antibodies or antigen-antibody complexes. As the number and variety of agents that modify immune reactivity increases, many do not clearly fit into either of these categories. An ancillary classification of practical value in the clinical utilization of these agents discriminates between agents, such as bacille Calmette-Guerin (BCG) and Cornybacterium parvum, that primarily stimulate relatively intact immune mechanisms and those that act to reconstitute impaired or deficient immunologic function. The latter category includes agents such as levamisole, transfer factor, and thymus extracts. As our knowledge of the mechanism of action of newer agents expands, this functional classification may be expanded to include natural and synthetic immune effectors or mediators, agents that act by changing the antigenicity of tumor cells, agents that affect malignant transformation or the maturation of tumor cells, and agents that may increase the capacity of the host to tolerate immunotoxic modalities of cancer treatment.

Of the large number of trials of immunotherapy in man that have been completed, few have been prospective randomized studies and few have been conducted in patients with head and neck cancer. The majority of immunotherapy trials in head and neck cancer have utilized nonspecific immunostimulants, such as BCG or C parvum, following surgery or radiotherapy. Some have used immunorestorative agents such as levamisole or thymosin either alone or combined with BCG. The results of these trials are summarized in Tables 29-12 and 29-13 and discussed in the following sections.

BACILLE CALMETTE-GUERIN

Nonspecific immune stimulation with BCG has been extensively investigated with variable results both in patients with nonsquamous malignancies and in patients with squamous carcinoma of the head and neck. The results of Mathe's initial clinical trials of BCG immunotherapy suggested that prolongation of the disease-free interval could be achieved with BCG immunotherapy in children with acute lymphocytic leukemia.[67] Encouraging results have been reported subsequently in studies of patients with ovarian cancer[1] and nodular lymphoma.[46] Although the systemic mode of action of BCG is unclear, it appears to be effective as a local immunotherapeutic agent when injected into skin nodules of immunologically competent patients with malignant melanoma[69] or intrapleurally following resection of stage I lung carcinoma.[64] The earliest trial with BCG in patients with head and neck squamous carcinoma reported a significant increase in tumor response rates to methotrexate when BCG and INH were added to the treatment regimen.[30] These provocative results, however, have not been reproducible. Numerous randomized trials of BCG as an adjuvant to chemotherapy in patients with unresectable or recurrent tumors[12, 79] and to chemotherapy combined

TABLE 29-12. RANDOMIZED TRIALS OF ADJUVANT IMMUNOSTIMULANTS IN PATIENTS WITH HEAD AND NECK SQUAMOUS CARCINOMA

Investigator	Evaluable Patients (stage)	Agents and Schedule (Immunotherapy arm)	Results of Immunotherapy Immunologic	Clinical
Taylor et al.[110]	39 (II–IV)	MTX (240 mg/m² + C.F.) × 3 pre-surg. +/or RT then MTX (60 mg/m²) q 3 mos. + BCG (Tice) q 2 weeks × 6, then monthly × 1 yr.	No signif. inc. in skin tests, PHA, % T cells, no correlation with prognosis.	No difference in recurrence rates. Follow-up 1 yr.
Cunningham et al.[26]	22 (III–IV)	After RT/surg., MTX (40 mg/m²) × 6 then monthly × 1 yr + BCG (Tice) and neuriminidase treated tumor cells monthly, some patients.	No improvement in DNCB, PHA or % T cells.	5/11 recurred on MTX alone. 2/11 recurred on immunotherapy, length follow-up not stated.
Richman et al.[93]	34 (recurrent)	BACON q 8 wks + BCG (Pasteur) weekly between chemotherapy.	Inc. positive skin tests (controls not tested).	Signif. inc. survival (13.5 wks vs. 30.5 wks). No difference in response rates or duration response.
Buechler et al.[12]	23 (recurrent)	HDMTX (15 mg/kg + C.F.) q 3 weeks + BCG (Tice) day 8 + 15 each cycle.	No correlation of initial skin tests with tumor response.	No difference in response rate, median duration response, or survival.
Papac et al.[79]	35 (inoperable)	MTX (0.8 mg/kg) biweekly + BCG (Tice) q 3 mos.	No difference in PPD, Candida, mumps skin tests. Inc. % T cells in responders.	No difference in response rate, duration or survival. Significant toxicity.
Terz[113]	99 (I–IV oral cavity)	C parvum intralesional pre-op then subq. monthly × 1 yr, then bimonthly.	Inc. monocyte chemotaxis.	No difference in recurrence or survival (3 mos. minimum follow-up). Suggested decreased recurrence in immuno. group having negative nodes.

TABLE 29-12. CONTINUED

Investigator	Evaluable Patients (stage)	Agents and Schedule (Immunotherapy arm)	Results of Immunotherapy	
			Immunologic	Clinical
Amiel et al.[5]	127 (I–IV)	BCG (Pasteur) weekly × 1 yr. after curative surg. + / or RT.	Not reported.	Inc. disease-free interval and survival but not statistically significant.
Szpirglas et al.[108]	95 (I–IV oral cavity)	C parvum q 2 wks × 2 yrs vs. MTX (400 mg) monthly, after surg. + / or RT vs. surg. + / or RT alone.	Not reported.	Signif. inc. survival for Stage I–II with either chemo. or immuno. No difference overall survival by stage or adjuvant therapy

with surgery or radiation therapy in those with potentially curable tumors[26, 110] have failed to demonstrate a significant clinical benefit for this form of immunotherapy. Richman and associates, however, reported that BCG combined with intensive chemotherapy in patients with recurrent tumors resulted in a significantly increased survival rate compared with chemotherapy alone, although no differences in tumor response rates or response duration were noted among the treatment groups.[93] A trial in which BCG was administered weekly following curative local therapy suggested that BCG immunotherapy was associated with increased disease-free interval and survival compared with controls, but the differences were not statistically significant.[5]

There have been major problems with the interpretation of data from clinical trials of BCG immunotherapy. These trials used a variety of crude products of differing viability and dosages prepared from a variety of bacterial strains with each preparation differing in biologic and immunologic characteristics. Furthermore, the results from animal investigations suggested that the effect of BCG may vary depending on tumor burden. In these studies, BCG was generally ineffective when administered systemically after a tumor had been established but was effective prophylactically and occasionally when given in conjunction with chemotherapy. However, enhanced tumor growth has also been reported with BCG in animal models in which minimal tumor challenge was employed.[66]

In man, the effects of BCG immunotherapy on immune reactivity have not been correlated with the clinical effects of the agent. BCG appears to stimulate bone marrow stem cells and the reticuloendothelial system. It increases lymphocyte cytotoxicity in vitro and increases the delayed hypersensitivity reaction to some antigens. Of significant importance are observations suggesting that immunocompetence may be a prerequisite to effective immunostimulation with BCG. Therefore, if BCG therapy is to be effective in patients with head and neck carcinoma, the impaired immune reactivity associated with advanced tumors may require correction prior to BCG immunotherapy.

CORNYBACTERIUM PARVUM

Cornybacterium parvum is an immunostimulatory vaccine consisting of phenol-killed bacteria. Like BCG, it produces a variety

TABLE 29-13. RANDOMIZED TRIALS OF ADJUVANT IMMUNORESTORATIVE AGENTS IN PATIENTS WITH HEAD AND NECK SQUAMOUS CARCINOMA

Investigator	Evaluable Patients (stage)	Agents and Schedule (Immunotherapy arm)	Results of Immunotherapy	
			Immunologic	Clinical
Olivari et al.[76]	134 (I–IV)	Levamisole (150 mg/day × 3) biweekly after surg. +/ or RT, until relapse.	Signif. inc. DNCB after local therapy both groups.	No overall difference in recurrence or survival at 36 mos.
			Signif. inc. recall skin tests in immunotherapy group.	Signif. inc. recurrences in Stages I + II.
				Suggested benefit for immunotherapy in Stage IV.
Olkowski et al.[78]	57 (II–IV)	BCG (Tice) q 2 wks × 4 then monthly × 1 yr + levamisole (150 mg) twice a week after RT.	Delayed recovery of % T cells, B cells and PHA reactivity after RT. No difference in recall skin tests.	Not reported.
Wanebo et al.[117]	53 (I–IV)	Levamisole (150 mg × 3) biweekly × 2 yrs after surg. +/ or RT.	No correlation of initial DNCB tests with clinical results either group.	Suggested inc. disease free interval (P<.06).
			No signif. change in lymphocyte levels, DNCB or PHA reactivity.	Signif. decreased recurrence in Stage II oral cavity (P<.01).
				Follow up<1 yr most patients.
Wara et al.[120]	82 (not stated)	Thymosin Fr. V (60 mg/ m² subq.) × 10 then twice weekly during and after RT, for 1 yr.	No difference in total T cells, B cells, PHA reactivity between groups.	No difference in disease-free interval, follow-up<1 yr.
			? inc. MLC reactivity.	

of immunopotentiating effects on macrophages, the reticuloendothelial system, and lymphocytes. Studies in animal tumor models indicate that C parvum can produce not only immune stimulation but also suppression of some immune functions. These observations suggest that the design of rational clinical trials using C parvum may depend on a better understanding of the dual effects of this agent on immune function.

A few randomized trials of C parvum in patients with head and neck cancer have been completed. A preliminary report of C parvum administered intralesionally prior to surgery and then subcutaneously monthly following surgery in patients with oral cavity tumors suggested a decreased recurrence rate in patients without lymph nodal metastases who received C parvum.[113] No differences were reported in the overall recurrence rate or survival although the follow-up period in this trial was brief. A similar trial in which patients with oral cavity tumors were randomized to receive either C parvum therapy, combination chemotherapy with methotrexate-bleomycin, or observation following definitive surgery or radiotherapy reported significantly increased survival in surgically treated patients with stage I or II tumors who received either C parvum or chemotherapy compared with controls.[108] In this study there were no overall differences in recurrence or survival rates when all patients were considered. In fact, patients with advanced tumors who were treated with surgery and radiation therapy had earlier and more frequent recurrences with either adjuvant treatment compared with controls. The results of these two studies could be interpreted as supporting the concept that immune competence is necessary for C parvum immunostimulation to be effective, since the only patients to apparently benefit from the immunotherapy were those with limited disease and therefore relatively intact immune reactivity.

Levamisole

Levamisole is an antihelminthic imidazole that has immune reconstituting activity believed to be due to biochemical properties similar to the thymic hormone, thymopoietin.[36] Levamisole may act by a variety of chemical mechanisms, e.g., by altering lymphocyte cyclic nucleotide levels, altering haptene binding for the induction of delayed hypersensitivity, or influencing the expression of thymocyte antigens on precursor cells. Observations in a number of animal systems indicate that levamisole is capable of enhancing immune reactivity only when immunity is impaired.

Clinical trials of levamisole in patients with breast and lung cancers show encouraging preliminary results.[4, 95] The results of the few randomized trials of levamisole immunotherapy in patients with head and neck squamous carcinoma, however, have been conflicting. The preliminary findings in a small trial by Wanebo and associates suggested that levamisole administered biweekly following surgery and/or radiation therapy resulted in a significant decrease in recurrences in patients with stage II oral cavity tumors. The results also suggested an overall increase in disease-free interval.[117] However, in a larger controlled trial in which the same levamisole schedule was used, significantly increased recurrences were reported for patients with stage I and II tumors who received levamisole compared with those receiving placebo.[76] In this trial, benefit from immune reconstitution was suggested only for those patients with stage IV tumors. In neither of these trials was clinical benefit from levamisole immunotherapy successfully correlated with improvements in in vivo or in vitro parameters of immune reactivity.

Thymic Hormones

Increasing interest in the role of the thymus in human immunocompetence and the regulation of the immune system followed the initial observations of the capacity of thymic extracts to restore immunocompetence in neonatally thymectomized mice. A number of thymic extracts with immunologic activity have been isolated by various investigators; however, the best characterized and most extensively studied clinically is thymosin fraction V. The effect of the thymic hormones on the immune response involves activities that promote lymphocyte maturation and the induction and functional expression of specific types of lymphocytes such as killer, helper, and suppressor cells. Thymosin fraction V has been shown to improve in vivo and in vitro immune reactivity in children with thymic-dependent immunodeficiency diseases.[118] Furthermore, in vitro improvements in cellular immunity have been correlated with in vivo improvements when thymosin was used clinically in both immunodeficiency diseases[119] and lung cancer.[60]

The preliminary results, thus far, of a single randomized clinical trial of thymosin fraction V in patients with cancer of the head and neck does not indicate a potential benefit of thymosin immunotherapy administration during and following radiation therapy.[120] Of potential importance in the interpretation of these results, however, is the fact that the immune reactivity of these patients did not significantly differ from normal subjects by the immunologic parameters measured. This may have clinical relevance, since previous studies of the in vitro and in vivo effects of thymosin suggest that immune enhancement is achieved only when immune reactivity is impaired.[60, 98] Furthermore, recent data from our laboratory on the effects of thymosin on leucocyte migration inhibition and T cell levels in normal subjects and patients with head and neck cancer suggest that thymosin may have a deleterious effect in patients with normal levels of these immune parameters.[51, 124] Thus, the immune modulatory role of the thymic hormones in restoring to normal levels either deficient or enhanced immune reactivity may be a critical factor in the interpretation and design of clinical trials in which immunorestorative agents are used.

OTHER AGENTS

A number of other immunotherapeutic agents are being studied in both animal tumor models and cancer patients but have not been utilized for trials in patients with cancer of the head and neck. These agents include the interferons, interferon inducers such as poly I:C and pyran copolymer, the lymphokines, tumor antigens, antitumor antibodies, and various chemical agents such as glucan, muramyl dipeptide, and isoprinosine. The rational and effective clinical utilization of the growing list of immunotherapeutic agents will depend on a better understanding of their mechanisms of action and the development of improved assays with which to monitor their effects,

predict response, and hopefully identify the population of patients who may be likely to benefit from such therapy.

Immune Reactivity and the Design of Immunotherapy Trials

The theoretic basis for immunotherapy in patients with squamous carcinoma of the head and neck is derived from the assumption that an immunologic response to neoplasia is important in tumor control and that correlations exist among host immunocompetence and the results of conventional therapy. These assumptions suggest several factors that may influence the results and design of immunotherapy trials. These factors include the assessment of the immune status of patients, the relationship of immune competence to tumor extent, and the effects of conventional therapy on the immune response.

In vitro studies in well-defined animal tumor systems have implicated a variety of immunologic mechanisms that appear to be important in host antitumor defense. A partial listing of these would include factors such as complement-dependent cytotoxic antibody, specific and nonspecific humoral factors (blocking factors, antigen-antibody complexes, lymphokines), and cytotoxic cell-mediated mechanisms attributed to T cells, killer cells, macrophages and possibly other effector and regulatory cell subpopulations of lymphocyte and monocyte lineage. Some of these mechanisms may also participate inappropriately by augmentation or induction of tumor tolerance. Despite increasingly sophisticated investigations, the in vivo mechanisms of effective tumor immunity and the mechanisms of failure in host defense are not well understood. Thus, the clinical effects of agents that modify these mechanisms in vitro remain largely speculative and the design of previous immunotherapy trials largely empirical.

A critical corollary to the theoretic basis of immunotherapy is that even in well-defined animal models, a clinically relevant approach to immunotherapy has been successful only for tumor prophylaxis or the eradication of small tumor burdens that would normally be undetectable in humans. These observations emphasize the importance of determining parameters of immune reactivity that accurately indicate the immune status of patients undergoing conventional therapy and predict clinical benefit from adjuvant immune modulation. Unfortunately, the currently utilized measures of immune reactivity in humans have not been sufficiently precise to allow the use of these parameters as indicators of therapeutic response or prognosis in *individual* patients. Despite this, a large amount of information is available suggesting a relationship among immune reactivity, tumor extent, the effects of conventional therapy, and prognosis.

One of the most consistent and potentially important observations made in patients with cancer of the head and neck is the assocation of impaired immune reactivity with advanced tumor extent. These observations, in which a variety of in vivo and in vitro assays were used, indicate that a major portion of the immunologic defect is due to local tumor burden, rather than regional lymph node or disseminated metastases.[22, 77, 117] Therefore, effective combinations of conventional and immune therapy for patients with head and neck squamous cancer may differ greatly from those employed for patients with other histologic types of tumors in whom immune reactivity is impaired only with tumor dissemination.[17] Furthermore, patients free of disease for sufficiently long intervals after treatment to be considered cured showed deficits in cellular immunity similar to untreated patients. These findings were in contrast to the results of studies in patients cured of tumors of other histologies in which cellular immunity did not differ from normals.[83, 114]

This suggests that control of the primary tumor and regional metastases may not be sufficient to correct the immunologic impairment in selected patients with ad-vanced disease. As discussed previously, consideration of the status of the immune system following conventional therapy may be as critical as initial tumor extent in the design of effective immunotherapy regimens. The relationship of immune reactivity with tumor extent is therefore complicated by the immunosuppressive nature of most, if not all, conventional therapeutic modalities. The immune depressive effects of surgery, radiation therapy, and chemotherapy are well documented. Following operative procedures under general anesthesia for a variety of benign and malignant conditions, patients showed inhibition of skin test responses to dinitrochlorobenzene (DNCB) and recall skin-test antigens, decreased levels of circulating T cells, diminished lymphocyte responsiveness to phytohemagglutinin (PHA), and loss of leucocyte migration inhibition in response to specific antigens.[17] Radiation therapy has been associated with significant decreases in T and B cell numbers and lymphocyte reactivity to mitogens, and these effects on cellular immunity may be long-lasting. Intermittent chemotherapy has been associated with profound transient immunosuppression and posttreatment rebound in immune parameters in patients whose tumors responded to therapy. Repeated treatment, however, may be associated with a cumulative immunosuppressive effect. Conversely, conventional treatment modalities may increase immunologic reactivity by reducing tumor burden thus eliminating a source of tumor antigen and immune complexes, and facilitating improved patient nutrition by reducing the size of obstructive lesions in the upper alimentary passage.

Thus, in the design of immunotherapy trials, considerations must be given not only to antecedent immune reactivity, which may be a reflection of tumor extent, but also to the timing, sequence, and long-term effects of immunosuppressive treatment modalities. The results of studies in which in vivo parameters of immune reactivity such as DNCB and recall antigen skin testing correlated with prognosis in patients with localized head and neck carcinomas[16, 65, 107, 116] suggest that clinical benefit would be derived by the administration of agents that correct or prevent the impaired immunity associated with advanced tumor extent and conventional therapy. The available data suggest that patients with stage I and II tumors that are associated with relatively normal levels of immune reactivity and high rates of local-regional tumor control with radiation or surgery may benefit from immune reconstitution during immunosuppressive therapy and immune stimulation following potentially curative therapy. Patients with advanced tumors that have associated impairments in immune reactivity and low cure rates would presumably benefit from immune reconstitution during and following conventional therapy. If such regimens restore immune competence, subsequent administration of immune stimulatory agents may be of benefit.

In summary, the future holds promise for the development of improved quantitative and qualitative indicators of immune reactivity, tumor persistence, and tumor recurrence that would allow timely and specific therapeutic intervention. Further investigation of the effects of conventional and immune therapy on immunologic mechanisms and the function of lymphocyte subpopulations may provide the insight necessary for the rational integration of these modalities for the treatment of individual patients. At the present time, however, carefully controlled clinical trials are needed to test the current concepts of immunotherapy and to identify those parameters and clinical situations that may correlate with benefit from these approaches.

REFERENCES

1. Alberts, D. S. 1977. Adjuvant immunotherapy with BCG of advanced ovarian cancer: A preliminary report. In Salmon, S. E., and Jones, S. E. Eds.: Adjuvant Therapy of Cancer. Elsevier/North-Holland Biomedical Press, Amsterdam, 327.

2. Al-Sarraf, M., Amer, M. H., Vaishampayan, G., Loh, J., and Weaver, A. 1979. A multidisciplinary therapeutic approach for advanced previously untreated epidermoid cancer of the head and neck: Preliminary report. International Journal of Radiation Oncology, Biology, Physics, 5: 1421.

3. Amer, M., Izbicki, R., Vaitkevicius, V. K., and Al-Sarraf, M. 1978. Combination of high dose cis-platinum, Oncovin and bleomycin in treatment of patients with advanced head and neck cancer. Proceedings of the American Society of Clinical Oncology, 19: 312.

4. Amery, W. K. 1978. Final results of a multicenter placebo-controlled levamisole study of resectable lung cancer. Cancer Treatment Reports, 62: 1677.

5. Amiel, J. L., Sancho-Garnier, H., Vandenbrouck, C., Eschwege, F., Droz, J. P., Schwaab, G., Wibault, P., Stromboni, M., and Rey, A. 1979. First results of a randomized trial on immunotherapy of head and neck tumors. Recent Results in Cancer Research, 68: 318.

6. Auersperg, M., Furlan, L., Marolt, F., and Jereb, B. 1978. Intra-arterial chemotherapy and radiotherapy in locally advanced cancer of the oral cavity and oropharynx. International Journal of Radiation Oncology, Biology, Physics, 4: 273.

7. Bagshaw, M. A., and Doggett, R. L. S. 1969. A clinical study of chemical radiosensitization. Frontiers of Radiation Therapy and Oncology, 4: 164.

8. Baker, L., and Al-Sarraf, M. 1979. A comparative trial of cis-platinum, Oncovin, and bleomycin vs. methotrexate in patients with advanced epidermoid carcinoma of the head and neck. Proceedings of the American Association for Cancer Research, 20: 817.

9. Berger, D. S., and Fletcher, G. H. 1971. Distant metastases following local control of squamous cell carcinoma of the nasopharynx, tonsillar fossa, and base of the tongue. Radiology, 100: 141.

10. Bertino, J. R., Mosher, M. B., and DeConti, R. C. 1973. Chemotherapy of cancer of the head and neck. Cancer, 31: 1141.

11. Bertino, J. R., Boston, B., and Capizzi, R. L. 1975. The role of chemotherapy in the management of cancer of the head and neck: A review. Cancer, 36: 752.

12. Beuchler, M., Mukherji, B., Chasin, W., and Nathanson, L. 1979. High dose methotrexate with and without BCG therapy in advanced head and neck malignancy. Cancer, 43: 1095.

13. Bonadonna, G., Tancini, G., and Bajetta, E. 1976. Controlled studies with bleomycin in solid tumors and lymphomas. Progress in Biochemical Pharmacology, 11: 172.

14. Bonadonna, G., Valagussa, P., Ross, A., Zucali, R., Tancini, G., Bajetta, E., Brambilla, C., and Delena, H. 1978. Are surgical adjuvant trials altering the course of breast cancer? Seminars in Oncology, 5: 450.

15. Bonomi, P. D., Slayton, R. E., and Wolter, J. 1978. Phase II trial of adriamycin and cis-dichlorodiammineplatinum (II) in squamous cell, ovarian and testicular carcinomas. Cancer Treatment Reports, 62: 1211.

16. Bosworth, J. L., Thaler, S., and Ghossein, N. A. 1976. Delayed hypersensitivity and local control of patients treated by radiotherapy for head and neck cancer. American Journal of Surgery, 132: 46.

17. Browder, J. P., and Chretien, P. B. 1977. Immune reactivity in head and neck squamous carcinoma and relevance to the design of immunotherapy trials. Seminars in Oncology, 4: 431.

18. Byers, R. M., Krueger, W. W. O., and Saxton, J. 1979. Use of surgery and postoperative radiation in the treatment of advanced squamous cell carcinoma of the pyriform sinus. American Journal of Surgery, 138: 597.

19. Cachin, Y., Jortay, A., Sancho, H., Eschwege, F., Madelain, M., Desaulty, A., and Gerard, P. 1977. Preliminary results of a randomized E.O.R.T.C. study comparing radiotherapy and concomitant bleomycin to radiotherapy alone in epidermoid carcinomas of the oropharynx. European Journal of Cancer, 13: 1389.

20. Carradonna, R., Paladine, W., Goldstein, J., Ruckdeschel, J., Hillinger, S., and Horton, J. 1978. Combination chemotherapy with high dose cis-diamminedichloroplatinum (II), methotrexate and bleomycin for epidermoid carcinoma of the head and neck. Proceedings of the American Society of Clinical Oncology, 19: 401.

21. Carter, S. K. 1977. The chemotherapy of head and neck cancer. 1977. Seminars in Oncology, 4: 413.

22. Catalona, W. J., Sample, W. F., and Chretien, P. B. 1973. Lymphocyte reactivity in cancer patients: Correlations with tumor histology and clinical stage. Cancer, 31: 65.

23. Clifford, P., O'Connor, A. D., Durden-Smith, J., Hollis, B. A., and Dalley, V. M. 1978. Synchronous multiple drug chemotherapy and radiotherapy for advanced (stage III and IV) squamous carcinoma of the head and neck. Antibiotics and Chemotherapy, 24: 60.

24. Condit, P. T. 1968. Treatment of carcinoma with radiation therapy and methotrexate. Missouri Medicine, 65: 832.

25. Cortes, E. P., Amin, V. C., Attie, J., Eisenbud, L., Khafif, R., Wolk, D., Aral, I., Sciubba, J., and Akbiyik, N. 1979. Combination of low dose bleomycin followed by cyclophosphamide, methotrexate and 5-fluorouracil for advanced head and neck cancer. Proceedings of the American Association for Cancer Research, 20: 259.

26. Cunningham, T. J., Antemann, R., Paonessa, D., Sponzo, R. W., and Steiner, D. 1976. Adjuvant immuno and/or chemotherapy with neuraminidase-treated autogenous tumor vaccine and bacillus Calmette-Guerin for head and neck cancers. Annals of the New York Academy of Sciences, 277: 339.

27. DeConti, R. C., and Schoenfeld, D. 1980. A randomized prospective comparison of intermittant methotrexate, methotrexate with leucovorin and methotrexate combination in head and neck cancer. An Eastern Cooperative Oncology Group Study. (personal communication).

28. Demard, F., Colonna d'Astria, J., Jausseran, M., Vallicioni, J., Gaillot, M., and Schneider, M. 1978. Intraarterial sequential chemotherapy in head and neck tumors. Meeting abstract, 4th Annual Meeting of the Medical Oncology Society, Nice, France.

29. Desprez, J. D., Kiehn, C. L., Sciotto, C., and Ramirez-Gonzales, M. 1970. Response of oral carcinoma to preoperative methotrexate infusion therapy. American Journal of Surgery, 120: 461.

30. Donaldson, R. C. 1973. Chemoimmunotherapy for cancer of the head and neck. American Journal of Surgery, 126: 507.

31. Donegan, W. L., and Harris, P. 1976. Regional chemotherapy with combined drugs in cancer of the head and neck. Cancer, 38: 1479.

32. Durkin, W. J., Pugh, R. P., Jacobs, E., Sadoff, L., Pajak, T., and Bateman, J. R. 1976. Bleomycin therapy of responsive solid tumors. Oncology, 33: 260.

33. Elias, E. G., Chretien, P. B., Monnard, E., Khan, T., Bouchelle, W. H., Wiernik, P. H., Lipson, S. D., Hande, K. R., and Zentai, T. 1979. Chemotherapy prior to local therapy

in advanced squamous cell carcinoma of the head and neck. Cancer, 43:   1025.

34. Freckman, H. A. 1972. Results in 169 patients with cancer of the head and neck treated by intra-arterial infusion therapy. American Journal of Surgery, 124:   501.

35. Glick, J. H., Fazekas, J. T., Davis, L. W., Rominger, J. C., Breen, F. A., and Brodovsky, H. S. 1979. Combination chemotherapy-radiotherapy for advanced inoperable head and neck cancer. Cancer Clinical Trials, 2:   129.

36. Goldstein, G. 1978. Mode of action of levamisole. Journal of Rheumatology, 5:   143.

37. Gollin, F. F., Ansfield, F. J., Brandenburg, J. H., Ramirez, G., and Vermund, H. 1972. Combined therapy in advanced head and neck cancer: A randomized study. American Journal of Roentgenology, Radium Therapy and Nuclear Medicine, 114:   83.

38. Haas, C. D., Coltman, C. A., Gottlieb, J. A., Haut, A., Luce, J. K., Talley, R. W., Samal, B., Wilson, H. E., and Hoogstraten, B. 1976. Phase II evaluation of bleomycin. A Southwest Oncology Group Study. Cancer, 38:   8.

39. Halnan, K. E., Bleehan, N. M., Brewin, T. B., Deeley, T. J., Harrison, D. F. N., Howland, C., Kunkler, P. B., Ritchie, G. L., Wiltshaw, E., and Todd, J. D. H. 1972. Early clinical experience with bleomycin in the United Kingdom in series of 105 patients. British Medical Journal, 4:   635.

40. Heyn, R. M., Holland, R., Newton, W. A., Tefft, M., Breslow, N., and Hartman, J. R. 1974. The role of combined chemotherapy in the treatment of rhabdomyosarcoma in children. Cancer, 34:   2128.

41. Holoye, P. Y., Byers, R. M., Gard, D. A., Geopfert, H., Guillamondegui, O. M., and Jesse, R. H. 1978. Combination chemotherapy of head and neck cancer. Cancer, 42:   1661.

42. Hong, W. K., Shapshay, S., Bhutani, R., Craft, M. L., Ucmakli, A., Yamaguchi, K. T., Vaugn, C. W., and Strong, M. S. 1979. Induction chemotherapy in advanced squamous head and neck carcinoma with high-dose cis-platinum and bleomycin infusion. Cancer, 44:   19.

43. Hussey, D. H., and Abrams, J. D. 1975. Combined therapy in advanced head and neck cancer: Hydroxyurea and radiotherapy. Progress in Clinical Cancer, 6:   79.

44. Jacobs, C., Bertino, J. R., Goffinet, D. R., Fee, W. E., and Goode, R. L. 1978. Cis-platinum chemotherapy in head and neck cancers. Journal for Oto-Rhino-Laryngology and its Borderlands, 86:   780.

45. Johnson, R. O., Lange, R. D., Kiskin, W. A., and Curreri, A. R. 1964. Infusion of 5-fluorouracil in cylindroma treatment. Archives of Otolaryngology, 79:   625.

46. Jones, S. E., Salmon, S. E., and Fisher, R. Adjuvant immunotherapy with BCG in non-Hodgkins lymphoma: A Southwest Oncology Group controlled clinical trial. In: Adjuvant Therapy of Cancer, (in press).

47. Kagan, A. R., Nussbaum, H., Handler, S., Shapiro, R., Gilbert, H. A., Jacobs, M., Miles, J. W., Chan, P. Y. M., and Calcaterra, T. 1976. Recurrences from malignant parotid salivary gland tumors. Cancer, 37:   2600.

48. Kalnins, I. K., Leonard, A. G., Sako, K., Razack, M. S., and Shedd, D. P. 1977. Correlation between prognosis and degree of lymph node involvement in carcinoma of the oral cavity. American Journal of Surgery, 134:   450.

49. Kaplan, B. H., Vogl, S. E., Chiuten, D., Lanham, R., and Wollner, D. 1979. Chemotherapy of advanced cancer of the head and neck with methotrexate, bleomycin and cis-diamminedichloroplatinum in combination. Proceedings of the American Society of Clinical Oncology, 20:   384.

50. Kapstad, B., Bang, G., Rennaes, S., and Dahler, A. 1978. Combined preoperative treatment with cobalt and bleomycin in patients with head and neck carcinoma—a controlled clinical study. International Journal of Radiation Oncology, Biology, Physics, 4:   85.

51. Kenady, D. E., Chretien, P. B., Potvin, C., and Simon, R. M. 1977. Thymosin reconstitution of T cell deficits *in vitro* in cancer patients. Cancer, 39:   575.

52. Kirkwood, J. M., Miller, D., Weichselbaum, R., and Pitman, S. 1979. Predefinitive and postdefinitive chemotherapy for locally advanced squamous carcinoma of the head and neck. Laryngoscope, 89:   573.

53. Klopp, C. T., Alford, T. C., Bateman, J., Berry, G. N., and Winship, T. 1950. Fractionated intra-arterial cancer chemotherapy with methylbisamine hydrochloride: Preliminary report. Annals of Surgery, 132:   811.

54. Knowlton, A. H., Percarpio, B., Bobrow, S., and Fischer, J. J. 1975. Methotrexate and radiation therapy in the treatment of advanced head and neck tumors. Radiology, 116:   709.

55. Kramer, S. 1975. Methotrexate and radiation therapy in the treatment of advanced squamous cell carcinoma of the oral cavity, oropharynx, supraglottic larynx and hypopharynx. Canadian Journal of Otolaryngology, 4: 213.

56. Leone, L. A., and Ohnuma, T. 1979. Combined high dose methotrexate rescue, bleomycin and cis-platinum for untreated Stage III and localized Stage IV for advanced squamous carcinoma of the head and neck. Proceedings of the American Association for Cancer Research, 20:374.

57. Levitt, M., Mosher, M. B., DeConti, R. C., Farber, L. R., Marsh, J. C., Papac, R. J., Thomas, E. D., and Bertino, J. R. 1972. High dose methotrexate versus methotrexate-leucovorin in epidermoid carcinoma of the head and neck. Proceedings of the American Assocation for Cancer Research, 13: 20.

58. Levitt, M., Mosher, M. B., DeConti, R. C., Farber, L. R., Skeel, R. T., Marsh, J. C., Mitchell, M. S. Papac, R. J., Thomas, E. D., and Bertino, J. R. 1973. Improved therapeutic index of methotrexate with "leucovorin rescue". Cancer Research, 33: 1729.

59. Liotta, L. A., Saidel, G., Kleinerman, J., and DeLisi, C. 1977. Micrometastasis therapy: Theoretical concepts. In: Day, S. B. Ed.: Cancer Invasion and Metastases, Biologic Mechanisms and Therapy. Raven Press, New York, 249.

60. Lipson, S. D., Chretien, P. B., Makuch, R., Kenady, D. E., and Cohen, M. H. 1979. Thymosin immunotherapy in patients with small cell carcinoma of the lung. Cancer, 43: 863.

61. Livingston, R. B., Einhorn, L. H., Burgess, M. A., and Gottlieb, J. A. 1976. Sequential combination chemotherapy for advanced recurrent squamous carcinoma of the head and neck. Cancer Treatment Reports, 60: 103.

62. Lustig, R. A., DeMare, P. A., and Kramer, S. 1976. Adjuvant methotrexate in the radiotherapeutic management of advanced tumors of the head and neck. Cancer, 37: 2703.

63. Lyman, G. H. 1980. (personal communication).

64. McKneally, M. F., Maver, C., and Kause, H. W. 1976. Regional immunotherapy of lung cancer with intrapleural BCG. Lancet 1: 337.

65. Mandel, M. A. 1976. Skin testing for prognosis or therapy formulation in cancer patients: Caveat emptor. Plastic and Reconstructive Surgery, 57: 64.

66. Mathe, G., Florentin, I., Olsson, L., Bruley-Rosset, M., Schulz, J., and Kiger, N. 1978. Pharmacologic factors and manipulation of immunity systemic adjuvants in cancer therapy. Cancer Treatment Reports, 62: 1613.

67. Mathe, G., Amiel, J. L., Schwarzenberg, L., Schneider, M., Cattan, A., Schlumberger, J. R., Hayat, M., and DeVassal, F. 1977. Follow-up of the first (1962) pilot study on active immunotherapy of acute lymphoid leukaemia: A critical discussion. Biomedicine, 24: 29.

68. Moore, G. E., Bross, I. D. J., Ausman, R., Nadler, S., Jones, R., Slack, N., and Rimm, A. A. 1968. Effects of chlorambucil in 374 patients with advanced cancer. Cancer Treatment Reports, 52: 661.

69. Morton, D. L., Eilber, F. R., Joseph, W. L., Wood, W. C., Trahan, E., and Ketcham, A. S. 1970. Immunological factors in human sarcomas and melanomas. Annals of Surgery, 172: 740.

70. Muggia, F. M., and Louie, A. E. 1978. Five years of adjuvant treatment of osteosarcoma: More questions than answers. Cancer Treatment Reports, 62: 301.

71. Muggia, F. M., Cortes-Fures, H., and Wasserman, T. H. 1978. Radiotherapy and chemotherapy in combined clinical trials: Problems and promise. International Journal of Radiation Oncology, Biology, Physics, 4: 161.

72. Muggia, F. M., Rozencweig, M., and Louie, A. E. 1980. Role of chemotherapy in head and neck cancer: Systemic use of single agents and combinations in advanced disease. Head and Neck Surgery, 2: 196.

73. Myer, M. H., Axtell, L. M., and Asire, A. J., Eds. 1976. Salivary glands. In Cancer Patient Survival, Report No. 5. Department of Health, Education and Welfare, Publication No. 77-992, Bethesda, MD.

74. O'Connor, A. D., Clifford, P., Dalley, V. M., Durden-Smith, D. J., Edwards, W. G., and Hollis, B. A. 1979. Advanced head and neck cancer treated by combined radiotherapy and VBM cytotoxic regimen—four year results. Clinical Otolaryngology, 4: 329.

75. Olivari, A. J. 1979. MTX vs. high dose MTX/CF vs. CACP plus surgery and/or radiation plus MER immunotherapy for epidermoid carcinoma of the head and neck. In Compilation of Clinical Protocol Sum-

maries, DHEW publication No. 79-1116, Bethesda, MD, 469.

76. Olivari, A. J., Glait, H. M., Guardo, A., Califano, L., and Pradier, R. 1979. Levamisole in squamous cell carcinoma of the head and neck. Cancer Treatments Reports, 63: 983.

77. Olivari, A., Pradier, R., Feierstein, J., Guardo, A., Glait, H., and Rojas, A. 1976. Cell mediated immunity in head and neck cancer patients. Journal of Surgical Oncology, 8: 287.

78. Olkowski, Z., McLaren, J., and Skeen, M. 1978. Effects of combined immunotherapy with levamisole and bacillus Calmette-Guerin on immunocompetence of patients with squamous cell carcinoma of the cervix, head and neck and lung undergoing radiation therapy. Cancer Treatment Reports, 62: 1651.

79. Papac, R., Minor, D. R., Rudnick, S., Solomon, L. R., and Capizzi, R. L. 1978. Controlled trial of methotrexate and bacillus Calmette-Guerin therapy for advanced head and neck cancer. Cancer Research 38: 3150.

80. Petrovich, Z., Block, J., Barton, D., Casciato, D., Hittle, R., Rice, D., and Jose, L. 1979. Treatment of Stage IV carcinoma of the head and neck with radiotherapy and chemotherapy and radiotherapy combination. Proceedings of the American Society of Clinical Oncology, 20: 422.

81. Pitman, S., and Frei, E. 1977. Weekly methotrexate citrovorum with alkalinization: Tumor response in a phase II study. Proceedings of the American Association of Cancer Research, 18: 124.

82. Pitman, S. W., Minor, D. R., Papac, R., Knopf, T., Lowenthal, I., Nystrom, S., and Bertino, J. R. 1979. Sequential methotrexate-leucovorin and cis-platinum in head and neck cancer. Proceedings of the American Society of Clinical Oncology, 20: 419.

83. Potvin, C., Tarpley, J. L., and Chretien, P. B. 1975. Thymus-derived lymphocytes in patients with solid malignancies. Clinical Immunology and Immunopathology, 3: 476.

84. Presant, C. A., Ratkin, G., Klahr, C., and Brown, C. 1979. Adriamycin, BCNU plus cyclophosphamide in advanced carcinoma of the head and neck. Cancer, 44: 1571.

85. Price, L. A., Hill, B. T., Calvert, A. H., Dalley, M., Levene, A., Busby, E. R.,

Schachter, M., and Shaw, H. J. 1978. Improved results in combination chemotherapy of head and neck cancer using a kinetically-based approach: A randomized study with and without adriamycin. Oncology, 35: 26.

86. Probert, J. C., Thompson, R. W., and Bagshaw, M. A. 1974. Patterns of spread of distant metastases in head and neck cancer. Cancer, 33: 127.

87. Rafla, S. 1977. Malignant parotid tumors: Natural history and treatment. Cancer, 40: 136.

88. Randolph, V. L., Vallejo, A., Spiro, R. H., Shah, J. P., Strong, E. W., Huvos, A. G., and Wittes, R. E. 1978. Combination therapy of advanced head and neck cancer. Cancer, 41: 460.

89. Ratkin, G. A., Brown, C. A., and Ogura, J. 1978. Combination chemotherapy in head and neck cancer. Proceedings of the American Society of Clinical Oncology 19: 330.

90. Rentschler, R., Burgess, M. A., and Byers, R. 1977. Chemotherapy of malignant major salivary gland neoplasms. Cancer, 40: 619.

91. Richard, J. M., Sancho, H., Lepintre, Y., Rodary, J., and Pierquin, B. 1974. Intra-arterial methotrexate chemotherapy and telecobalt therapy in cancer of the oral cavity and oropharynx. Cancer, 34: 491.

92. Richards, G. J., and Chambers, R. G. 1969. Hydroxyurea: A radiosensitizer in the treatment of neoplasms of the head and neck. American Journal of Roentgenology, Radium Therapy and Nuclear Medicine, 105: 555.

93. Richman, S. P., Livingston, R. B., Gutterman, J. U., Suen, J. Y. and Hersh, E. M. 1976. Chemotherapy versus chemo-immunotherapy of head and neck cancer: Report of a randomized study. Cancer Treatment Reports, 60: 535.

94. Rogers, L. S. 1964. Cancer chemotherapy by continuous intra-arterial infusion. Cancer, 17: 1365.

95. Rojas, A. F., Feierstein, J. H., Glait, H. M., and Olivari, A. J. 1977. Levamisole action in breast cancer Stage III. In Terry, W. D., and Windhorst, D. Eds.: Immunotherapy of Cancer: Present Status of Trials in Man. Raven Press, New York, 635.

96. Rosen, G., Wollner, N., Tan, C., Wu, S. J.; Hadju, S. I.; Cham, W.; D'Angio, G. J.; Murphy, M. L. 1974. Disease-free survival in children with Ewing's sarcoma treated with radiation therapy and adjuvant four

drug sequential chemotherapy. Cancer, 33: 384.

97. Sako, K., Razack, M. S., and Kalnins, I. 1978. Chemotherapy for advanced and recurrent squamous cell carcinoma of the head and neck with high and low dose cis-diamminedichloroplatinum. American Journal of Surgery, 136: 529.

98. Schafer, L. A., Goldstein, A. L., Gutterman, J. U., and Hersh, E. M. 1976. *In vitro* and *in vivo* studies with thymosin in cancer patients. Annals of the New York Academy of Sciences, 277: 609.

99. Shapiro, D. M., and Fugmann, R. A. 1957. A role for chemotherapy as an adjunct to surgery. Cancer Research, 17: 1098.

100. Shigematsu, Y., Sakai, S., and Fuchikata, H. 1971. Recent trials in the treatment of maxillary sinus carcinoma with special reference to the chemical potentiation of radiation therapy. Acta Oto-Laryngologica, 71: 63.

101. Simpson-Herren, L., Sanford, A. H., and Holmquist, J. P. 1976. Effects of surgery on the cell kinetics of residual tumor. Cancer Treatment Reports, 60: 1749.

102. Smith, B. L., Franz, J. L., Mira, J. G., Gates, G. A., Sapp, J., and Cruz, A. B. 1979. Simultaneous combination radiotherapy and multidrug chemotherapy for Stage III and IV squamous carcinoma of the head and neck. Proceedings of the American Society of Clinical Oncology, 20: 394.

103. Spiro, R. H., Huvos, A. G., and Strong, E. W. 1974. Adenoid cystic carcinoma of salivary origin. American Journal of Surgery, 128: 512.

104. Spiro, R. H., Huvos, A. G., and Strong, E. W. 1975. Cancer of the parotid gland. American Journal of Surgery, 130: 452.

105. Spittle, M. F. 1978. Methotrexate and radiation. International Journal of Radiation Oncology, Biology, Physics, 4: 103.

106. Stefani, S., Eells, R. W., and Abbate, J. 1971. Hydroxyurea and radiotherapy in head and neck cancer. Results of a prospective controlled study in 126 patients. Radiology, 101: 391.

107. Stefani, S., Kerman, R., and Abbate, J. 1976. Serial studies of immunocompetence in head and neck cancer patients undergoing radiation therapy. American Journal of Roentgenology, Radium Therapy and Nuclear Medicine, 126: 880.

108. Szpirglas, H., Chastang, C., and Bertrand, J. C. 1979. Adjuvant treatment of tongue and floor of the mouth cancers. Recent Results in Cancer Research, 68: 309.

109. Tarpley, J. L., Chretien, P. B., Alexander, J. C., Haige, R. C., Block, J. B., and Ketcham, A. S. 1975. High dose methotrexate as a preoperative adjuvant in the treatment of epidermoid carcinoma of the head and neck. American Journal of Surgery, 130: 481.

110. Taylor, S. G., Sisson, G. A., and Bytell, D. E. 1979. Adjuvant chemoimmunotherapy of head and neck cancer. Recent Results in Cancer Research, 68: 297.

111. Taylor, S. G., Bytell, D. E., DeWys, W. D., Applebaum, E., and Sisson, G. A. 1978. Adjuvant methotrexate and leucovorin in head and neck squamous cancer. Archives of Otolaryngology, 104: 647.

112. Tejada, F. 1980. (personal communcation).

113. Terz, J. 1980. (personal communication).

114. Twomey, P. L., Catalona, W. J., and Chretien, P. B. 1974. Cellular immunity in cured cancer patients. Cancer, 33: 435.

115. Vogl, S. E., and Kaplan, B. H. 1979. Chemotherapy of advanced head and neck cancer with methotrexate, bleomycin and cis-diamminedichloroplatinum II in an effective outpatient schedule. Cancer, 44: 26.

116. Wanebo, H. J., Jun, M. Y., Strong, E. W., and Oettgen, H. F. 1975. T-cell deficiency in patients with squamous cell cancer of the head and neck. American Journal of Surgery, 130: 445.

117. Wanebo, H. J., Hilal, E. Y., Strong, E. W., Pinsky, C. M., Mike, V., and Oettgen, H. F. 1979. Adjuvant trial of levamisole in patients with squamous cancer of the head and neck: A preliminary report. Recent Results in Cancer Research, 68: 324.

118. Wara, D. W., and Ammann, A. J. 1978. Thymosin treatment of children with primary immunodeficiency disease. Transplantation Proceedings, 10: 203.

119. Wara, D. W., Barrett, D. J., Ammann, A. J., and Cowan, M. J. 1979. *In vitro* and *in vivo* enhancement of mixed leukocyte culture reactivity by thymosin in patients with primary immunodeficiency diseases. Annals of the New York Academy of Sciences, 332: 128.

120. Wara, W. M., Wara, D. W., Ammann, A. J., Barnard, J. L., and Phillips, T. L. 1979. Immunosuppression and reconstitution with thymosin after radiation therapy. International Journal of Radiation Oncology, Biology, Physics, 5: 997.

121. Wheeler, R. H., Earhart, R. H., and Bull, F. E. 1979. Bleomycin, Oncovin, mitomycin-C ± methotrexate for squamous cell carcinoma. Proceedings of the American Society of Clinical Oncology, 20: 348.

122. Wittes, R. E., Cvitkovic, E., Shah, J., Gerold, F. P., and Strong, E. W. 1977. Cis-dichloro-diammineplatinum (II) in the treatment of epidermoid carcinoma of the head and neck. Cancer Treatment Reports, 61: 359.

123. Wittes, R. E., Heller, K., Randolph, V., Howard, J., Vallejo, A., Farr, H., Harrold, C., Gerold, F., Shah, J., Spiro, R., and Strong, E. 1979. Cis-dichloro-diammineplatinum (II)-based chemotherapy as initial treatment of advanced head and neck cancer. Cancer Treatment Reports, 63: 1533.

124. Wolf, G. T., Kerney, S. E., Makuch, R. W., and Chretien, P. B. Thymosin improves impaired leukocyte migration inhibition in patients with head and neck squamous carcinoma. American Journal of Surgery, (in press).

125. Woods, R. L., Tattersall, M. H. N., and Sullivan, J. 1979. A randomized study of three doses of methotrexate in patients with advanced squamous cell cancer of the head and neck. Proceedings of the American Association for Cancer Research, 20: 262.

126. Yagoda, A., Mukherji, B., Young, C., Etcubanas, E., Lamonte, C., Smith, J. R., Tan, C. T. C., and Krakoff, J. H. 1972. Bleomycin, an antitumor antibiotic. Clinical experience in 274 patients. Annals of Internal Medicine, 77: 861.

30 | Methods of Pain Control

Warren C. Boop, Jr., M.D.
Janet A. Fisher, R.N., B.S.N.

BASIC CONSIDERATIONS

The Nature of Pain

A renewed interest in the problem of pain has been evident by the explosion of publications on the subject since the mid-1960s. This interest was generated by the fortuitous development of new surgical and psychological techniques, the opening of the Republic of China revealing their popular use of acupuncture, and the publication of the Melzack and Wall "gate control theory"[10] of pain perception. Many of the recent publications on pain deal with new concepts of neural modalities involved in the sensation of pain, as well as with the reactions to chronic pain including the emotional, adversive, and cognitive.

The broader concept of the patient in pain has resulted in a proliferation of multidisciplinary teams to treat pain. Both "organic" and "psychological" factors (an admittedly artificial separation) must be handled successfully to produce a satisfactory outcome. For example, in cancer on the head and neck it is likely that disfigurement from ablative surgery and difficulty with swallowing or speaking distress the patient. The pain of which he complains may be the result of a collection of stresses working within him, with pain serving as the focal point for complaint.

Pain is an uncomfortable sensation carrying the connotation of body damage. It is an unpleasant, subjective experience influenced by both stimulus response and central psychological mechanisms. The intensity or severity of the latter may vary from person to person and in the same person from time to time. Pain produced by cancer may be the result of invasion, pressure, or traction by the cancer or by secondary inflammation.

When treating pain in a cancer patient, one should first determine a clear relationship of the pain to the etiology. A careful physical examination to define the lesion, supplemented by appropriate investigations such as radiographs of suspicious areas, may support the idea that the cancer is causing the pain. It is as unconscionable for a surgeon to allow his patients to suffer when methods of pain relief are available as it is to allow a patient to become drug dependent if there is a simple therapeutic solution to his problem. It is also important to properly manage sensations stemming from emotional factors related to the diagnosis of cancer. Therefore, the first step in treating the patient with pain is to understand all aspects of his problem and formulate plans to deal with the whole patient.

Cancer and pain are two of the most dreaded medical problems. What the patient perceives and tolerates as pain is influenced by his emotional state, his past experience, and how he feels about the cause of his pain. Further factors that may contribute to the emotional upheaval that leads to uncontrolled pain are the financial drain that often accompanies treatment of the disease and the potential loss of job and income. Treatment of head and neck cancer many times requires radical surgery that greatly changes the person's appearance. The accompanying loss of pride and dignity increases the depression and intensifies the pain. The fear of death often haunts the patient. To alleviate the pain, these emotional components must be dealt with effectively.

One's awareness of pain can vary even when the painful stimulus remains the same. The distraction of enjoyable pursuits such as visiting with friends, watching television, or even taking part in fatiguing physical activity, may decrease awareness of pain. Although Melsak and Wall[10] discussed the soldier in battle often not feeling the pain of a wound and used this as clinical evidence to deny a "pain pathway," it is equally likely that the wounded soldier is simply distracted.

Conversely, emotions such as anxiety, fear, anger, depression, and dependency may enhance one's perception of pain.

Anxiety often accompanies pain, especially in the case of the cancer patient who believes that the disease is fatal, disfiguring, or accompanied by an expensive and painful cure. Anxiety decreases a person's ability to tolerate pain by adding to muscle tension. Muscle tension can actually increase the pain and contribute to the patient's exhaustion. Exhaustion, in turn, reduces a patient's level of tolerance and leaves him less reserve with which to handle his pain. A debilitating cycle of anxiety, pain, exhaustion, more anxiety, more pain, and more exhaustion is begun. To break this cycle requires treatment of the patient's anxiety as well as his physical source of pain.

For some patients, the fear of pain is more profound than the fear of death. Uncontrolled pain also brings fear that one may not have the courage or strength to cope with it. Such fear contributes to the patient's overall discomfort.

A frequent response to pain is anger. "Why me?" and, "What did I do to deserve this?" are questions that spring from the anger brought on by uninvited pain. When pain becomes the overriding factor in the patient's life and the determinant of whether or not he can function, he may become angry over this loss of freedom and control of his life. Although his anger would seem to be a natural response to the continued effects of painful stimulus, it may be directed toward family, friends, or the health care team.

Depression is also a common reaction when one's life is interrupted by pain. Pain allows the depression to become the major mental effect of the illness. Depression and pain are mutually potentiating. This relationship between depression and pain is also demonstrated by the fact that measures used to relieve one often may relieve the other. Indeed, we have seen patients essentially relieved of "pain" when only their depression has been treated, without change of analgesics.

The quality of one's life depends on one's emotional as well as physical state. It may at times be difficult to distinguish between the contributions of each to the sensation of pain. Both the body and the psyche need to be treated as important factors because the pain-free condition is dependent upon the satisfactory resolution of emotional as well as physical problems. An adequate medical program to handle anxiety, depression, and fear is as important as proper use of analgesics or surgery for the control of pain.

ANATOMY

The pain produced by neoplasms of the head and neck is often a difficult problem to treat effectively. The tumors often infiltrate deeply into the nose or throat or other areas of overlapping cranial or cervical innervation. Regions are involved that may be supplied by the 5th cranial nerve or by the nervus intermedius; by the 9th and 10th cranial nerves; or by the first, second, and third upper cervical nerves. If the pain is exclusively in the distribution of one of these nerves, especially the trigeminal, the problem may be easier to manage. In any case, it is advisable to consider the application of simple surgical methods to alleviate pain prior to initiation of narcotics.

The trigeminal nerve provides much of

the sensory supply to the skin and mucous membranes of the head. The nerve is divided into three primary sensory divisions: the ophthalmic, maxillary, and mandibular. In addition to these sensory branches, the trigeminal nerve also has a motor component, which accompanies the mandibular sensory division. The sensory ganglion of the trigeminal nerve lies in a small depression in the temporal bone near the petrous tip. The three large peripheral divisions arise from the anterior margin of this ganglion. The central process, or root, of the nerve arises from the posterior margin of the ganglion and then proceeds to the pons.

The ophthalmic division of the trigeminal nerve is the smallest of the three divisions. It originates in the dorsomedial aspect of the ganglion and passes forward, lying in the lateral wall of the cavernous sinus. At the superior orbital fissure this division subdivides into three branches: the frontal, nasociliary, and lacrimal. These three branches all continue into the orbit through the superior orbital fissure. The branches are also joined by sympathetic fibers from the carotid plexus, which is in the cavernous sinus. The frontal branch divides into supraorbital and supratrochlear nerves. The supraorbital nerve leaves the orbit through the supraorbital notch (or foramen) and supplies sensation to the upper eyelid as well as the skin of the forehead and anterior scalp.

The supratrochlear nerve exits from the orbit about one fingerbreadth medial to the supraorbital nerve and serves the medial upper eyelid and a small area of forehead above the nose.

The nasociliary branch of the ophthalmic division runs obliquely to the medial wall of the orbit and there passes through the anterior ethmoidal foramen. It continues on to supply the sensation to the mucous membrane of the ethmoid, anterior part of the nasal septum, and lateral wall of the nasal cavity. The posterior ethmoid branch supplies the mucous membrane of the posterior ethmoids as well as part of the sphenoid. The nasociliary nerve finally

emerges from the nasal cavity as the external nasal nerve to supply sensation to the skin of the nose as far down as the tip.

An infratrochlear branch leaves the nasociliary in the orbit to supply the skin around the upper or lower eyelid and adjacent part of the nose. The third branch of the ophthalmic division of the trigeminal nerve, the lacrimal, supplies the lacrimal gland and receives sensory input from the lateral part of the upper eyelid and conjunctiva.

The ophthalmic division also subserves pain sensation from a large part of the meninges over the cerebral hemispheres. Tumors infiltrating the cranium and anterior base of the skull often produce ophthalmic division pain described by patients as being located in the retro-orbital area.

The maxillary division of the trigeminal nerve begins between the ophthalmic and mandibular divisions of the trigeminal ganglion. It is also found in the lateral wall of the cavernous sinus until it leaves the cranial cavity via the foramen rotundum. Immediately upon exiting from this foramen, it is found to lie within the pterygopalatine fossa and supplies the sphenopalatine ganglion. It continues on to subserve the sensory fibers to the mucous membrane of the maxillary sinus, a portion of the sphenoid sinus, the anterior-inferior nasal septum, the hard palate, the lower eustachian tube, the upper gum, the teeth, and the palate, as well as the skin of the face from immediately below the nose, the upper lip and the cheek area. It also supplies the dura of the middle cranial fossa, and pain from tumors invading the skull in this region is often referred to the upper teeth or maxilla. However, great variation in pain radiation patterns from the dura has been documented by Wirth and Van Buren.[26] These authors concluded that "head pain of dural origin has limited clinical usefulness in localizing a lesion because of this lack of consistency of pain patterns."

Also compounding the problem of determining the origin of pain is the varied pattern from other areas of the head. Robertson, Goodell, and Wolff[14] stimulated teeth in normal, as well as diseased, patients with a noxious stimulus and studied the pain patterns produced. They reported that pain from teeth of the upper jaw was local and spread to the eye, orbital ridge, and temple. In the lower jaw, pain could be local or radiate to the zygoma, the temple, and to the top of the ear. It would seem that a lesion localized to one area of the trigeminal nerve can induce discomfort in the region supplied by other divisions.

The mandibular division arises from the most lateral and inferior portion of the trigeminal ganglion. After its exit through the foramen ovale, which lies just lateral to the ganglion, the nerve branches and supplies pain fibers to the mucous membrane of the anterior two-thirds of the tongue via the lingual nerve. The lower teeth and gums, as well as the mucous membrane in the adjacent portion of the mouth, are supplied by the inferior alveolar nerve. The skin over the lower face and chin are supplied by the mental nerve of the mandibular division. A small area of skin of the ear and external auditory canal, including a part of the tympanic membrane as well as some mastoid air cells, is served by the auriculotemporal nerve of the mandibular division. Virtually no overlap exists between the skin areas supplied by the three peripheral divisions of the trigeminal nerve. This is unusual in comparison to the extensive overlapping of areas for nerves in the remainder of the body.

The sensory distribution of the facial (7th) nerve, generally called the nervus intermedius, shows marked individual variation. In general, however, it is thought that this nerve carries pain sensation from part of the external auditory canal, the tympanic membrane, and the lateral surface of the pinna as well as from a small area behind the ear and over the mastoid process (Fig. 30-1).

From the middle ear and medial aspect of the tympanic membrane, pain is carried over the tympanic branch of the 9th cranial nerve (glossopharyngeal). Known as Jacobson's nerve, this branch also subserves pain

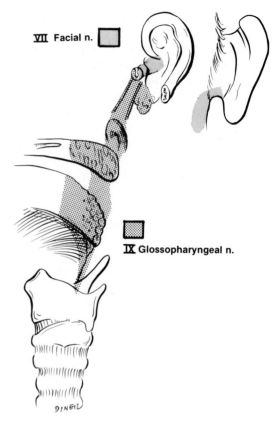

Fig. 30-1. Sensory distribution of the facial (VII) and glossopharyngeal (IX) nerves.

sense from the mastoid cells and upper eustachian tube. Other sensory fibers carrying pain in the glossopharyngeal nerve are derived from the soft palate, tonsillar region, posterior one-third of the tongue, and posterior pharynx down to the epiglottis (Fig. 30-1).

The vagus (10th) cranial nerve conveys sensation via the superior laryngeal nerve from the epiglottis and adjacent region of the pharynx and from the vallecula. The recurrent laryngeal nerve supplies the larynx below the vocal folds (Fig. 30-2).

The vagus also conducts pain sensation from a small area of the external auditory canal posteriorly and from adjacent skin of the external ear (Fig. 30-2).

One may readily see that pain in the ear may be a very difficult problem to eliminate because of the many nerves supplying the

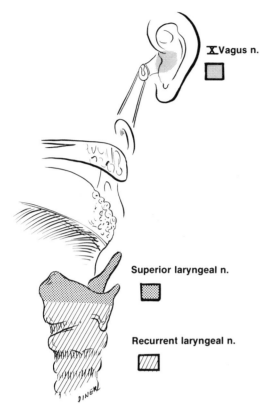

X Vagus n.

Superior laryngeal n.

Recurrent laryngeal n.

Fig. 30-2. Sensory distribution of the vagus (X) nerve.

area. Not only the vagus and glossopharyngeal nerves, but the facial (nervus intermedius), the trigeminal (auriculotemporal), and also the cervical plexus branch, the great auricular, carry pain sensation from this area. In addition, Sachs[15] presented evidence that "pain" fibers of the nervus intermedius may join the 8th nerve via anastomosing branches.

Most of the innervation of the back of the head and neck is supplied by the second and third cervical nerve roots. The first cervical nerve root has been demonstrated to have some sensory function also,[5] but this is apparently of a poorly localized nature. The cervical plexus is formed of the upper four cervical nerves (Fig. 30-3). The superficial branches are primarily sensory. They consist of the small occipital, supplying the skin of the side of the head behind the ear; the great auricular, subserving pain sensation

from the skin of the face in the region of the angle of the jaw and the lower ear lobe and skin over the mastoid; and the superficial cervical, which is distributed to the anterior and lateral parts of the neck. The great occipital nerve is a part of the posterior primary ramus of C2 and C3 and is sensory to the occipital portion of the neck and to the scalp as far forward as the vertex.

It is of interest that the pain fibers of all these nerves, 5th, 7th, 9th, 10th, and upper cervical, enter the CNS in a common tract of descending fibers and grey matter that is continuous down to the C4 level of the spinal cord. This tract is labeled the spinal tract of the trigeminal. As these fibers in the tract descend they give collaterals to all levels of the nucleus. There is, therefore, ample opportunity for these sensory nerves of the head and neck to overlap in function on a central basis. Referred pain patterns as well as similar somatic and visceral responses may be explained on this basis. Alteration of the input to this central neural pool may result in changes in other areas. For example, cervical nerve blocks have sometimes reduced the pain of an atypical facial neuralgia. Surgery to interrupt the descending fibers of the spinal tract has been advocated to alleviate pain of cancer of the head and neck.

PAIN MECHANISMS AND IMPLICATIONS IN THE CONTROL OF PAIN

Concepts of the neural mechanisms of pain are changing rapidly.[23] At present there is an inclination to believe that a specific system of pain receptors and their corresponding centrally coursing fibers activate "pain neurons" in the CNS. Although some of the CNS neurons respond only to noxious stimuli, a considerable number served by "pain fibers" respond to nonpainful input as well. This overlap in function between pain and nonpainful response tends to obscure the specificity of response expected from the cells. There are interactions between pain

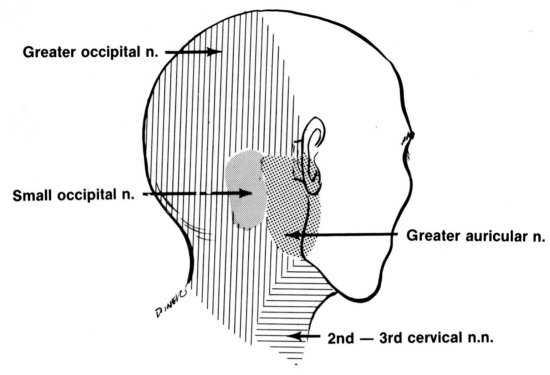

Fig. 30-3. Sensory distribution of the cervical plexus nerves.

and other sensations, both somatic as well as visceral, and these interactions make the identification of "pain pathways" and separation of the pain sensation difficult in experimental conditions.

More recently a complex modulating system of descending control has been demonstrated to operate against this background of pain input. There is a well-known descending system, originating from the cortex, that modulates transmission of "pain" through the dorsal horn. In addition, a powerful descending influence from the *nucleus raphe magus* of the brainstem reticular system appears to have an important function in analgesia produced by systemic morphine. The relationship of the naturally occurring morphine-like enkaphalin to morphine and stimulus-produced analgesia has been of great interest. The stimulation of the area of the midbrain periaqueductal grey and associated reticular system region results in marked elevation of the pain threshold. This area is an opiate receptor of high intensity.[16] Enkephalin concentrations are also high in this area. The importance of this area in pain processing and control in the brain is just beginning to be understood. Rapid developments in pain research hold the promise of new approaches to help the patient in pain.

CLINICAL CONSIDERATIONS

Determining the Etiology of Pain

Patients with cancer of the head and neck have complicated management problems when pain enters the clinical area. The physician must be competent in assessing the problem of pain in the most definitive manner possible. The etiology of the pain should be carefully analyzed and appropriate treatment undertaken when factors other than the tumor itself are the cause of pain. Just because a patient carries a diagnosis of cancer does not necessarily mean that the malignancy is responsible for the pain. This point cannot be overemphasized: we have seen patients treated with excessive medication because of the "incurable cancer" who later have been shown to have a source of pain from quite another problem—one that often times is remedied by simple procedures. For example, the pain of sinusitis caused by an obstructed sinus ostium may be relieved by appropriate treatment and should not just be masked by using narcotics.

The location and nature of the pain, whether it is constant or intermittent, and what makes it worse, are all characteristics that must be assessed prior to the institution of therapy. A careful clinical examination supplemented by x-ray or other laboratory diagnostic aids should be used in the evaluation of pain.

The tumor itself may, of course, be the cause of pain, especially when inflammation develops. Tumors of the intraoral and pharyngeal region are particularly prone to develop ulceration and infection, thereby producing pain. Tumors may invade or compress sensory nerves. Invasion alone usually does not produce pain, but compression of a nerve by the bulk of the tumor itself may result in pain.

Possible causes for the development of pain should be reviewed periodically in each case. The development of tension headache is not an unusual finding in the patient who has been treated for cancer of the head and neck. The headache is often described as either a sensation of tightness like a constricting band about the head or as an ache or sensation of pressure constantly present during the day and commonly located in the neck muscles and suboccipital region. The headache frequently radiates forward from the occiput to the frontal region. The recognition and alleviation of tension headache may require extensive efforts on the part of the physician. An aid in diagnosis may be obtained by use of the Minnesota Multiphasic Personality Inventory. This is a test consisting of statements covering many aspects of one's bodily health, interpersonal

relationships, and attitudes. Although this may serve as a guideline to psychological contributions of the pain, one often can make this assessment without such elaborate testing. Most often, pain that the patient can describe in a simple and crisp manner is organic in origin, whereas pain described more elaborately, and perhaps vaguely, may be a result of psychological factors that have come into play. For tension headaches, sedatives, analgesics, and even strong narcotics may not give complete relief of pain. Biofeedback and other similar methods for teaching autorelaxation have been found to be of some use in relieving these headaches. Good rapport between patient and therapist and reassurance are essential in gaining control of this cause of discomfort.

Sinusitis, especially of the sphenoid or ethmoid sinuses, may generate a diffuse and vague headache. This should be evaluated radiographically to demonstrate the fluid levels or opacification that is characteristic of these problems. Appropriate institution of drainage and antibiotic therapy usually gives complete relief of the pain.

Herpes zoster (shingles) occurs with increased frequency in association with tumors in and about nerve ganglia. The trigeminal nerve distribution is no exception to this. In the occasional patient, persistent pain may exist long after the disappearance of the herpetic rash. The patient complains of severe stabbing pain occurring spontaneously and also with a light touch rather than firm pressure on the skin involved. This has long been a difficult problem in which to achieve pain control but in recent years we have found the Yale Regimen to be helpful.[20] A combination of amitriptyline and fluphenazine is an effective remedy in a large proportion of the patients. Some of those not responding to this combination of drugs may obtain relief by treatment with transcutaneous neurostimulation. A variety of neuroablative procedures have been tried but have failed to control the postherpetic neuralgia of the face.

Traumatic neuritis, in the broadest sense, is not an infrequent cause of pain in the neck or head following tumor removal. The pain may be constant or intermittent in nature, but is usually constant in its neural distribution. If no remedial cause can be uncovered (e.g., suture involving nerve or bone spicule impinging on the nerve), one should analyze the problem with use of anesthetic blocks of the area. Subsequent neurectomy often gives permanent relief. Rhizotomy or tractotomy rarely need to be employed.

Dental problems may cause diffuse head and face pain not necessarily localized to the mouth. In the postoperative patient with a change in usual habits of mouth hygiene, tooth decay and abscess will only rarely be a confusing source of pain. Extraction of obviously diseased teeth at the time of surgery will prevent pain and problems from this source.

Trismus is produced when the masticatory muscles are invaded by tumor. This problem must be differentiated from common dental problems, as well as from Costen syndrome, or temporomandibular neuralgia. This latter entity, frequently occurring as a result of imbalance in dental occlusion, may be the etiology of preauricular pain with diffuse distribution to the mandible and tongue areas. Diagnostic block of the temporomandibular joint with Xylocaine may help in this differential diagnosis.

Cervical spine lesions may be a cause of both neck and head pain, especially orbital, forehead, or vertex pain. The anatomic and physiological basis for this has been amply demonstrated.[5, 6] Unusual positioning at surgery or surgical trauma to the upper cervical nerve roots can be a cause of continued or recurrent postoperative pain. Cervical degenerative disease with narrowed disc and vertebral spurring may be a predisposing factor associated with the onset of these pains. Occipital or paraspinous muscle tenderness when associated with limited range of motion of the neck may be clues leading to proper diagnosis. Simple treatment with cervical traction or a cervical collar may af-

ford considerable relief of head and neck pain in these individuals.

IMPORTANCE OF LOCATION OF PAIN

One of the more difficult pains with which to deal is pain in the ear. It has been pointed out that pain in the ear may be mediated by the trigeminal nerve, the nervus intermedius, the 9th nerve, the auricular branch of the vagus nerve (10th), and branches of the cervical plexus, and possibly by the 8th nerve. Trying to differentiate the nerve or nerves involved in relaying pain sensation from the ear is, therefore, often a taxing chore. Indeed, in an attempt to relieve ear pain, Grant[2] has sectioned the 7th, 8th, 9th, and 12th cranial nerves together with the upper three cervical posterior roots "without the slightest relief in the pain."

On the other hand, pain limited to the distribution of a portion of the trigeminal nerve, such as anterior maxillary pain or anterior tongue pain, is rather easily eliminated by interruption of the 5th nerve. There is little, if any, overlap of peripheral distribution of the 5th cranial nerve and its branches, and effective pain relief by surgery may be expected in the majority of cases.

Midline areas of multiple innervation such as the nose and the pharynx present serious technical problems for alleviation of pain by denervation. Analgesic medication and other techniques for pain control must be relied upon more often for the midline pain problems.

PRINCIPLES OF PAIN RELIEF

Establishing rapport with the patient is the first requirement in providing effective pain relief. It is often difficult for the patient to describe his pain adequately, and for that reason, it is important that specific questions be asked to allow the professional to properly assess the pain and to understand its components. The manner in which such questions are asked and the way the answers are received can be supportive. Having insight into the patient's self-perception is necessary to build a trusting relationship. This trust can help to control the patient's pain by decreasing anxiety and insecurity. Simply believing that the pain is going to get better oftentimes helps it do just that.

It is important that the patient be given as much responsibility as possible for his own pain relief. A patient who participates in working toward his own pain relief is much more likely to achieve that goal.

General Measures

Many large necrotic tumors in the pharyngeal and intraoral regions present as painful lesions. The establishment of drainage of any loculation of purulent matter and use of appropriate antibiotic therapy will often bring the inflammatory response under control, thereby alleviating the pain. Some of these tumors have secondary anaerobic infections that can frequently be controlled by giving clindamycin (Cleocin), 150 mg three or four times a day, with observation for the danger of colitis. Lactinex granules (a viable mixed culture of *Lactobacillus acidophilus* and *L bulgaricus*) may be helpful in controlling the diarrhea from Cleocin. One packet of granules in milk or water is given three or four times a day. Appropriate culture and sensitivity tests may guide further therapy. *Monilia* infection, producing pain in the mouth or pharynx, may be a problem during radiation or long-term antibiotic therapy. This may be effectively treated by using nystatin (Mycostatin) oral suspension held in the mouth, swished around, and then swallowed.

Topical anesthesia using viscous Xylocaine as a gargle or swished about the mouth on an "as needed" basis may be helpful to relieve pain. This has been effective in reducing the discomfort associated with radiation and chemotherapy mucositis or ulcerative disease in the mouth and pharynx.

Proper oral hygiene must be emphasized. The institution of vigorous measures to maintain cleanliness of the oral-pharyngeal areas aids in minimizing uncomfortable inflammatory response. If the usual measures of cleanliness (brushing and mild mouth wash) do not appear adequate, irrigation with salt and soda solution is a useful method for cleaning the mouth. Maintenance of adequate nutrition and hydration is also an aid in overall comfort to the patient.

Shoulder pain is experienced by most patients following radical neck dissection with resection of the spinal accessory (11th) nerve. Standard measures to relieve this pain have consisted of a shoulder sling for support and for elevation of the affected arm. More recently, Johnson et al.[4] have reported significant or total relief of pain in all 16 patients in their series treated with a program of (1) infrared heat from a 250 watt bulb, (2) strengthening exercises for the rhomboid and levator scapular muscles, (3) stretching of the serratus anterior, and (4) active range of motion exercises to increase shoulder joint motion. They believe that the shoulder pain results from limited shoulder motion in the postoperative stage, resulting in development of an adhesive capsulitis.

SPECIFIC PAIN THERAPY

It is evident from any review of the literature (and certainly it has been our experience) that there is no one form of treatment for the pain of cancer of the head and neck that is universally effective.

Radiation

Some patients develop painful bony metastasis, especially when the metastasis involves a vertebra. If the life expectancy is at least 2 months and the pain is severe, radiation therapy to that site may be of value in stopping the pain. If it is effective, pain relief is usually seen within 2 to 3 weeks of onset of treatment. The poorest results occur when vertebrae are involved with nerve compression.

Malignancies that are ulcerative when initially seen may be painful. If they respond to radiation therapy, the pain is usually controlled.

Chemotherapy

There is no question that some squamous cell carcinomas are sensitive to chemotherapy. Most of the difficult pain problems associated with head and neck cancer are in those patients who have recurrent and/or advanced cancers and have been treated with surgery and/or radiation therapy. In this group of patients, approximately 35 percent will respond to methotrexate or cis-platinum, and if severe pain is present, marked pain relief may be seen within 1 or 2 weeks.

Chemotherapy may offer excellent pain relief and is frequently well tolerated even in elderly, debilitated patients. The benefits must be weighed against the side effects. Methotrexate, 25 to 50 mg/m², administered intravenously once weekly is usually well tolerated by most patients.

Analgesic Drug Therapy

It is important to realize that acute and chronic pain are two entirely different entities. Keeping in mind that pain consists of both stimulus and affective response, the goal in control of pain associated with malignancy must still depend on the prognosis. With the modern techniques that control cancer for long periods of time, the effects and risks of drug addiction must be kept in mind. No one questions that the patient with a short life expectancy should be kept comfortable and that addiction to narcotics in this group is of little consequence. For those patients with longer life expectancy, and especially for those cured of cancer, it is still a failed treatment if the patient ends up hopelessly addicted.

A general guideline is to supply ample strength and quantity of drugs to the patient with uncontrolled cancer, while, on the other hand, substituting various nonaddicting medications to the patient who is free of disease. Because of the problem of developing drug tolerance and the need for stronger, more effective pain relief as the cancer progresses, the milder analgesics are used first even in the patient with known residual cancer. The mild analgesics that are often sufficient for a long period include aspirin, acetaminophen (Tylenol), propoxyphene (Darvon), and ethoheptazine (Zactirin). Aspirin tolerance is usually better when it is buffered by food or antacids and is probably the most effective of the commonly used mild analgesics. The tolerance and relief obtained by many patients using nonnarcotic drug combinations allows switching from one to another as confidence in one drug form fails. After the effectiveness of these mild drugs begins to subside, combinations of drugs are used, such as acetaminophen and propoxyphene (Darvocet), propoxyphene and phenacetin, aspirin, and caffeine (Darvon compound), orphenadrine with aspirin, phenacetin, and caffeine (Norgesic), and chlorzoxazone with acetaminophen (Parafon Forte).

Once the above category of drugs is no longer effective, consideration is given to proceeding to the next group of intermediate strength analgesics. This group includes codeine, usually in combination with acetaminophen or APC compound. The hazard to the kidney with excessive use of the phenacetin in the various "compound" drugs must be kept in mind with long-term use. Pentazocine (Talwin) may fit into this group of intermediate strength analgesics, but many patients seem unable to function with this drug when taken orally because of the hallucinations and dizziness occurring as side effects. It does seem to be more effective as an injection, but the subcutaneous and muscular fibrosis produced with chronic use of this drug has led to our rejection of it as a useful drug for chronic pain control.

Somewhat more potent than the codeine-containing compounds is a combination of acetaminophen and oxycodone (Tylox) and also a combination of oxycodone, homatropine, aspirin, phenacetin, and caffeine (Percodan). These drugs seem more addicting than the codeine-containing drugs, and in our pain clinic, represent some of the more difficult drugs from which to wean the addict. They are quite effective in relieving pain associated with cancer but should be used cautiously in the patients with long survival expectancy.

When the above category of drugs becomes ineffective, we must once again assess the patient's ability to cope with his condition and environment. Depression and anxiety are apt to become apparent when these drugs are not providing the desired relief. More complex treatment forms such as psychotropic drugs, behavioral modification, biofeedback, and/or autogenic relaxation techniques may be chosen for use. An effective regime often instituted at this time is a combination of (1) amitriptyline (an antidepressant, probably with some primary effect to raise the pain threshold) and (2) fluphenazine (Prolixin) or another phenothiazine such as chlorpromazine (Thorazine), along with (3) one of the mild or moderate class of analgesics. This combination therapy will often provide comfort even for the terminal patient.

If a decision is made that additional pain relief must be provided, we prefer to administer oral medication as long as this is feasible. When the patient has limited life expectancy but still can function if pain is controlled, we urge the use of neuroablative procedures when there is good expectancy of achieving pain relief.

The class of strong analgesics relieve pain but tend to produce apathy, somnolence, decreased appetite, and altered behavior. These drugs, generally, are unsatisfactory if the patient is to continue to be productive. The first drug in this group that we suggest is methadone (Dolophine) given orally. Fewer side effects are seen with this drug when compared to meperidine (Demerol) or morphine, and the duration of the analgesic effect is longer. A dosage of 5

or 10 mg every 6 to 8 hours will often suffice. It is especially important to administer these analgesics on a routine basis that has been predetermined by the professional managing the patient. Twycross[22] and others have pointed out that analgesic medication must be given before the effect of the previous dose has worn off and, therefore, often before the pain recurs. Generally, this will mean administration every 4 hours. If the pain is allowed to reemerge before administration of the analgesic, as on an "as needed" basis, higher dosage is required and the anxiety induced by this leads to more rapid drug tolerance and addiction.

Combinations of drugs may be more effective than a single analgesic. For the patient with progressive cancer and pain, the "Brompton's solution" may provide relief with oral dosage through the terminal stage. This mixture bearing the name of the Brompton Chest Hospital in Britain has been standardized for use in hospices there. The solution contains 10 mg of cocaine, 2.5 ml of pure ethyl alcohol, and a variable amount of chloroform water to make a solution of 20 ml when mixed with 2.5 mg morphine or up to 120 mg morphine. This solution should always be given with a phenothiazine.[12] While the Brompton's mixture has been satisfactory for some patients, for others it has not given adequate relief, and it is not well tolerated by many. A recent report by Melzak et al.[11] documents a double-blind study concluding that oral morphine alone is as effective as the Brompton mixture.

For a synopsis of useful drugs, see Table 30-1.

The parenteral use of strong narcotics is, of course, the last stage of progression of drug use for pain control. When combined with a phenothiazine (Thorazine), most patients will have relief of their pain. The usual drug doses recommended for the postoperative relief of acute pain are generally not adequate for the treatment of the chronic pain of cancer. Doses of narcotics such as morphine, meperidine, and butorphanol may be increased to the point of res-

TABLE 30-1. TABLE OF USEFUL DRUGS

Drugs	Notes
I. Mild Analgesics	
Aspirin	Better tolerated when buffered
Acetaminophen	Well tolerated
Propoxyphene with aspirin	May produce gastric upset
Propoxyphene napsylate	Better tolerated and may be mildly addictive
Ethoheptazine	Occasionally effective
Orphenadrine	Occasionally effective
Chlorzoxazone	Occasionally effective
II. Moderately Addictive Drugs Producing Moderate Analgesia	
Codeine	Good when used with aspirin
Pentazocine	More valuable injected, but many side effects
Oxycodone	Effective orally, but more addictive than others in this category
III. Strongly Addictive Drugs Producing Analgesia	
Methadone	First choice and inexpensive; effective orally
Meperidine	Not so good in severe pain
Morphine	Many side effects
Dilaudid	Produces euphoria
Butorphanol	May be less rapidly addictive and more like Pentazocine
Nalbuphine	May be less rapidly addictive and more like Pentazocine

piratory depression and in a few patients, adequate comfort still may not be obtained. The physician usually wishes that for these patients he had sought surgical relief of the pain at an earlier stage. The dosage of these medications at this stage can only be increased until agitation is overcome, at which point the patient spends most of his time sleeping and withdrawn. It seems infinitely better to resort to pain-relieving neural ablative procedures prior to this stage of development, even with the knowledge that total relief will not be obtained in all cases with surgery.

Surgical Therapy

The institution of surgical measures to attempt to relieve pain should not be relegated to the "last resort" category. Often a simple surgical maneuver may give excellent relief and may restore confidence and security to the patient and his family. In general, one should follow the rule of selecting the simplest procedure likely to produce pain relief. If a simple peripheral neurectomy or alcohol injection will produce adequate pain relief, one need not consider a central tractotomy. On the other hand, if we cannot reasonably expect a single procedure to be effective, we should not minimize our surgical approach but should ablate all the neural structures expected to convey pain from the lesion (e.g., perform multiple rhizotomies). However, the patient must have a life expectancy exceeding 3 months to advocate a major surgical denervation procedure.

While performing primary resection one should keep in mind the potential for later development of painful neuromas. Nerves should be cross-clamped, freed to the edge of the dissection, crushed, and a vascular clip placed across the proximal end. We often follow this by attempting to induce fibrosis with the injection of absolute alcohol through a 26 gauge needle. Next, the nerve end should be buried as deeply in the tissue as possible, preferably beneath a muscle. This procedure is particularly important for peripheral branches of the cervical plexus. The branches of the trigeminal nerve seem much less prone to produce neuromas. Avulsion of these branches at the time of operative intervention seems as good a maneuver as any to retard regrowth, although regeneration will occur if the patient survives long enough.

LOCAL BLOCKS AND PERIPHERAL NEURECTOMY

It has already been pointed out that when neoplastic disease lies within the trigeminal distribution, denervation may readily stop pain impulses. Local blocks in the trigeminal nerve distribution, therefore, may usually be expected to give pain relief if the tumor is in a circumscribed area in the distribution of that nerve branch. The technique of injection of alcohol into these branches may be found in many standard textbooks on nerve blocks, Injections into branches such as the infraorbital and supraorbital branches of the trigeminal nerve are simple and relatively safe. Anesthesia after such blocks may be expected to last for 6 months to a year. Neurectomy is an alternative modality of producing prolonged analgesia in specific areas. Although quite useful in trigeminal neuralgia, the limited areas of analgesia make this of limited use for pain from malignancies. The procedures, however, are generally innocuous and can be done with local anesthesia. The infraorbital nerve may be approached through an intraoral incision over the canine fossa or directly over the infraorbital foramen. The nerve is identified, grasped with a straight hemostat, and rolled about the instrument to avulse the nerve from the infraorbital

canal. The supraorbital nerve may be removed in similar fashion through a small incision just beneath the eyebrow.

Mental neurectomy may be done through a small mucoperiosteal flap, dissecting down to the mental foramen and avulsing the nerve there. The severe pain of cancer of the tongue may be controlled by resecting the lingual nerve in the floor of the mouth (Fig. 30-4). To determine the effectiveness of this procedure, local anesthesia can be used first, followed by resection of the nerve if adequate pain relief is obtained.

Results of neurectomies reported have varied, but in general the duration of analgesia is about twice that of the alcohol injections. Peripheral neurectomy is of particular value if alcohol injection fails, or when reinnervation occurs after initial successful alcohol block.

We no longer utilize the deep injection of major peripheral nerves with alcohol. It is preferable to the patients and to us to use percutaneous radiofrequency rhizotomy of the trigeminal ganglion. This procedure, which has been described in detail by Sweet and Wepsic,[19] is well tolerated by patients, more certain of producing the desired nerve block, and may be selective in producing hypalgesia while preserving touch sensation. The procedure is less predictive in neoplastic disease than in trigeminal neuralgia (tic douloureux) but is still effective in reducing pain in a majority of the patients with tumor in the trigeminal distribution.

Percutaneous radiofrequency Gassarian rhizotomy is accomplished by passing a temperature sensitive probe through an 18 gauge needle that has been guided through the foramen ovale into the region of the ganglion lying in Meckel's cave. Through radiographic control and electrical stimulation, the tip of the probe is adjusted within the ganglion until the desired portions are identified. A temperature-controlled lesion is then produced in the neural tissue in a graded fashion.

A similar percutaneous technique may be used to produce a lesion of the 9th and 10th nerves at the jugular foramen for relief

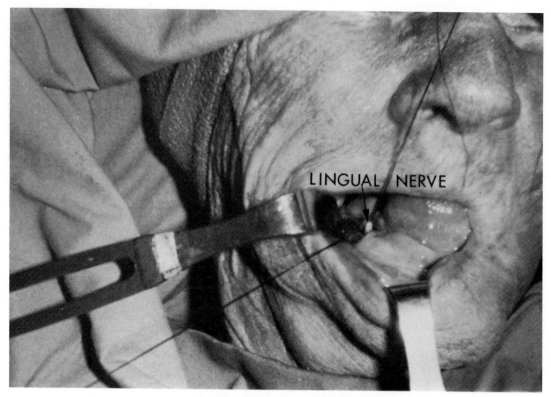

Fig. 30-4. Lingual nerve exposed in the floor of the mouth.

of throat pain[21] and to block the cervical nerve roots at the intervertebral foramina for relief of neck pain. Although this technique is not always successful, it is safe and relatively painless. We use intravenous Brevital to do this and find the procedure to be well tolerated by patients.

When the tumor lies in midline nonneural head or neck tissues, multiple innervation may make effective denervation very difficult. Neuroanatomic dissections have shown that cranial nerves VII to XII inclusive may interconnect with each other peripherally and with the upper cervical nerves.[25]

MAJOR SURGICAL NEUROABLATIVE PROCEDURES

If the patient has a life expectancy of 3 months or longer, operative neural ablative procedures may be considered for a few pa-

tients in whom the percutaneous procedures, relaxation techniques, and adequate oral analgesics do not give sufficient relief. The incidence of required operative intervention for pain in cancer of the head and neck varies from one institution to another. E. Harry Botterell from Toronto[1] reviewed the records of 1,813 patients receiving irradiation therapy for malignancy of the tonsil, tongue, lip, or jaw in the years 1953 to 1960. He found that 50 of these patients had been treated surgically for the relief of pain (2.7 percent). There were 31 intracranial sections of the 5th and 9th cranial nerves and the upper cervical sensory roots in various combinations.

Grant's report[2] of both peripheral alcohol block, sensory root avulsion, and intracranial neurectomy in 218 patients with cancer of the head and neck demonstrates the effectiveness of these treatment modalities. Of 58 patients referred for treatment of pain from cancer of the maxillary antrum and upper jaw, 9 required intracranial neurectomy and most of the others were given second or third division alcohol injection. Only 38 of the 58 cases had total relief of pain. Of 7 patients with cancer of the ethmoid and sphenoid sinuses, pain was not relieved in 3. Pain was relieved in 19 of 24 patients with tumors of the skin of the cheek. With cancer of the mandible, pain was relieved in 25 of 37 patients and partially relieved in 9 others. In cancer of the tongue, pain relief was obtained in only 12 of 21. Overall, Grant obtained pain relief in 60 percent and partial pain relief in another 14 percent. He could not achieve relief in 21 percent, and 5 percent died. The duration of follow-up was not given.

White and Sweet[25] have presented their analysis of 36 cases of tumors of the head and face treated exclusively by trigeminal rhizotomy. Half of the patients had recurrent pain and the average duration of relief when pain recurred before death was 4 months. They cautioned against doing only trigeminal rhizotomy when other nerves should be cut in cases when the lesion is situated so that the pain would soon spread outside the region innervated by the trigeminal. In a later review in 1977, Sweet[18] reported his results in 20 patients treated by percutaneous thermal rhizotomy in which he achieved anesthesia in 16 patients. In 4 patients he was unable to gain significant benefit, but the others had relief until death, and he could use the procedure in very poor risk patients who had a short life expectancy.

Multiple rhizotomy, including section of cranial nerves V, IX, and the upper part of X and upper cervical posterior roots, is advocated by many surgeons. Extensive rhizotomies such as these are more apt to give the desired result, as White and Sweet[25] have documented. Of 23 patients treated since their first report, only 2 did not have any immediate relief of pain. They conclude that especially in the patient with a slowly advancing cancer, the risk of the extensive rhizotomy required to give long, sustained relief may be well worthwhile.

TRACTOTOMY

The enthusiasm for incision into the descending spinal tract in the brain stem for relief of pain in the face and head seems to wax and wane. Weinberger and Grant[25] reported one of the early series for relief of tumor pain and had good success in six of nine patients, with partial relief in the other three. On the other hand, White and Sweet[25] reported early relief of pain in 12 of 19 patients but recurrence of pain later in 7 of the 12, which is unsatisfactory for such a major undertaking. They have now apparently abandoned the procedure in favor of either thalamotomy or frontal leucotomy. Others, however, have refined the technique and still advocate its use in selected cases. Speigel and Wycis[27] made stereotaxic lesions in the midbrain for various problems of pain. Their result of 31 percent successful relief of pain was rather discouraging. More recently Nashold[13] has pointed out that the midbrain procedure also has a significant complication rate.

FRONTAL LEUCOTOMY, CINGULUMOTOMY, AND THALAMOTOMY

The procedures on the cerebrum itself for relief of pain such as radiofrequency frontomedial leucotomy and cingulumotomy and sterotoxic frontothalamic section are available only in a few institutions. These procedures receive little general support in part because of the few opportunities to use them and in part because of the fear of producing major personality changes. The patients are often described as remaining indifferent to their pain, relieved of mental suffering but apathetic—an end result that can usually be obtained with large doses of phenothiazines and narcotics.

Similarly, Vernon Mark[25] has reported relief of pain from cancer of the head and neck with thalamotomy. Nineteen of 38 patients had excellent or good relief of pain and "in only one patient was there persistent apathy, confusion, and disorientation." Yet he admits that the complete relief of suffering in a patient with such disability as a fungating cancer of the mouth implies a certain inappropriateness of the patient's behavior. Some have felt that the good early results after thalamotomy have deteriorated with the passage of time.

Stimulation Techniques

The "rediscovery" of the beneficial effects of pulsed electrical impulses in alleviating pain has undergone extensive investigation since 1967.[24] We have used transcutaneous electrical stimulation to a limited extent about the head and neck with an occasional report of benefit. In general, this technique is too cumbersome and distracting to the patient for it to be used effectively on the head. Neurosurgical research interest in control of pain by electrical stimulation presently involves implantation of electrodes in the periventricular and periaqueductal areas. Hosobuchi[3] has reported that whereas this technique may be effective for pain in the caudal portion of the body, it does not often control pain in the head and neck. He also quotes Gybel's experience of failure with implanted stimulators to relieve pain in five of six cases with head and neck area pain.

PATIENT TEACHING AND PLAN FOR PAIN MANAGEMENT

Patient teaching is extremely important. The patient needs to understand what is wrong, why he hurts, and how long the pain may last. Patients want to know about their disease and are often afraid to ask. Their fantasies are often worse than the realities of their situation. It is better to encourage questions from the patient with the assurance that an honest answer is his right and that no question will be considered stupid. Reduction of anxiety is apparent when the avenues of communication are open.

The patient must be included in planning pain management and establishing realistic goals of treatment. The patient's input, cooperation, and participation are necessary for a pain-controlled state to be accomplished. The patient needs to be an active participant on the team rather than just a passive recipient of the team's efforts. A positive attitude on everyone's part helps to alleviate anxiety and improve the patient's quality of life.

Using several different, well-chosen methods of pain control is usually more effective and satisfactory than using one method, such as adding a new analgesic. Many adjunctive techniques of pain control are being explored in multidisciplinary pain clinics through the country. These include behavioral and environmental modification, relaxation, biofeedback, hypnosis, and acupuncture. Often the team approach is used involving anesthesiology, neurosurgery, radiology, physiology, psychology, sociology, and nursing. The time and cost factors are often high. Behavioral modification places emphasis on positive behavior that is incompatible with pain responses. Environmental modification is concerned with making the environment as conducive to comfort and pain relief as possible. Diversional activities are important and include "someone to talk to," hobbies, radio, etc. In the hospice experience it has been shown that "pain feels worse when it occupies the patient's whole attention."[22] Relaxation techniques can be taught to the patient, allowing him to loosen up and think pleasant thoughts. Cassette tapes are available for the patient to use while he is alone.

Biofeedback is being used successfully with some patients. It appears to give the patient an effective technique for self-regulation of pain. Four variables involved in biofeedback are shown to contribute to pain relief: distraction from the painful body site, suggestion that the pain will diminish, relaxation, and a sense of control over the pain.

Hypnosis is one of the oldest forms of treatment. Many theories attempt to explain hypnosis. No special personality attributes identify the hypnotist, nor is the person who can be hypnotized a typical type. It is widely accepted among hypnotists that "normal" people are easier to hypnotize than neurotics. Hypnosis may be specially adapted for the control of pain by using a set of instructions on relaxation techniques. Attention is directed at relaxing specific groups of muscles and controlling breathing. This may then be followed by special techniques to enhance feelings of better health, greater energy, and peacefulness. Some patients have obtained substantial pain relief with hypnosis.

Acupuncture, which has been used by Chinese physicians for over 5,000 years, is the practice of placing needles at certain acupuncture points on the body to achieve anesthesia. There seems to be little relationship between these points and the autonomic nervous system, and the effectiveness may be through "counterirritation."[7] The successful use of acupuncture to relieve pain is yet to be documented as being superior to the placebo effect. The placebo effect, however, should not be considered an artifact of pain control, but rather a useful adjunct when harnessed effectively. We have alluded to the importance of establishing rapport and a trusting relationship. With this accomplished, many more of our attempts at pain control seem to be effective. It may well be that the common factor in these alterations of motivational and cognitive components of pain is attributable to the influence on the powerful descending inhibitory neural pathways. The investigations of this inhibitory mechanism provide the framework for new approaches to control of pain. These psychological methods may decrease the intensity of pain and make it bearable.[9] Certainly it is evident that a response to a "placebo" does not mean the pain is "imaginary."

Cancer carries the connotation of prolonged pain and death. Once pain relief is accomplished, the health team tends to turn its attention to other problems of cancer control. However, the patient does not immediately forget his painful experience, especially if it was severe and frightening. If he is abandoned at this point, he may feel guilty or rejected because of his behavioral response to the pain he has suffered. Often this is a good time to provide information to the patient about his current status. He has been expected to assimilate a tremendous amount of information under very stressful conditions. He may cope with the emotional impact of his pain and disease by blocking out information rather than by understanding and accepting what he has been told. The patient should be given an opportunity to ask questions and express his feelings and discuss his pain. Talking about his feelings helps to put them into perspective and enables him to cope with reality.

Some patients will suffer pain for the rest of their lives. Some patients "need" to feel pain to manipulate others in their environment or for other secondary gain. The best therapy for these patients is to help them live with their pain—to be as comfortable as they will allow themselves to be and to make them feel they have achieved some quality and productivity in their lives.

The health professional must help the patient with his pain for as long as it exists. Albert Schweitzer once said, "But that I might save him from days of torture, *that* I consider my great and ever new challenge."

SUMMARY

The pain response to cancer will vary from patient to patient and in any particular patient from time to time. The professional team treating pain must take the time to evaluate the various physical and affective aspects of pain as well as to outline a comprehensive treatment plan. Irradiation, chemotherapy, analgesics, nerve blocks, or neural ablative procedures form the foundation for building a treatment plan. The complete plan, however, must include the assessment and successful support of personality factors that lead to a happier and more bearable life.

REFERENCES

1. Botterell, E. H. 1961. Second International Congress of Neurological Surgery. Excerpta Medical International Congress Series, 36: E26.

2. Grant, F. C. 1943. Surgical methods for relief of pain. Bulletin of the New York Academy of Medicine, 19: 373.

3. Hosobuchi, Y. 1978. Neurostimulation newsletter. Medtronics, 1: 1.

4. Johnson, E. W., Aseff, J., and Saunders, W. 1978. Physical treatment of pain and weakness following radical neck dissection. Ohio State Medical Journal, 74: 711.

5. Kerr, F. W. L. 1961. A mechanism to account for frontal headache in cases of posterior fossa tumors. Journal of Neurosurgery, 18: 605.

6. Knight, G. 1963. Post-traumatic occipital headache. Lancet, 1: 6.

7. Lipton, S. 1975. The treatment of intractable pain. Practitioner, 215: 461.

8. McCaffery, M. 1972. Nursing Management of the Patient with Pain. J. B. Lippincott, Philadelphia.

9. Melzack, R. 1973. The Puzzle of Pain. Penguin Books, Harmondsworth, England.

10. Melzack, R., and Wall, P. D. 1965. Pain mechanisms: a new theory. A gate control system modulates sensory input from the skin before it evokes pain perception and response. Science, 150: 971.

11. Melzack, R., Mount, B. M., and Gordon, J. M. 1979. The Brompton mixture versus morphine solution given orally: Effects on pain. Canadian Medical Association Journal, 120: 435.

12. Mount, B. M., Ajemian, I., and Scott, J. F. 1976. Use of the Brompton mixture in treating the chronic pain of malignant disease. Canadian Medical Association Journal, 115: 122.

13. Nashold, B. S., Wilson, W. P., and Slaughter, D. G. 1969. Stereotaxic midbrain lesions for central dysesthesia and phantom pain. Journal of Neurosurgery, 30: 116.

14. Robertson, S., Goodell, H. and Wolff, H. G. 1947. Headache. The teeth as a source of headache and other pain. Archives of Neurology and Psychiatry, 57: 277.

15. Sachs, E., Jr. 1968. The role of the nervus intermedius in facial neuralgia. Journal of Neurosurgery, 28: 54.

16. Snyder, S. H. 1977. Opiate receptors and internal opiates. Scientific American, 236: 44.

17. Spann, J. L., Sandlin, M. E., and Van-Wormer, D. 1977. A surgical technique for resecting malignancies invading the facial nerve and petrous pyramid. Journal of Surgical Oncology, 9: 315.

18. Sweet, W. H. 1977. Trigeminal neuralgias. In Alling, C. C., and Mahan, P. E., Eds.: Facial Pain. 2nd edn. Lea and Febiger, Philadelphia, 89.

19. Sweet, W. H., and Wepsic, J. G. 1974. Controlled thermocoagulation of trigeminal ganglion and rootlets for differential destruction of pain fibers. 1. Trigeminal neuralgia. Journal of Neurosurgery, 40: 143.

20. Taub, A. 1973. Relief of postherpetic neuralgia with psychotropic drugs. Journal of Neurosurgery, 39: 235.

21. Tew, J. M., Jr., and Keller, J. T. 1977. Percutaneous rhizotomy in the treatment of intractable facial pain. In Lee, J. F., Ed.: Pain Management. Williams and Wilkins, Baltimore, 145.

22. Twycross, R. G. 1975. Diseases of the central nervous system. Relief of terminal pain. British Medical Journal, 4: 212.

23. Wall, P. D. 1978. The gate control theory of pain mechanisms. A re-examination and restatement. Brain, 101: 1

24. Wall, P. D., and Sweet, W. H. 1967. Temporary abolition of pain in man. Science, 155: 108.

25. White, J. C., and Sweet, W. H. 1969. Pain and the Neurosurgeon: A Forty-Year Experience. Charles C Thomas, Springfield, Ill.

26. Wirth, E. P., Jr., and Van Buren, J. M. 1971. Referral of pain from dural stimulation in man. Journal of Neurosurgery, 34: 630.

27. Wycis, H. T., and Spiegel, E. A. 1962. Long-range results in the treatment of intractable pain by stereotaxic midbrain surgery. Journal of Neurosurgery 19: 101.

31 | Nursing Care of the Head and Neck Cancer Patient

Karen Jean Hannahs, R.N., B.S.N.
Jill A. Hooper, R.N., B.S.N.
Barbara A. Sigler, R.N., M.N.Ed.

INTRODUCTION

Care of the head and neck cancer patient is one of the most challenging aspects of oncology nursing. Advances are being made that influence the treatment and rehabilitation of these patients, providing the opportunity for a longer life while improving the quality of that life.

People are identified by their appearance and their speech. Cancer of the head and neck and/or its treatment may affect these areas resulting in physical alterations that cannot be hidden well.

The nurse working with these patients must have the self-assurance that comes from knowledge of oncology in general and specific knowledge of the upper air and food passages. The care provided must reflect an attitude of compassion without pity, optimism without false hope, and support without dependence.

THE SURGICAL PATIENT

Preoperative Considerations[5]

On the patient's admission to the hospital, the nurse should thoroughly assess the patient's symptoms, his health habits and practices, occupation, living conditions, and support systems. Some insight should be gained about the patient's use of his voice in his job,

the financial status of the patient and family, and the patient's future potential in the same job. While taking the health history, the nurse should question the patient and family about smoking and drinking habits, which are common to most head and neck cancer patients. The nurse may also use this interview to evaluate the knowledge that the patient and his family have about the patient's condition and their feelings about cancer. These feelings will affect their acceptance of the diagnosis and treatment and may also alter the postoperative and rehabilitative course. The nurse utilizes this data to formulate a problem list and initiate referrals to other health team members who may help to meet the patient's needs.

DIAGNOSTIC EVALUATION

Preoperative teaching begins upon admission. The patient and support persons should be informed of all testing that will be necessary, why the tests are being performed, and what is involved in the evaluation. Routine evaluations are performed on all patients prior to surgery. These include a chest x-ray to establish a baseline and to rule out pulmonary disease. A more detailed diagnostic workup may begin prior to the biopsy or may be deferred until a positive histologic diagnosis is made. Additional radiographic studies may be ordered to further evaluate tumor size and involvement.

These may be plain films, tomograms, or contrast dye studies. Alleviation of fears related to overexposure to radiation is usually the only teaching required prior to extensive radiologic studies. The patient requiring contrast dye studies such as laryngograms must be informed that in order to prevent aspiration he will be allowed nothing to eat or drink for 6 to 8 hours before the study. The contrast dye is given by drip following topical anesthesia, with repeated x-rays taken to evaluate the tumor. Most of the dyes used contain iodine; therefore, if the patient has a known allergy to this the radiology department must be notified. Following the dye studies, the patient is observed for aspiration and delayed allergic reactions. Once the gag reflex has returned, the patient may begin oral feedings. Cine-esophagram or a barium swallow test may be ordered to evaluate the patient's swallowing and to determine the extent of the tumor.

Scans of bone, brain, liver, and spleen may be indicated for patients with advanced lesions if distant metastasis is suspected. These scans employ radioisotopes that emit gamma rays identified by the scanner. Patients are informed prior to the procedure that a radioactive material will be either ingested or injected 2 to 3 hours prior to the scanning. The amount of radioactivity absorbed from the isotope is negligible, producing about the same radiation exposure as a chest x-ray. Patient allergies, especially to iodine preparations, are investigated and if an allergy exists, the nuclear medicine department is notified. The patient will be required to maintain exact positions for the scanning procedure, which may prove uncomfortable. The positions are important in obtaining the results and must be maintained to avoid repeating the procedure. The patient is instructed to report any discomfort to the technician. The only anticipated discomfort occurs at the venopuncture site, where slight burning may be felt at the time of radioisotope injection. Once the patient returns to the nursing unit, he is observed for signs of respiratory distress and allergic reactions. These symptoms are rare

and are not routinely expected following the scan. The patient's family and visitors should not be concerned about radiation hazard from the materials used to scan the patient.

Computerized tomography (CT scan) may be requested to localize intracranial lesions or extension of head and neck tumors. The procedure is completed in 30 to 60 minutes and contrast medium may be used, although the CT scan can be done without the contrast medium. The patient must remain immobile during the procedure to ensure accurate recordings. Sedation may be given if the patient cannot cooperate. Patient discomfort is minimal, and there are no restrictions following the procedure.

Complete blood counts including differential and platelet count, along with serum electrolytes, nitrogen compounds, liver function studies, and urinalysis provide a baseline survey as well as an evaluation of systemic pathology. The patient's blood should also be typed and crossmatched prior to surgery if a large blood loss is anticipated.

An immunologic survey and more extensive blood chemistry evaluation may be required for patients receiving chemotherapy or immunotherapy. These additional studies will be discussed later in this chapter in conjunction with these modes of treatment.

The biopsy may be done before or after the diagnostic procedures previously discussed. Prior to admission to the hospital, the physician prepares the patient and family for the biopsy, but the information must be reinforced by the nursing staff.

The biopsy may be done under local or general anesthesia depending upon physician choice and patient condition. It may be performed in the physician's office, the nursing unit, or in the operating room. A small piece of tissue is removed for histologic evaluation. If the biopsy is to be performed under general anesthesia, the patient is instructed to take nothing by mouth for 6 to 8 hours prior to the procedure. Once he has recovered from the anesthesia, the patient may begin taking feedings by mouth. Some discomfort may be present at the biopsy site or the throat may be sore from the endotracheal tube. Analgesics should be made available, with acetaminophen or aspirin usually offering sufficient relief.

MULTIDISCIPLINARY TEAM REFERRALS

Referrals to other members of the health care team are made during the preoperative period according to hospital protocol, anticipated surgical procedure, and identified patient needs. An audiologic evaluation, with or without eustachian tube function tests, is ordered for patients who will have procedures affecting their speech or hearing. This evaluation is also important to compare changes in hearing that occur following the procedure or following the administration of certain ototoxic antibiotics or chemotherapeutic agents.

Good oral hygiene is imperative to the head and neck cancer patient anticipating any of the treatment modalities. Preoperative referrals to the maxillofacial prosthodontist and the dental hygienist will provide the patient with the service as well as the instruction on future oral hygiene. The maxillofacial prosthodontist is also responsible for taking the appropriate impressions, both intraoral and facial, if the fabrication of prostheses and fluoride carriers will be necessary.

The hospital's social service department is another area that should provide preoperative consultation. The social worker can begin early during the hospitalization to identify and help solve existing or potential psychosocial problems of the patient and family. By developing rapport with the patient prior to treatment, the social worker will be able to help the health care team develop plans for discharge of the patient. The social worker can evaluate the financial status of the patient, determine employability, and offer resources available to the patient and family and may also help with the bewildering array of forms to be filled out for insurance and other benefits.

Due to a common history of heavy alcohol consumption, in addition to symptoms of pain and difficulty in swallowing, the patient may exhibit a substantial weight loss. A nutritional assessment, performed by the staff nurse, a clinical nurse oncologist, or a nutritionist, should be completed early in the hospital period. Daily weights, anthropometric measurements, and caloric and protein intake recordings should be routinely kept on all patients. The nutritionist can work directly with the patient and family but must also participate in patient conferences to update the health care team about the patient's progress.

The speech pathologist will obtain preoperative recordings of the patient's "normal" or pretreatment voice. This will provide an opportunity to know the patient while he can still communicate orally and will aid in developing a plan for postoperative speech rehabilitation.

Patients who will be undergoing a radical neck dissection should be referred to a physical therapist or occupational therapist for range of motion and muscle strength evaluation. These measurements will be utilized during the postoperative period in developing a specific exercise program to decrease the severity of shoulder drop and limitation of movement following a radical neck dissection. The physical therapy or respiratory therapy department may also be requested to do chest physiotherapy for the patient prone to pulmonary problems due to cigarette smoking.

All preoperative consultants work as part of the health care team to provide the patient and family with psychosocial support and counseling to enable them to cope with the anticipated treatment regime. In addition, the team can begin rehabilitative plans early in an attempt to return the patient to as normal a life as is possible.

PSYCHOLOGICAL PREPARATION

Education of the patient and family regarding the anticipated surgery is as important as the testing and referrals. Information concerning the surgical procedure, equipment to be used, and postoperative appear-

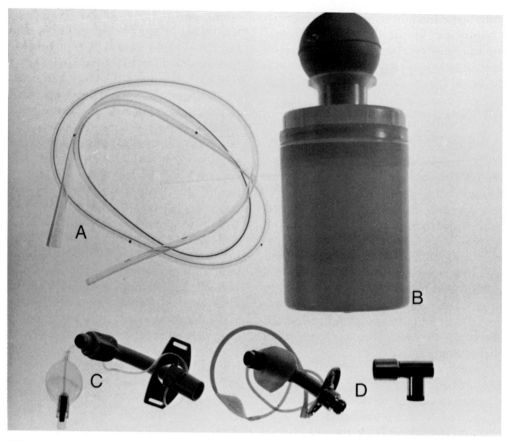

Fig. 31-1. Equipment on teaching tray for head and neck cancer patients includes: A, naso-gastric tube; B, feeding set; C, Shiley tracheostomy tube, and; D, cuffed metal tube with adaptor.

ance is furnished in as much detail as is required by the patient and family. The physical aspects of care are discussed using diagrams, illustrations, models, and teaching trays. Most patients have a difficult time visualizing the anatomic variations that will be created by surgically removing or altering a structure. Posters illustrating normal and surgically altered anatomy will make the learning easier for the patient and will allow for more coordinated teaching on the part of the nurse. If a model is used, incisions can be indicated, drainage catheters and tracheostomy tubes can be inserted, and dressings can be applied. The teaching tray may contain samples of tubes, catheters, and dressings so the patient can see and feel the equipment he will be using following sur-

gery (Fig. 31-1). Explanations of nursing procedures which will be performed post-operatively and the sensations the patient will feel are included in the preoperative teaching and are also reinforced prior to performing the procedure.

The psychological aspects of the patient are integrated with all care provided from the moment the patient is first seen by a health team member. Initial areas of concern to patients and families are usually related to the diagnosis of cancer. *Cancer* continues to be a term associated with pain, mutilation, punishment, and death. The health care team must work individually with each patient and family member to help each one cope with the diagnosis. We must offer hope but be careful not to cultivate unrealistic expectations. In addition to the diagnosis, there may be great concern regarding the treatment modality selected. Fears of mutilation, pain, loss of control, and death are associated with all modes of cancer therapy and these fears must be handled on an individual basis.

Loss of normal communication skills, fear of not being able to eat regular foods, altered body image, and problems of sexuality are other sources of anxiety for the patient and family. Ways of communicating after surgery must be reviewed with the patient. Initially, every effort will be made to anticipate the patient's needs. Later in the postoperative period, communication by writing will be encouraged. If the patient is illiterate, flash cards should be developed and used by the patient to indicate his needs. Even with permanent speech loss, other methods of verbal communication can be available to the patient (Fig. 31-2).

The ability to eat normally after surgery will be dependent upon the extent of the tumor and the surgical procedure anticipated. If the possibility of normal postoperative swallowing is limited, other ways of taking in nourishment should be thoroughly discussed with the patient. In some cases, the status of postoperative deglutition cannot be anticipated prior to surgery.

The alteration of body image and sexuality may be an area of concern to both the patient and family. During the preoperative phase, most patients are concerned about "surviving the operation" and eliminating the cancer; consequently, fear of body image alteration is usually not expressed until after surgery. Body image changes will occur with many head and neck cancer operations. It must be stressed to the patient that every possible rehabilitative measure will be taken to minimize the change but that removing the cancer is the primary goal. Ex-

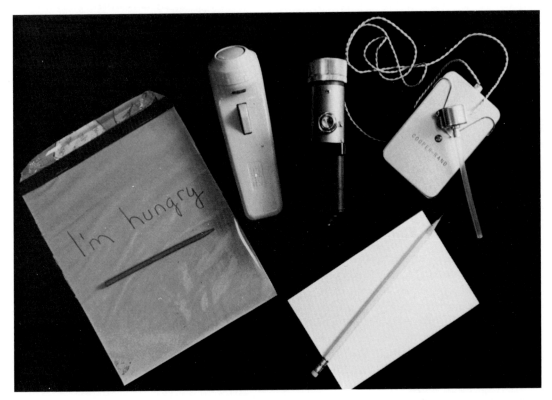

Fig. 31-2. Communication devices used for the postoperative tracheostomy and aphonic patient: Magic Slate, two models of neck-type artificial larynges, the Cooper-Rand electrolarynx, and pad with pencil.

planations regarding body parts that will be removed may also be helpful in minimizing the fear. Reinforcement should be offered to the patient and spouse regarding appearance and the ability to function. Through displaying affection, the spouse can do much to alleviate the fear expressed by the patient. The patient is still the same person loved prior to the diagnosis. Special counseling may be necessary to help the spouse cope with this problem.

Operating room and postanesthesia room procedures should be reviewed with the patient and family. This may be done by the staff nurse or a nurse from these specialized areas. If the patient will be transferred to a specialized unit or intensive care area after surgery, the patient and family should be notified. Explanation of procedures and policies in these areas may be discussed by any health team member. A nurse from the transfer unit may assist in the preoperative teaching regime to help alleviate fears the patient may have regarding transfer.

Prior to surgery, the patient is allowed nothing to eat or drink for at least 8 hours. A bedtime sedation is encouraged to help alleviate anxiety. Nurses will find it advantageous to plan the evening and night duties to allow for extra time to be spent with the patient preoperatively. Verbalization of fear may be held until the last moment and the nurse will need time to provide the patient with reassurance and explanation.

Postoperative Considerations

Immediately after surgery, the head and neck cancer patient requires very specialized care and, therefore, is on occasion admitted to an intensive care setting where the emphasis will be placed on airway maintenance, wound care, mouth care, fluid balance, and general comfort. While the patient is in this environment nursing goals include keeping the patient free of any preventable complications, minimizing pain and discomfort, and providing emotional support.[1a]

Specialized equipment is necessary to attain these goals. In addition to the routine intensive care unit (ICU) equipment, oxygen nebulization and sources of negative pressure are required because tracheostomy suctioning, wound drainage, and nasogastric tube drainage are expected. These devices may be either portable or wall-mounted units and are usually necessary for a minimum of 24 hours. The wound suctioning pressure should be approximately 80 to 120 mmHg and the negative pressure for tracheostomy and nasogastric suctioning should be approximately 40 to 60 mmHg.

TRACHEOSTOMY CARE*

The care of the airway is the most demanding of the special procedures, since many of these patients have a tracheostomy and are very apprehensive. Keeping the airway free of secretions is essential and accomplished most effectively by encouraging the patient to cough. This not only clears the airway but expands the lungs to prevent atelectasis and pneumonia. When secretions are present and coughing is ineffective—a situation that occurs in the presence of a tracheostomy—the secretions must be suctioned from the trachea. The need for this procedure can be evaluated by placing the hand 1 inch from the patient's tracheostomy and assessing the amount of air exhaled. When suctioning the trachea, sterile equipment should be used and the following rules adhered to: apply suction only upon withdrawal of the catheter; rotate the catheter as it is being withdrawn; and apply suction for no more than 10 seconds and then allow the patient to ventilate to replenish the oxygen supply (oxygen or resuscitation bag may be necessary). Gentle suctioning of the oral and nasal cavities may be beneficial; however, if performed prior to tracheostomy suctioning, catheters must be changed.

The choice of tracheostomy tube will

---

*Throughout this chapter, the authors refer to tracheostomy as the temporary or permanent surgical opening in the trachea.

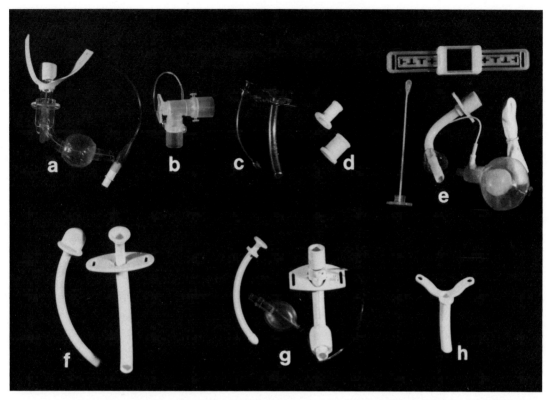

Fig. 31-3. Tracheostomy tubes commonly used after head and neck surgery: a, American tracheostomy tube; b, Swivel connector for a; c, Jackson metal tracheostomy tube; d, stoma buttons; e, Lanz controlled-pressure cuffed tracheostomy tube; f, Dow Corning Silastic tracheostomy tube—Moore design; g, Shiley low-pressure cuffed tracheostomy tube; h, Dow Corning Silastic tracheostomy tube—Aberdeen design.

vary according to the physician's preference (Fig. 31-3). Initially, it will be necessary to use a tracheostomy tube with an inner cannula for easy cleaning and an outside extension to keep the airway patent if bulky dressings are used. A tracheostomy tube with a high-volume, low-pressure cuff may be used to prevent aspiration and to provide a seal between the tube and trachea for assisted and controlled ventilation. It is extremely important that the cuff be inflated just enough to seal the leak. Overinflation of the cuff may result in necrosis of the tracheal mucosa and stenosis of the trachea.

While the patient is in the intensive care unit, tracheostomy tube and stoma hygiene is limited if a large neck dressing is present. It should be noted that these dressings may overlap even an extended tracheostomy tube and occlude the airway, and thus require strict observation to prevent this occlusion. The inner cannula should be cleansed at least every 4 hours to maintain the patency of the airway. Various solutions may be used to clean the tracheostomy tube, including hydrogen peroxide with or without water. A nylon-bristle brush is safest to use within the inner cannula as it does not leave a residue. After thorough scrubbing, the inner cannula should be rinsed with water and replaced within the outer cannula. Once the neck dressings are removed, more thorough cleansing of the skin and outer cannula is possible. The neck plate of the outer cannula and skin around the tracheostomy are cleansed with hydrogen peroxide and cotton-tipped applicators to loosen any crusts. The area is then rinsed well with water or saline to prevent skin irritation. An antibiotic ointment may be applied if skin irritation is observed. A dry gauze sponge may also be used under the neck plate of the tracheostomy tube to prevent irritation from the tube and excess secretions.

In changing the ties of the outer cannula, the nurse must secure the ties to prevent the tube from sliding up and down in the trachea but must leave them loose enough to allow fingertips under the ties, thereby avoiding excess pressure and facilitating cleansing of the skin beneath the tube collar. New ties should be secured before the soiled ties are removed in order to prevent dislodging of the tube, which may precipitate a medical emergency.

The initial removal of the entire tracheostomy tube is the responsibility of the physician. Future changes of the tube as a nursing function are dependent upon the hospital policy and physician's preference.

Stoma covering provides filter, humidi-

fication, and cosmesis for the patient. Various covers may be used including crocheted covers, gauze pads folded over cord tape, and commercially made foam rubber shields (Fig. 31-4).

Because the normal humidification system of the body is bypassed in a tracheostomy patient, supplemental humidification is essential. This can be accomplished by using oxygen nebulization or a portable humidifier. If secretions tend to be tenacious or if the patient forms mucous crusts, several drops of sterile normal saline solution can be placed directly into the stoma to loosen crusts and moisten the mucosa.

When the patient is able to observe the tracheostomy site, the nurse should begin teaching the patient to perform tracheostomy care. At this time, the procedure is performed using a clean technique rather than a sterile procedure, but aseptic methods must be emphasized. The patient can be taught to clean the inner cannula as well as

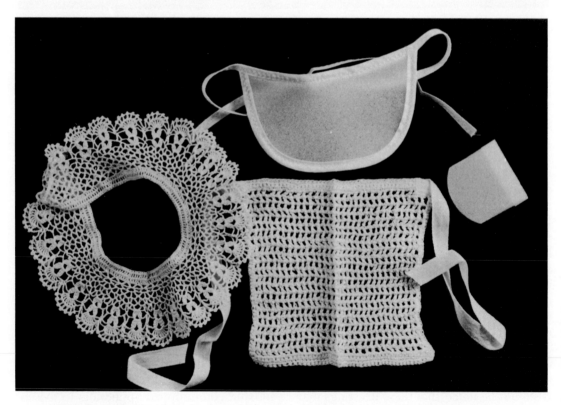

Fig. 31-4. Handmade and commercial stoma shields to be worn after laryngectomy.

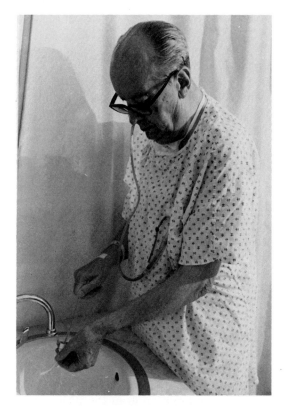

Fig. 31-5. Self-care is encouraged after head and neck surgery including cleaning inner cannula of tracheostomy tube.

the skin around the stoma (Fig. 31-5). If the patient has had a laryngectomy and a tube is required, changing and cleaning of the entire tube can be started after the initial tube removal.

Teaching the patient tracheostomy suction techniques will depend upon physician preference and hospital policy. Deep tracheal suctioning should be performed only by a professional health care worker, as trauma to the tracheal mucosa may occur. It is advisable to emphasize deep breathing and coughing techniques rather than suctioning to the patient.

WOUND CARE

Proper wound care in the immediate postoperative phase requires astute nursing observation. Large neck dressings applied after surgery prevent direct wound care. The neck dressing must be observed for excessive drainage and the wound catheter for adequate drainage. Hematoma and seroma formation, loss of flap viability, infection, chylous fistula, and carotid rupture are some of the major wound complications. The skin flap should be warm, natural in color, and without drainage. If the flap is accessible for observation, its viability may be checked by pressing on the flap to blanch it and then observing the length of time it takes to return to its natural color. Observation for infection involves careful monitoring of the patient's vital signs, laboratory data, and the appearance of the wound, noting the presence of any odor or drainage. A chylous fistula is the result of a lymphatic leak (usually from the thoracic duct on the left side) and can frequently be detected by observing the amount and characteristics of wound drainage. Lymph fluid is clear if the patient is not being fed but is opaque and milky in appearance if the patient is being fed. Fluid and electrolyte imbalances occur in the presence of a chyle leak; therefore, monitoring of the laboratory data is essential.

Nursing intervention in the management of the surgical site involves care of the neck drains and dressings. The hemovac tubes usually drain blood or fluid in the first 48 to 72 hours. Their patency is maintained by continuous suctioning and routine straightening, "milking," and aspirating (using a blunt-tipped needle). The amount and characteristics of the drainage should be monitored and recorded. The catheters remain in the wound until minimal or no drainage is noted.

The outer dressings will be removed by the physician on the second or third day. Until that time, drainage on the dressing should be noted. Reinforcement of the dressing may be required if loosening or increased drainage is observed. Once the dressing is removed, the suture line may be cleansed with hydrogen peroxide and water and an antibiotic ointment applied.

Edema can become a problem even in the early postoperative period. Proper positioning is helpful. The head of the bed should be elevated at least 45°, and the patient should avoid sleeping on the operated side in order to prevent fluid accumulation. If a pedicle skin flap is present, it usually is immobilized by the pressure dressing, and the patient's head is tilted toward the flap to avoid tension. Sometimes pillows, sand bags, and towel rolls help in maintaining the proper position comfortably and can aid in supporting skin tube pedicles to avoid "kinking" or pressure that can decrease the blood supply. Edema can also be increased as the result of an excessively tight dressing that may need to have its edges cut, according to physician's orders or hospital policy.

If skin grafts have been used during surgery, the graft and donor sites will require care. Care of the graft site includes keeping the edges clean, reinforcing the outer dressing as indicated, and assessing for fluid under the graft site. The donor site will be covered with fine mesh gauze, or a similar dressing, with a larger outer dressing in place. A bed cradle should be placed over the foot of the bed to prevent pressure from the bed linens. In addition, pajama bottoms can be cut to prevent irritation to the donor site. Once the outer dressing is removed, the inner dressing is exposed to the air for drying. A heat lamp can also be used to enhance this process. Once the donor site is healed (10 days to 2 weeks), the dressing is removed. If this cannot be done easily, the patient can soak in a warm bath to aid removal. The inner dressing should never be forcibly removed.

COMPLICATED WOUNDS

The patient with a fistula is a complex nursing care challenge. Fistulas are a "let down" to the patient, as they create a lengthier hospitalization. Therefore, nursing care of the patient with a fistula includes reassurance. Fistula care entails cleansing with hydrogen peroxide, packing, inserting a drain, and covering adequately with external dressing. This may vary within institutions, as most physicians write orders specifically for their own technique of fistula care. The primary objective is to promote fistula closure from within.

Open wounds require cleansing, packing, and covering in a manner similar to fistula care. Packing may be soaked in various solutions such as antibiotic, acriflavine, Dakin's, or normal saline, thus providing atraumatic debridement and cleansing of the wound.

Paraoral defects often require innovative coverings during the intermediate postoperative period. The threat of grave change in appearance is very real to the head and neck cancer patient. It is important that the nurse gradually introduce the patient to the defect, utilizing the patient's input as a guideline to readiness. The nurse's own reaction to the defect must be self-acknowledged, since acceptance or rejection from the nurse will be observed by the patient. Any expression of revulsion or shock by the nurse could be detrimental to the patient.

Rupture of the carotid artery becomes a potential complication in the presence of wound breakdown, fistula, necrosis, loss of flap, and exposure of the vessel. A mere trickle of blood may be the first warning signal and it can occur from days to weeks postoperatively. Specific nursing precautions can prevent a devastating experience. The patient who has a potential for carotid rupture should be close to the nursing station, be typed and crossmatched, and have at the bedside the following items: hemostats, intravenous (IV) administration set with solution, cut-down tray, suture set, and cuffed tracheostomy tube. If carotid rupture occurs, the nurse should apply firm pressure, start an IV or increase the fluid rate of the present IV, remain with the patient, and call for help.[4]

MOUTH CARE

When the surgical site is in the oral cavity, irrigations are vital in keeping the operative area free from debris. Frequent gentle oral cleansing is vital to the maintenance of a clean surgical area and promotion of healing.

The technique of mouth irrigations varies in institutions; however, the goals are universal: keeping the mouth clean, stimulating blood supply, reducing edema, alleviating pain and discomfort, controlling unpleasant odors, and aiding in prevention or resolution of infection.

The nurse should assist the patient in avoiding trauma to exposed tissue. Dentures should be removed prior to irrigations. When irrigating the mouth, the nurse should keep in mind the following: the objectives of the irrigation, the location of the surgical wound, and any special considerations peculiar to this patient.

Types of irrigation solutions include: hydrogen peroxide solution (one-half hydrogen peroxide, one-half water), salt and soda solution (1 teaspoon salt and 1 teaspoon soda per liter of warm water), and antibiotic solutions.

Equipment used in routine mouth care for the patient with a surgically treated oral cavity includes the irrigation set-up, comprising an enema bag and a rubber catheter (Fig. 31-6A). The more complex the wound or reconstruction of the oral cavity, the more complex the irrigation. Defects may be cleaned with a power spray apparatus, using saline or an antibiotic solution (Fig. 31-6B). The nurse should avoid displaying apprehension concerning the use of any of the equipment, as the patient may sense the nurse's anxiety and become more apprehensive of the procedure. Thorough explanation prior to power spraying will contribute immeasurably to the patient's acceptance and allay anxiety. Power spray should be performed in the treatment room so that the patient will not associate the treatment with his pleasant hospital room environment. This also provides additional privacy and prevents soiling the patient's room.

Water Piks are often used for mouth irrigations in the head and neck cancer patient. When utilizing the Water Pik, the nurse should be aware that the pulsation of the water is piercing and forceful and may injure a suture line or a skin graft. Therefore, the apparatus should initially be on a low setting unless otherwise ordered by the physician. Often upon discharge, the patient is sent home with this irrigation apparatus, so initial instructions regarding this type of irrigation will orient the patient toward self-care (Fig. 31-7).

The patient with an oral surgical defect poses another challenge to the nurse. In the early postoperative phase, the defect may be

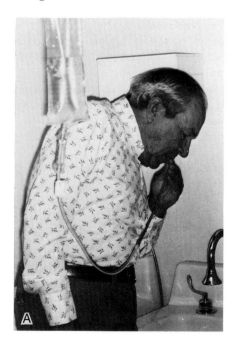

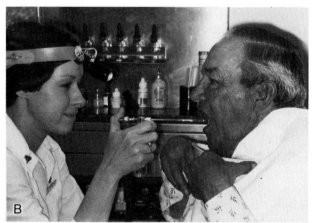

Fig. 31-6. (A) Salt and soda irrigations for oral hygiene. (B) Power spraying for additional prophylaxis.

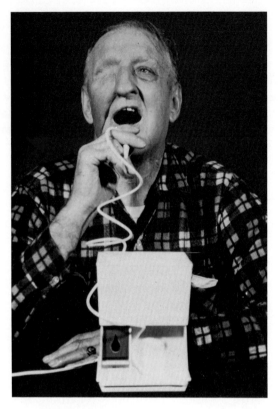

Fig. 31-7. Patient using a Water Pik to clean maxillary cavity following radical maxillectomy.

without a prosthesis and may require packing. The purpose of packing may be twofold: debridement and occlusion (the latter of which improves speech and facilitates oral intake). A wet-to-dry dressing is primarily utilized for packing; however, this is usually at the physician's discretion. The patient should be taught to insert the packing as soon as possible, so as to accomplish self-care.

The patient with an intraoral prosthesis should be taught the basic principles of prosthesis care. These include removing the prosthesis at night, keeping the prosthesis in water when out of the mouth to prevent drying or warping, and avoiding exposure to extreme temperature.

GENERAL CONSIDERATIONS

Additional care for the head and neck cancer patient is routine during the postopera-

tive period (monitoring of vital signs, intake and output, weight, etc.). The administration of IV alcohol may be indicated, since a significant number of these patients have a history of heavy alcohol consumption.

A word should also be said about the general comfort of the patient when he first arrives from the operating room. Generally he has very little pain but when medication is needed, it should be given immediately. *Caution should be used, however, in the case of a restless, struggling patient, since he may be suffering from hypoxia instead of pain.* Prompt nursing action is vital. The patient's airway should be evaluated and blood gas levels obtained. Sedation is *not* indicated until hypoxia is ruled out. Another aid to the patient's postoperative comfort is getting him out of bed (usually within 24 hours) and ambulating. His physical strength will return sooner, he coughs more productively, and his physical and psychological sense of well being is greatly enhanced.

NUTRITION

Proper nutrition of the head and neck cancer patient is vital for tissue healing. It may consist of parenteral therapy, enteral therapy, or both.

Intravenous Hyperalimentation (Total Parenteral Nutrition). The primary purpose of intravenous hyperalimentation (IVH) is to achieve and maintain normal body composition. In the head and neck cancer patient, this requires the infusion of sufficient calories and protein to maintain daily requirements, to correct preexisting deficits in the body, and to develop positive nitrogen balance in the patient. This nutritional solution is infused through a catheter inserted into the subclavian vein. This may result in the indwelling catheter becoming a potential source of infection. Nursing considerations of the patient receiving hyperalimentation include avoiding contamination of the catheter entry site, maintaining sterility by use of an occlusive dressing, maintaining patency of IV tubing, and maintaining proper infusion rate.

In preparing the patient for hyperalimentation it is important that the nurse explain the procedure. The patient should be placed in the Trendelenberg position and remain as motionless as possible during the procedure. The patient should be told that he will feel a local anesthetic agent injected into the skin and a sensation of pressure as the catheter is inserted. The patient also should be instructed not to touch the sterile drapes that will be placed on his shoulder during the procedure.

After the subclavian catheter is in place, the nurse should place an occlusive, sterile dressing over the entry site. This dressing must remain dry, and should be changed at least every other day. Sterile dressing changes will aid in preventing infection and promote longevity of the catheter.

For cleaning the catheter site, the following suggestions may be helpful. The patient should be in bed and the dressing removed by the nurse. Observation of the insertion site and examination for leakage, edema, skin reactions, and kinks in the catheter are necessary. The skin should be cleansed with a solvent such as acetone or ether that removes adhesive as well as skin oils and then scrubbed with a 2 percent iodine tincture or Merthiolate solution. An antibiotic ointment and small sterile dressing are then placed on the entry site. Tincture of benzoin is placed around the dressing, the IV tubing changed, and a large occlusive dressing replaced. The patient with a subclavian catheter can be active and ambulatory during this period of therapy.[2]

The nurse must be aware that IVH is a potentially dangerous method of nutritional therapy. The prescribed rate of infusion must be maintained in order to prevent complications. In addition, laboratory evaluations must be done frequently to determine the patient's metabolic needs. Urine specimens for glycosuria must be obtained every 6 hours to determine glucose usage.

Pain in the shoulder, swelling and/or edema over the puncture site, and swelling of the neck and/or face are signs of infiltration and the physician should be notified if they occur. A fever may indicate allergic reaction, infected catheter site, contaminated solution, or sepsis. Any temperature greater than 101°F should be reported to the physician.

Enteral Therapy is often the mechanism of nutrition utilized for the head and neck cancer patient. This mode of treatment involves a nasogastric (NG) tube, feeding esophagostomy, or gastrostomy.

If an NG tube is to be placed, a small (e.g., size 14 Levin) tube should be used. The nurse should confirm the position of the tube either by aspirating the stomach contents, or by placing a stethoscope on the abdomen, injecting air into the NG tube, and listening for air injection in the stomach. The depth of insertion varies with the individual patient, but the following guideline may be used: the NG tube should be inserted to a depth approximately equal to the length of an imaginary line running horizontally from the tip of the patient's nose to his ear and from the ear diagonally down to the xiphoid process of the sternum. Placement of the tube in the distal end of the esophagus rather than through the gastroesophageal sphincter usually prevents reflux and esophageal irritation. If the patient complains of epigastric pain and/or burning, the NG tube may be in too far. This can be corrected by pulling the tube back into the esophagus, which should cause the discomfort to disappear rapidly.

Nasogastric tube feedings should be administered while the patient is in a sitting position (Fig. 31-8). The food should be stored in the refrigerator to avoid spoilage and warmed to room temperature prior to administration in order to prevent abdominal cramping and diarrhea. The patient should be observed for aspiration from regurgitated feedings. This can be prevented by proper tube and patient positioning and by keeping the cuff of the tracheostomy tube inflated prior to, during, and immediately after the feeding procedure. Symptoms of aspiration include cyanosis, unexplained tachycardia, dyspnea, tachypnea, and cough.[3]

A cervical esophagostomy has certain advantages over an NG tube; however, it is not generally utilized unless a longer dura-

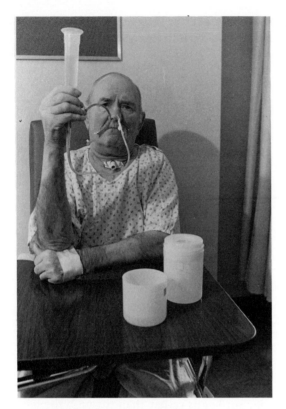

Fig. 31-8. Another aspect of self-care is administering tube feedings.

tion of tube feeding is anticipated. A feeding esophagostomy does not irritate the patient's nose or postcricoid area, and the patient can conceal the tube with clothing, because the tube enters the esophagus at a level below the cricoid cartilage. After the end of the first postsurgical week, a tract usually forms and the patient can insert the tube as needed for foods or medication. If the patient has had previous radiation therapy to the site of the feeding esophagostomy, the resulting alteration of tissues and blood supply may delay healing and possibly lead to wound breakdown or carotid artery rupture. There is little difficulty with food leakage or skin excoriations with a feeding esophagostomy. The type of tubing utilized is the same as the NG tube and can be secured around the neck with a cord-like tie.

Gastrostomy tube feeding is another method of enteral therapy for the head and neck cancer patient. This type of feeding tube requires the surgical placement of a Si-

lastic or rubber tube into the stomach through an abdominal incision. Gastrostomy placement is usually reserved for patients anticipating the need for long-term enteral feeding or for those whose neck is not suitable for a feeding esophagostomy.

Regardless of the type of feeding tube used, the following nursing measures should be taken:

1. Evaluate placement of the tube prior to administering feeding.

2. Check for residual food from previous feeding by aspirating stomach contents.

3. Place patient in sitting position.

4. Administer tube feeding slowly over 20 to 30 minutes to prevent diarrhea and bloating.

5. Follow tube feeding with 50 to 100 ml of water to rinse tube and prevent tube-feeding high sodium syndrome.

6. Warm tube diet to room temperature to prevent abdominal cramping and diarrhea.

Various types of diets are available for the patient receiving tube feedings. Blenderized diets are the least expensive and can be prepared easily in the home by the patient or family but may not contain sufficient calories and protein to meet the patient's requirements. If this diet is to be used, the patient and family should be counseled by a dietician and given special recipes to assure proper nutrition.

Commercial products are available as a total feeding program or as a supplement to a blenderized diet. Most commercial products contain 1 calorie per ml, thus providing more calories in a smaller volume than do blenderized foods. Both commercial products and blenderized foods can be given by bolus feeding or continuous drip infusion, depending on the patient's tolerance. Prior to choosing a commercial product, it is important to determine whether or not the patient has a lactose intolerance caused by a lack of the enzyme lactase in the small bowel mucosa. If the patient has the intolerance, it is important to choose a product that is lactose-free to prevent malabsorption, bloating, and diarrhea.

Oral feedings may initially be difficult to tolerate due to the extent of surgery and previous radiation. Oftentimes, the nurse must improvise in order to facilitate resumption of oral intake. Such improvisations may include the use of a straw, a syringe with flexible catheter or rubber tubing to eject food further into the oropharynx, spoon feeding, and tilting the head in various directions to facilitate swallowing. It is important to note that no one approach is appropriate for every patient and that several techniques should be tried until one is devised that is workable, acceptable, and practical for the individual patient.

Regardless of the technique or type of feeding, certain nursing measures can aid the patient nutritionally. These include:

1. Obtaining a nutritional assessment including information regarding food allergy, intolerance, and dislikes.

2. Setting realistic goals and stressing the importance of nutrition and exercise.

3. Weighing the patient daily.

4. Maintaining an accurate intake and output record.

5. Aiding the patient in selecting a menu.

6. Teaching the principles of tube feedings (if indicated).

7. Stressing the importance of self-care.

COMMUNICATION

Communication may be greatly hindered either by the surgical procedure or by the edema and/or tracheostomy that accompany the surgery. The nurse may initially attempt to anticipate and evaluate the patient's needs by asking questions requiring a yes or no answer. Written communication through use of a paper and pencil or Magic Slate is encouraged. For the illiterate patient, flash cards depicting various aspects of care or sign language can be devised.

Resuming communication may initially be frustrating to the patient. Frequently, he must repeat his message several times to be understood. The progression of speech is to be encouraged as tolerated by the patient;

however, dwelling on communication is not indicated. Adjustments by the patient and family will take time and patience.

When an oral defect is present, a prosthetic device or a packing may facilitate better speech, swallowing, and physical acceptance by the patient and family.

The patient with a tracheostomy can resume speech in the usual manner once the edema subsides. This may be accomplished by occluding the cannula with the finger or by plugging the tracheostomy tube with a cork.

The patient who has a laryngectomy will have a permanent loss of normal speech. The communication techniques used for the patient with a temporary speech loss are used for the laryngectomy patient. Prior to hospital discharge, the laryngectomy patient should begin working with the speech pathologist to learn an alternate method of speaking. Many physicians and speech pathologists are encouraging the use of an artificial larynx early in the postoperative period. This will provide the patient with a means of communication prior to mastering esophageal speech. The artificial larynx is also used for the patient who lacks the motivation or ability to learn esophageal speech. The nurse should reinforce the teaching of the speech pathologist and encourage the patient to use either the artificial larynx or esophageal speech to communicate. Emotional support provided by the family and health care team will help the laryngectomy patient during the learning process.

The nurse must convey a caring, supportive, and accepting attitude towards the patient. Nonverbal communication such as listening, touching, and just being there can be very effective. A positive, optimistic approach to communication is essential.

EMOTIONAL CONSIDERATIONS

It is not unusual for the head and neck cancer patient to become depressed before surgery, during the hospital stay, or after returning home. This is a normal reaction to the impact of the diagnosis of cancer and the threat of disfigurement. It is vitally important that the nurse understand the patient's emotions, personality, and values. The significance of the illness to the patient and family and their support systems should be evaluated. It is natural that the patient and family grieve over the loss of body parts and over the change in body image. They may respond initially to the crisis in a stunned manner, possibly utilizing denial; then a period of confusion and anxiety may be noted. During the recovery period, the family must adjust with the patient. Families have different ways of dealing with depression. Some pick up their spirits by taking a short trip, being with family and friends, or attending their houses of worship. The nurse's role with the family is that of an educator, listener, and supporter.

Approaches to emotional support include: allowing the patient and family to verbalize emotional fears and anxieties; facilitating patient-family interaction; involving family members with patient care; assisting in attainment of an acceptable quality of life as a family unit and reestablishment of values and goals; and giving imaginative, unhurried care with attention to detail and performing tasks with patience and devotion.

Body Image

Coping with an altered body image after head and neck surgery is often difficult for the patient. The reaction of the nurse to the patient's body image is important and may make a permanent impression upon the patient. The patient should be aware of the possibilities of masking defects and deformities with prosthetics. Referral to the maxillofacial prosthodontist should be obtained when indicated.

Concerns about sexuality should be discussed with the patient. Sexual adjustment is a common concern for people who have had head and neck surgery. They are afraid that they have become unattractive; therefore, unlovable. In our society, great emphasis is placed on physical appearance, and the defects produced by head and neck surgery are difficult to camouflage. The nurse's emphasis should be placed on conveying the concept that people are loved for themselves and not for their appearance.

The patient and his family should have patience with each other, since it takes a while to adjust to these physical changes. It is important for the family unit to be open about their feelings, as communication is vital. Sharing feelings and being honest enables the family members to express themselves and may foster a better family relationship.

If the nurse detects family difficulty, it is her responsibility to suggest the intervention of other health team members. A psychiatric social worker, psychologist, or psychiatrist may be indicated. This intervention may be facilitated by nursing rounds or multidisciplinary patient care conferences. Ongoing referrals and follow-up may be indicated.

Discharge Planning

Discharge planning should begin on the day of admission. When the patient is ready to be released from the hospital, discharge teaching requires a final assessment of the patient's ability to care for himself. If the patient has been performing the altered activities of daily living satisfactorily during the postoperative phase, the nurse should focus her teaching upon the adaptation process that will occur between the hospital and the home. All instructions should be written for the patient and family, since once the patient leaves the hospital most of the oral instructions will be forgotten. A discharge booklet or other written instructions will serve as a reminder (Fig. 31-9). Telephone numbers of the physician, clinical nurse oncologist, and clinic should be furnished for easy reference. The family should be encouraged to call should any problems be encountered. Even the smallest problem can cause unnecessary anxiety. Follow-up appointments with the physician and any rehabilitative service should be given to the

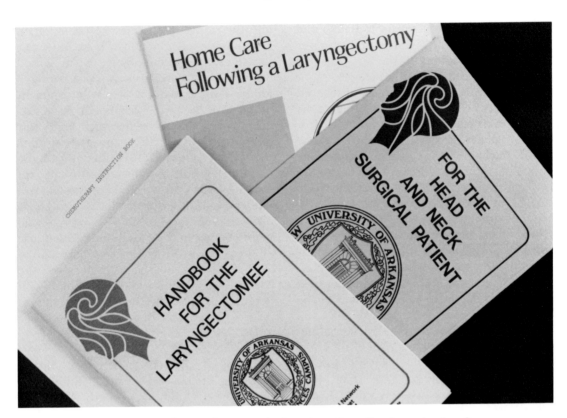

Fig. 31-9. Discharge instructions must be in written form for the patient's reference.

patient before he leaves the hospital. Routine visits to the physician are important to evaluate wound healing and possible complications and to check for persistent or new primary tumors.

Community services may be consulted in anticipation of discharge. A referral to the Public Health Nurse or the Visiting Nurse Association will provide the patient with a health care professional to help with routine or extended care that may be needed in the home. If unusual dressings, feedings, or care is required, the home nurse should have an opportunity to observe the hospital nurse perform the procedures. If this is not possible, detailed instruction sheets should be included with the referral.

Other referrals that may be necessary are the Bureau of Vocational Rehabilitation; the American Cancer Society for possible assistance with medications, dressings, or appliances required for home care; the community Lost Chord Club for support

services from other people who have had a laryngectomy; and Make Today Count for supportive measures provided by health professionals and other patients. Local social service agencies may be consulted to aid in the transition from hospital to home as well as in the evaluation of the home situation.

Stoma Care. Any patient discharged with a tracheostoma must receive information regarding hygiene and care of the stoma. The skin around the stoma is washed with mild soap and water. A thin layer of water soluble jelly or of petroleum jelly should be applied around the stoma to protect the skin and decrease crusting. The protective stoma cover should be worn at all times.

The tracheostomy patient no longer has a natural moisturizing system; therefore, supplemental humidification is beneficial. This can be accomplished by using a humidifier or vaporizer at the bedside or in the room in which the patient spends most of his time. Pans of water on radiators and wearing a moistened tracheostomy cover will also add humidity to the air breathed. Many times, patients will form crusts or plugs of mucus in spite of these measures. If the patient complains of this problem, he can be instructed to instill a few drops or sprays of normal saline solution into the stoma to loosen the plug and stimulate coughing. Sitting in a steam-filled bathroom or leaning directly over a vaporizer will also add highly concentrated humidity to help loosen crusts. Most people will experience this problem more in the winter, when the home heating system is used, than at any other time.

If the patient is discharged with a tracheostomy tube or stoma button in place, he and the family must be instructed in its care. Patients with permanent tracheostomas should be taught complete care of the tube, which includes removal, cleansing, and replacement of the entire tube daily. The cleaning techniques are the same as discussed in the section on postoperative care. The patient should be discharged with an extra tracheostomy tube set.

By the time of discharge, most patients will not require a suction machine to remove mucus. Proper coughing techniques learned during the postoperative period are continued and will rid the trachea of secretions. For those patients requiring a home suction unit, instruction and practice of proper technique should be provided in the hospital. The equipment can be rented through a surgical supply company and is similar to units used in the hospital. Altered techniques particular to the machine will be included when the equipment is obtained. Cleanliness of the tracheostoma and any equipment used in or around the stoma must be stressed.

Body hygiene must be maintained; however, alterations in customary bathing habits may be necessary. If showers are taken, a shower stoma covering may be used and care must be taken to aim the water flow low on the chest to avoid getting water into the stoma. Baths may be taken, again avoiding the introduction of soap and water into the stoma. Shampooing the hair should be done over a sink or using a sink spray.

Mouth Care.　Many patients will complain of halitosis following head and neck surgery. Frequent oral cleansing using a soft toothbrush, toothpaste, and dental floss should be encouraged. Brushing the tongue may be helpful. Mouthwashes of salt and soda or hydrogen peroxide and saline are used periodically during the day to eliminate a buildup of debris. Commercial mouthwashes may be used but frequent use of them is discouraged. If surgery of the oral cavity has not been performed, the edentulous patient should be fitted with dentures or have any necessary alterations made to his current dentures. Routine visits to the dentist are also added to the follow-up protocols.

Nutrition.　Adequate nutritional intake following discharge is essential for wound healing and regaining strength. Many patients will tolerate small frequent meals during the initial healing state with the diet advanced as tolerated. Supplemental high caloric liquids can be used to increase the caloric intake. If tube feedings are required after discharge, instructions regarding the liquefaction of foods must be provided. Normal table food can be used by placing the food in a blender with enough liquid to convert the food into a form that can pass through the tube. All feedings should begin and end with a few ounces of water to clear the tube and maintain its patency.

Some patients may complain of aspiration when swallowing. This will occur more often in patients who have had a supraglottic laryngectomy, oropharyngeal surgery, or glossectomy. The patient can employ various body positions or head positions to decrease or prevent aspiration. Semisolid foods rather than those with a more liquid consistency are usually better tolerated.

Occasionally, patients will complain of reflux esophagitis. Symptoms can be minimized by using antacids, eating a small evening meal, and sleeping with the head of the bed elevated.

If the patient is an alcoholic, encouragement should be focused on decreasing the alcohol intake and adhering to a nutritious diet. Malnutrition is an important concern with most alcoholic patients.

Wound Care. Care of incisions must continue after discharge. External wounds should be cleansed three or more times a day and ointment applied to keep the area free of crusts. If a fistula persists, packing and dressings, as discussed in the postoperative nursing care section, should continue. This may be done by the patient, an instructed family member, or a visiting nurse.

Intraoral wounds must be cleansed frequently. In addition, irrigations using a salt and soda or hydrogen peroxide solution following meals and at bedtime will remove crusts and debris not removed by ordinary procedures. These irrigations can be done with a Water Pik, syringe and catheter, or bag-type irrigating set. Low pressure should be used to avoid traumatizing the area.

Swelling of the face and neck may occur following surgery, especially after a radical neck dissection due to decreased lymphatic drainage. The patient is instructed to sleep with the head elevated and to avoid sleeping on the surgical side.

Additional Instructions. Most presurgical activities can be resumed following head and neck cancer surgery. Swimming and boating are two activities that are restricted for any patient with a tracheostoma. Extra bibs or other stoma covers should be used during cold weather to prevent the introduction of cold air into the stoma. This cover will also provide a method of warming and humidifying the air breathed.

The sexual relationship of the patient and spouse may resume as it was presurgically. The patient is still the same person as before and requires the same emotional relationship, if not more. Special attention to personal appearance and hygiene, which includes all the things discussed thus far, are helpful in maintaining closeness.

THE RADIATION THERAPY PATIENT

Radiation therapy can be used alone as a treatment modality or in combination with surgery or chemotherapy. The treatment can be given by external beam or by direct implantation of radioactive needles or seeds into the tumor. Patient teaching begins with thorough explanations of the treatment. The equipment should be described and the procedure explained. The frequency of treatments will be dependent upon the intent of treatment and the radiation oncologist's preference. Treatments are usually scheduled on a daily basis extending from 4 to 6 weeks, depending upon the dose and how the patient tolerates the treatments. The actual treatment takes only a few minutes; therefore, patients are encouraged to receive them on an outpatient basis unless this is impractical for medical or geographic reasons. The health care team should be aware of community resources available to aid the patient with transportation arrangements.

The assessment procedure and referral patterns for the patient receiving radiation therapy are the same as for the surgical patients. The nursing care required by these patients is geared to psychological support and prevention and treatment of the side effects that may occur with radiation therapy.

Preirradiation Considerations

Prior to beginning radiation therapy, the patient is referred to the maxillofacial prosthodontic department and the dental hygienist. A thorough oral examination and any required treatment is performed. Restorations are made and teeth that are unable to be saved are extracted. Any extractions that are necessary must be done prior to the commencement of treatment in an attempt to prevent osteoradionecrosis. Oral prophylaxis is done and instructions on the use of a soft-bristled toothbrush, fluoride toothpaste, and dental floss are given. The dentulous patient will also have impressions taken for the fabrication of fluoride carriers (see Ch. 8). These devices, used daily with topical fluoride after oral cleansing, are employed to prevent radiation caries. The nurse must encourage the patient to continue the oral hygiene routine both during the treatment regime and for the rest of his life.

Treatment Considerations

MUCOSITIS AND STOMATITIS

Mucositis, an inflammation of the mucous membranes (stomatitis, when describing the oral cavity), is a common side effect of radiation therapy and results from damage to the normal cells (Fig. 31-10). The degree of mucositis or stomatitis is related to the portals used to administer radiation and the dosage and type of radiation used. Good oral hy-

giene is essential for comfort, as well as to protect the oral mucosa from infection. The oral hygiene protocol taught by the dental hygienist is reinforced and irrigations or rinses of the oral cavity are encouraged. Solutions of hydrogen peroxide and water or saline, or soda preparation, can be used to cleanse the oral cavity, as well as to add needed lubrication. The patient's fluid and caloric intake must be maintained. Foods that are extremely hot, spicy, or acidic should be avoided, as they can irritate the already inflamed tissue. Alcohol intake and tobacco use in any form are discouraged because they will add to the intensity of the mucositis and stomatitis. The patient may find the use of viscous Xylocaine or a liquid antacid beneficial in soothing the irritation. These substances are used to rinse the mouth and then may be swallowed. Another preparation that may be helpful is a combination of equal parts of antacid, viscous Xylocaine, benadryl elixir, and glycer-

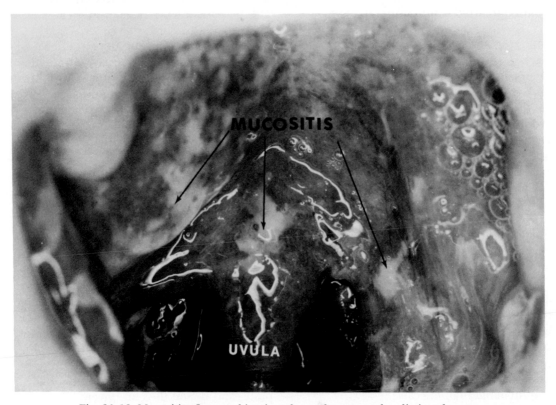

Fig. 31-10. Mucositis after combination chemotherapy and radiation therapy.

ine. This mixture is used to rinse the mouth and provides a topical anesthesia, as well as a lubricant, to the mucous membrane.

XEROSTOMIA

A few weeks after radiation therapy is started, the patient may begin to complain of dryness of the mouth (xerostomia). Radiation to the head and neck usually affects the salivary glands, resulting in the saliva becoming scant and very tenacious. This side effect may be temporary or permanent. Those nursing measures discussed in relation to inflammation of the oral cavity should be continued. In addition, the patient must maintain adequate fluid intake. Sugarless chewing gum and candy, such as lemon drops, may provide some relief of dryness. Special preparation of oral lubri-

cants, such as Orex* or Xero-Lube** may be used (Fig. 31-11). These mixtures help lubricate the oral cavity. Effects of these preparations last longer than water. A vaporizer or humidifier will provide increased humidification and if used routinely may offer temporary relief.

NUTRITIONAL PROBLEMS

Due to the previously discussed side effects and the general physical condition of most head and neck cancer patients, inadequate nutritional intake is another problem the patient may encounter. The fluid, caloric, and protein intake must be maintained

*Orex is available through Kings Specialty Co., Fort Wayne, IN, 46801.
**Xerolube is available through First Texas Pharmaceuticals, Inc., Dallas, TX, 75240.

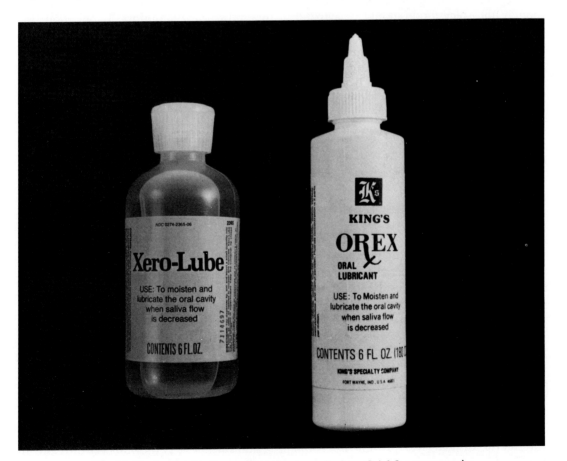

Fig. 31-11. Artificial saliva preparations may be beneficial for xerostomia.

throughout treatment. Small frequent meals containing food high in calories and protein are encouraged in addition to supplemental feedings between meals. Commercially prepared products or home-made preparations (e.g., eggnogs, milkshakes, and custards) will add the extra calories and grams of protein so important to this patient. Cold foods or foods served at room temperature may be better tolerated than hot foods. If mastication is a problem, chopped, blended, or pureed foods are required. Once xerostomia develops, food served with gravies or sauces may be swallowed with less discomfort than drier foods. Providing analgesics and antiemetics prior to meals may also be helpful.

Alterations in taste may cause the patient to decrease his dietary intake. Most patients describe their food as tasteless. Changes in seasoning can be suggested, although hot, spicy foods should be avoided. The patient may limit his diet to those foods that are tolerated but only if adequate caloric intake is maintained. If adequate intake is unable to be maintained, an NG tube may be necessary. The patient and family are instructed in the use of this tube as described in the section of this chapter on the postoperative period.

SKIN REACTIONS

Some patients may experience skin reactions during and following radiation therapy. These can range from erythema to actual desquamation with drainage. Erythema is a mild reaction. The patient is instructed to keep the skin dry, to avoid soap, and to expose the skin to the air as much as possible. Tight, constricting clothing should be avoided. An ointment containing vitamins A or D or a corticosteroid cream may be used to decrease the symptoms. In caring for the skin, caution must be taken to avoid removal of the radiation markings. The most severe skin reactions are best treated using sterile, moist compresses and antibiotic ointments with sterile dressings to prevent infection. Severe skin reactions may necessitate alter-

ations in or interruption of the treatment program. Dry, atrophic skin is a common sequela of radiation therapy. This can be helped by the use of lanolin-based creams and avoidance of exposure to temperature extremes. For those patients anticipating sun exposure, instructions should be given regarding the use of sun screens containing PABA.

EDEMA

Swelling of the face and neck may occur during radiation therapy, especially in patients who have had radical neck dissections. The patient should be instructed to sleep with the head of the bed elevated and to avoid sleeping on the treated side.

Laryngeal edema is another possible side effect of irradiation. Voice rest and the use of supplemental humidification will minimize the discomfort. In addition, the patient and family must be instructed to seek immediate medical attention in the event of airway distress.

OSTEORADIONECROSIS

Osteoradionecrosis has been mentioned in relation to oral hygiene and preirradiation dental care. Prevention of this side effect is of utmost importance. Dental extraction should be avoided following radiation therapy. If performed, the patient should receive antibiotics prior to, during, and following the procedure. When osteoradionecrosis develops, pain is the major problem. The area may require packing, debridement, and high doses of antibiotics. In severe cases, surgery to remove sequestered bone may be required.

RADIATION SICKNESS

Radiation sickness is unusual in the patient receiving radiation only to the head and neck. Anorexia, nausea, vomiting, and lethargy are the symptoms associated with radiation sickness. If they do occur, treatment of the specific symptom is necessary. These constitutional side effects usually subside upon completion of treatment.

FIBROSIS

Fibrosis is characterized by a hardening of the skin and structures underlying the radiated field. Mobility of the face and neck can be hindered, resulting in discomfort to the patient. An exercise program prescribed by an occupational or physical therapist is indicated. If there is pain involved, it should be properly controlled.

Radiation Implants

Implantation is another method of administering radiotherapy. The implants are inserted into the tumor in the operating room by the radiotherapist. The number of implants used is recorded in the patient's chart and sutures are attached to each implant for easy counting. Following implantation, the patient is placed in a private room with a bathroom.

During the time the implants are in place, direct contact with the patient should be minimal in order to avoid radiation exposure. The nurse should organize her care of the patient so that unnecessary exposure is avoided. All equipment used should remain in the room. Visitors or personnel entering the patient's room should observe isolation precautions by wearing a gown, mask, hair covering, and gloves. Restrictions of people coming in contact with the patient should be strictly enforced. No one under the age of 18 should be allowed in the room. Pregnant women are not permitted in the room of the patient with radiation implants.

The implants are removed by the radiation oncology team. If accidental displacement occurs, the radiation team should be notified immediately. Nothing in the room is to be removed or discarded until the implant is located. Once the implants are removed, isolation is no longer required and the patient may resume his activities of daily living.

The side effects experienced by the patient with implants are the same as those discussed for patients with external beam therapy. Local swelling and pain may be severe.

Psychological support of these patients is essential. In addition to all the emotional reactions previously discussed, the patient with radiation implants experiences isolation. Time must be provided to explain the reasons for being alone during the treatment and the rationale for the precautions being taken. Reassurance can be given during the planned nursing activities and time can be spent, at a distance, with the patient.

THE CHEMOTHERAPY AND IMMUNOTHERAPY PATIENT

Chemotherapy

Chemotherapy for the head and neck cancer patient is an additional type of treatment in which the nurse can participate; however, involvement with this activity will vary according to each professional setting and the requirements by the physician. With the age of specialization rapidly affecting nursing, there has been an increase in the number of nurse practitioners, clinicians, and specialists in head and neck oncology. This has resulted in more nurses becoming involved in the chemotherapy programs.

Chemotherapy for the head and neck cancer patient is still in its infancy. Continued research studies are being conducted in order to determine the optimal use for this type of treatment. Presently, chemotherapy is used with several purposes in mind. For the patient with advanced cancer, it is used for palliation because it may decrease pain and discomfort from the tumor and dry up those tumors that ulcerate. Probably its use adjunctively with other treatments (surgery and radiation therapy) is the most popular. Sometimes it is given before the more conventional treatment in order to decrease tumor size and/or to test the tumor's susceptibility to the drug. If the tumor reacts favorably to the drug and the patient is in a high risk category for recurrence, chemotherapy may be given prophylactically after the conventional therapy for as long as a year in some institutions.

Various drugs are used for head and neck cancer, including methotrexate, 5-fluorouracil, bleomycin (Blenoxane), cyclophosphamide (Cytoxan), cis-platinum (Platinol), and doxorubicin (Adriamycin). There are various pretreatment studies and assessments required in which the nurse can be helpful: (1) preparation for and obtaining the biopsy; (2) photography of the tumor when possible; (3) drawings, descriptions, and measurements of the tumor and nodal involvement; (4) baseline physical findings (weight, height, body surface in meters squared, blood pressure, and general physical and laboratory data).

There are usually psychological overtones involved for the patient and his family throughout the chemotherapy phase. Initially they must have a chance to verbalize their positive and negative feelings regarding the diagnosis and treatment plan. It is at this time that misinformation and misconceptions concerning chemotherapy can be explored and corrected. One of the more common attitudinal problems is that chemotherapy is most frequently used in terminal patients. Patients undergoing chemotherapy who do not fall into this category may be negative towards the treatment program because of this and the situation must be fully explained. A detailed discussion of the drug(s) and their side effects must be conducted with emphasis on the fact that the patient will probably not experience all of these side effects and that some of the side effects are not uncomfortable (for example, the red color of the urine after Adriamycin is given). After the discussion and question and answer session, a consent form is signed. It is important to assist the patient with financial concerns and problems associated with extensive traveling if the treatment facility is a long distance from his home. Whenever problems such as these arise, the aid of resource personnel should be solicited. The social worker can assist in exploring the financial supports for which the patient is eligible. A local physician could give some of the treatments to avoid frequent return visits. If a patient has unusual information requests concerning the drugs, a pharmacist can be utilized for the information. Also in any aspect of the treatment, a public health nurse or visiting nurse may be helpful with home care problems resulting from the chemotherapy.

The frequency of administration of the chemotherapy varies with each drug, although most are given intermittently. At each treatment, the patient must have a physical assessment to evaluate the occurrence and severity of any side effects and the response of the tumor to the drug (if a tumor is present and visible). This assessment usually involves weight, vital signs (temperature and blood pressure), examination of the oral cavity, palpation of the neck, and a discussion of the patient's appetite, toleration of the chemotherapy, and general condition. For those drugs that produce leukopenia and thrombocytopenia, blood must be drawn before each dose is given to make sure the patient has adequate neutrophils and platelets. In addition, any patient receiving chemotherapy should have electrolytes and liver and renal function studies every 4 to 6 weeks as well as a routine chest x-ray every 2 to 3 months.

The majority of the drugs are administered intravenously. For those drugs that do not cause tissue damage if extravasated, choosing a vein is not a problem. Lower arm and hand veins are desirable, but sometimes the patient receives some discomfort when these veins are punctured; therefore, the anticubital veins are also acceptable. However, for the drugs that do create tissue damage if extravasated, a large vein in the lower arm or hand should be utilized (a small vein would increase the risk of extravasation and the large anticubital veins are preferable for blood drawing).

For specific information on chemotherapeutic agents, refer to Table 31-1.

TABLE 31-1. SUMMARY OF CHEMOTHERAPEUTIC AGENTS

Agent	Major Side Effects	Interventions
Methotrexate	1. Bone marrow suppression (leukopenia and thrombocytopenia)	a. Reduction or elimination of dosage until WBC and platelet counts return to adequate levels b. Avoidance of infections c. Avoidance of severe bruising or body injury d. Blood components as indicated
	2. Mucositis	a. For hygiene: oral irrigations using a mixture of baking soda and water or hydrogen peroxide and water b. For pain: oral washings using either liquid antacids or viscous Xylocaine, Benadryl elixir, and glycerine separately or in combination in equal portions. May be swallowed. c. Diet alterations (e.g., soft or liquid meals, Popsicles, and ice cream)
	3. Anorexia, nausea, and vomiting	a. Diet alterations (e.g., frequent small amounts of mostly starches, sweets, and cold, clear liquids) b. Medication such as Compazine (oral or suppository), Combid (oral) c. Relaxation techniques (especially before and after meals) d. Frequent measuring of body weight
	4. Malaise and fever (101° to 104°F)	a. Rest b. Nonaspirin antipyretic c. Increased fluid intake
	5. Partial alopecia (more noticeable in high dose)	a. Application of scalp tourniquet (questionable effectiveness) b. Use of wigs, scarves, hats, etc. c. Reassurance about regrowth of hair
Blenoxane (sterile bleomycin sulfate)	1. Mouth ulcers	Same as with methotrexate
	2. Skin changes (hyperpigmentation, ulceration, redness, tenderness, pruritus, thickening, hyperkeratosis, and rash)	a. Medicated topical creams, lotions, or ointments b. Systemic antipruritic medication c. Avoidance of scratching d. Avoidance of irritating clothing e. Discontinuation of drug when severe skin changes occur

TABLE 31-1. CONTINUED

Agent	Major Side Effects	Interventions
Blenoxane (continued)	3. Pneumonitis, occasionally progressing to pulmonary fibrosis	a. Baseline chest x-ray study and test of pulmonary functions before beginning drug b. Periodic chest x-ray during therapy c. Patient alertness to early signs (shortness of breath, chest pains, etc.) d. Discontinuation of drug when pulmonary toxicity has been determined
	4. Anorexia, nausea, and vomiting	Same as with methotrexate
	5. Malaise and fever (101° to 104° F)	Same as with methotrexate
	6. Partial alopecia	Same as with methotrexate
	NOTE: The occurrences and severity of side effects for bleomycin are related to the total cumulative dose	
Cytoxan (cyclophosphamide)	1. Bone marrow suppression	Same as with methotrexate
	2. Anorexia, nausea and vomiting	Same as with methotrexate
	3. Hemorrhagic cystitis	a. Forced fluid intake and frequent voiding b. Observation for early warning symptoms such as hematuria and dysuria
	4. Partial alopecia	Same as with methotrexate
Adriamycin (doxorubicin)	1. Cardiac toxicity	a. Prevention—caution in exceeding recommended cumulative dose b. Discontinuation of drug when cardiac toxicity is noted
	2. Bone marrow suppression	Same as with methotrexate
	3. Anorexia, nausea, and vomiting	Same as with methotrexate

	4. Complete alopecia	Same as with methotrexate
	5. Skin tissue necrosis if drug is extravasated	a. Proper choice of vein for administration and cautious technique during entire procedure
		b. Immediate discontinuation of any intravenous administration if there is any indication of extravasation (example: swelling and pain at site of injection). Another site can be sought to continue infusion.
		*c. When extravasation occurs: immediate subcutaneous and intradermal injections of Solu-Cortef given to entire infiltrated area, then dressing with steroid cream and 4 × 4 gauze. Ice applied for 24 hours. Continued application of steroid cream twice a day until redness is gone.
Platinol (Cis-platinum)	1. Nephrotoxicity	a. Confirmation of normal renal status prior to and throughout therapy
		b. Forced fluid intake and frequent voiding to prevent retention
		c. Accurate intake and output measurement
		d. Avoidance of other nephrotoxic drugs
		e. Discontinuation of drug if nephrotoxicity occurs
	2. Ototoxicity	a. Careful monitoring by audiometry prior to initiating therapy and prior to subsequent doses
		b. Avoidance of other ototoxic drugs
		c. Hydration
	3. Anorexia, nausea and vomiting	Same as in methotrexate (Note: the intensity of this side effect may be severe and necessitates stringent prophylaxia and control
	4. Bone marrow suppression	Same as with methotrexate
	5. Complete alopecia	Same as with methotrexate
	6. Mucositis	Same as with methotrexate

*This approach is still experimental.

Immunotherapy

Immunotherapy for the head and neck cancer patient, although still in the experimental stage, holds great promise for improving the cure rate. It would be futile to go into much detail in this chapter since theories, procedures, and agents are always changing. Immunotherapy is usually used as an adjuvant.

Immunopotentiation is one method of immunotherapy and utilizes agents such as bacillus of Calmette-Guerin (BCG) and Corynebacterium parvum. BCG is the most commonly used of these two and may be administered in many ways, such as by intradermal injection, by scarification, by multiple puncture gun, by intratumor injection (especially for melanoma), and by mouth. For further information on the status of immunotherapy, see Chapter 29.

Although its value in oncology is unresolved, skin testing is sometimes used as an evaluative tool of a patient's immunocompetence before and during the therapy phase. Antigens such as mumps, intermediate purified protein derivative (IPPD) varidase, dermatophytin, and *Candida* are commonly used, along with dinitrochlorobenzene (DNCB) sensitization and challenge (Fig. 31-12). Bates et al.[1] have reviewed immunologic skin testing and interpretation in detail.

PAIN MANAGEMENT

The head and neck cancer patient experiences pain in all different phases of his disease and treatment, and management of this pain is frequently the most frustrating aspect of his care. This topic is discussed in great detail in Chapter 30; however, the role of the nurse in pain management merits mentioning here.

Careful assessment of the patient's pain will aid in effective treatment. It is important to know whether the pain is dull, piercing, shooting, etc. Other questions that should be answered include: where is the pain? how long has it been there? how strong is it? and how is it affecting the patient? The patient's pain threshold and coping mechanisms are important to evaluate. Patients with essentially the same type of pain could require different pain management approaches depending on their coping mechanisms. Finally, evaluation of previous analgesic attempts, whether they be internal or external, is a necessary guide in helping the patient with his pain.

Once the assessment is accomplished, the nurse can begin to intervene with a very basic and simple approach. When feasible, the patient should be encouraged to verbalize his feelings about his pain. This helps him to cope better and also allows the nurse to develop the all important "therapeutic nurse-patient relationship." The nurse will be able to convey to the patient that she really understands and cares about his pain; and, therefore, through confidence in the nurse, the patient will have some pain relief

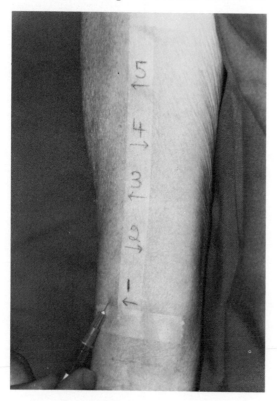

Fig. 31-12. Skin testing for evaluation of immunocompetence.

from the knowledge that very serious and conscientious attempts will be made toward total pain management.

The components of nursing care for pain management are comfortable positioning of the body, environment manipulation, relaxation techniques, and administration of pain medication. The first rule to follow is to always continue with any remedy that has proved its worth. Environmental manipulation includes arranging for a nonirritating roommate, proper ventilation and lighting, and a comfortable temperature. Scheduled administration of analgesics without undue concern of addiction should be carried out. The recent philosophy of "staying on top of the pain" by giving pain medications on a scheduled basis instead of as circumstances may require (p.r.n.) has proven extremely effective with very little resultant addiction. Once the pain is relieved, the patient usually does not require as much medication.

The final step in pain management for the nurse is constant documentation and evaluation of the remedies being used. One must always be aware of the present situation and be ready with another approach should one method fail.

THE TERMINALLY ILL PATIENT

As with many other disease entities, there are some patients in which the disease takes over, and the medical goals then change from cure to palliation. Regardless of whether the palliation takes the form of conservative surgery, radiation therapy, or chemotherapy, good basic nursing care is of great value.

The patient's comfort is the nurse's primary concern. Pain control is probably the most important and usually the most difficult aspect of the patient's care because there is the constant challenge of medicating the patient adequately without interfering excessively with his mentation and alertness (the exception to this problem is the

patient in the very final stage of dying). Other nursing care priorities for the terminally ill patient are maintaining body hygiene, skin integrity, adequate hydration, and a tranquil environment. If the mouth is involved, extra mouth care will be required. An ulcerating tumor near a tracheal stoma also creates additional problems in that the possibility of aspiration and choking is present. Vaseline gauze wrapped around the tracheostomy or laryngectomy tube or stoma button can reduce this problem.

Tumor hygiene is another concern especially when ulceration has occurred. Gentle washing using soap and water, hydrogen peroxide, etc., irrigating with salt and soda, neomycin, etc., and, at times, power spraying or use of the Water Pik are very helpful procedures but must be done with care to avoid bleeding in the tumor area. Odor control can be achieved by these cleansing techniques as well as from room deodorizers, medicinal packings, and systemic medications. Cleocin and Lactinex granules may result in remarkable odor control if anaerobic organisms are the cause. Dressings can be applied for drainage problems and for cosmetic purposes. It is advisable, however, to use an ointment or nonadhering gauze, since the wound tends to dry and dressing changes can be difficult and irritating to the area. For dressings that must be changed often, the use of Montgomery straps would be helpful in preventing skin damage from frequently removed tape.

The nurse plays an important role in the psychological support of the patient and family. The qualities a nurse needs in order to give good emotional support are self-confidence, calmness, composure in an emergency, a positive cheerful approach, and the ability to be a good listener with empathy for the patient and his family.[6] People's reactions, values, and priorities vary greatly, and it is very important for the nurse to individualize support according to the patient's and family's wishes without personal judgment on these wishes. The stress that everyone is experiencing makes psychological support difficult at times, but the nurse can help somewhat by assuring privacy but not isolation, allowing time for verbalization of feelings, and assisting in home care arrangements as the patient and family desire. Home care for the head and neck cancer patient who is dying is usually very complex because most of the vital functions are involved and impaired (especially breathing and eating), thus requiring various equipment and causing extreme anxiety on the part of the family and friends. If home care is not feasible, the nurse needs to facilitate patient-family interaction and to involve the family in the health care setting as much as possible and to the degree they desire.

Usually the head and neck cancer patient's direct cause of death is pneumonia, systemic infection, total body function collapse due to "tumor load," or carotid rupture due to tumor invasion or wound slough. At this point, the nurse's attention turns to the family as she facilitates the grieving process, assists with funeral arrangements, and makes contact periodically with them in the weeks and months to come to check on their adjustment to the death and to offer any final assistance. If the nurse has been working with the patient and family for a long time, there will probably always be some ties with the family, but it is at this time that the intense therapeutic relationship is terminated.

SUMMARY

The complexities involved in the care of the head and neck cancer patient create a great challenge for the nurse. The nurse must combine many functions, including providing physical and emotional support as well as teaching. As a catalyst, her involvement results in coordination of care leading to improved quality of life for not only the patient but the entire family.

With some patients the nurse can fight the long, hard battle and share the glorious victory. With the patients whose battles end in defeat, one shares the tears and the knowledge that their lives were better because of the nurse and the nurse's life has been enriched because of them.

REFERENCES

1. Bates, S. E., Suen, J. Y., and Tranum, B. L. 1979. Immunological skin testing and interpretation: A plea for uniformity. Cancer, 43: 2306.

1a. Chrzan, D. J. 1975. O.R./R.R. and special nurses. Hospital Topics, 53: 48.

2. Grant, J. 1973. Patient care in parenteral hyperalimentation. Nursing Clinics of North America, 8: 165.

3. Millen, D. 1978. Aspiration: Foiling a silent killer. RN, 41: 34.

4. O'Dell, A. J. 1973. Objectives and standards in the care of the patient with a radical neck dissection. Nursing Clinics of North America, 8: 159.

5. Rickel, L. H., Watson, P. G., and Sigler, B. 1978. Solid neoplasms. In Jones, D. A., Dunbar, C. F., and Jirovec, M. M., Eds.: Medical Surgical Nursing: A Conceptual Approach. McGraw-Hill, New York, 162.

6. Zavertnik, J. 1967. Emotional support of patients with head and neck surgery. Nursing Clinics of North America, 2: 503.

32 | The Incurable Patient

James M. Dowaliby, II, M.D.

INTRODUCTION

A life in medicine, like a life in any other field of endeavor, is studded with triumphs and defeats. What makes medicine different from most other fields is that our triumphs are human lives saved and our defeats are human lives lost. This is particularly true for the physician or surgeon who treats cancer. Each life saved and each life lost is the life of an individual: a person whom we have come to know well personally, a person for whom we may have provided medical care for several years and for whom we have developed considerable affection.

We are taught, as medical students and as young physicians, that we should not become "involved" with our patients. There were hints that our judgment might be clouded, and that we might not be able to make the correct decisions regarding their treatment. Most of us, however, became physicians precisely because we wished to care for the sick. It is our hope that we can make each of our patients well; however, we can continue to care for those patients whom we cannot make well. In order to do this effectively, we must become involved with them. We must be willing to listen to them carefully and we must know enough about them and their families that we can hear what they are saying. If we refuse to do this, if we insist upon *not caring* about the patients for whom we provide medical attention, then we are denying the very qualities in ourselves that impelled us into medicine in the first place. This kind of involvement need not cloud judgment nor deflect decisions.

Fortunately, we are living in a time of renewed interest in the humanitarian aspects of medical care, including the care of the dying patient and the patient who is living with incurable disease. Much credit for this renewed interest is due to Elizabeth Kübler-Ross.[2, 3] Her meticulous and moving description of her work with dying patients has been the pivot point around which the ideas of many of us have changed. The care of these patients is demanding, but it is also rewarding. It gives us unusual opportunities to learn from them about their living and their dying, and, therefore, perhaps an opportunity better to understand our own living and our own dying. This chapter will deal with some of the questions and problems that arise in caring for the patient with cancer, especially incurable cancer.

THE MATURE PHYSICIAN AND THE CONTEMPLATION OF DEATH

The diagnosis of cancer raises the specter of death in the patient's mind. We must recognize that the specter is also raised for the physician. Physicians are not necessarily better prepared to face the idea of death than their patients. Our denial mechanism is only as good as anyone else's. Indeed, there is evidence[1] that physicians as a group have a greater fear of death than nonphysicians. Death strikes at the doctor's very foundation, his power to heal. If we cannot heal, of what use are we to our world, our patients, or ourselves?

The fact is, life is a fatal condition. No

869

doctor saves every patient. Each of our patients will eventually die. Each of us will eventually die. These things are not easy for us to contemplate, but we must contemplate them nonetheless. If a doctor is unable to consider or discuss death, he cannot be open and supportive with his cancer patients.

The contemplation of death is not necessarily a morbid activity. It may help us to recognize and to accept our own vulnerability. It may help us to realize that we are more like our patients than we once thought—our fears and our deaths are just a few steps behind theirs. This realization can bring a sense of renewed sweetness and heightened urgency to every day of life that we have. It may also help us to free ourselves of some old fears and taboos so that we can discuss death with our dying patients, giving them and their families the emotional support and the ability to communicate that they need—and indeed, that we need, too.

THE DOCTOR-PATIENT RELATIONSHIP WHEN THE PATIENT HAS CANCER

The relationship between the doctor and the patient who has cancer is by its nature a more profound relationship than the usual relationship between doctor and patient. Because cancer is a potentially fatal disease, the cancer patient needs more support from the relationship than does the average patient. This means that the doctor must give his cancer patient more time, as well as closer and more sympathetic attention. The effectiveness of the relationship and its value to the patient depends upon the doctor's physical and emotional availability to the patient. The doctor must be willing to see the patient when the patient needs to be seen. He must be willing to listen to the patient and to discuss whatever troubles the patient, without permitting his own anxieties to come between them. The tone of the relationship is largely set by the tone of the

first encounter. The relationship between the doctor and the cancer patient divides itself into three phases: the phase of diagnosis, the phase of treatment and remission, and the phase of recurrence and death.

Phase of Diagnosis

Nobody really wants to visit the doctor. Every person visiting a doctor's office for the first time is a prisoner, forced to be there against his will. Often the patient is anxious and afraid. He must be met with consideration and kindness. These things are true of every patient but are especially true of the patient who thinks he may have cancer.

If the patient does indeed have cancer, then the physician is confronted with three questions: Shall I tell him he has cancer? How shall I tell him? and "Doctor, am I going to die?"

Shall I tell him he has cancer?

This question is largely rhetorical now, because in our time the legal right of the competent patient to know his diagnosis has been made clear. Many hospitals now publish policies concerning the rights of patients. At the Yale-New Haven Hospital in New Haven, Connecticut, the policy concerning the rights of patients is posted on all patient-care divisions and in out-patient areas, and is available in each patient's room. The second article of this policy states, in part, that the "patient has the right to obtain from his physician complete current information concerning his diagnosis, treatment, and prognosis in terms he can be reasonably expected to understand."

Nonetheless, the patient's family may wish to hide the diagnosis from him. The doctor, especially if he is an old family friend, may wish to acquiesce in this plan. The temptation, however, must be resisted. A competent patient must be told his diagnosis—once, and perhaps more than once. There is no need to bludgeon the patient with facts until he is driven into despair. It is, however, the doctor's responsibility to ensure that there is communication between the patient and the other family members, and among the doctor, the patient, and the family.

Communication and mutual support must be based on truth. Lies, whether outright lies or lies of omission, are inappropriate. The patient sees through them, but if he has not been told the truth he may not say that he sees through them. He may play the game of not knowing because doctor, family, and friends play the game of not knowing. The patient thus ends up carrying his burden of fear and grief alone in order to protect the survivors. The lies benefit the doctor, the family, the hospital staff—everyone except the patient. Furthermore, Kübler-Ross[2, 3] has shown that all of her hospitalized cancer patients are aware of the diagnosis, whether they have been specifically told or not.

The following case histories illustrate the kind of situation in which we may involve ourselves if we fail to be truthful with our patients.

CASE HISTORY 1

J.R. was a 28-year-old father of two who ran a gasoline station in New Haven, Connecticut. In August of 1969 he presented to a colleague of mine with a lump in the neck, difficulty in swallowing, nasal stuffiness, and unilateral middle ear effusion. Medical evaluation led to a biopsy that confirmed the diagnosis of non-Hodgkin lymphoma involving the nasopharynx and the neck. He was treated with radiation therapy, but was not cured. Two months after the completion of radiotherapy, he was readmitted to the hospital with inability to swallow, dehydration, and airway distress. He underwent an emergency tracheotomy and a feeding pyriformostomy in order to stabilize his condition.

At that point, Mr. R. was a patient whose tumor had failed to respond to radiation therapy. The question of chemotherapy was raised by the physician and it was this issue that forced the truth. His pretty young wife said, "Let him go in peace. Do not give him any chemotherapy." His mother said, "No, no. Please keep him alive as long as you can. Treat him." Both said, "Don't let him know he has cancer." In their frustration with the entire situation, the two women became enraged with each other and ended by not speaking to each other at all.

We called in a psychiatric consultant, who wrote on the chart, "He already knows the worst." The family called in consultation an oncologist who was an old friend. He wrote, "I feel we should consult only the patient" in regard to chemotherapy.

Early one morning the attending surgeon, a resident, and two medical students walked down to Mr. R's room. The attending surgeon warned Mr. R's wife and his mother that Mr. R. had to make his own decision in regard to chemotherapy, and, therefore, he had to be told his diagnosis. With that, the mother burst into tears and fled down the corridor. The wife half fell into an arm chair at the patient's bedside and sat very still. The surgeon stepped to the patient's bedside and said, "Mr. R., what do you understand to be the nature of the problem?" Mr. R. picked up his clipboard and in a shaky hand wrote, "CANCER." He had known the diagnosis all along.

The surgeon then discussed chemotherapy briefly and asked Mr. R. if he was interested in it. Again Mr. R. picked up his clipboard and pen. This time he wrote, "I want to wait." This seemed to be a curiously revealing and satisfactory answer. It was neither an acceptance nor a refusal. It closed no doors. It allowed recognition of the finality of his disease, but preserved a tiny door of hope.

Within 24 hours the patient's wife and his mother were friends again. They could not say enough nice things about each other. The patient and his wife were able to discuss his impending death and make plans for the education of their children. The air had cleared. Lines of communication were established that were maintained until the patient's death.

CASE HISTORY 2

Al was 72. He had a long history of cigarette smoking and emphysema. On a routine chest x-ray he was noted to have hilar adenopathy. Laminograms showed a nodular density in the right midlung field. Mediastinoscopy led to the diagnosis of bronchogenic carcinoma with metastasis to the paratracheal nodes. On the day that the biopsy report was to be given to Al, brother A. drove Al to the specialist's office. The specialist told Al and brother A. that Al would be fine. When they had left his office, the specialist telephoned brother B. and told him that Al had cancer. Brother B. immediately telephoned brother C., saying that the specialist had just reported to him that Al had a lung cancer. Brother A. then called brother C. and told him that the specialist had said that Al would be fine. There was instant uproar among the brothers. A flurry of telephone calls ensued, leading to increasing confusion and consternation.

At this point brother B. called the family doctor and told him that the family was in an uproar. The family doctor then called the specialist. The specialist explained that Al indeed had cancer of the lung and went on to say, "I've known this family for a long time. I just couldn't bring myself to tell him."

The family doctor then visited Al, talked with him awhile, and explained that he had a cancer and that it would require treatment with radiation. Al replied, "I knew I was getting the runaround from those guys, but I didn't know why." The family doctor then spoke with each of the brothers in turn, stating the situation truthfully. By evening of that day, everyone in the family knew the facts. Communication had been established and the family members were able to meet together for dinner that night. As in the previous case, communication once established was maintained until the patient's death.

How shall I tell him?

There is of course no single answer to this question. The approach depends partly upon the patient, partly upon the doctor, and partly upon the dynamics of their relationship with each other. In reviewing my own experiences, I find that a general pattern emerges. What follows is based on this pattern.

In many, and perhaps most, cases of tumor of the head and neck, the tumor will be apparent at the time of the patient's first visit to the doctor. At this stage the doctor and the patient do not know each other very well and both may feel a little tentative in the relationship. It is important not to lie—the relationship must be based firmly upon truth from the beginning. However, there is no need to be either blunt or cruel. If, upon completion of the history and the physical examination, the physician finds a mass that will require biopsy, he may say, "Mr. Jones, I do find an abnormality. There is a mass here that may possibly be a tumor. We should make arrangements for a biopsy." At this point, the patient may wish to ask several questions. The physician must take the time to listen sympathetically and to answer honestly. The quality of the doctor-patient relationship is being established. Now is the first opportunity to make it a firm and comfortable relationship.

When the patient comes to the office or to the hospital for his biopsy, a second opportunity arises. This is often the appropriate time to use the word "cancer" first. The doctor may say, "Mr. Jones, I hope that this is a benign tumor, but you and I must both consider the possibility that it might be malignant—a cancer."

If the biopsy report indicates that the tumor is benign, the patient will not be angry with the doctor for having considered the possibility of cancer. However, if the report indicates that the tumor is a malignant one, then the patient has had a chance to consider in his mind that he might have a cancer. If the tumor is indeed malignant, the physician must report this to the patient, kindly but honestly. "Mr. Jones, I am sorry, but the news on the biopsy is not good. The tumor is indeed malignant. It is a kind of cancer."

Why use the word cancer? First of all there is no kindness in assuring the patient over and over before his biopsy that "everything will be fine, everything will turn out all right," if at the end you have to tell him he has a cancer. This approach has in it the elements of a terrible kind of joke—the patient has been guided and steered down a comfortable and fear-free pathway until suddenly at the last moment he is jerked around and presented with a nightmare. It is kinder to present the possibility of cancer early on so that the diagnosis does not come as a complete and sudden shock. If the biopsy report indicates a benign condition, then the patient will not be angry with the doctor for having raised the possibility of cancer. He will be relieved. If the biopsy report indicates a malignancy, the patient has been prepared for the possibility. Furthermore, it is the physician's obligation to discuss with the patient alternate modalities of treatment. Clearly the patient cannot participate in an informed manner in the selection of his treatment if he does not know the diagnosis.

"Doctor, am I going to die?"

This is a difficult question for many of us to answer, but it must be addressed. We do not, of course, know when the patient is going to die. And this is just as well, as it permits us to answer the question honestly without destroying the patient's hope. One approach to the answer is something like this: "Mr. Jones, we are all going to die. If you are asking me whether your tumor will kill you and if so when, then I cannot answer the question directly. We are going to treat you. We will cure you if we can, but even if we cannot, we will take care of you. Does this answer your question?" This opens a way for further discussion if the patient wishes it.

Phase of Treatment and Remission

At this point, the doctor-patient relationship enters into its second phase—the phase of treatment and remission. It is our hope, of course, that our treatment will be curative.

But even if it is not, the remission we induce by surgery or radiation therapy or chemotherapy or a combination of these usually gives the patient and his family time to become reconciled to the disease and time to mourn as well.

Kübler-Ross[2, 3] has elucidated five stages through which patients may pass in response to news of a fatal illness—denial, anger, bargaining, depression, and acceptance. As surgeons in temperament, as well as in fact, we are not likely to be as detailed in our analysis of our patient's emotional responses to his disease as is Kübler-Ross.

We need to be aware of the mechanisms patients use in dealing with fatal disease. Denial is used initially by almost all patients. It is for this reason that we must present the diagnosis of cancer to our patients gently, leaving them time to accept it at their own pace. Nothing will be accomplished by brutal frankness. The patient's anger may be directed at us, his family, or his friends. We must understand this and be able to explain it to the patient's family, so that anger and resentment do not build up on both sides.

Bargaining would appear to be an internal dialogue. It may not often be expressed to the physician. Depression can be accepted if it is mild, and treated if it becomes severe. Acceptance is to be hoped for, but cannot be demanded and will not be achieved by all patients. During the phase of treatment and remission, as always, the doctor must be available to the patient and to the patient's family. Family members, especially the spouse, may need office counselling from time to time. The doctor must ensure that the patient has at least one person with whom he can talk frankly and openly. This should be a family member, if possible. Ideally, it is the spouse.

Phase of Recurrence and Death

If treatment fails and the tumor recurs, this phase begins. It is during this phase that we must deal with what is euphemistically called the "management of death." In fact, we do not manage death. Death manages us.

However, we can often control the pain, nausea, anxiety, and depression that the patient encounters in this phase. Thus we can often prolong the patient's active period. As the disease progresses the patient may need a tracheostomy or gastrostomy or both. These procedures will not necessarily prolong the patient's life, but they may improve markedly the quality of his life. Respiratory distress is never tolerable and must be relieved. Gastrostomy will permit the patient to be fed and medicated and maintained free from intravenous therapy as long as possible. These two procedures—tracheostomy and gastrostomy—will permit many patients to remain at home and to die at home. Home and loved ones become increasingly important as death approaches. Death at home can be more dignified and more peaceful in most cases. This requires that the family, especially the spouse, be willing and able to accept the care of the patient during his last days or weeks.

For individual practitioners and small groups, visiting nurse or other agencies available through the hospital home care service can provide day-to-day care and dressing changes. The patient and the family must have access to the doctor for technical support and to each other for emotional support.

In the case of the large medical center or university head and neck cancer service, a multidisciplinary team can be established. The composition of such a team will vary from place to place. It should include surgeons, nurses, and social workers. In this situation nurses and social workers are usually the team members who work most closely with the patients. Primary care providers should have easy access to consultants in radiation therapy, chemotherapy, psychiatry, the clergy, physical therapy, and occupational therapy.

THE HOSPICE MOVEMENT

In recent years, with increased interest in the care of the dying patient, a number of hospices have been established in the United States for the care of the terminally ill. We, in New Haven, are fortunate to have in our community the first of these, Hospice, Inc. Based on St. Christopher's Hospice in England, it was established as a home care service for terminally ill patients and their families in 1974.[4] Its goals are

To keep the patient home as long as possible,

To educate health professionals and lay people,

To supplement existing services,

To support the family as the unit of care,

To help the patient to live as fully as possible,

To keep costs down.

A Hospice team consists of physicians, nurses, a social worker, a physical therapist, pastoral counselors, secretaries, and volunteers. Staff members visit their patients regularly and are available on call 24 hours a day, 7 days a week. The program seeks to control physical symptoms and to provide social, psychological, and spiritual support to the patient and his family. An inpatient facility is presently being built. The New Haven Hospice has been the model for some 170 similar facilities that are now being developed throughout the country.

PLANNING FOR DEATH

A few families whose loved ones die at home will make tentative funeral arrangements before the patient's death. In these instances the hospital can be by-passed. The physician can make the declaration of death and fill out the certificate at the patient's home. The funeral director can then be notified of the death.

More often, the family will call an ambulance and the patient will be taken to the hospital emergency room where the declaration of death is made. It is important that the physician not abandon the family at this time. Family members may need continued support and may need continued access to the physician for consultation. If the physician can make time in his schedule to attend the patient's funeral, the family will be lastingly grateful. Furthermore, the ceremony may provide some catharsis for the physician, helping him to terminate a relationship that at the least will have been a significant one and at the most may have been a very powerful one in his life.

REFERENCES

1. Feifel, H. 1969. Perception of death. Annals of The New York Academy of Sciences, 164: 635.

2. Kübler-Ross, E. 1969. On Death and Dying. Macmillan, New York.

3. Kübler-Ross, E. 1974. Questions and Answers on Death and Dying. Macmillan, New York.

4. Lack, S., and Buckingham, R. 1978. First American Hospice. Hospice, Inc., New Haven.

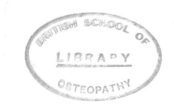

Index

Page numbers followed by f refer to figures and t to tables.